Pathology and Therapeutics
for Pharmacists

Pathology and Therapeutics for Pharmacists

A basis for clinical pharmacy practice

SECOND EDITION

Russell J Greene
BPharm MSc PhD MRPharmS
Senior Lecturer in Clinical Pharmacy
Head, Pharmacy Practice Group

Norman D Harris
BPharm PhD FRPharmS DIC
Emeritus Reader in Pharmaceutics

with contributions by

Larry I Goodyer
BPharm MPharm PhD MRPharmS

Department of Pharmacy
King's College London
University of London
UK

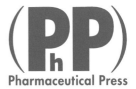

Pharmaceutical Press

Published by the Pharmaceutical Press
1 Lambeth High Street, London SE1 7JN, UK

First edition published by Chapman & Hall 1993
First published in paperback 1994
Reprinted 1995

Reprinted by the Pharmaceutical Press 1996, 1997, 1998
Second edition 2000

© Russell J Greene and Norman D Harris 1993, 2000

Text design by Barker/Hilsdon, Lyme Regis, Dorset
Typeset by J&L Composition Ltd, Filey, North Yorkshire
Printed in Great Britain by TJ International, Padstow, Cornwall

ISBN 0 85369 373 0

A catalogue record for this book is available from the British
Library

Disclaimer

**The drug selections and doses given in this book are for illustration only. The authors and publishers
take no responsibility for any actions consequent upon following the contents of this book without
first checking current sources of reference.**

All doses mentioned are checked carefully. However, no stated dose should be relied on as the basis for
prescription writing or monitoring. Recommendations change constantly, and a current copy of an official
formulary, such as the *British National Formulary* or the *Compendium of the Association of British Pharmaceutical
Industry*, should always be consulted. Similarly, therapeutic selections and profiles of therapeutic and
adverse activities are based upon the authors' interpretation of official recommendations and the literature
at the time of publication. The most current literature must always be consulted.

We trust that pharmaceutical manufacturers will appreciate our need to restrict ourselves to broad generalizations. The omission of a drug or product does not imply ineffectiveness or unsuitability, nor does the
mention of one constitute a recommendation. The listing of generic adverse effects does not imply that
every member of that class of medicines causes them. Listings of cautions, side effects and interactions are
not comprehensive.

Contents

Dedication and acknowledgements

WE DEDICATE this book to Minnie and Odilian, whose support, patience and forbearance over many years and two editions made the travails of authorship bearable, and to all our student readers, to whom we wish good fortune in their studies, and who we hope will find this book useful.

We must also record our gratitude to the numerous people whose invaluable help made this book possible, notably the clinicians and clinical pharmacists who kindly reviewed different parts of this book and provided many invaluable suggestions. For the first edition they were mostly clinicians from Riverside Health Authority and the NW Thames Health Region, namely Drs T. Cantopher, J. Curtis, M. Gore, J.M. Hunt, D. Jarrett, M. Johnson, A.C. Keat, S. Neill, R.J. Playford, and P. Wise. Dr David Anderson, District Pharmaceutical Officer, Bloomsbury Health District, reviewed the whole manuscript with diligence and patience. Several pharmaceutical companies kindly supplied us with reference material or illustrations, for which we express our gratitude.

For the second edition reviewers were experienced clinical pharmacists primarily from London teaching hospitals, namely Jo Coleman, Care of the Elderly Pharmacist, Royal Free Hospital; Jatinder Harchowal, Senior Pharmacist, renal services, King's College Hospital, King's Healthcare; Alison Hole, Drug Information and Audit Pharmacist, Royal Marsden NHS Trust, Sutton, Surrey; Barry Jubraj, Teacher Practitioner and Training Pharmacist, King's College London and Chelsea and Westminster Hospital; Andrzej Kostrzewski, Principal Pharmacist for education and training, Guy's and St Thomas's Hospital Trust; Julie Mycroft, Principal Pharmacist for clinical services, Royal Marsden NHS Trust; Duncan McRobbie, Principal Clinical Pharmacist, Guy's and St Thomas's Hospital Trust; Jonathan Simms, Senior Clinical Pharmacist, Chelsea and Westminster Hospital; Tamsin Stevenson, Teacher Practitioner and Senior Pharmacist for education and training, King's College London and Basildon and Thurrock General Hospitals Trust, Essex; David Taylor, Chief Pharmacist, Maudsley Hospital and Honorary Senior Lecturer, Institute of Psychiatry.

We greatly value their advice but of course take complete responsibility for the opinions and judgements expressed throughout the book.

We are once again particularly indebted to Larry Goodyer for his contribution of Chapters 2 and 13, which considerably lightened our load.

Many other individuals and companies have assisted in providing information, illustrations or permission to reproduce material and are specifically acknowledged as appropriate. The staff of the Pharmaceutical Press, notably Charles Fry, Paul Weller, John Wilson, Jane Weir and Linda Horrell, all worked immensely hard to convert our updated manuscript into the second edition. We are also grateful to our copyeditor, Bill Down, and especially to our proofreader, Dr Millie Davis, whose eagle eye and attention to detail have ensured consistency and accuracy in the final text. However, some errors and omissions are inevitable in a book of this size which are the authors' responsibility.

Finally, we must not forget the generations of pharmacy students who have passed through the King's College (formerly Chelsea) Department of Pharmacy. They have provided us with much useful feedback on the suitability of our treatment of the material. Through their interest, enthusiasm and hard work in the face of a very full and difficult course, they have kept alive our faith in the importance and relevance of the subject throughout the writing of this book.

Figure acknowledgements

Figure 12.4 and Plates 1, 3, 4, 5, 8, 9, 11, 14 and 16 are reproduced with permission from Dr J.J.R. Almeyda, Enfield Health District, London, UK.

Plates 2, 6, 7, 12, 13 and 15 are reproduced with permission from Dr J.W. Woodward, Sidcup Health Centre, Kent, UK.

Plate 10 is reproduced with permission from the Photographic Library, St John's Hospital for Diseases of the Skin, London, UK.

Preface to the second edition

WE WERE DELIGHTED when responsibility for this book was taken over by the Pharmaceutical Press midway through the numerous reprints of the first edition. We feel that the book thus has gained a larger, but also more targeted, audience. We are most grateful to them for their enthusiastic encouragement, support and assistance in producing this second edition.

Few areas match medical knowledge in the pace of scientific advance, and the task of updating this book was daunting. As far as possible we have included only those extensions to pathology which have been sufficiently well proven as to have become accepted improvements to our understanding of disease states. Similarly, we have reflected modern therapeutic practice using – where they have been published – consensus statements based on sound evidence of efficacy. As before we have indicated potential growth areas of research but this has not been our focus. Because of the pace of change, we have to accept that inevitably some of our information will have become dated between the proofs leaving our desks and the finished book leaving the printer. We urge readers routinely to check in a current reference source such as the *British National Formulary* when considering prescribing or advising in specific situations.

The text has been extensively rewritten to improve clarity, coherence and uniformity. We have taken the opportunity for significant re-organization and harmonization of sections and headings in attempt to make them more consistent, using a consistent headings structure to facilitate comprehension and internal cross-referencing. The overall design has been improved, figures and tables have been redrawn, and the text has benefited greatly from the use of a second colour. The References and further reading lists have been updated. We have introduced rINNs for drug nomenclature, following the *British National Formulary* wherever possible. The index has been rewritten. We have however retained the term 'clinical pharmacy' to describe the area in which this book will be applied. We believe that despite the interest 'pharmaceutical care' has recently generated, in essence it encompasses no more than clinical pharmacy in its widest, original sense.

As before, in describing adverse drug reactions we have drawn attention mainly to the most common or the most serious effects, particularly in relation to their presumed mechanisms, rather than simply reproducing exhaustive lists of adverse effects and interactions which can be readily obtained elsewhere. The reader's attention is drawn to the disclaimer (see p. iv).

We have been pleased to note that sales of the first edition extended beyond the undergraduate audience originally targeted, and also far beyond these shores, there having been sales in over 50 countries. We hope the new edition will serve as useful a purpose as the first evidently has, and also that it will be found of interest outside of the confines of pharmacy, reflecting the more integrated nature of modern health care.

Russell J Greene
Norman D Harris

February 2000

Extract from preface to the first edition

CLINICAL PHARMACY has been defined in many different ways, according to the interests and outlook of the practitioner. We take a very broad definition, encompassing all aspects of the use of medicines in patients and of responding to patients' concerns about their health. It is thus an essential component of the practice of virtually all pharmacists, whether working in the community, in hospital or in industry, and must be based on a sound knowledge of the mechanisms of disease and the principles of drug selection. It has been a principle of our teaching that clinical pharmacy practice requires an understanding of the medical process and of the nature of serious diseases and their treatment. This must underlie any involvement of pharmacists in contributing to the management of patients, or in the diagnosis and management of minor illness. Since pharmacists have to work with clinicians, and there are well-established intellectual disciplines in medicine for diagnosis and management, aspiring clinical pharmacists need to understand the way in which doctors approach the diagnosis of disease and the treatment of patients.

Since starting clinical teaching, we have always lacked a suitable single basic text. Existing textbooks stress diagnosis, drug treatment or the pharmacist–patient interaction, but are often too detailed or cumbersome in some areas, while lacking sufficient detail about the pathophysiological origin of the abnormalities and the ways in which this knowledge leads to correct diagnosis and, finally, to management and treatment. Thus, it has been necessary to refer students to a variety of texts on pathology, immunology, clinical medicine, clinical pharmacology and therapeutics.

Hence the present book. Our ideas were first collated as a series of lecture notes for Chelsea students. This text represents a considerable expansion of these notes, intended to serve as a basis from which clinical pharmacy practice can be developed, both for students and as a basic introduction for all practising pharmacists. We also hope that many other groups of health care professionals, including nurses and doctors, will find the book useful.

This book is not intended to be a textbook of clinical pharmacy, nor is it intended to replace basic biomedical science texts. We assume that the reader will have an understanding of the principles of physiology and pharmacology, and the concepts of clinical pharmacology. We are not trying to compete with detailed texts on drug therapy and so have omitted prescribing detail, about proprietary forms, precise doses, etc., unless it is necessary to an understanding of drug selection or drug use. Similarly, we have not usually included any formal consideration of the mechanisms of adverse drug reactions or interactions, but deal with these as they arise as one of several factors which constrain the prescribing and use of a drug.

Our aim is to show the rationale and role of drug therapy in the management of some common diseases through a consideration of the mechanisms of disease processes in relation to normal function. Most chapters concern a single body system, e.g. the renal system or the gastrointestinal tract. Occasionally, we felt it necessary to depart from this pattern, and to consider a single disease group (e.g. infections), or a particularly important symptom (e.g. pain). The normal physiology of the whole system is first reviewed briefly, sufficient anatomy being included to give an appreciation of where symptoms arise. This is followed by a comparative discussion of the mechanisms and measurement of the principal malfunctions (aetiology, pathology, pathogenesis and investigation), and the relationship between the pathology and the resulting signs and symptoms. Each disease is described in sufficient detail to give an understanding of what it means to the patient and how it affects their lifestyle. Finally, there is an outline of management, stressing the aims and general strategy and showing the role of drugs as one of the therapeutic options, with an emphasis on the rationale and criteria for medicine selection, including biopharmaceutic and qualitative pharmacokinetic considerations.

Although, as pharmacists, we are convinced of the value of drugs and medicines, we are conscious of the fact that medicines are often used empirically and may provide only symptomatic relief. Although cure is often impossible, medicines can usually provide relief from suffering, and a good quality of life, while the normal processes of repair and recovery proceed. Further, social change, e.g. in nutrition, education and wealth, may have contributed more to the conquest of diseases such as tuberculosis than has medical practice. We believe this book provides, in a single compact volume, succinct, integrated information about major diseases and the principles of their management, either as a primer or as a quick refresher, without the need to refer to several different texts.

Recommended reference sources

WE LIST BELOW some of the major tertiary reference sources in pathology and therapeutics for the reader who needs to delve more deeply. These general sources will provide detail on all of the topics covered in this book. Further specific reading (usually textbooks or recent reviews) is suggested at the end of each chapter, which will represent a consensus view of the topic. Clinical pharmacists will also need to refer elsewhere for detailed information on responding to symptoms, counter-prescribing, counselling, the interpretation of pharmacokinetic parameters, and the many other specialisms which comprise modern pharmacy practice.

Berkow R, ed. (1999) *The Merck Manual of Diagnosis and Therapy*. 17th edn, Rahway, NJ: Merck & Co.
A comprehensive and inexpensive general medical practitioners' handbook, especially useful for understanding American practice.

DiPiro JT, *et al.*, eds (1996) *Pharmacotherapy, a Pathophysiological Approach*. 3rd edn. New York: Elsevier.
A detailed and comprehensive coverage of specific diseases and their treatment.

Katzung BG (1997) *Basic and Clinical Pharmacology*. 7th edn. Stamford, Connecticut: Lange.
Up to date and largely successful attempt to correlate a basic pharmacological approach with the clinical.

Guyton AC (1995) *Textbook of Medical Physiology*. 9th edn. Philadelphia: WB Saunders.
The seminal work relating normal to abnormal physiology.

Kumar PJ, Clarke ML, eds. (1998) *Clinical Medicine – a Textbook for Medical Students and Doctors*. 4th edn. London: Balliere Tindall.
A compact, inexpensive and very clearly written basic medical text.

Parfitt K, ed. (1999) *Martindale – the Complete Drug Reference*. 32nd edn. London: Pharmaceutical Press.
The most comprehensive single reference source on drugs and preparations.

Roitt IM, Brostoff J, Male D (1997) *Immunology*. 5th edn. London: Mosby.
A well illustrated account of medical immunology.

Schmidt RF, Thews GH (1989) *Human Physiology*. 2nd edn. Berlin: Springer Verlag.
An excellent, thorough, basic physiology book, with splendid graphics.

Speight TM, ed. (1997) *Avery's Drug Treatment*. 4th edn. Auckland: Adis Press.
A prime source of information on drug usage.

Stockley IH (1999) *Drug Interactions*. 5th edn. London: Pharmaceutical Press.
A comprehensive review of most specific interactions, evaluated for clinical significance.

Taussig P (1995) *Processes in Pathology and Microbiology*. 3rd edn. Oxford: Blackwell.
A comprehensive, readable book on the biology of disease.

Toghill PJ, ed. (1994) *Examining Patients. An Introduction to Clinical Medicine*. 2nd edn. London: Edward Arnold.
A simple introduction to basic medical techniques.

Walker R, Edward C, eds (1998) *Clinical Pharmacy and Therapeutics*. 2nd edn. London: Churchill Livingstone.
A comprehensive multi-authored British clinical pharmacy textbook.

Weatherall DJ, Ledingham JGG, Warrell DA, eds. (1996) *The Oxford Textbook of Medicine*. 3rd edn. Oxford: Oxford University Press.
One of the most thorough and authoritative general medical texts.

In addition, the following journals and bulletins

are recommended for up-to-date comparative discussions of disease and drug selection.

Drugs. Adis Press.

In effect, a monthly update of the comparative therapeutics found in Avery's *Drug Treatment*. It also gives detailed reviews of new drugs and retrospective evaluations of older ones.

Drug and Therapeutics Bulletin. Consumers Association.

Gives regular critical assessments of drug treatment and new drugs in relation to existing therapies.

MeReC Bulletin. Medicines Resource Centre.

Regular reviews of comparative therapeutics produced by NHS.

Medicine International. The Medicine Group.

Regularly updated on a 3- to 4-year cycle, this reviews, with excellent graphics, advances in all fields of medicine, using a grouping similar to that used in this book.

Abbreviations

μg	microgram
AAC	antibiotic-associated colitis
AC	anticonvulsant
ACE(I)	angiotensin converting enzyme (inhibitor)
ACh	acetylcholine
ACP	serum acid phosphatase
ADH	antidiuretic hormone
AFP	alpha-fetoprotein
AHPT	antihypertensive (drug)
AIDS	autoimmune deficiency syndrome
ALP	serum alkaline phosphatase
ALT	alanine aminotransferase
ANA, ANF	fluorescent antinuclear antibody test
APN	acute pyelonephritis
AS	ankylosing spondylitis
ASO	anti-streptolysin antibody
AST	aspartate aminotransferase
ATN	acute tubular necrosis/nephropathy
ATP	adenosine triphosphate
AZT	zidovudine
BBB	blood–brain barrier
BDA	British Diabetic Association
BG	basal ganglia
BNF	*British National Formulary*
BP	blood pressure
BSP	bromsulphthalein retention test
BUN	blood urea nitrogen, blood urea
CAPD	continuous ambulatory peritoneal dialysis
CAT	computerized axial tomography
CAVH	continuous arteriovenous haemofiltration
CAV-HD	continuous arteriovenous haemodialysis
CCU	coronary care unit
CEA	carcinoembryonic antigen
ChE	cholesterol
CK	creatine phosphokinase
cm	centimetre
CMI	cell-mediated immunity
CNS	central nervous system
CO	cardiac output

COAD	chronic obstructive airways disease
COMT	catechol *O*-methyl transferase
COPD	chronic obstructive pulmonary disease
CPK	*see* CK
CPN	chronic pyelonephritis
CRF	chronic renal failure
CRP	C-reactive protein
CSF	cerebrospinal fluid
CSI	continuous subcutaneous infusion
CT	computed tomography, computerized axial tomography
CTZ	chemoreceptor trigger zone
CVP	central venous pressure
CVS	cardiovascular system
Da	dalton
DA	dopamine
DBP	diastolic blood pressure
DNA	deoxyribonucleic acid
DSM	Diagnostic and Statistical Manual of Mental Disease
DU	duodenal ulcer
Dx	diagnosis
EAA	essential amino acid
ECF	extracellular fluid
ECG	electrocardiogram
ECT	electroconvulsive therapy
EDP	end-diastolic pressure
EDRF	endothelium derived relaxing factor
EDV	end-diastolic volume
EEG	electroencephalogram
EF	ejection fraction
EFA	essential fatty acid
EGF	epidermal growth factor
EPS	extrapyramidal syndromes, symptoms
ERCP	endoscopic retrograde cholangiopancreatography
ESR	erythrocyte sedimentation rate
ESRD	end-stage renal disease
ESWL	extracorporeal shock-wave lithotripsy
Fab	antigen-binding fragment of immunoglobulin
FANA	*see* ANA
FBC	full blood count
Fc	crystallizable fragment of immunoglobulin
FEV_1	forced expiratory volume in 1 second
FEV_1/FVC	forced expiratory ratio of the lungs
FFA	free fatty acid
FVC	forced vital capacity (of the lungs)
GABA	gamma-aminobutyric acid
G-CSF	granulocyte colony stimulating factor

GFR	glomerular filtration rate
GHb	*see* HbA$_{1c}$
GI(T)	gastrointestinal (tract)
GM-CSF	granulocyte-macrophage colony stimulating factor
GnRH	gonadotrophin-releasing hormone, gonadorelin
GT	gammaglutamyl transpeptidase
GTN	glyceryl trinitrate
GTP	guanosine triphosphate
Hb	haemoglobin
HbA$_{1c}$	glycosylated haemoglobin
2HBSS	2-h blood sugar screen
HD	haemodialysis
HDL	high-density lipoprotein
HDN	haemolytic disease of the newborn
HF	heart failure
5-HIAA	5-hydroxyindole acetic acid
HIV	human immunodeficiency virus
HLA	human leukocyte locus-A gene/antigen
HMG CoA reductase inhibitor	3-hydroxy-3-methylglutaryl coenzyme A reductase inhibitor (statin)
HPT	hypertension
5HT	5-hydroxytryptamine, serotonin
h	hour/hours
IBD	inflammatory bowel disease
IC	immune complex, inspiratory capacity of the lungs
ICD	International Classification of Disease
ICF	intracellular fluid
IDDM	insulin-dependent diabetes mellitus
Ig	immunoglobulin
IgA	immunoglobulin A, secretory immunoglobulin
IgE	immunoglobulin E, reaginic antibody
IgG	gamma-globulin
IgM	macroglobulin
IHD	ischaemic heart disease
IL	interleukin
IM	intramuscular
IPD	intermittent peritoneal dialysis
IV	intravenous
IVU	intravenous excretory urogram
Ix	investigation(s)
JCA	juvenile chronic arthritis
JGA	juxtaglomerular apparatus
JVP	jugular venous pressure
K	T lymphocyte killer cells
kcal	kilocalorie

kJ	kilojoule
K, K$^+$	potassium (ion)
L	litre
LDH	lactic dehydrogenase
LDL	low density lipoprotein
L-dopa	L-dihydroxyphenylalanine, levodopa
LST	lateral spinothalamic tract of the spinal cord
LT	leukotriene (plus type number)
LVEDP	left ventricular end-diastolic pressure
LVF	left ventricular heart failure
MAF	macrophage activating factor
MAO(I)	monoamine oxidase (inhibitor)
MAP	mean arterial pressure
MBC	minimum bactericidal concentration
mg	milligram
MHC	major histocompatibility complex
MHPG	3-methoxy-4-hydroxy-phenylethyleneglycol
MI	myocardial infarction
MIC	minimum inhibitory concentration
MIF	macrophage inhibitory factor
min	minute
mL	millilitre
MPTP	methylphenyltetrahydropyridine
MRI	(nuclear) magnetic resonance imaging
MRSA	methicillin-resistant *Staphylococcus aureus*, multi-resistant *Staph. aureus*
MW	molecular weight
NA	noradrenaline (norepinephrine)
NAC	*N*-acetylcysteine
NIDDM	non-insulin-dependent diabetes mellitus
nm	nanometre
NMR	*see* MRI
NSAID	non-steroidal anti-inflammatory drug
OA	osteoarthritis
OAD	oral antidiabetic drug
OTC	over-the-counter
OT	occupational therapy
P_aCO_2, P_ACO_2	partial arterial/alveolar pressure of carbon dioxide
PAF	platelet activating factor
PAH	*para*-amino hippuric acid
PAN	polyarteritis nodosa
P_aO_2, P_AO_2	partial arterial/alveolar pressure of oxygen
PCO_2	partial pressure of carbon dioxide
PCV	packed cell volume, haematrocrit
PD	Parkinson's disease, peritoneal dialysis
PDGF	platelet-derived growth factor

PEF	peak expiratory flow
PG	prostaglandin (plus type letter and number)
PH	portal hypertension
PID	prolapsed intervertebral disc
PMH	past medical history
PMN	polymorphonuclear leukocyte
PND	paroxysmal nocturnal dyspnoea
PO_2	partial pressure of oxygen
PR	peripheral resistance to blood flow
PRF	peptide regulatory factors
PT	prothrombin time, physiotherapy
PTCA	percutaneous transluminal coronary angioplasty
PUVA	psoralen plus ultraviolet radiation therapy
RA	rheumatoid arthritis
RAP	right atrial pressure
RAS	reticular activating system
RAST	radioallergosorbent test
RBC	red blood cell
RF	renal failure, rheumatoid factor
Rh	rhesus
RhD	rhesus D antigen
RLD	restrictive lung disease
RP	Raynaud's phenomenon
RV	residual volume of the lungs
RVF	right ventricular failure
Rx	treatment(s)
SAA	serum amyloid-A protein
SAD	seasonal affective disorder
SSRI	selective serotonin re-uptake inhibitor
SBP	systolic blood pressure
SCI	stem cell inhibitor
SBE	subacute bacterial endocarditis
SG	substantia gelatinosa of the posterior horn of the spinal cord
SGOT	serum glutamic-oxaloacetic transaminase, *see* AST
SGPT	serum glutamic-pyruvic transaminase, *see* ALT
SLE	systemic lupus erythematosus
SRS	slow reacting substance
SSx	symptoms and signs
TB	tuberculosis
TBW	total body water
T_C	cytotoxic T cells
T_H	T helper cells
TENS	transcutaneous electrical nerve stimulation
T_S	T suppressor cells
TIBC	total iron-binding capacity
TLC	total capacity of the lungs
TSH	thyroid-stimulating hormone, thyrotropin
TV	tidal volume of the lungs
Tx	thromboxane (plus type letter and number)

UGPD	University Group Diabetes Programme
UT(I)	urinary tract (infection)
UV	ultraviolet radiation
UVA	longer wavelength ultraviolet radiation, 320–400 nm
UVB	shorter wavelength ultraviolet radiation, 290–320 nm
VC	vital capacity
VLDL	very low density lipoprotein
WBC	white blood cell
WCC	white cell count

Note on drug nomenclature

WE HAVE USED rINN throughout for drugs. However, certain substances are referred to primarily in their physiological or pharmacological role, especially *adrenaline* and *noradrenaline*. There has been no move towards changing pharmacological and physiological terms such as *adrenergic* and so to reduce confusion the names *epinephrine* (for adrenaline) and *norepinephrine* (for noradrenaline) have not been adopted as primary names in this edition.

Where the British Approved Name (BAN) differs from the rINN we have listed the differences below, for easy reference. Lists 1 and 2 have been extracted from the current recommendations published in the *British National Formulary* (39) and *British Approved Names 1999: British Pharmacopoeia Commission* (published by the Stationery Office). The reader is referred to these publications for additional information and updates. Within the text, for drugs from List 1 we have used the rINN followed by the BAN in parentheses. For drugs from List 2 we have used the rINN only.

Where the United States Adopted Name (USAN) or United States Pharmacopeia (USP) name differs from the rINN, the USAN/USP name has been included in the text in parentheses, after the rINN. A list of the differences is supplied below (List 3).

List 1 – Both rINN and BAN have been used

rINN	BAN
alimemazine	trimeprazine
bendroflumethiazide	bendrofluazide
chlormethine	mustine
dicycloverine	dicyclomine
dosulepin	dothiepin
epinephrine	adrenaline
fludroxycortide	flurandrenolone
formoterol	eformoterol
furosemide	frusemide
hydroxycarbamide	hydroxyurea
levothyroxine	thyroxine
lidocaine	lignocaine
methylthioninium chloride	methylene blue
mitoxantrone	mitozantrone
norepinephrine	noradrenaline
tetracaine	amethocaine
trihexyphenidyl	benzhexol

List 2 – The rINN has been used exclusively

rINN	BAN
amoxicillin	amoxycillin
beclometasone	beclomethasone
benorilate	benorylate
busulfan	busulphan
cefalexin	cephalexin

List 2 (cont.)

rINN	BAN
cefaloridine	cephaloridine
cefradine	cephradine
ciclosporin	cyclosporin
clomethiazole	chlormethiazole
colecalciferol	cholecalciferol
cefalotin	cephalothin
colestyramine	cholestyramine
dantron	danthron
desoximetasone	desoxymethasone
diethylstilbestrol	stilboestrol
ethinylestradiol	ethinyloestradiol
etamivan	ethamivan
flupentixol	flupenthixol
indometacin	indomethacin
lisuride	lysuride
oxetacaine	oxethazaine
oxyphenisatine	oxyphenisatin
phenobarbital	phenobarbitone
sodium amidotrizoate	sodium diatrizoate
sodium cromoglicate	sodium cromoglycate
sulfamethoxazole	sulphamethoxazole
sulfapyridine	sulphapyridine
sulfasalazine	sulphasalazine
sulfinpyrazone	sulphinpyrazone
tioguanine	thioguanine
trimethadione	troxidone

List 3 – Both rINN and USAN/USP name have been used

rINN	USAN or *USP name
aciclovir	acyclovir
azapropazone	apazone
calcipotriol	calcipotriene
ciclosporin	cyclosporine
cinchocaine	dibucaine*
dextropropoxyphene	propoxyphene*
dithranol	anthralin*
glibenclamide	glyburide
hydroxycarbamide	hydroxyurea
isoprenaline	isoproterenol*
lauromacrogol 400	laureth 9
oxybuprocaine	benoxinate*
paracetamol	acetaminophen*
pethidine	meperidine*
phenazone	antipyrine*
pizotifen	pizotyline
sodium cromoglicate	cromolyn sodium
tioguanine	thioguanine
trioxysalen	trioxsalen

1

Therapeutics: general strategy

This book is about the rationale of therapeutic decision making, and in particular the logic of drug selection. Thus, it must start with an account of where drug therapy fits into the general management of a patient, and the factors which govern the selection of a drug regimen. What may be called the **medical process** starts with the taking of a case history. In its broadest sense this includes examination, investigation and diagnosis, and culminates in a decision about management. A similar if less elaborate process must be followed by a pharmacist to respond to symptoms presented by a patient. All this information is gathered together to provide a systematic classification of knowledge about a patient.

However, before considering the structure of a case history, the terminology and systematic description of disease must be introduced. Just as knowledge about a drug is classified by pharmacists into such categories as 'indications' and 'adverse effects', etc. so knowledge about disease is systematically described using special categories.

The medical process and the systematic description of disease form the framework for the discussion of specific conditions and disease groups in subsequent chapters.

Terminology of disease

Definition

An account of a disease starts with a description of its general nature, including the organ system affected and important features which differentiate it from similar conditions. The following are two examples:

- *Essential hypertension is a chronic slowly progressive cardiovascular condition in which the mean diastolic blood pressure is consistently above the population normal range for the patient's age, but below 130 mmHg and not rising rapidly.*
- *Rheumatoid arthritis is a chronic progressive inflammatory erosive polyarthropathy, primarily articular synovitis, but with systemic features.*

Aetiology and pathology

These categories are sometimes difficult to distinguish, especially when the cause of a disease is uncertain (Table 1.1). **Aetiology** is concerned with general causes of a disease and the circumstances ('risk factors') which predispose an individual to suffer from its effects: it may be thought of as answering the question, 'why?'. Aetiology makes no assertions about the processes by which these factors bring about the condition. Thus, the aetiology of tuberculosis involves public hygiene, patient immune status and the mycobacterium; that of cancer may include genetic predisposition, viral infection and environmental toxins; that of essential hypertension involves obesity, salt intake and stress, etc.

Pathology is concerned with the mechanisms of the disease process, what the disease does, and how it does so. It describes the changes caused in body function and the body's response to this. The **pathophysiology** of a disease relates its effects to the disruption of normal physiological functions; e.g. the pathophysiology of essential hypertension involves a raised peripheral vascular resistance and possibly an expansion of the intra-vascular fluid volume. **Pathogenesis** describes the development or progression of the disease process. Thus, the pathogenesis of rheumatoid arthritis involves synovial hyperplasia followed by inflammatory cell infiltration, then articular erosion. Where immunological processes are known to be involved in the disease, e.g. the autoimmune pancreatic destruction in type 1 diabetes mellitus, the term **immunopathology** is used.

There are a few general pathogenic mechanisms, such as **inflammation** and **ischaemia**, which occur as fundamental bodily responses to very many diseases. These are described in Chapter 2.

Epidemiology

It is important to know how common a condition is, and whether any particular population group is more susceptible by virtue of birth or environment. There may also be significant differences in frequency between the sexes, different ethnic groups and ages. The **incidence** is the number of new cases of the disease; it is usually expressed as per million of a population per year. The lifetime incidence is the proportion of the population which is likely to suffer at some time in their life, e.g. the lifetime incidence of duodenal ulcer among British males is about 1 in 10.

Prevalence refers to the number of active cases at any one time, e.g. the overall prevalence of Parkinson's disease is about 1 in 1000, affecting men and women equally, but is 1 in 200 among those over 70 years of age. The term **morbidity** is sometimes used more loosely to describe the prevalence of a disease; thus heart disease has a relatively high morbidity, renal cancer a low morbidity.

The relationship between incidence and prevalence depends on the natural history (usual course) of the condition. Although the annual incidence of the common cold may be up to

Table 1.1   Terminology used in disease and its management

Term used		Description
Definition		Brief summary
Aetiology	*Why?*	Causes; risk factors
Epidemiology	*Who?*	In population as whole, and in specially susceptible groups
Incidence		Frequency of new cases
Prevalence		Number of sufferers at any time
Pathology	*How? What?*	Mechanisms of malfunction
Pathogenesis		Underlying disease process
Pathophysiology		Disorder of normal function
Clinical features		
(Presentation)		
Symptoms		Features noticed by patient:
		Subjective ('complains of')
Signs		Features noted by clinician:
		Objective ('on examination')
Investigations		Most appropriate methods
Natural history	*When?*	Onset, progression, duration, resolution
(Course)		Severity
		Complications
		Mortality
Management		
Aims		Symptomatic relief
		Arrest disease
		Reverse disease (cure)
		Prevent disease
Treatment modes		Medication
		Nursing care
		Surgery
		Occupational therapy
		Radiotherapy
		Physiotherapy
		Social support, etc.
Monitoring		Progress of disease
		Side effects of treatment
Prognosis		Probable outcomes

1 in 2 in the UK, the prevalence at any given time will vary between perhaps 10 million and merely several hundred thousand, depending on the season, as colds are acute in onset and short-lived. On the other hand, the prevalence of chronic renal failure depends on the annual incidence and the average survival time following diagnosis.

A knowledge of the epidemiology of a disease may provide clues about its aetiology. For example, the incidence of stomach cancer is higher in Japan than the USA, but the prevalence among Japanese immigrants to the USA is similar to that of native Americans. This strongly suggests that environmental factors (e.g. diet) are more important than genetic ones.

Clinical features

Signs and symptoms, often thought to be synonymous, are distinct terms. **Symptoms** are subjective; they are noticed by the patient and either reported (the things a patient 'complains of') or elicited on questioning. **Signs** are usually found objectively 'on examination' by the clinician, although occasionally may be noticed by the patient. Both are important: the former emphasize what are likely to be the patient's major concerns; the latter aid precise diagnosis.

The typical pattern of clinical features caused by a disease is called its **presentation**. Many diseases have such consistent presentations as to be almost diagnostic, e.g. a spiking fever, stiff neck and photophobia in meningitis; such definitive features are called **pathognomonic**. A well-defined group of clinical features which commonly occur together is sometimes called a **syndrome**, e.g. proteinuria, hypoproteinaemia and oedema together are known as the 'nephrotic syndrome'.

Investigations

It is helpful to describe the most useful tests or procedures for confirming a diagnosis, distinguishing between closely related conditions (**differential diagnosis**) or monitoring progress. For example, although the measurement of urinary glucose is not a very good method of assessing control in diabetes mellitus, it is quite suitable for screening large groups for possible diabetes.

Natural history

Knowledge of the usual course of a disease from its onset to its final outcome is important for several reasons. It enables predictions to be made about a patient's likely recovery or degree of eventual disability, i.e. the **prognosis**. It also helps in judging whether improvements in a patient's condition are due to treatment or to natural remission. Many chronic diseases progress by a series of exacerbations, remissions and relapses, and improvements cannot with certainty be ascribed to any treatment which is being given. The patient may have improved despite the treatment rather than because of it.

Different disease subgroups may be differentiated by different natural histories. For example, rheumatoid arthritis typically has an insidious onset, but if there is an acute onset of multi-joint inflammation the prognosis is better. Furthermore, some two-thirds of rheumatoid arthritis patients will have such a slowly progressive disease that they can expect little disablement within a normal life-span.

The average duration of the disease must also be recorded, as well as its pattern of activity. Does it remain stable or tend to deteriorate steadily (**progressive disease**) and if so, at what rate? Is it continuous or fluctuating, with remissions and exacerbations? Is there any residual disability after the disease has resolved, or can it be cured? Many diseases also have typical secondary complications, e.g. haemorrhage in peptic ulceration; what is their prevalence, especially in different age or sex groups?

The likelihood of a fatal outcome is the **mortality**, usually expressed as the proportion of patients expected to die after a specified time. Conversely, **survival** is the proportion of patients alive at a specified time after diagnosis. Both are commonly cited as medians; e.g. a 3-year median survival means that half of patients are expected to be still alive after 3 years. Alternatively one may speak of, for example, mortality at 5 years being x%, or an annual mortality rate of y%. It is important to distinguish between the mortality and morbidity of a particular disease, in order to compare the suitability of different treatments. Thus, skin diseases generally have a high morbidity but very low mortality, so toxic therapy is rarely indicated. However, malignant melanoma, while having a low morbidity, has a very high mortality, so aggressive therapy is warranted.

Management and treatment

Management embraces all the decisions made to deal with the patient's complaint; it defines the strategy. Its first task is to decide realistic aims, based on a knowledge of the presentation, investigations and natural history. Within the broad area of management, **treatment** comprises the range of interventions, like drugs, surgery or physiotherapy, that can be used to achieve these aims. Of course, this can include doing very little if the condition is self-limiting on the one hand, or so advanced as to be incurable on the other: management might then involve no more than simple reassurance and appropriate counselling, i.e. palliative care.

The assessment of the risk-to-benefit ratio of different treatments must be based on a knowledge of the severity and mortality of the condition and the toxicity of the treatment.

Aims

The various possible aims of management may be set in a hierarchy (Table 1.1). Prevention may be the ultimate aim of medicine, but symptomatic relief is frequently all that can be offered. Only by having clearly defined aims can it be judged to what extent the treatment has been successful, and thus whether such treatment should be continued or changed.

Prevention
This can only follow from an understanding of the aetiology and pathology, but that alone is not always sufficient. Some infectious diseases have been almost completely eliminated in some countries by a systematic combination of public health measures and vaccination, e.g. diphtheria. Smallpox is the only disease which has been completely eradicated world-wide. Yet although much is known about the causes of chronic bronchitis and ischaemic heart disease, prevention here probably resides more in the domains of education and social and economic policy than in medicine. On the other hand, there is at present little hope of preventing most cases of chronic renal failure or cancer because so little is understood of their aetiology.

Reversal
Prevention has clearly failed if a patient presents with symptoms. Some diseases are intrinsically temporary, self-limiting and reversible, such as minor gastric upset. For others, the ideal would be to reverse the disease process and leave the recuperative powers of the body to restore health

completely. This amounts to a **cure**, and it is depressing to reflect how few important diseases there are for which this is a realistic aim. When patients have recovered from an infection, they are usually physiologically just as they were before their illness. In almost all other common serious chronic diseases the sad truth is that we do not do a very good job. Consider heart disease and cancer, which together account for over 50% of all premature deaths in the West. This is not to obscure the fact that immense good is done by modern medicine, and medicines, in the relief of the misery associated with serious illness, in particular the damaging effects of acute exacerbations of chronic diseases.

Transplantation is a growing area which can be said to reverse some diseases (although immunosuppressant therapy prevents completely normal life) and in the future gene therapy promises tremendous advances in this direction.

Arrest progress
Many measures may arrest or stabilize a condition, preventing deterioration and minimizing exacerbations or relapses. Thus in chronic bronchitis, stopping smoking will avoid further lung damage, and prompt antibiotic treatment will minimize infective exacerbations. Anticonvulsant drugs will prevent most epilepsy seizures but without rectifying the underlying disease process. Replacement therapy in endocrine deficiency diseases such as diabetes will restore normal function, although it cannot restore the original organ. In many chronic diseases, by the time diagnosis is made there is often fixed, irreversible organ damage.

Symptomatic relief and palliation
Finally, there are some circumstances in which there exists no hope at all of influencing the disease process, and all that can be done is to treat the symptoms as they arise, or more generally make the patient feel better. Terminal cancer is the prime example. Analgesics, parenteral nutrition, surgery to relieve intestinal obstruction: these are all directed at improving the patient's quality of life, and not at controlling the disease.

Some would claim that the majority of medical and pharmaceutical efforts do no more than meet this aim: for example, do anxiolytic or anti-inflammatory drugs really do more than suppress symptoms? Yet the relief of suffering and improvement in the quality of life are surely worthwhile benefits in themselves.

Modes

Having decided on a realistic aim, it is necessary to make appropriate selections from the many available modes of treatment. Thus serious joint disease may need social and economic help, as well as support from a multidisciplinary team including clinicians, nurses, pharmacists and social workers, to alleviate the condition. Treatment may involve surgery, and nearly always physiotherapy, to achieve or maintain joint mobility. Nursing skills are of paramount importance both in hospital and in the home if the rheumatoid patient is to return as quickly as possible to their normal activities.

Drugs play an important part in the management of many diseases, but they must be seen as only one part of the patient's whole treatment. When individual diseases are discussed in later chapters, the role of drug therapy – and its limitations – will be emphasized in relation to the other important modes of therapy.

Monitoring

Decisions about aims are meaningless without ways of determining to what extent they are being achieved. The method of monitoring will depend on the nature of the abnormality (e.g. blood glucose level in diabetes, blood pressure in hypertension) and the aims of therapy (e.g. symptoms, imaging or a biochemical marker in cancer). Similarly, certain choices carry with them the obligation to watch for adverse effects (e.g. regular blood counts in cytotoxic chemotherapy). Pharmacists are playing an increasing role in these monitoring processes.

Case history

A case history is a systematic report of the progress of a patient's disease, including the information and reasoning behind diagnosis and management decisions. It is the core of the medical process and provides a central database for all concerned with the care of the patient. Taking a history and making a coherent record of it are two of the most fundamental skills of medicine, and they are being increasingly adapted for use by paramedical professions such as nursing and pharmacy.

Taking a 'good history' involves more than simply obtaining information and examining the patient. It is a subtle mixture of communication skills such as listening and questioning, comprehensive clinical knowledge, lateral thinking and detective work. Unless the results are systematically recorded in a standardized way, its purpose may be largely defeated.

The way that these data fit into the general flow of information gathering is shown in Fig. 1.1. The categories of information reported in a case history will be considered next. This will introduce some further essential medical terminology and should help the pharmacist to understand case reports in the medical literature (Table 1.2).

Although in some cases the complete work-up will not seem immediately appropriate – the accident victim admitted through the Accident and Emergency Unit need not be questioned about childhood illnesses – a thorough history prevents important facts such as a drug allergy possibly being missed, or less obvious diagnoses being overlooked.

Patient details

A case history report is conventionally prefaced by a brief description of the patient and his or her complaint. This serves to orientate the reader and also to summarize data that will subsequently be important for both diagnosis and treatment.

Age, sex, ethnic origin and occupation are recorded because certain diseases are more prevalent in particular groups (e.g. type 2 diabetes in the elderly, haemoglobinopathies in people of Mediterranean origin), and numerous diseases are occupationally related. Exotic disease might be suggested by the ethnic group or recent travel: in the UK, fever in a non-travelling Londoner would be regarded differently from that in a

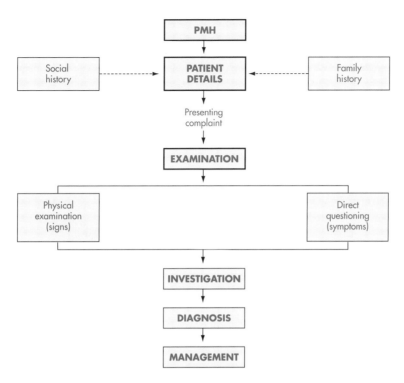

Figure 1.1 Case history and the medical process: the inter-relationship of the various data recorded in a case history. PMH, past medical history.

newly arrived African or Asian immigrant. Decisions about treatment may also be affected by such data, e.g. pharmacogenetic differences in drug handling, religious or ethnic dietary preferences.

It is usual to note how the patient came to medical attention and with what complaint; this gives an idea of the urgency of the problem and how it is perceived by the patient. An experienced clinician can also tell a lot from the patient's general appearance. The section might conclude with circumstantial observations such as a walking stick, medication or cigarettes at the bedside. Thus, a case history might start:

Mr M, a 45-year-old slightly obese Caucasian business man, was admitted 3 days ago through casualty after collapsing at work, complaining of a crushing chest pain of 3 h duration. On admission he appeared pale, anxious and in great pain.

Past medical history

Certain childhood diseases, and recent or current chronic illnesses, may have a bearing on the present illness. For example, rheumatic fever often causes heart disease in later life, chickenpox may manifest later as shingles and hay fever suggests an allergic predisposition. After using open questions (e.g. 'tell me about any serious illnesses you have had'), the patient will be asked specifically about the more common chronic conditions such as epilepsy, asthma, hypertension, diabetes, jaundice, rheumatic fever and tuberculosis (TB).

A **medication history** should ideally comprise a list of current medication and recent medication used for the presenting complaint, including self-medication bought over-the-counter (OTC) and remedies recommended by a pharmacist. The effectiveness of each medication and any adverse effects encountered, including allergy or

Table 1.2 Format of typical case history report, including common abbreviations

Patient details	Age, sex, occupation
	Race, ethnic group
	Place of normal residence; recent travel
	Build, weight
	Route of admission
	Main complaint
	General appearance
Past medical history (PMH)	Illnesses since childhood
	Medication history
Family history (FH)	Relatives' (living and dead) medical history
Social history (SH)	Social drug use
	Domestic and financial situation
	Mobility
	How is patient coping (at work, leisure)?
History of presenting complaint (HPC, 'complains of')	Onset, nature and intensity of symptoms
	Changes; provoking and relieving factors
	Referrals
	Medication
Systematic examination (Review of systems)	Directed questioning: each body system
	Physical examination: each body system
Investigations (Ix)	Blood, urine analysis
	Radiography
	Etc.
Diagnosis (Dx)	Differential, provisional or confirmed
Management (Rx)	For each current problem
	Aims
	Modes
	Monitoring
	Outcome(s)

sensitivity, need to be recorded. Patients may need prompting, especially for self-medication; even certain prescription items are frequently not regarded as medicines, e.g. oral contraceptives. Patients also tend to be rather unreliable or imprecise on adverse effects; e.g. the term 'allergy' may be used colloquially to describe almost any adverse effect, even mild dyspepsia. Unfortunately, an accurate and complete record is seldom easy to obtain, even when there is access to medical notes.

There is some evidence that pharmacists can obtain more complete medication histories than physicians, possibly owing to their wider product knowledge.

Family history

Because many diseases have a significant genetic basis, a knowledge of any chronic illness in siblings and parents, and the causes of death if appropriate, may give vital clues. The connection may be direct, e.g. type 2 diabetes, or indirect, e.g. hay fever in the sibling of someone with dermatitis or a wheeze, implying a familial allergic predisposition.

Social history

Enquiries about a patient's circumstances and way of life ('lifestyle') have a number of aims. Clearly, (anti-)social habits such as smoking, drinking and illicit drugs have a bearing on illness, although patients seldom give a reliable estimate (as a general rule, double the number of drinks or cigarettes admitted to). Excessive tea or coffee consumption may also be significant. Special dietary habits are important, especially with ethnic minorities, in vegans, obsessive slimmers, etc.

Equally important is information about a patient's financial and domestic circumstances. Can they afford to be ill? Are they the sole breadwinner, or a single parent? What will be the economic impact of hospital admission, or attendance at a clinic? Is unemployment a factor? Are their living conditions contributing to their illness? What can be done for a patient with heart failure living on the tenth floor and with unreliable lifts? Who does the shopping?

If a patient has a chronic condition, how are they coping? It must also be ascertained whether the patient is psychologically and intellectually able to comprehend the diagnosis and treatment, and to give genuinely informed consent to surgery or other invasive procedures.

History of presenting complaint

So far, little has been said about the patient's actual problem, but a comprehensive picture has been built up which will be useful both for the diagnosis of the current condition and for future reference. There is now an opportunity for the patient to relate their 'story'. Patients should, as far as possible, be allowed to express themselves at their own pace and in their own words, although occasionally some pertinent prompting or 'constructive interruption' is required. The aim is discover how the symptoms arose, what

they are like, how they have developed, and what has been done so far.

Consider pain, for example. The nature and intensity of pain are often significant, such as the difference between crushing cardiac chest pain and the burning retrosternal pain of gastrointestinal origin. How did it start? Is the pain constant, short-lived, episodic or predictable? What makes it better or worse, e.g. warmth, cold, a particular posture? Has the patient already consulted a relative, pharmacist or general practitioner, and what was their advice? Has any treatment been tried, and if so, to what effect?

Note that the clinician need not yet have actually seen the patient. Indeed, much of the history could have been obtained by an assistant or a computer; in fact, in trials computers are sometimes quite effective. It is estimated that up to 75% of diagnoses in primary care can be made correctly by this stage, so consistent is the presentation of most illness. This explains how some doctors are sometimes able temporarily to 'diagnose' and prescribe by telephone, although it is hardly the technique of choice.

Systematic examination (review of systems)

The next stage is to look in detail at each body system. Although it is impossible to avoid this examination being influenced by information obtained so far, ideally it should be objective and complete, so that nothing obscure or unusual is overlooked and the data can be used later for reference. The examination usually starts with general observations of the patient's appearance and condition, in particular his or her coloration, body surface markings, etc. Traditionally, the presence or absence of jaundice, anaemia, cyanosis, clubbing and oedema are noted.

The details relevant to each body system will be discussed as appropriate in the following chapters. For each there are five stages:

1. Directed questioning (functional enquiry) about symptoms likely to follow malfunction of that system.
2. Observation for physical signs.
3. Palpation (feeling).
4. Auscultation (listening with a stethoscope).

5. Percussion (tapping an area and listening to the sound).

Thus, for the cardiovascular system the patient will be asked about tiredness, swelling, palpitations and shortness of breath – especially at night. He or she will then be observed for objective signs such as exercise tolerance, gasping and oedema (ankles, abdomen). The pulses will be felt at different parts of the body, and the extent of any peripheral oedema estimated by local pressure. Auscultation employs the stethoscope to check cardiac rhythm and valve sounds, and also any evidence of pulmonary oedema. Percussion of the chest shows the extent of pulmonary oedema.

Obviously, history and examination must be guided by urgency and the presence of obvious symptoms or signs: a road traffic accident victim with head and chest injury is not asked about their bowel habit or the presence of athlete's foot. Nevertheless, a full review of systems would always be performed at some stage after hospital admission, as part of the clerking process.

Investigations

By this stage, a further 20% of diagnoses will have been made. This leaves perhaps 5% which require further investigation. Simple investigations may be done in a general practitioner's surgery, e.g. ophthalmoscopy, peak flow and blood pressure measurement and urine dipstick tests. Many practices now have ECG equipment. Blood biochemistry and microbiology samples are collected in the surgery and usually sent to a local laboratory. The most common test for which the patient will be referred to a hospital (in the UK) is simple X-ray imaging.

If the diagnosis is still in doubt, investigations of increasing sophistication and expense are gradually employed, so that an ever greater complexity of test is used to diagnose a diminishing proportion of cases.

Diagnosis

A definitive diagnosis is usually clear by this stage; alternatively, it will be provisional, awaiting confirmation from investigations. If several possible diagnoses seem to fit the facts, this differential diagnosis will be resolved by further investigations. Sometimes, the diagnosis remains provisional. If the patient recovers, there may be no benefit in subjecting him or her to invasive, uncomfortable and possibly dangerous further investigation. This sometimes happens with acute moderate chest pain, where a patient is discharged with a final diagnosis of '?myocardial infarction', but without definitive test results, and subsequently managed non-invasively (with counselling, dietary recommendations, etc.) as if the patient had had a mild myocardial infarction.

Management

Each history should conclude with a management plan, which summarizes the aims and the modes prescribed to meet them. In the **problem-orientated** approach, the record of management starts with a summary of all the patient's present problems, which appears at the front of the patient's notes. The summary includes:

- The current complaint (an 'active problem', e.g. hypertension).
- Important past medical history (either active, e.g. peptic ulcer disease, or inactive, e.g. a past myocardial infarction).
- Behaviour which requires modification (e.g. smoking, poor diet).
- Possibly, psychological and social problems.

For each active problem a plan is outlined. This includes any further investigations required for diagnostic confirmation or assessment of severity, the aim of management, the recommended treatment, the means of monitoring and the period of follow-up, e.g. a further appointment in so many weeks. Progress reports recorded in the patient's notes will then be based on this management plan, dealing with each problem for which treatment has been recommended, and the management strategy may be modified according to the patient's response. This systematic approach is also sometimes known by the acronym SOAP:

- **S**ubjective: patients reported or perceived problems.

- Objective: data recorded by clinician or obtained from investigations.
- Assessment of problems.
- Plan of action.

Whether or not such a formal approach is explicitly used, the history always includes progress notes. The outcome or progress of each management aim is recorded and the reasoning behind any changes in treatment explained, e.g. adverse drug effects.

For a hospital admission, the final component is the discharge summary, usually in the form of a letter to the patient's general practitioner.

Drug selection

This introduction concludes with a general review of the factors which determine or influence the choice of drug therapy following diagnosis. In the succeeding chapters the way these principles are applied in common diseases is demonstrated.

The decision process

The typical sequence is illustrated in Fig. 1.2. Clinical findings may suggest several appropriate groups of drugs (or none at all). This must then be progressively narrowed down to one group, then a particular member of that group; finally a route of administration and dose must be chosen.

Consider, for example, managing hypertension. Precise diagnosis of the condition may suggest a particular drug group; quite different strategies will be needed depending on whether the condition is benign primary (essential) hypertension or hypertension secondary to some other disease state, e.g. renovascular disease or to adrenal tumour. Clinical findings will also indicate the urgency of treatment. In primary hypertension the choice would be from among the thiazides, the beta-blockers or the vasodilators; in renovascular disease an angiotensin converting enzyme (ACE) inhibitor may be indicated (if the problem is unilateral); in the

third case, surgery might be feasible. In a patient with essential hypertension and concurrent ischaemic heart disease, beta-blockers may be indicated, but should this be selective or non-selective, short- or long-acting, lipophilic or non-lipophilic? Finally, having selected the most appropriate drug entity, what should be the preferred route of administration, dose and formulation?

In making these decisions, clinical factors such as precise diagnostic class, drug factors such as mode of action and half-life, and patient factors such as age and renal function, are all important. The choice from among the various drugs indicated at each stage is determined initially by **drug factors** (i.e. drugs of choice for the particular disease, independent of the particular patient). Early in the decision process the considerations are principally pharmacodynamic (pharmacological, including toxicological). As the choice becomes more focused, biopharmaceutical and pharmacokinetic factors become more relevant. Thus for essential hypertension there are several types of drugs indicated, related to their pharmacological effect on blood pressure. Once a drug group has been decided upon,

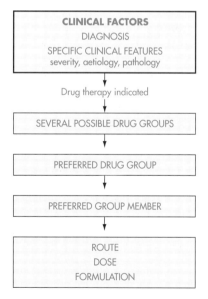

Figure 1.2 Factors affecting choice in drug therapy. This is a generalized scheme showing the sequence of decisions taken when pharmacotherapy is decided following diagnosis of a new disease.

selecting a particular member would need to take account of the spectrum of pharmacokinetic properties of the group, or the formulations available.

At each stage the selection based on drug factors may then be modified or constrained by **patient factors**, such as the patient's response to the agent (pharmacodynamics), their handling of it (pharmacokinetics), or possibly concurrent disease or drug therapy. Thus the choice of a renally cleared drug might have to be changed in a patient with renal impairment; a patient with compliance problems might benefit from a modified-release preparation; a patient with diabetes should avoid thiazides. Finally, one should not forget cost: from a number of comparably efficacious and safe drugs the most economic one must always be first choice.

There are also what may be described as **prescriber factors**, i.e. the clinician's own preference, exercised on the basis of familiarity and experience, and these may be as good a guide as any when choosing from among a range of very similar preparations. On the other hand this may occasionally be based on unsystematic anecdotal evidence or outdated habits. In their new role as pharmaceutical advisers, pharmacists are now assisting GPs in making evidence-based choices and constructing rational formularies to facilitate drug selection.

Drug factors

Pharmacodynamics and toxicity

These are the primary criteria. Occasionally the diagnosis will indicate a unique drug group or even one specific drug (e.g. levothyroxine (thyroxine) in hypothyroidism), but usually there are a number of approximately equivalent strategies available at this stage. Precise pharmacological properties then become important, the choice depending on the clinical presentation. For example, an arterial vasodilator may be more useful than a venodilator in certain types of heart failure; a cough suppressant rather than a decongestant may be preferred for a cough unproductive of mucus. Receptor subtype specificity may also be relevant, e.g. cardioselectivity

of beta-blockers, specific amine re-uptake block in antidepressants.

A drug's therapeutic index must also be considered: what is the risk-to-benefit ratio of treatment? The severity of the condition may indicate the need for a more potent but more toxic agent, but can the plasma level or adverse effects be easily monitored? If so, does the plasma level correlate with the concentration at the presumed site of action or the therapeutic benefit, or with the intensity of adverse effects?

Biopharmaceutics

Formulation is frequently important, e.g. for intravenous preparations, where stability and pharmaceutical compatibility are crucial, and dermatological preparations, where penetration, skin hydration, miscibility, etc. can influence effectiveness. Formulation can also affect bioavailability, which is particularly important for drugs with a narrow therapeutic index used to stabilize serious chronic conditions, e.g. phenytoin in epilepsy, aminophylline in asthma.

Some drugs are unsuitable for certain routes, e.g. benzylpenicillin is destroyed by gastrointestinal enzymes and so is unsuitable for oral administration, theophylline requires too high a dose mass for aerosolization, and phenytoin is too irritant for intramuscular use.

Pharmacokinetics

A drug's physicochemical properties, especially its hydrophilic/lipophilic balance, pKa and molecular size, affect its absorption, distribution to the required site of action, mode and rate of clearance and route of elimination.

Hydrophilic/lipophilic balance
The characteristics conferred by predominant hydrophilic or lipophilic properties (summarized in Table 1.3) are particularly noticeable within a series of otherwise similar drugs, e.g. the beta-blockers. Most drugs need both properties: lipophilic to cross membranes, hydrophilic to enable transport and distribution in aqueous media such as plasma. For lipophilicity the drugs will need some non-polar groups in their structure and, if such drugs are ionic, they will exist

Table 1.3   Effects of hydrophilic and lipophilic tendencies on the biological properties of drugs

Predominantly lipophilic	Predominantly hydrophilic
Good membrane penetration	Poor membrane penetration
Good oral absorption	Poor oral absorption
Distributed in body fat	Distributed in body water
Cross blood–brain barrier	
Hepatic metabolism	Cleared renally unchanged
Longer half-life	Shorter half-life
First-pass effect possible	
Clearance dependent on liver function	Clearance dependent on renal function
Biliary excretion of hydrophilic metabolites (MW >400 Da)	
Possible interaction with other hepatically metabolized drugs	Increased plasma protein binding
	Possible interaction with other bound drugs

MW, molecular weight.

to a significant extent in unionized form at body pH, i.e. their pKa should be near 7.4. Strongly hydrophilic drugs are often highly polar, and those that are ionic have pKa values significantly less than or greater than 7.4.

Membrane permeability, which determines many biological properties, is highly dependent on polarity. Lipophilic drugs (e.g. most general anaesthetics) pass biological membranes easily, whereas ionized molecules (e.g. aminoglycoside antibiotics) generally penetrate membranes poorly in the absence of specific transmembrane pumps.

Hydrophilic drugs (e.g. atenolol) are cleared mainly by renal excretion, which often tends to give them a shorter half-life especially if they undergo tubular secretion. Lipophilic drugs (e.g. propranolol) are likely to be metabolized rapidly by the liver to produce a more hydrophilic molecule that can then be more easily excreted by the kidney. This is an important purpose of hepatic 'detoxification', in addition to simple chemical deactivation. Taken orally, lipophilic drugs are more likely to suffer first-pass hepatic metabolism, with consequent reduced bioavailability (e.g. propranolol). Highly lipophilic drugs partition into body fat, and so may have a high volume of distribution and prolonged half-life (e.g. diazepam).

Although lipophilic molecules are freely filtered at the glomerulus, they are equally freely reabsorbed from the tubules, so their net renal clearance is inherently low. In contrast, hydrophilic molecules are less efficiently reabsorbed and are more likely to pass out in the urine.

pKa

Acidic drugs (e.g. aspirin) are generally more highly bound to plasma albumin, giving a lower volume of distribution, i.e. they tend to stay in the plasma rather than distribute to the tissues (Table 1.4). Basic drugs (e.g. many CNS-acting agents, such as phenothiazines) are, theoretically at least, more prone to binding to acid glycoprotein, an acute phase inflammatory plasma protein; however, albumin also has binding sites for basic drugs. Plasma protein binding reduces the free (unbound) drug plasma concentration, and thus both drug activity and clearance, because it is this fraction which is available for pharmacodynamic effect, and also for hepatic extraction and renal excretion.

Table 1.4 Effects of pKa on the biological properties of ionizable drugs

pKa	Effect
<7.4	Hydrophilic; acidic Absorbed in stomach (fastest) Bound to plasma albumin Reduced solubility in normal urine
About 7.4	Lipophilic
>7.4	Hydrophilic; basic Absorbed in ileum (delayed) Bound to plasma acid glycoprotein Increased solubility in normal urine

Interactions may occur intrarenally owing to competition for the special tubular secretory transport mechanisms that exist for weak acids and bases. The pH of the urine can affect clearance: a more acid urine promotes the clearance of basic drugs, and vice versa. This is the basis of forced acid or alkaline diuresis to treat poisoning, e.g. urinary alkalinization for barbiturate or aspirin overdose.

Molecular size

Membrane permeability is also affected by molecular size. Ionized or highly polar molecules greater than 100 daltons do not cross membranes. Hydrophilic hepatic metabolites greater than 400 daltons are likely to be excreted in the bile, while smaller molecules are excreted renally.

Overall effect

The sum of all the pharmacokinetic properties of a drug will determine important parameters of its use:

• The half-life.
• The time a single oral dose will take to reach peak concentration, which affects the usefulness in an emergency and the best timing of plasma level sampling.
• The time to reach steady state, which may in turn affect the time to initial onset of useful action, and the minimum advisable interval between dose changes.
• Peak and trough plasma levels.

• The frequency of dosage, which may affect compliance.

As an example of how these factors affect choice, consider drugs for the oral prophylaxis of recurrent urinary tract infection. If they are to be effective they must be well absorbed, should not be significantly deactivated by the liver and should be excreted in antimicrobially significant concentrations in the urine. Because prophylactic therapy is often associated with compliance problems, a long-acting drug or formulation with a once-daily dosage regimen would be preferred.

Toxicity may also be influenced by physicochemical factors, e.g. the more lipophilic beta-blockers readily cross the blood–brain barrier and may cause adverse CNS effects.

Patient factors

There is often a wide interpatient variation in response, both therapeutic and toxic, to a standard dose of a drug. Thus, despite careful attention to all the above factors, there is still a need to review carefully the drug and dose choice for an individual patient. This variation arises owing to a combination of differing pharmacological responses (pharmacodynamics; Table 1.5) to the drug and differing drug handling (pharmacokinetics; Table 1.6).

Response

Drug response varies with **age**. The elderly and the very young may have atypical responses to many drugs. These may be due to anomalous or exaggerated sensitivity, especially to drugs acting on the CNS, e.g. aggression in some elderly patients taking benzodiazepines. Alternatively, there may be impaired physiological or homeostatic mechanisms, e.g. an exaggerated hypotensive effect with vasodilators, or hyponatraemia with diuretics. In some cases there are genetic or **racial** differences in drug response, e.g. thiazide diuretics are much more effective antihypertensives in Blacks, who respond less favourably than Whites to beta-blockers.

In attempting to explain unexpected responses, particularly apparent ineffectiveness, the possibility of patient **non-compliance** should always

Table 1.5 Reasons for variation in patient response

Age
Race
Compliance
Concurrent disease
Concurrent medication
Pregnancy, breast feeding
Tolerance, hypersensitivity
Genetic variability in metabolic enzymes

Table 1.6 Variations and constraints in drug handling

Absorption	Interactions with diet or other drugs
	Site of absorption:
	– gastrointestinal disease
	– regional perfusion
	– airways patency
	– etc.
	Parenteral:
	– fluid volume
	– venous access
	– local perfusion
Distribution	Age
	Weight/build
	Fluid and electrolyte balance/ hydration
	Systemic/regional perfusion
	Internal barriers
	Plasma protein level
	Interactions with other drugs
Elimination	Renal and hepatic function:
	– age
	– race
	– disease
	Interactions with other drugs

be borne in mind. The possible reasons for non-compliance are many and pharmacists have an essential role in detecting it and improving the situation. In some cases a change in drug or formulation may encourage better compliance, e.g. a long-acting, once-daily form for essential hypertension. In other cases, an inappropriate dose or exaggerated sensitivity to adverse effects may be to blame. Sensitive enquiry of the patient will often uncover an innocent or perfectly reasonable explanation, frequently deriving from poor communication or imperfect patient understanding. The currently recommended ideal is to develop a **concordance** between prescriber and patient, i.e. mutually agreed objectives and constraints and mutually agreed treatment.

Concurrent diseases may increase the patient's sensitivity to some drugs; for example, the myocardium is more sensitive to digoxin after infarction, or in thyroid imbalance. Other diseases may indirectly make a patient less tolerant of the drug, e.g. beta-blockers are contraindicated in asthma. The patient's biochemical and physiological status is often important, e.g. digoxin toxicity is greatly increased in the presence of potassium imbalance.

Previous or sustained exposure to a drug may produce an unexpected **tolerance** to either the therapeutic effect (e.g. prophylactic nitrates in ischaemic heart disease) or an adverse effect (e.g. anticholinergics). The patient may be taking *other drugs* which have an antagonistic effect (e.g. corticosteroids and thiazides antagonize oral hypoglycaemic drugs) or synergism may occur (e.g. two CNS depressants given concurrently, such as an OTC antihistamine and an anxiolytic).

For reasons that are poorly understood some patients have anomalous or **idiosyncratic** adverse reactions to certain drugs, the penicillins being the best example. These are often immunologically based, non-dose-dependent Type B adverse effects.

Finally, with women, the possibility of the drug having an effect on **conception, pregnancy** or **breast feeding** must be considered.

Handling

Interpatient variation in pharmacokinetic parameters may be inborn or acquired, and is particularly important in dosage and route selection, but also sometimes affects which drug group is selected.

Absorption
Many diseases can affect oral absorption. Disease of the gut itself may of course affect absorption

(e.g. vomiting, diarrhoea, inflammatory bowel disease), but so too can cardiovascular disease, which may compromise gastrointestinal perfusion. The elderly are more prone to such diseases, especially heart failure. Oral absorption is little affected by age itself. Oral intolerance, e.g. gastric upset, is a common adverse effect and a reason for both non-compliance and serious morbidity.

There may be unwanted interactions with the patient's diet or other drug therapy, e.g. tetracycline absorption being impaired by concurrent milk or antacid consumption.

Absorption from any site depends on an adequate blood supply. Subcutaneous or intramuscular injections may be ineffective if the circulation is compromised, because blood is redirected to the core visceral circulation. Thus, following myocardial infarction, morphine must always be given intravenously. Diabetics should understand that insulin absorption from a limb injection site is more variable than an abdominal one, because limb perfusion will depend on physical activity.

There may be other barriers to absorption. Bronchodilators will not easily penetrate constricted airways, and transdermal absorption will vary according to the skin thickness of the area to which a dermatological or transdermal preparation is applied and to the local blood flow (e.g. increased in inflammation).

If intravenous infusion is planned, the condition of the patient's veins must be considered, and whether the patient can tolerate the fluid load of the vehicle or any associated ions, e.g. sodium with benzylpenicillin.

Distribution

Distribution is affected by the proportion of adipose tissue to lean body mass (which is aqueous), and by the plasma protein level which may affect the free drug plasma level, depending on its kinetics. This can affect both the overall volume of distribution, the distribution between different compartments, and access to the organs of elimination, chiefly the liver and kidney.

The elderly have a lower lean body mass and a relatively smaller aqueous compartment than middle-aged adults, and the very young have a higher proportion of body water. Both the elderly and the very young have reduced plasma albumin. The patient's nutritional state and hydration will similarly affect drug distribution between various compartments, as will a large volume of oedema fluid. A large volume of distribution will result in lower plasma levels.

Delivery to the target site is dependent primarily on the regional blood perfusion. This may be seriously impaired in heart failure, shock, peripheral vascular disease or diabetic blood vessel disease. For example, it is difficult to treat an infection in a diabetic's foot with systemic antibiotics.

Distribution may be further modified by the body's internal barriers. For example, the blood–brain barrier impedes polar molecules, but this effect is much reduced if it is inflamed, e.g. in meningitis. Pus is poorly penetrated by some antibiotics, and sputum concentrations of antibiotics are frequently far lower than plasma concentrations.

Other drugs that a patient may be taking may compete for plasma protein binding sites, causing an increase in the free drug levels of the one displaced. However, despite the many theoretical possibilities of such interactions, relatively few are clinically significant and only a small number are serious. One drug will only cause a significant elevation in the free concentration of another by displacement if both are avidly bound to the same site, are in high concentration in the plasma, and have a low volume of distribution, i.e. most of the drug in the body is in the plasma.

Moreover, clearance of the displaced drug may be increased, and this tends to counteract any rise in plasma level. Only certain drugs are likely to cause clinically significant problems by this mechanism: these include potentially toxic drugs with a narrow therapeutic index, and those whose doses are carefully titrated to stabilize a chronic condition, e.g. anti-epileptics, oral hypoglycaemics and anticoagulants.

Concurrent disease may also influence binding. Endogenous metabolites such as bilirubin, which is elevated in jaundice, may compete for binding sites. A high blood urea level, i.e. renal failure or 'uraemia', impairs protein binding, and hypoproteinaemia in liver failure, malabsorption and the nephrotic syndrome, will reduce available sites.

Elimination

The function of either of the main organs of elimination may be impaired by disease, age or concurrent drug therapy. A knowledge of the patient's renal and hepatic function, their medication history and the mode(s) of elimination of the drug to be used, is essential when selecting therapy. This complex subject cannot be dealt with in any detail here, and the reader is referred to the References and further reading section for texts on clinical pharmacology.

Pharmaceutical care

As stated in the Preface, this is not a textbook of clinical pharmacy. However, it is relevant to note at this point the most recent developments in the involvement of pharmacists in patient care. Pharmacists are increasingly taking more responsibility for the management and optimization of the entire spectrum of a patient's pharmacotherapy. This has extended the concept of clinical pharmacy beyond validating indications and screening contraindications, interactions and dosage regimens. Pharmacists now have a commitment to anticipate or identify all possible drug-related problems. Pharmaceutical care involves devising an appropriate pharmaceutical care plan and specifying how this will be implemented and monitored for success and adverse events. This is similar to the problem-oriented model of medical management, and the pharmaceutical care plan has adapted the SOAP approach (p. 10).

References and further reading

Graeme-Smith DG, Aronson JK (1992) *Oxford Textbook of Clinical Pharmacology and Drug Treatment.* 2nd edn. Oxford: Oxford University Press.

Hope RA, Longmore JM, Moss PAH, Warrens AN (1993) *Oxford Handbook of Clinical Medicine. Chapter 2: History and physical examination.* 3rd edn. Oxford: Oxford University Press.

Petrie JC, ed. (1999) Clinical pharmacology. *Medicine* **27** (3): 1–16.

Speight TM, ed. (1997) *Avery's Drug Treatment. Section I: Clinical pharmacology.* 4th edn. Auckland: Adis Press.

2

Major pathological processes in disease

Just as physiology is the study of the way in which the body works, pathology is the scientific study of abnormal physiology, i.e. disease.

There are many ways in which physiological processes can be upset, and knowledge of the cause of a disease (aetiology) may give valuable clues to diagnosis and management. The physician will rely on the signs and symptoms resulting from the derangement of normal physiology to reach these decisions. In this chapter we will examine how physiological processes are altered by disease.

PHYSIOLOGICAL PROCESSES are delicately balanced to maintain a stable internal environment, i.e. homeostasis. This includes, for instance, maintaining a constant temperature or blood pressure, ensuring that the body is properly hydrated and adjusting levels of electrolytes. Homeostasis involves complex inter-related positive and negative feedback mechanisms. It is the mechanism by which the body can defend itself both externally and internally against a changing and sometimes hostile environment. This concept of homeostasis as a defence mechanism plays a key to understanding pathology.

One reason why physiology becomes abnormal is that the various homeostatic mechanisms have been overwhelmed, e.g. being severely injured in a road accident could overwhelm all of the various physiological responses to injury. Similarly, bacteria may enter the bloodstream in such numbers as to overwhelm the immune system. However, this only explains a relatively narrow range of diseases. Most appear to be due to defective adaptive mechanisms (defensive or homeostatic) which, instead of maintaining a stable internal environment, actually disrupt normal function. Table 2.1 lists some general causes of disease and how they can give rise to four major pathological processes: inflammation, degeneration, neoplasia and inherited disease. Running through each of these is the recurrent theme of failure in adaptive mechanisms; this is **maladaptation.**

For example, with infection, it is often the response of the body in trying to eliminate the organism rather than the presence of the organism, or even its toxins, which cause the major problem. Immunological processes themselves can be more harmful than beneficial under certain circumstances. Antibodies can attack and damage the body's own tissues.

However a tissue is damaged, the body attempts to remove the source of the injury and

Table 2.1 Classification of pathological processes

Pathological process	Aetiology	Examples of results
Inflammation (tissue response)	Infection Immunological Physical • trauma • toxins • radiation	Any '-itis' Fibrosis
Degeneration (cellular response)	As for inflammation Ischaemia	Cell/tissue destruction • myocardial infarction • renal failure • stroke
Neoplasia	Predisposing factors Carcinogens	Tumours
Inherited disease	Faulty genetic codes	Disease with strong family history • malformation • inborn errors of metabolism

repair the tissue. The fundamental tissue response to injury is known as **inflammation**, but if it is inappropriate or excessive it may do more damage than the original injury. The consequences of inflammation are far-reaching and underlie many different disease states. For this reason much of this chapter is devoted to a consideration of inflammation and the closely related **immunological** processes.

Degeneration is another major pathological process and can be considered as a cellular response to injury. Radiation, toxins, infections, immunological defects and ischaemia may all lead to cellular damage, degeneration and eventually tissue death (**necrosis**).

Many diseases are caused through cardiovascular problems. If blood loss is very severe, circulatory collapse (**shock**) may result. Conversely, **thrombosis** (a blood clot in a vessel) can be viewed as a defect in the homeostatic mechanisms that normally prevent blood loss.

The results of thrombosis, shock and related phenomena can all lead to a reduction in blood flow to an area of tissue, i.e. **ischaemia** (literally 'blocking blood'), which may cause degeneration or death of the tissue supplied (ischaemia is discussed in some detail later, pp. 46–50).

Many of these disease processes are interrelated. For instance, an inflammatory response evoked by a widespread burn will lead to a large exudation of protein-rich fluid from the bloodstream. The resulting low blood pressure (shock) will cause kidney ischaemia. As a result, the kidney nephrons may degenerate and, once the number of functioning nephrons falls below a critical level, renal failure will result. Thus one pathological process may lead to another, and often does so.

Immunology

Specific and non-specific immunity

We have discussed the concept of disease as a breakdown in the internal or external defence mechanisms. There are three general lines of defence against a hostile environment: the simple barriers provided by the skin and mucous membranes; the complex but non-specific inflammatory reaction; and the specific immune defence mechanisms. We concentrate here on the last two.

Following exposure to infection, defence will usually develop against the organism concerned and the chance of re-infection is slight. This is known as **specific acquired immunity**. Immunology is the study of the way in which the body develops specific immunity and its various consequences. Specific immunity may be due to circulating antibodies (**humoral immunity**), or to specific sensitized cells (**cell-mediated immunity**).

There are also systems of innate **non-specific immunity**, which do not depend on contact with a foreign organism, protein, etc. The key cells here are neutrophils and macrophages which engulf and digest any microbe or foreign material with which they come into contact, regardless of whether it has previously encountered the immune system or not. However, the action of these cell types is greatly enhanced if the body has developed acquired immunity to the organism. Similarly, **complement** (p. 28) provides a non-specific immunity, but can also act to potentiate acquired immunity.

Antigens

An antigen is any foreign substance, of whatever origin, that is capable of initiating the production of a specific protein – called an immunoglobulin (Ig, antibody) – which will act against it. The immunoglobulins so formed will react preferentially with that particular antigen. However, other antigens possessing a sufficiently similar chemical structure may cross-react with the immunoglobulin. The antigen–antibody reactions involve close intermolecular binding and depend on a 'lock and key' steric fit, similar to the binding of drugs to receptors.

Most antigens are proteins. Once these have been recognized by the immune system as 'non-self' (foreign) an immune response is initiated. Microorganisms always express several antigenic groupings (determinants, epitopes) on their surface, so a number of different immunoglobulins may be produced against a particular organism.

A vast number of non-microbial proteins are also capable of stimulating antibody production, including the numerous substances to which allergies are developed. Macromolecules other than proteins can also lead to the production of antibodies, e.g. lipopolysaccharides. Smaller molecules or ions, e.g. heavy metals, may act as antigenic determinants if they combine with normally non-antigenic proteins; in this case they are termed **haptens.**

Cell types involved in the immune system

White blood cells (leucocytes) of three classes are the chief components of the immune system (Fig. 2.1).

Lymphocytes

These comprise two main classes, the **B cells** and **T cells.** B cells are responsible for the production of immunoglobulins, i.e. humoral immunity. They originate in the bone marrow but mature in lymphoid tissue, probably within the alimentary tract, and are stored in the cortical region of lymph nodes. They are capable of producing immunoglobulins only when mature. Only about 0.1% of B cells are found in the bloodstream, and those that produce immunoglobulins are called **plasma cells.**

T cells mature within the thymus and are stored in the paracortical area of the lymph nodes. They have two important roles: **cell-mediated immunity** (CMI) directly against certain types of microorganisms and viruses, and regulation of the activity of B cells. There are two important classes of T cells: **T helper cells** (TH) which have a general regulatory function and **cytotoxic T cells** (TC), which identify and eliminate virus-infected host cells as well as certain bacteria.

TH cells are able to recruit TC cells, and they can also stimulate B cells to form antibodies. TH cells perform these functions through the production of **cytokines,** some of which have a stimulatory action and others an inhibitory effect on lymphocytes. It has been postulated that a third type of cell, T suppressor cells, have

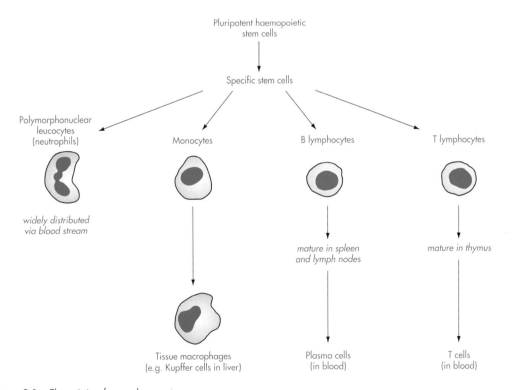

Figure 2.1   The origin of some leucocytes.

a general inhibitory function, but it is now widely held that there is no separate lineage, simply that TH cells will in certain circumstances produce inhibitory cytokines.

Different types of T cells can be distinguished by the use of monoclonal antibodies (pp. 24–27) to distinguish specific groups of cell surface antigens, the so-called cluster of differentiation (CD) number. TH cells possessing CD4 receptors are able to bind to **major histocompatibility complex** (MHC) class II molecules on the surface of antigen-presenting cells (pp. 34–35). TC cells possessing CD8 receptors are able to bind with MHC class I molecules, thus identifying cells that have been infected by a virus. Over 30 CD antigen types have been identified on a wide variety of cells from platelets to macrophages.

Monocytes

Monocytes are formed in the bone marrow and migrate via the bloodstream to various body tissues, where they are termed macrophages. Some macrophages have specific names according to the particular tissue they inhabit, e.g. a macrophage in the liver is called a **Kupffer cell**. Macrophages are scavengers, capable of phagocytosing (engulfing) a wide variety of foreign matter or microorganisms. Once the particle or organism has been taken up by the macrophage, it may be destroyed by the action of superoxides, free radicals and lysosomal enzymes.

There has recently been great interest in the secretory function of macrophages, particularly of the interleukin (IL) group of cytokines. IL-1 and IL-6, when secreted by macrophages, are believed to play an important part in some of the generalized symptoms of systemic inflammatory reactions, e.g. septic shock (p. 48), particularly fever. The role of macrophages as antigen-presenting cells (pp. 24–27) is also partly facilitated by the action of interleukins. Many other substances are secreted by macrophages, some of which have an important role in chronic inflammation (pp. 44–46).

Polymorphonuclear leucocytes (polymorphs, neutrophils, PMNs)

Like the macrophages, these are phagocytic. However, there are important differences: poly-morphonuclear leucocytes are shorter-lived than macrophages, play no part in cell-mediated immunity, and are important in acute rather than chronic inflammation. However, like macrophages, they will readily ingest antigens that have been coated with antibody (**opsonized**).

Cellular messengers: the cytokine network

In recent years much attention has focused on the way in which the various cells involved in the immune system are controlled and interact. The principal cellular messengers involved comprise the cytokine network, which is being intensively researched to provide immunological treatments for a wide range of diseases.

Cytokines are produced by a range of leucocytes; those produced by T cells are referred to as **lymphokines**, those by monocytes as **monokines**. The cytokines that have the particular property of inducing chemotaxis are sometimes called **chemokines.** Various cytokines have a number of overlapping actions, and the exact role in the immunological response is not always easy to define, often being dependent on the initial reason for stimulation. For instance, some cytokines produced by TH cells to stimulate macrophages will in other circumstances also inhibit B cell function. The most important cytokines are the **interleukins**, **interferons**, **colony stimulating factors** and **tumour necrosis factors**; these are listed in Table 2.2 with their cells of origin and range of actions. Some cytokines are already used in clinical practice:

- Both **interleukin 2** and **interferon-alpha** are used in the management of certain types of tumour.
- The immunosuppressive effects of **beta-interferon** are utilized in multiple sclerosis to reduce the incidence of acute attacks in the relapsing/remitting form of the disease.
- **Granulocyte colony stimulating factor** (G-CSF) and **granulocyte-macrophage colony stimulating factor** (GM-CSF) are employed as adjuncts to chemotherapy in order to stimulate white blood cell production after treatment with myelosuppressive agents (*see* Chapter 11).

- Inhibitors of interleukins and tumour necrosis factors are also being investigated for use in the management of a variety of autoimmune diseases, e.g. rheumatoid arthritis.

Humoral immunity: antibody formation

When antigens first appear in the body they are taken up by monocytes (which reside in the lymph nodes) and expressed on their surfaces; these are then known as **antigen-presenting cells** (APCs). After expression of an epitope of the immunogen on the surface of the APC, and in combination with an MHC (as described on pp. 34–35), the antigen can be readily recognized as foreign by TH cells. These in turn stimulate B cells to produce immunoglobulins. Although most antigenic responses require the involvement of T cells in this way, some bacterial antigens are T cell-independent and B cell clones can be stimulated directly. Communications between T and B cells are mediated by interleukins (Fig. 2.2).

A single B cell cannot form all the varieties of immunoglobulin (Ig) that may ever be required. A clone of B cells will produce antibody against a single antigen. When the antigen is presented to B cells belonging to the correct clone, the cells multiply, mature and produce the appropriate Ig. Cells belonging to a particular clone can recognize the specific antigen, owing to the presence on the cell surface of the Ig that it will eventually synthesize, i.e. the Ig acts as a surface receptor. Reaction between antigen and immunoglobulin

---

Table 2.2   The cytokines

Type	Cellular origin	Main action
Interleukins		
IL-1	APC/macrophages	Clonal proliferation of TH cells
IL-2	TH cells	Activation of other T, B and K cells
IL-3	Stem cells	Stimulates lymphocyte growth in marrow
IL-4, 5, 6	T cells	B cell growth and differentiation
	Macrophages	Inflammation
IL-7	Marrow and thymus	Stimulates B and T cell growth
IL-8	Macrophages	Attracts neutrophils
IL-9	T cells	Growth factor
IL-10, 13	TH cells	Inhibitory action
IL-11	Bone marrow	Stimulates stem cells
IL-12	B cells	Stimulates T and K cells
Interferons		
IFNα	Macrophages	Suppresses cell growth
IFNβ	Fibroblasts	Stimulates K cells
IFNδ	T cells	Blocks viral mRNA transcription
Colony-stimulating factors		
GM-CSF (+G-CSF, M-CSF)	Marrow	Granulocyte/macrophage production
Erythropoietin	Kidney	Erythrocyte production
Tumour necrosis factors		
TNFα	Macrophages	Inflammation
TNFβ	Lymphocytes	Healing
		Vascular shock

APC, antigen-presenting cell; G-CSF, granulocyte colony stimulating factor; GM-CSF, granulocyte-macrophage colony stimulating factor; IL, interleukin; K, killer cell; M-CSF, macrophage colony stimulating factor; TH, T helper cell.

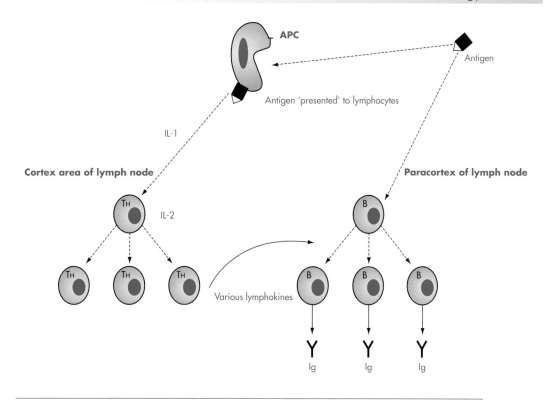

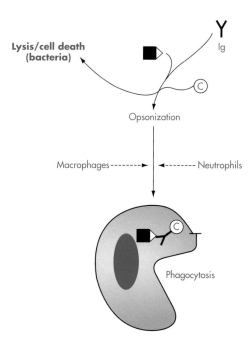

Figure 2.2   Humoral immunity. APC, antigen-presenting cell; B, B lymphocytes; C, complement; Ig, immunoglobulin; IL, interleukins; T$_H$, T helper cells.

acts as a signal for the clone to proliferate. A microorganism may activate a number of clones, but a specific antigen will only stimulate a single clone, to produce **monoclonal antibodies**. The latter are an important research tool, e.g. as markers for certain cancer cells. They also have useful clinical application, such as immunosuppression to prevent graft rejection, where monoclonal antibodies have been raised against the T lymphocytes causing rejection of the graft. The same principle is being investigated for the treatment of a variety of autoimmune diseases by using monoclonal antibodies against CD4 to inhibit the function of Tᴴ cells. Fab fragments of monoclonal antibodies that can complex digoxin (e.g. **Digibind**) have been used for some time to treat overdoses of this drug. The use of Fab fragments in the treatment of cancer has been less successful, because penetration of the antibody into the tumour mass appears to be a limiting factor.

Immunoglobulin production is modulated by Tᴴ cells, which promote or suppress Ig production. This introduces the concept of **immune tolerance**, i.e. when potentially antigenic material fails to elicit an immune response. Natural tolerance to host (self) tissues is acquired during fetal development. The mechanisms by which the immune system distinguishes between 'self' and 'non-self' are not clear, but may be by the elimination of clones of B cells capable of producing self-antibodies (anti-host antibodies) early in fetal development. This clonal elimination is not the only mechanism that safeguards the body tissues from immunological attack – the HLA system (described later) also plays an important part in distinguishing self from non-self. Failure of the body to recognize self-antigens causes a variety of **autoimmune diseases**. An acquired tolerance to other antigens can also develop later in life if the body is subjected to progressively larger doses of antigen. This is the basis of **hyposensitization therapy** for allergic diseases, although this technique is not yet very effective therapeutically, and is potentially hazardous.

Antigenic material can make contact with the host defence system wherever white blood cells are found, e.g. the bloodstream, lymphatic system and in epithelial tissues. Antibodies can be detected approximately 2 weeks after the first exposure to an antigen, corresponding to the time required for the B cells to multiply and differentiate into plasma cells. This is the **primary response**. On subsequent contact with the same antigen, antibodies are synthesized almost immediately and in far higher concentrations than during the primary response.

The basic structure of immunoglobulins comprises two types of polypeptide chain (heavy and light), which together comprise a crystallizable fragment (Fc) and an antigen binding fragment (Fab). There are five groups of immunoglobulins (IgA, IgG, IgM, IgD and IgE), distinguished by the type of heavy chain. The general structure of IgG, of which there are at least 45 subclasses, is illustrated in Fig. 2.3. The Fc portion is responsible for non-specific cell binding to macrophages or polymorphs. The Fab fragment binds to specific antigens and has the highly variable structure responsible for the specificity of antibodies. Each Fab fragment is a particular 'lock' which matches just one antigen 'key'. Antibodies combine with the antigens so that opsonization by phagocytic cells can more readily take place. Some antibodies are also directly toxic to cells after subsequent combination with complement. A brief description of each type of immunoglobulin is given in Table 2.3.

We can now complete the picture of humoral

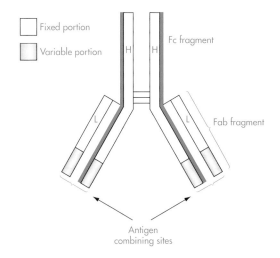

Figure 2.3   Structure of gamma-globulin (IgG). H, heavy chain; L, light chain.

Table 2.3 The principal properties of the immunoglobulins

Immunoglobulin	% of total pool	Function	Action
IgG	73%	Most antibody responses	Opsonization Antiviral Antitoxin
IgM	7% (mostly in blood)	Many (initial) antibody responses	Opsonization Bacterial agglutination
IgA	20% (mainly in secretions)	Secreted by epithelia, e.g. intestines, lung Protects mucosa from infection	Antitoxin Prevents adherence of bacteria and viruses to mucosa
IgE	0.001%	Opposes helminth infection Binds to mast cells if present	Allergy
IgD	0.02% (on surface of B cells)	Unknown	–

immunity. After production by plasma cells, an immunoglobulin links to the antigen via the variable end of the Fab moiety. Complement sometimes binds to the Fc moiety. This **immune complex** is now available for opsonization. The immune complex binds strongly to the surface of a phagocytic cell, again by the Fc fragment, and is then easily drawn inside the cell where it can be destroyed. Antigenic determinants on the cell surface of a bacterium would bind Igs, resulting in opsonization and phagocytosis in a similar way.

Although opsonization is the primary mode of action of Igs, they can also act directly on bacteria by causing them to clump together (**agglutinate**). Additionally, certain Igs (antitoxins) can neutralize bacterial toxins. The overall scheme is shown in Fig. 2.2.

Cell-mediated immunity (CMI)

Bacterial, fungal and viral infections may be combated via CMI, but CMI is far slower-acting than humoral immunity. Even the secondary response may take days to appear. The cells chiefly responsible are T cells and macrophages.

Initial contact with a bacterial antigen causes the proliferation of sensitized lymphocytes similar to the process seen with B cells. Extremely long-lived **memory T cells** are also produced, ensuring that sensitized T cells are available on subsequent exposure to the antigen. The initial recognition of antigens by TH cells is achieved by expression of the antigen by an APC, as previously described, usually in combination with an MHC class II molecule. Bacteria eliciting this response are generally the larger ones, e.g. *Mycobacterium tuberculosis*. Fungi such as *Candida albicans* are also dealt with via CMI. The process in summarized in Fig. 2.4(a).

CMI can also combat viral infections if the virus has altered the surface of the cell it has invaded, so as to confer new antigenic properties on the cell. This commonly occurs because the virus contains genetic material affecting cell surface structures. In this case the host cell is recognized and attacked by TC cells via MHC class I molecules on the host cell surface (Fig. 2.4(b)). The proliferation of some cancer cells may be inhibited similarly, if the neoplastic change renders them recognizable as foreign by the immune system (*see* Chapter 11).

Interleukins also play an important part in the process of stimulating the various cell types involved in CMI. For instance, IL-1 is released from APCs to stimulate TH cells to produce IL-2, which in turn stimulates TC cells. Furthermore, some cytokines produced by TH cells are able to stimulate and attract macrophages.

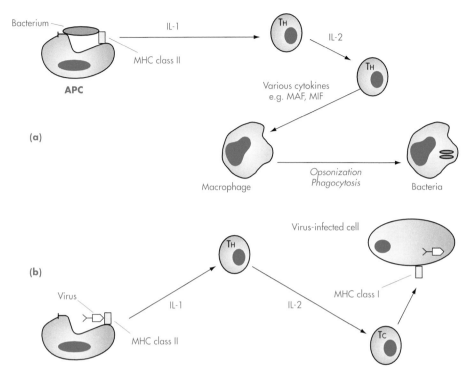

Figure 2.4 Cell-mediated immunity. (a) Bacteria; (b) viruses. APC, antigen-presenting cell; IL, interleukin; MAF, macrophage activating factor; MIF, macrophage inhibiting factor; Tc, cytotoxic T cell; TH, T helper cell.

The complement system

This system has already been mentioned in connection with opsonization and will be encountered later in connection with inflammation. The complement system is an example of a nonspecific immune mechanism in that a similar process occurs, regardless of the type of stimulus.

About 20 different, naturally occurring plasma proteins make up this system; the steps involved in the activation of the complement system are summarized in Fig. 2.5. In practice, the individual complement components combine with each other at various stages of the cascade. C1 is activated by the presence of an immune complex, and then acts as an esterase to cleave C4 into C4a plus C4b, and C2 into C2a plus C2b. These complement factors then combine and cleave others to continue the cascade as shown. Finally, C8 and C9 binds with C567 which lyses

cell membranes, either bacterial or host. This sequence of events is known as the **classical pathway** for complement activation. In certain situations, e.g. in some viral infections, the **alternate pathway** may be invoked and C3 can be activated directly without the production of C3 (C42) convertase.

Two important aspects of the complement system should be noted. First, sequential activation results in amplification of the system. Thus one bimolecule of C3 convertase will produce many C3b molecules, and one molecule of C8 can bind up to six molecules of C9. Also, many of the individual components of the system have intrinsic immunological and inflammatory properties in their own right.

The complement system also plays a part in blood clotting by a complex process which is linked to the activation of Hageman factor and the kinin system.

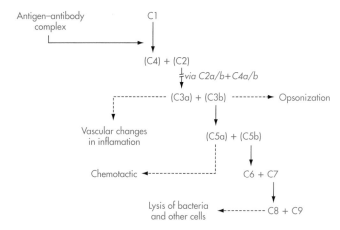

Figure 2.5   Classical complement pathway (simplified).

Potential problems with the immune system (immunopathology)

If part of the immune system simply fails to work (immunodeficiency), the consequences may be disastrous. Rarely, the failure is the result of a hereditary lack of a particular immunological process or component. In **hypogammaglobulinaemia** the patient fails to produce adequate levels of immunoglobulins because of B cell defects, so children with this condition will suffer recurrent bacterial and other infections. There are many other examples of hereditary immunodeficiency. Children born with the more serious forms will often fail to thrive.

Most drugs used to treat cancer suppress the immune system by inhibiting cell division in the bone marrow. This leaves the patient very susceptible to serious infections, often by organisms which are not normally pathogenic, e.g. *Pseudomonas*, *Candida* or *Pneumocystis*. Some diseases may also suppress the immune system. The clinical consequences of HIV infection are not only potentially fatal infections but also the occurrence of certain tumours; this emphasizes the importance of T cells in limiting the growth of cancers.

Much of immunopathology is concerned with an inappropriate or maladaptive immune response. For convenience these have usually been divided into four classes, summarized in Fig. 2.6. In each class, one or more of the immune responses that have already been

described (both humoral and cell-mediated) are involved, but the responses are often out of proportion to the stimulus eliciting them. Such **'hypersensitivity reactions'** will result in inflammation as they all involve some tissue damage.

Although hypersensitivity is sometimes described as an inappropriate or exaggerated response by the immune system, it should be considered more correctly as an immune reaction that happens to damage body tissue. The four classes of inappropriate immune response/ hypersensitivity are described below. However, a reaction to a particular stimulus may involve more than one of these, e.g. serum sickness can involve both type II and type I reactions.

Type I hypersensitivity: anaphylactoid

Many **allergic** reactions involve the excessive formation of IgE, produced in response to primary contact with an antigen (called in this case an **allergen**). The IgE binds strongly to mast cells by the Fc portion. Subsequent contact with the same allergen results in a reaction between the allergen and bound IgE on the cell surface. The cross-linking of IgE molecules by the allergen causes destabilization of the mast cell membrane and the release of **histamine** and other mediators from granules within its cytoplasm. These mediators play an important part in the process of inflammation (pp. 35–46). The consequences of this mediator release can vary from very mild

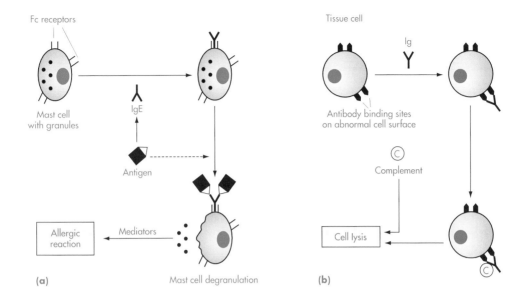

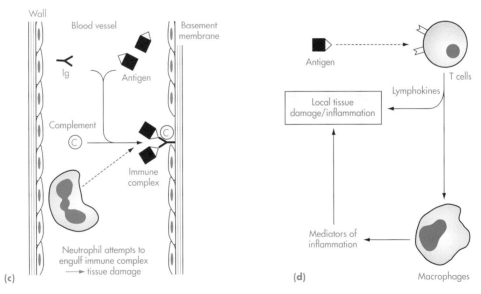

Figure 2.6 Types of hypersensitivity. (a) Type I. (b) Type II. (c) Type III. (d) Type IV. Fc, crystallizable fragment of immunoglobulin; Ig, immunoglobulin; IgE, immunoglobulin E.

reactions to life-threatening ones. The most extreme form is **anaphylactic shock**, with acute bronchoconstriction, rash, gastrointestinal disturbance, profound hypotension and collapse.

Less dramatic anaphylactoid reactions are asthma, hayfever and eczema. However, the link between these conditions and mast cell degranulation is not always clear.

Children will sometimes develop one or more anaphylactoid reactions, and such individuals are said to be **atopic**. There is usually a family history of atopic disease and a positive skin prick reaction to a variety of allergens. Both the tendency to produce high levels of IgE and the presentation of symptoms are genetically determined. Many different allergens trigger this type of reaction; the better known ones include pollen and housedust mite. Various classes of drugs also act as haptens to induce type I hypersensitivity, e.g. penicillins and non-steroidal anti-inflammatory drugs.

Type II hypersensitivity: cytotoxic

In this type of reaction, antigens become attached to or are part of cell surfaces. Subsequently, immunoglobulins react with antigens and activate complement, which then causes cell lysis. Complement components (C3a,C5a) may also attract phagocytes which are unable to engulf the large cells of the body, and so release enzymes which actually cause much of the damage. In addition, a class of lymphocytes known as **K (killer) cells** may have a cytotoxic action on the tissue cells. K cells belong to a group of lymphocytes called **null** cells, being neither T nor B type, whose immunological role has not been fully identified. The reaction often involves red blood cells, and autoantibodies directed against the cell surface will cause a **haemolytic anaemia**. This may be due to the binding of a foreign molecule to the red blood cell surface, conferring new antigenic properties. Methyldopa may cause the formation of such autoantibodies, which are detectable by a Coombs test, although a positive test does not always mean that haemolytic anaemia will occur.

Transfusion reactions are one form of type II reactions. If red blood cells carrying A, B or both antigens on their surfaces are transfused into individuals whose red cells do not carry these antigens, i.e. blood group O, the transfused red blood cells are haemolysed by anti-A and anti-B antibodies already in the recipient's blood. Blood group O individuals can donate blood to anyone without initiating a reaction, whereas those of blood group AB can receive any blood group because they have no antibodies in their serum.

Unusually for immunological reactions, the immunoglobulins against blood group antigens are normally present even if the individual has not been previously exposed to the foreign blood group, so a reaction will occur on the first transfusion. People with genetically determined group O red cells, which do not possess A or B antigens, will not eliminate clones of plasma cells that produce anti-A or anti-B Igs.

An individual's **Rhesus status** and certain other antigens must also be considered when cross-matching blood. This is a consequence of the immune tolerance already described. **Haemolytic disease of the newborn** occurs where a Rhesus-negative mother, who does not possess the Rhesus D (RhD) erythrocyte antigens, has a child by a Rhesus-positive man. The child will also be Rhesus-positive. If the child's red blood cells come in contact with the mother's circulation, as usually happens during birth, the mother will produce anti-RhD antibodies. The child of the first pregnancy will usually be unaffected, but in subsequent pregnancies anti-RhD antibodies cross the placenta to cause fetal/neonatal red cell destruction in the Rhesus-positive child. This may be prevented by the use of an antiserum containing anti-RhD antibodies, which is administered prophylactically to the mother within 72 h of the first birth. Thus, any Rhesus-positive fetal erythrocytes reaching the bloodstream of a mother so treated are destroyed before they can stimulate the production of endogenous anti-RhD antibodies. Subsequent pregnancies will then occur normally, similar to a first pregnancy.

Organ transplants (of which blood transfusion is a simple form) can also initiate a type II reaction. Antibodies directed against a transplanted organ and pre-existing in the recipient's blood, may contribute to a **hyperacute graft rejection** almost immediately after the transplant is in place (*see* Chapter 4).

Type III hypersensitivity: immune complex

When an antigen combines with an antibody an immune complex is always formed, which is normally cleared by the reticuloendothelial system. Complement may make small complexes soluble within the bloodstream, whereas the larger immune complexes are removed by phagocytes. Small complexes tend to be formed if the antigen is in excess, whereas antibody excess produces larger complexes. Under certain circumstances, relating to the size and number of these complexes, the clearance mechanisms are overwhelmed and circulating levels of immune complexes may increase. These become trapped in body tissues, causing local inflammation.

The immune complexes often penetrate vessel walls and attach to the basement membrane which separates the endothelial cells from the tissues of the vessel wall. Subsequent complement activation causes recruitment and activation of neutrophils which release enzymes that cause collateral damage to the vessel wall. In addition, platelets adhere to the inflamed site and complete vascular occlusion may result in smaller vessels.

A similar situation may occur in the skin if an antigen is injected intradermally. The resulting localized inflammation, known as an Arthus reaction, reaches its peak after 4–10 h. Its intensity is greatest when antigen and antibody are present in approximately equivalent amounts.

Antigenic material from streptococcal infections is responsible for some forms of glomerulonephritis (see Chapter 4) in which the immune complexes lodge in the basement membrane of the kidney glomeruli. Immune complex formation is also involved in certain autoimmune diseases such as systemic lupus erythematosus (SLE) and rheumatoid arthritis (see Chapter 8), which explains the multisystem damage seen in these conditions.

In the early days of immunotherapy, large doses of antiserum obtained from horse sera were used to treat infections such as diphtheria and tetanus. However, the horse immunoglobulins are antigenic to humans and induce antibody formation. The resultant immune complex of horse antitoxin and human antibody led to the development of a systemic type III reaction known as **serum sickness.** Consequently, antisera produced in horses are now only rarely used. Instead, human immunoglobulins, e.g. tetanus, are now used and these carry a far lower risk of serum sickness.

When certain antigenic material is inhaled, immune complexes may form in the lung alveoli. Thus in farmer's lung and bird fancier's lung (see Chapter 5), immune complexes with IgG are formed in the alveoli, causing **extrinsic allergic alveolitis** leading to a form of irreversible **restrictive airways disease**, with a delayed allergic type of response to antigen inhalation.

Type IV hypersensitivity: cell-mediated

Antibody production plays the major role in all of the three classes of hypersensitivity so far described. The reactions occur fairly rapidly, often appearing within minutes to a few hours after contact with the antigen. However, in many types of hypersensitivity, symptoms may not occur for days or even weeks after antigenic exposure. This is seen quite frequently in **contact dermatitis**, for example, where the offending material, such as a metal ear-ring, may have been in contact with the skin for many days before any inflammation is observed. The process is similar to that discussed under CMI (p. 27). The production of sensitized cytotoxic T cells plays a central role, but as they take some time to appear in the bloodstream the term **delayed hypersensitivity** is often used to describe this type of reaction, which takes more than 12 h to appear. The lymphokines released by sensitized T cells contribute to the overall tissue damage and also recruit macrophages which release lysosomal products and enzymes, causing further tissue damage. The result is **chronic inflammation**, and often the end result is the formation of scar tissue to repair the damaged area (pp. 41–43).

Tuberculosis is a good example of the link between this class of hypersensitivity and chronic inflammation. The actual tissue damage in the lung and formation of the tubercle (a granuloma) is not caused directly by the bacteria but by the body's attempts to deal with it via CMI. In the Mantoux or Heaf test, tubercular antigens are injected intradermally. In individuals previously sensitized to the mycobacterium by infection or immunization, a cell-mediated hypersensitivity reaction causes inflammation at the injection site, the result being read 72 h after injection. The induration and red weal sometimes persist for up to a year. For this reason, a

Mantoux or Heaf test is always performed before Bacillus Calmette–Guérin (BCG) vaccination, because immunization of positive subjects may result in an extensive, deforming, local inflammatory reaction. Other stimuli eliciting this type of hypersensitivity include insect bites, fungal infections and certain chemical haptens.

Autoimmune disease

In the most extreme case of maladaptation, the body turns its immunological defences against its own tissues. This can involve any of the types of hypersensitivity reaction described above and causes a wide variety of diseases. However, the immunopathological mechanisms for many of the autoimmune diseases are not well understood, and may involve more than one type of immune response. In general, autoimmune diseases may be associated with a number of different underlying abnormalities.

Sometimes, as in **contact dermatitis** (*see* Chapter 12), normal proteins may be altered and rendered antigenic by the presence of haptens. The attachment of drugs such as methyldopa to red blood cells may induce the formation of autoantibodies by altering red cell surface proteins. Similarly, virus infections may alter the expression of surface proteins of the cells they infect, leading to a failure of self-recognition, although their exact role in autoimmunity is still uncertain.

If a protein is normally sequestered and thus not exposed to the immune system, it follows that tolerance cannot develop and if such cells subsequently come in contact with the immune system, they will be recognized as non-self. Spermatozoa are one example, and **mumps orchitis** (inflammation of the testes) may result in the abnormal contact between spermatozoa and the immune system, leading to infertility.

Sometimes, antibodies produced against a pathogen may cross-react with normal healthy tissue. The organisms most often associated with this type of problem are certain types of streptococci, especially in **rheumatic fever**. Although this disease is less common since the introduction of penicillin, the late complications are still sometimes encountered among the older popu-

lation. The intense pain and inflammation of the joints experienced after an untreated streptococcal infection result from the formation of an antibody that is active against both the organism and most synovial membranes. Presumably the surface proteins of the *Streptococcus* bear some resemblance to those of certain human tissues. A more serious and long-term problem is the damage caused to cardiac tissues by such antibodies. The effects on heart valves will eventually lead to an impairment in cardiac function that may only become apparent in later life.

By far the largest group of autoimmune diseases are due to a breakdown in self-tolerance. In many diseases of uncertain aetiology the immune system has failed to recognize certain tissues as self. We have seen that the immune system normally distinguishes self or non-self by the nature of the cell surface, because surface proteins determine its antigenic properties. There are two possible broad mechanisms for developing a lack of tolerance: the immune system fails to recognize these surface proteins as being self or, owing to an intrinsic property of the surface proteins, there is a tendency for them to become antigenic under certain circumstances. The reasons for the development of autoimmunity in any particular disease are usually unknown. An understanding of the HLA system, described below, goes some way towards clarifying the problem. If failure of self-recognition is responsible, subsequent failure in T cell regulation may give rise to an autoimmune reaction, e.g. in SLE (*see* Chapter 8, pp. 511–514), which is characterized by the development of autoantibodies to nucleoproteins.

There are other examples in which autoantibodies, possibly resulting from defective T cell regulation, play a major role. **Hashimoto's thyroiditis** is a well-recognized autoimmune disease in which the antibodies produced attack both thyroid cells and thyroglobulin. Similarly, almost all patients with **pernicious anaemia** possess anti-parietal cell autoantibodies and 50% also have antibodies against intrinsic factor.

The role of immunoglobulins is less certain in other autoimmune diseases. Rheumatoid arthritis is often associated with the production of IgMs known collectively as **rheumatoid factor**. These do not attack the synovial membrane directly but combine with IgG to form immune complexes which subsequently trigger inflammation.

Although **inflammatory bowel disease** and the **seronegative arthropathies** have a possible autoimmune aetiology, no autoantibodies or abnormal immunological processes have been identified. Nevertheless, both conditions possess a strong association with certain HLA types. **Insulin-dependent diabetes**, **myasthenia gravis** and **multiple sclerosis** also have an autoimmune basis.

Increasing numbers of diseases are thought to involve autoimmunity, and our understanding of the mechanisms involved – although imperfect – is improving. With greater knowledge of the immune mechanisms and various trigger factors involved, prophylactic measures and better treatments may eventually become available.

The HLA system

The limiting factor in organ transplantation is the phenomenon of **rejection**. The organ is recognized as non-self and the immune system is activated to attack it. However, transplantation between identical twins is certain of success. The chances are reduced in inverse relation to the closeness of the relationship between donor and recipient. If the recipient is a sibling, the success rate might be 80–90%, but this falls to 60% or less between unrelated individuals, even though strenuous efforts are made to find a suitable match. This is because there are surface antigens on the cells of transplanted organs which are genetically determined and can be recognized by the immune system of the recipient (host) as foreign. There must be a finite variety of these groups of antigens because transplants between unrelated individuals do not always lead to rejection.

These surface antigens are described as histocompatibility antigens. The most important antigens are determined by the major **histocompatibility complex** (MHC) genes found on chromosome 6 in man. They are termed **human leucocyte antigens** (HLA) because they were originally discovered on the surface of human leucocytes, although they are now known to be present on many other tissue cells. The antigens themselves are trans-plasma membrane glycoproteins.

There are six important MHC gene loci. Any individual may possess two of a number of possible gene types (alleles) from each locus, each gene expressing a particular MHC molecule. The three D region genes (DP, DQ and DR) code for the MHC class II molecules, and those of the A, B and C regions code for the class I molecules. A third region, sometimes referred to as class III molecules, codes for certain complement factors. Each gene locus is therefore identified by a letter, and the individual alleles within each series are given a number, e.g. A1–A41, although these numbers are not necessarily consecutive. New antigens are constantly being discovered and are at first given the letter W (e.g. DW3) to denote that they are antigens whose existence has yet to be officially recognized. It is also common for certain antigens to occur together, a phenomenon known as **linkage disequilibrium**. For instance, DR3 and B8 will occur together more frequently than might be expected from chance alone. Also some types are more common in certain races, e.g. A1 is less common in black Africans, and Bw6 is only found in the mongoloid race.

MHC class I molecules play an important part in the recognition of cells that have been affected by viruses, as such cells express viral antigens on their surface. They are attacked by T cells only in the presence of an MHC molecule. The reason for this could be that T cell binding sites are not taken up by free viral antigens, maximizing the antigens' potential for attacking infected cells. Class II molecules are important in the recognition by T cells of antigens taken up by antigen-presenting cells.

The HLA system therefore partly explains transplant rejection. Only transplants between individuals with identical HLA antigens can be performed without recourse to immunosuppresive therapy, and this is only likely to occur between close relatives.

The link between the HLA system and disease, in particular autoimmune disease, has a wider significance. Some known associations between the occurrence of certain HLA types and various diseases are listed in Table 2.4. However, with the exception of narcolepsy, this represents only an increased risk of developing the disease, e.g. there is a strong link between HLA-B27 and ankylosing spondylitis, so that those individuals who carry the B27 gene have a higher risk of developing this disease than those without it. Whether or not they do presumably depends on other factors, such as contact with an exogenous trigger, e.g. infection or a dietary toxin.

MHC molecules allow the body to distinguish between self and non-self, and the link between HLA type and autoimmunity could involve cross-reactions between MHC molecules and an antigen or microorganism, resulting in immunological activity directed against body tissues. Several explanations have been proposed, although a single cohesive theory has yet to be established. For instance, some HLA groups may bind antigens better than others, resulting in a more intense reaction. Alternatively, possession of a particular HLA group may involve an increased immunological response to a particular antigen. It has also been suggested that in some cases there may be an inappropriate expression of MHC class II molecules on tissues where they are not normally found.

Inflammation

Definition

This important pathological process is defined as the 'reaction of the living microcirculation and its contents to injury'.

The term **microcirculation** describes the system of arterioles, venules and capillaries that are in direct contact with the body tissues. Within the microcirculation (blood) are the various classes of white blood cells of particular interest. The term 'injury' refers to any damage to tissues, e.g. trauma, extremes of temperature, radiation, immunological or infectious.

The function of an inflammatory reaction is to limit and eventually to resolve any damage caused through an injury. In physical injury, direct damage to vascular tissue initiates the reaction. Following infection, the immune system is responsible for detecting the invader and initiating the inflammatory process, but the growth of microorganisms within tissues may also cause some physical damage. Sometimes, inappropriate stimulation of the immune system initiates the reaction, as in autoimmune disease, or hypersensitivity reactions, e.g. to pollen in hayfever. Part of the purpose of the vascular responses in inflammation is to facilitate the access of blood-borne defence mechanisms to the site of injury. In physical injury these defences may simply be agents for healing and repair. In the case of infection, antibodies or lymphocytes must gain access initially to enable them to deal with the infection, before healing can take place.

Acute inflammation

The stages and processes involved in acute inflammation are readily seen if the forearm is

Table 2.4   HLA and disease

Disease	Gene coding for antigen	Relative risk (%)
Narcolepsy	DR2	100
Ankylosing spondylitis	B27	87.8
Reiter's disease	B27	35.9
Rheumatoid arthritis	DRw4	4.0
Multiple sclerosis	A3	1.8
	B7	2.0
	Bw2	1.9
	DRw2	3.8
Myasthenia gravis	B8	3.4
	DRw3	3.0
Psoriasis	A1	2.1
	B13	8.7
	Bw37	8.1
	Cw6	4.3
Addison's disease	Dw3	8.8
Grave's disease	B8	2.5
	Bw35	5.0
	Dw3	5.5
Coeliac disease	B8	8.6
	Dw3	73.0
Chronic active hepatitis	B8	9.2
	DRw3	4.6

scratched with some force. Almost immediately, a narrow red line will be seen on the skin along the line of the scratch. This is quickly followed by a more diffuse reddening around the line of injury. After a while the red area will become slightly raised. This sequence of events is the **Lewis triple response**, the three components of which are flush (central red area), flare (more diffuse red area) and weal (raised area). Furthermore, the inflamed area is somewhat warmer than the surrounding skin and, if the scratch was too vigorous, pain will also be experienced. This skin reaction displays the four so-called cardinal signs of inflammation (redness, heat, swelling and pain) described by Celsus in the first century AD. If the injury has been excessive, a fifth sign – loss of function – may occur. Two important points should be noted: the same sequence of events occurs no matter what the cause of the injury, and the reaction would be similar no matter what tissue was damaged, although any functional impairment would clearly depend on the organ involved.

The triple response resolves completely in a few hours and is therefore an example of **acute inflammation**, major features of which are: hyperaemia, exudation and leucocyte migration. If the inflammation is inappropriate, particularly when the cause is immunological, or the reaction is out of proportion to the potential damage caused by the stimulus or persists when the stimulus is removed, it becomes maladaptive and pathological. As tissue damage plays a large part in many disease processes it is not surprising that many diseases have an underlying inflammatory pathology. Such conditions or diseases are normally suffixed with 'itis', e.g. dermatitis is inflammation of the skin, arthritis is inflammation of the joints.

Hyperaemia

An essential function of inflammation is to provide an increased blood flow to the damaged area, facilitating the transport of agents involved in defence or repair. After a brief reflex vasoconstriction to minimize local bleeding etc. the local arterioles dilate, flushing the capillary network with blood. An axon reflex mechanism is responsible for the initial local reaction (Fig. 2.7). Substance P may be the neurotransmitter released from nerve endings to initiate this part of the response. This involvement of the nervous system may partly explain the emotional link often observed with exacerbations of certain inflammatory conditions, e.g. eczema and ulcerative colitis. A more diffuse and prolonged vasodilation is achieved by the release of chemical mediators (Table 2.5). This vasodilation explains the redness associated with inflammation: the rise in local temperature is partly the result of an increase in local blood flow and partly of a higher rate of metabolism in the inflamed area.

Exudation

The swelling observed is caused by leakage of protein-rich fluid through the vessel wall into the tissue interstitial space (oedema) (Fig. 2.8). In normal capillaries the hydrostatic pressure of

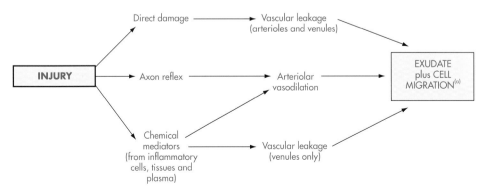

Figure 2.7 Effects of injury on the microcirculation. [a]*See* Figs 2.8 and 2.9.

the blood forces fluid into the interstitial space, and this pressure is partly offset by the **oncotic pressure** exerted by plasma proteins. Plasma proteins are too large to pass through normal capillary walls and so are retained in the bloodstream. During inflammation this balance is upset. Arterial vasodilation results in an increased capillary hydrostatic pressure and hence an increased volume of interstitial fluid. In addition, the blood vessel walls become leaky and allow some plasma proteins to enter the tissue space, thus increasing tissue oncotic pressure and further facilitating the movement of fluid from the blood to the interstitial space. The increased permeability of the vessels is believed to be due to the formation of leaky junctions between the endothelial cells. A more diffuse vascular leakage from venules distant from the site of injury is caused by chemical mediators. The exudation, which results in tissue swelling, is offset by an increase in lymphatic drainage. However, if microorganisms are responsible, the infection can spread into the lymphatic system resulting in a **lymphangitis** (inflamed lymph channels) and **lymphadenopathy** (swollen lymph glands). Some of the pain experienced in local inflammation may also be due to swelling.

The increased blood flow to the region and the exudation bring antibodies to the site of infection and may also dilute any bacterial or other toxins. Exudation may also result in tissue fibrinogen which, on conversion to insoluble fibrin by the action of thrombin, is an important element of the blood clotting mechanism. The formation of a blood clot is essential if physical trauma has resulted in haemorrhage, but fibrin

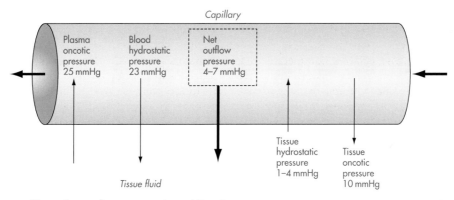

Normal: net outflow pressure to tissues 4–7 mmHg

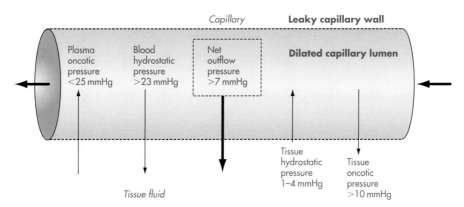

Inflammation: net outflow pressure to tissues increased

Figure 2.8   Exudation from capillaries.

deposition in other circumstances may cause more problems than it resolves (p. 41). The initial exudate has a similar consistency to plasma, i.e. it is a clear, cell-free fluid. However, eventually white blood cells will appear in the exudate, particularly in the presence of infection.

Various forms of exudation can occur which may have important consequences should the inflammation fail to resolve quickly (p. 41). The clear exudate seen under a blister is known as **serous exudate**, whereas the thick exudate from mucous membranes, e.g. a runny nose, is termed as **mucinous**. If white blood cells enter the exudate, as described below, it is described as **purulent**. Often a mixed picture is seen, e.g. a cold would initially produce mucinous and then later a **mucopurulent** exudate.

Leucocyte migration

Humoral and cell-mediated immunity are not the only mechanisms of defence against microorganisms; white blood cells of all classes are also involved. The **neutrophils (polymorphonuclear leucocytes)** are responsible for engulfing and digesting microorganisms. Neutrophils migrate from the bloodstream to the site of inflammation (Fig. 2.9) and appear first in the area of acute inflammation.

Loss of fluid from the bloodstream tends to increase blood viscosity locally and slow its flow rate. The white blood cells, which are normally distributed evenly throughout the blood, then tend to collect along the endothelium (**marginate**) outside the central axial stream. They then adhere to the inner surface of blood vessels and, by mechanisms not fully understood,

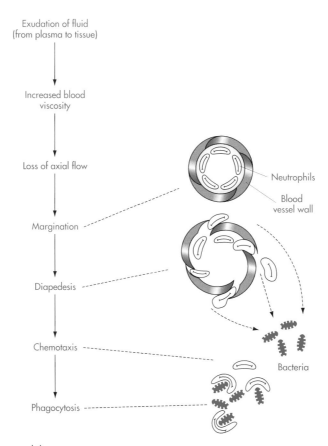

Exudation of fluid
(from plasma to tissue)

Increased blood viscosity

Loss of axial flow

Margination

Diapedesis

Chemotaxis

Phagocytosis

Neutrophils

Blood vessel wall

Bacteria

Figure 2.9   Migration of neutrophils.

squeeze through the endothelial gaps and enter the tissue space. This movement of phagocytes is known as **diapedesis**.

Leucocytes are attracted to the site of inflammation by chemotaxins, some of which are components of the complement system (C3a, C5a). Certain bacteria, e.g. staphylococci and *Klebsiella*, also seem to exert a highly chemotactic effect, attracting very large numbers of neutrophils to the site of infection. Neutrophils engulf and digest the microorganisms, particles of tissue debris, etc. During phagocytosis, proteolytic enzymes may be released from the white blood cells, causing further local damage. After a day or so the number of neutrophils falls, to be replaced by macrophages (p. 45).

Systemic inflammation

The preceding discussion has considered examples of local inflammation, i.e. the acute inflammatory response does not involve the generalized activation of the immune system and is restricted to a specific organ/tissue. In systemic inflammation the reaction is more widespread and usually involves stimulation of the immune system generally. This is seen especially if an infection reaches the general circulation, i.e. **septicaemia**. Rheumatoid arthritis is a good example of systemic inflammatory disease; the main problem for the patient may be with the joints, but there is a general inflammatory process involving many other parts of the body remote from the affected joints (*see* Chapter 8, pp. 484–485).

A number of generalized clinical features usually accompany systemic inflammation. These include:

- A rise in white blood cell count.
- Raised body temperature (pyrexia).
- Lethargy and tiredness.
- Anaemia, which is especially seen in the more chronic systemic inflammatory conditions such as rheumatoid arthritis.

Another useful index is the erythrocyte sedimentation rate (ESR). If anticoagulated blood is placed in a glass tube, the red blood cells tend to clump and sediment to the bottom. The greater the clumping the faster the sedimentation; the length of the column of clear supernatant plasma remaining after 1 h (in mm) gives the ESR. The presence of globulins and fibrin will tend to cause an increased clumping of the red blood cells and hence raise the ESR. It is therefore a non-specific sign of systemic inflammation and/or immune stimulation.

Mediators of inflammation

The list of chemical mediators believed to be involved in the various stages of inflammation increases inexorably. The following is a brief review (*see also* Table 2.5 and References).

Mediators can be classified according to whether they are derived either from tissue or plasma. The principal tissue-derived mediators are the **prostaglandins** and **vasoactive amines** (histamine and serotonin). Histamine is found widely distributed in the body, particularly in specialized white cells resident in tissue called **mast cells**. Histamine release from mast cells is believed to be important in type I hypersensitivity reactions. Serotonin occurs in platelets and there is increasing interest in the role of platelets in inflammatory reactions.

There are many types of prostaglandins, which are derived from the action of cyclooxygenase enzymes on arachidonic acid, which in turn is formed from membrane phospholipids. The most important ones involved in inflammation are PGE_2 and PGI_2. Together with the **thromboxanes** (derived from a similar source), these constitute the class of mediators known as the **acidic lipids**. A further group of mediators, derived from arachidonic acid via the 5-lipoxygenase pathway, are the **leukotrienes**, and the previously termed Slow Reacting Substance A (SRSA) is a mixture of these mediators. Leukotriene antagonists have been developed for the treatment of asthma.

The other two major classes of mediators, the **vasoactive polypeptides** (e.g. kinin and bradykinin) and complement, are both derived from plasma, so it is not surprising that they are closely linked to the clotting system, with which they have certain elements in common. Their release and control further mirrors that of clotting mechanisms in that it involves a cascade

Table 2.5   Some mediators involved in inflammation

Mediator	Source	Effect
Vasoactive amines • histamine • serotonin	Mast cells Platelets	Vascular dilation Vascular leakage
Platelet activating factor	Various white blood cells	Chemotaxis
IL-8	Monocytes Lymphocytes	Chemotaxis
C-reactive protein (an 'acute phase protein')	Liver	Opsonization
Prostaglandins and leukotrienes	Tissue phospholipids	Vascular leakage Chemotaxis Pain Anti-inflammatory
Vasoactive polypeptides	Plasma	Vascular dilatation Vascular leakage Pain
Complement	Plasma	Chemotaxis Vascular leakage Cell lysis Opsonization

IL, interleukin.

mechanism which amplifies the effects (Fig. 2.10). The complement system itself, as we have seen, is most commonly activated by infection. The C3a and C5a fragments seem to be the most active in the inflammatory process, and the C5a fragment also appears to initiate histamine release. The actions of both kinins and histamine are potentiated by prostaglandins.

There is thus a highly sophisticated system of interactions, not only between the various classes of mediators but also between the clotting system and immunological mechanisms. This degree of complexity enables the body to initiate and maintain the inflammatory reaction long enough to deal adequately with the original injury and also to switch it off when the response is no longer required. Histamine and serotonin are responsible for the initial reaction, but their effect is short-lived, about 2 h. The reaction is then maintained by the kinins. Prostaglandins may extend the reaction still further, although their main role may be to control

the extent and intensity of the process because certain classes of prostaglandins have been shown to be anti-inflammatory. Lysosomal enzymes released from neutrophils may further help to maintain the reaction. The close links between the inflammatory and immunological processes ensure that invading microorganisms are dealt with effectively. The links with the blood clotting/fibrinolytic system also aid in the healing process.

The relative importance of particular mediators may vary between tissues. Thus, rhinitis and hayfever seem largely (but not entirely) mediated by histamine, but histamine plays only a minor role in asthma.

The therapeutic agents employed in modifying the inflammatory process usually interfere with the action of chemical mediators. The antihistamines have a limited, and in many cases short-lived, activity. Two classes of agents that are widely used, and which have inhibition of prostaglandins as their mode of action, are the

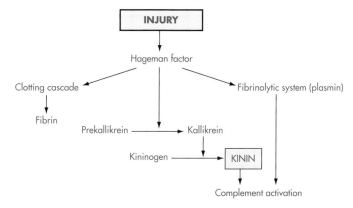

Figure 2.10 Vasoactive polypeptides and their relationship to the clotting/fibrinolytic system.

corticosteroids, which inhibit the conversion of phospholipids to arachidonic acid, and the **non-steroidal anti-inflammatory agents**, which inhibit cyclooxygenase activity. The steroids in particular are useful in controlling most types of inflammation, although they have a delayed onset of action.

Sequels to inflammation

Acute inflammatory reactions are usually beneficial and do not always lead to major medical problems. However, there may be serious problems when organ function is severely compromised, e.g. in meningitis, hepatitis and asthma. However, these reactions also usually soon subside and the inflammation is unlikely to cause permanent damage if treated promptly. It is the sequels to inflammation, that is the resolution and healing processes, which may sometimes cause permanent damage (Fig. 2.11).

Resolution

The most favourable outcome to inflammation would be the complete removal of the causative agent without any residual deleterious effects on the tissue involved. However, complete resolution is possible only if there has been very little tissue damage and minimal cell death (necrosis). In the example of a simple triple response these criteria are obviously fulfilled.

If the cause of inflammation is an infection, the offending organism would have to be removed quickly. Prompt treatment of an infection of a vital organ using antibiotics will prevent inappropriate resolution (see below) and the potential loss of function of that organ. For example, in kidney infection (**pyelonephritis**), prompt effective treatment prevents **fibrosis** of kidney tubules and eventual renal failure.

In addition to elimination of the initial trigger, exudate and dead cells must also be removed promptly, because delay may also result in fibrosis. To do this efficiently the inflamed area needs to be well supplied with capillary and lymphatic vessels. In pneumonia (infection and inflammation of the lung alveoli), once the causative organism has been dealt with there is no lasting damage providing the initial infection is not too serious. The alveoli themselves have a very good blood supply and any fibrin which has been laid down and subsequently dissolved by plasmin can be readily removed via the circulation. The remaining debris is cleared by macrophages and the tissue then usually reverts to its normal state. In more serious bacterial infections there may be pus formation, necrosis and permanent tissue damage.

Organization, healing and fibrosis

If there is an excessive amount of exudate which cannot be easily removed or a large amount of necrotic tissue is present, organization or 'healing' of the damaged tissue may take place. The result may be the formation of **scar tissue**.

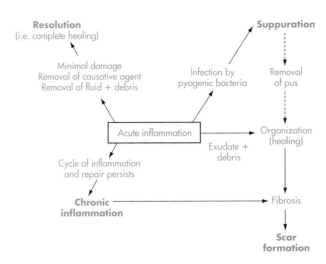

Figure 2.11   Sequels to inflammation.

Exudation carries fibrinogen into the inflamed area where it will eventually be converted into insoluble fibrin. Capillary buds then begin to grow into the area of dead tissue and inflammatory exudate as part of the healing process, and these further facilitate the migration of macrophages and fibroblasts into the area. The fibroblasts then lay down connective fibrous tissue (collagen), which gradually replaces the fibrin. This immature fibrovascular tissue is known as **granulation tissue**, and the process by which it is formed as **organization**. The formation of excessive amounts of abnormal connective tissue (scar tissue), leading to impaired tissue or organ function, is called **fibrosis.**

A good example of this is when exudate forms in the pleural cavity, e.g. following lung infection. The blood supply to this area is quite poor, so exudate tends to remain, granulation tissue is formed and organization occurs. The lungs then become stiff, making breathing painful and difficult – a condition known as **pleurisy**. The fibrin laid down within the pleural cavity has effectively formed an **adhesion** between the two surfaces. Progressive fibrosis may lead to severe restrictive lung disease. Adhesions may complicate the healing process in many tissues, e.g. they may cause considerable pain and discomfort if they form following abdominal surgery.

Fibrosis is an important pathological process in a wide variety of disease states (Fig. 2.12). For example, if scarring occurs in the pyloric sphinc-ter (between the stomach and duodenum) as a result of the chronic inflammation associated with peptic ulceration, the sphincter may become incompetent and large amounts of acid will be lost from the stomach. A further possible complication of peptic ulceration is shrinkage of the scarred area, or **cicatrization.** This can grossly alter the shape of the stomach, giving it an 'hour-glass' appearance if it occurs in the fundus.

The development of scar tissue during organization frequently leads to impaired function in the affected organ. Following myocardial infarction, part of the ischaemic area dies and is replaced by scar tissue. Normal function is lost, perhaps leading to heart failure if myocardial cells are affected, or to arrhythmias if the damage is in the conducting tissue.

Therefore in a vital organ, such as the heart, kidney or liver, the development of scar tissue may be fatal, whereas in others, e.g. a joint, loss of function will result.

Wound healing

The degree of scarring following organization depends on the extent of previous damage and inflammation. This is particularly true of wound healing, which is a special case of organization. Although a wound can be inflicted on any tissue, wound healing commonly refers to repair of the skin.

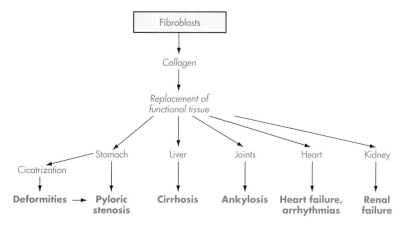

Figure 2.12   Fibrosis.

Following injury or laceration of the skin, blood vessels are damaged and a clot forms, consisting of coagulated blood and other debris, including microorganisms. The healing which follows is classically divided into healing by 'first intention' and 'second intention'. The former refers to a clean cut, e.g. as with a knife, or one that has been brought together promptly by suturing. Healing by second intention occurs when the edges of the cut are not in close proximity and granulation tissue forms within it. In practice, the only difference between the two is that healing by first intention results in a smaller scar. In both types the following sequence takes place (Fig. 2.13):

- Initially, macrophages will enter the wound area, to digest the debris.
- New blood vessels start to grow inwards from the edges of the wound, initially as solid cords of cells but soon becoming canalized, allowing blood to flow through them.
- The ingrowing blood vessels eventually join within the wound forming 'loops and arcades'.
- The young vessels are leaky, allowing both blood cells and plasma to seep out. This is the serous fluid which is often visible in healing wounds.
- The new capillaries differentiate into arterioles and venules.
- Fibroblasts appear in the serous fluid, and lay down connective tissue.

- This mixture of newly formed blood vessels, connective tissue and serous fluid forms **granulation tissue**, usually heralding good wound healing.
- After the laying down of connective tissue and removal of any remaining debris, the epithelium begins to regenerate. This is achieved by mitosis of the epithelial cells surrounding the wound, which gradually migrate to cover the wound surface.

If the wound is small, the underlying scar tissue eventually merges with surrounding tissues, but in larger wounds scarring may become permanent. Wound healing is indistinguishable from the other forms of fibrosis and organization discussed earlier, except that the organ affected is the skin.

Suppuration

The bacterium *Staphylococcus aureus*, implicated in many types of infection in man, is **pyogenic** (pus-producing). The presence of pus can also lead to fibrosis and the formation of scar tissue. The best example of suppuration is seen in boil formation, which is usually caused by *Staph. aureus*. Although leucocytes are attracted into the area to deal with the organism in the usual way, in this case they are initially largely unsuccessful and die at the site of infection. The creamy pus so formed is a mixture of dead leucocytes, bacteria, lipid, exudate and necrotic tissue.

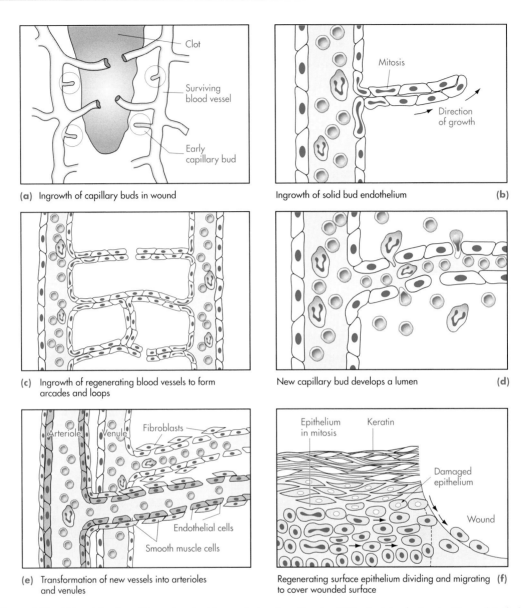

(a) Ingrowth of capillary buds in wound

Ingrowth of solid bud endothelium   (b)

(c) Ingrowth of regenerating blood vessels to form arcades and loops

New capillary bud develops a lumen   (d)

(e) Transformation of new vessels into arterioles and venules

Regenerating surface epithelium dividing and migrating (f) to cover wounded surface

Figure 2.13 Wound healing. (Reproduced with permission from Spector WG. *An Introduction to General Pathology*: 2nd edn (1980). Edinburgh: Churchill Livingstone.)

The bacteria are prevented from spreading throughout the body by the formation of a capsule or pyogenic membrane composed of partially organized coagulated plasma which surrounds the area of suppuration. When the infection has eventually cleared, this connective tissue remains and, depending on the size of the boil, scar tissue may be visible.

Chronic inflammation

The persistence of an inflammatory reaction for months or even years implies that the cause of the inflammation has not been removed, although this is not always the case. Chronic inflammation may, or may not, be preceded by an acute phase.

Features

Two main features distinguish chronic from acute inflammation: the type of leucocyte involved and the occurrence of fibrosis.

The most important class of leucocyte involved in chronic inflammation is the **macrophage**, whereas in the early stages of acute inflammation it is the neutrophil. The neutrophils are soon replaced by macrophages, which are not only longer-lived than neutrophils, but are also extremely robust. Even if bacteria which have been engulfed by macrophages are not killed outright, the macrophage itself may remain unharmed or even allow the organism to multiply within the cell, as in tuberculosis. In this way a microorganism can persist for years at the site of infection. Furthermore, macrophages have the ability to change in function: they can become **epithelioid cells**, or they can combine to form multinucleate **giant cells.**

If the reaction is prolonged, healing and repair will often accompany the inflammation, rather than follow it. Thus **fibroblasts** have an important role in chronic inflammation, and **fibrosis** is the main cause of damage, as in organization and repair. The laying down of connective tissue may be a lengthy process, with years elapsing before any loss of organ function is noted. There may also be alternating cycles of inflammation and repair. Damage may again not be apparent until after many cycles.

Chronic inflammation following acute inflammation

There is considerable overlap in the various sequels to acute inflammation. If suppuration and abscess formation predominate this is sometimes termed **chronic suppurative inflammation**, whereas the organization and repair (resulting in fibrosis) described earlier is termed **chronic fibrous inflammation**. A further example of chronic suppurative inflammation is encountered following staphylococcal bone infection (**osteomyelitis**), in which some bone may be destroyed by the bacteria during the initial acute phase. This necrotic tissue is poorly penetrated by blood, and so protects the surviving bacteria from the body's defence mecha-

nisms. Thus the infection becomes chronic and large numbers of macrophages and fibroblasts continue to enter the area, which becomes chronically inflamed.

Certain other types of tissue seem prone to chronic inflammatory changes following an acute phase, the classic example being **peptic ulceration** (*see* Chapter 6). Small acute erosions in the duodenum or stomach may be visible after slight trauma, e.g. ingestion of alcohol. It is only if the mucosal protection is deficient or if the trauma is prolonged or repeated frequently that a chronic sequel occurs. The connective tissue subsequently formed results in a weakening of the stomach wall with the danger of gastric bleeds or even perforation during a subsequent acute episode. Other parts of the gastrointestinal tract can be similarly affected. Cholangitis (inflammation of the bile ducts) may result from infection, often precipitated and aggravated by the presence of bile stones. If the stones are not removed, repeated episodes of infection (and acute cholestasis, *see* Chapter 6) may eventually lead to chronic inflammation and atrophy of the bile ducts.

Chronic inflammation without previous acute inflammation

In both biliary tract disease and peptic ulceration there is a discernible phase of acute inflammation, and prolongation of the acute phase eventually leads to chronic changes. However, there is frequently no evidence of an initial acute reaction and inflammation is chronic from the outset. Even in such conditions as rheumatoid

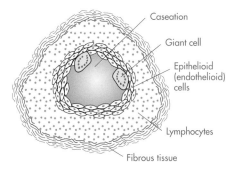

Figure 2.14 Structure of a tubercle (as an example of a granuloma).

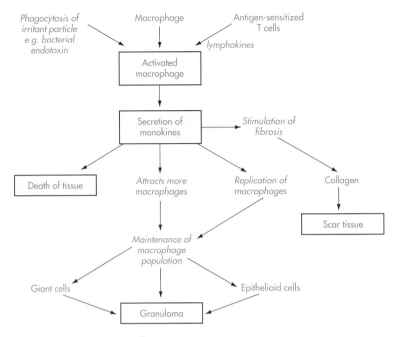

Figure 2.15   Role of macrophages in chronic inflammation.

arthritis, where an 'attack' exhibits all the signs of acute inflammation, the underlying process is chronic in character, although of variable severity. Sometimes no acute phase is seen but there is often the formation of a dense mass of tissue known as a **granuloma**, which should be distinguished from the granulation tissue in wound healing described earlier. A granuloma may be produced by an infection or aseptic foreign bodies such as asbestos, or may be of unknown origin, as in sarcoidosis.

The classical example of granulomatous chronic inflammation is tuberculosis (TB). The bacillus is able to survive within the macrophage providing a focus for granuloma formation, known as a tubercle (Fig. 2.14). At the centre of the tubercle is an area of caseated ('cheese-like') necrotic tissue. Surrounding this are epithelioid and giant cells derived from macrophages. The structure is enclosed in a layer of T lymphocytes. Granulomas are also seen in Crohn's disease, sarcoidosis and rheumatoid arthritis (as rheumatoid nodules).

Cell-mediated immunity is often associated with chronic granulomatous inflammation because of the sensitizing or stimulatory effect that T cells have on macrophages. Because tuberculosis invokes a cell-mediated immune response, it is not surprising that chronic inflammation plays such a large part in its pathology. Figure 2.15 illustrates the central role that macrophages play in granuloma formation.

Ischaemia

Causes

Ischaemia is a deficiency of blood supply to tissues, resulting in damage and, if the deficiency is sufficiently severe and prolonged, the eventual death of that tissue (**necrosis**). The most common general cause is a failure of blood flow resulting from obstruction or cardiovascular insufficiency. Table 2.6 classifies the general causes of ischaemia, with examples of resulting clinical conditions. These various conditions are discussed in the appropriate chapters.

When arteries are chronically inflamed (**arteri-**

Table 2.6 Causes and consequences of ischaemia

General cause	Examples of associated diseases or conditions
Local vascular obstruction	
Inflammation (vasculitis)	Collagen-vascular diseases
Vasoconstriction	Variant angina[a]
	Transient ischaemic attack[a]
	Raynaud's disease
Arteriosclerosis	Diabetes mellitus
	Hypertension
Atherosclerosis	Diabetes mellitus
	Hyperlipidaemia
	Hypertension
Embolism	
Fat	Bone fracture
Air	Faulty IV administration
	Diver's decompression
	sickness (bends)
Thrombotic	Venous stasis
	Atheroma
Hypoperfusion	
Systemic – reduced cardiac output	Chronic heart failure
	Shock:
	• cardiogenic
	• hypovolaemic
	• septic
Local – haemorrhage or thrombosis	Stroke[a]

[a] Consequences of ischaemia; all others are causes.

very small arterioles may become occluded. By contrast, **atherosclerosis** affects the **intimal** lining of the artery wall, particularly in the medium to large arteries. Atheromatous **plaques** are laid down which occlude the lumen partially and become sites for thrombus formation. The distinction between these two conditions is discussed further in Chapter 3 (pp. 116–129).

A **thrombus** (intravascular blood clot) may be formed over the site of an atheromatous plaque in an artery. Thrombi may also form in large veins usually owing to stasis of blood. If a thrombus, or a fragment of it, breaks away from its site of formation in a vein, it will travel downstream through veins of increasing diameter, through the heart and into the arterial tree, until it lodges in a small vessel. This obstruction to the circulation is known as an **embolus**. An embolus derived from a blood clot formed at one site, which lodges in another, is known as a **thromboembolus**. The site of formation of an embolus often determines the organ eventually affected, which may be predicted on the basis of the anatomy of the vascular tree. For example, thrombosis in a leg vein (**deep vein thrombosis**) can lead to pulmonary embolism, resulting in rapidly fatal respiratory failure if it is sufficiently large.

Emboli can also be due to air introduced into the bloodstream inadvertently during intravenous therapy (**air embolus**) and fat droplets released from the site of a fracture (**fat embolus**). Fat emboli do not cause an infarction as such, but can result in a severe interruption of gas exchange if deposited in the lung.

A thrombus formed in a coronary artery may throw off emboli which travel further into the arterial tree to cause a myocardial infarction. Emboli formed on damaged heart valves can reach the retina, whereas those resulting from atrial fibrillation tend to cause strokes by occluding a cerebral artery. Platelet clumps are quite quickly dissolved by factors in the blood. Small emboli originating from atheromatous arteries in the brain are often composed largely of platelets. The consequent interruptions of central nervous system (CNS) function, known as transient ischaemic attacks (TIA), are therefore temporary.

Constriction of the vascular smooth muscle (**vasospasm**) may occur in coronary arteries, as

tis) the artery wall may be permanently damaged by the neutrophil infiltration and necrosis. If this involves small arteries the entire arterial wall is affected and complete occlusion of the lumen may occur. If a larger artery is affected, only part of the wall is damaged and blood is still able to pass. Healing will then occur with the formation of scar tissue which may weaken the artery wall and an **aneurysm** (bulge) may result, which may eventually rupture.

A common cause of vascular obstruction is **arteriosclerosis**, in which the **media** of the arterial wall becomes hard and inelastic. Once again, in variant angina, or in peripheral arteries, as in Raynaud's disease (*see* Chapter 8, pp. 516–517).

Poor perfusion of tissue may also arise from circulatory insufficiency. If cardiac output is low, e.g. because of heart failure or arrhythmia, the blood supply to many tissues will be reduced. This may also occur if the blood volume is low, perhaps following severe blood loss, causing the syndrome known as shock.

Shock

Shock is a syndrome of severely compromised peripheral blood flow with very low cardiac output and blood pressure. Severe blood loss causes a fall in blood pressure and hypovolaemic shock. Other forms of shock include a sudden fall in cardiac output due to cardiac damage (**cardiogenic shock**; *see* Chapter 3) and the production of certain bacterial endotoxins which causes profound vasodilation (**septic shock**).

However, a precipitate fall in blood pressure invokes homeostatic mechanisms to conserve blood flow to vital organs, such as the heart, lungs and brain, which would be irreversibly damaged by even short periods of ischaemia. This **central conservation** may be at the expense of other organs or tissues, when vasoconstriction, mediated by sympathetic stimulation, diverts blood away from the periphery. This restricts blood flow to skeletal muscle, liver, skin, intestines and kidneys. The resultant renal ischaemia may cause the most serious long-term problems.

The features of shock may therefore include reduced blood pressure, increased heart rate, cold extremities and a pale appearance. The patient may also feel disorientated and/or lose consciousness. Hyperventilation, from stimulation of the respiratory centre caused by a metabolic acidosis and hypoxaemia, may further add to the overall state of distress. The exact combination of signs and symptoms will depend on the cause of the shock and the degree to which the compensatory mechanisms have been activated.

In severe shock, even the heart, lungs and brain may eventually succumb to the effects of ischaemia. When coronary perfusion is compromised, cardiac output is further reduced, adding to the vicious cycle of shock.

Other serious problems may occur in the lungs (**shock lung**) resulting in a dramatic reduction in lung function. This is probably caused by changes in the capillaries and alveoli resulting from a combination of poor perfusion and the release of prostaglandins or other mediators. The result is a form of alveolitis with exudate flooding the air sacks, causing pulmonary oedema and congestion, impairing gas exchange and increasing the risk of infection (pneumonia).

Effects of ischaemia on body tissues

The significance of local ischaemia will depend on the physiological importance of the organ affected and the extent of the damage caused. Providing blood flow is not completely obstructed, the tissue may survive, although its function may be compromised. When the blood supply is so reduced that necrosis occurs, permanent damage or failure of the organ may result. An area of necrosis of an organ resulting from ischaemia is termed an **infarct**, which may occur in any organ or tissue. The extent of the damage caused through ischaemia will depend on a number of factors. Highly vascular tissues and those which can draw blood from other sites can develop a **collateral blood supply** and survive periods of ischaemia more readily than poorly vascularized ones. Extensive damage results if a major vessel is obstructed or if the obstruction is of long duration. Furthermore, some tissues are more sensitive to the effects of hypoxia and others have a reduced ability to regenerate after infarction. Some organs also lose their ability to function properly, even if only partially damaged. If an infarcted area becomes infected i.e. in the limbs, immunological and other healing factors will be unable to reach the area, resulting in the tissue destruction known as gangrene. How these factors apply to various organs and the clinical consequences of hypoxia and infarction are shown in Table 2.7.

Ischaemia in any muscle results in anaerobic metabolism to obtain energy. The lactic and other acids so formed lead to the symptom of **cramp**; angina pectoris is a form of myocardial

Table 2.7 Results of ischaemia on specific organ systems

Organ/tissue	Significance	Clinical effects of:	
		Ischaemia[a]	Anoxia[b]/infarction
Less important			
Limbs/periphery	— Non-vital function — Many collaterals — Bone has a low oxygen demand — Muscle regenerates readily	• Poor healing • Local cyanosis • Cold • Pain (cramp)	• Gangrene
Lungs	— Dual circulation (bronchial + pulmonary) — Direct O_2 supply — Low intrinsic oxygen demand — Spare capacity	• Pulmonary congestion • Systemic hypoxia • Pulmonary hypertension	• Respiratory failure
More important – vital organ			
Brain	— No collaterals — Acutely sensitive to hypoxia — No regeneration	• Cognitive impairment (acute or chronic) • Loss of consciousness • Coma	• Stroke (acute) • Dementia (chronic)
Kidney	— Acutely sensitive to hypoxia (angiotensin/renin release)	• Fluid retention • Electrolyte disturbances • Heart failure • Hypertension	• Renal failure
Heart	— Few collaterals — Only perfused during diastole — High O_2 demand — Hypoxia sensitive — Little regeneration — Functions as integrated organ	• Angina pectoris • Heart failure • Arrhythmias	• Myocardial infarction • Cardiogenic shock (heart failure, arrhythmias)

[a] Ischaemia, relative lack of oxygen.

[b] Anoxia, complete absence of oxygen.

cramp. For the reasons listed in Table 2.7, periods of hypoxia in skeletal muscle are unlikely to result in any serious permanent damage. The opposite is true of the myocardium where, providing the patient survives the initial infarction, formation of scar tissue can result in arrhythmias and congestive heart failure (*see* Chapter 3, pp. 140–141). The general clinical effects of a poor peripheral circulation are reduced wound healing and the persistence of infections. In extreme circumstances this can lead to gangrene and loss of digits or even limbs, as in diabetes mellitus.

Obstruction of pulmonary arteries will not necessarily lead to infarction, but an embolus may occasionally obstruct blood flow to a large area of lung tissue and compromise lung function severely.

The brain is particularly sensitive to a reduction in blood flow and hypoxia because it has no reserves of either oxygen or glucose. Fainting (**syncope**), resulting from cerebral hypoxia, is often remedied by simply placing the head between the knees to increase blood flow to the head. Unfortunately, the consequences of a cerebral infarct cannot be as easily resolved because nerve cells have very little capacity for regeneration. Thus necrosis can occur after only 5–7 min of hypoxia and even small infarcts (**strokes**) can cause paralysis or permanent cognitive impairment.

We have noted that the kidney is also very sensitive to ischaemia and both acute and chronic renal ischaemia can lead to renal failure. Furthermore, any reduction in blood flow to the kidney will tend to activate the renin/angiotensin system, resulting in renal vasoconstriction and further ischaemia (*see* Chapter 4).

References and further reading

Govan AD, MacFarlane PS, Callander R (1995) *Pathology Illustrated*. 4th edn. Edinburgh: Churchill Livingstone.

Playfair JHL (1996) *Immunology at a Glance*. 6th edn. Oxford: Blackwell Scientific Publications.

Price SA, McCarty-Wilson L (1997) *Clinical Concepts of Disease Processes*. 4th edn. St Louis: Mosby.

Roitt I, Brostoff J, Male D (1998) *Immunology*. 5th edn. London: Mosby.

Spector WG (1989) *An Introduction to General Pathology*. 3rd edn. Edinburgh: Churchill Livingstone.

3

Cardiovascular system

In the West, cardiovascular disease is the most common cause of premature death in men, and a frequent cause of disability. Much of this illness is preventable because factors such as smoking and diet are strongly implicated. By understanding the mechanisms of the various disease processes it is easier for health professionals to contribute to helping patients avoid or cope with these illnesses.

Cardiovascular diseases and treatment frequently cause considerable confusion because there seem to be a number of closely related conditions and a wide range of drugs, many of which can be used in more than one condition. It is the aim of this chapter to explain how an understanding of the principles of haemodynamics in particular can clarify not only the relationship between cardiovascular diseases but also common threads running through their pharmacotherapy.

The first section discusses some important general principles of the normal function of the cardiovascular system. We will first consider the cardiovascular system (CVS) simply as a closed system of pump, tubes and fluid designed to perfuse the tissues. Energy handling in cardiac muscle, its oxygen demand and its oxygen supply will then be discussed. This haemodynamic approach allows predictions to be made about how the CVS responds to normal and abnormal circumstances, and how it responds to many drugs.

Physiological principles of the cardiovascular system

This section assumes a basic understanding of the physiology of the cardiovascular system (CVS). Appropriate background material for revision of the anatomy, physiology and pharmacology of the CVS is suggested in the References and further reading section.

Haemodynamics

Blood flow and blood pressure

The purpose of the cardiovascular system is to provide an adequate perfusion of blood to all body tissues under a variety of sometimes swiftly changing demands. The ability of the heart as a pump to maintain this perfusion may be termed the **pump performance**, usually expressed as **cardiac output** (CO).

Fluid flow through a rigid tube depends on the pressure gradient and inversely on the resistance to flow:

$$\text{Flow} \propto \frac{\text{Pressure gradient}}{\text{Resistance}} \qquad (3.1)$$

Because blood vessels are not rigid this relationship does not precisely describe blood flow, but it is a useful approximation. The pressure gradient is generated by the heart during contraction, i.e. when doing work and using energy. It is equivalent to the blood pressure (BP), or more precisely the **mean arterial pressure** (MAP), which is approximately equal to diastolic pressure plus one-third of the systolic–diastolic pressure difference. Note that the pressure is merely a means to an end: output is the primary goal.

Blood pressure is required to overcome the **peripheral resistance** (PR), which depends predominantly on the radius of the blood vessels (r) and the viscosity of the blood (Poiseuille's law):

$$\text{Resistance} \propto \frac{\text{Viscosity}}{r^4} \qquad (3.2)$$

Blood viscosity is approximately constant, although it may be altered pathologically, e.g. by increased red blood cell mass or acute dehydration. Thus variations in resistance usually reflect changes in the calibre of blood vessels. Not all vessels contribute equally. The arterioles are the main resistance vessels; together with the arteries they contribute about 70% of the PR.

Thus changes in systemic BP, or perfusion of any particular region of the body, are readily achieved by altering the calibre of the resistance vessels, especially because the resistance depends on the fourth power of the vessel radius. From Equations 3.1 and 3.2:

$$\text{Flow} \propto \text{Pressure} \times r^4 \qquad (3.3)$$

Thus very small changes in vessel diameter will produce large changes in flow if pressure is unaltered. For example, a small sustained constriction of all the body's resistance vessels will mean that a considerable increase in blood pressure is required if the same flow is to be maintained. This may be relevant to the aetiology of hypertension. Conversely, vasodilatation will permit increased flow.

Regional control of resistance and flow: autoregulation

The CVS exploits the flow/resistance relationship to increase the perfusion of specific areas temporarily at no extra cost in cardiac work. Blood is diverted from areas of lesser need, such as the skin, to those of greater need, such as muscle, by constricting vessels in the former and dilating those in the latter. Because the overall PR does not change, CO and BP also remain unchanged and there is no requirement for extra cardiac work.

How are these adjustments made? When activity in a tissue or organ increases, more oxygen is required. Initially blood flow does not increase, so oxygen demand outstrips supply and the tissue becomes hypoxic; consequently metabolic by-products, including acids and carbon dioxide, accumulate extracellularly. These have a direct dilating effect on local resistance vessels, facilitating increased perfusion. Conversely, when a tissue is receiving too much blood for its needs, the reverse mechanism mediates local vasoconstriction.

Here is an elegant example of the economy of the body, a sensitive self-regulating system which continuously monitors blood flow through all tissues and redistributes it according to need. Note that, initially at least, no interventions from the nervous or hormonal systems are required.

The lung is an important exception to this general rule of hypoxic vasodilation. Lung arterioles **constrict** when hypoxic, and it is not difficult to see why. Hypoxia in an area of lung implies inefficiency in gas transport, possibly as a result of local disease. Blood perfusing that area will be inadequately oxygenated and thus dilutes the total pulmonary oxygen output. Consequently, blood is directed away from damaged areas of lung by local vasoconstriction. However, this mechanism becomes counterproductive (i.e. maladaptive) when large areas of lung are involved (*see* Chapter 5).

Other local influences on blood vessel calibre include injury (causing constriction) and numerous local hormones and mediators, including **prostaglandins** (prostacyclin is a vasodilator), **thromboxanes** (predominantly constrictor), **endothelins** and **angiotensin** (constrictor) and **nitric oxide** (formerly called endothelium-derived relaxing factor, EDRF). Most are released from vascular endothelial cells and some may have a crucial influence on blood vessel growth and proliferation, which has a bearing on vascular obstructive disease (*see* p. 116).

Distribution of blood volume

The amount of blood contained in different components of the circulation is in inverse proportion to their resistance. Low-resistance veins and venules contain up to 75% of blood volume and are referred to as **capacitance vessels**. Although they have little effect on peripheral resistance

they have two other important roles in circulatory regulation: they exert a crucial influence on cardiac output and buffer modest untoward changes in blood volume (discussed below).

Because resistance vessels (arteries and arterioles) contain only a small proportion of the blood, changes in their calibre alter the blood volume only slightly. Moreover, they are committed to the maintenance of the blood pressure. Veins, on the other hand – being both compliant and muscular – can dilate or constrict to accommodate sudden changes in blood volume (e.g. intravenous infusions, fluid depletion), buffering the effect on venous return and pump performance (p. 57).

Cardiac output and blood pressure

Equation 3.1 can be expressed more familiarly as:

$$\text{Cardiac output} = \frac{\text{Blood pressure}}{\text{Peripheral resistance}} \quad (3.4)$$

This illustrates important relationships between the main haemodynamic parameters. For example, any rise in resistance requires an increased BP, generated by the heart, if CO is be maintained. If the situation is sustained, the extra work required will take its toll and eventually this may lead to heart failure. An increased PR is commonly found in most hypertensive patients, but rather than being the cause of the condition this could be a secondary autoregulation in response to an excessive CO (p. 97). Thus in treating hypertension, although reducing PR is the most obvious therapeutic target, strategies to reduce CO are equally appropriate; indeed, this is one of the ways that both beta-adrenergic blockers (beta-blockers) and diuretics are thought to act.

Pump performance

An appreciation of the way the heart behaves as a pump is crucial. To understand the pathogenesis of heart failure and the rationale for treating it, the factors which influence cardiac performance must be considered. Three variables determine the performance of a pump: (i) its

(a)

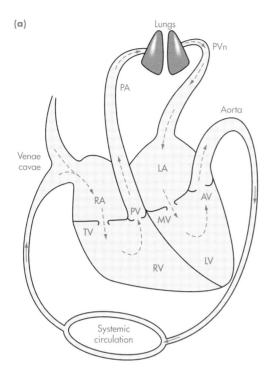

CIRCULATION (starting with return of blood to the heart from the peripheral circulation)

- Deoxygenated blood returns to the right side of the heart from venae cavae during **diastole (relaxation)**
- It enters the right atrium at a pressure of 0–10 mmHg
- Right atrial contraction increases pressure until the tricuspid valve opens
- Blood flows through the tricuspid valve into the right ventricle during diastole, partially assisted by atrial contraction (the 'atrial kick')
- As right atrial pressure rises, the tricuspid valve closes and the pulmonary valve opens
- Right ventricular **systole (contraction)** sends blood via pulmonary arteries to the lungs at a pressure of about 30 mmHg
- Blood is oxygenated in the lungs and returns to the left atrium via the pulmonary veins
- Left atrial systole increases pressure until the mitral valve opens
- Blood flows through the mitral valve into the left ventricle during diastole
- Left ventricular contraction during systole
- As pressure rises, the mitral valve closes ('lub') and the aortic valve opens
- Left ventricular contraction during systole sends blood via the aorta to the body at a maximum pressure of about 120 mmHg
- Ventricular pressure falls and the aortic valve closes ('dup')
- Blood perfuses the periphery and oxygenates tissues
- Mean pressure falls to 30 mmHg at the arterial end of capillaries and 15 mmHg at the venous end
- Deoxygenated blood returns to the heart via the veins; flow is facilitated by the peripheral muscle pump, and back flow is prevented by one-way venous valves

(b)

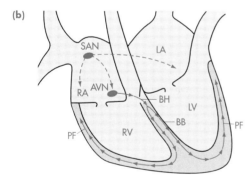

CARDIAC CYCLE (starting at end of diastole)

- Impulses originate in the sino-atrial node, which controls rhythm and causes atrial systole
- Impulses spread across the atrium to the atrioventricular node
- Impulses traverse the bundle of His and bundle branches in the septum (between Left and Right heart)
- Ventricular systole starts from the apex of the ventricles
- Intraventricular pressure rises, initially without change of size because the aortic and pulmonary valves are closed (isovolumic phase)
- Impulse spreads towards the base of the ventricles (valves) via Purkinje fibres
- Mitral and tricuspid valves close as pressure rises
- Aortic and pulmonary valves open as pressure exceeds systemic or pulmonary
- Blood propelled towards the aortic and pulmonary valves by contractile wave spreading from the apex and twisting deformation of the ventricles due to asymmetric myocardial muscle sheets (ejection phase)
- Blood flows to the lungs from the right ventricle, and to the rest of body from the left ventricle
- Pressure in the ventricles falls and the aortic and pulmonary valves close
- Blood flows from the aorta into the coronary arteries as the ventricles relax; ventricular diastole

Figure 3.1   Important components of the heart. (a) The main internal structural components of the heart. This diagram (not anatomically precise or to scale) also shows the blood flow through the different chambers, emphasizing the origins and destinations of blood on each side. (b) The main centres of electrical excitation and pathways of electrical conduction in the heart. N.B. All given pressures are approximate. AV, aortic valve; AVN, atrioventricular node; BB, bundle branches (right and left); BH, bundle of His; LA/RA, left/right atrium; LV/RV, left/right ventricle; MV, mitral valve; PA, pulmonary artery; PF, Purkinje fibres; PV, pulmonary valve; PVn, pulmonary vein; SAN, sinoatrial node; TV, tricuspid valve.

initial priming with fluid to be pumped; (ii) its intrinsic power; and (iii) the resistance which it must overcome in expelling fluid. In cardiac terms these are known as **preload**, **intrinsic contractility** and **afterload**.

Cardiac cycle

A brief summary of the main stages in the cardiac cycle is given in the text accompanying Fig. 3.1, and will be referred to in the subsequent discussion.

Preload

The force of contraction of a muscle is proportional to the degree to which it is stretched before contracting; this is the preload. In the heart it is equal to the degree of distension of the chamber at the end of diastole, the **end-diastolic volume** (EDV). This is the basis of the well-known **Starling's law**, which is often simply stated as: 'the cardiac output equals the venous return'. It may be restated more precisely as: 'the stroke volume is proportional to the EDV', where the **stroke volume** is the volume expelled in one systolic beat. Some readers may find the mechanical analogy given in Figs 3.2 and 3.3 helpful in understanding this concept (*see also* References and further reading).

An important implication of the Starling relationship is that **the heart is driven by the venous return** (VR). This is another example of economical self-regulation. Consider what happens when exertion such as running is initiated. The leg muscles need extra blood immediately, and the arterioles rapidly dilate as the tissue becomes hypoxic. But even as this happens there will be an increased VR, due to the **peripheral muscle pump**. As deep-lying peripheral veins in the leg are compressed by contracting muscles, an increased blood flow is immediately delivered to the right side of the heart (one-way flow being ensured by the non-return valves in veins). Thus as soon as vigorous activity starts, the preload is increased, raising the cardiac output by the Starling mechanism.

This does not require the intervention of any hormonal or neural mechanisms, the increased VR and CO being directly proportional to the increased activity. It also explains why one raises

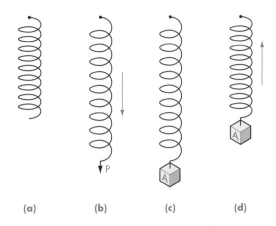

Figure 3.2 Spring model of the loading on a pump. (a) Spring in resting position. (b) Spring stretched (primed) by preload P. The degree of stretch, and therefore the energy stored for subsequent recoil, is proportional to the level of preload. (c) Afterload A applied to spring. (d) Spring recoils (contracts). Resistance to recoil depends on level of afterload, and force of recoil depends on physical nature of spring ('contractility').

the legs of someone who has fainted (it certainly does not 'increase the blood supply to the head' directly).

Filling pressure

The preload on a cardiac chamber can also be expressed as the pressure within it at the end of diastole, the **end-diastolic pressure** (EDP), which is approximately the **filling pressure** of the blood flowing into that chamber. A rise in either of these factors implies that a normal heart is being overloaded or that an ineffective heart requires an elevated preload to maintain normal output. The right atrial pressure (RAP) and the left ventricular EDP (LVEDP), measured by cardiac catheterization via peripheral arteries, give important information about the degrees of right- and left-sided heart failure respectively. The RAP also indicates whether the systemic circulatory volume is appropriate, and so can be used to monitor intravenous infusions and prevent the heart becoming overloaded.

The right heart preload may be determined more conveniently and less invasively by measuring the pressure in the great veins as they enter the right atrium The **central venous pressure** (CVP) is measured by passing an intravenous

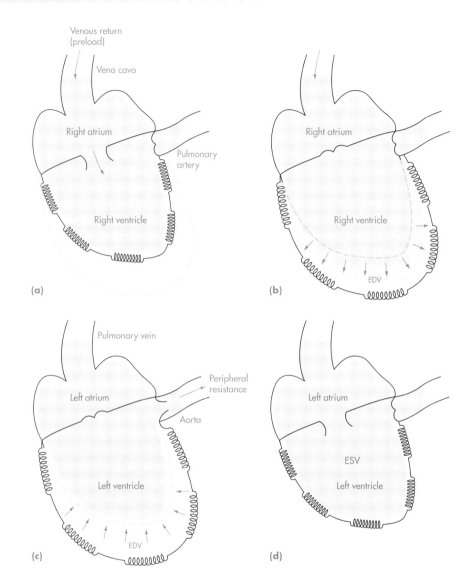

Figure 3.3   Stages in the cardiac cycle to illustrate loading, using the analogy of the spring. The effects of preload and afterload may be grasped more easily if it is imagined that there are springs in the ventricular wall which behave in a similar way to the those in previous figure. The **right** side is shown during diastole to illustrate preload and the **left** side during systole to illustrate afterload. This is because changes in preload (systemic filling pressure) usually affect the right side, while the left side is usually affected by changes in afterload (systemic vascular resistance). However, similar considerations apply to either side and they fill and empty simultaneously. (Volumes given below apply to average resting cardiac cycle, i.e. no exertion.) (a) Right side of heart at the end of systole (ESV, end-systolic volume; about 50 mL). Myocardial fibres are contracted ('springs' recoiled). Venous return starts to fill right atrium and then right ventricle, producing preload. (b) Right side at the end of diastole (EDV, end-diastolic volume; about 120 mL). Myocardial fibres are stretched, to a degree proportional to preloading (equivalent to volume of venous return). The potential force of subsequent contraction is proportional to the degree of myocardial stretch (equivalent to EDV). (c) Left side of heart at end of diastole. Myocardial fibres now start to contract. The afterload is equivalent to the resistance of the systemic arterioles (peripheral resistance) against which the left ventricle must eject the stroke volume (approx. 70 mL). The stroke volume will also be determined by the condition of the myocardium (contractility, perfusion, etc.). (d) Left side at end of systole; position is same as in (a). RV starting to fill. Stroke volume (SV) = EDV−ESV. Ejection fraction = SV/EDV (usually > 50%).

catheter percutaneously in the neck region so that its tip rests in the superior vena cava.

Filling is not a passive process; it is energy-dependent. This energy is derived partly from relaxation of the compressive deformation of the previous systolic contraction, elastic recoil aiding the restoration of diastolic shape. An important determinant of filling is ventricular **compliance** (distensibility, the inverse of stiffness). If it is reduced, a higher preload will be needed, possibly leading to **diastolic failure** (p. 93).

Ejection fraction

The ratio of the stroke volume to the EDV represents the effectiveness of cardiac emptying during systole. It is thus a good index of cardiac efficiency and is used as a quantitative measure of the degree of heart failure:

$$\text{Ejection fraction} = \frac{\text{Stroke volume}}{\text{End-diastolic volume}} \quad (3.5)$$

The average ejection fraction value in health, measured by echocardiography, is greater than 50%.

Intrinsic contractility

The biochemical and metabolic condition of heart muscle will influence its performance regardless of preloading – a unique property that is not found in skeletal or other smooth muscle. Contractility is affected by the autonomic nervous system, systemic hormones (e.g. adrenaline [epinephrine]) and disease (e.g. ischaemia due to obstructed coronary vessels), so that the same preload may produce a greater or lesser performance. Contractility also increases with increased heart rate (the force frequency effect). These represent further adaptive mechanisms available to the CVS.

Afterload

This is the resistance which the heart meets in contracting and doing work to drive blood through the arteries. A raised peripheral resistance will at first reduce CO, although normally a reflex increase in contractility will promptly restore it, at the expense of extra cardiac work.

For most purposes the afterload is approximately equivalent to the BP.

Summary

Within the normal physiological range, cardiac performance is directly proportional to preloading (EDV or filling pressure) and contractility and inversely proportional to afterload (vascular resistance). These relationships are illustrated and explained further in Fig. 3.4.

Factors affecting pump performance

Preload

This, the most complex of all determinants of cardiac performance, is usually taken as equivalent to the venous return. However, the more precise concept of filling pressure must be used to understand how preload varies (Fig. 3.5). The filling pressure at the right atrium is usually about 10 mmHg. It depends on three main factors:

1. The degree to which the circulatory system as a whole is 'filled' with blood, i.e. the blood volume.
2. The pressure exerted by the veins to accommodate this, i.e. the venous tone.
3. The contribution of muscular activity to venous return, i.e. the peripheral muscle pump (p. 55).

Blood volume

The renal control of body fluid volume is discussed in detail in Chapter 4. Fluid and electrolyte clearance by the kidney is varied to defend blood pressure. In particular, fluid is retained if renal perfusion is threatened. This is achieved through a variety of endocrine mechanisms including the renin/angiotensin system, vasopressin/antidiuretic hormone, prostglandins, kinins and possibly **atrial natriuretic peptide** (ANP). Urine output also varies with renal perfusion.

The physiological role of ANP is uncertain. Because it is a natriuretic and vasodilator hormone released from the atria in response to increased atrial pressure, it may serve as counter-regulatory hormone to limit excessive cardiac dilatation, peripheral vasoconstriction and renal

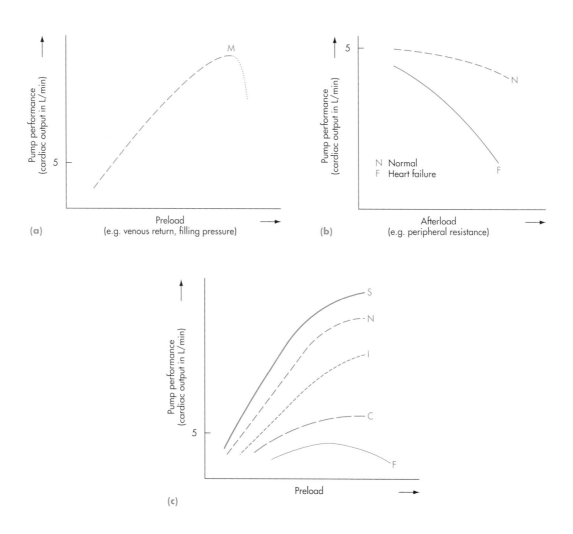

Figure 3.4   Variation of pump performance with preload, afterload and contractility. (a) **Preload**. Assuming afterload and contractility remain constant, the preload/output curve is normally steep up to a maximum M (which depends on fitness). M is seldom reached and above it performance declines steeply with increasing preload. Note that the average resting cardiac output is 5 L/min. These 'contractility curves' or Frank–Starling curves clearly show how cardiac output is driven by venous return. They are useful to illustrate variations in cardiac performance resulting from changes in other parameters. (b) **Afterload**. If contractility and preload remain constant, increases in afterload (usually peripheral resistance) reduce performance almost linearly, as shown in curve F. However, a curve such as this would only be found in heart failure. Normally, preload and contractility do not remain constant but increase reflexly to defend cardiac output (curve N), producing an almost flat relationship over a wide range. Comparison of curves F and N shows why arterial vasodilators, which reduce afterload, have little effect on output in health but can considerably improve it in failure. (c) **Contractility**. This family of contractility curves shows how different intrinsic contractilities affect the response of the heart to preload (assuming afterload is constant). Curve N is as in (a). Curve S, showing positive inotropic stimulation (e.g. sympathetic nervous system) is steeper and goes higher. Curve I shows the inhibitory effect of negative inotropic influences (e.g. parasympathetic nervous system). Curves S, N and I represent normal physiological variation. In compensated heart failure (C) the curve may barely rise above the minimum resting output. In decompensated failure (F), output actually falls with increases in preload beyond a certain point. This explains why preload reduction in heart failure can actually improve output (*see* p. 84).

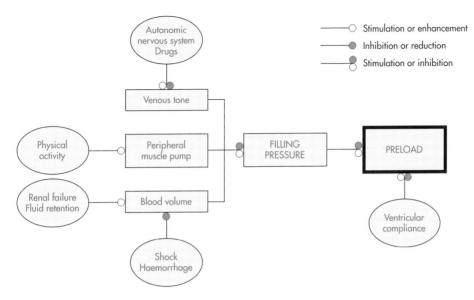

Figure 3.5 Factors affecting filling pressure and preload.

fluid retention, and as protection against fluid overloading.

Venous tone

The balance between the volume of fluid within blood vessels and its pressure is controlled by the tone of the vessels. If fluid volume is increased, e.g. by renal fluid retention, the pressure will tend to rise. The veins, being more compliant than arteries, will then dilate to accommodate the extra volume and hence buffer what would otherwise generate a dangerous rise in filling pressure and cardiac drive. Without this compliance the heart could easily be overloaded and fail. Conversely, sudden falls in blood volume, e.g. as a result of severe haemorrhage, can be partially compensated by venoconstriction.

However, venous compliance is limited and large rises in blood volume do increase filling pressure at first, although compensatory mechanisms eventually come into play, e.g. increased renal fluid clearance.

Venous tone is, like arterial tone, under autonomic control. Adrenergic drugs or stimulation of the sympathetic nervous system cause venoconstriction, which is consistent with the stress response ('fight or flight'): it increases the venous return and filling pressure and so CO. Conversely, extensive venodilatation is impli-

cated in the pathogenesis of circulatory shock because it causes a profound reduction in CO and BP.

Ventricular compliance

Resistance to filling is determined by the ease with which the shape and size of the ventricle are restored during diastole. The hypertrophy of ventricular muscle which accompanies some forms of cardiomyopathy (diseased heart muscle) and the diffuse fibrosis of chronic ischaemic heart disease can produce a stiff myocardium which significantly reduces ventricular compliance, preventing adequate filling (p. 74).

Afterload

The afterload is determined mainly by arteriolar tone, which is affected by both normal physiological mechanisms and disease (Table 3.1). In health, the overall tone is kept within narrow limits because there is rarely any physiological advantage in raising afterload. In hypertension, afterload is persistently raised, which means the heart must work harder to maintain normal output; the ultimate result may be left ventricular failure.

In health, blood viscosity is also constant. Persistent hypoxaemia (reduced blood oxygen level,

Table 3.1   Factors affecting afterload

	Increase afterload	Reduce afterload
Peripheral resistance		
Physiological		
Autonomic nervous system *via* vasomotor centre	Sympathetic tone ↑	Sympathetic tone ↓
Renal system	Renin/angiotensin	? Kinins
	Vasopressin	
Atrial endocrine function		Atrial natriuretic peptide
Local factors?	Endothelin	Endothelium-derived
		relaxing factor
Drugs	Alpha-adrenergic stimulants	Alpha-adrenergic blocker
	(e.g. *noradrenaline*	(e.g. *prazosin*)
	(*norepinephrine*))	Arterial dilators
		(e.g. *hydralazine*)
Pathological	Hypertension	Shock
	Arteriosclerosis	
Blood viscosity		
Pathological	Polycythaemia	

e.g. chronic obstructive pulmonary disease) causes a reflex rise in red blood cell count (polycythaemia). The resulting increase in blood viscosity increases the afterload and so contributes to right ventricular failure (*see* Chapter 5).

Contractility

Agents or circumstances which increase or decrease contractility are termed positively or negatively inotropic, respectively (Table 3.2). Small changes in perfusion demands are normally accommodated by changes in preloading and the Starling effect rather than in contractility. However, if necessary, positive inotropic effects can be activated rapidly by the sympathetic nervous system, and more slowly under hormonal influences, e.g. thyroxine.

The myocardial adrenergic receptors are mainly beta$_1$. However, the existence of a small but significant population of beta$_2$-receptors means that beta$_2$ selectivity among agonists such as the bronchodilators can never entirely free them from cardiac effects. This contrasts with highly selective beta$_1$-adrenergic blocking drugs, which will spare the lung and other beta$_2$-populated sites. The parasympathetic nervous system has negatively inotropic effects via muscarinic receptors, restricted mainly to the atria.

Among drugs, two main groups affect contractility: the beta-adrenergic agents (stimulants and blockers) act via their normal autonomic receptors, while the cardiac glycosides and other agents, e.g. the phosphodiesterase inhibitors, affect myocardial cells directly.

Myocardial pathology
Numerous conditions cause a deterioration in myocardial contractility. Hypoxia (low tissue oxygen level) is one of the most important. It is usually the result of impaired coronary perfusion, i.e. ischaemic heart disease. However, reduced blood oxygenation (hypoxaemia) will have a similar effect, e.g. severe chronic anaemia or chronic obstructive pulmonary disease.

Subtle problems may be caused by excessive myocardial hypertrophy. A modest increase in myocardial mass is usually a beneficial adaptive response to chronically increased cardiac loading, as in any well-exercised muscle. However, if the myocardium grows too quickly it may outpace the formation of new coronary vessels, causing relative ischaemia. In addition, a thick myocardium is less compliant (impairing filling)

Table 3.2 Factors affecting intrinsic myocardial contractility

	Contractility increased	Contractility reduced
Physiological		
Cardiovascular centre and autonomic nervous system	Sympathetic tone ↑ (atria and ventricles) Heart rate ↑ (*adrenaline* (*epinephrine*))	Parasympathetic tone ↑ (mainly atria) Heart rate ↓ (*acetylcholine*)
Endocrine	Levothyroxine (*thyroxine*), *adrenal hormones*	
Compensation	Myocardial hypertrophy	
Drugs	*Digoxin* Beta$_1$-adrenergic stimulants e.g. *dopamine, noradrenaline* (*norepinephrine*)	Beta$_1$-adrenergic blockers e.g. *atenolol*
Pathological		Hypoxia Excessive hypertrophy Excessive loading, etc. (*see* pp. 74–76)

and the extra cardiac work required to contract it during systole will also reduce efficiency.

Overloading, e.g. excessive afterload in chronic hypertension or excessive preload in fluid retention, can damage the myocardium by forcing it to operate beyond its ability to compensate, causing heart failure. This and the various other pathological processes which directly affect the myocardium are discussed in more detail on pp. 74–76.

Heart rate

This represents yet another compensatory option for the CVS because CO can quickly be changed with no change in stroke volume or intrinsic contractility:

$$\text{Cardiac output} = \text{Stroke volume} \times \text{Heart rate} \quad (3.6)$$

Heart rate is under broadly similar physiological influences to contractility. However, while the sympathetic nervous system exerts an excitatory influence on contractility, the predominant physiological control on resting rate is inhibitory parasympathetic tone via the vagus

nerve (i.e. negatively **chronotropic**). When the heart rate is increased the diastolic interval is reduced but the systolic time is generally unchanged. Generally speaking, the CVS will use changes in rate only to produce rapid temporary changes in output. Medium-term output changes require altered contractility, and chronic changes involve renal compensation and possibly myocardial hypertrophy.

Summary

The relationship between the factors discussed above is summarized in Fig. 3.6. This emphasizes the multifactorial nature of CVS adjustments, involving coordination of haemodynamic, neural and endocrine feedback loops and control paths.

Coronary circulation

Because the heart pumps continuously and has little reserve metabolic substrate (e.g. glucose), its blood supply is critical. Moreover, it has the highest oxygen extraction of any organ in the body (i.e. the arteriovenous oxygen difference is greatest). This means that increases in oxygen

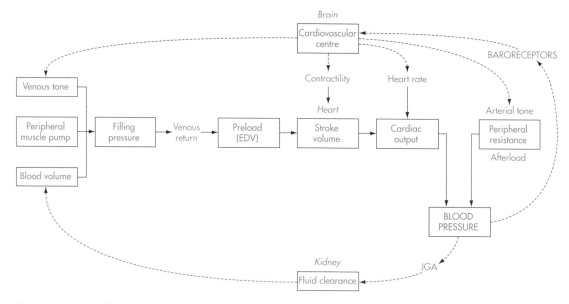

Figure 3.6 Main determinants of cardiovascular function. The solid arrows represent relationships between physiological variables. The broken arrows show hormonal or neuronal feedback loops and control paths. EDV, end-diastolic volume; JGA, juxtaglomerular apparatus.

demand need to be met mainly by increases in perfusion. Many common cardiac diseases result from impaired coronary perfusion.

Coronary perfusion

Flow into the coronary arteries is driven by the elastic recoil of the aorta immediately following systole, as the myocardium relaxes (Fig. 3.7). Perhaps surprisingly, the ventricles are only effectively perfused during diastole, because myocardial contraction during systole causes compression of the coronary vessels, especially in the highly compressed inner layer (endocardium).

Thus the perfusion pressure driving blood into the coronary arteries is the difference between the pressure in the aorta and the pressure within the heart chamber during diastole (Equation 3.7).

| Coronary perfusion pressure | = | Mean arterial pressure | − | Left ventricular end-diastolic pressure | (3.7) |

Thus both low BP and a raised EDP (e.g. during heart failure) can compromise coronary per-

fusion. Note also that blood has to change direction and flow back towards the heart during diastole to enter the coronary arteries, which branch off the aorta just after the aortic valve. This tends to produce turbulence, which may be a factor in the peculiar sensitivity of the coronary arteries to atherosclerosis.

Control and compensation

The principal physiological controls on coronary vasculature are autoregulatory, with dilatation occurring in response to increased demand as metabolic by-products accumulate in the stimulated myocardium. Autonomic control plays a minor role via alpha-adrenergic constrictor and beta$_2$ dilator nerves. These may however play a role in coronary vasospastic diseases such as variant angina (pp. 129–137). Further, non-cardioselective beta-blockers could theoretically impair coronary flow. However, the heart normally compensates by locally mediated coronary vasodilatation.

The heart does not have a well-developed system of collateral vessels; thus it is more compromised by vascular obstruction than other tissues. Therefore atheromatous plaques which occlude

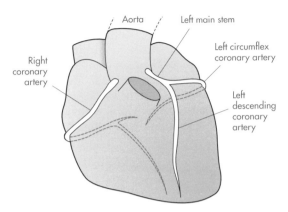

Figure 3.7 Main coronary arteries. The left main stem and right coronary arteries arise near the origin of the aorta. The left main stem coronary artery divides early, giving three principal coronary arteries. Atherosclerosis is commonly found in any of these arteries or their branches; disease of all three is known as 'three-vessel disease'. Myocardial infarction is commonly associated with occlusion of the left descending artery.

coronary arteries in ischaemic heart disease (p. 115) will have a disproportionately large effect. Regular exercise stimulates the continual development of coronary collaterals.

A fixed obstruction such as an atheroma not only reduces the lumen but also impairs the vessel's ability to dilate, and may abolish it completely. Furthermore, during ischaemia dilatation occurs normally in vessels adjacent to the obstructed one; this may actually divert blood away from the area served by the obstructed vessel if that area does not have a collateral supply. This phenomenon, known as **coronary steal**, is sometimes seen when vasodilators are used in acute angina; the pain actually increases as blood is redirected away from the ischaemic area.

Myocardial energetics

Oxygen demand

The work done by the heart is given approximately by the product **cardiac output × blood pressure**. Clearly, oxygen demand is related to the work done. This relationship is governed by several variables. One way of expressing it is:

$$O_2 \text{ demand} = \text{Contractility} \times \text{Myocardial wall tension} \times \text{Time in tension} \qquad (3.8)$$

Contractility depends on the contractile state of the myocardium (p. 57), time in tension is related to heart rate, and wall tension is related to mean arterial pressure (for the left ventricle). Thus adrenaline (epinephrine), hypertension and tachycardia (increased heart rate) all increase oxygen demand if other factors remain unchanged. This is particularly important to remember when the coronary supply is compromised, because increases in such factors may precipitate acute angina.

If contractility is approximately constant, Equation 3.8 simplifies to:

$$O_2 \text{ demand} \propto \text{Heart rate} \times \text{Blood pressure} \qquad (3.9)$$

This semi-quantitative approximation, known as the 'rate–pressure product', is convenient for clinical studies because the variables are easily measured. It can be used to predict the effect of various strategies or drugs on oxygen demand. In the treatment of certain conditions the aim is to reduce the rate–pressure product, e.g. in ischaemic heart disease, where oxygen supply is restricted.

Efficiency

This may be taken as the work the heart does in relation to its oxygen consumption. Although absolute values do not concern us here, relative changes do. A number of specific consequences affecting efficiency follow from the fact that the heart is a hollow chamber.

First, for reasons not fully understood, 'volume work' is more efficient than 'pressure work'. That is, work done to increase CO requires a smaller increase in oxygen demand than does the same amount of work done raising BP. Thus volume overloading is less harmful to the heart than sustained high BP. Consequently, heart failure or angina develop far more readily from hypertension or aortic stenosis (narrowing of the aortic valve) than from fluid retention or aortic incompetence (incomplete closure of aortic valve). Conversely, strategies to reduce afterload might be expected to be more effective at reducing cardiac workload than strategies reducing preload.

A second and even more important problem relates to myocardial wall tension, a major determinant of oxygen demand. The ability to expel blood during systole depends on the tension generated in the ventricular wall and this is determined by the diastolic stretch imparted by preloading. However, the effect is not linear and as preload increases there are disproportionately greater increases in oxygen demand. Thus doubling the preload will require more than double the oxygen demand if output is also to be doubled.

The explanation is given by **Laplace's law**. Clearly, the walls of a hollow container need to develop or maintain tension in order to generate or withstand pressure within. Laplace's law states that this tension is proportional not only to the magnitude of the required pressure but also to the size of the container. In the cardiovascular context the 'containers' we are interested in are blood vessels and heart chambers.

$$\text{Wall tension} \propto \text{Internal pressure} \times \text{Radius} \qquad (3.10)$$

This explains why large arteries need much thicker walls than smaller ones, despite their internal pressure being similar. (Similarly, thin bicycle tyres, because of their small radius, can withstand much higher pressures than much thicker car tyres.)

Thus the larger the size from which a heart has to contract, i.e. the greater the diastolic volume, the greater will be the wall tension required to generate the same internal pressure needed to overcome the afterload. This means an increased oxygen demand for the same output (Equation 3.8). So, for a given individual, the larger the heart, the less efficient it is. 'Larger' in this context means an increase in chamber size and should be distinguished from 'hypertrophy', which is an increase in muscle mass (p. 66).

The significance of this may be gauged when it is recalled that cardiac enlargement by the Starling mechanism is a prime strategy for accommodating extra haemodynamic demands.

Normally it causes no problem because there is sufficient cardiac reserve. However, in the failing or ischaemic heart this reduced efficiency can mean the difference between compensation (i.e. coping) and decompensation. It also explains the rationale for the use of vasodilators, which reduce preload or afterload and therefore ventricular wall tension, in heart failure.

Cardiovascular reserve

The cardiovascular (cardiac) reserve is the degree to which the CVS can increase its performance to meet extra circulatory demands, or can maintain performance in the face of increased afterload or impaired contractility. Changes in systemic cardiovascular demand (as opposed to local autoregulation) are detected by a comprehensive system of receptors (*see* Fig. 3.6). Baroreceptors in the aortic arch, the carotid body, the atria and the ventricles detect changes in intravascular or intracardiac pressure and relay these to the cardiovascular/vasomotor centre in the medulla. This then mediates an appropriate response via adjustments in sympathetic and parasympathetic outflow, principally to the vasculature and myocardium, and also via antidiuretic hormone (ADH; vasopressin) secretion. Intracardiac baroreceptors also mediate ANP secretion. The renal juxtaglomerular apparatus is another important detector of reduced perfusion, mediating its response principally via the renin/angiotensin system. The kidney may increase erythropoietin secretion, expanding red blood cell numbers. Chemoreceptors in the carotid body and the aortic arch detect oxygen tension, which would fall if lung perfusion were compromised.

At rest, the average CO is approximately 5 L/min. Because absolute values depend on body size, the CO is sometimes adjusted for body surface area: the resting **cardiac index** is approximately 3 L/min/m^2. In a fit adult, CO can be increased on demand up to 20–30 L/min; there may also be a rise in BP. The difference between resting and maximum CO is the **cardiac reserve**. With a diseased heart, the cardiac reserve will be less. In mild heart failure the reduction may be small and therefore only noticeable on vigorous exertion, when the patient will become unusually fatigued. As heart function deteriorates, the degree of exertion which produces the same level of fatigue becomes progressively smaller. This reduced **exercise tolerance** is a measure of diminishing cardiac reserve.

As long as the patient can maintain an adequate CO at rest the heart failure is termed **compensated**. However, as the condition deteriorates the patient will eventually be unable to sustain an adequate CO for normal activity, or may even be breathless at rest; this is **decompensation**.

The various haemodynamic, neural and endocrine mechanisms and strategies of cardiovascular compensation are summarized in Table 3.3; many have already been discussed. They are classified according to the speed with which the CVS can mobilize them. Note that medium- and long-term compensation mechanisms resemble

normal physiological responses to exercise training.

Acute compensation

The CVS can respond very rapidly to acutely increased demand. Cardiac output may be raised through the Starling mechanism following increased venous return and/or venoconstriction. The cardiovascular centre and sympathetic nervous system also contribute by acting on the myocardium and pacemaker, giving positive inotropic and chronotropic responses. Falls in BP are also compensated by a sympathetic nervous system vasoconstrictor response.

ANP may be secreted by the right atrium when atrial baroreceptors detect an increase in atrial filling, as a counter-regulatory response to limit or buffer these actions. This suppresses excessive activity of the sympathetic nervous system.

Table 3.3   Mechanisms of cardiovascular reserve

Mechanism	Effect
Acute	
Starling effect: preload ↑	End-diastolic volume ↑ (= heart size ↑)
Inotropic: sympathetic nervous system ↑	Contractility ↑
parasympathetic nervous system ↓	
Chronotropic: parasympathetic nervous system ↓	Heart rate ↑
sympathetic nervous system ↑	
Vasomotor: sympathetic nervous system ↑	Arteriolar constriction → blood pressure ↑
	Venous constriction → preload ↑
Medium-term	
Persistence of acute mechanisms above	(May become down-regulated)
Renal compensation:	
• juxtaglomerular apparatus:	Fluid retention, vasoconstriction
renin/angiotensin/aldosterone ↑	
• pressure natriuresis ↓	Fluid retention
Endocrine:	
• adrenaline (epinephrine) ↑	Positively inotropic, chronotropic
• ADH (vasopressin) ↑	Fluid retention, vasoconstriction
Long-term	
Cardiac hypertrophy	Contractility ↑
Polycythaemia	↑ O_2 to tissues
Renal compensation	As in 'medium-term'

The role of **atrial natriuretic peptide** (ANP) in normal physiology is unclear (*see* p. 57 and p. 64).

Medium-term compensation

If the stress is more prolonged many acute compensatory mechanisms may persist, but other ones also have time to come into play. Renal compensation (*see* Chapter 4, p. 161) involves the renin/angiotensin system and fluid retention to expand or maintain circulating fluid volume. There may also be secretion of ADH. More directly, if renal perfusion pressure is reduced there will be reduced urine output owing to reduced filtration and increased reabsorption.

Long-term compensation

Chronically increased demand induces myocardial hypertrophy, an increase in myocardial muscle mass which increases contractility (note that this differs from 'cardiac enlargement', which means an increased EDV). If there is persistent hypoxaemia as a result of poor pulmonary perfusion, an increased red cell count will eventually be induced, possibly resulting in polycythaemia. The kidneys continue to retain fluid.

Constraints on cardiac reserve

There are limits to most of these mechanisms; the CVS cannot accommodate increasing demands indefinitely (Table 3.4). Eventually these essentially beneficial haemodynamic and neuro-endocrine mechanisms come to be employed in circumstances beyond their design limits: they then become maladaptive (counterproductive). This accounts for many of the features of heart failure.

Starling/renal

The kidneys will attempt to support a failing circulation by retaining fluid, increasing the filling pressure and thus CO. However, because of the Laplace limitation (p. 64), a failing myocardium cannot benefit indefinitely from this. As the heart becomes progressively more stretched not only does it become less oxygen efficient but the cells also become fatigued and unable to respond. There is a limit to the degree of stretch (cardiac enlargement) that the muscle fibres can tolerate, dependent at the ultracellular level on the degree of interdigitation of the actin and myosin filaments. Beyond this, fluid retention becomes maladaptive. There is also the more tangible constraint of the indistensible pericardial sac around the heart.

Sympathetic nervous system

Adrenergic receptors on myocardial or vascular smooth muscle eventually become desensitized (accommodated) to prolonged and unrelieved stimulation, and therefore less responsive, possi-

Table 3.4   Limitations on cardiovascular compensation (cardiac reserve)

Compensation	Limitation
Starling	Overstretch → myocardial cell damage
	Laplace-related inefficiency
Sympathetic nervous system	Overactivity → depletion of cardiac transmitter stores and down-regulation of cardiac beta-receptors
Vasomotor	Accomodation of baroreceptors
Heart rate	Arrhythmias: impaired filling
Endocrine	ANP response blunted
Renal fluid retention	Becomes maladaptive when heart cannot respond to dilatation by increasing contractility
Hypertrophy	Chamber size ↓
	Coronary perfusion ↓
	Myocardial compliance ↓

ANP, atrial natriuretic peptide; although level raised, effectiveness appears to be diminished.

bly through down-regulation or post-receptor uncoupling. This may induce reflex sympathetic over-activity which, among other things, produces an unsustainable increase in myocardial oxygen demand and encourages arrhythmia.

At this stage, which is found in early chronic (compensated) heart failure, a further protective mechanism is activated. Atrial and arterial baroreceptors (stretch receptors) signal the CVS centre to *limit* sympathetic activity and promote increased vagal activity. This reduces myocardial wall stress by reducing excessive cardiac stimulation and peripheral vasoconstriction; arrhythmias are also inhibited. Thus as cardiac function declines the heart is protected against excessive demands. As we will see below, later still this mechanism becomes blunted; baroreceptor failure signals the onset of decompensation and overwhelming maladaptive stimulation of heart and arteries.

Renal/endocrine

Renin secretion may also become excessive, partly mediated by the sympathetic nervous system, and angiotensin then contributes to the decompensation. A failure in the counter-regulatory ANP and nitric oxide (EDRF) mechanisms exacerbates the situation. It will allow excessive fluid retention and vasoconstriction by no longer attenuating the actions of aldosterone, angiotensin and endothelin.

If the **heart rate** increase is excessive, co-ordination becomes disrupted and arrhythmias develop that compromise the efficiency of ventricular ejection. The practical maximum heart rate in a fit person is about three times the resting rate. Even before this stage efficiency may be reduced because of inadequate time for complete emptying or refilling within each cardiac cycle.

Finally, myocardial hypertrophy is not without disadvantages (Fig. 3.8):

- The heart becomes stiffer, i.e. less compliant, and so more work and more oxygen are required for each contraction.
- The muscle growth will be partly inwards reducing the effective chamber size.
- The thicker walls will produce unequal stresses at different levels within the thickness

during contraction so more energy will be expended in deforming them.
- Muscle development may outstrip new coronary vessel growth.

It must be remembered that the main purpose of the Starling mechanism is to **maintain** stroke volume under conditions of increased loading. Even under maximal exercise stimulation stroke volume rarely increases by more than about 25%. The increase in CO during exercise is principally due to increased heart rate. The main cardiovascular effect of **training** is to increase resting stroke volume and EDV and reduce resting heart rate. This increases cardiac reserve by a allowing greater latitude for increased heart rate and ejection fraction.

Thus although the CVS is beautifully designed to compensate most economically for wide variations in physiological demands, there are certain stresses with which it cannot cope and these

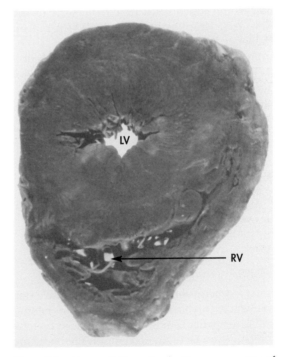

Figure 3.8 Myocardial hypertrophy. Transverse section of a hypertrophied heart showing gross thickening of the left ventricular wall. Note how the chamber size is reduced. This leads to increased stiffness and restriction of coronary perfusion. LV, left ventricle; RV, right ventricle. (Reproduced with permission from *Muir's Textbook of Pathology*, 10th edn.)

can lead to cardiovascular disease, particularly heart failure. An understanding of cardiovascular mechanisms shows how these problems arise and indicates possible modes of treatment.

Clinical features of cardiovascular disease

Symptoms

Because the CVS supplies all organs, symptoms may arise in any one, and the cause may not be obviously cardiovascular, especially to a patient. Further, because most CVS disease is chronic, symptoms may at first be noticeable only on exertion. As the disease progresses, the point at which symptoms develop comes earlier. The severity of many acute cardiovascular symptoms can often be graded empirically by the application of the widely used functional scale of the New York Heart Association (NYHA) based on challenge to the cardiac reserve. This can be approximately linked to the ejection fraction (EF) as an objective index, but symptoms are not directly related to objective measures of ventricular dysfunction:

- Grade I. No symptoms at ordinary physical activity (abnormality detected only on investigation; EF <45%).
- Grade II. Symptoms evident on strenuous exertion (EF <40%).
- Grade III. Symptoms evident on moderate exertion (EF <30%).
- Grade IV. Symptoms at rest (EF <25%).

Fatigue

Impaired perfusion to body skeletal muscle due to reduced myocardial function (heart failure) will cause patients to tire easily. Reduced exercise tolerance can be estimated empirically by asking how far a patient can walk, climb stairs, etc. or quantified by formal exercise testing on a treadmill or exercise bicycle (with ECG monitoring). Of course, fatigue can have numerous other causes, both physical and mental. Common iatrogenic causes include beta-blocker therapy

and, in the elderly especially, diuretic-induced electrolyte imbalance (sodium, potassium).

Dizziness; fainting (syncope)

Temporarily interrupted CNS perfusion (transient ischaemic attacks, TIA) commonly result from, among other causes, sudden temporary ventricular arrhythmias (e.g. Stokes–Adams attacks) or postural hypotension. It is usually reversible within a few minutes (contrast epilepsy, stroke, etc.). Possible iatrogenic causes of syncope are CNS depressants, vasodilator therapy or diuretic-induced hypovolaemia. Simple faints in otherwise healthy individuals are not uncommon and usually are due to increased parasympathetic activity causing transient hypotension (vasovagal attack).

Dyspnoea

Shortness of breath or difficulty in breathing is a subjective feeling which may or may not be associated with objectively reduced blood oxygenation. Possible causes are mainly cardiovascular (in left ventricular failure, via pulmonary oedema), primary pulmonary disease (*see* Chapter 5) and anaemia. Postural variation is common in cardiovascular dyspnoea: it is worse when supine, so that the patient breathes more easily when erect or sitting (**orthopnoea**). This is because intrathoracic pressure becomes increased when the patient is recumbent, raising pulmonary venous pressure and thus promoting the formation of alveolar oedema (see below).

Palpitations

An abnormal awareness of the heartbeat is usually caused by an arrhythmia, particularly an extrasystole. Patients may also notice severe tachycardia or bradycardia.

Pain

Pain arising in the chest region can have many origins, including the upper gastrointestinal tract, the lungs and the chest wall, as well as acute anxiety. The typical cardiac ischaemic pain associated with coronary artery disease is characteristically described as 'crushing' or 'choking', but seldom as 'sharp' nor 'momentary'. Patients may illustrate it by making a fist against their sternum or describing it as "like someone bear-hugging you from behind". The pain may radiate down the left arm or up to the jaw. The most important differential diagnosis for a pharmacist is dyspeptic pain from the oesophagus, stomach or duodenum, which is classically described as sharp ("like a knife") and patients illustrate by pointing (*see* Chapter 6). However, it may not be possible from the patient's description to distinguish between cardiac pain and that of epigastric origin, and such symptoms should not be used in isolation to diagnose cardiac events.

Examination: signs and history

Pulse

Palpating the pulse indicates cardiac rate and rhythm. If vascular obstructive disease is suspected, it is customary to take the pulse at several sites on either side of the body (both wrists, elbows, ankles, knees) to check for possible impaired or asymmetric perfusion. (Thus, for example, a diabetic may have normal pulses at the knee but weak ones at the ankle owing to angiopathy.) The **pulse pressure**, the difference in pressure between systole and diastole, can be detected by palpation and yields useful semi-quantitative information: e.g. both the arterial rigidity of arteriosclerosis in the aged, and an incompetent aortic valve, cause a sharp difference with each beat (i.e. wide pulse pressure).

Palpation of the left chest at the fifth rib, about half-way between the sternum and side of body, will reveal the **apex beat**. This is where the left ventricle impacts on the chest wall during systole, yielding information about the rhythm and strength of the heart beat. In an enlarged heart this point is shifted leftwards (away from the sternum).

Blood pressure

Measurement of **systemic arterial blood pressure** is discussed on pp. 93–115. The pressure is at or near systolic level for only a short part of the cardiac cycle: for most of the cycle, pressure is nearer diastolic. Thus **mean arterial pressure** (MAP), which gives an indication of the average stress put on the arterial system, is not a simple average: it is calculated as a weighted average of the two, with the greater weight given to the diastolic:

$$\text{Mean arterial pressure} = \text{Diastolic} + 1/3\,(\text{Systolic} - \text{Diastolic}) \qquad (3.11)$$

This is why emphasis is often put on raised diastolic pressure when defining and treating hypertension. The long-term damage to blood vessels that untreated hypertension causes is proportional to the elevation of mean pressure, but to save calculation, approximation to the diastolic is more reliable than the systolic.

The BP rises with age, the systolic faster than the diastolic as arteriosclerosis (p. 116) reduces arterial compliance. Between the ages of 20–60 years the approximate normal values are given by:

$$\text{Systolic blood pressure} = 100 + 2/3\,\text{Age} \qquad (3.12)$$

$$\text{Diastolic blood pressure} = 67 + 1/3\,\text{Age} \qquad (3.13)$$

Thereafter, the diastolic stabilizes at about 90 mmHg whereas the systolic continues rising, up to 180–200 mmHg at age 80. However, these rises are much less marked in non-industrialized societies.

The **central venous pressure** (CVP) is the BP at the point where the great veins enter the right atrium and is normally between 0 and 10 mmHg. The CVP represents the right atrial pressure or preload and is a good index of cardiac performance, because reduced ventricular performance will cause it to rise. It may be used to monitor possible fluid overload in heart failure or intravenous fluid therapy. The **jugular venous pressure** (JVP) is a non-invasive external indicator, detectable by examining for possible swelling of the jugular vein in the neck. It is measured by estimating the height of this swollen portion above the line of the clavicle (with the patient sitting with his or her thorax at 45°). Normally it is undetectable; in (right) heart failure it is raised.

Cyanosis

This blue coloration of blood is due to reduced oxygen saturation of blood (increased deoxy-haemoglobin). It is particularly noticeable in highly vascular areas such as lips, tongue or nailbeds. The terms central and peripheral in relation to cyanosis refer to its origin and not where it is observed – a common source of confusion. **Central cyanosis** is caused by generalized arterial hypoxaemia, due for example to pulmonary oedema. In **peripheral cyanosis** the arterial oxygen saturation may be normal but perfusion of a particular area is compromised. In heart failure this commonly occurs in the skin where vasoconstriction diverts blood away to more important areas. Local blood flow is slowed, more oxygen is extracted, the arteriovenous oxygen difference is raised, and the blood becomes abnormally deoxygenated and blue-tinged. The area will be cold, but if it is massaged to improve local perfusion then normal colour may be restored (contrast this with central cyanosis).

Oedema

The origins of oedema are complex. The conventional explanation is given in Fig. 3.9, although recent evidence has questioned the completeness of this. In this model the oedema of heart failure is primarily due to a combination of raised total body water (owing to renal fluid retention) and the preferential redistribution of an abnormal amount of this water to the extravascular extracellular compartment, i.e. tissue fluid (owing to raised peripheral venous pressure). As will be discussed below, hydrostatic factors also contribute. Generally, pulmonary oedema results from left heart failure, and peripheral oedema (in ankles, sacrum, abdominal organs) from right heart failure. If the oedematous area is compressed firmly with the thumb for about 10 sec (this is usually painless for the patient), the impression remains as a pit for very much longer than would be the case for normal skin – hence the term **pitting oedema**.

Investigation

Catheterization

A fine plastic catheter may be introduced into the heart via a peripheral artery (left side of the heart) or vein (right side) so as to lie with its tip in a chamber or great vessel. Radiocontrast medium may then be injected, pressure at that point measured or blood withdrawn for gas analysis. Particularly useful pressures to ascertain are right atrial pressure (equivalent to CVP or preload), pressure drop across a valve, and pressure in the pulmonary vein (pulmonary 'wedge' pressure, equivalent to left atrial pressure).

Imaging

A plain chest **radiograph** (*see* Fig. 3.13) will show the size of the heart and whether or not the lung fields are clear. Shadowing at the bases of the lungs along the lower margin (defined by the diaphragm) usually indicates accumulation of fluid (pulmonary oedema). Radiography may be enhanced by using radio-opaque contrast material.

In **ventricular angiography**, heart movement throughout the cardiac cycle can be visualized by injecting radio-opaque material into the general circulation. In **coronary angiography**, much smaller quantities of contrast medium are precisely injected via a catheter at the root of a coronary artery to visualize possible obstructive lesions. This is becoming a standard investigation of cardiac ischaemic symptoms for deciding whether bypass or angioplasty is indicated, and if so where.

Nuclear imaging is used in two ways. In radionuclide ventilography, Thallium-201 taken up from coronary blood by healthy myocardial tissue leaves 'cold' spots which identify underperfused (ischaemic) areas. Technetium-99-labelled red blood cells enable visualization of the heart chambers and their movement; the ejection fraction can be measured accurately.

Less invasive imaging is generally to be preferred if appropriate. **Echocardiography** provides a continuous timed record of all cardiac

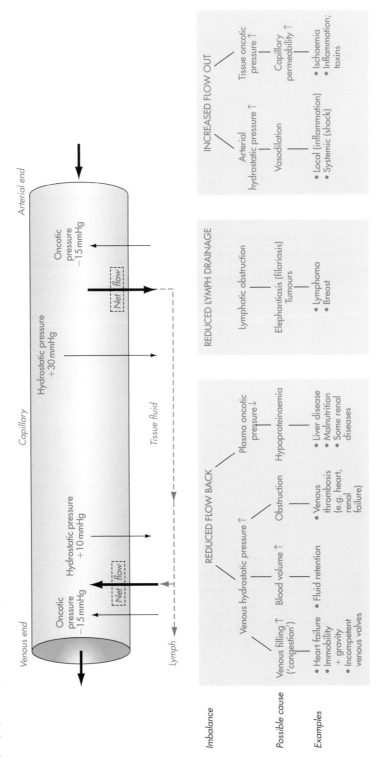

Figure 3.9 Formation of oedema. Tissue fluid is formed by ultrafiltration of plasma at the arterial end of capillaries, carrying with it nutrients and O_2. The motive force is the excess of hydrostatic pressure within the vessel forcing fluid out, over the oncotic (osmotic) pressure of the plasma proteins drawing it in. At the venous end, hydrostatic pressure has fallen but the oncotic pressure is little changed because plasma proteins do not pass out. Thus tissue fluid drains back, carrying with it waste products and CO_2. A small excess (2.5 L daily for the whole body) forms the lymph. Excess tissue fluid will accumulate if this balance is disturbed by either excess formation, impaired flow back to veins or lymphatic obstruction. The major ways in which this balance is upset are shown. Note: tissue pressures ignored.

movements and dimensions of the chambers (including thickness and lumen size) and valves, and so can be used to measure ejection fraction. **Magnetic resonance imaging** (MRI) and **computed tomography** (CT) scanning may also be used.

ECG

An electrocardiogram reveals to the trained eye both qualitative and quantitative information about the heart's activity and electrical conduction system. The multiplicity of leads enables localization of certain lesions (e.g. where an infarction has occurred). Exercise provocation and 24-h recording may be useful modifications. The trace as it most commonly appears in generic ECG illustrations (similar to lead II) is shown in Fig. 3.10, together with an account of the origin of each component. A number of basic ECG traces will be used in the relevant sections below to illustrate some typical abnormalities.

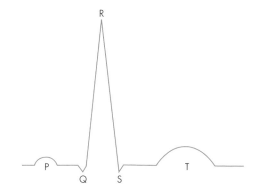

Figure 3.10   Normal electrocardiogram. The P wave represents atrial depolarization, the QRS complex ventricular depolarization, and the T wave ventricular repolarization. The PQ interval represents impulse speed between atrium and ventricle, altered in heart block. The height of the R wave represents ventricular mass, increased in hypertrophy. Myocardial ischaemia often manifests as abnormalities of the ST complex.

Heart failure

Heart failure (cardiac failure) is not a disease but a syndrome, with many possible aetiologies and a complex pathogenesis. Yet it may be simply defined as the **failure of the heart to meet the normal perfusion demands of the body**. Many diseases can impair cardiac performance and all are usually serious. Consequently, chronic cardiac failure has a poor prognosis, comparable with that in many forms of cancer.

Whatever the cause of failure, the clinical picture resulting from reduced contractility is due to a combination of the haemodynamic consequences of impaired perfusion and the secondary consequences of maladaptive attempts by the CVS to compensate. The latter frequently involve the neuroendocrine mechanisms we met in discussing cardiac reserve (p. 64; Table 3.3). In heart failure these can exacerbate the situation as one or more components fail to respond satisfactorily (e.g. a failure to increase myocardial contractility following increased sympathetic nervous system activity). The sequence of events is illustrated in Fig. 3.11. The heart failure syn-

drome may also involve peripheral organ damage not directly due to reduced blood supply, especially in skeletal muscle.

Terminology

Terms commonly used to describe different aspects of heart failure are given in Table 3.5. Most cases of heart failure would be properly classified as 'chronic compensated low-output left ventricular systolic failure'. The clinical features of left and right failure differ in certain crucial aspects, but many patients present with bilateral failure. The distinction between acute and chronic is important for management. The difference between systolic and diastolic failure is discussed below.

Epidemiology

Determination of the prevalence of heart failure depends upon which grade, ejection fraction cut-off point and population are being considered. Estimates for symptomatic heart failure vary between 0.5% and 2%, but among those aged over 80 years this rises to 10%. If asymptomatic cases (Grade 1) are included, overall preva-

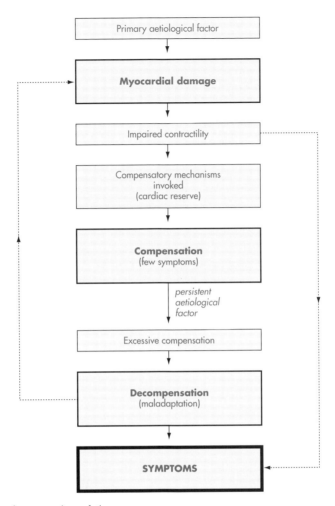

Figure 3.11   Sequence of events in heart failure.

lence is almost 10%. The annual incidence in the UK is approximately 0.3%, representing over 150 000 cases.

Aetiology

The causes of heart failure may be considered in two broad groups:

1. **Pump failure**, with primary reduction in myocardial contractility.
2. **Overloading**, with either excessive afterload (pressure overload) or excessive preload (volume overload), which arise outside heart and reduce contractility secondarily.

Specific causes within these groups may give rise to failure acutely or chronically and may initially affect one specific chamber or side of the heart. However, in chronic heart failure both sides are usually affected eventually. Table 3.6 shows common causes in each category.

Despite this wide range of possible aetiologies, in industrialized countries by far the most common cause of left ventricular failure is ischaemic heart disease; the second most common is untreated systemic ('essential') hypertension. With improved public health and sanitation, valve disease resulting from childhood rheumatic fever is now uncommon. However, in developing countries the picture quite different, with infective and nutritional causes being far more common.

Table 3.5   Terminology of heart failure

Term	Typical causes/comments
Acute	Myocardial infarction (sudden onset)
Chronic	Valve disease (gradual onset, usually progressive course)
Right	Lung disease (cor pulmonale)
Left	Untreated essential hypertension
Bilateral	Almost any cause (usually chronic)
Low output	Reduced contractility – most causes (usual variety)
High output	Anaemia, thyrotoxicosis – due to excessive cardiac drive
Systolic	Reduced contractility → impaired emptying (usual variety)
Diastolic	Reduced ventricular compliance → impaired filling (less common)
Compensated	Compensation prevents symptoms at rest but cardiac reserve diminished
Decompensated	Cardiac reserve exhausted
Congestive (CHF, CCF)	Imprecise traditional term describing generalized oedema; usually implies bilateral failure
Cardiogenic shock	Acute severe decompensation: very low BP and CO; poor tissue perfusion
LVF/RVF	Left/right ventricular failure

BP, blood pressure; CCF, congestive cardiac failure; CHF, congestive heart failure; CO, cardiac output.

Pathogenesis

Primary pump failure

Damage to the myocardium usually results in **systolic failure**. Ischaemic heart disease (restriction of the coronary blood supply) is the most common cause; it usually affects just one chamber, most commonly the left ventricle. Ischaemic failure may develop suddenly without prior warning, following **myocardial infarction**, or there may be slowly progressive **diffuse fibrosis** with multiple minor and possibly asymptomatic infarcts, especially in the elderly. Alternatively, chronic ischaemia may induce asymptomatic **myocardial hibernation**, with progressive decline in systolic function, though potentially this is reversible by coronary surgery. However, it must be remembered that ischaemic heart disease is a separate disease entity from heart failure and does not invariably lead to it. Heart failure rarely results from stable angina pectoris.

The cardiomyopathies are a miscellaneous group in which diffuse damage occurs throughout the myocardium. They are either idiopathic or secondary to conditions such as infection, toxins (e.g. alcohol), inflammation or autoimmune disease. Interestingly, cardiac **tumours** are rare. In **dilated cardiomyopathy** the myocardium becomes thin, weak and excessively enlarged, with a raised EDV and a low ejection fraction. In **hypertrophic cardiomyopathy** there is excessive thickening of the myocardium, leading to poor ventricular filling and obstructed ejection particularly due to structural distortion around the valves, whereas in **restrictive cardiomyopathy** there is increased ventricular stiffness but little hypertrophy.

In the ageing heart a diffuse ('senile') **fibrosis** can occur and a number of systemic diseases such as sarcoid and amyloidosis may have diffuse cardiac complications that lead to eventual failure. Arrhythmias may also cause pump failure.

While most forms of pump failure cause reduced contractility and systolic failure, some diffuse diseases of the myocardium can lead to it becoming fibrosed and stiff, with reduced compliance. This results in difficulty in filling the heart adequately during diastole, and leads to **diastolic failure**. This has been recognized in about one-fifth of patients with symptoms of failure (i.e. low output) but a normal heart size and ejection fraction (and thus normal systolic function), and may be present in up to half of all heart failure cases. Causes include patchy ischaemic or senile fibrosis, restrictive cardiomy-

Table 3.6 Aetiology of heart failure

Haemodynamic defect	Cause	Side affected[a]	Acute or chronic
Pump failure			
Systolic failure	Ischaemic heart disease	L usually	Acute, chronic
	Cardiomyopathy	L and/or R	Chronic
	Arrhythmias	L + R	Acute, chronic
	Infection, inflammation, alcohol	L + R	Acute, chronic
	Systemic disease (e.g. amyloidosis)	L + R	Chronic
	Diffuse fibrosis (senile, ischaemic)	L + R	Chronic
Diastolic failure	Ischaemia, cardiomyopathy, fibrosis	L + R	Chronic
Excessive afterload			
	Hypertension – systemic	L	Chronic
	– pulmonary (COPD)	R	Chronic
	Valve stenosis	L or R	Chronic
	Polycythaemia	R	Chronic
Excessive preload			
Hypervolaemia	Fluid retention e.g. renal failure, aldosteronism, Excess IV infusion, Polycythaemia	R	Usually chronic
Excessive demand	Hyperdynamic: anaemia, thyrotoxicosis	R	Chronic
	Regurgitation: valve incompetence	R or L	Chronic
Obligatory	Vasodilation: beri-beri, septicaemia	L + R	Chronic

[a] Initial side of heart affected (L, left; R, right); in chronic disease usually both sides eventually fail.

COPD, chronic obstructive pulmonary disease; MI, myocardial infarction.

opathy and hypertrophic cardiomyopathy (owing to, for example, untreated hypertension).

Overloading

Both over-work and over-stretch cause structural and biochemical abnormalities in the myocardial cells, such as the deposition of fibrils and impaired calcium utilization. The result is in a decreased force and velocity of contraction and delayed relaxation. These effects are usually irreversible.

Excessive afterload

If the systemic vascular resistance is abnormally high, i.e. systemic hypertension, the raised afterload on the **left** ventricle may eventually cause it to fail; the right ventricle will initially be unaffected. The heart is far more prone to damage from pressure overloading than from volume overloading, although the former is now relatively uncommon, because hypertension is detected earlier by screening and is treated far better by less toxic drugs. However, it is possible that failure diagnosed as ischaemic or cardiomyopathic may have been aetiologically related to chronic undetected hypertension.

In an analogous way, sustained rises in pulmonary vascular resistance (pulmonary hypertension, e.g. secondary to many chronic lung diseases) can eventually lead to **right** ventricular failure, known as **cor pulmonale**.

Theoretically, the afterload on both sides may be increased significantly by abnormally high blood viscosity, such as in polycythaemia, but this is unlikely to cause failure in the absence of other abnormalities.

Excessive preload

This is an uncommon general cause of failure. Whether or not excessive increases in venous return lead to failure depends on the cause and other factors. The heart tolerates volume overload well, and because the output initially is high, symptoms are not at first evident. The left side of the heart receives the same volume of venous return as the right, at approximately the same preloading (the lungs usually offering little resistance). Because the left ventricle is by far the more powerful, if decompensation is caused by raised systemic filling pressure the **right** side will be first to fail.

If moderate hypervolaemia develops, the initially raised output will be surplus to the perfusion needs of the body. Owing to autoregulation there will be vasoconstriction throughout the body and a rise in peripheral resistance: blood pressure will increase and output will return to normal (remember, BP = CO × PR). Thus, the raised preload is converted to a raised afterload and, if not corrected, this may itself lead to failure. (This could also have a bearing on the pathogenesis of essential hypertension, *see* p. 98.)

Precisely the opposite occurs in diseases where widespread vasodilation results in a severely reduced peripheral resistance, e.g. in septicaemic shock. This produces an obligatory requirement for raised CO to maintain BP, leading eventually to what is known as **high-output failure** (although this is a misleading term since by definition it does not become failure until the myocardium can no longer sustain the output). Other conditions create an excessive (hyperdynamic) systemic demand for output, stimulating the heart via the usual CVS reflexes. Examples include chronic severe anaemia – low blood oxygen being the stimulus – and thyrotoxicosis, where basal metabolic rate is increased.

Although not usually primary causes of heart failure, anaemia, severe infection, fluid retention (including that from drugs such as NSAIDs and corticosteroids) or over-enthusiastic intravenous infusion can be causes of decompensation in patients with otherwise stable and compensated heart failure.

Valve disease

Stenosis (narrowing or failure to open fully) causes an outflow obstruction which increases afterload; thus mitral stenosis can cause left atrial failure. Alternatively, valve incompetence (failure to close fully) will permit regurgitation which causes volume overload in the chambers on either side of the valve. On this basis we can predict the consequences of stenosis or incompetence of the mitral, tricuspid, aortic and pulmonary valves, i.e. which chamber(s) will fail and whether this is the result of excessive afterload or preload.

Pathophysiology

Haemodynamic changes

Heart failure is a dynamic process rather than a single event, even when acute. Whatever the aetiology, the process is similar and the changes in cardiac effectiveness can be represented by pump performance curves (Fig. 3.12).

As contractility falls the stroke volume is reduced; this leaves a higher EDV after ejection. This means an increased preload for the next contraction so that contractility is increased appropriately (by the Starling mechanism). Consequently **output is restored,** but as long as the myocardium is impaired then output is being maintained only **at the expense of increased diastolic size,** i.e. the EDV is increased. Because the heart is now 'larger' it is less efficient (according to Laplace's law). In health this is usually insignificant, but in heart failure this compensation seriously reduces efficiency and erodes the cardiac reserve.

In Fig. 3.12, curve **N** represents normal contractility. Point **n** represents the resting cardiac output of 5 L/min (that which is sufficient to maintain resting organ function and renal fluid clearance); the distance between **n** and **n-max** represents the cardiac reserve. If output falls much below 5 L/min there will be symptoms of hypoperfusion, notably fatigue. Alternatively, should perfusion demands exhaust the cardiac reserve by requiring preload to rise beyond point

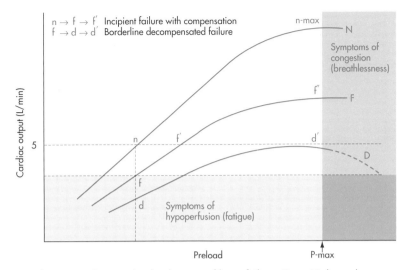

n → f → f'   Incipient failure with compensation
f → d → d'   Borderline decompensated failure

Figure 3.12   Contractility curves showing the development of heart failure. Curve N shows the pump performance (contractility) curve of the normal heart with cardiac output plotted against preload in arbitrary units (e.g. end-diastolic volume). Curve F shows compensated failure and curve D decompensated failure. P-max is maximum preload. See text for further details.

P-max, output will not increase, and may fall. Consequently venous pressure will rise causing congestive symptoms, i.e. oedema. On the left side of the heart this will result in pulmonary oedema and breathlessness.

Acute failure

Suppose that a patient with normal cardiac function suddenly were to suffer a moderate myocardial infarction (MI). Contractility immediately drops and output may quickly fall below the normal resting minimum, to point **f** on a new, less-steep contractility curve (**F**). The patient experiences extreme fatigue at rest, among other symptoms, and the CVS initiates compensation.

The heart enlarges until a new equilibrium is attained at a higher preload (point **f'**). The cardiac reserve is now reduced, as is the maximum output that can be reached by maximal preload (**f''**). At rest, the patient may be unaware of any disability but he or she will have reduced exercise tolerance, becoming breathless earlier than before the MI. This situation (**n → f → f'**) is termed **compensated failure**. Note that a higher preload than before is needed to sustain even resting cardiac output (**f'**), so the heart is permanently less efficient.

If the infarction is very severe, the output may drop precipitately to point **d**, putting the patient on curve **D**. After maximum compensation to point **d'** normal resting output can only just be attained at maximal preload; the patient may even be beyond this, on the falling arm of the curve. There is now zero cardiac reserve and the patient will be fatigued at the slightest exertion and may be breathless even at rest: this is **decompensated failure**.

Chronic failure

A gradual reduction in cardiac contractility produces a similar pattern, except that the patient's haemodynamics would be represented by a series of progressively declining contractility curves, rather than a sudden fall.

A patient could remain in chronic compensated failure indefinitely if the disease progression is arrested or is sufficiently slow. However, a supervening severe stress, e.g. a serious infection, sudden fluid overload, excessive exertion or (more chronically) anaemia, often drives them into decompensation.

Severe heart failure is dramatically visualized by a plain chest X-ray. Figure 3.13(a) shows a normal chest: the heart shadow occupies about

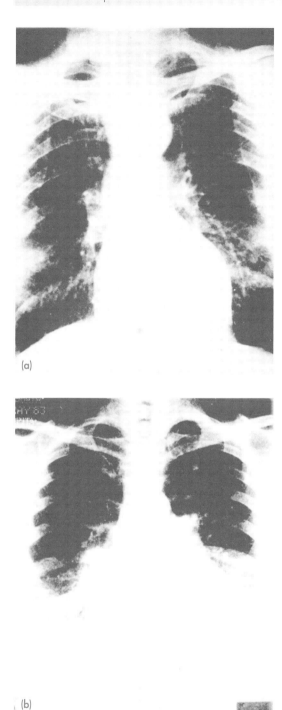

(a)

(b)

Figure 3.13   Chest X-ray in heart failure. (a) Normal pattern. (b) Patient with severe heart failure. Note the increased width of the heart shadow indicating cardiac enlargement, and the diffuse shadowing at the lung bases indicating pulmonary oedema.

half the width of the thorax, i.e. the **cardiothoracic index** is 0.5. In Fig. 3.13(b) (severe failure) the cardiac enlargement is easily seen; the index is nearer 0.7. The increased size is not due to cardiac hypertrophy, which does not show up on plain X-ray (the absolute increase in size in hypertrophy being relatively modest and growth predominantly inwards). What is shown is the result of an increased EDV.

Compensation and consequences: decompensation

Heart failure is more than simply a reduction in CO and accompanying tissue hypoperfusion. As was shown above (p. 64), when the cardiac reserve is mobilized in circumstances where its main effector system – the heart itself – cannot respond, it soon becomes maladaptive. Cardiac enlargement, driven in part by excessive fluid retention and possibly by venoconstriction, brings inefficiency and over-stretch as muscle fibres lose mutual adherence. Excessive hypertrophy interferes with ventricular filling and ejection. The maladaptive changes in ventricular shape due to dilatation and hypertrophy, especially when they follow myocardial infarction, are termed **remodelling**; angiotensin may contribute to this.

At this stage the protective baroreceptor-mediated inhibition of sympathetic outflow becomes blunted, and unrestrained sympathetic drive results in excessive inotropic stimulation of the myocardium and widespread peripheral vasoconstriction. Both conditions place further loads on the heart. Circulating levels of noradrenaline (norepinephrine), angiotensin, aldosterone and ADH (vasopressin) are raised, and ANP secretion falls.

Decompensation thus occurs as these mechanisms combine to reduce CO, rather than to increase or even just maintain it. The heart has passed the maximum on its contractility curve, as shown above (Fig. 3.12). Irreversible myocardial cell damage and necrosis follow. Clearly, treatment must target not only low CO but also these maladaptive mechanisms.

Cardiogenic shock
If contractility falls below that which can sustain the resting CO, producing widespread hypoper-

fusion, this counterproductive cycle deteriorates rapidly. Peripheral arterioles throughout the body respond to local hypoxia by autoregulatory dilatation, overcoming the centrally mediated vasoconstriction which attempts to defend BP. The result is a disastrous fall in BP (cardiogenic shock), low venous return and poor coronary perfusion; together these result in even worse contractility and lower CO. At the same time, hypoxic lung vessels constrict, thereby increasing right ventricular afterload.

Despite the most aggressive management, the whole devastating vicious cycle can be rapidly fatal, especially if irreversible multi-organ damage occurs before circulation is restored.

Clinical features

The classical symptom triad of heart failure is exercise limitation (fatigue), shortness of breath and oedema. However, the clinical picture, although fairly consistent, is often more complex. Many of the clinical features result from impaired flow ahead of the heart or the single affected chamber (the **forward component** or **hypoperfusion**); others from an increase in pressure in the veins draining into the affected

chamber (the **backward component** or **congestion/oedema**). Both conditions usually coexist – they are different aspects of failure, not different forms of it. However, they give rise to different features (Fig. 3.14) and may also vary according to which side of the heart is affected. The picture is further complicated by the neuroendocrine compensatory mechanisms.

Forward component (hypoperfusion)
The effects of hypoperfusion are independent of which side of the heart fails because the outputs from either side are always equal, even when reduced. The principal feature is **fatigue**, but numerous other symptoms follow from poor peripheral perfusion. The extremities will be **cold** and **pale** as the CVS attempts to redirect the reduced CO away from skin and muscle by peripheral vasoconstriction, conserving it for the brain, heart and other central organs. Reduced renal perfusion pressure will cause fluid and electrolyte retention, partly via activity of the renin/angiotensin system, contributing to **oedema**. Over-activity of the sympathetic nervous system produces symptoms such as **tachycardia** and **tachypnoea** (increased respiratory rate).

It is possible that fatigue is not due just to

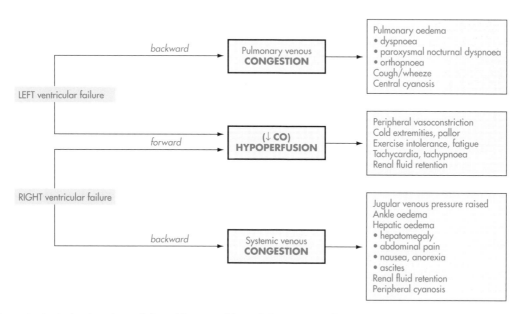

Figure 3.14 Pathophysiology of clinical features of heart failure. See text for definitions of terms. CO, cardiac output.

skeletal muscle hypoperfusion but is part of a generalized **myopathy** secondary to heart failure. It may result from impaired energy handling and subsequent atrophy, or rises in catabolic cytokines, possibly of cardiac origin, such as tumour necrosis factor. Both myocardial and respiratory muscle would also be affected, exacerbating the cardiac problems and contributing to the breathlessness.

Backward component (congestion/oedema)
Right-sided failure. The raised pressure within the great veins draining into the right side of the heart, i.e. systemic venous congestion, will be communicated back to the venous end of systemic capillaries where it impairs the venous drainage of tissue fluid, causing peripheral oedema (p. 70). A further factor in acute failure is the haemodilution caused by expansion of the blood volume. This reduces plasma protein concentration and thus oncotic pressure, contributing to further loss of fluid from the vascular compartment.

Not all areas are affected equally. The additional effect of gravity will make oedema first noticed in the **ankles** of erect patients, or in the sacral area of the bed-bound. The liver, being highly vascular, is also affected early, causing **hepatomegaly** (enlarged liver), and the patient may then feel **bloated**, **nauseous** and **anorexic**. Congestion of the stomach and duodenum may impair nutrient and drug absorption. Later, **ascites** (free oedema fluid in the abdominal cavity) may develop.

A raised **jugular venous pressure**, seen as distension and pulsation of the external jugular veins in the neck, gives an accessible, approximate clinical index of the severity of right heart failure. The CVP (p. 55) is a more precise indicator for monitoring the progress of severe failure, but measuring it is invasive.

The raised systemic venous pressure reduces the arteriovenous pressure difference, slowing peripheral blood flow and causing **peripheral cyanosis**.

In the kidney, raised venous pressure has more far-reaching consequences. It reduces the glomerular filtration rate (owing to raised efferent arteriolar pressure; *see* Chapter 4), thus exacerbating the **fluid and electrolyte retention**.

This is counterproductive because the resultant increased intravascular volume further raises venous pressures, exacerbating excessive preload and oedema.

In summary, right-sided failure alone causes fatigue, fluid retention, peripheral oedema, abdominal congestion and peripheral cyanosis.

Left-sided failure. This is more common and usually more serious. The rise in pulmonary venous pressure causes pulmonary congestion and **pulmonary oedema** by a similar mechanism to that causing peripheral oedema in right-sided failure. However, unlike most other tissues, lungs do not normally have any tissue fluid; they are 'dry'. In the lung, the equivalent of the extravascular space is the alveolar space. Thus even a small imbalance in transcapillary pressure can allow fluid into the alveoli, which seriously interferes with gas diffusion and also reduces pulmonary compliance (increasing the work of breathing). The resulting hypoxaemia causes severe breathlessness (**dyspnoea**) and **central cyanosis**. Severe pulmonary oedema can be rapidly fatal (*see also* Chapter 5).

The dyspnoeic effects of mild pulmonary oedema are particularly noticeable when the patient is supine because the oedema fluid then spreads throughout the lungs When erect, i.e. sitting or standing, venous filling pressure is reduced as intravascular fluid is redistributed to lower parts of the body, reversing the conditions which produce pulmonary oedema. **Orthopnoea** means breathing adequately only when erect. Even a moderate change in posture such as propping a patient up in bed with pillows promotes redistribution of the fluid, which collects at the lung bases to leave the apexes relatively clear and permitting adequate ventilation at rest. (This is easily visualized by X-ray; Fig. 3.13.) However, in all but the mildest pulmonary oedema, changes in posture alone are insufficient and drug therapy is needed. In addition to oxygen and diuretics, opiates are used, which work in part by venodilation, causing a rapid reduction in filling pressure.

A typical history given by patients with untreated left heart failure is of waking breathless, wheezy and coughing after a few hours sleep. They go to the window for a 'breath of fresh air', and quite soon feel better: not because of the air, plainly, but owing to the change in posture. This phenomenon, because it may recur throughout the night, is called **paroxysmal nocturnal dyspnoea** (PND). It is a classical, almost pathognomonic sign of left ventricular failure. Such patients are advised to sleep with three or four cushions, or in a chair, which usually improves matters at least in the early stages.

To summarize, left ventricular failure causes severe fatigue, pulmonary oedema, severe breathlessness and central cyanosis.

Predominant pathophysiological pattern

The backward and forward components can occur to different extents in the same patient. Which predominates – congestive or a hypoperfused – depends on the shape of the patient's contractility curve and the position of its maximum. Figure 3.15 shows left ventricular contractility curves in heart failure. The 'dyspnoea threshold' represents the preload above which pulmonary venous pressure is so high as to cause breathlessness. Below the 'fatigue threshold', output is so low as to cause severe tiredness.

If the maximum output attainable is below the dyspnoea threshold (curve **H**, hypoperfused pattern), fatigue will occur after even moderate exertion, but before breathlessness. On the other hand, the patient with curve **C** will become breathless before their muscles actually become fatigued (congestive pattern).

Bilateral (biventricular) failure

Unilateral chronic failure is uncommon. Usually, patients present with bilateral failure and have mixed symptoms because failure of one side eventually compromises function on the other. The hypoperfusion which follows single-sided failure affects the pulmonary and systemic circulations equally. Coronary hypoperfusion will ensue, leading eventually to chronic ischaemic ventricular failure on the opposite side. Conversely, following left ventricular failure pulmonary congestion will increase the afterload on the right ventricle and if this is untreated, right ventricular failure will result.

Asymptomatic left ventricular dysfunction

The early stages in slowly deteriorating chronic heart failure are initially fully compensated and therefore asymptomatic (Grade I on the NYHA scale). It can only be detected by investigation, but there is evidence that early detection and

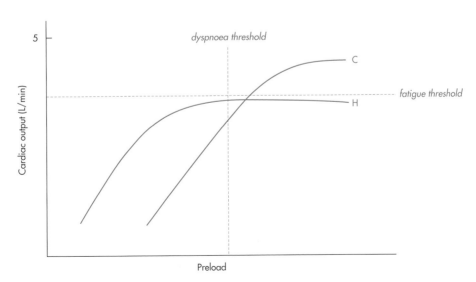

Figure 3.15 Different contractility patterns in heart failure. Hypoperfusive pattern; exercise is limited by fatigue. Congestive pattern; exercise is limited by breathlessness. See text for details.

treatment – before irreversible myocardial damage develops – improves prognosis.

Presentation

A few common examples of heart failure patients will serve to illustrate typical presentations. One might be an undiagnosed hypertensive male in his mid-forties, probably somewhat obese, possibly living a stressful life, perhaps starting to suffer from angina pectoris. His heart failure may be precipitated acutely by MI or may develop slowly along with ventricular hypertrophy. Another example might be an older smoker with chronic bronchitis, slowly developing cor pulmonale. A third example might be an elderly woman with underlying asymptomatic ischaemic heart disease and developing valve disease, perhaps following childhood rheumatic fever.

Most will complain at first of increasing fatigue and a reduced exercise tolerance: climbing stairs, running for a bus, working or going shopping, etc. They will find breathing particularly difficult at night and may have obvious ankle oedema after a day on their feet. They may complain of palpitations. Eventually they will see their GP, when the diagnosis will usually be straightforward.

Prognosis

The seriousness of heart failure can be judged from its poor prognosis, which the advent of angiotensin converting enzyme inhibitor (ACEI) therapy has only modestly improved. For NYHA Grade IV heart failure the median survival is only 1 year, while for Grades III and II it is 3–5 years. The annual mortality rate from asymptomatic left ventricular disease (Grade I) is about 5%.

Investigation

Investigations are used in heart failure to determine the cause, to grade the extent of dysfunction, and to monitor the progress of treatment.

It is important to try to determine the cause of heart failure because it may be reversible or correctable, and extensive investigation is not usually required. A chest X-ray will show the extent of cardiac enlargement and the existence of lung congestion, i.e. pulmonary oedema. The stethoscope may reveal the characteristic sounds of valve disease or the crackles on breathing (crepitations) that are characteristic of pulmonary oedema. The pulse may indicate an arrhythmia. An ECG will reveal any cardiac hypertrophy (usually from long-standing hypertension), ischaemia, the possibility of MI and any arrhythmia.

More sophisticated tests and instruments are available for the few cases which present diagnostic problems, including echocardiography, isotope imaging, cardiac catheterization and coronary angiography.

A variety of semi-quantitative bedside methods and scales are employed for grading. The patient is asked about limitations on daily activities such as walking distance or stair climbing before the onset of fatigue or dyspnoea, or how many pillows they sleep with. These questions may be supplemented by formal exercise testing in suitable cases. Examination of the jugular venous pressure and the extent of oedema are important. Such observations can be used to grade the patient on the NYHA scale.

For more severe disease greater precision is needed. The single most useful index of ventricular dysfunction and the best predictor of prognosis is the ejection fraction: this is measured by echocardiography. Angiography and scans can be used to measure the extent of myocardial damage. Except in acute severe failure invasive haemodynamic measurements are rarely indicated. Currently the potential of plasma noradrenaline (norepinephrine), ANP or renin levels as indices of severity and progress is being evaluated.

Symptomatic improvement correlates poorly with changes in haemodynamic indices. Thus for monitoring therapy and progress generally, subjective assessments by the patients, global measures of exercise tolerance and estimations of the 'quality of life' are often the most useful methods. For patients on medication these must be supplemented by regular clinical biochemistry monitoring for urea and electrolytes.

Management

The management of heart failure involves not only attempting to correct the consequences of low cardiac output and congestion, but also addressing the consequences of the various maladaptive pathophysiological responses which have complicated the clinical picture. The general approaches will first be reviewed, before discussion of the therapeutic and management strategies. Only properties pertinent to heart failure are covered here. A fuller account of many of the drugs mentioned in this section is given on pp. 107–115; Hypertension.

Aims

The various aims in managing heart failure are listed below. They overlap in sequence, objectives and methods and are not in order of precedence.

- Identify and correct any causative or contributory factors.
- Improve cardiac efficiency and effectiveness:
  - Reduce cardiac workload.
  - Increase cardiac output.
  - Counteract maladaptive responses.
- Relieve symptoms.
- Reduce progression and prolong survival.

Ideas about improving declining cardiac performance have changed. Rather than attempting to force the heart to increase its diminished output, current practice favours two alternative strategies:

1. Reduce the load on the heart to match its reduced pumping ability rather than attempting to force it to maintain an unrealistic output whilst decompensated.
2. Limit the counterproductive compensatory mechanisms.

Stimulation, unloading or cardioprotection?

The traditional treatment for heart failure has been inotropic agents, notably cardiac glycosides. However, treatment concepts have advanced through two further stages. First, reducing cardiac load to match pump performance; and second, breaking the vicious circle of maladaptive compensatory reflexes.

Careful trials showed that simple **inotropic** agents do not improve prognosis, and indeed most worsen mortality. The possible exception is digoxin, the value of which probably rests on various actions other than its inotropic activity (see below).

Unloading is theoretically more attractive than simple stimulation because it is more physiological. If the heart cannot sustain an adequate output to meet current demands, it is appropriate to reduce those demands. Put more prosaically, in order to open a stiff door on rusty hinges a few drops of oil are preferable to brute force. This approach often produces haemodynamic improvement, but little survival benefit, so has now given way to cardioprotection.

Most recently, attention has focused on the failing myocardium and the high level of endogenous stimulation it undergoes via compensatory mechanisms. Particularly important are the neuroendocrine mechanisms involving the renin/angiotensin system and the sympathetic nervous system, together with cardiac beta-receptors. For example, in heart failure there is excessive sympathetic drive to which the myocardium can no longer respond, and high renin and aldosterone levels. It was subsequently shown that blocking these mechanisms with ACEIs and beta-blockers **protects the heart** against further damage, retards progression of the failure, and significantly improves prognosis.

These new insights might also explain why extra stimulation by inotropic drugs might be superfluous and possibly harmful. Moreover, increasing contractility increases oxygen demand, which is counterproductive, particularly in ischaemic failure.

Correct causative or contributory factors

Although attending to the underlying cause of the failure would seem to be a priority, it may not be immediately feasible, whether obvious (e.g. MI) or only revealed on investigation (e.g. valve disease, coronary artery disease). Both causal and potential contributory factors (e.g. hypertension, anaemia) may have to wait until the patient is stabilized before appropriate, possibly long-term, corrective measures are initiated, e.g. attention to CVS risk factors, salt restriction, stopping smoking, antihypertensive therapy, weight reduction, valve replacement, haematinics.

Reduce cardiac workload

A basic form of unloading has always been practised. Rest is imposed by the exercise limitation of the condition and patients are often fatigued. However, excessive bedrest can be detrimental to exercise tolerance as well as predisposing to thromboembolic complications. Thus there is a trend to moderate physical training in chronic failure which is likely to improve quality of life, even if it does not benefit survival. Our better understanding of haemodynamics now enables us to intervene positively to reduce the myocardial workload either by reducing afterload with arterial dilators or by reducing preload with venodilators or diuretics (Fig. 3.16).

Preload reduction

Starling's law predicts that reducing preload will reduce CO. If so, would reducing the preload not exacerbate the hypoperfusion (forward component) of heart failure? This would be true if the failing myocardium were not operating on the falling limb of its contractility curve (*see* Fig. 3.3(a)) and so no longer governed by Starling's law. In this situation reducing preload may actually increase output, as well as decreasing oxygen demand by reducing diastolic volume (Laplace's law).

Diuretics. Dietary sodium and fluid restriction and natriuresis are the first-line strategy in all patients with evidence of fluid retention. Diuretics have several diverse but interdependent effects. They mobilize the excess fluid retained by the kidneys, reducing intravascular fluid (blood) volume, which lowers preload. Consequently, venous end-capillary pressure is lowered, an effect enhanced by the venodilator action of diuretics (Table 3.7). This reduces oedema by facilitating the return of oedema fluid to the circulation, to be cleared by kidneys. Kidney function benefits from the improved cardiac function. Diuretics are usually given with ACEIs in heart failure.

The principal danger is dehydration, especially if loop diuretics are needed, because this would further compromise cardiac and renal function. Clearly, diuretics are contraindicated in hypovolaemic, low-output states. Potassium, and per-

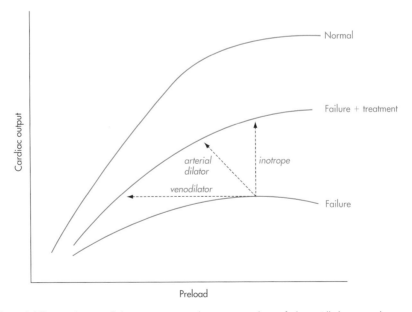

Figure 3.16 Effect of different classes of drugs on contractility curves in heart failure. All drugs act by moving patients onto a more favourable contractility curve. Venodilators reduce preload, maintaining reduced output more efficiently (before compensation). Inotropes increase output for the same preload (before compensation). Arterial dilators have an intermediate effect (after compensation; see also Fig. 3.3(b)). (Adapted with permission from Balakumaran *et al.* (1986) *Drugs* **32**: 372.)

haps magnesium, plasma levels need to be monitored carefully because of the arrhythmogenic effects of hypokalaemia and hypomagnesaemia on the myocardium, especially in the presence of cardiac glycosides. (For a more detailed discussion of diuretics, *see* pp. 108–109.)

Venodilators. Increased venous capacitance leads to reduced pressure in the venous system, lowering filling pressure and venous end-capillary pressure, as with diuretics. Either *nitrates* (predominantly venodilator) or venous-arteriolar dilators (e.g. *alpha-adrenergic blockers, ACEIs*) may be used. The main problems with nitrates are tolerance and untoward falls in CO and BP causing syncope. They may be used alone or in combination with arterial dilators in both acute and chronic failure, but nowadays are most often used in acute failure.

Afterload reduction
Almost invariably, as CO and BP fall the body responds with increased sympathetic drive and renin/angiotensin levels. This may defend BP, but only at the expense of raised peripheral resistance – further overloading an impaired myocardium. If the BP continues to fall, attempts to restore it with vasoconstrictor drugs will have the same effect.

Although changes in peripheral resistance have little effect on the output of the normal heart (*see* Fig. 3.3(b)) owing to reflex compensation, the performance of the diseased heart can be markedly improved by reducing afterload. Thus, ideally, if afterload is reduced output will rise while BP is preserved. Moreover, because pressure work is the most energy-consuming component of cardiac performance, reducing the afterload is a very effective way to reduce

myocardial oxygen demand. This may be particularly important in ischaemic failure.

Balancing the benefits of reduced resistance against the possible problems of hypoperfusion of vital organs may be very difficult, and in acute severe failure this strategy is restricted to specialist units.

Arterial vasodilators (p. 107). These are a heterogeneous group (Table 3.7) that act by several different mechanisms. In theory, this group is most appropriate for patients with hypoperfusion or heart failure secondary to hypertension. However, they are often helpful in severe or resistant failure.

Although the older *sympatholytic* (e.g. prazosin) and direct-acting (e.g. *hydralazine*) agents are still used, the *ACEIs* are now first-line vasodilators, having both arterial and venodilator effects as well as several other actions (p. 89). Further, the ACEIs are free from adverse effects of postural hypotension, tolerance and reflex compensation. The simple arterial and/or venodilators do not have a beneficial long-term effect, probably because of reflex activation of the renin/angiotensin system, which ACEIs block. Thus combined dilator therapy (e.g. hydralazine plus nitrates) has been replaced by monotherapy with ACEIs unless contraindicated. However, vasodilators may be added in where severe failure is not controlled with diuretics and ACEIs.

Calcium blockers are generally avoided because they are potentially negatively inotropic. However, those with a predominant vasodilator action (*see* Table 3.25) may be useful in ischaemic failure or where there is hypertension, particularly the newer *amlodipine* and *felodipine*.

Beta-adrenergic agonists, e.g. salbutamol, are occasionally used in acute failure as vasodilators,

Table 3.7   Predominant vascular sites of action of vasodilators used in heart failure

Arterioles	Arterioles and veins	Veins
Hydralazine	ACEIs	Nitrates
Calcium channel blockers	Alpha-adrenergic blockers	
Beta$_2$-adrenergic agonists	Thiazide/loop diuretics	
Dopaminergic agonists	Nitroprusside	

ACEI, angiotensin converting enzyme inhibitor.

with the additional potential for positive inotropic action, presumably on cardiac beta$_2$-receptors.

Improve effectiveness: increase cardiac output

In severe heart failure, symptoms may persist despite the measures mentioned, especially if shock has supervened. Inotropic drugs are then needed. The three main groups, each of which acts at different sites, are the traditional cardiac glycosides, the sympathomimetic amines, and the phosphodiesterase inhibitors. They have different roles, advantages and drawbacks and none is regarded as a first agent. All improve symptoms, although only digoxin has been shown to reduce mortality.

Cardiac glycosides

Action. The traditional role of digitalis glycosides has been as inotropes, mediated by the action in increasing intracellular calcium through inhibition of membrane Na/K-ATPase. The observation that they improve contractility without an increase in myocardial oxygen demand is probably explained partly by their multiple other actions (Table 3.8). These actions may also account for their superiority over conventional inotropes.

Digoxin has a negative chronotropic effect, owing partly to increased vagal activity. This is invaluable when the failure is complicated by atrial fibrillation, and generally it tends to limit oxygen demand. The action on conduction is complex, and includes a negative dromotropic action (slowing conduction times). The negative chronotropic effect is distinct from the positive inotropic effect, the latter usually being observed first.

Note that by contrast the sympathomimetic amines are both positively inotropic and positively chronotropic and so almost always increase oxygen demand. For detailed accounts of the pharmacology of the cardiac glycosides the References and further reading section should be consulted.

Side effects. The principal drawback of glycoside therapy is the narrow therapeutic index, with toxicity sometimes resembling the symptoms being treated, i.e. various arrhythmias (Table 3.9). This problem is compounded by the sensitivity of plasma level and receptor activity to diverse pharmacokinetic and pharmacodynamic factors (Table 3.10). Routine plasma level monitoring is not essential for safe and effective use if there is close monitoring of clinical and toxicological signs. However, it is invaluable

---

Table 3.8   Actions of digoxin and other cardiac glycosides

Pharmacological action	Effect on cardiovascular function	Site or mode of action
Positive inotropic	↑ Contractility	↓ Na/K-ATPase in myocyte
Negative chronotropic	↓ Conduction velocity	Direct (AV nodes, etc.)
	↓ Heart rate	↑ Parasympathetic activity (vagus)
Reduced sympathetic activity[a]	↓ Excessive myocardial stimulation	Restored baroreceptor sensitivity →
	Peripheral vasodilatation	• ↓ central sympathetic activity
		• ↓ noradrenaline (norepinephrine) level
Reduced renin secretion[b]	↓ Fluid retention	Kidney (juxtaglomerular apparatus)
	↓ Peripheral vasoconstriction	• ↓ sympathetic stimulation?
		• ↓ Na/K-ATPase reduces renin release?

[a] ↓ noradrenaline (norepinephrine).

[b] ↓ angiotensin.

where the response is unexpected, or when renal impairment is known or suspected.

Digitoxicity is managed by drug withdrawal and use where appropriate of:

- Plasma level measurement of digoxin, potassium and creatinine.
- Oral potassium.
- Digoxin-specific antibody fragment.
- Oral binding agents (e.g. cholestyramine).
- Occasionally anti-arrhythmics.

The recent DIG trial has convincingly indicated that digoxin is far safer than was previously thought. This implies that previous fears of digoxin toxicity have been exaggerated, or else that the toxicity which occurred could have been due to inadequate monitoring.

Role. Glycosides are of no benefit in shock or cor pulmonale (possibly because of hypoxaemia) and are rarely useful after MI. Until recently their recommended use has been limited to moderate failure complicated by supraventricular (especially atrial) tachycardia. This was because of concern over toxicity and the lack of evidence from good clinical trials of benefit in mild to moderate compensated failure in sinus rhythm.

Digoxin has seemed perennially to be on the verge of popular revival, without ever quite making it. Recent well-organized trials (e.g.

Table 3.9   Adverse drug reactions of digoxin

Gastrointestinal	Nausea, anorexia, dyspepsia, vomiting, diarrhoea
Central nervous system	Blurred vision, other visual disturbances
	Confusion, drowsiness
Cardiovascular	Bradycardia, premature ectopic beats, heart block, almost any other arrhythmia

---

Table 3.10   Problems with digoxin therapy

Low therapeutic index – may require plasma level monitoring

Pharmacokinetics
- absorption depends on gut perfusion (may be reduced in heart failure)
- long half-life; easily accumulated but difficult to remove
- highly tissue-bound (myocardial and skeletal muscle) – high volume of distribution
- renal clearance, but renal function may be reduced in heart failure and in the elderly

Interactions, including with other drugs used in cardiac disease
Pharmacokinetic (alter plasma levels), e.g.
- ↓ absorption – *cholestyramine, sulfasalazine*
- ↓ non-renal clearance – some *calcium channel blockers*
- ↓ renal clearance – *quinidine, verapamil*
Pharmacodynamic (on the myocardium), e.g. *anti-arrhythmics, calcium channel blockers*

Toxicity
Serious cardiac toxicity
Enhanced by hypokalaemia (e.g. from diuretic treatment), hypomagnesaemia, hypercalcaemia

Myocardial sensitivity increased in:
- ischaemia, e.g. after infarction, in lung disease and cor pulmonale
- hypothyroidism (but sensitivity decreased in hyperthyroidism)
- elderly and infants

RADIANCE, DIG) have improved its image, having demonstrated significant reductions in signs and symptoms with fewer adverse effects than expected, definite deterioration when discontinued and a small reduction in heart failure deaths, but no reduction in all-cause mortality. While digoxin may once again be due for a renaissance, its arrhythmogenic potential is still worrying. The precise position of digoxin in the protocol remains uncertain, but it is unlikely to be better than third-line, especially as its benefit in combination with beta-blockers is not proven.

Sympathomimetic inotropic amines

Prolonged reflex stimulation of the failing myocardium by the sympathetic nervous system may become counterproductive, resulting in depletion of catecholamines and down-regulation of myocardial beta-receptors, with the paradoxical result that although beta-agonists are helpful in some situations, beta-blockers are preferred in others.

Inotropic amines, usually given parenterally, have traditionally been a last resort in refractory failure and shock. They affect a variety of receptors, producing a mixed spectrum of effects (Table 3.11). This is especially true of natural mediators such as *adrenaline* (*epinephrine*) and *noradrenaline* (*norepinephrine*), which cause unwanted arterial vasoconstriction that increases afterload and reduces cardiac output. *Isoprenaline* (*isoproterenol*), an early synthetic agent, causes hypotension and arrhythmias. All raise heart rate and myocardial oxygen demand, sometimes excessively, although this may eventually be offset by increased efficiency.

Dopamine has dose-dependent receptor selectivity. In low doses it stimulates vasodilator dopaminergic receptors, a most useful property in shock. At higher doses it also stimulates inotropic $beta_1$-receptors. However, further dose increases result in alpha receptor-mediated vasoconstriction; it also liberates noradrenaline (norepinephrine). *Dobutamine* only affects $beta_1$-receptors and this pure inotropic effect is sometimes preferable. *Dopexamine* has a greater affinity for both cardiac and peripheral $beta_2$-receptors, and there is evidence that in chronic failure, although $beta_1$ myocardial receptors may be down-regulated, the $beta_2$-receptors are not. Its main action is likely to be vasodilatory.

Predominant $beta_2$-agonists, more commonly used in obstructive airways disease, e.g. *salbutamol*, also have peripheral vasodilator actions,

Table 3.11   Pharmacological properties of cardioactive sympathetic agonists and antagonists, including receptors affected

	Positively inotropic (β_1) ISA	Positively chronotropic (β_1) Arrhythmias	Vasodilate[a] (β_2, DA)	Vasoconstrict (α) BP ↑	Negatively inotropic (β_1 block)
Adrenaline (epinephrine)	++	++	+	++	
Noradrenaline (norepinephrine)	+	++		++	
Isoprenaline (isoproterenol)	++	+++	+		
Dopamine[b]	++	+	+	++	(+)
Dobutamine	++	+		+	
Dopexamine	++		++		
Salbutamol[c]	(+)		++		
Xamoterol	++	++			+
Pindolol	+		++		
Carvedilol			++		+

[a] 'Inodilators'.

[b] Levodopa, ibopamine also used.

[c] Pirbuterol is similar.

α, alpha-adrenergic receptor; β_1, beta$_1$-adrenergic receptor; β_2, beta$_2$-adrenergic receptor; DA, dopaminergic receptor; ISA, intrinsic sympathomimetic activity.

and this is particularly useful in cor pulmonale. These agents offer more choice in their route of administration, including oral and inhalation, which is beneficial in chronic failure. A particular risk of these drugs is hypokalaemia.

Phosphodiesterase inhibitors

Aminophylline, a (methyl)xanthine, has traditionally been used in acute failure complicated by pulmonary oedema, where reflex bronchoconstriction ('cardiac asthma') is common. As well as bronchodilator activity it has inotropic, diuretic and respiratory stimulant properties. However, xanthines are also arrhythmogenic and increase oxygen demand, and are no longer used.

The bipyridines are a new group with inotropic and vasodilator actions. *Milrinone* and *enoximone* act by a novel mechanism, increasing CO and reducing peripheral resistance with little or no increase in oxygen demand. They improve symptoms and exercise tolerance but increase mortality. They can only be used parenterally. Their role has not yet been defined.

Pimobendan, which is still under investigation, has additional calcium-sensitizing actions but once again, while providing symptomatic improvement, it reduces survival.

Other methods

In severe heart failure that is resistant to drug treatment, an intra-aortic balloon pump (counterpulsation) may be temporarily placed in the thoracic aorta. Synchronized with the ECG, the balloon is inflated during diastole to improve systemic and coronary perfusion. Cardiac transplantation is being seen increasingly as a realistic option in otherwise untreatable end-stage heart failure, especially that caused by cardiomyopathy. Although a satisfactory completely artificial heart still awaits development, a number of sophisticated ventricular assist devices are proving useful on a temporary basis for patients awaiting transplantation. Alternatively, these may relieve the damaged heart of its workload for few months, which in some cases may enable a degree of recovery to occur.

Alternative, potentially simpler surgical procedures are currently undergoing development. In cardiac myoplasty a muscular pouch surround-ing the heart is fashioned using local chest wall muscle tissue. Surprisingly, this skeletal muscle acquires the structural characteristics of cardiac muscle. Where there is gross ventricular dilatation (dilated cardiomyopathy) the Batista procedure involves remodelling (by excision of a wedge of ventricle), producing a smaller, less-stressed chamber. (This has inescapable echoes of the historical technique of venesection for severe failure, or bloodletting for 'the dropsy' as it was known.)

Counteract maladaptive responses

We have seen that the consequences of maladaptive neurohumoral activation include excessive sympathetic drive, vasoconstriction, fluid retention and cardiac hypertrophy with ventricular dilatation. Several of the agents already discussed mitigate these effects.

Angiotensin converting enzyme inhibitors

The action of these drugs is complex. Inhibition of the production of circulating angiotensin causes both venous and arterial dilatation and reduced aldosterone levels. They also reduce the local production of angiotensin in many tissues, notably the kidney (where it normally inhibits glomerular filtration) and the heart and blood vessels (where it has growth-promoting action). The action of ACEIs is not reduced by tolerance or reflex sympathetic compensation.

The renal action of ACEIs counteracts the aldosterone hypersecretion found in some heart failure patients and reduces fluid retention in most, with no risk of hypokalaemia. Indeed, when used with potassium supplements or potassium-sparing diuretics there is a risk of hyperkalaemia. Nevertheless, the combination of ACEIs with diuretics is logical and synergistic and is indicated in all but mildest failure. (Interestingly, spironolactone, the direct-acting aldosterone inhibitor, is not very successful in this situation.) It is also likely that reduced local tissue angiotensin production leads to reduced vascular and myocardial hypertrophy (remodelling), including that which usually follows MI.

Most importantly, several large trials such as SOLVD, CONSENSUS and V-HeFT have demonstrated that ACEIs prolong survival, even in mild heart failure (by on average 12%). They also reduce disease progression, hospitalization and MI, though higher doses than originally recommended are necessary. (For a discussion of ACEI therapy generally, *see* p. 111.)

Beta-blockers and partial sympathetic agonists

Recent trials have convincingly, if rather surprisingly, demonstrated beneficial effects of conventional beta-blockers such as *metoprolol* in most grades of heart failure. Newer beta-blockers also shown to be beneficial include *bisoprolol*, *carvedilol*, which also has an alpha-blocking vasodilator action, and *bucindolol*, a direct vasodilator. These drugs have been shown to reduce hospitalization, disease progression and symptoms, and to reduce significantly all-cause mortality. The resultant increase in survival is greater than that conferred by ACEIs. Possible mechanisms include reduction of sympathetic stimulation, heart rate and oxygen demand, and up-regulation of receptors.

In chronic severe heart failure (Grade IV) or acute severe decompensation the myocardium relies on sympathetic drive, so the well-known negative inotropic problem of beta-blockers in heart failure may be dangerous. There may also be in all cases an initial transient worsening of symptoms. Thus in heart failure beta-blockers need to be introduced at low doses and with great care. They are particularly indicated in failure associated with ischaemia, but at present their use in the elderly, and in failure with normal systolic function, has not been demonstrated.

The seemingly anomalous use of beta-blockers in heart failure, although it goes against conventional teaching which has always warned of the hazard in this situation, is not without precedent. Beta-blockers are indicated in hypertrophic cardiomyopathy, in which grossly thickened, fibrosed ventricular walls obstruct outflow if systolic contraction is too vigorous; this condition is exacerbated by inotropic agents and venodilators.

However, the realization that beta-blockers can improve the prognosis of most cases of mild to moderate heart failure is likely to change clinical practice and heart failure management protocols significantly (*see* p. 91). At present it is likely that primary carers will seek consultant cardiological opinion before starting patients on this mode of therapy. The fact that both ACEIs and beta-blockers are effective only in systolic dysfunction make it important that suspected heart failure is always investigated echocardiographically to measure the ejection fraction.

Another seemingly logical approach to reducing excess sympathetic drive is to use a partial sympathomimetic agonist, i.e. an adrenergic beta-blocker with intrinsic sympathomimetic activity (ISA). *Xamoterol* is a beta$_1$-agonist with about 50% of the agonist activity of the natural mediator adrenaline (epinephrine). When sympathetic tone is low, xamoterol has an inotropic action, but when there is maximal endogenous mediator secretion it acts as a competitive beta-blocker. This may protect the myocardium against excessive oxygen demands, particularly in ischaemic failure. Unfortunately, xamoterol causes excess deaths in more severe disease, and so in the UK it is only indicated for mild heart failure and is little used. (For a discussion of beta-blocker therapy generally, *see* p. 109.)

Digoxin

The recent recognition of the neuroendocrine complications in heart failure have indicated how the diverse actions of digoxin (*see* Table 3.8) may contribute to its beneficial effect. The precise mechanisms have not been fully elucidated but an important component is the restoration of baroreceptor activity.

As heart failure develops, baroreceptor responses to increased atrial and arterial pressure rises serve to dampen sympathetic outflow and increase parasympathetic activity, protecting the heart from excessive stimulation and loading (p. 66). However, these responses eventually become blunted due to stretch receptor damage from prolonged activation, permitting excess sympathetic activity. Digoxin appears to improve baroreceptor function and thus mitigate this counterproductive development. Consequently, noradrenaline (norepinephrine) levels fall, vagal activity increases (contributing to the negative chronotropic action), and myocardial wall stress and peripheral vasoconstriction are both reduced. The activity of the renin/angiotensin system is also depressed, limiting fluid retention and vasoconstriction.

Reduce symptoms

The above strategies bring about symptomatic improvement such as reductions in oedema, fatigue and dyspnoea, an improved sense of well-being and quality of life, and possibly an increased exercise tolerance. However, objective haemodynamic improvement may be difficult to demonstrate. In mild failure the main aim of diuretic therapy may be simply to reduce uncomfortable or unsightly oedema.

The *opiates* are frequently used in pulmonary oedema, having venodilator, anxiolytic and respiratory depressant actions. This last action is useful in suppressing the inefficient, fast, shallow respiration (tachypnoea) commonly found in pulmonary oedema. In addition, a severely hypoxaemic patient will be given *oxygen*, provided that there is no chronic pulmonary disease present (*see* Chapter 5, pp. 291–294).

Reduce progression and prolong survival

Recently, it has become feasible to anticipate increased survival and retarded progression. Several trials have now shown that ACEIs and beta-blockers can improve survival in chronic heart failure patients, and that this is due in part to a cardioprotective action inhibiting further myocardial damage.

Drug selection

An overview of the current consensus for drug selection in systolic failure, as recommended by the European Society of Cardiology (1997), is given in Fig. 3.17. The main criterion is severity, the strategy being gradually to increase intervention with the addition of more drugs. Few patients are managed by monotherapy. Although most chronic cases can be managed in the community, particular complications such as arrhythmia and pulmonary oedema will require specific additions, while acute failure may require management in a specialist coronary care unit where parenteral therapy and close monitoring of haemodynamic and ECG parameters are available.

Recent trends include the almost obligatory use of ACEIs in most cases (except where contraindicated), the recommendation for the wider if cautious use of beta-blockers, and the use of digoxin in severe cases (even in sinus rhythm).

Asymptomatic (Grade I)

ACEIs should be used alone where evidence of systolic dysfunction is discovered, to reduce progression. Systolic dysfunction is indicated by a dilated heart and an ejection fraction below 35% (normal = 50%).

Patients with atrial fibrillation should be started on *digoxin* straightaway, usually with *warfarin* to protect against stroke from an atrial-originating embolism. Ventricular or supraventricular arrhythmia may require *amiodarone* (care must be taken with digoxin–warfarin interactions).

Mild–moderate (Grade II)

Where there are no signs of fluid retention *ACEIs* can be used alone, increasing the dose to attain effect if necessary. Oedema is more usually present and *diuretics* are used in combination with ACEIs. Although *thiazides* can be used in mild failure, and are still occasionally used in the elderly (where they are less likely to cause dehydration than loop diuretics), *loop diuretics* are more usual. Because of the combination with ACEIs, potassium-sparing adjuncts are not required.

Where fluid retention is particularly resistant (possibly due to a low glomerular filtration rate [GFR] with poor delivery of diuretic to the tubule), a synergistic diuretic combination may be required for a few days. A loop diuretic with the thiazide *metolazone* is often successful ('sequential nephron blockade'), although any thiazide should work as well. For pulmonary oedema, high doses of loop diuretic may be given along with morphine and oxygen and the patient is nursed sitting almost erect. With high-dose and combination diuretics, attention should also be paid to the serum potassium level.

On the other hand, if the patient improves the diuretics may be stepped down, though ACEIs should always be retained.

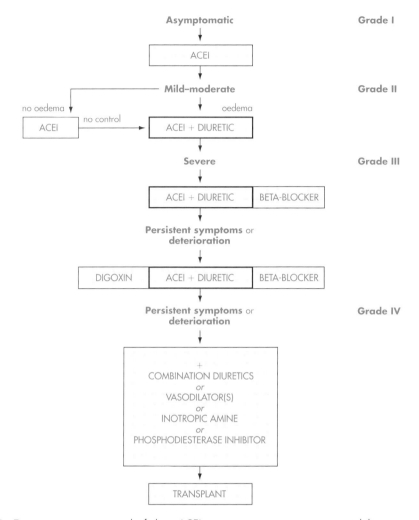

Figure 3.17   Treatment strategy in systolic failure. ACEI, angiotensin converting enzyme inhibitor.

Severe (Grade III)

If symptoms persist or the patient deteriorates, *beta-blockers* or *digoxin* can be added; eventually, both may be needed. Which is used first will depend on the experience of the clinician, but evidence of ischaemia would indicate beta-blockers. Further therapy would involve diuretic combinations and high-dose diuretics if they have not already been tried.

End-stage (Grade IV)

This stage represents irreversible myocardial damage and the only curative measure is *trans-plantation*, now a realistic option. The prognosis is otherwise very poor, with a median survival of less than 1 year. Medical therapy is mainly palliative while awaiting surgery. Various schemes have been devised for the optimum combination of *diuretics*, *arterial dilators* and *venodilators*, based on haemodynamic parameters such as filling pressure and pulmonary venous pressures (*see* References and further reading).

Intravenous sympathomimetic or dopaminergic *inotropes*, or oral inotropes such as the bipyridines, may be tried but their potential for increasing myocardial oxygen demand must always be remembered. None is beneficial in long-term use.

Diastolic failure

This form of heart failure is especially difficult to treat, and there is as yet no reliable trial evidence. Efforts to increase diastolic time with cardiodepressants such as beta-blockers, or with calcium channel blockers such as verapamil, may be tried. Drugs which reduce preload (and hence diastolic filling) need to be used with great caution: this includes nitrates and diuretics. Xamoterol and the less cardiodepressant calcium channel blockers, e.g. nicardipine, may have a role where ventricular compliance is low. In general, ACEIs and inotropes, including digoxin, are counterproductive.

Hypertension

Definition and epidemiology

For most diseases a population can usually be divided into two distinct groups, 'normal' or 'ill', on the basis of a defining characteristic or measurement. Unfortunately, it is less easy to define normal or abnormal blood pressure (BP) because within a given population there is a continuous distribution of BP about a single modal value, although this value varies with age, ethnic group, etc. Figure 3.18 shows the distribution of diastolic pressure for a Western industrialized population: it can be seen that it is almost uniform, but is skewed towards the higher levels. Clearly, the oft-cited 'normal' levels of 120 mmHg systolic blood pressure (SBP) and 80 mmHg diastolic (DBP) are only a statistical approximation for a majority around the modal value. The majority do lie between 70–90 mmHg diastolic, but there is a substantial minority above 90 mmHg.

A clear distinction would be invaluable in identifying those who need treatment, because untreated high BP is associated with long-term morbidity and premature mortality. Although the risk to an individual cannot be precisely predicted from their BP, actuarial data confirm that excessive BP is harmful. We know that different population groups with different mean BPs have different prevalences of diseases thought to be caused by hypertension (HPT). However, these risks are also graded continuously, and the challenge is to know at which point the benefits of treatment (reduced long-term complications) outweigh the risks of treatment (adverse effects, reduced quality of life, etc.). The balance will vary between individuals according to numerous other factors including age and the presence of other disease (Table 3.12). Generally, the cut-off point has tended to be reduced gradually over the years as less toxic drugs have been developed which reduce the risk of treatment.

Variations in blood pressure

In developed countries, BP rises with age. Systolic pressure is affected more than diastolic, continuing up to the age of about 70 years and reaching an average of 140–150 mmHg. Diastolic pressure rises less steeply to around 90 mmHg at age 60 years, and then flattens out. Blood pressure is normally a little lower in younger women but tends to rise faster post-menopausally so that pressures converge and older women have higher systolic pressures than men. In less developed and rural areas there is little change with age, but

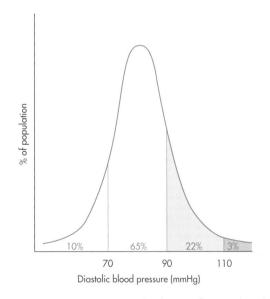

Figure 3.18 Approximate distribution of mean diastolic blood pressure in Western urban population. The curve shows the skewed but smooth distribution of blood pressure, with a greater proportion above the modal value.

Table 3.12   Risk factors and aetiological influences in hypertension

Risk factor or aetiological influence	Possible rationale and comment
Major	
Family history	Inherited tendency – probably polygenic
Dietary Na high	Fluid retention; vascular wall oedema; ion pump defect (p. 98)
Obesity	Artefact of measurement (problem with arm cuff)?
	Greater perfusion demands of increased body mass
	Reducing weight can reverse borderline HPT
Alcohol	Unknown mechanism; possibly 30% of HPT related to alcohol abuse
Sedentary life	Unknown mechanism; regular exercise lowers BP
Renal disease	Overt or occult renal disease often implicated
Minor	
Age	See text
Stress or Type A personality	Overactive sympathetic nervous system $\rightarrow$ vasoconstriction and/or raised CO.
	Difficult to quantify; effect may have been exaggerated
Dietary	
Ca, K, Mg $\downarrow$	Some evidence, especially for K
Saturated fat $\uparrow$	May induce vasoconstriction via endothelial interactions
Animal products	Vegetarians may have lower BPs
Smoking	No sustained effect on BP itself but greatly exacerbates atherosclerotic complications of HPT
Glucose intolerance	Complex interaction between insulin resistance, hyperlipidaemia and HPT
Race	Increased average BP in urban Blacks: $\uparrow$ response to stress or dietary salt?

BP, blood pressure; Ca, calcium; CO, cardiac output; HPT, hypertension; K, potassium; Mg, magnesium; Na, sodium.

often migrants from rural areas to industrialized ones tend to acquire the rising pattern, suggesting the existence of strong environmental factors.

Twenty-four-hour monitoring of BP shows that it varies constantly throughout the day owing to both regular diurnal variation (lower overnight and higher in the morning) and irregular physical and mental stress, as might be predicted from physiology. Thus it is important to standardize the conditions of measurement (see below). Even so, large-scale epidemiological studies have shown a close correlation between single random BP measurements and cardiovascular risk.

Definition

Most definitions of HPT accommodate the greater proportional rise in SBP and include intermediate classifications to recognize the continuous variation. Because increased risk is associated with pressures sometimes regarded as normal, an 'optimal' classification has been proposed (Table 3.13).

SBP is inversely proportional to arterial compliance, which seems to decline with age owing to smooth muscle fibrosis and calcification (arteriosclerosis). DBP reflects the peripheral resistance, a measure of the average size of blood vessel lumens against which the heart has to develop and maintain a pressure.

Because the vasculature is exposed to diastolic pressure for the greater part of the cardiac cycle, it has been assumed that DBP was the main marker for vascular damage (the main complication of HPT). Thus most early trials monitored DBP and aimed at reducing it. However, systolic pressure is increasingly being accepted as an equally or more important prognostic indicator. Because both tend to be elevated in hypertension this is not so important. However, more

Table 3.13   Gradations of blood pressure and hypertension

	Systolic pressure (mmHg)		Diastolic pressure (mmHg)
Optimal	<120	and	<80
Normal	<140	and	<90[a]
Mild hypertension (grade 1)	140–160	and/or	90[a]–100
Moderate hypertension (grade 2)	160–180	and/or	100–110
Severe hypertension (grade 3)	180–210	and/or	110–120
Very severe hypertension (grade 4)	>210	and/or	>120

[a] A recent WHO–International Society of Hypertension report (1999) has proposed reducing this figure to 85 mmHg, except for the elderly.

recently a group of patients with **isolated systolic hypertension** and normal diastolic pressure has been identified. It appears that such patients are at greater risk, but also benefit more from treatment. Nevertheless, since these tend to be older patients there remains some doubt about the wisdom of aggressive treatment because resultant excessive hypotension or reduced perfusion to vital areas may increase mortality (discussed below).

Prevalence

The estimation of prevalence depends crucially on how hypertension is defined, i.e. what thresholds are assumed. Based on a definition of HPT with a diastolic pressure above 95 mmHg or systolic pressure above 150 mmHg, it has been estimated that there may be 4 million mild hypertensives in the UK. If a level of 140/90 mmHg is taken, the figure will be nearer 20% of the population, i.e. up to 12 million. This shows the difficulty of defining a condition solely on the basis of a physiological measurement which varies throughout the population. The definition of HPT is essentially statistical and epidemiological. All that can be done is to mark off certain pressures on either side of the median as bounding the 'normal' limits, and class all others as 'abnormal'.

Exactly where this borderline is drawn has changed as understanding of the risks of untreated HPT has grown, and as more effective, less toxic treatments have been developed. Formerly, active treatment was considered only if the DBP was consistently above 100 mmHg.

Now, with better and safer drugs the borderline has dropped to 95 mmHg, or even 85 mmHg for those with most more cardiovascular risk factors, if not all patients.

Hypotension

The definitions of blood pressure in Table 3.13 imply that no harm is believed to be associated with pressures below 'normal' (i.e. 70–80 mmHg diastolic). This is indeed the case in the UK and the USA. In mainland Europe however a distinct diagnostic category of what is in effect essential **hypotension** is commonly employed, and this condition is usually treated with various drugs including inotropic and pressor agents. Interestingly, evidence is emerging of an adverse prognosis for persons with low blood pressure – symptoms are vague and subjective, including depression, tiredness, etc. – although as yet it is not a recognized illness in the UK. This phenomenon must be distinguished from BP low enough to affect normal function or consciousness (as in postural hypotension or shock), but should be considered in relation to the problem of possible over-treatment of borderline hypertension in the elderly (see below).

Course and prognosis

Hypertension is a chronic condition with a variable rate of progression and a highly variable prognosis. Being insidious in onset and initially symptomless, it may go undetected for years, and is often discovered incidentally. Yet if untreated the patient will eventually develop one or more of the complications, frequently leading to premature death.

What then are the risks of having too high a blood pressure? After all, if a layman asked what blood pressure was for, you might reply that it drove blood round the body. He might then justifiably retort that surely then you could not have too much of it – the more the better. This credibility gap needs to be bridged when a diagnosis is first made, and reinforced when adverse drug effects occur in a previously asymptomatic 'patient'.

For although HPT is almost invariably symptomless for many years there are subtle, sinister pathological processes at work causing long-term damage to the heart and blood vessels and so also to other vital organs, especially the kidney. A middle-aged patient with a DBP above 110 mmHg has a one in five chance of dying within 5 years: a 35-year-old patient with DBP over 105 mmHg has his life expectancy reduced by 15 years.

The list of conditions from which hypertensives may ultimately suffer reads like a recitation of the ills of civilized man: myocardial infarction and angina, stroke, heart failure, renal failure, blindness. Death is usually from stroke or myocardial infarction, far more commonly than in normotensives. These risks are related to the duration and severity of the elevated BP. Adequate, early treatment reduces the incidence of complications by two-thirds or more.

Aetiology

Heredity

Hypertension occurs about equally in men and women, although younger men in particular are more prone to atherosclerotic complications. There is often a family history, but it is probably a susceptibility to HPT that is inherited and this is only expressed if certain environmental factors are present. Immigrant populations with low mean blood pressures tend to assume the prevalence of the host country. On the other hand, certain races have a higher prevalence of HPT even in mixed societies (e.g. Blacks in the USA), although environmental variables such as diet and response to stress may still contribute to this. There are almost certainly several genes involved.

Many factors may complicate epidemiological studies. In making cross-cultural and international comparisons there are difficulties in ensuring control for all environmental factors, and in the reliability and comparability of BP measurement. Nor, in following the fate of migrant communities, can we always assume that the migrant population is representative of the area of origin (e.g. migrants may include a higher proportion of those with higher BPs). On the other hand, even prenatal influences may be environmental (e.g. maternal diet or smoking) so that a positive family history does not necessarily imply a genetic mechanism.

Environmental factors

Whatever the genetic contribution to susceptibility, environmental factors are extremely important in the manifestation of the disease (*see* Table 3.12). All these factors have to be addressed in the assessment, education and management of the hypertensive patient. Because the precise pathogenesis of hypertension is still unresolved the way in which most aetiological factors contribute to raised BP is usually unknown.

Controversy still surrounds the various 'salt hypotheses' (p. 98). Salt intake is difficult to measure accurately, and a general correlation both within and between populations is difficult to demonstrate. Dietary salt restriction, although generally beneficial, usually produces disappointingly small reductions in BP. However, some individuals and some races (e.g. Blacks) do have a 'salt-sensitive' HPT, where blood pressure is very responsive to changes in sodium intake.

Other factors, particularly smoking and hyperlipidaemia, exacerbate the complications of HPT (especially atherosclerosis), but probably do not contribute directly to permanently raised BP. Hyperlipidaemia, and by extension a high fat/cholesterol diet, has recently been implicated as an independent causal factor for raised BP, possibly through interaction with vascular mediators such as endothelin at the vascular endothelium. Some factors contribute to both hypertension and atherosclerosis, e.g. stress, a sedentary life. Whether glucose intolerance, hyperinsulinaemia and insulin resistance contribute directly to the raised BP or merely exacerbate the potential for complications is unclear (*see* Chapter 9, p. 543).

Obesity and lack of exercise are important factors in modern life which have a significant hypertensive effect. Alcohol intake, considerably in excess of that providing the putative beneficial effect on reducing atheroma, is a major contributor to the overall hypertensive load. A number of drugs are hypertensive agents (Table 3.14).

Pathophysiology

Underlying haemodynamic defect

Blood pressure can be expressed as the product of cardiac output and peripheral resistance (i.e. BP = CO × PR), so an elevated BP implies that one or both of these factors must also be raised. Attention has traditionally focused on the PR. This is almost invariably raised in hypertension,

and most early theories of HPT tried to account for this increase through an underlying increased vascular tone.

More recently, attention has turned to the possibility of a raised CO as a prime cause. Fluid retention is known to be an occasional cause of secondary HPT. This is readily explained in haemodynamic terms: blood volume is increased, venous return and preload are raised and cardiac output rises, at least initially. However, systemic peripheral resistance would then increase, as part of the normal autoregulation of blood flow to limit the resulting excessive perfusion. CO would then return to normal. When the patient finally presents, these compensations will have reached equilibrium and only a raised PR is found. Thus, possible causes for an initially high CO or circulating fluid volume are currently being investigated; this links with the 'salt hypotheses'.

Primary (essential) and secondary HPT

In about 10% of cases there may be obvious reasons for an elevated PR or CO (Table 3.14).

Table 3.14   Causes of secondary hypertension

Possible cause or underlying disease	Raised haemodynamic parameter	
	Peripheral resistance	Cardiac output
Renal/endocrine		
Glomerular damage → ↓ GFR → fluid retention	–	+
Increased renin secretion → angiotensin ↑	+	+
(e.g. renal artery disease)		
Endocrine		
Phaeochromocytoma → adrenaline (epinephrine) (very rare)	+	+
Cushing's disease/Conn's syndrome → aldosterone ↑	–	+
Vasomotor		
Increased intracranial pressure (e.g. trauma, tumour)	+	–
Anatomic		
Aortic coarctation (constriction)	+	–
Iatrogenic, e.g.:		
NSAIDs, corticosteroids, oral contraceptives, sympathomimetics, MAOIs	+	+

GFR, glomerular filtration rate; MAOI, monoamine oxidase inhibitor; NSAID, non-steroidal anti-inflammatory drug.

Secondary HPT is often associated with a high pressure and rapid progression, but appropriate therapy (possibly surgical) will often correct the problem. However, in most cases there is usually only a mild or moderate elevation of BP for which no obvious cause can be found. Moreover, the body resists attempts to lower the pressure. It seems that one of the body's pressure control mechanisms (e.g. baroreceptors) has been reset at a higher level: hence the term **essential hypertension**.

Benign and malignant HPT

Hypertension is called malignant or accelerated (terms not strictly synonymous but often used so) when the DBP is above 120 mmHg and usually rising rapidly. Urgent reduction of the pressure is essential to prevent stroke, cardiac failure or renal failure. The prognosis for the 5% or so of hypertensive patients who present with or who develop this form of the condition is much poorer than for the majority with benign (mild or moderate) HPT. Malignant HPT commonly has an underlying renal cause.

Pathogenesis

Most theories of essential HPT implicate the kidney. This creates a difficulty because renal damage is commonly also a consequence of prolonged HPT owing to damage to renal arterioles. Thus renal damage found in a patient with HPT of indeterminate duration could be either a cause or a consequence. Indeed, by that stage a vicious cycle will have been initiated: renal damage raises BP which in turn causes further renal damage. In early HPT an identifiable renal lesion or functional impairment can rarely be found, but this does not mean that subclinical or microscopic damage has not already occurred.

Figure 3.19 illustrates one theory of how renal damage can initiate, and then sustain, hypertension. In Fig. 3.20 there is reference to one way in which sodium is implicated, via a generalized defect in the transmembrane sodium pump. In the kidney this would impair sodium and water clearance, and in blood vessel smooth muscle it

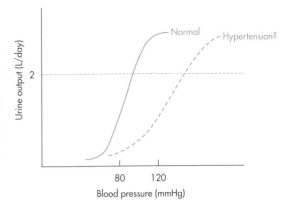

Figure 3.19 'Pressure natriuresis' theory of hypertension. The solid curve represents the normal response of the kidney to changes in arterial pressure (equivalent to renal perfusion pressure). This is the prime mechanism for the maintenance of blood pressure and body water. Assume normal urine output is about 2 L/day. The steepness of the curve shows the brisk diuresis caused by a small elevation in BP, and the rapid fluid retention following any fall in BP. In some hypertensive patients (broken curve) there may be a renal lesion resulting in the kidney needing a higher pressure to clear the same daily fluid load. The CVS then resets baroreceptors to maintain a sufficiently elevated pressure.

could lead to calcium accumulation and vasoconstriction.

The major theories are summarized in Table 3.15, and Fig. 3.20 provides an overview of how some of these proposed mechanisms may interact to change CO or PR. There may be several subgroups of hypertension, in each of which a different mechanism operates. For example, some patients have high renin levels with perhaps silent renal damage caused by subtle intrarenal ischaemia, but most have normal or low levels. A low renin level would be an expected response to HPT if the renal mechanisms were intact, because of feedback inhibition. Then again, only some patients experience reduced BP following salt restriction. Not all hypertensives are highly stressed type A personalities, but some undoubtedly are.

Further details are not given here because there is alas still no firm evidence for the most likely mechanism. Thus, in the absence of a clear pathogenesis the management of essential HPT generally, and drug selection specifically, are

Table 3.15   Pathogenetic theories of essential hypertension

Site	Lesion	Possible consequences
CV centre	↑ Activity	SNS outflow → vasoconstriction and/or ↑ contractility Arterial baroreceptors reset
Kidney	↓ Na/water clearance (? occult malfunction)	Fluid retention → ↑ CO Higher pressure set by CV centre to maintain normal fluid/electrolyte clearance (*see* Fig. 3.19)
	↑ Renin	Vasoconstriction and fluid retention
Circulating Na pump inhibitor	↑ Intracellular [Na]	Vascular wall oedema → ↓ lumen Intracellular Ca availability and/or ↓ resting membrane potential → ↑ constriction
Endocrine	↑ Renin/angiotensin/aldosterone ↓ Bradykinin/prostaglandin ↓ Atrial natriuretic peptide ↑ ADH	Vasoconstriction and fluid retention ↓ Vasodilatation Vasoconstriction and fluid retention Fluid retention
Arterial structure	Hypertrophy (↑ growth factors?)	↓ Vascular lumen → ↑ PR → ↑ BP → further vascular damage

ADH, antidiuretic hormone; BP, blood pressure; Ca, calcium; CO, cardiac output; CV centre, cardiovascular centre in medulla; [Na], Na concentration; PR, peripheral resistance; SNS, sympathetic nervous system.

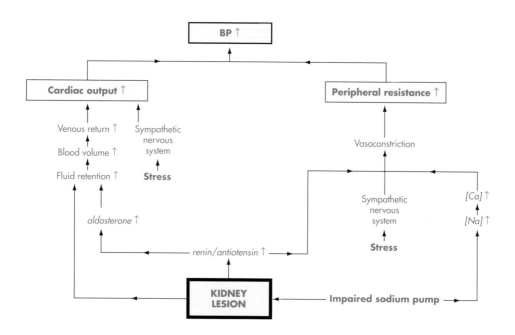

Figure 3.20   Possible pathways in the pathogenesis of hypertension. [Ca], intracellular calcium concentration; [Na], intracellular sodium concentration.

directed empirically at reducing pressure rather than at supposed underlying pathological targets.

Diagnosis and investigation

Measurement

BP should be measured in a consistent and standardized manner. The British Hypertension Society's recommendations include:

- The patient sitting or lying, as long as the cuff is at heart height.
- The patient should have rested for 10 min beforehand; the procedure should have been explained (this is rare, but obviously sensible).
- The average of two or three readings at any one time should be taken.
- The effects of anxiety, time of day, smoking, alcohol and room temperature should be minimized.
- The so-called phase 5 recording of the DBP is recommended (i.e. when sounds completely disappear, rather than just being muffled, as there can be a 5–10 mmHg pressure difference according to the method of recording).

Unless a very high pressure is discovered, i.e. DBP greater than 115–120 mmHg, depending on age, little need be done at once. Measurements as outlined above should be repeated twice, at intervals of a few weeks. Often the pressure will settle down as the patient becomes familiar with the procedure and their 'white-coat hypertension' subsides. Simply being labelled as hypertensive is stressful, so the diagnosis should not be made lightly, and care taken when explaining it to the patient.

In certain cases where the pressure seems erratic, borderline or resistant to therapy, or when a more objective and reproducible measurement is required, it may be helpful to arrange 24-h ambulatory monitoring. A permanent cuff is connected to a portable, battery-powered electronic manometer which samples pressure throughout the day at approximately hourly intervals to determine the diurnal pattern and compute a mean.

Investigation

There are three reasons for investigating a newly diagnosed hypertensive:

1. To identify significant risk factors.
2. To discover any primary, perhaps treatable cause.
3. To assess the current extent of end organ damage.

Clinical examination, simple blood chemistry (urea, electrolytes and lipids), urinalysis (protein, glucose, cells), chest X-ray and ECG will suffice in most patients. A basic grading derives simply from the blood pressure itself (*see* Table 3.13). However, a global grading that takes into account not just elevation but also duration and thus potential organ damage, can be made by ophthalmoscopy (fundoscopy), which assesses the degree of retinal arterial damage. A drug history is also important. These data will serve as a baseline for subsequent monitoring and also reveal clinical signs or biochemical abnormalities suggestive of secondary HPT. In such cases more invasive investigation would then be needed, including renal function tests and urography, and additional blood analysis (corticosteroids, aldosterone, cathechols, renin).

At the same time an assessment is made of risk factors both for HPT and for arterial complications, e.g. smoking, alcohol, body-weight, exercise habits, diet, diabetes, stress and family history, so that an initial plan of general advice for the patient may be drawn up.

Clinical features and presentation

Moderate diastolic HPT is symptomless. Complaints of nose bleeds, tiredness or vague headaches usually derive not from raised pressure but from popular misconceptions about hypertension, or possibly concern about the diagnosis itself. However, malignant HPT certainly may cause severe headaches and other neurological phenomena (hypertensive encephalopathy).

Consequently, patients are usually identified opportunistically during routine screening or life insurance or employment medical examinations. Increasingly, screening by general practitioners is identifying cases much earlier. Any genuine presenting symptoms will usually have been caused by one of the complications, e.g. angina, visual problems. Thus all cases of heart failure, ischaemic heart disease, etc. are investigated for HPT.

Complications

The problems caused by a chronically elevated arterial pressure can be largely anticipated from a consideration of the disturbed haemodynamics (Table 3.16). In general, the extent of the damage will be proportional to the increase in pressure and its duration before detection. There are two broad groups of complications. If pressure is greatly raised there will be direct organ or vascular damage, including heart failure, renovascular disease/malignant hypertension, hypertensive encephalopathy and haemorrhagic stroke. The benefits of blood pressure-reducing interventions are most easily demonstrated in this group. For more modest elevations, the problems are caused indirectly by the promotion and acceler-

ation of atheroma formation. The genesis of these complications is significantly exacerbated by interaction with other common atherogenic risk factors, notably smoking and hyperlipidaemia.

Heart failure

Hypertension was a common cause of heart failure before safe and effective treatment was available. The persistently increased afterload on the left ventricle initially leads to compensatory hypertrophy (remodelling), often seen on the ECG of newly diagnosed hypertensive patients as a higher R-wave (*see* Fig. 3.10). Eventually there is left ventricular dilatation and decompensation.

Arteriosclerosis

Excessive stress on the walls of resistance vessels exposed to elevated pressure stimulates the development of thicker muscular walls in order to withstand it (Laplace's law; *see* p. 64). Hypertrophy of all arterial walls, especially arteriolar ones, has several consequences:

- It encroaches on the lumen, narrowing it (remodelling), which reduces end-organ

Table 3.16   Complications of untreated hypertension

Pathology	Pathogenesis	Clinical consequence
Direct effects		
↑ Peripheral resistance	Elevated LV afterload	LV failure
Arteriosclerosis	↑ Wall stress, medial hypertrophy	Renovascular disease → renal failure
		Haemorrhagic stroke, multiple infarcts, dementia → hypertensive encephalopathy
		Retinal damage → visual defects
Indirect effects		
Atherosclerosis	Possible: ↑ fat penetration, vessel wall damage, turbulent flow	Ischaemic heart disease
		Peripheral vascular disease
		Renal failure
		Cerebrovascular disease → thrombotic stroke, dementia

LV, left ventricular.

perfusion, causing ischaemia, especially in the kidney.

- Peripheral resistance is further raised.
- Arterial compliance falls, which increases afterload and hastens ventricular failure.
- Damaged vascular walls are more prone to aneurysm (bulging) and haemorrhage, especially cerebral vessels.

Atherosclerosis

Perfusion problems are exacerbated by an increased tendency to arterial atheroma which is encouraged by high pressure and associated blood turbulence. In atherosclerosis (not to be confused with arteriosclerosis; p. 116) there is focal deposition of lipid-rich fibrous lesions (atheromas) in the inner lining layer of certain arteries. Atheroma, atherosclerosis and thrombosis are all accelerated by HPT.

Morbidity and mortality

Almost any organ can be affected by these problems, but the heart, brain, kidney, eyes and (particularly if the patient smokes) lower limbs are especially prone. The results may be heart failure, angina, myocardial infarction, stroke, renal failure, blindness or possibly limb amputation: the most common causes of death among hypertensives are stroke and myocardial infarction. These complications can be prevented or retarded by effective antihypertensive therapy although stroke, heart failure and renal impairment seem to be far more effectively prevented than atheromatous complications such as myocardial infarction. Ventricular and possibly vascular hypertrophy are reversible with optimal treatment.

Assessments of the effect of different treatments on prognosis have sometimes been inconclusive, perhaps because many of the complications are advanced at first diagnosis owing to the silent pre-clinical progression. Moreover, common antihypertensive drugs (especially beta-blockers and thiazides) may have atherogenic adverse effects.

Management

Decision to treat

In a patient with mild HPT the most important decision to be made is at what point to initiate drug treatment. In addition to the level of the BP itself, the patient's age and the presence of risk factors or any established end-organ damage must be taken into account in balancing the likely benefits of intervention against the adverse effects and reduced quality of life attendant on lifelong drug therapy (Table 3.17). Unfortunately, the many well-established risks of untreated disease are not precisely quantifiable for individuals, while treatment has far more predictable adverse effects and is lifelong.

Numerous protocols exist for determining the threshold for starting drug treatment, notably from the World Health Organization (WHO), the British Hypertension Society, and the American Joint National Committee. Table 3.18 represents an approximate consensus. At the borderlines of different grades the recommendation is that the patient should be monitored closely over 3–6 months and treatment started if the pressure remains high thereafter. In general, the US rec-

---

Table 3.17 Factors indicating need for early drug treatment in hypertension. Risk factors for producing end-organ damage and evidence of established end-organ damage

Risk factor[a]	Organ damage
Hyperlipidaemia	Retinal damage
Smoking	Renal impairment
Diabetes mellitus	Cardiac enlargement
Family history of	Cardiac ischaemia
cardiovascular	Angina/past myocardial
disease	infarction
Male sex	Past stroke
Older patient	Peripheral vascular disease

[a] Risk factors considered here are unmodifiable, difficult to modify or already likely to have caused or contributed to some organ damage. See also Table 3.12.

Table 3.18   Drug treatment thresholds for hypertension

Blood pressure (mmHg)	No other risk factors[a] or no end-organ damage	One risk factor or moderate organ damage	Multiple risk factors and/or severe organ damage
SBP >180	✓	✓	✓
SBP >160	(✓)	✓	✓
DBP >110	✓	✓	✓
DBP >100	(✓)	✓	✓
DBP >95	?	?	✓
DBP >90	?	?	✓

[a] See Table 3.17.

✓, always treat; (✓), treat if still high after 3–6 months' observation and non-drug therapy; ? observe and monitor regularly.
DBP, diastolic blood pressure; SBP, systolic blood pressure.

ommendations are to start a little earlier than in the UK, at a DBP about 5 mmHg lower.

Severe hypertension

Very severe hypertension, above 210/120 mmHg, represents a medical emergency with the risk of encephalopathy, renal damage or haemorrhagic stroke. Nevertheless, this is not corrected too aggressively because a rapid fall in BP can compromise cerebral perfusion. Parenteral therapy is generally avoided, a smooth fall over a number of hours being preferred, and this can be attained effectively with oral therapy (e.g. *ACEI, hydralazine, labetalol*). Intravenous *nitroprusside* is reserved for established hypertensive encephalopathy and other situations of immediate danger.

For pressures consistently above 110 mmHg diastolic and/or 180 mmHg systolic, the normal treatment protocol (see below) should always be initiated.

Moderate hypertension

A DBP between 100 and 110 mmHg and/or SBP 160–180 mmHg should probably always be treated, but in the absence of risk factors a period of 3–6 months' observation is suggested to see if the pressure can be reduced with conservative measures. It must be remembered that there is clear evidence that older patients benefit as much from treatment as younger ones, especially in the reduction of stroke.

Mild hypertension

The current UK consensus (British Hypertension Society) is that DBPs between 95 and 100 mmHg only need immediate attention in those already showing complications or with specific risk factors, and drug treatment is rarely justified below 95 mmHg (in the USA, 90 mmHg). The benefit of treating young women with mild HPT and no risk factors has also yet to be proven.

Some cardiologists caution against over-vigilance. Patients with marginal or illusory disease, especially the elderly, are perhaps being over-diagnosed and over-treated. In older patients there may be less time for the complications to become significantly limiting, and in the meantime reduced pressure might compromise cerebral or coronary perfusion. Thus therapy might cause more problems immediately than it might prevent in the future, and lowering BP below 80–85 mmHg may be associated with an increased mortality from ischaemic heart disease. There is some evidence for a J-shaped mortality curve for blood pressure, with mortality lowest around 80 mmHg diastolic and rising at pressures not only higher but also lower than this. This might explain the failure to demonstrate a reduction in ischaemic heart disease mortality in some hypertension trials. However, this relationship has not been conclusively demonstrated and other evidence supports similar treatment of the elderly to younger persons, with comparable benefit.

Isolated systolic hypertension

Although raised SBP without a raised DBP was formerly regarded as less dangerous, recent trials have shown that it is also associated with increased mortality. In particular the SysEur trial showed a significant benefit in treating SBP above 150 mmHg in the elderly; there is less stroke and less dementia.

Aim and strategy

From a community perspective the management of hypertension, although improving, is still far from ideal. Detection rates are increasing but it is still believed that up to half of cases remain undiagnosed at any given time. Of those diagnosed, half may be sub-optimally treated. Of those prescribed optimal treatment perhaps no more than half are normotensive, owing to inadequate compliance or other problems. Thus active screening and follow-up monitoring are crucial. Furthermore, pharmaceutical care is important in ensuring optimal prescribing, patient comprehension and concordance.

Strategy

The general strategy in managing hypertension follows the following stages:

- Ensure that blood pressure is genuinely elevated by repeated measurement.
- Decide a target for reduced pressure.
- General measures: reassurance; health education; advice on lifestyle.
- Non-drug interventions.
- Optimal drug monotherapy.
- Combined drug therapy.
- Regular monitoring.

Target blood pressure

The recommended objective for HPT treatment has, as already noted, gradually been reduced as the risk–benefit ratio changes. New studies with safer drugs, such as the HOT (Hypertension Optimal Treatment) trial, have produced greater reductions in morbidity and mortality by targeting lower pressures, with no significant increase in adverse effects. At the time of writing the British Hypertension Society is revising its protocol: it is likely to recommend aiming for below 150/90 mmHg in patients without complications

(currently 160/90 mmHg), 140/85 mmHg after MI and 140/80 mmHg for hypertensives with diabetes. The most recent guidelines of the WHO–International Society of Hypertension (WHO-ISH) recommend 130/85 mmHg for diabetic and young or middle-aged hypertensives, and 140/90 mmHg for the elderly. Whether these guidelines will be observed eventually in the UK cannot yet be predicted.

Because HPT is a chronic progressive disease, lifelong monitoring and usually a progressively increasing level of intervention will be required. In such an insidious, symptomless condition the patient's cooperation and compliance are essential, and patient education is an important means of securing this. Imposed medical edicts are no longer acceptable. The initial plan should be to counsel and to educate the patient about his or her disease, but perhaps suggest nothing positive at first. A mildly elevated BP, discovered incidentally, will often return to normal within a few months and may remain so for several years.

General measures

The notion of a general change in habits and way of life should next be introduced. Simple psychotherapy is sometimes helpful, e.g. engendering the idea of a combined effort of health workers and patient to conquer the condition. Continuous encouragement and reassurance are important. Scare tactics are almost invariably unhelpful: the history of anti-smoking propaganda teaches us this, even though the connection between smoking and its respiratory consequences is far more obvious.

Suitable advice and recommendations at this stage are summarized in Table 3.19. Measures are included to reduce both BP and the risk of arterial complications. Alas, this is not a list to endear the clinician to an otherwise healthy, apparently fit and symptomless patient.

A moderate reduction in sodium intake is a realistic goal, especially if done by simply cutting down on added salt. The ideal is about 6–9 g sodium chloride daily (100–150 mmol Na). As with sugar intake and the 'sweet tooth', the subjective saltiness of food may be relative, determined in part by average consumption: if intake is reduced, eventually less salt will taste equally salty. However, very low-salt diets are unappetiz-

Table 3.19 Non-drug measures to reduce blood pressure or hypertensive complications

	Reduce blood pressure	Reduce complications
Reduce salt intake; increase potassium intake	✓	
Hypnosis, biofeedback	✓	
Reduce stress: relaxation techniques, yoga, meditation	✓	✓
Moderate alcohol intake	✓	(✓)
Aim for ideal body weight	✓	✓
Moderate exercise	✓	✓
Reduce saturated fat/cholesterol intake	(✓)	✓
Stop smoking		✓

✓, definitely desirable; (✓), possibly beneficial.

ing, result in poor compliance and are of arguable benefit. Salt reduction rarely produces BP falls greater than about 5 mmHg and is more successful in some patients than others ('salt-sensitive' hypertension). An overall reduction in the salt added to processed foods might be more beneficial in reducing HPT prevalence than individual targeting. A moderate increase in potassium intake (e.g. in fresh fruit and vegetables) may also be helpful: the most important factor could be a lowering of the dietary Na/K ratio.

The role of calcium and magnesium supplements is still controversial. Diets low in fat and cholesterol may be both anti-atherogenic and hypotensive. The role of pharmacists in smoking cessation is becoming well established.

Non-drug interventions

Encouraging results have been obtained with non-invasive techniques to reduce BP. Some may act by reducing stress: for example, moderate routine aerobic exercise (such as walking a few miles a day), biofeedback (where the patient monitors his or her own BP and consciously tries to lower it), relaxation therapy, hypnotherapy and meditation. The usefulness of these approaches very much depends on patient preferences and health beliefs.

Drug therapy

Despite the best efforts of clinician and patient, the above measures rarely produce more than a modest fall of about 5–10 mmHg, even when combined. Blood pressure then starts to rise again and most patients eventually require drug therapy. Furthermore, many drug regimens – after working effectively for some time – eventually fail to control the condition. This may be because of poor compliance with drug therapy or general measures, progression of the condition, or the body's reflex (if maladaptive) defence of the abnormal pressure.

General principles. The philosophy of 'stepped care' in using antihypertensives (AHPTs) means a progressive increase in intervention to maintain control. At one time it also implied a fairly rigid sequence of specific drugs at specific stages: nowadays a more tailored approach is used. The general sequence and important general considerations are summarized in Table 3.20.

Patients are likely to be taking AHPTs for the rest of their lives so it is important to use agents with the fewest adverse effects first, at the minimum effective dose, and to monitor therapy regularly. Compliance is further encouraged by minimizing the number of daily doses using long-acting agents or modified-release formulations.

Table 3.20 Principles of drug therapy in hypertension

- As few drugs as possible
- As few daily doses as possible
- Start with most suitable initial drug[a]
- Increase the dose gradually until adequate effect achieved
- If primary failure, substitute another suitable drug from different group
- If effectiveness declines, add another agent rather than substitute
- Combine agents acting by different mechanisms
- Combine agents tending to reduce each other's adverse actions
- Monitor adverse reactions and patient compliance regularly

[a] No contraindications, least toxic, best tolerated, most suitable to established organ damage (see text).

Any new dose level must be given for several weeks to achieve both pharmacokinetic and, more importantly, biological steady state. Some drugs, notably the thiazide diuretics and the beta-blockers, have a non-linear or almost flat dose–response curve, so that maximum clinical effect is achieved at little above the minimum effective dose. Thus, because adverse effects are usually dose-dependent it is counterproductive to increase the dose if adequate control is not achieved.

Details of specific drug selection, indications and contraindications are considered below (p. 115).

Combination therapy. AHPTs act on many different sites or mechanisms which the body uses to maintain BP (Fig. 3.21). Thus, if control is not achieved by the maximum tolerated dose of one type there are several advantages to combining two or failing that even three agents:

• Additive or possibly synergistic effect.
• Reduced individual adverse effects.
• Mutual antagonism of adverse effects.

When choosing a drug to be added, one from a different group should be added to the regimen to give an additive or possibly synergistic effect, ensuring that adverse interactions are avoided (see below).

The possibility of minimizing adverse effects is twofold: partly by keeping individual doses low but also by specific antagonism. Because the body's BP control mechanisms have been reset to maintain an abnormally high pressure, when a drug lowers pressure by interfering with one mechanism, e.g. by dilating arterioles, the body responds by recruiting another, e.g. tachycardia or fluid retention, in an attempt to raise pressure again. Thus diuretics can cause palpitations (tachycardia) and renin release, and vasodilators can cause fluid retention (with possible oedema) and tachycardia. However, diuretics will counteract oedema and beta-blockers will prevent tachycardia and renin release. Furthermore vasodilators will counteract the peripheral vasoconstriction (causing cold hands and feet) that occurs with beta-blockers. Thus the combination of all three is logical if blood pressure warrants it.

Fixed-dose proprietary combination products are only occasionally indicated owing to the usual problems of being unable to manipulate

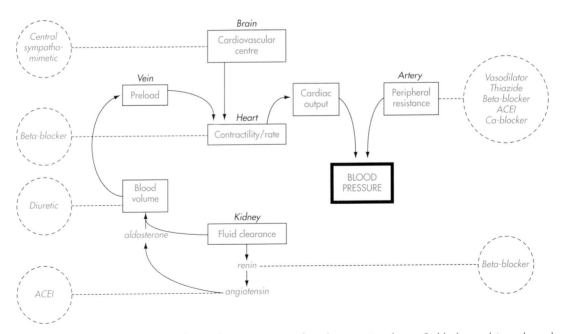

Figure 3.21   Proposed targets and haemodynamic actions of antihypertensive drugs. Ca-blocker, calcium channel blocker; ACEI, angiotensin converting enzyme inhibitor; Central sympathomimetic, e.g. methyldopa.

the doses of components independently, and the difficulty of ascribing adverse effects. One strategy is first to stabilize the patient on the individual components separately and then to introduce a combined product, if a suitable one is available, to aid compliance.

Monitoring

Regular follow-up is essential to monitor compliance with therapy, possible adverse drug effects and disease progression, especially complications. Pharmacists have a role in promoting and reinforcing this process.

Drugs used in hypertension

In this section we consider the properties of the various groups of AHPTs, concluding with a review of the rationale for selection.

Mode of action

Figure 3.21 shows the possible sites of action of common AHPTs; their general haemodynamic actions are summarized in Table 3.21. However, their modes of action in HPT are often uncertain and some may act by more than one mechanism.

All AHPTs affect either CO or PR either directly or indirectly. However, CO is rarely raised in essential HPT, and long-term reduction would compromise exercise tolerance or even resting systemic perfusion. So when we reduce CO we rely on subsequent vascular autoregulation to dilate vessels and decrease resistance reflexly, in response to the reduced perfusion, thus restoring normal output. Recall that the effect on CO of reducing the afterload varies according to whether the myocardium is unimpaired or in failure (*see* Fig. 3.4).

Diuretics

Diuretics cause a small sustained reduction in blood volume, and as a consequence also in CO, but how far this contributes to their action remains unclear. They also promote vasodilatation, but this could be partly due to autoregulation. The *thiazides* seem to be more effective in HPT than the more powerful *loop* diuretics, partly because they generally have a longer duration of action (although loop diuretics may be given twice daily). None has any significant hypotensive effect in normotensive subjects.

Table 3.21   Antihypertensive drugs classified haemodynamically

Cardiac output reduced	Peripheral resistance reduced	Examples
Beta-blocker	Beta-blocker	*Atenolol*
Diuretics	Thiazide diuretic	*Bendrofluazide*
ACEI	ACEI	*Captopril, enalapril*
	Angiotensin-II receptor antagonist	*Losartan*
	Calcium channel blocker	*Nifedipine, diltiazem*
	Direct-acting vasodilator	*Hydralazine, nitroprusside, minoxidil, diazoxide*
	Alpha-blocker	*Prazosin, doxazosin, labetalol, phentolamine*
	Centrally acting sympathomimetic	*Methyldopa, clonidine*[b]
	Centrally acting selective imidazoline receptor agonist[a]	*Clonidine*[b], *moxonidine*
	Adrenergic neurone blocker[a,b]	*Guanethidine*

[a] Often classed together as vasodilators.

[b] Rarely used now.

ACEI, angiotensin converting enzyme inhibitor (angiotensin receptor antagonists have similar actions).

Diuretics promote compensatory reflex activation of the renin/angiotensin system but this does not significantly impair their overall activity.

Beta-blockers

By inhibiting the intracellular adenylate cyclase/kinase system, beta-blockers effectively prevent calcium entry into cells, so reducing sarcoplasmic calcium concentration. This inhibits both smooth muscle contraction and tissue conduction, and explains the similar spectrum of activity to calcium channel blockers. The negative inotropic action of the beta-blockers will certainly reduce CO, but there are other possibilities. Thus beta-blockade reduces renin release and peripheral adrenergic (vasoconstrictor) tone and there may also be central actions. Long-term reduction in peripheral resistance is an important overall effect.

Angiotensin converting enzyme inhibitors

ACEIs act at several sites crucial to BP maintenance, which probably accounts for their considerable success, although doubt still surrounds the principal antihypertensive mechanism. The most likely explanation is that inhibition of angiotensin production causes both a direct reduction of arteriolar vasoconstriction and a secondary reduction of aldosterone-induced fluid retention. At least two other mechanisms contribute. Angiotensin converting enzyme (ACE) is also responsible for the breakdown of vasodilatory bradykinin, so kinin levels rise when ACE is inhibited (this may also contribute to the cough associated with ACEIs; see below). There may also be a direct vascular action inhibiting local angiotensin-induced vessel wall hypertrophy; in untreated HPT this contributes to the long-term vascular complications.

Angiotensin receptor antagonists are assumed to have almost identical therapeutic actions.

Calcium channel blockers

The mode of action of these agents is complex because the different calcium channels and associated receptors have not been fully characterized. There are at least two types of calcium channel, associated with different tissues: the L-type (smooth muscle, including myocardium) and the T-type (nodal/neuronal tissue). Most existing agents block either the former only, or both. (The only T-specific agent to reach clinical use, *mibefradil*, was withdrawn soon after its first being marketed owing to toxicity.)

A further distinction between target tissues is in the post-receptor excitation coupling involving calcium. In cardiac muscle cells, adrenergic stimulation of adjacent beta-adrenergic receptors opens the calcium channel, leading to an increase in intracellular calcium concentration. This promotes the Ca^{++}-troponin C interaction which eventually leads to contraction. Thus beta-blockers and calcium channel blockers have similar, synergistic inhibitory effects; in the heart, this negative inotropism can lead to severe depression of contractility. By contrast, in peripheral vascular smooth muscle, intracellular calcium interacts with calmodulin to promote contraction, whereas beta-stimulation inhibits this. Thus beta-blockers cause vasoconstriction but calcium channel blockers promote relaxation; indeed, calcium channel blockers will antagonize the peripheral constriction sometimes experienced with beta-blockers (*see* Table 3.25).

The three calcium channel blocker groups, the benzothiazepines (*diltiazem*), the phenylalkylamines (*verapamil*), and the dihydropyridines (or DHPs, e.g. *nifedipine*) each bind to a different receptor site within the calcium channel. More importantly, they have different affinities for target tissues. The dihydropyridines are more active on cardiac and nodal tissue, the other groups preferentially target vascular smooth muscle.

Other vasodilators

This diverse group of drugs acts on arteriolar tone at a variety of different sites, both locally and through the autonomic nervous system (Fig. 3.21 and Table 3.21). Thus vasodilators from different groups may be combined.

Clinical use

Diuretics

Thiazide diuretics have long been first-line drugs, owing principally to their low toxicity and the fact that they (along with beta-blockers) have been convincingly shown to reduce mortality in HPT (Table 3.22). However, their use is

Table 3.22   Advantages and disadvantages of diuretics in hypertension

Advantages	Disadvantages
Cheap	Metabolic effects – altered blood chemistry:
Effective	• ↓K, ↓Ca, ↓Mg
Proven to reduce mortality	• ↑glucose
Well tolerated	• ↑lipid
Single daily dose	• ↑urate
Little acute toxicity	• hyponatraemia/dehydration (especially in elderly)
Suitable in:	Impotence
• Blacks	
• elderly	
• renal impairment[a]	

[a] Use loop diuretics in severe renal impairment; otherwise, thiazides usually used.

being re-appraised as an adverse effect on plasma lipids has been added to their other well-known biochemical disturbances (Table 3.22). The contribution of these adverse effects to cardiovascular morbidity and mortality via arrhythmias, glucose intolerance and atheroma may be more serious than formerly suspected. In addition they cause impotence in males, seriously impairing the quality of life.

Nevertheless, thiazides are still recommended by some authorities, e.g. by the British Hypertension Society, as first-line drugs for mild to moderate HPT. One reason may be the trend to very low doses (e.g. *bendrofluazide* 1.25–2.5 mg daily), which are almost equally effective but cause significantly fewer adverse effects. Moreover potassium supplementation, which used to be routinely co-prescribed although poorly tolerated and poorly complied with, is rarely needed. Thiazides are increasingly used in combination with potassium-sparing diuretics or ACEIs. If potassium supplements are used in these circumstances the risk then is of hyperkalaemia rather than hypokalaemia.

Choice. There is little to choose between the available thiazides; *bendrofluazide* is among the cheapest. Most may be given once each morning. They seem particularly beneficial in Blacks, whose hypertension is often volume-dependent, and in the elderly because of their freedom from acute toxicity in low doses. In renal impairment loop diuretics are required, but these diuretics are otherwise avoided because they act briefly and so do not provide sustained control; they also lack the direct vasodilator effect of thiazides.

Beta-blockers
The generally mild or predictable adverse effects and wide choice in this group mean that they are often used as first-line therapy, particularly for hypertensives with arrhythmias or ischaemic heart disease. They also reduce mortality in hypertensives.

Dose. As with diuretics, recommended doses of beta-blockers have been reduced (e.g. atenolol 50 mg daily) with no loss of antihypertensive action, but reduced adverse effects. Once- or twice-daily dosing is usually sufficient because the effect of beta-blockade is not directly related to plasma level. For once-daily dosing, to improve compliance, drugs with a longer half-life (e.g. *atenolol*) or modified-release formulations may be used. The dose should start low and be increased gradually. Should it be necessary to stop therapy, the dose must be tapered off equally slowly, especially in those with ischaemic heart disease, because of the risk of rebound adrenergic over-stimulation causing tachycardia, angina, hypertension, etc.

Side effects, contraindications and cautions. The well-understood dose-related adverse effects are summarized in Table 3.23. Probably as a

Table 3.23 Side effects and contraindications of the beta-adrenergic blocking drugs

Site	Side effect	Caution or contraindication[a]
Bronchial smooth muscle[b, c]	Bronchoconstriction	C/I in obstructive airways disease; depends on severity
Peripheral arterioles[b, c]	Vasoconstriction: cold hands and feet; muscle weakness; fatigue	C/I in peripheral vascular disease, Raynaud's syndrome; use agent with intrinsic sympathomimetic activity
Myocardium[c]		
• negative inotropic	Fatigue, reduced exercise tolerance	Use with caution in heart failure[d]
• negative chronotropic	Bradycardia	C/I in bradycardia, heart block
Systemic beta receptors[b]	Atherogenic dyslipidaemia ($\uparrow$ triglyceride; $\downarrow$ HDL)	Care in dyslipidaemia
	$\downarrow$ Response to hypoglycaemia	Care in diabetes or impaired glucose tolerance
Pancreas[b]	Reduced insulin secretion; possible hyperglycaemia	Care in Type II diabetes
Central nervous system[e]	Nightmares, confusion, depression, psychotic reactions	Avoid evening dose; avoid lipophilic agents
	Impotence and reduced libido – may reduce compliance	Counsel

[a] Contraindication (C/I) may be relative or absolute.
[b] β_2 blockade; effect more prominent with non-selective agents.
[c] Effect offset in agents with intrinsic sympathomimetic activity.
[d] May be used in certain circumstances; see p. 91.
[e] Effect more common or severe with lipophilic agents.

result of a combination of these, beta-blockers can significantly reduce the quality of life of some patients. Cautions and contraindications can be predicted from the adverse effect profile. Beta-blockers must be used with extreme caution in obstructive airways disease, and probably not at all in asthma. They should also be avoided in peripheral vascular disease, Raynaud's syndrome, bradycardia and heart block. Their cautious use in heart failure is discussed on p. 91.

In diabetic patients given beta-blockers, early physiological responses to developing hypoglycaemia (hunger, tachycardia, etc.) and the patient's perception of these effects are diminished, with potentially disastrous results. In type II diabetics, insulin release may be inhibited, aggravating hyperglycaemia and impairing control (see Chapter 9).

Choice. All beta-blockers have equivalent antihypertensive activity. Three main properties yield criteria for differentiating beta-blockers (Fig. 3.22) and choice is further qualified by possible adverse effects and precautions (Table 3.23).

Cardioselectivity is conferred by a greater affinity for beta$_1$-receptors, located mainly on the myocardium, compared with beta$_2$-receptors (most other beta-adrenergic sites). Cardioselectivity is relative and is less marked at higher doses. Nevertheless, selective agents are preferred in all but those few indications where information on their use is inadequate, such as hypertrophic cardiomyopathy, thyrotoxicosis, migraine and immediately after a MI. Respiratory, metabolic and peripheral vasoconstrictor effects (via beta$_2$-receptors) are still seen, and even selective agents are potentially hazardous in asthmatics.

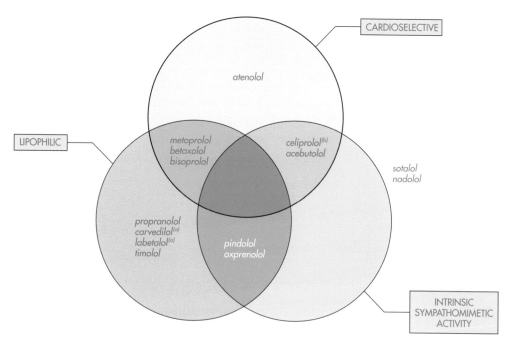

Figure 3.22   Classification of adrenergic beta-blockers. The list is not exhaustive. Only common representatives of each class are shown. [a] alpha- and beta-blockade; [b] beta$_2$-agonist.

Intrinsic sympathomimetic activity (ISA, partial agonist activity) may offset bronchoconstriction, peripheral vasoconstriction and myocardial depression in some patients. The vasodilator action is perhaps the most useful. *Pindolol* has the greatest ISA. A similar effect is achieved in agents which have additional alpha-blocking activity (*labetalol, carvedilol*). *Celiprolol* combines highly selective beta$_1$-blocker with selective beta$_2$-stimulant activity, which also counteracts peripheral vasoconstriction.

Lipophilic drugs have two important general properties: they cross the blood–brain barrier and they require hepatic metabolism before elimination. Central beta-blockade can cause CNS disturbances, most marked with *propranolol*. Hepatic clearance means potentially low bioavailability (owing to first-pass metabolism) and a shorter half-life (unless there are active metabolites). It also makes dose titration more difficult because steady state takes longer to achieve. *Pindolol, timolol* and *betaxolol* are cleared both renally and hepatically, making their elimination less susceptible to impairment of either system. *Betaxolol* is unusual in being both long-acting and lipophilic.

ACEIs

ACEIs appear to interfere less with quality of life than other AHPTs, which is particularly important in lifelong HPT treatment. They are now often used as first choice in moderate HPT in combination with a diuretic, as well as in severe resistant HPT regardless of renin levels because they effectively combat the raised renin levels induced by diuretics. Combinations with calcium blockers or beta-blockers are also successful. ACEIs may be especially useful in diabetic hypertension because they seem to protect against nephropathy (*see* Chapter 9). ACEIs have an undisputed place as sole therapy in the reno-vascular, high-renin hypertension.

Using newer agents or lower doses of captopril, the ACEIs are proving to be remarkably free of the adverse effects common with other potent AHPTs, both serious (central, postural, dysrhythmic, metabolic, etc.) and simply troublesome (fatigue, sexual and mental impairment).

Side effects, contraindications and precautions (*see* **Table 3.24**). The main problems with ACEIs are related to their potent antihypertensive and anti-aldosterone actions. Severe first-dose

Table 3.24   Side effects of the angiotensin converting enzyme inhibitors

Side effect	Comment
Hypotension	Common, especially first dose effect Especially hypovolaemic, hyponatraemic, on diuretics
Renal impairment/failure	Especially with renal artery stenosis, pre-existing renal disease, cardiac failure or on NSAIDs
Hyperkalaemia	Avoid potassium-sparing diuretics, potassium supplements, NSAIDs
Dry cough	If persistent, change to angiotensin receptor antagonist
Angio-oedema	Rare; bradykinin-related?
Neutropenia/agranulocytosis	Rare
Proteinuria, impaired taste, skin rash	Rare; only *captopril* in high doses?

NSAID, non-steroidal anti-inflammatory agent.

hypotension may occur, particularly in volume- or salt-depleted patients such as those already on diuretic therapy. Sometimes patients are initiated on a low dose of the short-acting captopril given at night to test their reaction, and switched to a longer-acting preparation if successful. If possible, diuretics should be stopped a day before starting ACEI therapy, and reintroduced if necessary under careful medical supervision. Significant hyperkalaemia may follow concomitant use of potassium-sparing diuretics or potassium supplements. Severe hypersensitivity reactions (angio-oedema, with fatal laryngeal obstruction) have occurred.

Related to hypotension is the possibility of severe renal impairment, especially if there is pre-existing renal disease, owing to reduced renal perfusion pressure. A particular problem is bilateral renal artery stenosis (usually atherosclerotic in origin). In such cases the BP is being kept high by elevated renin levels in order to maintain renal perfusion. Inhibition of the renin/angiotensin system may then produce a disastrous fall in BP, even precipitating acute pre-renal failure. Caution is even advised with ACEIs in unilateral stenosis in the elderly, or any evidence of peripheral vascular disease.

Persistent dry cough affects up to 20% of patients. It is probably due to excess bradykinin (which is usually metabolized by ACE) and sometimes proves intolerable, in which case an angiotensin receptor antagonist can be substituted (this being the primary advantage of this group). Alternatively, inhaled sodium cromoglycate can be tried, because its action is thought to be mediated via bradykinin inhibition.

Initial reports of bone marrow toxicity (neutropenia) with captopril resulted from the use of unnecessarily high doses. Moreover, these and some other adverse effects, e.g. taste disturbance and skin rash, may be immunologically based, and related to the sulphydryl group found in captopril but not newer ACEIs (see also *penicillamine*, Chapter 8). Rarely, neutropenia can occur with any of the ACEIs.

The principal drug *interaction* of the ACEIs, apart from that with potassium-sparing diuretics (see above), is with NSAIDs. Partly through their action on intrarenal prostglandins, NSAIDs used in combination with ACEIs can result in a reduced antihypertensive effect, increased renal toxicity and increased potassium retention.

Calcium channel blockers

These are increasingly used as initial therapy in HPT because they cause less adverse cardiovascular, bronchial and metabolic problems than the beta-blockers. Careful selection within the group is needed for specific indications (Table 3.25). Predominantly vasodilator agents are preferred in HPT, but anti-arrhythmic and negative inotropic activity is useful in hypertensive patients with ischaemic heart disease. The non-cardiodepressant calcium blockers can be usefully and safely combined with a beta-blocker.

Side effects. Most problems are minor, namely flushing and headaches, and are due directly to vasodilation, particularly with the dihydropyridines. Similarly, reflex tachycardia with possible palpitations may occur. This is undesirable in ischaemic patients since it increases myocardial oxygen demand, in which case, in the absence of ventricular dysfunction, the use of a non-dihydropyridine or combination with a beta-blocker is recommended. Peripheral oedema, usually in the ankles, is due to leakage from pre-capillary vessels subjected to higher pressures owing to arteriolar dilatation. As this oedema is not due to fluid retention, it does not respond to diuretics but it may respond to an ACEI.

By contrast, non-dihydropyridines (e.g. *verapamil*) have little effect on blood vessels but are cardiodepressant, with the risk of heart failure or bradycardia.

A number of recent reports have linked certain calcium channel blockers to an increased incidence of cancer, depression and suicide, gastrointestinal haemorrhage and excess cardiac morbidity and mortality. The evidence for the cardiac effects has mainly involved *nifedipine*, but related drugs are also suspected (Table 3.25). Patients with hypertension and diabetes appear particularly prone. Considering the widespread use of calcium channel blockers these reports are worrying and their validity is still being hotly debated and re-investigated. It is postulated that a rapid clinical effect provokes myocardial ischaemia, either from too rapid a fall in BP (and coronary perfusion) or from the consequent reflex sympathetic activation.

Cautions and contraindications. Discontinuation has been associated with exacerbated ischaemic events in those with ischaemic heart disease, and so should be performed gradually. (Discontinuation of *mibefradil* caused hypotension and fatal cardiogenic shock in some patients, necessitating its withdrawal.) Combination of the negatively inotropic agents verapamil, diltiazem and nifedipine with beta-blockers is absolutely contraindicated because it can cause heart failure

or heart block. Enzyme inhibition by grapefruit juice enhances the action of most calcium channel blockers, except *verapamil* and *amlodipine*. As yet, the only firm recommendation to emerge regarding possible cardiovascular toxicity has been to avoid the shorter-acting dihydropyridine derivatives in hypertension (or acute ischaemic events), especially in diabetic patients.

Modified-release preparations of calcium channel blockers are not interchangeable and should not be prescribed or supplied generically.

Vasodilators

This large heterogeneous group (*see* Table 3.21) has had a chequered history in HPT treatment. Not surprisingly, the first antihypertensive agents used targeted the peripheral arterioles. Predominant arterial dilatation is preferred (*see* Table 3.7), but this can cause postural hypotension by inhibiting natural reflex vasoconstriction. Early sympatholytic vasodilators, including ganglion blockers (e.g. *hexamethonium*) and non-specific alpha-blockers (e.g. *phentolamine*), had limited effectiveness and serious adverse effects, chiefly postural hypotension, impotence and reflex tachycardia. The adrenergic neurone blockers (e.g. *guanethidine*), although somewhat more successful, still have serious adverse effects and are reserved now for resistant HPT.

Newer vasodilators cause less postural problems and most produce less lipid abnormalities than beta-blockers or thiazides. Other common vasodilator drawbacks such as headaches, dizziness, palpitations, flushing and reflex fluid retention are less serious. A miscellaneous 'reserve' group of the more toxic direct-acting vasodilators (e.g. *minoxidil*) is still sometimes needed.

Centrally acting sympatholytics (e.g. *methyldopa, clonidine*) have long been used as third- or fourth-line drugs, but now have little place owing to central effects such as impotence and depression. However, methyldopa remains a useful alternative in a variety of special circumstances where standard drugs are contraindicated: for example in diabetes, in the HPT of pregnancy and when postural hypotension is especially hazardous, such as in the elderly or in those with cerebrovascular disease. *Clonidine* is now known to act partly via central imidazoline

Table 3.25   Comparative properties of calcium channels, related to different groups of calcium channel blockers

Primary site	Vascular smooth muscle	Myocardial muscle	Myocardial conducting tissue
Clinical effect of blockade	Arterial dilatation	Negative inotropic: ↓ O_2 demand	Inhibit SA and AV node; slow heart
Related side effects	Flushing, headaches, oedema	Myocardial depression; CHF	Bradycardia
Related indication	Hypertension, variant angina	Ischaemic heart disease	Supraventricular tachyarrhythmia
Excitation-contraction coupling	Calmodulin-linked	Troponin C-linked	Troponin C-linked
Examples of blockers[a]			
Short-acting DHP *nifedipine, isradipine, nicardipine*	+++	-/+	-/+
Longer-acting DHP *amlodipine, felodipine, lacidipine*	+++	-	-
Non-DHP *verapamil, diltiazem*	+	+++	+++

[a] Drugs are grouped for clarity, but there may be detailed differences – check in reference source for individual properties.

AV, atrioventricular; CHF, coronary heart failure; DHP, dihydropyridine; SA, sinoatrial.

+++, major effect on these tissues; +, minor effect; -/+, possible effect; -, no effect.

receptors, and the newer more specific *moxonidine* may have fewer adverse effects.

The direct-acting spasmolytic *hydralazine* lost favour owing to its tendency to precipitate a lupus-like syndrome, especially in slow acetylators. However it has recently been reprieved: at doses below 200 mg daily – possibly below 100 mg – the risk is small. The selective (post-synaptic alpha$_2$) adrenergic blockers, e.g. *prazosin, terazosin, doxazosin*, seem to cause less tachycardia and, except for the first dose, less postural hypotension. They also reduce plasma cholesterol and produce a favourable change in the HDL/LDL ratio (pp. 120–122).

Drug selection

So far, only diuretics and beta-blockers have been shown in long-term controlled trials to reduce overall mortality in hypertension and are still usually recommended as first-line therapy in the absence of contraindications. The benefits of other groups have until recently been demonstrated only indirectly using logical but essentially surrogate end-points such as BP lowering. Such trials cannot identify the possibility of long-term adverse effects which may eventually outweigh potential benefit. Several long-term trials with calcium channel blockers and ACEIs are under way. The most recent to report, the Hypertension Optimal Therapy trial (HOT, 1998) did produce better evidence in support of these two groups.

Almost all existing AHTPs have comparable BP-lowering efficacy. The optimal order of selection in a given patient is governed primarily by adverse effects, precautions and contraindications. Factors which modify choice in common conditions or patient groups are summarized in Table 3.26. Recent concerns over the long-term safety of the beta-blockers and diuretics and the emergence of the relatively safe calcium channel blockers and ACEIs has widened the choice for initial therapy. A new consensus has not yet emerged, but it may now be advisable to try a number of different monotherapies if control is not achieved, before starting dual therapy. The scheme in Fig. 3.23 represents one possible approach. Numerous other combinations are of course possible, particularly in refractory HPT, when up to four drugs may be needed. Even then, there need usually be no resort to the more toxic ('reserve') drugs.

Attention must be paid to potential drug interactions which may involve AHPTs. Table 3.27 illustrates the general principles with some representative examples. Details will be found in standard texts (*see* References and further reading).

Ischaemic heart disease

Ischaemia means literally 'to hold back blood'. Ischaemic heart disease (IHD) is the collective name for a number of conditions in which obstructive lesions of the coronary arteries restrict myocardial blood flow. IHD is also called 'coronary artery disease' or simply 'heart disease'. The main clinical manifestations are **angina pectoris** and **myocardial infarction**, but **heart failure** and **arrhythmias** also occur. IHD is the greatest single cause of death, especially premature death, in industrialized societies: in the UK it is responsible for about 30% of all male deaths and causes considerable morbidity. This is especially significant because IHD is largely preventable.

There are wide geographic, ethnic and national variations in prevalence, e.g. the male mortality from IHD per 100 000 varies between 400 in Finland and 30 in Japan. However, immigrant groups tend to assume the same prevalence as their host country when fully assimilated, showing the importance of environmental risk factors.

Table 3.26   Specific indications, side effects and contraindications of antihypertensives

Situation	Drugs to avoid/caution	Specific alternatives or recommendations[a]
Elderly	Sympatholytic (*postural effect*)	Thiazide, beta-blocker, methyldopa
Young male	Thiazide, beta-blocker	ACEI, Ca-blocker
Black ethnic group	Beta-blocker, ACEI	–
Peripheral vascular disease	Beta-blocker, ? ACEI	Vasodilator
Angina	Vasodilator	Beta-blocker *or* Ca-blocker
Myocardial infarction	–	Beta-blocker *or* ACEI
Heart failure	Beta-blocker, verapamil, diltiazem	Thiazide, ACEI
Heart block	Beta-blocker, Ca-blocker	–
Hyperlipidaemia	Beta-blocker, thiazide[b]	ACEI, Ca-blocker, selective alpha-blocker
Diabetes (especially Type 1)	Thiazide[b], beta-blocker[c]	ACEI, selective alpha-blocker
Obstructive pulmonary disease	Beta-blocker[c]	–
Pregnancy	Thiazide, ACEI	Methyldopa, labetalol, furosemide (frusemide)
Hepatic impairment	Ca-blocker	Methyldopa
Renal impairment: early	Thiazide	ACEI
severe	ACEI	Furosemide (frusemide), beta-blocker
Renal artery stenosis	ACEI	–
Vascular disease in elderly	ACEI	–
High renin	–	ACEI
Thyrotoxicosis	–	Beta-blocker
Depression	Lipophilic beta-blockers, methyldopa, clonidine	–
Gout, hypokalaemia	Thiazide	–

[a] Where no alternative indicated, any group other than those contraindicated is equally suitable.

[b] Thiazides have significant effects on lipid and glucose levels only at doses higher than required in treating hypertension.

[c] Except possibly cardioselective agents.

ACEI, angiotensin converting enzyme inhibitor; Ca-blocker, calcium channel blocker.

Epidemiological and pathological studies and large-scale intervention trials strongly suggest that the causes lie in the industrialised or developed way of life.

Atherosclerosis and vascular obstructive disease

The pathology and treatment of IHD can best be understood in the general context of vascular obstruction (partial block) and occlusion (complete block). Therefore this will be reviewed first.

Classification

The main chronic processes responsible for chronic arterial obstruction are arteriosclerosis and atherosclerosis. In addition, thrombosis may occur as an acute complication, in both veins and arteries (Fig. 3.24).

Arteriosclerosis

Although this term is commonly used to describe all degenerative or proliferative arterial lesions, it should be reserved for the symmetrical thickening of the middle **muscle layer** (**media**)

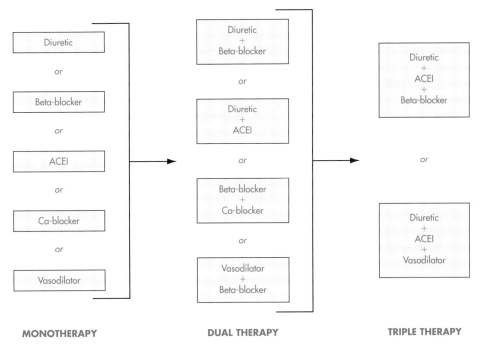

Figure 3.23 Drug selection in hypertension.

Table 3.27 Potential interactions with antihypertensive therapy[a]

Drugs that elevate blood pressure	
Vasoconstrictor sympathomimetics	Oral decongestants (phenylephrine), bronchodilators especially non-specific[b] amphetamines
Drugs causing fluid retention	Corticosteroids, oral contraceptives, non-steroidal anti-inflammatory drugs

Drugs that lower blood pressure	
CNS depressants	Tranquilizers, alcohol
Vasodilators	Nitrates, specific bronchodilators[b]

Specific interactions	
Beta-blockers	Verapamil, diltiazem → cardiac depression, failure
Alpha-blockers	Beta-blockers, diuretics → exaggerated first-dose hypotension
ACEIs	Potassium-sparing diuretics, potassium supplements → hyperkalaemia

[a] This table only lists the overall interference with blood presure control and mutual interactions of antihypertensives. Interactions of antihypertensive agents with other specific drugs can be found in the *British National Formulary*.

[b] Bronchodilators: non-specific, e.g. ephedrine; specific, e.g. salbutamol.

ACEIs, angiotensin converting enzyme inhibitors.

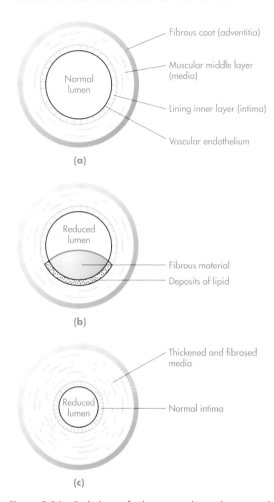

Figure 3.24   Pathology of atheroma, atherosclerosis and arteriosclerosis. A diagrammatic representation emphasizing distinctions between arteriosclerosis and atherosclerosis. (a) Normal arteriolar wall. The middle layer (media) is composed of muscle and elastic tissue. (b) Simple atheroma. An asymmetrical deposit of fat and fibrous tissue in the inner layer (intima) invades the arterial lumen. New endothelium has overgrown the lesion. Should there be further damage, with mural thrombosis, it would be termed atherosclerosis. (c) Arteriosclerosis. Symmetrical thickening of the media in most arterioles, usually in response to chronically raised arterial pressure. (Reproduced with permission from Burt *et al.* (1982) *Chemist Drugg* **217**: 867.)

of arterioles throughout the body. It usually arises in response to hypertension, when it may be partially reversed by treatment, but it also seems to be a normal consequence of ageing. Because it is widely disseminated it increases peripheral resistance, thus aggravating HPT and perpetuating a vicious circle. The lesions are often fibrosed and calcified especially in the elderly. It is popularly known as 'hardened arteries'.

At first there may be no significant impairment of perfusion. However, in the elderly there may be chronically reduced cerebral or renal perfusion. Moreover, the stiffened, non-compliant vessels are weakened and eventually may bulge (aneurysm) and rupture, particularly in cerebral vessels where the result is acute haemorrhagic stroke.

Arteriosclerosis is described here to differentiate it from atherosclerosis. It will not be considered further and all that follows will apply specifically to atheroma/atherosclerosis.

Atherosclerosis

In this condition, fatty-fibrous plaques or **atheromas** are deposited asymmetrically within the **innermost layer (intima) of certain (not all) arteries**. Sites such as bends, branches or bifurcations seem especially prone. This patchy (focal) distribution means that there is little effect on total peripheral resistance, but local perfusion may be crucially impaired. Atherosclerosis can occur in many different organs, the result being a wide spectrum of clinical manifestations (Fig. 3.25).

Thrombosis

Thrombi result from abnormal triggering of the coagulation process within intact **arteries** or **veins** (rather than, as is normal, after damage or rupture). This causes sudden occlusion. Small particles (**thromboemboli**) may break off and lodge further downstream, with similar outcome. Arterial thrombi frequently form at the sites of coronary or cerebral atherosclerotic lesions, with potentially fatal consequences (Fig. 3.25).

Aetiology

Classes of contributory factors

An understanding of the formation of atheroma and thrombosis is important for prevention and

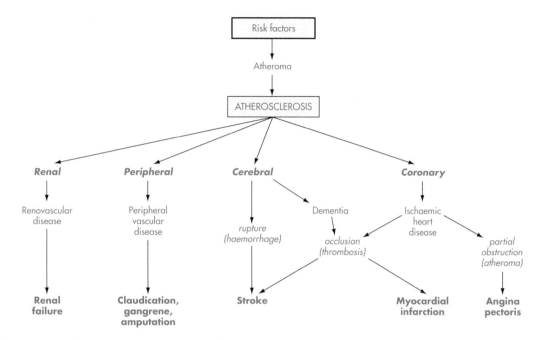

Figure 3.25   Clinical manifestations of atherosclerosis.

treatment. The contributory factors are usually grouped into three categories: histological (endothelial damage), rheological (abnormal blood flow) and biochemical (abnormal blood or tissue constituents). These may occur independently or together (Table 3.28). The **response to injury** theory proposes that atherosclerosis arises from a maladaptive chronic inflammatory reaction in which an attempt is made to repair the vascular wall or to limit chronic damage. This reaction persists at the expense of obstructing the vessel lumen and possibly promoting further damage.

Vascular endothelial damage

An **atheroma** is probably initiated by factors which breach the arterial endothelial defences exposing underlying tissue. Constituents of tobacco smoke undoubtedly contribute to this. It is also possible that partially oxidized components of the plasma lipid particle **low density lipoprotein** (LDL) irritate the endothelium, with more significant oxidation occurring within the wall. Recent findings, yet to be confirmed, implicate chronic inflammatory damage from systemic microbial colonization, possibly with

Chlamydia or *Helicobacter* species. Finally, hyperlipidaemia itself may be directly damaging to the vessel wall.

Thrombosis may be triggered by a sudden split or ulceration of a previously stable atheromatous plaque, with acute effects. More chronically, the atheroma may become the focus of a **mural (wall) thrombus**, which complicates and extends it. This may occur without major symptoms, or the condition may present as unstable angina. Inflamed venous or heart valves are also foci for thrombosis.

Abnormal flow

In **arteries**, atheromas are most commonly found where flow is turbulent and wall shear forces high. Presumably this causes endothelial cell dysfunction. (It may interfere with shear-triggered, nitric oxide-mediated vascular relaxation, which alters LDL flow through the vessel wall, or causes enlargement of intercellular gaps allowing abnormal access of irritants.) Atheromas are not found in veins but rather in the normally low pressure pulmonary arteries in cases of pulmonary hypertension.

In **veins**, it is abnormally sluggish flow that

Table 3.28   Factors initiating atheroma and thrombosis

Abnormality	Arterial atheroma	Arterial thrombosis	Venous thrombosis
Histological	Chronic inflammation (? oxidized LDL, smoking) Infection (*Chlamydia, Helicobacter*) Hypoxia (smoking)	Ruptured atheroma? Heart valve (i) inflamed (ii) vegetation (endocarditis)	Inflamed venous valve (phlebitis)
Rheological	High pressure (i.e. hypertension) High wall stress (i.e. hypertension) Fast turbulent flow (bend, branch)	Atrial fibrillation	Venous stasis, e.g. prolonged bedrest, recumbency
Biochemical	Dyslipidaemia ($\uparrow$ LDL, $\downarrow$ HDL) Platelets (growth factors) Diabetes (dyslipidaemia)	Clotting factors ($\uparrow$ fibrinogen) Platelets (adhesiveness, growth factors)	Clotting factors Platelets Drugs, e.g oral contraceptives

HDL, high density lipoprotein; LDL, low density lipoprotein.

causes problems, e.g. prolonged bedrest predisposes to venous ('deep vein') thrombosis, usually in the leg. This is one reason why patients are mobilized rapidly after surgery. In atrial fibrillation, static pools of blood develop within the heart and may clot. In either case thrombi may be carried downstream as emboli. From the leg the path taken by thrombi is through widening veins and the right heart, ultimately to lodge in a pulmonary artery. Thrombi originating from the right atrium also lodge in the lungs, while those from the left atrium lodge in the brain or coronary arteries.

Abnormal constituents. Endothelial damage can trigger platelet adhesion and aggregation or the clotting cascade, especially if there is an imbalance between platelet promoter and inhibitor factors. For example, certain prostaglandins (e.g. prostacyclin released from vascular endothelium) tend to inhibit platelet activation and aggregation while others, notably the thromboxane series, are pro-aggregatory. Clotting factor abnormalities, e.g. high levels of fibrinogen, have been found in IHD patients. Coagulation is also disturbed following severe trauma, e.g. major surgery, and by certain drugs, e.g. oral hormonal contraceptives.

Risk factors

The four primary modifiable risk factors for atherosclerosis are **hypertension**, **smoking**, **diabetes** and **hyperlipidaemia** (dyslipidaemia). Diabetes may act partly though the associated dyslipidaemia. These four act synergistically, so that for example possessing any two poses more than twice the risk. Numerous other less crucial factors have been implicated (Table 3.29), some of them associated with industrialized societies and modifiable by changes to lifestyle. A possible protective effect of moderate alcohol intake is still widely debated. There is also evidence of prenatal influences on the fetus. Maternal nutritional deprivation may cause not just low birthweight but also a predisposition in later life to atherosclerosis, hypertension and diabetes. The prevalence in younger males is about three times that in females, but the rates converge later in life because the incidence among postmenopausal women is greatly increased.

The lipid hypothesis
The lipid hypothesis of atherogenesis traces the causal links between dietary lipid, plasma lipid, atherosclerosis and IHD. An outline of the steps in the argument is given in Table 3.30. Patients

Table 3.29   Risk factors for atherosclerosis

Primary modifiable	Secondary modifiable	Unmodifiable
Hyperlipidaemia	High sugar and low fibre intake	Family history
Smoking	Obesity	Ethnic group
Hypertension	Sedentary life	Age
Diabetes[a]	Industrialized society	Male sex
	'Stress'[b]	Type A personality[b]
	Heavy alcohol intake	
	? Fetal deprivation due to	
	maternal malnutrition	
	? Chronic infection[c]	
	? Raised plasma urate	
	? Raised plasma homocysteine	
	? Soft water	

[a] Modifiable in so far as it can be well controlled.

[b] Striving, highly motivated individual.

[c] e.g. *Chlamydia, Helicobacter*.

Table 3.30   Lipid hypothesis of atherosclerosis

Summary of the argument for the central role of lipids in the pathogenesis of atherosclerosis

- The risk of atheroma formation is related to total plasma cholesterol (ChE)
- Total plasma ChE is related to (but is not dependent entirely upon) total dietary lipid but more to saturated (animal) fat intake than to dietary cholesterol. It is inversely related to unsaturated (vegetable) fat intake
- ChE is transported in the blood in solubilized form as lipoprotein (along with triglyceride, phospholipid and protein)
- Low and very low density lipoprotein fractions (LDL, VLDL) carry ChE from the gastrointestinal tract or liver to the tissues; high density lipoprotein (HDL) carries it away from the tissues and back to the liver
- Atherogenesis is most closely correlated with VLDL/LDL levels and inversely related to HDL (i.e. high HDL is protective): the HDL/LDL ratio may be the most important parameter
- Triglycerides (TG) are not an independent risk factor; the correlation between atherosclerosis and raised TG is probably accounted for by an associated link with reduced HDL
- Coronary risk correlates more closely with total plasma ChE than any one fraction
- Diets high in total lipids and with a high ratio of saturated to unsaturated fats raise plasma ChE levels, especially the VLDL/LDL fraction, and this favours the formation of atheroma
- Diets low in saturated fats and ChE and relatively high in unsaturated fats reduce atherogenic plasma lipids and this reduces an individual's susceptibility to atheroma formation
- Lowering plasma lipids by diet or drugs will not only retard progression of atherosclerotic lesions but may also reverse them
- Retarding or reversing lesions will reduce the mortality and morbidity from the associated clinical syndromes, including ischaemic heart disease

Terminology

Dyslipidaemia – abnormality in one or more of blood lipid fractions

Hyperlipidaemia – elevation of one or more of blood lipid fractions with familial hyperlipidaemia have long been known to suffer a high incidence of premature atherosclerotic disease. A similar pattern is seen in diabetics, whose lipid metabolism is also disturbed. However, the relationship between dietary lipid and plasma lipid, especially cholesterol, and the mechanisms controlling the metabolism, transport and interconversions of lipid within the body, are incompletely understood. Note that plasma cholesterol derives from the body pool of cholesterol, which itself comes mainly from hepatic synthesis (75%), with only a quarter from dietary cholesterol. This is why although dieting often helps to reduce lipid levels moderately in many patients, even the most rigorous diet may not reduce plasma lipids sufficiently in some. Moreover, dietary saturated fat has more influence on plasma cholesterol than dietary cholesterol itself.

Saturated fats (SFA, from animal sources) raise LDL levels, partly by stimulating cholesterol synthesis, and both cholesterol or saturated fats may stimulate the synthesis of aggregatory prostaglandins. Of course, some dietary SFA intake is essential.

By contrast, unsaturated fats in general (mostly oils from plant sources, also fish oils) appear to have a protective effect, possibly by increasing the breakdown of LDL. Polyunsaturated fatty acids (PUFA) are thought to be beneficial in both reducing LDL and increasing synthesis of antithrombotic anti-aggregatory factors. PUFA however, and particularly those of the n-6 series, are prone to oxidation and in large amounts may reduce HDL. Mono-unsaturated fats (MUFA; found especially in olive oil and rape oil) do not have these disadvantages. Polyunsaturates in the n-3 series (especially fish oils) appear to be protective, probably by an antithrombotic action. It is known that fish-eating populations such as the Eskimos and the Japanese have a low incidence of atherosclerosis.

Other factors

Regular exercise is protective, partly by raising plasma HDL levels and possibly by encouraging the development of collateral blood vessels. Both exercise and low-fat diets may reduce BP, and hypertension is an independent atheroma risk factor. A large number of other substances have been implicated in the aetiology and pathogenesis of IHD, including dietary factors (e.g. folic acid and flavinoids) and other plasma constituents (e.g. lipoprotein a, homocysteine, fibrinogen).

The evidence

The lipid hypothesis is supported by such epidemiological observations as: (i) the correlation between the mean plasma cholesterol levels of different population groups (even those with relatively low mean levels) and their prevalence of atherosclerosis; and (ii) the decline in heart disease among large population groups who have reduced dietary lipid intake, e.g. in the USA and Finland.

The role of pharmacological intervention with lipid-lowering drugs in secondary prevention is now well established, even in patients without initially high lipid levels, and their use in primary prevention is justified in risk/benefit terms for those at a high risk of developing IHD. Three major intervention trials reporting from different parts of the world in the past 5 years have provided persuasive evidence of the benefits of reducing lipid levels on morbidity and mortality from IHD (and stroke). They have also shown that using *statin* lipid-lowering drugs to do so significantly improves the outcome, with very little added risk.

The Scandinavian **4S** trial targeted secondary prevention in over 4000 patients with hyperlipidaemia and existing IHD (angina or MI); the **CARE** trial 4000 was similar, but patients had near-average lipid levels. The Scottish **WOSCOPS** trial involved primary prevention in over 6000 men with hyperlipidaemia but no ischaemic symptoms. In all cases the beneficial effects were correlated with the reduction in lipid levels.

The only step in the lipid hypothesis not yet firmly supported by major clinical trial evidence is whether reducing lipid levels can bring about regression of established atheromatous plaques. Empirically this might seem unlikely because atheromas are organized structures, and not simple fatty deposits; nevertheless, some lipid-lowering trials have appeared to demonstrate increased arterial patency.

Pathogenesis

The precise sequence of events leading to the development of an atheromatous plaque is complex and incompletely understood. In an evolving plaque there are chronic immuno-inflammatory cells such as T lymphocytes, macrophages and fibroblasts, together with a wide variety of mediators and cytokines with chemotactic, cytotoxic, growth promoting, pro-aggregatory and pro-inflammatory actions. This supports the concept of atheroma being primarily a protective mechanism. In addition, in the latest modification to the lipid hypothesis, a primary causative role is given to an abnormally oxidized form of LDL. It is as yet uncertain exactly how and where the LDL becomes oxidized, but it is likely to be after uptake into the intima; macrophages, endothelial cells

and smooth muscle cells may be involved. The process may in part result from an imbalance between pro-oxidant factors and natural anti-oxidant substances such as tocopherol (vitamin E), carotene (vitamin A) and ascorbate (vitamin C). This of course has important implications for possible preventative measures.

Figure 3.26 integrates current knowledge to give an overall picture of the process. It is necessarily a simplified summary of complex and poorly understood events, but will serve to identify potential targets for therapeutic intervention.

Following endothelial damage, LDL particles gain access to the intima. Here their components are oxidized by peroxidase enzyme and thereby are rendered immuno-active (particularly the oxidized apoprotein component) as well as perhaps doing further direct damage. Part of the

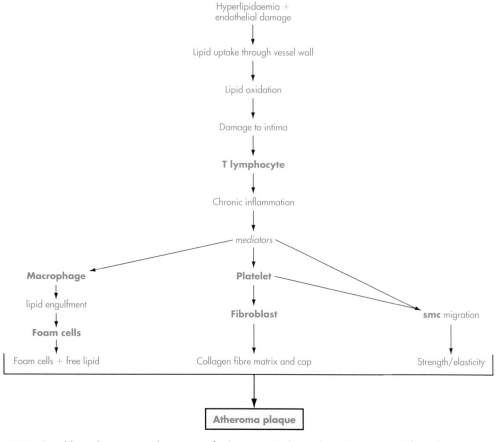

Figure 3.26 Possible pathways in pathogenesis of atheroma. Mediators have been omitted from the diagram. smc, smooth muscle cell.

protective action of HDL may be in antagonizing this process, or removing oxidized LDL particles before they do harm. Otherwise, T lymphocytes recognize the particles as foreign and secrete mediators that recruit other immune cells, as well as causing further local inflammatory damage. Macrophages displaying receptors for oxidized LDL scavenge it by phagocytosis, forming 'foam cells', some of which break down to release free lipid.

The process may cease at this point, resulting in relatively innocuous 'fatty streaks' of little haemodynamic consequence within arteries. Such lesions are often found in young otherwise healthy adults, but there is still debate over whether they are early signs of clinical atherosclerosis or a separate harmless phenomenon.

If the risk factors persist, the defence mechanisms may be overwhelmed. Platelets are attracted and secrete chemotaxins and platelet-derived growth factor (PDGF). This induces smooth muscle cells to migrate from the media into the intima, and fibroblasts to start producing collagen fibres. Local angiotensin may also contribute to growth promotion, providing one possible prophylactic role for ACEIs. The con-

nective tissue matrix of the developing atheroma is thus strengthened, and eventually a protective fibrous cap forms over the lipid and foam cells, and this becomes overgrown by new endothelial cells. A stable plaque will have a high proportion of fibrous components whereas an unstable one – which is liable to rupture and thrombosis – has more macrophages and lipid.

Progression and outcome

Chronic vascular obstruction may follow a number of courses (Fig. 3.27). The most benign outcome is repair or resolution, with perhaps a small degree of residual obstruction. New blood channels may eventually be formed (recanalization). However, slow progression of the flow restriction is more usual, with gradually worsening symptoms, e.g. angina or **intermittent claudication**.

Sometimes there will be an acute exacerbation, with complete arterial occlusion. This may be the result of platelet aggregation, thrombosis or perhaps the rupture and haemorrhage of a weakened atheroma cap. This usually occurs in coronary or cerebral vessels, resulting in myocardial

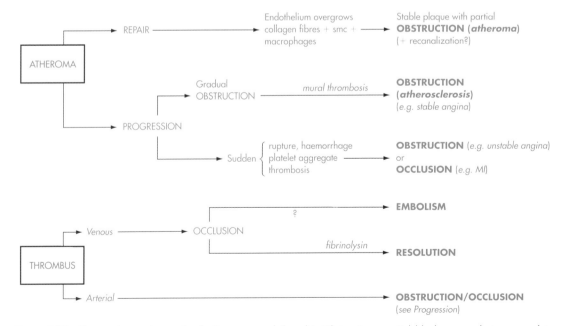

Figure 3.27   Progression and sequels of atheromas and thrombi. Obstruction, partial blockage; occlusion, complete blockage. MI, myocardial infarction; smc, smooth muscle cell.

or cerebral infarction (MI or stroke). Figure 3.28 shows the transverse section of an artery severely obstructed by an atherosclerotic plaque.

Myocardial ischaemia

Why the heart?

The general clinical consequences of ischaemia were discussed in Chapter 2 (pp. 48–50). The factors which make the heart particularly sensitive are:

- The myocardium has a high O_2 demand and high O_2 extraction.
- The heart works continuously.
- There are relatively few coronary collateral vessels.

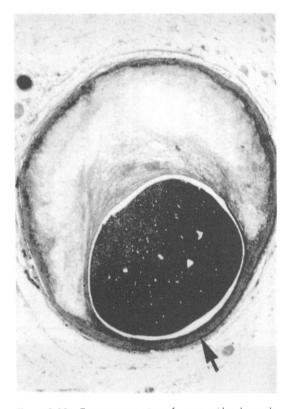

Figure 3.28 Transverse section of artery with atherosclerotic lesion. This photomicrograph shows a much thickened asymmetrical intimal lesion and considerable narrowing of the lumen. The arrow points to normal arterial wall. The dark mass within the lumen is an artefact. (Reproduced with permission from Davies (1985) *Med Int* **20**: 1.)

- Myocardial cells regenerate poorly after damage.
- The heart is an integrated organ.

Unlike the brain and kidney – the other main organs that are sensitive to ischaemia – the whole heart functions in an integrated manner so that malfunction of any part will have a disproportionate effect on overall efficiency. As it is not composed of many identical functional subunits, the heart cannot divert function from damaged areas to healthy ones. The efficient ejection of blood requires coordinated contraction, and the process uses the whole myocardium to conduct the electrical excitation, so even small areas of ischaemia or necrosis can severely reduce pump performance.

Thus the heart is a prime target for circulatory insufficiency, and because it is such a vital organ the results are almost always serious. This is why IHD is such a problem. Furthermore, atheromas seem to be preferentially deposited in the coronary circulation. This may be a consequence of the anatomy because coronary flow is retrograde (backwards towards the heart) and thus potentially turbulent (p. 62). Because the left ventricle has the greatest oxygen demand and the most vasculature, coronary atherosclerosis usually affects the left ventricle.

Myocardial oxygen balance

The degree of ischaemia in a tissue depends on the balance between oxygen supply and oxygen demand. Myocardial oxygen **demand** varies according to circulatory requirements. Assuming that blood is adequately oxygenated, myocardial oxygen **supply** is normally determined by the calibre of the coronary vessels and coronary perfusion pressure. The calibre is altered mainly by reflex autoregulation. The perfusion pressure is the difference between pressure in the left ventricle at the end of diastole (LVEDP) and mean aortic pressure. This balance between supply and demand can be disturbed by either excessive demand or reduced supply.

Excessive myocardial demand
The fixed lesions of atherosclerosis limit the extent of the dilatation that can be induced by

autoregulation (or drugs). Thus while coronary perfusion may be adequate at rest, at some point during escalating effort blood flow will be unable to increase sufficiently to meet the rising demand. Because normally the myocardium has few collateral vessels, the area beyond a lesion will become ischaemic.

Symptoms only become evident after 75% of the lumen of a major coronary vessel has become obstructed. There will be no permanent damage to the myocardium if effort, and thus cardiac workload, are promptly reduced. The ischaemia is partial and is reversed when oxygen demand falls. This produces the typical clinical picture of acute predictable onset and rapid reversibility that is characteristic of classical angina pectoris (often called 'angina of effort').

Restricted oxygen supply

If an event such as thrombus formation produces complete occlusion, or greater than 90% obstruction, then myocardial anoxia occurs. The precipitating event may be unrelated to excessive effort or exertion. If this occlusion is not reversed within about 6 h the anoxic myocardial tissue will die: this is myocardial infarction (MI). Alternatively, there may be severe but transient, reversible spasm of one or more sections of either atheromatous or apparently normal coronary artery. This may account for 'variant' or Prinzmetal angina. (Intermediate stages, known as the acute coronary syndrome, can also occur; see below.)

Clinical consequences

Angina and MI, although very similar pathologically, represent two distinct clinical entities which can exist independently. Angina is not invariably a precursor of MI and not all angina patients go on to suffer MI. Their differential pathogenesis is illustrated in Fig. 3.29.

Other cardiac abnormalities may follow from myocardial ischaemia, possibly without even causing symptoms. Numerous small, subclinical infarcts can produce a widely disseminated patchy

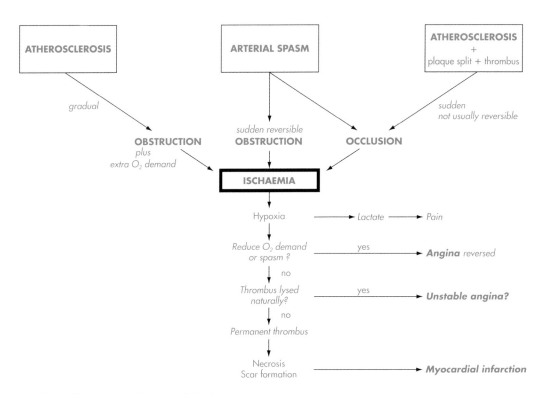

Figure 3.29   Pathogenesis of myocardial ischaemia.

fibrosis of the myocardium leading to dilated cardiomyopathy and chronic **heart failure**, without the patient ever complaining of typical ischaemic pain. Twenty-four-hour ECG monitoring has shown that this so-called 'silent ischaemia' may be more common than was formerly supposed. Heart failure also frequently follows frank MI.

Ischaemia may affect conducting tissue as well as cardiac muscle, either acutely (during MI) or chronically leading to **arrhythmias**. Ventricular fibrillation may account for many cases of unexplained sudden death.

Less commonly, ischaemic symptoms may occur unassociated with any coronary obstruction, not even vasospasm. Examples include:

- Excessive cardiac oxygen demand (e.g. thyrotoxicosis).
- Severely reduced supply (e.g. severe anaemia).
- Reduced coronary perfusion pressure, as in hypertrophic cardiomyopathy, aortic stenosis (raised LVEDP) and cardiogenic shock (inadequate aortic pressure).

Ischaemic pain is probably related to the accumulation of the products of anaerobic metabolism, e.g. acid or lactate. However, the picture of angina or MI pain as a type of muscle cramp, although adequate for most purposes, is probably an oversimplification.

Prevention and treatment

Primary prevention theoretically implies preventing the atherosclerotic process from starting whereas **secondary** prevention means taking measures to limit or perhaps reverse damage that is discovered subsequently. In practice however, primary prevention is usually extended to mean preventing the appearance of signs or symptoms of ischaemia, even though clinically silent atheromas may be present. Unfortunately, most patients only discover they have atherosclerosis when symptoms (which may not be cardiovascular, but usually are) first occur, in which case secondary prevention is the best that can be offered. Nevertheless, much effort is being put into attempting to change the habits of whole communities so as to reduce the prevalence of the disease and its multi-organ consequences.

Tables 3.29 and 3.31 indicate the general approach. Of the primary modifiable risks, diabetes is discussed in Chapter 9 and hypertension on pp. 93–115 of this chapter. Smoking and its cessation are issues that are too broad for

Table 3.31   Reducing risk factors for atherosclerosis

Recommendation	Rationale – pathological factor targeted
Stop smoking	Vascular endothelium, platelets
Reduce salt intake	Blood pressure
Reduce cholesterol intake	Cholesterol absorption
Reduce saturated fat[a]	Cholesterol synthesis
Increase unsaturated fat[a]	LDL level; *also* encourage anti-aggregatory mediators, etc.
Increase fibre intake[b]	Lipid absorption?
Increase fresh fruit and vegetable intake	Lipid level; *also* provide anti-oxidants
Moderate alcohol intake	Blood pressure; *also* protect against atheroma?
Moderate exercise	Blood pressure and lipid level; *also* encourage coronary collateral vessel development
Reduce sugar intake	Calorie intake/weight
'Reduce stress'	Reduce atheroma formation?
Aim for ideal body weight	Lipid level, cardiac load, blood pressure

[a] Fats to provide no more that 30% total energy intake: 10% as saturated fat, 10% as n-3 polyunsaturated fat, and 10% as monounsaturated fat.

[b] Non-starch polysaccharide (NSP), 'soluble fibre'.

consideration here, but are discussed briefly in Chapter 5 (Respiratory disease) and Chapter 11 (Neoplastic disease). We will focus here on the management of hyperlipidaemia.

Hyperlipidaemia

The pathology of this complex issue was discussed above (pp. 120 and 123). The current non-drug prophylaxis recommendations are summarized in Table 3.31, and the reader is directed to the References and further reading section for detailed reviews.

The current target is to reduce total plasma cholesterol below 5 mmol/L, and there is a trend to aim for even lower levels. Earlier fears that reducing plasma lipid, especially LDL, to too low a level is associated with an increase in non-cardiac morbidity and mortality, mainly from depression, suicide and other violent death (e.g. accident), have not been borne out by large-scale trials.

Primary prevention

The major problem with interventions to reduce the lipid level lies in identifying the threshold of risk. As with blood pressure (see Fig. 3.18), total plasma cholesterol varies unimodally throughout the population, and an increased risk can be demonstrated at levels near or even below the population average (6 mmol/L for middle-aged males in the UK). Thus a risk stratification approach analogous to that used for managing hypertension has to be adopted. The intervention threshold for a given patient must be based not just on their lipid level but also on the presence of other atherosclerosis risk factors and existing ischaemic symptoms. This is balanced against the inherent risk of the intervention. However, universal lipid screening is not currently cost-effective; thus opportunistic screening needs to be targeted on high-risk groups (Table 3.29).

As with hypertension, the initial approach is for abnormal readings to be repeated; if hyperlipidaemia is confirmed, possible underlying secondary causes must then be eliminated. The risk/benefit analysis is then done. This is aided by an algorithm such as the 'Sheffield table', which recommends evidence-based treatment

thresholds for hyperlipidaemic patients of different ages with various combinations of major coronary risk factors (see References and further reading).

Unless the cholesterol level is dangerously high (>10 mmol/L approx.) or there are other risk factors, the first step is to initiate non-drug methods and to try them for 3–6 months. Simple risk factor reduction (lifestyle recommendations and dietary measures) would be suitable for an asymptomatic younger non-smoking patient with normal BP, no family history and a total cholesterol level under 6.5 mmol/L (7.8 mmol/L in younger women). If this fails, or there are other risk factors, then drug therapy is the next stage, as shown by the WOSCOPS trial. A cholesterol level greater than 8 mmol/L will usually require drug treatment eventually in all patients.

Secondary prevention

The decision is simpler if a patient already has ischaemic symptoms or has suffered a MI or stroke. There is now ample evidence of the benefits of lipid-lowering drugs in almost all patients after MI or unstable angina whether the lipid level is high (4S trial) or not (CARE trial).

The presence of disabling ischaemic symptoms would indicate the need for prompt surgical intervention.

Risk factor reduction

The individual risk and community load of IHD in particular and atherosclerosis in general can be reduced by targeting known risk factors through health promotion and regular screening. Most of the advice coincides with the general tenets of a healthy life, and is in many ways similar to specific recommendations for reducing hypertension (pp. 93–115); of course keeping BP within normal limits itself reduces atherosclerosis. However, hypertension screening and medication compliance are notoriously poor. The difficulties of smoking cessation are well known. Dietary habits also are difficult to change, but average reductions of 10–15% in serum cholesterol can be achieved in this way.

There is still a long way to go in changing public perceptions and practices regarding a healthy lifestyle, but there is epidemiological evidence from, for example from the USA and Finland, that population-wide changes can produce significant falls in atherosclerosis prevalence. A prolonged reduction of no more than 0.6 mmol/L – which can be achieved by dietary means alone – has been shown to reduce the incidence of coronary disease by 30%.

Drug therapy

Drug therapy is indicated in secondary prevention and for primary prevention of IHD in high-risk individuals.

Lipid-lowering therapy

The *hydroxymethyl-glutaryl-CoA reductase inhibitors* (HMGIs, or 'statins') have emerged as the drugs of choice, and appear to have few serious adverse effects. Although currently expensive, these agents cause a significantly reduced rate of coronary events and slow progression of atherosclerotic lesions. There are few significant adverse effects. Other agents such as the *fibrates* and the *bile-salt binding resins* may be added if necessary. For the detailed pharmacotherapy of hyperlipidaemia the reader is directed to the References and further reading section.

Antiplatelet therapy

Secondary prevention of MI and stroke routinely involves *aspirin*. The recent understanding of the role of inflammation in atheroma has further validated this approach and newer less gastro-toxic and broader-spectrum platelet inhibitors are being developed or undergoing trial. *Ticlopidine* and *clopidogrel* are more effective than aspirin, blocking a different pathway to platelet aggregatory factor synthesis. The former has a relatively high incidence of neutropenia and blood counts are essential; the latter is safer.

The final common aggregation pathway involves the platelet membrane fibrinogen receptor, glycoprotein gIIb/IIIa, and blockers of this have been developed. Chimeric glycoprotein receptor antibody fragments such as *abciximab*, and direct inhibitors such as *eptifibatide*, are promising, and may be used more widely when oral preparations become available. Other uses for these drugs include post-angioplasty situations and in unstable angina.

Future possibilities include the use of *antibiotics*, if an aetiological role for chronic infection in atherosclerosis is eventually defined, and *angiogenic growth factors*, which promote the growth of new collateral blood channels around the obstruction. Older antiplatelet drugs rarely used now include dipyridamole and sulfinpyrazone.

Vascular surgery

Revascularization is only indicated in secondary prevention or emergency treatment. Coronary bypass and angioplasty will be discussed in the sections on angina and MI below.

Angina pectoris

Definition and classification

Angina is both defined and diagnosed by clinical criteria. Typical ischaemic cardiac pain is retrosternal (behind the breastbone), intense, diffuse rather than sharp, and gripping, constricting or suffocating: patients describe the sensation of having their chest crushed by a bear-hug. Yet even when it radiates to the upper arms, neck or jaw on either side it may be difficult to distinguish from severe dyspepsia, 'heartburn' or oesophageal pain (*see* Chapter 6), or pericarditis, so other signs must also be sought.

In **classical angina** pain comes on acutely following exertion, and is relieved within a few minutes by resting or by taking buccal or sublingual *glyceryl trinitrate* (GTN). Attacks occur predictably at the same level of effort. Coronary atherosclerosis is almost invariably present. A minority (about 10%) of patients suffer from a **variant** (**Prinzmetal**) form, where attacks are unpredictable and may occur even at rest, although commonly under emotional stress. In such cases there may be no permanent coronary obstruction, the attacks being due to reversible vasospasm.

Clinical features, investigation and diagnosis

Angina can be triggered by any circumstances which acutely increase cardiac workload (Table

Table 3.32   Trigger factors, symptoms and signs of an angina attack

Trigger factors

Exertion, e.g. climbing stairs, sexual intercourse
Emotion – increased heart rate
Heavy meals – increased gastrointestinal perfusion
Getting into a cold bed
Going out in cold windy weather } peripheral vasoconstriction raises peripheral resistance

Symptoms

Onset: pain builds up over seconds or minutes (not instantaneous)
Crushing, constricting, dull central chest pain
Relieved by rest or glyceryl trinitrate
Radiation of pain into throat, left jaw and arm, occasionally into back and right arm
Tachycardia, sweating, anxiety
Breathlessness

Signs

ECG[a]   between attacks – normal
          during attack   – classical: ST segment depressed
                              variant: ST segment elevated

[a] See also Fig. 3.30.

3.32). The clinical features are highly suggestive and rapid relief with GTN is almost conclusive. However, in ambiguous cases an exercise ECG, e.g. on a treadmill, will usually show reversible ST segment changes (Fig. 3.30). The resting ECG is usually normal but may show evidence of a past, possibly silent MI (Fig. 3.30(d)) or of myocardial hypertrophy (possibly resulting from untreated hypertension) which would show as an elevated R-wave. In variant angina, ST elevation is more common but the exercise test may not cause an attack, and 24-h ambulatory ECG monitoring can be valuable.

More invasive tests are rarely justified in moderate stable disease. Angiography (Fig. 3.31) or isotope scans are reserved for unstable angina or evaluation before surgery because their results would otherwise not affect management. Moreover, patients with little objective obstruction may have severe symptoms, while evidence of extensive atherosclerosis is sometimes found in patients who complain little. Angiography indicates objective severity and provides a baseline

for assessing progress. In general, the elderly seem less likely to experience ischaemic pain, and neuropathy in diabetics can disguise it.

A functional assessment is essential – at what point does the pain occur and what does it prevent the patient doing? Angina can be graded using the NYHA functional scale (p. 68).

Course and prognosis

Many angina patients have such slowly progressive disease that it causes little disability. Nevertheless, their mortality rate is on average about four times that of those without coronary disease, some eventually dying of MI. The rate of progression depends partly on how early the disease is detected and partly on what measures are taken to reduce risk factors, although the effectiveness of such measures once symptoms have become evident is uncertain. The 5-year mortality rate for moderate stable uncomplicated angina involving only one main coronary vessel

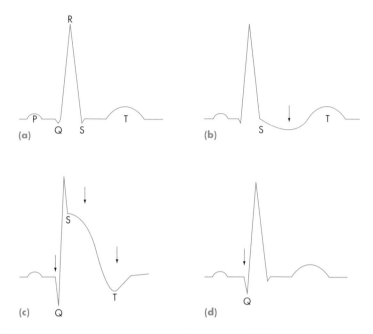

Figure 3.30   ECG changes in myocardial ischaemia. (a) Normal trace. (b) Myocardial ischaemia typical of an angina attack, the ST segment is depressed. (c) Early myocardial infarction (MI), with Q depression and ST elevation; the latter gradually returns to normal over the course of weeks. (d) Months or years after MI; the abnormal Q wave, indicative of permanent infarct, persists long after the patient has recovered from acute symptoms. Note: In myocardial hypertrophy the R-wave is elevated.

is less than 10%, but this may be doubled if more risk factors are involved.

Some patients experience an acceleration of symptoms with a rapidly reducing exercise tolerance and unpredictable attacks, often unassociated with exercise or their accustomed trigger factors. This is **unstable angina**, also termed crescendo or pre-infarction angina or acute coronary insufficiency. It is likely that at this stage the plaque is starting to rupture, and platelet aggregates or small thrombi (or both) are forming transiently but being cleared naturally before frank infarction supervenes; there may also be some spasm. This represents a medical emergency, because without aggressive prophylaxis in a coronary care unit, half such patients would go on to develop MI.

Many **MI**s are preceded by similar, if perhaps accelerated, phenomena and this dynamic process continues after symptoms develop. Thus infarction is to be viewed not as a one-off event but as a process evolving over 12–24 h, so that

antithrombotic and fibrinolytic therapy may be beneficial over a longer period than was at first thought.

Management

Aims and strategy

The overall aim in the management of angina is to minimize myocardial ischaemia. There are three objectives:

1. To abolish the symptoms of an acute attack.
2. To prevent or minimize the frequency of symptomatic or silent myocardial ischaemia.
3. To reduce the progression of the underlying atherosclerosis.

In prophylaxis and acute management the main strategy is to manipulate favourably the oxygen supply/demand balance (Table 3.33). For long-term management, coronary risk factors must also be reduced.

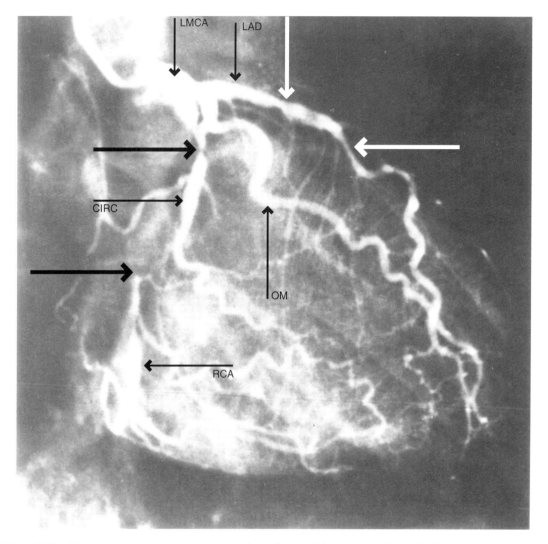

Figure 3.31   Coronary angiogram showing severe atherosclerosis. Obstructions, indicated by heavy arrows, occur on three main coronary arteries ('three-vessel disease'). Those in the left anterior descending (LAD) and circumflex (CIRC) coronary arteries reduce perfusion. The right coronary artery (RCA) shows retrograde filling distal to the obstruction, via collaterals. Also labelled are the left main (LMCA) and oblique marginal (OM) coronary arteries. (Reproduced with permission from Gotto (1977) *Atherosclerosis*. Upjohn, Kalamazoo: Scope Publications.)

Reducing oxygen demand

As in heart failure, drug therapy is mainly aimed at 'unloading' the heart. However, there are important differences. Negative inotropes (especially the *beta-blockers*), although usually contraindicated in heart failure, are very useful in angina. On the other hand, care is needed with simple arterial dilators. If used alone they can produce reflex tachycardia which will increase cardiac work, and so combination with beta-blockers is preferable. Alternatively, a cardiodepressant *calcium channel blocker* can serve both functions. The *nitrates* mainly act indirectly (both acutely and in prophylaxis) by peripheral venodilation: they dilate the great veins and reduce venous return, so rapidly reducing CO and thus cardiac work; they also dilate arteries.

It is equally important to improve overall car-

Table 3.33   Rectifying myocardial oxygen imbalance

Strategy	Methods	Example
Reduce oxygen demand		
Reduce cardiac workload		
Reduce perfusion demands	Rest	
	Avoid stress	
	Stop smoking	
	Reduce weight	
Reduce preload	Venodilator	Nitrate
Reduce afterload	Arterial dilator	Ca-blocker, nitrate[a]
Reduce rate/contractility	Negative inotrope	Beta-blocker, Ca-blocker
Improve cardiac efficiency	Improve fitness	Exercise, stop smoking
Improve oxygen supply		
Increase coronary flow	Arterial dilator	Ca-blocker, nitrate[a]
	Surgery	Bypass, angioplasty
Prevent further obstruction		
Reduce progression of atherosclerosis	↓ Risk factors	Diet, stop smoking, etc.
	Antiplatelet?	Aspirin
	Lipid-lowering?	Statin, fibrate

[a] Nitrates are predominantly acute venodilators, but in chronic use also affect arteries.
Ca-blocker, calcium channel blocker.

diovascular efficiency. Regular moderate exercise enables the best use to be made of reduced myocardial capacity. Stopping smoking improves oxygen carriage in the blood by reducing carboxyhaemoglobin levels, and this reduces cardiac output requirements. Thus despite drug treatment which apparently reduces cardiac performance, i.e. reducing preload and contractility, there may be no fall in absolute exercise capacity.

Improving oxygen supply
This is generally more difficult because most angina is caused by fixed lesions. If the atheroma occupies less than about 60% of the arterial circumference, which is uncommon in symptomatic angina, *arterial dilators* may be beneficial by direct action on the obstructed part of the coronary vessel. However, there will usually be maximal physiological autoregulatory dilatation. Indeed, vessels near the diseased artery may be preferentially dilated by autoregulation or vasodilators, thereby diverting blood away from the deprived region and exacerbating symptoms ('coronary steal').

In variant angina, caused mainly by vasospasm, vasodilators work mainly by direct action on the coronary arteries. Recent angiographic studies also suggest that transient vasospasm superimposed on fixed obstructions may contribute more to classical angina pain than has been assumed, thus providing a role for coronary vasodilation.

In severe advanced angina, with almost complete blockage of one or more main coronary arteries, surgery becomes necessary. In **coronary bypass** a length of vessel, taken from a leg vein or from the more conveniently located internal mammary artery, is grafted between the aorta and a site beyond the obstructing lesion. This can produce dramatic improvements in symptoms but unfortunately atherosclerosis at the same site tends to recur after 5–10 years.

Percutaneous transluminal coronary angioplasty (PTCA) is a much less invasive technique.

In this method a special coronary catheter is inserted via a peripheral artery until a small balloon at its tip rests adjacent to the plaque. Inflation of the balloon either breaks up the plaque, flattens or stretches it, or stretches the surrounding vessel wall. The patient is *heparinized* for the procedure; this is followed by a short course of intensive antiplatelet therapy (e.g. *aspirin + ticlopidine*), then aspirin indefinitely. Subsequent microembolization occasionally causes further obstructions (less than 1% of cases).

Angioplasty has few other complications and avoids the need for open-heart surgery. Recurrence of plaque occurs in about 35% of cases, but the procedure may be repeated. The technique is also used for other stenosed arteries, including the femoral and renal arteries.

A technique which is rapidly becoming standard procedure following coronary angioplasty is to place a rigid net-like tubular supporting structure or **stent** intra-arterially at the site of the lesion. Costing around £1000, these alloy devices are up to a few centimetres long and about the diameter of the vessel being remodelled. After insertion, the stent eventually becomes overgrown with new endothelium. The use of stents has led to a significant reduction in the restenosis rate.

Prevent further obstruction

General measures such as stopping smoking, losing weight, keeping fit, modifying diet, etc. are an essential part of initial angina management, and are aimed at either directly inhibiting further atheroma (e.g. smoking) or reducing other risk factors (e.g. obesity, hypertension or hyperlipidaemia). The onset of angina symptoms renders the patient receptive to such advice.

As noted above (pp. 127–129), the risk–benefit ratio at present also favours giving *lipid-lowering agent*s to all symptomatic angina patients. Lifelong low-dose *aspirin* (75–150 mg daily) has also proved to be beneficial in preventing further complications, and should also be used if tolerated.

Acute attack

Glyceryl trinitrate

The tradit ional sublingual GTN has yet to be bettered for rapid symptomatic relief (Table 3.34). Patients should be encouraged to anticipate situations which will provoke an attack, and use GTN prophylactically immediately beforehand, which keeps the ischaemic burden to a minimum.

If a patient complains of worsening or accelerating symptoms, with declining effectiveness of

---

Table 3.34   Use of glyceryl trinitrate for acute angina attacks

Mode of action	Peripheral venodilatation → reduced preload Coronary vasodilation?
Rapid effect	Buccal/sublingual absorption • avoids delay in absorption • effect within 1 min; lasts 30 min • may be chewed for more rapid effect • avoids hepatic first-pass metabolism • sublingual aerosol available
Side effects (vasodilaton)	Hypotension – patients advised to sit when taking Flushing Headache (often regarded as an index of effectiveness)
Stability	Volatile, easily absorbable – use tightly sealed glass containers, with foil lined closures To be discarded 8 weeks after dispensing Buccal m/r and aerosol formulations more stable – longer shelf-life

his or her tablets, poor storage rather than unstable angina may be to blame (Table 3.35). The absence of side effects such as headache and flushing is a marker for either non-compliance or inactive tablets. For patients who use GTN only infrequently, the buccal aerosol formulation is preferable because it has greater stability and thus a longer shelf-life after dispensing. It also has a more prompt action.

Calcium blockers
Some patients, presumably with a component of coronary spasm, obtain relief by biting nifedipine capsules and swallowing the fluid contents to speed gastric absorption. (There is no point is keeping the contents in the mouth because nifedipine is not absorbed buccally.)

Prophylaxis

Atherosclerosis prophylaxis. This was discussed on pp. 120–122.

Beta-blockers. These are first choice unless contraindicated (*see* Table 3.23). In addition to the details given on pp. 109–111, a number of specific points about the use of beta-blockers in angina should be noted:

- Their action in secondary protection following MI has been clearly demonstrated.

- They improve exercise capacity.
- They are contraindicated in coronary spasm (e.g. Prinzmetal angina) because they permit unopposed coronary alpha-constrictor tone.
- Withdrawal, if necessary, should be slow (over 4 weeks) to avoid rebound exacerbation or even MI (owing to up-regulated receptors).
- Cardiospecific drugs are preferred.
- Drugs without intrinsic sympathomimetic activity are preferred (reduced likelihood of reflex tachycardia).

Formerly, a resting heart rate of about 60–70 beats/min was the therapeutic target, but a more reliable predictor of effectiveness might be the limitation of exertional tachycardia to 100 beats/min. This permits higher doses.

Calcium blockers. These are often successful if beta-blocker therapy fails or is inappropriate (*see* pp. 112–113); they are the first choice for variant angina. Those with considerable negative chronotropic and inotropic action as well as vasodilation, e.g. *verapamil*, *diltiazem*, which may be beneficial provided that ventricular function is adequate (and not in combination with a beta-blocker). Otherwise, a dihydropyridine (e.g. *nifedipine*) is used, although these can cause reflex tachycardia. Calcium blockers are perhaps better tolerated than beta-blockers and are suitable for a wider variety of patients. At present it would seem wise to avoid using any short-acting formulations of the dihydropyridines (p. 113).

Nitrates. These act as in heart failure to reduce preload, with lesser effects on afterload and coronary vessels. Various formulations of organic nitrates are available to help counteract the problems of this group, which are related to vasodilatation or tolerance (Tables 3.34 and 3.35). The former may prevent up to a quarter of patients from using nitrates. The latter requires a daily 'washout' period of low plasma level; e.g. overnight, in the absence of nocturnal attacks, and *vice versa*. It occurs because sulfhydryl (-SH) groups on receptors become saturated and can no longer produce NO from the nitrate for dilatation.

Topical GTN patches are expensive and offer little advantage except the psychological benefit

Table 3.35 Problems with nitrates in angina prophylaxis, and possible solutions

Problems	Solutions
Poor bioavailability First-pass metabolism Variable absorption Brief action	Alternative dose forms: • sublingual metered-dose aerosol • high-dose sustained release • chewable sustained release • percutaneous (patch) Use mononitrates (primary metabolite)
Ready tolerance	10-h daily washout period

of direct application to the chest, or other patient preference. Unless used with care they may even exacerbate tolerance, which is encouraged by a stable plasma level. Buccal m/r preparations provide a combination of prompt and sustained action.

Because there is no convenient clinical index of plasma levels, such as bradycardia with beta-blockers, dose adjustment is imprecise.

Potassium channel openers. These drugs, e.g. *nicorandil*, combine nitrate-like venodilator action (due to NO production) with calcium blocker-like arterial dilatation. Theoretically they could replace a combination of nitrate and calcium channel blocker, with the potential advantage that nitrate intolerance would be masked by the arterial dilator action. They have not yet found their optimal role in therapy and tend to be reserve drugs.

Drug selection

All patients have regular aspirin and GTN as required. Those with hyperlipidaemia have this addressed (*see* pp. 127–129). If prophylaxis is indicated, then beta-blockers are preferred. Other choices for monotherapy are shown in Fig. 3.32. It is rare that a patient is unable to take either beta-blockers or calcium blockers. If either of these alone fails, a variety of synergistic dual therapies are available. Some have particular advantages, e.g. a beta-blocker plus calcium channel blocker counteracts the peripheral constriction induced by the former, and the tachycardia induced by the latter. A dihydropyridine calcium blocker should be chosen to avoid myocardial depression. The tendency to tachycardia induced by nitrates is countered by the bradycardia induced by diltiazem or beta-blockers. Hypotension can occur with a nitrate plus a calcium blocker (in which case the dihydropy-

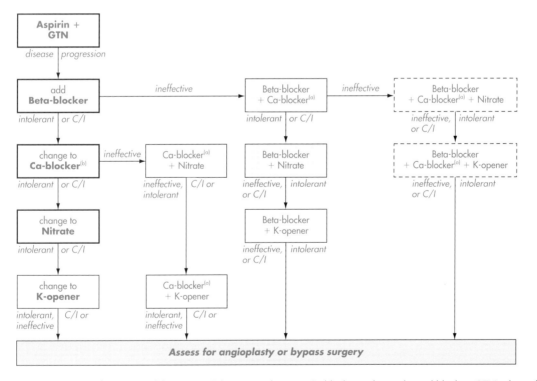

Figure 3.32   Drug selection in stable angina. C/I, contraindication; Ca-blocker, calcium channel blocker; GTN, glyceryl trinitrate; K-opener, potassium channel opener. [a] Dihydropyridine group. [b] Verapamil.

ridines should be avoided). The role of potassium openers in combinations is not yet established.

Most patients will be well-controlled on dual therapy, but triple therapy is sometimes used. Otherwise, failure of dual therapy is an indication that the patient is a candidate for angioplasty or bypass surgery.

Unstable angina

Prompt attention is required to prevent an MI developing. Admission to a coronary care unit should be arranged and management is much as for a suspected MI (pp. 138–139). The therapeutic aims are:

- To reduce cardiac oxygen demand – *nitrate and beta-blocker*.
- To provide anti-platelet therapy – *aspirin*.
- To provide antithrombotic therapy – *heparin*.

The patient should take sublingual GTN and 300 mg aspirin immediately. Low-dose aspirin is continued; if aspirin is not tolerated, or if a patient is awaiting revascularization, more expensive alternatives include *ticlopidine, clopidogrel* and *abciximab*. The use of *low molecular weight heparin* (e.g. *dalteparin*) permits much easier anticoagulation than unfractionated heparin. A more predictable and consistent effect is obtained with regular twice-daily dosing without the need for syringe pumps and anticoagulant

monitoring. *Nitrate* is given intravenously at first, as is a *beta-blocker*; therapy is continued orally. If the patient does not respond within 48 h, angioplasty is indicated.

Myocardial infarction

Myocardial infarction (MI, 'heart attack', 'coronary thrombosis') occurs when a coronary vessel becomes occluded for more than about 6 h, whether or not the occlusion is subsequently relieved. However, dilatation of neighbouring vessels by autoregulation may protect the area adjacent to the ischaemic core from complete anoxia, thereby limiting infarct size. Exertion is not the most common trigger, and although MI is frequently associated with current stress or general 'life events' the patient may be unable to recall a particular precipitating event.

Angina and MI

MI is not simply an intensification of angina: it differs in a number of crucial respects (Table 3.36). Many patients have stable angina for many years and never develop an MI. For others a fatal MI is their first and last experience of myocardial ischaemia – about 50% of MIs occur without previous ischaemic symptoms.

Table 3.36   Comparison of classic angina and myocardial infarction

Angina	Myocardial infarction
Caused by atherosclerosis	Caused by atherosclerosis
Pain: severe, crushing, retrosternal, possibly radiating	Pain: severe, crushing, retrosternal, possibly radiating
Triggered by exertion	Triggers often unknown
Pain reversed on resting in a few minutes	Pain persistent
Pain relieved by GTN	Pain unrelieved by GTN
↑ Oxygen demand	↓ Oxygen supply
Partial obstruction	Complete occlusion
Myocardial hypoxia	Myocardial anoxia
Reversible	Irreversible

GTN, glyceryl trinitrate.

Pathogenesis

Role of thrombosis

Post-mortem examinations after MI almost invariably show advanced coronary atherosclerosis with a thrombotic occlusion in one vessel. 'Sudden ischaemic death' within an hour or so of the onset of symptoms – before infarction proper can develop – is probably due to ventricular fibrillation. However, these patients usually also have obstructive lesions.

Thrombi are not always found, and because early trials with anticoagulant prophylaxis were unsuccessful the original thrombosis theory was discredited. It was argued that when thrombi were found they had formed behind some other primary obstruction which had caused haemostasis and promoted secondary clotting. However, isotope studies have now identified thrombi very early in the process and the success of modern thrombolysis has confirmed the central role of thrombosis. Thus the popular term 'coronary thrombosis' has renewed validity.

Initiating event

Why should an apparently stable atheromatous plaque suddenly precipitate thrombosis and occlusion? Stress-induced acute abnormalities in both clotting factors and platelets have been proposed, but it is currently thought that a particularly lipid-rich ulcerated plaque, with low amounts of smooth muscle and fibrous support, may fissure or rupture. This exposes lipid and subendothelial structures, triggering massive platelet aggregation and thrombosis.

In the few cases where no substantial atheroma is found on angiography or at post-mortem examination the cause may be severe vasospasm or a primary platelet or clotting abnormality.

Severity

The process of infarction in general was described in Chapter 2 (pp. 46–50). If a tissue undergoes a period of anoxia, then irreversible damage occurs, followed by wound healing and organization of scar tissue. This scar tissue cannot fulfil the functions of the tissue it replaces. In the heart this means that as well as being non-contractile, the tissue is inelastic and poorly conducting. This has the following potential consequences:

- Poor contractility leads to poor ejection, i.e. systolic failure.
- Poor elasticity (reduced compliance) leads to poor filling, i.e. diastolic failure.
- Poor conductivity leads to arrhythmias.

The consequences in individual cases depend primarily on the size of the area of myocardium served by the coronary vessel that is occluded. The mildest form involves a small arteriole, resulting in a clinically silent (symptomless) infarction; however, when repeated over a long period this results in widespread 'patchy fibrosis' and eventual cardiac failure. Occlusion of larger arterioles will cause a classical presentation of MI, but if the area damaged is not too extensive the patient will survive, possibly with a degree of permanent cardiac failure. At its most severe an MI may involve one of the main coronary arteries (often the left anterior descending, which supplies most of the left ventricle; *see* Fig. 3.7, causing an **anterior infarct**), and death is likely if more than about 50% of the left ventricle is damaged. An important factor is how well developed are the patient's collateral coronary vessels.

The other factor determining outcome is how much conducting tissue is involved. Conduction across the whole myocardium is necessary for coordinated contraction, and ischaemic muscle may conduct erratically. In addition, damage to nodal tissue or nerve tracts may have a disproportionate effect because arrhythmias can compromise the function of the entire heart.

Course and prognosis

About 40% of all patients developing symptoms of MI die in the first 24 h, with half of the deaths occurring in the first hour from ventricular fibrillation, before medical help is usually available. Subsequent deaths are mainly from heart failure. The median survival time (i.e. after which only half of patients survive) is 1 year, and the 10-year survival rate is about 30%.

In the immediate post-infarction period the myocardium surrounding the developing lesion becomes hyperexcitable owing to excess sympathetic tone and the high local levels of potassium released from the damaged cells. The patient is then at great risk of a fatal arrhythmia. Some community 'coronary first aid' programmes have significantly reduced mortality. Lay people are instructed in elementary resuscitation, and the emergency services, e.g. ambulance staff and firemen, are taught the 'blind' use of defibrillators, parenteral anti-arrhythmics and in some cases thrombolytics.

The patient who survives this critical period has a reasonable prognosis: ironically, those who get to hospital include those who least need it. Many patients with uncomplicated MI require only supportive therapy and are soon discharged. Such patients may do better at home in familiar, unthreatening surroundings rather than in a stressful high-technology coronary care unit (CCU). However, the consensus view is that all suspected MI patients should preferably be assessed initially in a hospital. Poorer prognosis is indicated by older age, past history of IHD and the development of heart failure or arrhythmias.

Clinical features

Some MIs may be so mild as to be dismissed by the patient, relatives and sometimes even doctors as indigestion, especially if the patient has not had ischaemia before. It may be some time before the persistent pain brings a patient to medical attention. Angina patients, however, will recognize an MI because although the pain is familiar it persists, tends to be more severe, and is not relieved by normal medication (i.e. GTN). With large areas of myocardial damage the patient may collapse from acute heart failure or cardiogenic shock.

On admission, patients are usually cold and pale (owing to central conservation of reduced CO), clammy (due to sympathetic discharge), nauseated and breathless with rapid shallow breathing. Their great distress is due not only to severe pain but also to profound fear and anxiety.

This heightens the perception of pain because patients are literally mortally afraid. There may be hypotension, tachycardia or profound bradycardia, and signs of pulmonary oedema (crackles heard through the stethoscope).

Investigation

All patients with suspected MI are closely monitored for 72 h to confirm the diagnosis and anticipate complications. Precise diagnostic criteria vary, but generally the diagnosis depends on significant findings in at least two of three main areas:

* Clinical presentation and history.
* Progressive ECG changes.
* Progressive serum enzyme changes.

In many cases the 'classical' clinical features are absent and it can be very difficult to ascribe a cardiac cause. This is especially true of milder attacks with minimal myocardial damage and no cardiac failure, and in diabetics and the elderly. Objective criteria then become important.

ECG

Certain characteristic changes occur after a typical **transmural** MI (affecting the full myocardial thickness). The ST segment quickly becomes markedly elevated, only settling down to normal after several weeks (Fig. 3.30(d)). A 'pathological' Q-wave occurs early and persists as a permanent marker of a past MI. The particular ECG leads which detect these changes indicate the position of the infarct within the myocardium, while the magnitude of such changes indicates the severity of the MI. Less commonly, if the infarct does not affect the entire thickness of the cardiac wall, the Q-wave remains normal and the ST segment is depressed (*non-Q-wave* or subendocardial infarction).

In hospital, these time-dependent changes can be followed by continuous monitoring. A more important reason for such monitoring is the early detection of serious arrhythmias. Modern equipment will sound an alarm automatically when this happens.

Cardiac enzymes

Measurement of the serum levels of certain enzymes typically found in myocardial cells but released on injury or death, provides additional evidence (Fig. 3.33). A particular range, quantity and sequence of enzyme release is characteristic of MI. Elevation more than 15% above the normal range is diagnostic. Recently, a test for a more specific serum marker, troponin-T, has been developed. This enzyme is a component of cardiac muscle fibrils and it is detectable earlier than others and persists for about 2 weeks. In addition its presence during unstable angina indicates a greater likelihood of subsequent infarction.

Despite these simple investigations a definite diagnosis may still not be possible in mild or borderline cases. In non-Q-wave infarction there are few enzyme changes. Even so, more sophisticated invasive tests, such as angiography or isotope scanning, are rarely justified. Formerly, in doubtful cases there was little risk in assuming a genuine uncomplicated MI for which management was supportive, symptomatic and generally non-invasive. Now, the higher risk and greater expense of thrombolytic therapy, and the fact that it cannot easily be repeated in the short term (pp. 142–144), means more care has to be taken so as not to expose patients unnecessarily to thrombolysis.

Complications

About half the patients with MI who survive the first 2 h develop one or more of the complications shown in Table 3.37, mostly within the first few days. The frequency and severity of these are the best arguments for the existence of CCUs, where continuous monitoring and prompt attention are assured. If such complications do not develop, the patient is at less risk and may do better at home. The occurrence of heart failure is the single most accurate predictor of long-term outcome.

A transmural infarct may be overly compliant, bulging during systole (aneurysm), reducing ventricular output and thus causing heart failure. A septal infarct may rupture into the right ventricle. Rupture into the pericardial cavity is usually fatal but the risk is reduced by early beta-blockade. Ventricular aneurysm may persist after the infarction has healed. Non-Q-wave infarction is initially less serious but has a poorer prognosis; there is a likelihood of a full MI in the near future with a higher overall mortality than normal.

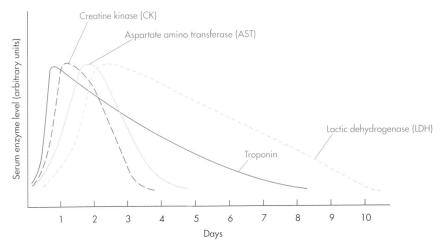

Figure 3.33 Plasma enzyme changes following myocardial infarction. Myocardial necrosis releases a characteristic group of intracellular enzymes in a characteristic sequence over the first 2 weeks. The creatine kinase MB enzyme isoform (CK-MB), more specific for cardiac muscle, is now measured.

Table 3.37 Complications of myocardial infarction

Complication	Comment
Early	
(Left) ventricular failure	Common
Pulmonary oedema	If LV failure severe
Cardiogenic shock	10% MI patients; if ventricular damage >33%
Arrhythmias, especially ventricular fibrillation, asystole	Potentially fatal; monitoring essential
Thromboembolism	Hypercoagulable state
• further infarct, stroke	• transmural infarcts (endocardial damage)
• deep vein thrombosis	• prolonged immobilisation
Hypotension/bradycardia	Autonomic imbalance
Late	
Pericarditis	First few days
Systolic stretch; ventricular aneurysm	Causes ventricular failure
Ventricular rupture	
• cardiac tamponade[a]	10% hospital MI deaths
• septal defect	Rare
Post-MI autoimmune syndrome	Pericarditis, fever, effusion

[a] Fluid within pericardium, inhibiting cardiac filling.

LV, left ventricular; MI, myocardial infarction.

Ventricular **remodelling** by dilatation and hypertrophy gradually compensates for the loss of functional myocardium, a process which may continue for up to 6 months after the infarction. Although this may be beneficial in many patients, progressive dilatation can lead to chronic ventricular failure, and cardiac enlargement is a poor prognostic factor. There is evidence that ACEIs limit this process.

Weeks or months after an infarct, and particularly after a second or third such occurrence, an autoimmune reaction to necrotic cardiac tissue (Dressler's syndrome) may develop, though this is managed with steroids.

Management

The aims in managing MI are:

- To act promptly to save life and reduce complications.
- To treat acute symptoms.
- To minimize subsequent infarct size.
- To treat complications.

- To rehabilitate.
- To ensure secondary prevention of subsequent attack.

Routine acute management

The acute management of MI is primarily symptomatic and supportive (Table 3.38). The intravenous route is preferred because reduced peripheral perfusion delays uptake from intramuscular sites, and frequent injections are more conveniently given via an *in situ* intravenous line.

Opioids are invaluable as analgesics, tranquillizers and venodilators. Paradoxically, their respiratory depressant action is also useful: it reduces the ineffectual fast respiration associated with panic. In the UK, *diamorphine* (*heroin*) is routinely used, but *morphine* or *pethidine* (*meperidine*) are also suitable; an anti-emetic (e.g. *prochlorperazine*) may be required. High-concentration *oxygen* (40% or more by mask) is often needed. Heart failure and shock are discussed below.

For many patients no more may be required. If heart failure does not develop and investigations

Table 3.38   Routine acute management of myocardial infarction symptoms

Target	Management
Pain	GTN, opioid plus anti-emetic
Distress, anxiety	Opioid
Hypoxaemia	Oxygen
Heart failure	Bedrest, diuretic, nitrate, ACEI
Pulmonary oedema	Diuretic, opioid
Cardiogenic shock	Inotrope, vasodilator

ACEI, angiotensin converting enzyme inhibitor; GTN, glyceryl trinitrate.

are inconclusive, a patient may be discharged after a few days with a final diagnosis of 'Chest pain ?MI'.

Myocardial salvage: reducing infarct size

Until recently, it was thought that little could be done to prevent myocardial damage, which was assumed already to have occurred irreversibly. However, several interventions have recently been developed. They are best initiated within 6 h of the onset of symptoms, although evidence is emerging that the thrombotic process in some infarctions evolves continuously over the first 24 h, so that later interventions may still be beneficial. Broadly, these techniques involve attempts to reduce myocardial oxygen demand, which spares less severely hypoxic areas, and methods of improving oxygen supply.

Cardiac workload reduction

Surrounding an evolving infarct there are relatively hypoxic, but not completely anoxic, areas. Reducing the oxygen deficit of these might be expected to aid their recovery, reduce the size of the subsequent infarct, and thus improve prognosis. In addition this contributes to the management of any heart failure. The strategies used are similar to those in angina:

- Reduction of heart rate and contractility using beta-blockers.
- Reduction of afterload using arterial dilators, e.g. ACEIs.
- Reduction of preload using venodilators, e.g. nitrates, ACEIs.

Early intravenous *beta-blockers* have been shown to reduce infarct size, arrhythmias and cardiac rupture. Because the usual cardiac contraindications to beta-blockers are all common after MI – especially serious heart failure, bradycardia, heart block and hypotension – many patients who might benefit are excluded. Although the most successful agents so far have been metoprolol and atenolol, there is no evidence that cardioselectivity or any other specific property is to be preferred. However, on theoretical grounds those with intrinsic sympathomimetic activity, which increase heart rate, should be avoided. Therapy is continued orally for secondary prevention (below).

Oral *ACEIs* started 24–48 h after infarction have also been shown to improve outcome, especially when there is frank failure, impaired ventricular function or hypertension. They appear to counter the ventricular enlargement (remodelling) which occurs after infarction and worsens ventricular function and prognosis. Obviously they are particularly useful when beta-blockers are contraindicated. ACEIs are routinely used for at least 6 weeks if not contraindicated, e.g. by hypotension, and are continued if heart failure persists.

There is no consensus on the routine use of early intravenous *nitrates* in the absence of ischaemic pain or heart failure. In addition to reducing oxygen demand they will counter any primary or reflex coronary spasm. Calcium channel blockers are not beneficial.

Metabolic support

A number of trials have indicated that early infusion of glucose with insulin and potassium (GIK therapy) may limit ischaemic damage, and interest in this essentially simple and cheap treatment is being revived. It has been shown definitely to benefit diabetics after MI but its more general application is not yet accepted. It is based on the theory that the ischaemic myocardium cannot extract enough glucose to fuel anaerobic glycolysis, which could maintain basic functions. Instead, it switches to free fatty acid metabolism and in excess this produces toxic metabolites which lead to failure or arrhythmia. Providing glucose, plus insulin to accelerate cellular uptake, might inhibit this process; the potassium may contribute an anti-arrhythmic effect.

Reperfusion: thrombolysis

The key to improving outcome in MI is to restore blood flow to the ischaemic area by opening up the occluded coronary artery as soon as possible. In some areas (especially the USA) it is possible to organize balloon angioplasty or even bypass surgery sufficiently rapidly as a primary intervention, but this is uncommon in the UK. Instead, pharmacological **fibrinolysis (thrombolysis)** is the treatment of choice.

The natural endogenous fibrinolysin (thrombolysin) is plasmin, a proteolytic enzyme which lyses fibrin clots forming accidentally within the normal circulation, or following repair of any vessel damage (Fig. 3.34). It also destroys other clotting factors, inhibiting further thrombosis. Both blood and tissue factors activate its precursor, plasminogen. The delicate dynamic equilibrium between clotting and anti-clotting factors is overwhelmed following pathological thrombosis. **Thrombolytic (fibrinolytic)** drugs activate plasminogen artificially (Fig. 3.34 and Table 3.39).

Available agents. *Streptokinase* (SK) is a foreign and therefore antigenic protein which acts directly on plasminogen anywhere in the circulation. *Anistreplase* (APSAC) is a complex of SK with an inactive form of plasminogen. Unlike SK itself, the plasminogen component has a greater affinity for fibrin than its precursor fibrinogen

and so the complex accumulates at the coronary clot. There the plasminogen is deacylated and subsequently activated by the streptokinase. *Alteplase* (rt-PA) and *reteplase* are plasminogen activators of human origin which are also clot-specific because they are selective for plasminogen in the presence of fibrin.

Indication and use. Pharmacological thrombolysis is now considered for all patients seen with symptoms strongly suggestive of MI and confirmed by ECG. Thrombolysis recanalizes up to 50% of patients and reduces mortality rate by 25%. Patients with anterior infarcts benefit most, the benefit being greatest for those patients treated earliest. Ideally, this should be within 2 h of onset of symptoms (i.e. usually before reaching hospital), but 6 h is probably more realistic

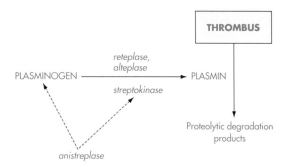

Figure 3.34 Action of fibrinolytic agents. *alteplase*, tissue-type plasminogen activator (rt-PA); *anistreplase*, APSAC.

Table 3.39   Comparison of fibrinolytic agents[a]

Streptokinase	Alteplase	Reteplase	Anistreplase
Infusion (1 h)	Infusion (3 h)	**Bolus** (2 min × 2, 30 min apart)	**Bolus** (5 min)
Antigenic	**Non-antigenic**	**Non-antigenic**	Antigenic
Haemorrhagic[b]	**Less haemorrhage?**	**Less haemorrhage?**	**Less haemorrhage?**
Cheap	Expensive	Expensive	Expensive
	Short half-life	Longer half-life	Longer half-life
Proven in large trials	**Proven in large trials**	–	–

[a] Relative advantages are emphasized in bold type.

[b] Especially stroke.

Alteplase, genetically engineered human tissue plasminogen activator, rt-PA; anistreplase, anisoylated (acylated) plasminogen–streptokinase activator complex (APSAC); reteplase, recombinant tissue plasminogen activator.

and 12 h is the maximum for significant benefit; there are small gains for longer delays. Outcome is greatly improved if oral *aspirin*, presumably as prophylactic antiplatelet therapy, is started as soon as possible, beginning with 300 mg taken as soon as possible after symptoms develop.

Early *heparin* infusion alone does not reduce infarction size or prevent reinfarction. Heparin is used routinely as an adjunct to alteplase therapy. It also is indicated in patients with a tendency to thrombosis, to reduce venous thrombosis and pulmonary embolism.

Choice. *Streptokinase* is currently the cheapest agent. Intravenous use of SK has proved as effective as the intracoronary route (which requires the complexity of coronary catheterization) without causing the serious systemic haemorrhagic effects initially feared. Because both SK and *anistreplase* are foreign proteins, antibodies form within 4 days. This may cause allergic reactions, but fortunately anaphylaxis is uncommon. The outstanding problem is the lack of effect if treatment is repeated after 4 days, because the antibodies bind the drugs and prevent them from acting. *Alteplase* or *reteplase* must be used if a patient has a second infarct after treatment with either of the other two drugs.

Alteplase and reteplase, although more expensive, permit lower doses and hence reduction of systemic bleeding by targeting the coronary clot. However, this is generally exploited to use higher doses for a better vessel opening rate. Used this way the clot-specific agents are more likely to produce haemorrhagic stroke as a complication. Either way, the advantage of selectivity is not translated into as large an increase in survival as expected, possibly because these agents permit a greater tendency to early re-occlusion.

The activation stage required by anistreplase gives it a longer half-life so that it may be administered as a bolus; this makes it potentially useful for emergencies outside hospital, though it is still antigenic. The newer reteplase is also longer acting to permit bolus dosing.

Overall, differences in efficacy are small and of far less significance in survival terms than variations in the time between symptoms and thrombolysis ('pain to needle time') or admission and thrombolysis ('door to needle time'). Thus research continues for a thrombolytic agent closer to the ideal. In the UK at present, SK is the drug of choice in the absence of contraindications.

Contraindications and cautions. The principal general consideration is the patient's tendency to haemorrhage. Obviously any active bleeding will prevent thrombolysis. Current or recent problems contraindicating use or indicating the need for particular care are listed in Table 3.40.

Complications

Arrhythmias
Ventricular fibrillation needs prompt electrical defibrillation. Early prophylactic *lidocaine* (*lignocaine*) or procaine enjoyed a vogue, but are not used now in the UK. Other specific arrhythmias are treated as usual when they occur. Early prophylactic *magnesium* infusions are not useful.

Heart failure and shock
These are managed as usual (pp. 72–93). They require careful haemodynamic monitoring because of the autonomic imbalance and unstable homeostatic control after MI.

Table 3.40 Contraindications and cautions with thrombolytic therapy

---

Active problems
Anticoagulation therapy
Peptic ulceration
Oesophageal varices
Severe liver disease (varices)
Diabetic retinopathy
Severe systolic hypertension
Pregnancy
Severe menorrhagia

Recent history of:
General surgery
Stroke
Subarachnoid haemorrhage
Major head injury

Thromboembolic complications

These may be deep vein, pulmonary, cerebral or endocardial (mural) and are prevented by a short course of *heparin*, perhaps followed by *warfarin* for a few weeks. Long-term oral anticoagulation is not needed if aspirin is being given.

Rehabilitation

Patients without complications are mobilized within 2–3 days and discharged soon after. This reduces the chance of venous thrombosis, and is good for morale. Other aspects of rehabilitation are summarized in Table 3.41. Patients may eventually lead near-normal lives. Although most do eventually die of IHD, nothing indicates that a life of self-imposed semi-invalidism improves their chances and the quality of such a life is inferior. By following simple positive health recommendations, to which infarct survivors are especially receptive, by 6 months after their infarct many patients say that they feel better than for many years before.

Secondary prevention

Antiplatelet therapy

The long-term benefit of regular low-dose aspirin is clear, especially following thrombolysis. However, even large-scale trials have failed to resolve uncertainty over the optimal dose: recommendations range between 50 mg and 300 mg daily. Several new approaches are under development (*see* p. 129).

Beta-blockers

Routine prophylactic cardiospecific beta-blockade, for at least 2–5 years – and perhaps for ever – is beneficial. Even patients with moderate heart failure can be treated. On the other hand, very low-risk patients are unlikely to benefit. Pooled data suggest an overall 25% reduction in mortality rate.

ACE inhibitors

In the presence of heart failure or demonstrable ventricular dysfunction, regular ACEIs are recommended, particularly if beta-blockers are contraindicated (about 25% of patients). The optimum duration of treatment is not yet clear, but is at least 5 years.

Lipid-lowering agents

These have recently been clearly demonstrated to be of benefit even in patients with only moderate elevations of plasma lipids (p. 129). A target would be to use a statin when total cholesterol is >5 mmol/L (or LDL cholesterol >3 mmol/L) after an optimal trial of diet modification.

Anticoagulants

Because early anticoagulant trials were flawed and used imprecise monitoring methods, toxicity seemed to outweigh any potential benefit. Despite re-analysis, more consistent monitoring methods and even revival of the thrombosis theory, these drugs are unlikely to be used routinely for the majority of patients after MI.

Figure 3.35 summarizes the various treatment options for a wide spectrum of possible presentations and clinical opinions. Note that this is not a flow chart for management, but an overall framework for comprehending the many possible eventualities and remedies.

Table 3.41 Rehabilitation and general health education after myocardial infarction

---

Gradual re-establishment of normal activity including work and sex
Counselling and reassurance
• little interference with normal activity expected
Improve general fitness
• stop smoking
• moderate routine aerobic exercise
• attain ideal body weight
• join 'post-MI' self-help group
Stress reduction?
• simple psychotherapy, relaxation therapy

MI, myocardial infarction.

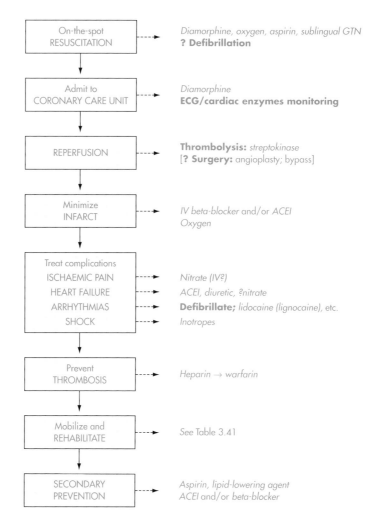

On-the-spot **RESUSCITATION**	*Diamorphine, oxygen, aspirin, sublingual GTN* **? Defibrillation**
Admit to **CORONARY CARE UNIT**	*Diamorphine* **ECG/cardiac enzymes monitoring**
REPERFUSION	**Thrombolysis:** *streptokinase* [**? Surgery:** *angioplasty; bypass*]
Minimize **INFARCT**	*IV beta-blocker and/or ACEI* *Oxygen*
Treat complications **ISCHAEMIC PAIN** **HEART FAILURE** **ARRHYTHMIAS** **SHOCK**	*Nitrate (IV?)* *ACEI, diuretic, ?nitrate* **Defibrillate;** *lidocaine (lignocaine), etc.* *Inotropes*
Prevent **THROMBOSIS**	*Heparin → warfarin*
Mobilize and **REHABILITATE**	*See* Table 3.41
SECONDARY PREVENTION	*Aspirin, lipid-lowering agent* *ACEI and/or beta-blocker*

Figure 3.35   Overview of management of myocardial infarction. Precise treatment will depend on the severity of infarction and occurrence of complications. ACEI, angiotensin converting enzyme inhibitor; GTN, glyceryl trinitrate; IV, intravenous.

References and further reading

Beevers DG, MacGregor GA (1995) *Hypertension in Practice.* 2nd edn. London: Martin Dunitz.

Cohn JN (1997) Overview of treatment of heart failure. *Am J Cardiol* **80**: 2L–6L.

Connor WE, Bristow JD, eds (1985) *Coronary Heart Disease.* Philadelphia: Lippincott.

Doughty BN, Sharpe N (1997) Beta-adrenergic blockers in the treatment of congestive heart failure. *Ann Rev Med* **48**: 103–114.

European Society of Cardiology (1997) The treatment of heart failure. *Eur Heart J* **18**: 736–753.

Geoghardis M, *et al.* (1997) Pharmacotherapy for systolic dysfunction. A review of randomised clinical trials. *Am J Cardiol* **80**: 14H–27H.

Hudson S, *et al.* (1998) Pharmaceutical care: essential hypertension. *Pharm J* **260**: 411–417.

Mason P (1997) Diet and coronary heart disease – an update. *Pharm J* **258**: 170–173.

Mehta HM, Kim AE (1998) Secondary prevention of acute myocardial infarction. *Br Med J* **316**: 838–842.

Mohrman DE, Heller LJ (1997) *Cardiovascular Physiology.* 4th edn. New York: McGraw-Hill.

National Prescribing Centre (1996) Hyperlipidaemia. *MeReC Briefing* 10; Liverpool.

Opie LH, ed. (1997) *Drugs for the Heart*. 4th edn. Philadelphia: WB Saunders.

Opie LH (1992) *Angiotensin Converting Enzyme Inhibitors*. New York: Authors' Publishing House.

Packer M (1997) End of oldest controversy in medicine. Are we ready to conclude the debate on digoxin? *N Engl J Med* **336**: 575–576.

Packer M (1992) Pathophysiology of chronic heart failure. *Lancet* **340**: 88–91.

Packer M (1992) Treatment of chronic heart failure. *Lancet* **341**: 91–95.

Robertson JIS, Ball SG (1994) *Hypertension for the Clinician*. London: WB Saunders.

Ramsey LE, *et al.* (1996) Targeting lipid-lowering therapy for primary prevention of coronary artery disease: an updated Sheffield table. *Lancet* **348**: 387–388.

Sani M, Jackson G (1997) Angina. *Pharm J* **258**: 841–845.

Sani M, Jackson G (1997) Myocardial infarction. *Pharm J* **258**: 203–206.

Stanton AV (1998) Calcium channel blockers. *Br Med J* **316**: 1471–1473.

Thelle DS (1996) Salt and blood pressure revisited. *Br Med J* **312**: 1240–1241.

Timmis A (1997) *Essential Cardiology*. 3rd edn. Oxford: Blackwell Scientific.

Wiltzum JL (1994) The oxidation hypothesis of atherosclerosis. *Lancet* **344**: 793–795.

4

Renal system

Renal disease and its ultimate consequence – renal failure – represent important issues in the health debate. Although it is now technically feasible to relieve or reverse renal failure, limits to what can be done in practice arise from ethical issues surrounding the allocation of health care resources and the organization of organ donation – issues which are in constant flux.

Chronic renal failure (CRF) is potentially fatal and may condemn a patient to years of dialysis with a substantially reduced quality of life. Although successful renal transplantation provides an almost complete solution and is now extremely reliable, society has not yet fully adjusted to the implications of organ donation. Regular controversies on the persistent vegetative state ('brain death') testify to this.

This chapter first reviews the normal function of the kidney. Subsequently, the consequences of impairment of these functions, i.e. homeostatic imbalances and renal failure, are explained. Finally, the common clinical conditions which cause these abnormalities are discussed.

Physiological principles of the renal system

The kidney is both structurally and functionally complex, and plays a central role in homeostasis. Thus, many possible varieties of renal malfunction can cause a wide range of clinical conditions. Manifestations of renal disorder include fluid, electrolyte and pH imbalance, haemodynamic imbalance, the accumulation of drugs, toxins and waste metabolic products, loss of essential metabolites, and endocrine abnormalities such as anaemia and bone disease.

Structural damage can occur to the glomeruli, the tubules or the urinary tract, such damage resulting from pathological processes such as infection, inflammation, auto-immunity, neoplasia and toxins. Systemic or local circulatory insufficiency can also seriously compromise renal function. The most common pathologies are glomerular inflammation, urinary tract infection and drug-induced nephrotoxicity. In this section we review the physiological principles of normal renal function, so that abnormality of the renal system may be better understood.

Anatomy

The gross anatomy of the renal system is shown in Fig. 4.1. It is important to distinguish between the **kidneys**, which are structurally complex, and the **lower urinary tract**, the function of which is essentially the storage and transport of fluid. Three main regions are distinguished within the kidney: the cortex, the medulla, and the pelvis. The **cortex** contains the glomeruli and the proximal and distal tubules, and the **medulla** contains the loops of Henle. Glomeruli in different areas have different-length loops of Henle to permit differential control over urine concentration. The loops of the juxtamedullary nephrons, nearest the medulla, extend almost to the **pelvis**, the area into which the formed urine drains from the collecting ducts. Throughout the

kidney there are interstitial cells, probably concerned with endocrine functions.

Although kidney disorders are almost always serious, disorders in the lower urinary tract are often symptomatically troublesome but seldom are serious in themselves. However, chronic problems in the lower urinary tract may eventually cause damage to the kidneys.

The importance of the kidneys may be judged from the fact that although they together weigh just 500 g (less than 1% of body weight) they receive 25% of the cardiac output. Like many other organs, the kidneys are modular, each having about one million functional subunits or **nephrons**. This represents considerable functional over-capacity, and life can continue quite normally with less than one-half of a functioning kidney. Thus when the kidneys are diseased, symptoms do not appear until there has been over 90% damage; moreover, such damage is often irreversible, making treatment difficult.

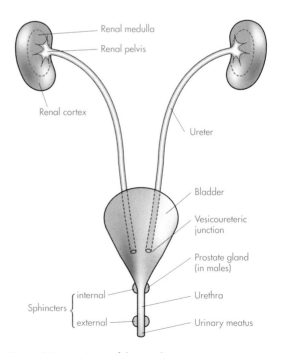

Figure 4.1   Anatomy of the renal system.

Renal functions – summary

The kidney is the key organ of overall homeostatic control and its functions may be considered in three main groups (Table 4.1). Elimination of waste is normally first associated with the kidneys, but their regulatory functions are equally important. The kidneys also are involved in several major endocrine systems.

Elimination

The potentially toxic by-products of metabolism must be excreted, along with excess nutrients and any exogenous toxins absorbed from the gut, and their subsequent metabolites. Generally, elimination is passive, although some selected substances are actively secreted.

Carbohydrate metabolism, the major energy pathway of the body, produces carbon dioxide and water. Most carbon dioxide is eliminated passively by the lungs, but the kidneys have far more control in secreting it as acid. Much of the water produced by metabolism, along with that taken in the diet, is lost through sweating and insensible losses, but once again the kidney can exercise selective control to maintain balance.

The predominant nitrogenous waste product is urea from protein metabolism; as such, its level in the blood provides a useful approximate index of renal function. Nucleic acid breakdown produces urate, which is actively secreted, and muscle metabolism produces creatinine (also used as an index of kidney function). Some sulphate and phosphate are also released by protein metabolism. Urea is not as harmful as is commonly believed; guanidine, amines and other metabolites (phenols, hydroxyacids, etc.), are more toxic.

The kidney also has a role in the metabolism of peptides, including e.g. insulin.

Fluid and electrolyte balance

The kidney plays a crucial and active role maintaining the correct ionic, osmotic, pH and fluid balances throughout the body. It detects imbalances, secretes local regulatory hormones, and actively excretes or retains substances as necessary. One of the drawbacks of its interaction with so many different systems is that there may occasionally be conflicting demands, which can be resolved only by compromises. For example, chloride may be variously regarded as an anion, an acid or simply an osmotically active particle, depending on circumstances. Controlling chloride to preserve electrical neutrality or osmotic balance may compromise pH balance.

Water balance

The body is normally in positive water balance, the kidney adjusting for varying intakes and losses by altering water clearance. Certain irreducible constraints enforce a minimum average daily intake of about 1 L (Table 4.2).

Table 4.1   Functions of the kidney

Elimination of waste/surplus	Carbohydrate-derived	Water, acid
	Nitrogenous	Urea, creatinine, uric acid, guanidine, amines, etc.
	Other	Sulphate, phosphate, exogenous toxins, etc.
Control of fluid and electrolyte balance	Total body water	
	Plasma osmotic pressure	
	pH	
	Na, K, Ca, Mg, etc.	
	Chloride, bicarbonate	
Hormonal homeostasis	Blood pressure	
	Calcium and bone metabolism	
	Red blood cell production	

Table 4.2   Approximate average daily water balance[a]

Obligatory losses		Sources of replacement	
Kidneys[b]	500	Metabolism of glucose	500
Skin[c]	500	Diet[b]	1000
Lungs[c]	400		
Faeces	100		
TOTAL	1500		1500

[a] Only minimum values given (mL); there are considerable daily variations.

[b] Normally about 1000 mL greater than obligatory minimum.

[c] 'Insensible losses'.

The kidney requires at least 500 mL of water to excrete the average daily load of osmotically active waste products at maximal urinary concentration, i.e. under maximal antidiuretic hormone stimulation. This is just about balanced by the water produced by metabolic oxidation. The minimum dietary intake is then that which will replace insensible losses in breath and faeces, and through the skin, excluding additional or exertional perspiration.

Fluid compartments
The main fluid compartments of the body and their predominant ionic concentrations are given in Fig. 4.2. The intravascular and extravascular components of the extracellular fluid (ECF) are in equilibrium by free diffusion, except that plasma proteins generally cannot leave the blood. Although water diffuses across cell walls passively under osmotic forces, there are membrane pumps effecting the flow of most other substances to and from the intracellular fluid (ICF). However, the activity of these pumps is largely dependent on concentration gradients. Thus the kidney, by controlling ECF composition, effectively influences all compartments.

There is a complex and subtle interplay between the maintenance of ECF osmotic pressure (mainly through control of sodium concentration) and the total volume and relative distribution of fluid between the compartments. The kidney also controls plasma potassium level and thus total body potassium. By selectively varying the secretion of hydrogen ions and reabsorption or regeneration of bicarbonate the kidney can significantly alter plasma pH, and thus body pH.

Endocrine functions

The kidney is involved in at least three important systemic hormonal systems.

Blood pressure
Renal involvement in blood pressure (BP) control operates via a number of mechanisms (p. 160). This is partly 'enlightened self-interest' because the kidney cannot operate without an adequate perfusion pressure, but it also contributes to the systemic BP control mechanisms.

Calcium
The kidney is vital to calcium and bone metabolism. In addition to being a target organ for vitamin D and parathormone, the kidney is responsible for the final stage in the activation of vitamin D by hydroxylating 25-hydroxycholecalciferol to 1,25-dihydroxycholecalciferol.

Erythropoiesis
In response to hypoxaemia, the kidney secretes erythropoietin, which promotes red blood cell production in the bone marrow. Without erythropoeitin, erythropoiesis cannot proceed efficiently and haemoglobin levels stay below 10 g/100 mL. In certain renal conditions (e.g. polycystic kidney, renal tumour) there is erythropoietin over-production, with consequent polycythaemia.

It can now be appreciated why renal failure is so serious. In acute renal failure it is mainly elimination and fluid/electrolyte control that are affected. The patient suffers particularly from retention of excess water, acid and potassium. In

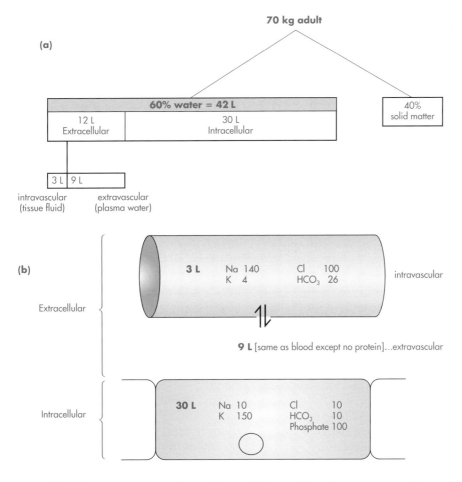

Figure 4.2   Body fluid compartments. (a) Relative volumes. (b) Principal electrolyte composition of intracellular and extracellular compartments (mmol/L).

chronic renal failure, endocrine malfunction adds other problems, including hypertension, bone disease and iron-resistant anaemia.

Mechanisms of elimination

The kidney goes about elimination in a seemingly perverse and inefficient manner. Instead of selectively excreting unwanted substances it filters almost everything, and then selectively reabsorbs what needs to be conserved. About 10% of the total renal blood flow, i.e. 120 mL/min, is filtered at the glomeruli, along with most low-molecular weight constituents: this is the **glomerular filtration rate** (GFR). Some 99% of

this 180 L/day is then actively reabsorbed, leaving an average daily urine volume of only about 1.5 L. (This system may be a relic of the aquatic era of evolution, when the large amounts of fluid and sodium that were lost could easily be replaced.)

There are three main phases of elimination (Fig. 4.3):

1. Size-selective but otherwise indiscriminate **ultrafiltration** across the glomerular membrane from plasma into the tubular lumen to produce filtrate.
2. Active **reabsorption** into plasma of useful substances in bulk, mostly from the proximal tubule.

3. Selective **secretion** from plasma or reabsorption into plasma of certain critical substances in small amounts to maintain the fluid and electrolyte balances, mainly in the distal tubule and collecting duct.

In order to understand how certain diseases affect renal function, the factors which affect filtration and the patterns of reabsorption and secretion must be briefly reviewed. This simple discussion will not distinguish between the cortical and juxtamedullary nephrons; unless otherwise stated, the former are implied.

Filtration

During glomerular ultrafiltration blood cells and colloidal macromolecules (i.e. plasma proteins) are retained but smaller molecules (crystalloids) are carried through the glomerular basement membrane (GBM) under hydrostatic pressure by solvent drag. Substances with a molecular weight less than 5000 daltons pass freely. Passage decreases with increasing molecular size, especially above about 25 kDa; only 3% of haemoglobin (64 kDa) would pass if it were free in plasma, and less than 1% of albumin (minimum size approx. 70 kDa) passes. Anions pass less easily than cations because the GBM is negatively charged, but again this effect is only significant for larger molecules.

Factors affecting glomerular filtration rate

The GFR is the key index of renal function because if there is no filtration then none of the regulatory mechanisms which act on the filtrate can operate. Figure 4.3 is a functional diagram of a nephron: within the illustration are identified the sites where factors which influence the GFR operate. Table 4.3 summarizes the clinical conditions under which these factors can become altered. This usually happens due to changes in filtration pressure (especially the systemic arterial pressure). The integrity of the basement membrane is another important factor.

Perfusion. The kidney strives to maintain systemic arterial blood pressure, but failing that, filtration pressure at the glomerulus is defended by intrarenal mechanisms. Probably the most common cause of acute renal failure is systemic hypotension (e.g. from haemorrhagic or cardiogenic shock) when such mechanisms are overwhelmed. Long-term damage to renal arteries (e.g. arteriosclerosis and/or atherosclerosis from untreated hypertension) can cause chronic renal failure.

Renal **autoregulation** maintains renal blood flow, filtration pressure and GFR over wide variations in renal perfusion pressure, principally by alterations in the calibre of afferent and efferent

---

Table 4.3   Factors that can reduce glomerular filtration rate

Factor	Clinical condition where altered
Impaired renal perfusion	
Reduced systemic blood pressure	Heart failure, shock (e.g. MI, haemorrhage)
	Drugs, toxins, etc.
Renal arterial obstruction	Renal thrombosis, atherosclerosis
	Untreated hypertension
Damaged glomerular basement membrane	Inflammation (glomerulonephritis)
	Connective tissue disease
	(e.g. systemic lupus erythematosus)
	Diabetic nephropathy
	Nephrotoxic drugs (e.g. penicillamine)
Reduced glomerular number	Ageing, chronic renal failure, nephrectomy
Increased tubular back pressure	Urinary tract obstruction (e.g. stones, tumour)
	Tubular inflammation ('tubular nephropathy')
	Tubular infection (pyelonephritis)

MI, myocardial infarction.

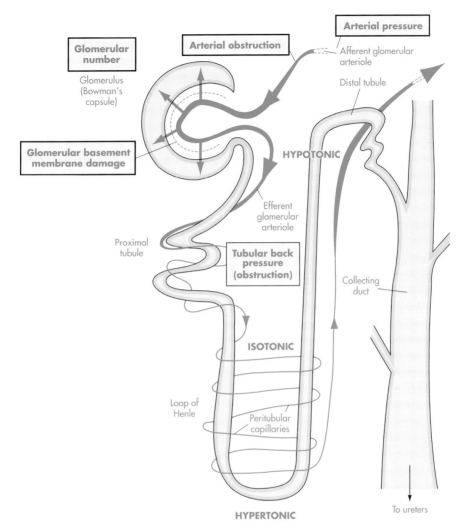

Figure 4.3 Diagram of single nephron showing main functional components and factors which influence filtration (boxed).

glomerular arteries. The afferent arterioles are dilated by intrarenal prostaglandins, while the efferent ones are constricted by intrarenal angiotensin. In this way the transmembrane hydrostatic pressure, and hence GFR, is defended. One input to this system is **tubulo-glomerular feedback**. If the GFR is altered, the consequent changes in the solute load of the glomerular filtrate are detected in the distal tubule by the juxtaglomerular apparatus (p. 159), which is involved in intrarenal hormone systems.

Another important intrarenal regulatory mechanism is the potentially confusingly named **glomerulotubular balance**. This is a second line of defence if GFR is compromised beyond the ability of the primary compensatory mechanisms. It serves to preserve excretion of water, sodium and other solutes in the face of reduced GFR. It thus provides one aspect of renal reserve, delaying the onset of azotaemia and symptomatic uraemia if renal function declines chronically. Its physiology is poorly understood.

The operation of these control mechanisms is illustrated by the adverse effect of angiotensin converting enzyme inhibitors (ACEIs) when used to treat hypertensive patients with obstructive lesions in both renal arteries (bilateral renal artery stenosis), or patients in whom renal perfusion is otherwise compromised by hypovolaemia or cardiac failure. In such cases optimal renal perfusion is maintained partly by raised levels of angiotensin originating from the renal response to the hypoperfusion. Angiotensin maintains renal blood flow by causing intrarenal efferent arteriolar constriction and also, possibly, by elevating systemic BP. ACEIs, by blocking this protective mechanism, may precipitate renal failure by causing a significant reduction in renal perfusion. Similarly, prostaglandin inhibitors, e.g. non-steroidal anti-inflammatory drugs (NSAIDs), can have an adverse effect on renal haemodynamics, causing renal impairment and fluid retention.

Glomerular basement membrane.   The GBM is a sensitive structure that is exposed to high flow rates and high concentrations of potential toxins and mediators. It can be damaged by numerous pathological processes, and this forms the basis of many chronic renal diseases. If the GBM is damaged, its permeability to large particles – especially smaller colloids such as albumin – may be increased, causing proteinuria. In more severe cases there may also be, paradoxically, retention of water and sodium owing to a degree of renal impairment (reduced GFR).

Simple changes in pore size cannot account for these changes; pore size may be partly related to a loss of the negative membrane charge, which normally repels the similarly charged plasma albumin. Some proteins smaller than about 60–100 kDa are normally filtered, but are almost completely reabsorbed. However, the reabsorptive capacity is low and soon exceeded if there is an increase in tubular protein concentration. The catabolism of filtered protein within the renal tubules, which is normally minimal, may be increased in the presence of proteinuria.

Glomerular number.   In chronic renal failure, diminishing renal function is believed to result from a reduced number of fully active nephrons rather than to a general decline in the function of all nephrons (the 'intact nephron hypothesis').

The main reason why the elderly have reduced renal function is the loss of functional nephrons – a process which continues at a steady rate throughout adult life. Normally about half of the nephrons are lost by the age of 80 years.

Tubular back pressure.   Obstruction anywhere along the urinary tract will inhibit filtration by increasing the pressure within the tubule, reducing the filtration pressure across the GBM. Obstruction can occur within the tubules themselves, if they are damaged; in the renal pelvis (in pyelonephritis and some forms of nephrotoxicity); or in the lower urinary tract, owing to the presence of a ureteral stone or bladder outflow obstruction.

Reabsorption and secretion

Clinically, the important features here are the consequences of the interlinked exchange mechanisms which the kidney employs.

Overall pattern through nephron

Proximal tubule.   The glomerular filtrate contains essential nutrients as well as waste matter. Most of the former are returned to the circulation by reabsorption from the proximal tubule into the peritubular capillaries (Figs 4.3 and 4.4). Water follows osmotically and chloride electrochemically. There are specific pumps for most substances, such as sodium, potassium, bicarbonate, amino acids, glucose, etc. These pumps have a maximum transport capacity and if the filtrate concentration of a substance exceeds the capacity of the pump some of the substance appears in the urine. The plasma concentration of the substance is then said to exceed its **renal threshold**. The most common example of this is glycosuria in diabetes mellitus.

Most nutrients, and about 70% of the filtered water and electrolytes, are reabsorbed proximally. Reabsorption depends largely on non-selective bulk transport, necessitated by the profligacy of glomerular filtration. *Osmotic diuretics* act in this region by increasing the osmotic pressure of the filtrate, which inhibits water reabsorption.

Some substances, especially acids and bases,

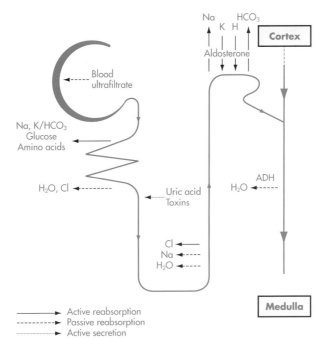

Figure 4.4   Reabsorption patterns in the renal tubule. HCO$_3$, bicarbonate; Cl, chloride; Na, sodium; H, acid; ADH, antidiuretic hormone. (From Greene R, Harris N (1984) *Chemist Drugg* **222**: 683. Reproduced with permission of Benn Publications.)

are actively secreted in the opposite direction, from the peritubular capillaries into the proximal tubule, e.g. uric acid and many toxins and drugs. This increases the clearance of molecules which have escaped filtration.

Loop.   The main function of the loop of Henle is not to reabsorb water and electrolytes but to generate an osmotic gradient between the renal cortex (hypotonic) and the medulla (hypertonic) by a countercurrent mechanism. This enables the collecting ducts, which pass through this gradient, to adjust urine concentration under the influence of **antidiuretic hormone** (ADH). No more than 10–15% of sodium, chloride and water are reabsorbed here. The powerful loop diuretics, e.g. *furosemide (frusemide)*, act by inhibiting this mechanism, preventing subsequent attempts at concentration by the collecting ducts.

Distal tubule.   In the distal tubule, and to a lesser extent in the collecting ducts, there is the potential for fine adjustments. Although the

total amounts of solutes reabsorbed are not great – no more than the final 10% of sodium and water – this is where the kidney exerts its main control of electrolyte balance.

Selective control in distal tubule
The distal tubule is crucial to the homeostasis of a number of important systems. If body sodium, blood volume or blood pressure is low, the distal reabsorption of **sodium**, with **chloride** or **bicarbonate** and some water, can be increased by the action of the mineralocorticoid **aldosterone**. Here, sodium does not carry with it an iso-osmotic load of water, so the immediate effect is a net increase in plasma osmotic pressure.

Aldosterone also inhibits the secretion of potassium into the urine, in response to body requirements, reabsorbing it in exchange for sodium. **Potassium** secretion is closely linked to that of **acid** (hydrogen ion) because the same transport mechanism is used for both. However, acid secretion is under a different, and therefore potentially conflicting, control mechanism. Variations in plasma pH affect the activity of tubular carbonic anhydrase which alters acid production and secretion (p. 161).

Total body water.   If the body is fluid-depleted or relatively hypertonic, ADH is secreted. This hormone permits passive diffusion of water from the filtrate in the distal tubule and collecting duct back into the peritubular capillaries. This is possible because the ducts pass through the hypertonic region of the renal medulla. Conversely, when the body is relatively hypotonic or fluid overloaded, ADH secretion is inhibited, water is prevented from leaving the ducts, and a dilute urine is produced. In diabetes insipidus there is an deficiency in the ADH secretion, resulting in severe polyuria.

Consequences of tubular exchanges

There will be occasions when conflicting demands on the kidney mean that one adjustment needs to be compromised to serve another. In general, the maintenance of osmotic pressure seems to be paramount, but in severe hypovolaemia the defence of blood pressure takes precedence. Three consequences need to be emphasized, because they have important implications for electrolyte imbalance and its management (Fig. 4.5):

1. Sodium is reabsorbed with *either* chloride *or* bicarbonate.

2. Sodium is exchanged for *either* acid (hydrogen ion) *or* potassium in the distal tubule.
3. All acid secreted results in an equivalent amount of bicarbonate being reabsorbed.

Potassium and pH balance

The amount of potassium which can be reabsorbed in the distal tubule, where fine control is exercised, is related to the amount of acid secreted (Fig. 4.5, 2). To secrete acid in exchange for sodium, the tubule must forgo the secretion of potassium because potassium and acid use the same transport mechanism; at the same time the tubule must also reabsorb bicarbonate (Fig. 4.5, 3). Thus, as far as the kidney is concerned, **potassium moves with alkali** (this is easy to remember if one associates K with KOH). Therefore, when the body requires alkali, in the form of bicarbonate, it tends to accumulate potassium and when it wants to eliminate excess alkali, potassium tends also to be lost.

Ordinarily this causes no problems, but the transport mechanism may become saturated if the demand is excessive. Competition between potassium and acid then forces a compromise to be made so that dyskalaemias (potassium imbalances) are frequently associated with pH imbalances. Thus, for example, if hypokalaemia is not corrected alkalosis will eventually occur as the kidney attempts to retain potassium by using

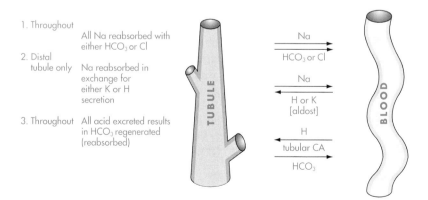

Figure 4.5   Important exchanges between blood in the peritubular capillaries and the filtrate in the renal tubules. Aldost, aldosterone; CA, carbonic anhydrase; Cl, chloride; H, acid; HCO_3, bicarbonate; Na, sodium.

this exchange pump, and in doing so it secretes acid. Conversely, acidosis is often complicated by hyperkalaemia. Similar considerations apply to alkalosis and hyperkalaemia.

Chloride and pH balance

Because alkali conservation (bicarbonate reabsorption) is linked to chloride excretion, in effect **chloride moves with acid**. However, plasma pH is determined primarily by the carbon dioxide/carbonic acid/bicarbonate equilibrium (p. 161), the only anion here being bicarbonate. Thus, if bicarbonate is displaced from the plasma by another anion, such as chloride, the resulting fall in bicarbonate will cause acidosis.

Similarly, if there is a high tubular load of chloride then it may be used non-specifically as the anion to accompany the reabsorption of important cations, which compromises bicarbonate reabsorption and produces a loss of alkali (Fig. 4.5, 1). Hence the tendency to **hyperchloraemic acidosis** when chloride intake is abnormally high.

This has important implications for fluid therapy with 0.9% sodium chloride solution (physiological saline). Compare its ionic composition with extracellular fluid (e.g. plasma):

- *Physiological saline*:   Na, 150 mmol/L; Cl, 150 mmol/L (approx.).
- *Extracellular fluid*:   Na, 150 mmol/L; Cl, 100 mmol/L (approx.).

Thus 0.9% NaCl is by no means 'normal', and the term *Normal Saline* is now outmoded. Although iso-osmotic, it is relatively chloride-rich and prolonged intravenous administration, in the standard 3 L/day regimen, eventually produces hyperchloraemic acidosis. Conversely, prolonged diuretic therapy, by increasing chloride loss, may produce hypochloraemic alkalosis (in addition to a hypokalaemic alkalosis). One benefit of simple physiological saline infusion is that it will correct mild metabolic alkalosis, so that acidic solutions, e.g. ammonium chloride, are rarely needed.

Sodium, potassium and pH

In a similar way, sodium imbalance is also likely to be associated with both pH imbalance and dyskalaemia (Fig. 4.5, 2). The rationale for these associations is left to the reader to elucidate, applying the same principles as used above.

Homeostasis

Total body water and osmotic pressure

Control

The mechanisms for the control of fluid volumes and extracellular osmotic pressure are complementary and interdependent. The volume of water in the body – **total body water** (TBW) – is determined by the total amount of osmotically active substances. Normally, water is retained to maintain a uniform osmolar concentration approximately equivalent to twice the plasma sodium level. Sodium levels are controlled by the renal regulation of tubular reabsorption. The distribution of water between the intracellular and extracellular compartments (plasma plus tissue fluid) is also primarily determined by osmotic forces, the osmotic pressure within cells normally being about the same as that of plasma.

Because TBW is usually distributed optimally, it is only necessary for the body to monitor one compartment for it to regulate all. Blood volume is the most 'accessible' because this is reflected in blood pressure. This is monitored in several ways with feedback to renal control mechanisms (p. 160).

The inter-relationship between adjustments of plasma osmolarity and body water is shown in Fig. 4.6. Note that aldosterone controls sodium reabsorption, but does not affect blood pressure directly. Aldosterone serves only to change plasma osmotic pressure, because the sodium reabsorption under aldosterone control is not accompanied by an iso-osmotic amount of water. The feedback loop is completed by ADH, which adjusts water reabsorption as appropriate.

Thus volume imbalance causes changes in electrolyte reabsorption via aldosterone, whereas osmotic imbalance causes changes in water reabsorption via ADH. This interdependence of the two systems permits very fine control.

Imbalance

The juxtaglomerular apparatus (JGA) is an area of specialized tissue strategically located between

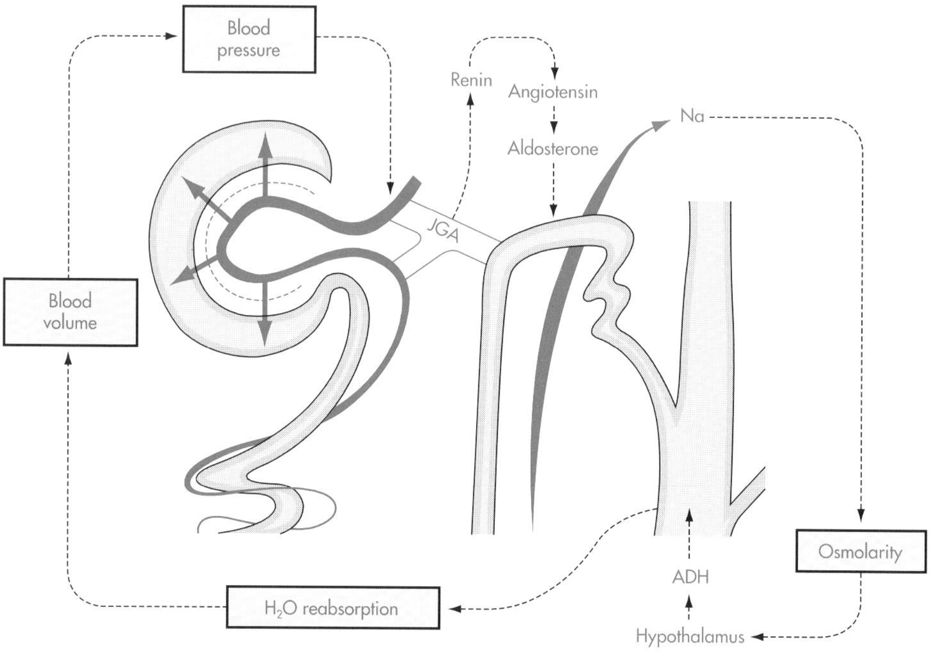

Figure 4.6 Inter-relationship of mechanisms controlling total body water and osmotic pressure. ADH, antidiuretic hormone; JGA, juxtaglomerular apparatus.

the afferent and efferent glomerular arterioles and beginning of the distal tubule in each nephron, and in contact with all three (Fig. 4.6). The JGA can thus detect changes in pressure in the afferent arteriole (usually proportional to systemic arterial pressure) and consequent changes in tubular filtrate flow and concentration. It can then attempt to rectify any fall in BP by the secretion of renin, which causes the activation of both systemic (plasma) angiotensin and local mechanisms involving intrarenal angiotensin and vasodilatory prostaglandin.

Consider the consequences of haemorrhage or severe diarrhoea. The iso-osmotic volume loss (hypovolaemia) causes a fall in BP. In response, the JGA secretes renin, aldosterone increases sodium reabsorption, and plasma osmotic pressure rises. This promotes ADH secretion, increasing tubular water reabsorption and restoring TBW. Conversely, in hyponatraemia the osmotic imbalance initially causes reduced water reabsorption and increased urine volume (via ADH), tending to normalize osmotic pressure at the expense of TBW, blood volume and BP. Subse-

quently the systems once again interact gradually to restore both factors.

Thirst is a relatively crude mechanism for replenishing both electrolyte and fluid loss. This loosely controlled process requires the kidney to make the appropriate fine adjustments.

Blood pressure control

The main ways in which the kidney is involved in maintaining BP are briefly summarized here (*see* Chapter 3, pp. 52–68 for a fuller discussion).

Simple pressure natriuresis

As BP changes, a complex interplay of autoregulatory variations in glomerular blood flow and/or tubular reabsorption makes compensatory changes in urine volume. Thus, a fall in BP will cause an automatic fall in urine volume, the fluid retained tending to restore BP. Generally the GFR is maintained constant so as not to compromise excretory functions; the principal mechanism for this is a change in tubular reabsorption.

Renin/angiotensin/aldosterone and the osmoreceptor/ADH systems
These are discussed on pp. 159–160.

Atrial natriuretic factor
Rises in blood volume can be detected by increased pressure in the atria of the heart, which secrete a peptide, atrial natriuretic factor (ANF) that acts in the kidney to inhibit water reabsorption. ANF seems to play an important role in supporting cardiac output in heart failure (*see* Chapter 3, p. 72–93).

Acid–base balance

Plasma pH is determined by the ratio of bicarbonate to total carbon dioxide, including free carbon dioxide and carbonic acid:

$$pH \propto \frac{[\text{bicarbonate}]}{[\text{carbon dioxide}]} \qquad (4.1)$$

This effect depends on the hydration of carbon dioxide, which is catalysed by carbonic anhydrase in kidney tubules and all body cells:

$$CO_2 + H_2O \overset{\substack{carbonic \\ anhydrase}}{\rightleftharpoons} H_2CO_3 \rightleftharpoons HCO_3^- + H^+$$

Although other ions, e.g. phosphate and ammonium, become involved, this is essentially the process that occurs in the tubules as acid is secreted and bicarbonate reabsorbed or, more correctly, regenerated. Further, both fat metabolism and the anaerobic metabolism of carbohydrate produce ketoacids (acetoacetate, lactate, etc.) and protein metabolism results in the production of sulphate and phosphate. These non-volatile acids must also be eliminated by the kidney.

Respiratory compensation
Most of the carbon dioxide produced by the aerobic metabolism of carbohydrate is eliminated routinely by the lungs (about 15 000 mmol of acid per day). Yet despite their massive capacity, the lungs can only be used temporarily to adjust for unwanted changes in acid level. Prolonged fast breathing is exhausting (and the extra energy used produces yet more carbon dioxide), and obviously respiration cannot be reduced without causing hypoxaemia. Moreover, the net effect is to produce absolute increases or falls in blood buffering capacity. Nevertheless, the lungs provide important rapid **primary respiratory compensation**. This can be judged from the fact that if respiratory rate were reduced to 25% of normal (in the absence of initial pH imbalance), blood pH would soon fall to 7.0. This is the pathogenesis of respiratory acidosis, which occurs when a respiratory abnormality impairs elimination of carbon dioxide.

Renal compensation
It is the kidney that makes the long-term adjustment for abnormal changes in pH (assuming it is not itself the primary cause of the problem) by appropriate changes in acid secretion and complementary bicarbonate regeneration. The kidneys normally secrete only a small amount of acid: on average about 100 mmol per day. However, this can be varied considerably to compensate for dietary or metabolic imbalance or respiratory impairment. This **secondary renal compensation** is delayed and slow, but can work indefinitely. A consequence is that metabolic acidosis is a major problem in renal failure.

Control of this important process is essentially autonomous and passive. Carbonic anhydrase in the tubular cells is simply responding to the law of mass action: as the plasma level of carbon dioxide rises, more is hydrolysed and consequently more acid is secreted and bicarbonate regenerated. There is no central or humoral control but the proper functioning of the tubules is of course essential. Respiratory function on the other hand is very tightly controlled by medullary receptors sensitive to pH. However, pH is used merely as an index of carbon dioxide accumulation: the principal role of this mechanism is the maintenance of blood oxygen level.

Maintaining pH homeostasis: the overall pattern
To maintain blood pH at 7.4 ± 0.05, these mechanisms work in concert, as follows:

- Small natural changes (most commonly falls) are initially countered by the blood buffer system.

- If this is insufficient, the respiratory centre responds rapidly by altering respiratory rate to increase the retention or elimination of carbon dioxide, thereby adjusting the bicarbonate/acid ratio and returning pH to normal. This happens whether or not the initial cause was actually a change in carbon dioxide level.
- Finally, renal compensation will slowly restore the absolute as well as the relative levels of acid and bicarbonate.

Clinical features and investigation of renal disease

The clinical features of renal dysfunction are either changes in urine flow and composition, or systemic features due to the failure of renal mechanisms.

Symptoms

Patients readily associate symptoms arising in the lower urinary tract as renal in origin. However, as a consequence of the imbalances caused by renal malfunction, symptoms may arise in any body system and may at first be obscure and seem unrelated to the renal system.

Urinary symptoms

Some of the common urinary symptoms and their possible clinical implications are summarized in Table 4.4. While micturition abnormalities usually result from the lower urinary tract, persistent abnormalities of urine volume usually imply a more serious aetiology. The significance of defining oliguria as less than 500 mL of urine per day is that this is the minimum volume required to carry the average daily osmotic load of waste matter at maximal urine concentration; any less implies a degree of malfunction. However, the precise value for an individual will vary somewhat depending on diet, body size and fluid intake.

Systemic features

Volaemic and osmotic imbalance
Fluid and electrolyte imbalance commonly result from renal impairment. Fluid imbalance generally has haemodynamic consequences with cardiovascular features such as changes in BP, oedema, shortness of breath, etc. Osmotic imbalance usually results in neurological features, e.g. drowsiness, convulsions, because of changes in the intracranial pressure.

'Uraemia'
This term is a traditional synonym for renal failure (implying high levels of blood urea); another

---

Table 4.4   Urinary symptoms

Abnormality	Symptom	Definition	Possible causes
Micturition	Dysuria	Painful	Urinary tract infection/inflammation
	Hesitation	Difficulty in starting	Outflow obstruction (e.g. prostatitis, stone)
	Frequency		Stress, polyuria, infection, prostatitis
	Incontinence	Difficulty in preventing	Stress, neuromuscular
	Nocturia	Frequency at night	Polyuria, heart failure, diabetes
Urine volume	Polyuria	>2.5 L/day	Diet, climate
			Renal tubular disease
			Chronic renal failure
			Diabetes (mellitus or insipidus)
	Oliguria	<500 mL/day	Obstruction, renal failure
	Anuria	<100 mL/day	Obstruction, renal failure

is **azotaemia** (high levels of nitrogenous products). Sometimes the former term is used more specifically for the clinical picture and the latter for the biochemical picture. The clinical consequences of renal failure extend far beyond the immediate effects of high blood levels of urea or other nitrogenous metabolic waste products. However, these undoubtedly contribute to the general malaise, lethargy, pruritus, cramps, peripheral tingling, nausea, vomiting and anorexia of which patients frequently complain. In addition, pH imbalance and abnormalities of sodium, potassium and other substances cause specific symptoms that will be discussed in the appropriate sections below.

Signs, examination and investigation

Urine

Much information on kidney function can be inferred by looking for the consequences of suspected malfunction. This is generally easier, less invasive and often more sensitive than examination of the kidneys directly. Useful qualitative and semi-quantitative information is given by microscopic or simple chemical examination of the urine. Simple biochemical urine tests, valuable for preliminary screening (Table 4.5), can nowadays be done using dipsticks, and should be part of a routine clinical examination.

Renal function

More accurate measurements are required for the diagnosis and monitoring of serious disease, or when drug dosage calculation is important.

Filtration and clearance

Since the principal function of the kidney is filtration, the rate at which this occurs is a crucial measure of its efficiency. However, direct measurement of this rate is difficult and so the concept of **clearance** is utilized. Clearance is defined as a hypothetical volume of blood from which a substance would be completely removed by filtration in 1 min. It is calculated by measuring the blood or plasma concentration of the substance, urine flow rate (usually measured over 24 h to minimize collection errors) and the urine concentration of the substance. The clearance is given by:

$$\text{Clearance} = \frac{\text{Urine concentration} \times \text{Urine flow rate}}{\text{Plasma concentration}}$$

We know that approximately 120 mL of filtrate is normally produced each minute. If a substance were completely filtered at the glomerulus and subsequently neither reabsorbed from the tubules nor secreted into them, then the equivalent of 120 mL of blood would be cleared of the substance each minute and its clearance would be 120 mL/min. Inulin fulfils these criteria, but it

Table 4.5   Simple semi-quantitative examination of urine

Test	Significance/implication
Specific gravity	Urine concentrating ability (tubular function)
pH (indicator method)	Generally not very helpful; a failure to acidify urine (renal tubular acidosis) requires detailed assessment
Abnormal constituents	
Protein (proteinuria; albuminuria)	Glomerular disease; vigorous exercise (transient)
Blood (haematuria)	Infection/inflammation/tumour
Haemoglobin	Haemolytic anaemia
Pus (pyuria)	Renal or urinary tract infection
Crystals (crystalluria)	Depends on identity of crystals
'Casts'	Clumps of protein and blood cells – often glomerulonephritis or pyelonephritis

is preferable to exploit creatinine, a natural body constituent, which very closely does so. **Creatinine clearance** is thus the usual index of GFR. (Creatinine is actually secreted to a small extent in the tubules, so its clearance gives a slightly high estimate of GFR; fortuitously however, current laboratory measurement slightly overestimates plasma creatinine, tending to cancel this out.)

Creatinine clearance measurement involves a tedious and error-prone 24-h urine collection. Hence, a single serum creatinine measurement will often suffice because the serum creatinine level depends on the balance between production (which is dependent on muscle mass, gender and age and is normally constant for an individual) and renal output (which is directly proportional to filtration rate). Creatinine clearance can be derived from the serum creatinine alone by correcting for age, sex and weight using tables or a simple formula:

$$\text{Creatinine clearance} = K \times \frac{(140 - \text{Age}) \times \text{Weight}}{\text{Serum creatinine}}$$

where age is in years; weight in kg, serum creatinine in micromol/L and the correction factor K is 1.04 for females and 1.23 for males.

Unfortunately, serum creatinine does not start to rise significantly until there is serious renal impairment, so early renal disease is easily missed if this method is relied upon. This is because early renal damage is often compensated by hypertrophy and hyperfiltration of remaining nephrons, which maintains clearance. Furthermore, the serum creatinine level is inversely related to GFR, and the effect of this reciprocal relationship, illustrated in Fig. 4.7, is that quite large early falls in GFR will cause only small absolute rises in creatinine. For example, when the GFR has fallen to 50% of normal (60 mL/min), creatinine level doubles to only about 200 micromol/L, not far outside the normal range. Subsequently it starts to rise sharply, e.g. fourfold normal when GFR falls to 25% and tenfold normal when GFR fall to 10%.

Thus serum creatinine cannot be relied upon to detect moderate renal impairment. Its main value in renal disease lies in monitoring the decline in renal function of a known sufferer from kidney disease, following a single full creatinine clearance measurement to establish the relationship to serum creatinine in that particular patient. This can best be followed by plotting the reciprocal of creatinine clearance: the slope of the resulting straight line indicates the rate of decline of renal function. Any change in this slope requires investigation. Furthermore, an extrapolation can be made to indicate the time when GFR will fall below 10 mL/min, and thus to predict when a patient will probably require some form of renal replacement therapy (Fig. 4.7).

Blood urea measurements suffer from similar limitations. Blood urea levels are affected acutely by dietary variations in protein intake, by skeletal muscle damage and by catabolic states, e.g. fever or starvation. Nevertheless, blood urea is a traditional general index of renal function and malfunction (the routine 'urea and electrolytes').

Tubular function

Urine concentrating ability can be tested by subjecting the patient to water deprivation. Inability to conserve water, manifested clinically as polyuria, may be an early sign of chronic renal disease. ADH can be used to establish whether it is of pituitary origin (diabetes insipidus) or is nephrogenic (e.g. tubular disease, nephrogenic diabetes insipidus). Giving an acid or base load can be used to test the kidney's ability to secrete or conserve acid, i.e. its urine acidifying ability.

General secretory function is tested with a substance which is completely cleared in one pass through the nephron owing to maximal tubular secretion, e.g. *para*-amino hippuric acid (PAH). The secretion of specific metabolites can if necessary be tested by giving known loadings. This might be helpful, e.g. in distinguishing diabetes mellitus from renal glycosuria, a rare condition of reduced glucose threshold.

Blood biochemistry

The above tests can give precise measures of discrete renal functions, but in practice it is the consequences of impaired function which are clinically important. The best indices are thus the plasma levels of the metabolites and toxins normally cleared renally. In addition to urea and

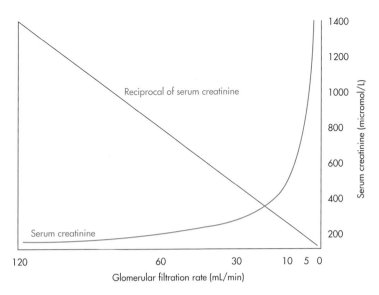

Figure 4.7 Changes in serum creatinine concentration and reciprocal creatinine concentration correlated with glomerular filtration rate.

creatinine, routine measurement of plasma sodium, potassium, bicarbonate, calcium, phosphate and pH is vital in estimating and monitoring renal function, although of course the plasma levels of these substances may be altered by other factors and disorders.

Imaging

Ultrasound will show the size and position of the kidneys; this technique has replaced plain abdominal X-ray as the first-line investigation as it is cheaper and less invasive. Enlargement of both kidneys suggests polycystic disease, while unilateral enlargement implies obstruction. Shrunken kidneys imply, non-specifically, advanced chronic renal disease. Calcified deposits in the kidney or ureters (stones) will also be visible. Doppler ultrasound can be used to visualize arterial supply and intrarenal blood flow; this is less invasive than the alternative, **angiography**, although the latter gives much more reliable and complete information. Computed tomography (**CT**) and magnetic resonance image (**MRI**) scanning are also used to examine intrarenal structures.

An **intravenous excretory urogram** (IVU; formerly intravenous pyelogram or IVP) uses an X-ray contrast medium to produce a series of images which will show any inequality of perfusion between the kidneys, the rate of renal filling, internal renal structural abnormalities, e.g. cysts, and the patency and completeness of voiding of the lower urinary tract (UT). However, patients may react badly to iodine-containing contrast media. Isotope renography yields similar information and is potentially less toxic, although less readily available. In the recently introduced technique of **antegrade urography** a needle is introduced into the renal pelvis (nephrostomy) and contrast medium injected, giving a picture of the whole urinary outflow pathway.

The lower UT can be visualized by **retrograde urography** to investigate possible obstruction; the contrast medium is administered via a urethral catheter. There is a significant risk of introducing infection, but the technique may still be used if the patient cannot tolerate contrast media. The lower UT may also be investigated with a fibreoptic **cystoscope**, which also permits biopsy samples to be taken. However, **biopsies** of the renal mass must be taken percutaneously. They are particularly useful in the differential diagnosis of nephritis and in assessing transplant rejection.

Fluid and electrolyte imbalance

Only a general outline of the principles of this complex topic are given here. The References and further reading section (p. 214) lists some excellent specialist texts.

Volume and osmotic imbalance

Because control of total body water and plasma osmolarity are closely linked there are often coexisting imbalances. There is seldom a simple loss or excess of either water or sodium, but if so the result would be a mixed disorder, e.g. primary (pure) water depletion would cause hypovolaemia with hypernatraemia. Moreover, a patient's observed biochemical status may be due to the primary problem, to inadequate or incomplete compensation, or to treatment. For example, water and sodium loss from excessive sweating, over-compensated by drinking hypotonic fluid (e.g. pure water), will at some stage cause both hypervolaemia and hyponatraemia.

Aetiology

Some of the possible combinations of volume and osmotic imbalance and their possible primary causes are summarized in Table 4.6.

Water imbalance
Water depletion occurs either through excessive losses or deficient intake. As water depletion causes severe thirst, it will usually only become serious when thirst cannot be satisfied. The degree of associated hypernatraemia will depend on salt intake and the effectiveness of renal compensation by fluid retention. The main causes of **water excess** are renal, although excess fluid intake may produce a hypervolaemic, hypo-osmolar state.

Sodium and osmotic imbalance
Sodium imbalance is rarely the direct result of either excess or deficient sodium intake. More usually it reflects either compensated primary water imbalance or a renal sodium handling defect.

Plasma sodium concentration gives a valuable index of the relative excess or deficit of sodium and water and thus of the underlying cause of any fluid or electrolyte imbalance. However, plasma sodium level must always be interpreted in association with the haemodynamic status and haematological parameters. Thus hypovolaemia from isotonic fluid loss (e.g. from burns) would not cause a sodium imbalance, but would raise packed cell volume, whereas predominant water depletion (e.g. from vomiting) would lead to **hypernatraemia**. Net sodium loss, e.g. dehydration and inappropriate (hypotonic) replacement, would result in **hyponatraemia**.

Generally, sodium imbalance implies an osmotic imbalance. However, in some circumstances other osmotically active substances can first appear in the plasma in abnormal amounts and the sodium level will then be adjusted accordingly. For example, in diabetic hyperglycaemia or severe uraemia, sodium will effectively be displaced from the plasma by glucose or urea, giving a secondary or appropriate hyponatraemia. Thus, abnormal plasma sodium measurements may reflect neither abnormal sodium balance nor true plasma osmolarity. Further complications can arise in hyperlipidaemia or hyperproteinaemia when the aqueous fraction of plasma is reduced. This is not taken into account by the usual sodium measurement techniques, and so the sodium level will appear low even though it is actually in isotonic concentration in the plasma water ('pseudohyponatraemia').

Pathophysiology

The consequences of fluid or osmotic imbalance are far-reaching, which is why the body defends normal balances so strongly. In general, fluid imbalance has haemodynamic consequences while osmotic imbalance causes neurological complications (Fig. 4.8).

Volume imbalance
Even small changes in the **intravascular (i.e. blood) volume** can affect BP, cardiac performance and tissue perfusion. In contrast, the intracellular and the extracellular (extravascular tissue) spaces can tolerate quite large changes. The tissues most affected will be those under least external pressure opposing redistribution. This includes soft tissues and areas where hydrostatic forces increase diffusion from the capillaries into the tissues, e.g. in dependent areas such as

Table 4.6   Disorders of osmotic and water balance

Imbalance	Possible causes	Comment
Hypervolaemia		
Hyperosmolar	Excess Na intake (e.g. HCO_3)	Rare
Normo-osmolar	Excessive intake	**True hypervolaemia**
	• diet	Excessive IV infusion
	Fluid retention	
	• renal failure	
	• drugs	e.g. corticosteroids
	• aldosteronism	Cushing's disease, heart failure
Hypo-osmolar	Excessive hypotonic fluid intake	**Water intoxication**
	• excessive thirst, beer intake	
	• excessive IV infusion	Especially dextrose 5%
	Impaired water clearance	
	• inappropriate ADH secretion	
	• prostaglandin inhibition (NSAIDs)	
Normovolaemia		
Hypo-osmolar	'Dilutional' hyponatraemia	
	• excessive hypotonic fluid intake	e.g. beer
	• dehydration + hypotonic replacement	Net Na loss
	'Sick cell syndrome'	Na-pump problem (severe illness)
Hypovolaemia		
Hyperosmolar	Predominant water loss	**Primary water depletion**
	• hyperventilation	
	• sweat, e.g. hot climates, fever	GI fluids and sweat are hypotonic
	• GI fluids (vomit, diarrhoea)	
	• osmotic diuresis	
	– hyperglycaemia (diabetes mellitus)	
	– mannitol	
	• reduced ADH secretion/action	
	– diabetes insipidus	
	– drugs, e.g. alcohol, lithium	
	Reduced intake	
	• coma, dysphagia, postoperative	
Normo-osmolar	Excessive isotonic fluid loss	**Dehydration**
	• as above with partial compensation	
	• burns, haemorrhage	
	• polyuric chronic renal failure	*See* pp. 184 and 180
	• diuretic phase of acute renal failure	
	• excessive diuretic use	

ADH, antidiuretic hormone; GI, gastrointestinal; NSAID, non-steroidal anti-inflammatory drug.

the ankles. This is one mechanism of oedema formation. Usually, oedema is without ill effect, except in the lungs, where pulmonary oedema is always dangerous.

Isotonic changes in total body water will usually be restricted to the ECF, i.e. plasma and tissue fluid, because sodium movement across cell membranes is restricted. Changes in free water, e.g. excess of

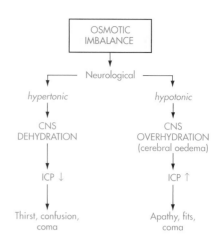

Figure 4.8 Pathophysiological consequences of volume and osmotic imbalance. CNS, central nervous system; ICP, intracranial pressure.

hypotonic fluid, or water with a solute such as glucose which is normally diffusible across cell membranes, will be distributed throughout all body fluid compartments. Thus the haemodynamic consequences will be buffered, delayed and less severe.

Osmotic imbalance

If there is an acute osmotic imbalance between the ECF and the ICF, water will diffuse passively under osmotic forces. Plasma and tissue fluid which is **hypertonic** relative to ICF will draw water from all body cells, causing intracellular dehydration. Conversely, **hypotonic** ECF will overload cells with water. Small changes in the intracellular volume of most tissues are of little consequence, but the brain is an exception. Because the brain is contained within the rigid skull, small changes in volume will alter intracranial pressure, and quite small alterations in this pressure can have serious neurological effects, potentially resulting in coma or death.

These effects only occur after acute changes; compensatory mechanisms eventually tend to correct the imbalance. Aldosterone and ADH will restore extracellular osmotic pressure by adjusting sodium clearance, and brain cells threatened with dehydration can manufacture osmotically active substances intracellularly to retain water.

If plasma oncotic (colloid osmotic) pressure is reduced owing to hypoproteinaemia, there will be a disproportionate loss of water to the tissues. Although the absolute osmotic differences are

relatively small the resultant oedema can sometimes be gross, as in nephrotic syndrome.

Clinical features

The combination of signs and symptoms presented by a patient will depend on the primary cause, the main volaemic (haemodynamic) or osmotic (neurological) consequences and secondary effects or compensations. The acute effects before compensation are summarized in Table 4.7.

Management

Degree and speed of intervention

The first step is to ascertain the cause of osmotic imbalance. If the situation is not critical, i.e. there are no severe neurological problems or pulmonary oedema, correction of the cause will often be sufficient. If there is no underlying renal disease the body is able eventually to reverse most imbalances. Otherwise, minimal intervention with the very simplest of corrections may suffice. More specific measures usually need be taken only when there is renal impairment.

Great care is needed, even with simple correction. All interventions, whether by the oral or the parenteral route, initially alter only the volume or concentration of the plasma. Equilibration between intravascular and extracellular fluid occurs quite rapidly, but several hours are needed for equilibration between the extracellu-

Table 4.7   Clinical features of volume and osmotic imbalance

Hypervolaemia	Hypertension
	Incipient heart failure ('high output')
	Oedema (especially pulmonary)
	Oliguria (if renal impairment is cause)
	Increased intraocular pressure, visual problems
	Weight gain
Hypovolaemia	Thirst, dry mouth, sunken cheeks
	Reduced intraocular pressure, visual problems
	Pale cold skin, with loss of turgor (dehydration of dermis)
	Low cardiac output, tachycardia
	(Postural) hypotension, collapse, shock
	Oliguria; incipient pre-renal failure
	Weight loss
Hypernatraemia/hyperosmolar	Confusion, hallucinations, convulsions, coma
	Muscular jerks
	Oliguria or polyuria (depending on cause)
Hyponatraemia/hypo-osmolar	Anorexia, nausea and vomiting
	Lethargy, apathy, confusion
	Headache, convulsions, coma
	Reduced intraocular pressure (osmotic loss), visual problems

lar and intracellular compartments. Thus, too rapid a correction will cause a disproportionate, potentially dangerous initial change in plasma osmolarity or blood volume and result in an overshoot, e.g. hyponatraemia treated too vigorously with hypertonic saline may cause an equally harmful hypernatraemia.

Conversely, if therapy is too delayed, compensation will have already been initiated – particularly in the brain – and correction may then have an opposite effect. For example, if plasma is hypertonic for too long, brain cells will also become hypertonic. At that stage, rapid attempts at correction with hypotonic fluids may then cause CNS over-hydration and raised intracranial pressure.

Dose estimation and monitoring

Various formulae are available for calculating fluid and electrolyte deficits and the amounts needed for correction from electrolyte measurements. However, these can only be used for initial guidance. Subsequently, it is far more important to observe the effect of initial therapy and make appropriate adjustments according to the patient's physical signs and haemodynamic and biochemical status.

The three main measures used in monitoring water balance and general hydration are:

- Sodium concentration.
- Blood pressure (or preferably central venous pressure).
- Packed cell volume.

All three measures must be considered together. Urine volume may also be significant. For all fluid and electrolyte imbalances, the possibility of coexisting potassium or pH imbalance must be checked.

Specific therapy

Dehydration and hypovolaemia. Mild volume deficit, especially of gastrointestinal origin, may be corrected orally with glucose–electrolyte solutions if the patient is able to drink. Severe volume depletion with circulatory insufficiency requires intravenous therapy, and physiological saline is usually satisfactory. Restoration of urine output is the best index of successful therapy. Physiological saline infusion should not be continued unnecessarily because it can lead to hyperchloraemic acidosis.

Hypernatraemia. If neurological involvement is threatened, the logical treatment would be a sodium-reduced fluid. Sodium chloride 0.45% or weaker solutions are available, but dextrose 5% is probably better. This is isotonic on injection but yields pure water once the dextrose is metabolized. Dextrose 4% plus sodium chloride 0.18% ('dextrose saline') is similar but provides some sodium. Nevertheless, sodium chloride 0.9% is often adequate if renal function is unimpaired. Because the aim is a gradual reduction of osmotic pressure, the small diluting effect produced is temporarily beneficial until the kidneys can make the necessary compensation.

Hypervolaemia. If mild, this can be treated by simple water restriction. In severe cases with pulmonary oedema or threatened cardiac failure, a diuretic is needed.

Hyponatraemia. Mild hyponatraemia can be treated orally with sodium chloride, but more aggressive action is needed if cerebral oedema develops. Temporarily, a poorly diffusing osmotic diuretic such as mannitol may be infused to elevate plasma osmotic pressure. Corticosteroids such as *dexamethasone* are also advocated but neither the mechanism nor the benefit is clear. Such cases can be treated cautiously with hypertonic sodium chloride, with a concentration of up to 5% being used.

Inappropriate secretion of ADH can be treated with *lithium* or *demeclocycline*. The treatment of diabetes insipidus is not considered here.

Potassium imbalance

Pathophysiology

Distribution of body potassium

Most body potassium (K^+) is either within the cells or in bone (Fig. 4.9). Extracellular fluid K^+, as measured in the plasma, represents only a very small proportion of total body load. Yet it is plasma K^+ which has the greatest physiological importance, being involved in maintaining the membrane potential of all cells. Changes in plasma K^+ of more than ± 2 mmol/L can have serious effects on nerve and muscle function, especially in the heart. The terms hypokalaemia and hyperkalaemia refer specifically to plasma level abnormalities, and say little about total body potassium balance.

Bone potassium is exchanged very slowly and so plays little part in acute changes. The ICF acts as a reservoir and buffers plasma potassium so that considerable variations in total body potassium can occur before the plasma level changes: up to 200 mmol can be lost from the cells with no appreciable change in plasma K^+. Despite plasma level being a poor index of potassium status it is the only easily accessible direct measure available. Any related pH imbalance must also be taken into account when interpreting plasma K^+ levels.

Homeostasis

Extracellular K^+ is in equilibrium with the ICF, an unequal distribution across the cell membrane being maintained by the sodium (Na/K^+ exchange) pump. Cellular uptake of K^+ is promoted by an alkaline plasma (pH >7.4), aldosterone, adrenaline ((epinephrine), via beta-receptors) and insulin.

A rise in plasma K^+ causes insulin release, which promotes the uptake of glucose and K^+ by cells. Whether this is a co-transport mechanism or simply the supply of extra energy for the pump itself is not known, but it provides a useful therapeutic strategy in hyperkalaemia. Conversely, acidic conditions, lack of insulin, beta-blockers and the absence of aldosterone, inhibit K^+ uptake and may cause hyperkalaemia.

These factors have a special significance in renal tubular cells where they control not only

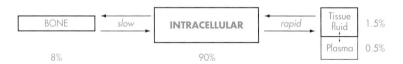

Figure 4.9   Distribution of body potassium.

the intracellular/extracellular distribution but also total body potassium, as follows: when the tubular filtrate reaches the distal tubule almost all potassium has been reabsorbed. If plasma K^+ is too high, aldosterone causes the distal tubule cells to remove K^+ from the plasma and secrete it into the tubular fluid (urine), in exchange for Na^+. Because this same transport mechanism mediates acid secretion, conflicts can arise (pp. 158–159).

Aetiology

Gross abnormalities in total body potassium, which may or may not be reflected in plasma level changes, must be recognized in addition to clinically significant hypokalaemia or hyperkalaemia. Because K^+ is not metabolized, total body imbalance arises from abnormalities in either intake or loss (Table 4.8). Acute changes will affect the plasma level, but more protracted changes will at first be compensated for by the intracellular pool. Acute plasma imbalances may also arise from disturbed intracellular/extracellular distribution, with no net change in total body K^+.

Hypokalaemia

Normally the body is in positive potassium balance. Daily renal, faecal and sweat losses rarely exceed 40 mmol, and a healthy diet provides 50–100 mmol.

However, a diet which is deficient in fresh fruit and vegetables can cause potassium deficiency.

Most **diuretics** cause some potassium loss, partly by presenting more filtered sodium to the distal tubule. The kidney tries to compensate for the enforced natriuresis by reabsorbing Na^+, and in doing so exchanges it for K^+. Neither diet nor diuretics alone usually cause clinically significant hypokalaemia but the combination may be serious, especially in the elderly.

Alkalosis affects the plasma K^+ level in two ways. It directly promotes cellular uptake of K^+ and it causes the kidney to conserve acid by reabsorbing it distally in preference to K^+. This increases K^+ loss and can exacerbate the hypokalaemia.

Aldosteronism (excess mineralocorticoid activity) can present in various ways, e.g. Cushing's disease, Conn's syndrome, corticosteroid therapy, heart failure or hypoproteinaemia (e.g. from hepatic disease or nephrotic syndrome). In the last two of these conditions, reduced BP and/or circulating fluid volume activate the renin/angiotensin system, causing excess aldosterone secretion with Na^+ retention and K^+ loss.

Gastrointestinal secretions contain high levels of K^+, and **laxative abuse** is sometimes a hidden cause of hypokalaemia. Liquorice, which is sometimes used as a laxative, has an aldosterone-like

Table 4.8   Causes of potassium imbalance

	Hypokalaemia	Hyperkalaemia
GI intake	Poor diet	Excess K salts/supplements
GI output	Laxative abuse	
	Vomiting, diarrhoea	
	Fistula, stoma	
Renal clearance	Drugs	Renal failure
	• loop and thiazide diuretics	Drugs
	• osmotic diuretics	• K-sparing diuretics
	• steroids, carbenoxolone	• aldosterone antagonists
	Alkalosis	Acidosis
	Aldosteronism	Adrenal insufficiency
Distribution	Alkalosis	Acidosis
	Adrenaline (epinephrine), SNS	Tissue trauma, exercise
	Insulin	Diabetes mellitus (uncontrolled)

GI, gastrointestinal; SNS, sympathetic nervous system.

action (as does the now obsolete anti-ulcer agent, carbenoxolone).

Hyperkalaemia

Potassium excess (hyperkalaemia) is less common than hypokalaemia, but is harder to treat. Renal failure is probably the most common cause of hyperkalaemia, and this is one of the main problems in managing renal patients. Dietary causes are rare, but over-zealous use of potassium salts, e.g. potassium citrate mixture in the self-treatment of cystitis, can be responsible. Over-use of potassium supplements is only a remote possibility, given patients' well-known lack of enthusiasm for the slow-release forms. More subtly, potassium-retaining diuretics, e.g. *amiloride*, can lead to excessive inhibition of K^+ secretion, especially in combination with the ACEIs. This situation can be exacerbated in the elderly, who usually have impaired renal function.

Clinical features

Dyskalaemias disturb the transmembrane ionic balance and the membrane potential, so muscle cells are particularly susceptible.

Hypokalaemia, depending on its duration and severity, can cause numbness, weakness, paralysis, low cardiac output, tachyarrhythmias and heart failure. The myocardial toxicity of digoxin is also enhanced. In the longer term, renal damage can occur, while inhibition of gastrointestinal activity can lead to bowel obstruction. Renal attempts at compensation with potassium conservation and acid loss leads to metabolic alkalosis, as in long-term diuretic overuse. Chronic severe hypokalaemia can impair renal concentrating ability, leading to ADH-resistant polyuria and polydipsia.

Hyperkalaemia, although more dangerous, causes fewer symptoms and indeed may be silent until cardiac arrest occurs. A characteristic ECG change of a spiked T-wave may be observed. Acidosis is a further complication.

Management

Correction of abnormal plasma levels is the immediate therapeutic target in potassium imbalance. Oral therapy is adequate for mild imbalances but severe dyskalaemia (<3 or >6 mmol/L) needs urgent attention, mainly to protect the heart. However, the total body excess or deficit will be many times larger than the simple correction of plasma level would imply.

For example, a plasma level of 2.5 mmol/L requires 2 mmol/L to restore a normal level of 4.5 mmol/L. For an average plasma water volume of 3 L this requires $3 \times 2 = 6$ mmol of K^+ (less than half a standard oral potassium tablet). But most of the administered potassium will be distributed extravascularly and diffuse rapidly into the tissue fluid (9 L) and then more slowly, over 24 h, into the cells (30 L). The plasma will retain less than one-fifteenth of the administered dose. However, because of the time this takes to occur, attempts at rapid correction with the calculated total body deficit (in this case, $6 \times 15 = 90$ mmol) would cause acute hyperkalaemia. Conversely, too rapid a reduction in raised plasma K^+ by dialysis will cause hypokalaemia. Gradual adjustment with frequent monitoring of plasma level is important.

Hypokalaemia

Generally speaking, it is easier to get potassium into a deficient body than it is to extract an excess.

Mild hypokalaemia. Here, dietary correction is preferred. The routine prescription of potassium supplements with diuretics is no longer thought necessary and should preferably only follow plasma level measurement of K^+.

Most potassium salts have an unpalatable, saline taste. Effervescent formulations disguise the taste, but they usually contain bicarbonate, which is often contraindicated because of the associated alkalosis. Liquid preparations of the chloride are perhaps underused. Very large oral slow-release forms are probably the least complied with of all medication, and there is the additional possibility of gastrointestinal irritation, ulceration or obstruction.

Fixed-dose combination preparations, e.g. diuretic and potassium, used to be popular but need particular care. In addition to the usual problems of preformulated combinations (inflexibility of individual component dosage, possible confusion over adverse effects, etc.), these preparations seem particularly likely to cause severe gastrointestinal lesions. They have now been superseded by potassium-sparing diuretics.

Severe hypokalaemia.   This needs parenteral potassium usually by IV infusion. Because of the time needed for equilibration it must not be injected too rapidly or in too high a concentration. Acceptable maxima are a 40 mmol/L solution given at no more than 20 mmol/h, with an 80 mmol daily maximum.

Hyperkalaemia

Mild hyperkalaemia.   It is possible to reduce plasma K level slowly by binding it in the gut lumen with a cationic ion exchange resin such as *polystyrene sulphonate*, used as the calcium or sodium salt. This is unpalatable and can be given rectally, but neither route is very efficient.

Severe hyperkalaemia.   The immediate need is to correct the plasma level: the overall body excess is less urgent. Calcium (10 mL of 10% *calcium gluconate*) is injected to provide a temporary physiological antidote to the cardiotoxic effect. This is followed (in the absence of renal impairment) by infusion of up to 200 mmol of *bicarbonate* (depending on the degree of acidosis), *insulin* (20 units) and *glucose* (50 g). This stimulates potassium uptake into all body cells, reducing the plasma level, but of course does not correct the total body excess. Beta-adrenergic agonists may also be used, e.g. nebulized or injected *salbutamol*, which presumably stimulate the sodium pump by activating Na/K-ATPase. The effect may be additive to that of insulin and glucose.

Measures to reduce body potassium level then follow. An ion exchange resin treatment is started, but dialysis may be necessary if plasma levels cannot be controlled satisfactorily. Otherwise, renal compensation is given time to work.

Acid–base imbalance

This potentially confusing topic will be dealt with here in a simplified way, to enable imbalances and therapy to be understood. One common problem with the terminology can be readily clarified. Any pH imbalance resulting from respiratory disorder is termed 'respiratory' (either acidosis or alkalosis); all other forms are 'metabolic', whether or not they are caused by a genuine metabolic defect. Thus the ingestion of battery acid is as 'metabolic' as lactic acidosis, although 'non-respiratory' might be a preferable term.

Aetiology

Acid–base imbalance can be conveniently visualized by considering the normal and possible abnormal routes for the intake, production and output of acid and bicarbonate in relation to the equation which controls pH (Fig. 4.10). Overactivity or under-activity of any of these pathways can cause pH imbalance (Table 4.9).

Because the body is normally in positive acid balance, acidosis is more common than alkalosis. **Respiratory acidosis** is usually predictable because of associated cardiorespiratory disease; **respiratory alkalosis** is rare. Among the vast number of possible **non-respiratory** disturbances gastrointestinal causes are common and acidosis is also a major problem in renal failure. The accumulation in the blood of lactate, ketoacids or acidic drug metabolites is another major cause. Biguanide-induced lactic acidosis is now rare.

Investigation and diagnosis

The first priority is to identify and correct the underlying cause. Initially this involves measurement of blood CO_2, HCO_3^- and pH, and a simplified guide is given in Fig. 4.11. The precise biochemical picture will depend on the nature and degree of compensation. Complex mixed disorders are possible, e.g. metabolic and respiratory acidosis in a poorly controlled diabetic with chronic bronchitis.

Anion gap

Normally total plasma cations (mainly Na^+ and K^+) exceed the measured anions (mainly Cl^- and HCO_3^-) by about 15 mmol/L. The difference –

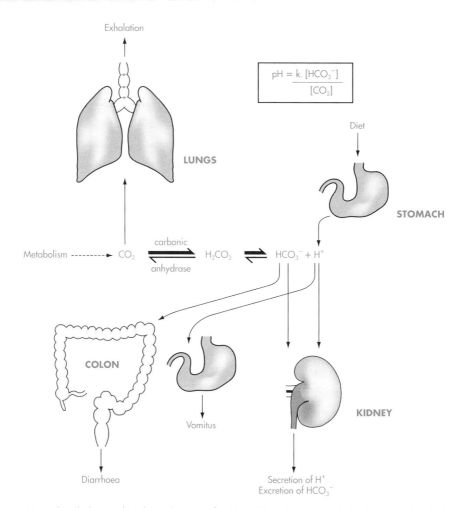

Figure 4.10   Normal and abnormal intake and output of acid and bicarbonate, related to the normal acid–base balance equation.

called the anion gap – is made up by phosphate, sulphate, protein and other organic acids:

$$\text{Anion gap} = ([Na^+] + [K^+]) - ([Cl^-] + [HCO_3^-])$$

In acidosis caused by the accumulation of endogenous or exogenous toxic organic acids (e.g. lactate, salicylate), these anions displace bicarbonate and the anion gap is increased. Conversely, in acidosis from simple acid accumulation (e.g. renal failure) or bicarbonate loss (e.g. diarrhoea), the bicarbonate is replaced by chloride so the gap is normal. Lactic acidosis is sometimes further subdivided into type A caused by tissue hypoxia and type B caused by abnormal production of acids, e.g. in uncontrolled diabetes mellitus.

Clinical features

The effects of pH imbalance are profound but non-specific, and diagnosis is usually made biochemically. Most systems in the body are affected (Table 4.10) but the main clinical problems are cardiovascular. Acidosis reduces cardiac contractility – an effect potentiated by beta-blockers – and dilates arteries and constricts veins; all have adverse haemodynamic effects. Oxygen dissociation from haemoglobin is increased, which may improve tissue oxygenation but impair pulmonary oxygen uptake.

The CNS is depressed by acidosis, but nerve and muscle excitability are increased by alkalosis, leading to seizures and tetany. In non-

Table 4.9   Possible causes of pH imbalance

Acidosis (pH <7.2)	Alkalosis (pH >7.6)
Carbon dioxide gain Respiratory failure Obstructive airways disease Respiratory depression (inc. drugs)	**Carbon dioxide loss** Hyperventilation (panic attacks)
Bicarbonate loss Diarrhoea Carbonic anhydrase inhibitors Renal tubular acidosis Aldosterone deficiency Hyperkalaemia Hyperchloraemia	**Bicarbonate gain** Antacid overuse ($NaHCO_3$) 'Milk alkali syndrome' Potassium citrate mixture Aldosteronism Hypokalaemia Hypochloraemia Diuretics
Acid gain Renal failure Ketoacidosis • starvation • diabetes mellitus Lactic acidosis • exercise • shock • hypoxia • biguanides • fructose/sorbitol IV Salicylate poisoning Reye's syndrome Ammonium chloride overuse	**Acid loss** Vomiting, pyloric stenosis Aldosteronism Hypokalaemia

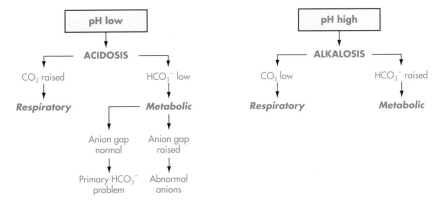

Figure 4.11   Biochemical parameters of pH imbalance.

Table 4.10   Clinical features of pH imbalance

Acidosis	Alkalosis
Hyperventilation	Hypoventilation
Impaired consciousness	Seizures, tetany
Hyperkalaemia	Hypokalaemia
Cardiovascular	
• reduced cardiac output	
• circulatory insufficiency	
• arrhythmias, arrest	

respiratory disorders the respiratory rate is altered to compensate for this. Urinary acid secretion is changed appropriately, with consequences for potassium balance.

The distribution and clearance of acidic and basic drugs is affected. This is the basis of forced diuresis for treating poisoning. Alkali loading causes an alkaline urine which encourages the clearance of acids such as salicylate. Conversely, acid will encourage the clearance of bases, e.g. many psychotropic agents, such as amphetamine. Some drug interactions are explained by this mechanism; for example, rheumatoid arthritis patients stabilized on salicylates can experience a loss of analgesic effectiveness if they consume too much antacid.

Management

Unless the severity of the imbalance is causing cardiovascular or CNS problems or the cause is irreversible, e.g. chronic renal failure, the best general strategy is simply to remove the cause and allow the body to carry out normal correction at its own pace.

Acidosis

Chronic **moderate acidosis** can be treated orally with *sodium bicarbonate*. In acute **severe metabolic acidosis** specific correction is avoided if the patient can be expected to recover spontaneously. The use of bicarbonate infusion is easily misjudged, causing an equally serious 'alkaline overshoot'.

Various strengths of bicarbonate injection are available. The preferred 1.4% preparation is isotonic and provides one-sixth of a mmol/mL. For urgent cases more concentrated solutions are available as boluses, but these must be injected very slowly. An 8.4% solution provides

1 mmol/mL, which facilitates dose calculation but is very hypertonic (six times normal). Intermediate strengths are also available. Lactate is no longer used because it acts indirectly and some acidotic patients may not be able to metabolize it to its active form (i.e. bicarbonate).

The total dose needed is usually 100–200 mmol of bicarbonate. An estimate in mmol can be made empirically from the patient's body weight (kg) and the measured plasma bicarbonate:

$$\text{Bicarbonate dose} = \tfrac{1}{3}\,\text{Body weight} \times (\text{Normal plasma } HCO_3^- - \text{Measured } HCO_3^-).$$

However, as with K imbalance, frequent monitoring and adjustment are better guides.

In **respiratory acidosis** the cause must be treated directly, if necessary by ventilation. Simple bicarbonate correction is inappropriate.

Alkalosis

Metabolic alkalosis can usually be treated with simple infusions of 0.9% sodium chloride (p. 159). Sometimes, however, direct infusion of acid is required. Hydrochloric acid has been used, but the *hydrochlorides* of *ammonium*, *lysine* or *arginine* are preferred. Ammonium chloride may be given orally.

Respiratory alkalosis is very rare and is almost invariably a temporary self-correcting condition. Rebreathing from a bag, which limits carbon dioxide loss, may speed recovery.

Renal failure

Renal failure denotes a global loss of renal function, but it occurs to different degrees. The body can maintain normal homeostasis with reduced renal function down to about half the normal GFR (60 mL/min). The term **renal impairment** is used when the GFR falls below this but remains above 30 mL/min; at this stage the patient may still be predominantly symptom-free. **Renal failure** may be defined as a GFR below 30 mL/min, when symptoms become evident. When the GFR falls below about 10 mL/min, the condition is termed **end-stage renal failure**.

Like heart failure, renal failure is not a specific disease but a complex syndrome with many possible causes and a fairly uniform clinical presentation. In **acute** renal failure (ARF) the impairment of regulatory and excretory functions predominates: in the **chronic** form (CRF) there is also an endocrine abnormality.

ARF most commonly occurs secondary to generalized circulatory failure. The condition develops rapidly and has a high mortality but is reversible if treatment is provided early enough: if the patient survives there may be no permanent sequelae. CRF has an insidious onset and is usually caused by direct damage to the renal tissue. The large natural renal reserve and the slow progression of CRF mean that considerable irreversible damage has usually occurred by the time the patient reports symptoms. There is then an inexorable decline towards end-stage renal failure, which is fatal without renal replacement therapy, i.e. dialysis or transplantation.

Classification and aetiology

The many factors which can impair renal function may be divided into three groups, depending on whether the primary fault is in renal perfusion, the kidney tissue itself or urinary outflow (Table 4.11).

Table 4.11 Aetiology of renal failure

General pathology	Examples
Pre-renal	
Circulatory shock	Hypovolaemia (burns, dehydration, haemorrhage)
	Cardiogenic (myocardial infarction)
	Septicaemia
	Liver disease, pancreatitis
	Obstetric (septicaemia, haemorrhage)
Intrinsic renal	
Glomerular	Autoimmune (e.g. glomerulonephritis)
	Connective tissue disease (e.g. SLE)
	Diabetic nephropathy
Tubular	Acute tubular nephropathy (vasomotor, nephrotoxic)
	Interstitial nephritis
Renovascular	Renal thrombosis, infarction
	Hypertension: essential, malignant
	Connective tissue disease (polyarteritis, etc.)
Infection	Pyelonephritis, malaria
Nephrotixicity	Glomerular (e.g. penicillamine, heavy metals)
	Interstitial (e.g. penicillin, NSAID)
Metabolic	Hypercalcaemia, hypokalaemia
	Hyperuricaemia
Congenital	Polycystic disease
Post-renal	
Stones	Usually oxalate
Structural	Tumour, stricture, prostatitis
Nephrotoxicity	Analgesic nephropathy (e.g. phenacetin)
	Crystal uropathy (e.g. sulphonamides)
	Urate deposition (cytotoxics, gout)
Outside the urinary tract	Abdominal tumour (e.g. ovarian)
	Retroperitoneal fibrosis (e.g. methysergide)

SLE, systemic lupus erythematosus.

Pre-renal failure

The kidney relies on a continuous supply of blood at sufficient pressure to maintain the glomerular filtration and endeavours to maintain systemic or intrarenal perfusion pressure. However, severe hypovolaemia and/or hypotension, owing usually to fluid depletion, cardiac failure or other shock states, overwhelmingly compromise this, and ARF commonly follows.

Intrinsic renal failure

The kidney is especially prone to immunological or toxic damage. This is probably because in its excretory role the kidney concentrates the products of the immune system (e.g. immune complexes) and of metabolism, and its high blood flow exposes the renal tissues to potential toxins far more than most organs. Nephrotoxicity is a common cause of renal failure, and a medication history is essential in investigating any unexplained renal impairment.

The glomeruli and the tubules and interstitial tissues may be affected independently by different causes, although some conditions affect both, e.g. ischaemia following circulatory failure. Intrinsic damage is usually a chronic process but toxic or ischaemic nephropathy can be acute.

Post-renal failure

Obstruction anywhere from the renal pelvis to the urethra is a less common and normally reversible cause of renal failure. Back pressure is raised in the tubules and this reduces the glomerular filtration pressure and hence the GFR. The obstruction is usually within the urinary tract, but external pressure from an abdominal mass may also be responsible.

Post-renal failure is usually chronic. Occasionally, acute forms may cause anuria. A common cause of this in elderly men is prostatic hypertrophy obstructing bladder outflow.

Acute tubular nephropathy (ATN)

This term describes acute reversible tubular damage and is sometimes called, somewhat inaccurately, 'acute tubular necrosis'. It can be an important consequence of acute pre-renal failure following circulatory insufficiency which is not rapidly reversed. Thus ARF and ATN frequently coexist and, confusingly, the terms are some-times used synonymously. ATN may also be the result of renovascular, glomerular or tubular disease or toxic damage.

It may be asked what difference there is for the kidney between renal ischaemia resulting from renovascular obstruction (nominally 'intrinsic ATN') and general systemic circulatory collapse (pre-renal). The conventional distinction, made on clinical grounds, is that pre-renal failure is rapidly corrected by restoration of circulation whereas once ATN has supervened recovery is usually much slower.

The precise pathology of ATN is not known. It seems to be precipitated by intense intrarenal vasoconstriction, which inhibits filtration because of the reduced afferent glomerular artery pressure. The nephrotoxicity of prostaglandin inhibitors (e.g. NSAIDs) is due to a similar effect. The vasoconstriction may simply be a response to injury, or it may be a maladaptive attempt to maintain renal perfusion pressure. In either case the subsequent ischaemic damage is counterproductive. Moreover, it may be perpetuated even after perfusion has been restored, owing to glomerular damage or tubular obstruction with inflammatory or necrotic debris.

Pathophysiology

The loss of renal function has complex and serious consequences. One useful distinction, which helps to account for the clinical pictures found in different types and stages of renal failure, is between glomerular and tubular dysfunction. Although both structures may be damaged, the trauma is often predominantly to one or other, e.g. glomerulonephritis primarily causes glomerular damage whereas aminoglycoside nephrotoxicity is mainly tubular. In pre-renal failure both types occur at different stages.

Glomerular dysfunction

The principal causes of this are pre-renally impaired perfusion, intrinsic glomerular inflammation and post-renal obstruction. As the main function of the glomeruli is filtration, there is a fall in GFR with retention of those substances usually cleared by filtration, including water (Table 4.12).

Table 4.12 Consequences of glomerular dysfunction

Clinical feature	Cause
Oliguria Hypervolaemia Uraemia Hyperkalaemia Hyperphosphataemia Hyperuricaemia	Reduced filtration plus increased reabsorption
Hyperkalaemia Acidosis	Reduced secretion owing to reduced distal [Na]

The consequent reduced volume of filtrate and slower tubular flow permits increased proximal tubular reabsorption, which reinforces these effects. Furthermore, the reduced amounts of sodium delivered to the tubules means that less is available for the distal exchange mechanism involved in acid and potassium secretion.

In some types of glomerular damage, despite a reduced GFR there may be an apparently paradoxical increased protein loss (proteinuria).

Tubular dysfunction
The main function of the tubules is the selective reabsorption of water, electrolytes and other useful substances. Thus, the main consequence of tubular failure is the voiding of large volumes of dilute urine (polyuria) of low specific gravity, along with electrolytes and nutrients (Table 4.13).

Table 4.13 Consequences of tubular dysfunction

Clinical feature	Cause
Polyuria	Reduced countercurrent and reduced Na/water reabsorption
Hypokalaemia Glycosuria Phosphaturia; hypophosphataemia Aminoaciduria	Reduced reabsorption
Acidosis	Reduced exchange/secretion

If the loop of Henle fails to generate an adequate intrarenal concentration gradient in the medulla, urine cannot be concentrated and passive reabsorption is compromised by the consequently increased tubular flow rate. Because of the proximal tubular failure there is a vast increase in potassium loss, which completely swamps the limited potassium retention that would be caused by the impaired distal sodium–potassium–acid exchange pump. On the other hand, the failure in distal acid secretion is significant and acidosis results.

Summary
Predominant **glomerular** damage results in reduced urine volume, retention of water, acid and electrolyte, and possibly protein loss. This is the syndrome of oliguric renal failure. **Tubular** damage leads to acidosis, urine of low specific gravity and, if the GFR is adequate, to polyuria with fluid and electrolyte depletion.

Acute renal failure

Aetiology and prognosis

Although most of the conditions listed in Table 4.11 can cause ARF, pre-renal causes such as hypovolaemia or shock are by far the most common (75% of cases). Less common are intrinsic causes such as nephrotoxicity and acute glomerulonephritis (20%); ARF as a result of post-renal obstruction is uncommon (5%).

ARF is a serious medical emergency which can develop very rapidly and has a high mortality. It may be defined as a sudden fall in GFR to below about 15 mL/min. Without treatment, survival is less than 10% – which shows the crucial role of correct renal function. With treatment in a specialist unit, mortality can be reduced to below 50% but oliguric forms have a poorer prognosis. These outcomes reflect the seriousness of the conditions which precipitate ARF and the rapidly progressive nature of the multi-organ damage caused, rather than inadequacy of management. With the increased availability of renal dialysis, the outlook for ARF has improved, and death now rarely results from biochemical derangement.

Course

Whatever the primary cause, untreated ARF usually follows a fairly well-defined and predictable course (Fig. 4.12). Onset is frequently associated with oliguria which continues for up to a month if the patient survives. Urine flow then recovers and the patient may become polyuric (up to 5 L per day) for 5–10 days. During the final recovery phase, which may last several months, urine flow and renal function gradually return to normal.

A simplified explanation of these phases is as follows:

* The early **oliguric** phase is caused by poor glomerular perfusion or tubular obstruction. Both result in a predominant pattern of glomerular dysfunction with reduced renal clearance and fluid and electrolyte retention. Any tubular impairment is masked by the reduced glomerular filtrate.
* In the **polyuric** ('diuretic') phase the glomeruli have recovered somewhat and are again producing filtrate, although the GFR remains low. However, tubular dysfunction persists, causing failure to concentrate and loss of fluid and electrolytes. The initial diuresis may be partly due to the accumulated fluid and osmolar load, but this could not alone account for the prolonged pattern sometimes seen.
* In the **recovery** phase the tubule cells slowly regenerate.

After recovery there is usually no overt residual renal damage. Although sensitive measures of clearance will almost certainly detect some degree of permanent impairment, this is well within the renal reserve. The effect of a single episode of ARF resembles a small acceleration of renal ageing, with additional nephrons having been lost prematurely.

In pre-renal ARF, ischaemia rapidly produces ATN. Intrinsic toxic tubular damage has the same effect. ATN is a serious complication which usually accounts for the oliguric phase, but may be avoided if the circulation is promptly restored or the offending toxin, usually a drug, is withdrawn (Fig. 4.13). Similarly, early and aggressive immunosuppression can minimize the seriousness of some types of acute glomerulonephritis.

Clinical features

In the more serious oliguric phase the clinical problems are mainly of fluid and electrolyte overload and accumulation of metabolic by-products. Secondary or indirect complications such as infection, pericarditis and bleeding may also occur. Other symptoms will depend on the initial cause and the stage at which treatment is started. For example, even though hypovolaemia may have caused pre-renal failure it could be masked by subsequent fluid retention. Table 4.14 summarizes most possible features, that are unlikely to occur simultaneously, along with a brief outline of their conservative management.

In the polyuric phase, dehydration and electrolyte depletion are possible, but are rare nowadays. Modern treatment has reduced the frequency with which ARF occurs, and may prevent it entirely.

Management

There is no specific remedy for ARF. Management is aimed at eliminating the cause and keeping the patient alive until the kidney function recovers naturally. Thus the aims are to:

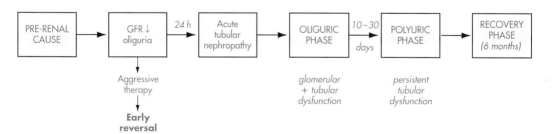

Figure 4.12   Typical clinical course of acute renal failure. GFR, glomerular filtration rate.

Table 4.14   Clinical features and conservative[a] management of oliguric acute renal failure

Pathology	Clinical finding[b]	Management[b,c]
Hypovolaemia	Hypotension	*Plasma, dextran, saline*
	Low cardiac output	
	(Shock)	*(Inotropes)*
Oliguria	Fluid overload	*Osmotic* or *loop diuretic* (high dose)
		Fluid/Na restriction
		Bladder catheter
		(*Dopamine?*)
Hyperkalaemia	Arrhythmias	See p. 173
Acidosis	Low plasma bicarbonate	*Bicarbonate* infusion
Uraemia	Nausea, vomiting	Protein restriction?
	Diarrhoea	
	Pruritis	
Non-specific azotaemia	Tiredness, lethargy	Adequate non-nitrogenous caloric intake

[a] Without dialysis.

[b] Parentheses indicate less common findings or treatments.

[c] See text.

- Discover and reverse or remove cause.
- Minimize renal complications, i.e. ATN.
- Correct fluid and electrolyte imbalances.
- Support the patient through the acute oliguric phase.
- Avoid fluid and electrolyte depletion in the later phases.

Many of these aims are met by renal dialysis, but conservative management may be adequate and is discussed first.

Discovering the cause

The cause of ARF – particularly if pre-renal – will usually be evident from clinical examination, but a medication history should always be sought (Table 4.15). Intrinsic renal damage may be more obscure as may some indirect forms of obstruction. A plain abdominal X-ray and an ultrasound scan are usually carried out if there is anuria. If the failure is advanced, supportive and symptomatic treatment are more important than immediate definitive diagnosis.

Restoration of function

In pre-renal failure, the first priority is prompt *fluid or blood* replenishment and restoration of the cardiovascular function, with monitoring of central venous pressure; this can prevent ATN from developing. If sudden anuria suggests obstruction (e.g. unimpaired cardiovascular function) the patient will be *catheterized*, which also enables accurate assessment of urine output. Aggressive *diuretic* therapy may sometimes restore urine flow, partly by clearing tubular obstruction. Osmotic or high-dose loop diuretics given intravenously increase tubular flow (e.g. mannitol 20%, 120 mg furosemide (frusemide)). Both may also cause local vasodilatation by inhibiting prostaglandins intrarenally, thus counteracting a contributory factor to the ATN. Another mechanism may be the reduction of ischaemia by inhibition of energy (oxygen)-dependent reabsorption pumps. Low-dose *dopamine* infusion may produce intrarenal vasodilatation, but it is uncertain whether this provides clinical benefit in ARF; other vasodilators such as *calcium channel blockers* have been tried experimentally. Failure to respond to the combination of volume expansion and diuretics rules out pre-renal failure or incipient ATN as the cause of the symptoms.

Fluid and electrolytes

A careful balance must be struck between the repletion of any volume deficit which might have first caused the failure, and the prevention of accumulation from subsequent oliguria. The

Table 4.15   Common drugs causing nephrotoxicity[a]

Drug		Type of damage				
		Glomerulonephritis	Interstitial nephritis	Tubular 'necrosis'	Obstructive uropathy	Other
Antimicrobial	Penicillin	+	++			
	Cephalosporins		+	++		
	Tetracycline					+
	Aminoglycoside		+	++		
	Co-trimoxazole		+			
	Sulphonamides	+	+	+	+	
	Erythromycin		+			
	Vancomycin			+		
	Amphotericin			+		
	Rifampicin	+	+			
Analgesic/antirheumatic	Phenacetin		+		++	
	Paracetamol (acetaminophen)[b]		+		+	
	NSAID[c]	+	++			
	Gold	++	+	+		
	Penicillamine	++				
Diuretic	Loop		++			
	Thiazide	+	+			
Radiocontrast media				++		
Cytotoxic	Many				+	
	Methotrexate			+		
	Doxorubicin	+				
	Cisplatin			+		
Heavy metals	Pb, Hg, etc.		+	+		
Antihypertensive	ACEI[b]	+	+			
	Methyldopa			+		
	Hydralazine	+				
	Propranolol		+			
Miscellaneous	Ciclosporin (cyclosporine), tacrolimus			++		
	Lithium		+	+		
	Allopurinol	+	+		+	+
	Phenytoin		+			
	Interferon	+				
	Methysergide				+	

[a] This list is neither comprehensive nor exclusive, but serves to illustrate likely problems with common drugs.

[b] In overdose.

[c] Also cause intrarenal glomerular blood flow 'dysregulation'.

+ damage; ++ serious damage.

ACEI, angiotensin converting enzyme inhibitor; NSAID, non-steroidal anti-inflammatory drug.

patient's fluid balance and haemodynamic status must be evaluated precisely before resorting to diuretics which might cause further volume depletion and exacerbate the condition. Similarly, diuretics are inappropriate in obstruction, e.g. in prostatic hypertrophy, and surgery or cautious catheterization are more appropriate. During the oliguric phase, sodium and fluid are restricted and fluid balance is monitored closely by weighing and meticulous charting of intake/output.

Hyperkalaemia is dealt with as usual (p. 172). Acidosis may be cautiously treated with sodium bicarbonate, taking care to avoid fluid and sodium overload.

Dialysis

If oliguria persists or ATN has supervened, or if plasma urea, creatinine or potassium are rising rapidly, patients are dialysed for short periods as required. This solves most of the problems and has the advantage of allowing a near-normal diet. Continuous arteriovenous haemofiltration is the preferred technique (p. 195), though haemodialysis or peritoneal dialysis are also used. Dialysis minimizes the restriction of fluid intake and may facilitate parenteral nutrition if needed.

General measures and support

Some protein restriction may be needed if gastrointestinal or cutaneous uraemic symptoms are severe (Table 4.14). However, over-zealous protein restriction is avoided as it can retard recovery, especially as patients may be hypercatabolic with increased protein breakdown and weight loss. If protein is restricted, caloric intake must be maintained by increased carbohydrate and fat. Parenteral feeding may be needed in the early stages. Daily fluid intake is restricted to the daily urine output plus 500 mL to replace insensible losses (*see* Table 4.2).

Infection is common. All drug therapy, including antibiotics, must be carefully evaluated to avoid toxic accumulation of renally cleared drugs or their sodium salts. Clinical pharmacists have an important role here.

Recovery

After the critical phase has passed, patients are soon discharged. They will need to be instructed about maintaining an adequate fluid and electrolyte intake and keeping a fluid balance chart.

For most patients the first episode of ARF will be their last. Survivors make an apparently complete recovery, but a few will develop chronic renal failure (CRF), the first attack representing an acute-on-chronic decompensation against a background of progressive renal disease.

Chronic renal failure

Chronic renal disease presents a very different picture from ARF. It usually has different causes, is insidious in onset, follows a slowly progressive course, and is irreversible. In addition to azotaemia and fluid and electrolyte problems there are serious endocrine abnormalities. On the other hand, there is usually time to consider the best management options before the patient reaches end-stage renal disease (ESRD) and the range of treatments available can provide the vast majority of patients with a reasonable quality of life.

Aetiology

It is difficult to quantify the relative frequencies of different causes of CRF. Patients usually present very late, with kidneys so shrunken and fibrosed that retrospective diagnosis is impossible. Table 4.16 gives one estimate of the distribution of probable causes among Europeans, but it is approximate, and varies geographically, ethnically and racially. For example, hypertensive nephropathy is more common among Afro-Caribbeans, and diabetic nephropathy more common among South Asians.

Generally, most CRF is due to intrinsic renal disease, usually glomerular in origin. Iatrogenic disease is an increasing problem, as are diabetes (the prevalence of which is rising) and the various multisystem disorders as advances in treatment prolong survival. Hypertension is now usually recognized earlier and treated better than previously. Renal neoplasms are uncommon.

No general preventative measures can generally be recommended, because the heterogeneous aetiologies of many of the most common causes, such as glomerulonephritis and pyelonephritis, are uncertain. Nevertheless, there is no excuse for the lack of vigilance which permits most iatrogenic renal disease to occur, especially in the elderly. Further, in diabetes it is to be hoped that improved control, and the use of ACEIs, will slow the rate of progression of CRF and reduce the prevalence of end-stage diabetic nephropathy. Fortunately, the management of advanced renal failure is relatively uniform, regardless of the aetiology.

Epidemiology

Because of national and regional differences in diagnosing, reporting and treating ESRD, precise figures for incidence and prevalence are elusive. Most available data derive from analyses of patients considered for renal replacement therapy and so are skewed by treatment policies. For the UK, the approximate most recently available data are given in Table 4.17. The significance of some of this information will be referred to when discussing renal replacement therapy.

Course

The slow decline in the number of functional nephrons, GFR and renal reserve may take decades to pass from normal to end-stage (Table 4.18), although the progression from early to end-stage may be rapid. Patients often first present with a history of several months of vague ill health, with tiredness, pruritus, sickness and loss of appetite and weight. Hypertension is often found and patients may have been ignoring moderate urinary symptoms, usually polyuria, for some time. The other common presentation is ARF following abnormal stress on the already

Table 4.16 Causes of chronic renal failure

Cause	Approximate frequency (%)
Glomerulonephritis	20–25
Diabetes[a]	15–20
Multisystem disease, tumour, miscellaneous[b]	10–15
Pyelonephritis	10
Hypertension/renovascular	10
Congenital (including polycystic)	10
Drug nephrotoxicity	5–10
Interstitial nephritis	5
Unknown	10–15

[a] Frequency as cause of renal disease varies with ethnic group.

[b] Including systemic lupus erythematosus, polyarteritis, scleroderma, haemolytic-uraemic syndrome, gout, tuberculosis, sickle cell disease, etc.

Table 4.17 Epidemiology of end-stage renal disease and renal replacement therapy[a]

	Annual incidence[b]	Total number in UK		
End-stage renal failure	80	4000	Home HD	1500
Patients on dialysis	400	8500	Hospital HD	3000
Transplanted patients	–	16000	PD	4000
Awaiting transplant	50	5000		
Transplants/year	–	2000		

[a] Approximate figures for UK, mid-1990s.

[b] Per million population, new cases.

HD, haemodialysis; PD, automated or continuous ambulatory peritoneal dialysis.

impaired kidneys ('acute-on-chronic' renal failure).

Following diagnosis, declining function is monitored by regular serum creatinine measurement, which correlates inversely with GFR (*see* Fig. 4.7). Careful management during this stage can minimize complications and may delay the onset of the end-stage decline. The patient then has time to review and discuss with the physician the ultimate treatment options, and to prepare psychologically.

Whatever form of renal replacement therapy patients undergo, there is a reduced life expectancy. The greatest mortality is from cardiovascular disease, mainly ischaemic heart disease and heart failure. Following transplantation there may be complications resulting from long-term immunosuppression, e.g. infection and neoplasia.

Pathology

In CRF there is usually a complete and permanent failure of increasing numbers of nephrons. This contrasts with ARF where there is usually a uniform reversible partial impairment of all nephrons. Consequently, in CRF the residual intact nephrons come under increased loading. Changes in intrarenal haemodynamics cause compensatory glomerular hypertension and increases in filtration rates (hyperfiltration). These cause or accelerate glomerular sclerosis and tubular atrophy, and the kidneys gradually shrink. One important exception is polycystic disease where gross enlargement occurs, although functional tissue is similarly reduced.

Renal reserve consists of there being far more nephrons than are needed to sustain life, but numerous adaptations and compensations operate when the number is so reduced as to threaten organ function. Adaptation to maintain water, acid, sodium and potassium levels is good, so hypervolaemia, acidosis and changes in plasma electrolyte levels only occur when the GFR falls below 5–10 mL/min, which determines the onset of the end-stage. However, both urate and phosphate will accumulate before then. Urea and creatinine levels also rise, in inverse proportion to the fall in GFR, because there are no compensation mechanisms for these molecules.

Before end-stage, the patients' reduced renal reserve makes them prone to decompensation if additional demands are made on the kidneys. Infection, surgery, fluid depletion (e.g. severe diarrhoea or vomiting), trauma, certain drugs (e.g. tetracyclines), excess potassium (e.g. potassium-retaining diuretics, foods with high potassium content), etc. can produce exacerbation, or an acute-on-chronic crisis which may be the first indication of severe renal disease.

Pathophysiology and clinical features

A summary of the main clinical problems of CRF is given in Table 4.19, with their presumed pathogenesis and the measures taken to retard progression or limit symptoms. When ESRD is reached, many of these features are mitigated or reversed by renal replacement therapy.

Fluid and electrolyte imbalance
Urine concentrating ability is often diminished in the early stages, causing dilute polyuria and the risk of dehydration and electrolyte

---

Table 4.18 Progression and nomenclature of chronic renal failure

Stage	GFR[a] (mL/min)	Symptom prevalence	Urine production
Diminished renal reserve	<120	–	Normal or mild polyuria
Renal impairment	30–60	+	Usually polyuria
Early renal failure	<30	++	Oliguria
End-stage renal failure	<5	++++	Oliguria/anuria

[a] Assumes normal GFR = 120 mL/min.

Table 4.19   Clinical features of chronic renal failure

Cause	Clinical feature	Conservative management
Retention		
Sodium/water	Hypertension	*Na/water restriction, diuretics,*
	Oedema, general and pulmonary	*antihypertensives*
	Heart failure	
Potassium	Hyperkalaemia, arrhythmia	Dietary restriction
Nitrogenous		
• urea	Nausea, vomiting, purpura	Careful adjustment of protein intake
• urate	Hyperuricaemia, gout	
• creatinine	? uncertain	
• others	? lethargy, anorexia, etc.	
Middle molecules[a]	Lethargy, anorexia, etc.	
Phosphate	Renal osteodystrophy	Dietary restrictions, *phosphate binders*
Melanin, etc.	Skin pigmentation	
Acid	Metabolic acidosis, dyspnoea	*Oral bicarbonate*
Endocrine		
Vitamin D and calcium	Renal osteodystrophy	Vitamin D analogues, calcium
deficiency	Myopathy	
	Peripheral neuropathy, cramps	
	Pruritis	
Erythropoietin deficiency	Anaemia	*Biosynthetic erythropoietin*
Other		
Glucose tolerance ↓	Hyperglycaemia; hyperlipidaemia?	Care with diabetics
Insulin metabolism ↓	Hypoglycaemia	
Lipoprotein lipase ↓	Hyperlipidaemia, atherosclerosis,	Dietary fat restriction;
	ischaemic heart disease	*lipid-lowering agent (statin)*
Immunodeficiency	Infections	*Antibiotics*
?	Pericarditis	
Platelet defect	Impaired coagulation	
Stress ulceration		*Histamine (H_2) antagonist*
Problems with drug therapy	(see text)	

[a] Various metabolites in the 500–5000 Da range (see text).

depletion, as in the polyuric phase of ARF. This is partly the result of an osmotic diuresis induced by raised urea levels in the tubular filtrate of the remaining intact nephrons.

In the later stages urine volume falls and the consequent retention of sodium and water is the main cause of the hypertension usually found in CRF patients. Other potential complications of hypervolaemia are oedema, including pulmonary oedema, and heart failure. At the onset of end-stage failure the patient may become anuric.

Uraemia
The major biochemical problems result from the accumulation not of urea itself but of various electrolytes and miscellaneous other, mainly nitrogenous, toxins. Nevertheless, urea can cause troublesome gastrointestinal symptoms and may be responsible for the capillary fragility and purpura (bruising) seen in renal patients.

Although urate levels are raised, clinical gout is rare. Various other 'middle molecules' (500–5000 Da, nitrogenous and otherwise) may contribute to the variety of non-specific symptoms.

Continuous ambulatory peritoneal dialysis is particularly efficient at clearing these substances, leading to an improvement in well-being.

Potassium and acid

These are not retained in dangerous amounts until end-stage. Before that, renal patients seem to tolerate mild hyperkalaemia and acidosis, or adapt to them. However, along with water retention these are the most serious acute problems at end-stage.

Metabolic features

There are several inter-related changes in lipid and carbohydrate metabolism (Table 4.19). The kidneys normally catabolize several hormones, including about one-third of all natural insulin, and this mechanism is diminished. Conversely, glucose tolerance is increased, so the effects are unpredictable, especially in diabetics. Dyslipidaemia results in a rise in atherogenic lipid fractions.

Cardiovascular disease

Hypertension is almost universal and there is an increased incidence of ischaemic heart disease and heart failure. Numerous factors contribute to a vicious cycle. Hypertension results from fluid retention and possibly renin/angiotensin abnormalities. Dyslipidaemia and hypertension accelerate atherosclerosis, which is a common feature. Heart failure is multifactorial, involving hypervolaemia, hypertension, ischaemia and anaemia. Cardiomyopathy is part of a generalized myopathy caused by calcium and phosphate imbalance. Pericarditis sometimes occurs.

Anaemia

The major cause of anaemia in renal patients is marrow hypoplasia due to reduced or absent erythropoietin (p. 152). The iron-resistant, normocytic, normochromic picture resembles that seen in many chronic diseases (though for a different reason); haemoglobin levels rarely exceed about $80\,g/L$ (normal = $120–180\,g/L$). Iron and folate deficiencies are often superimposed owing to anorexia, dietary restrictions, a bleeding tendency, and losses from haemodialysis and frequent blood testing. Renal anaemia significantly reduces the quality of life of renal patients, producing poor exercise tolerance and the risks of cardiac failure and exposure to multiple transfusions (p. 190).

Renal bone disease

The syndrome of **renal osteodystrophy**, which is still incompletely understood, includes complications associated with disturbed calcium and phosphate metabolism. Together they form perhaps the most serious group of chronic clinical problems because of their prevalence, their widespread, multisystem secondary effects and the difficulty of treatment.

The pathophysiology of osteodystrophy involves impaired bone mineralization (osteomalacia or 'renal rickets'), bone demineralization (osteitis fibrosa) and extraskeletal deposition of calcium phosphate, especially in blood vessels and joints (**metastatic** or **ectopic** calcification). The clinical consequences are fractures, bone pain, deformity, arthritis and atherosclerosis with regional ischaemia. In addition, abnormal calcium and/or phosphate levels may contribute to pruritus, anaemia, anorexia, muscle cramps, myopathy, tetany and peripheral neuropathy. Figure 4.13 shows a simplified account of these features in relation to normal calcium homeostasis.

Other features

The immune system is compromised. Impaired metabolism and/or urinary clearance of melanin and other pigments often gives a characteristic brown skin pigmentation. Abnormal plasma constituents may affect erythrocytes and coagulation factors, causing haemolysis and a haemorrhagic tendency that results in bruising, nose bleeds, gastrointestinal bleeding, etc. Some of these problems are ascribed to the retention of 'middle molecules'.

Lethargy, fatigue and general malaise occur more in patients who are poorly managed or who are less compliant with their treatment regimens or fail to comprehend them.

Drug-related problems

All drug therapy in renal patients needs close attention, as there are both pharmacokinetic and pharmacodynamic implications. The most obvious is a reduced clearance of hydrophilic drugs

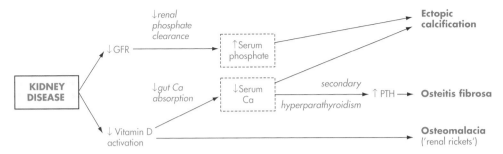

Figure 4.13   Possible pathogenesis of renal osteodystrophy. Impaired Vitamin D activation (normally a renal endocrine function) results in osteomalacia both directly (impaired mineralization) and via low serum calcium levels. Phosphate excretion is reduced initially by reduced renal clearance but later by parathyroid hormone (PTH); eventually the serum phosphate level rises sufficiently to cause the solubility product ([Ca] × [Phosphate]) to be exceeded resulting in ectopic calcification. The parathyroid gland attempts to correct both ionic abnormalities by secreting excess PTH (**secondary hyperparathyroidism**). The resulting increase in calcium gut uptake and reduced calcium renal reabsorption, with the opposite effects on phosphate, together with resorption of both from bone (demineralization) normalizes levels temporarily. As the GFR falls renal phosphate clearance eventually becomes impossible and phosphate levels rise. Ca, calcium; PTH, parathyroid hormone. (Adapted with permission from Greene R, Harris N (1985) *Chemist Drugg* **223**: 195.)

or drug metabolites, with a potential for toxic accumulation in inverse proportion to the reduced GFR.

Azotaemia impairs plasma protein binding, and protein levels may be low in glomerular disease owing to proteinuria; thus, drugs that are normally highly protein bound may have high plasma levels of free drug. Fluid retention can increase the volume of distribution of hydrophilic drugs, reducing effectiveness, but this should not occur if patients are adequately treated. Hepatic drug metabolism is generally depressed, possibly also as a result of azotaemia. The net effect is a need for carefully calculated reduced doses and/or increased dose intervals (*see* Chapter 1). The avoidance of all but the most essential drugs is even more important than usual. Because of reduced renal reserve, renal patients have a very low tolerance of nephrotoxicity, imposing another constraint on drug choice. Finally, the actions of drugs which rely on renal mechanisms, e.g. diuretics, is modified.

Management

The general management strategy and conservative treatment of the patient before ESRD are considered first. Renal replacement therapy is considered on pp. 191–203.

Aims and strategy

The aims in managing CRF are:

- Early detection.
- Identification and removal of cause.
- Retardation of deterioration in renal function.
- Identification and management of complications.
- Preparation of the patient for renal replacement therapy.

Early detection of CRF is unusual, and often a primary cause cannot be identified because the disease is advanced by the time it is detected. Problems such as untreated hypertension, urinary tract obstruction and the use of nephrotoxic drugs, which are potential causes or exacerbating factors, must first be excluded or eliminated.

'Acute-on-chronic' exacerbations of patients not yet at end-stage, resulting from infection, fluid depletion or overload, etc., must be promptly treated. Complications such as anaemia, hyperphosphataemia and secondary hypertension must be minimized. Precise dietary recommendations remain controversial, but appropriate dietary control may slow the progression of the renal damage.

Regular measurements of serum creatinine provide a reliable index of the decline in function and enable the onset of end-stage to be predicted. The rate of decline varies greatly between patients but is generally constant for a given patient. Patients must be encouraged to come to terms psychologically with the fact that they have an irreversible illness which eventually will require artificial or surgical intervention. How this idea is introduced will depend on the clinician's assessment of the patient's psychological resilience. The family must also be involved and encouraged to be supportive.

As patients approach end-stage they will, unless unsuitable, be tissue typed and entered on the transplantation register. Their home may be assessed for the suitability of home dialysis, and a subcutaneous fistula may be fashioned in preparation for haemodialysis.

The situation does not remain static once end-stage has been reached: treatment needs regular re-assessment. Patients may need to switch between different forms of dialysis, in and out of hospital, according to circumstances. Should a transplant prove unsuccessful, they must return to dialysis.

Fluid and electrolytes

Daily water intake is restricted to urine output plus 300–500 mL. Such restriction can be extremely unpleasant in the later stages because thirst is so troublesome. When there is severe oliguria or complete anuria, a restriction of total fluid intake to 500 mL including drinks, sauces, fruit, cleaning teeth and liquid medication may be almost impossible to maintain. However, the swift symptomatic penalties of incipient heart failure or pulmonary oedema are salutary correctives.

Salt intake is restricted, with no added salt and low-salt foods. High-potassium foods, such as fresh fruit and vegetables, chocolate, etc. (the very ones that used to be sought by non-renal patients on diuretics) are avoided. As this becomes less effective, gastrointestinal *ion exchange resins* may be added to reduce potassium absorption. Uncontrolled hyperkalaemia is one of the prime indications for starting dialysis.

Acidosis can be managed with oral *sodium bicarbonate*, but calcium carbonate is needed when sodium restriction is critical; the calcium may also benefit bone disease. The usual care is needed if bicarbonate infusion is used to treat acidosis (p. 176), and persistent severe acidosis is another indication for dialysis.

Diet

Adequate nutrition with high-quality protein in reduced amounts (40–50 g/day) will prevent a negative nitrogen balance and protein malnutrition, and also perhaps reduce the disease progression. High-protein diets are thought to encourage hyperfiltration, thus accelerating renal decline. Very low-protein diets in the early stages have their advocates.

Protein must be restricted when the GFR falls below about 50 mL/min, to minimize uraemic complications. Low protein diets have the beneficial side effect of reducing phosphate, potassium and acid intake, and this might account in part for their apparent effect in some trials of reducing degeneration of renal function. Adequate caloric intake is provided by increasing carbohydrate and unsaturated vegetable fats or oils, using dietary supplements.

The lower the protein content of the diet, the more important that it should be of high biological value so essential amino acid (EAA) supplements may be needed. A further way of minimizing nitrogen catabolism while maintaining protein synthesis is to include ketoacid analogues of EAAs in the diet, as these can be transaminated and thus provide EAAs without additional nitrogen intake.

Vitamin supplementation should not be needed, but many patients – even before dialysis – are given water-soluble multivitamins and iron to compensate for possibly poor nutrition and the loss of blood in frequent blood tests. Dietary compliance (including electrolytes and especially fluid) tends to be poor and the involvement of a renal dietician is highly recommended. The summation of the different restrictions can be difficult for a patient to comprehend, and malnutrition, anxiety or guilt may occur. Dietary restriction may be partially relaxed once the patient has started on dialysis.

Hypertension and other cardiovascular problems

Careful attention to fluid intake may at first be sufficient to control the hypertension which most patients suffer. Otherwise, the usual drugs are employed. While the patient is still producing urine, diuretics may be used. Loop diuretics e.g. *furosemide* (*frusemide*) are preferred because thiazides are ineffective when the GFR is below 30 mL/min: high-dose furosemide (frusemide) may be used when the GFR is very low. Vasodilators are also particularly useful. There is increasing evidence that ACEIs have the additional benefit of retarding the progression of CRF, possibly by causing intrarenal vasodilatation and thus reducing glomerular hypertension. Thus ACEIs and calcium blockers are the drugs of choice after diuretics, although the potential nephrotoxicity of ACEIs must not be forgotten.

Diuretics are also needed for pulmonary oedema and heart failure, and temporary dialysis may be necessary if these are unsuccessful. If dietary modification fails, hyperlipidaemia may require *HMG CoA reductase inhibitors* (*statins*), the clearance of which is less affected by renal impairment than other lipid-lowering agents.

Anaemia

Any iron or haematinic vitamin deficiency is treated in the usual way, but this never restores the normal haemoglobin level. The use of multiple transfusions presents a dilemma. On the one hand, the wide range of antibodies that the patient raises against the pooled blood received in this way throughout his or her illness may sensitize them against a future transplant. While this may be minimized by using washed packed red blood cells, there remain the possibilities of depressed erythropoiesis and iron overload. On the other hand, paradoxically, several units of blood in the months preceding a transplant may improve graft tolerance (p. 200).

Epoetin (recombinant human erythropoietin) has resolved this. The near-normal haemoglobin level which this drug can produce significantly improves the quality of life of patients on dialysis. However, if normalization of the haemoglobin level is attempted, complications may arise owing to the resulting polycythaemia (excessive red blood cell count) causing increased blood viscosity and blood volume. Hypertension may be exacerbated, possibly causing encephalopathy with convulsions, and thromboses may obstruct vascular catheters used for haemodialysis access. The ideal target haemoglobin level for each patient needs careful assessment. Nevertheless, the main constraint on the use of epoetin is economic because it is currently very expensive, although its true value is shown by an analysis which includes improved quality of life.

Epoetin therapy must be matched by appropriate iron intake, and iron supplementation is usually required. This is increasingly being given intravenously to accommodate the increased iron requirement generated by the epoetin. Moreover, careful optimization of iron status can reduce the demand for epoetin, thus conferring considerable economies.

Renal bone disease

Osteodystrophy is difficult to manage, partly because its pathology is incompletely understood and partly because it changes during the course of the illness and thus requires different treatments at different times. Moreover, renal bone disease is one of the complications that is least improved by dialysis.

For hypocalcaemia in the absence of hyperphosphataemia, raising the plasma calcium level will improve osteomalacia (Fig. 4.13). Initially, calcium supplements may be used, *calcium carbonate* being the most suitable as it will also counteract acidosis and complex some phosphate in the gut. Later, *1,25-dihydroxycholecalciferol* (*calcitriol*) or *1-alpha-hydroxycholecalciferol* (*alfacalcidol*) are needed, neither of which rely on renal hydroxylation for activation (as does vitamin D, cholecalciferol). Care must be taken not to elevate the plasma calcium level excessively, as this might exacerbate metastatic calcification.

Hyperphosphataemia is treated initially with phosphate restriction, but this is extremely difficult because phosphate occurs widely in foods (e.g. dairy products, many fish, eggs, liver, many vegetables, chocolate, nuts). Eventually, oral phosphate binders are required, to prevent dietary phosphate and also any phosphate in gastrointestinal secretions being reabsorbed. Formerly, *aluminium hydroxide* was the standard therapy; in the gut this forms insoluble aluminium phosphate which is lost in the faeces. Aluminium hydroxide is given in dry capsule form, e.g. 'Alu-Cap', the more usual antacid mixture being unsuitable for fluid-restricted patients. However, significant aluminium absorption occurs in renal patients who clear it inefficiently, and long-term use was associated with dementia, anaemia and a form of osteodystrophy. This was exacerbated by exposure to aluminium in dialysis fluids, derived from the water supply in certain areas.

Current practice favours *calcium carbonate* tablets with the incidental benefits mentioned above, though large doses are needed. Magnesium salts have also been used. Close monitoring of plasma phosphate and calcium are vital because doses are easily misjudged and dietary mismanagement by the patient may undo the most careful adjustment. If secondary hyperparathyroidism is troublesome and refractory to medical management, then partial or total parathyroidectomy may be indicated.

Other problems

Some of the miscellaneous problems such as neuropathy, gastrointestinal upset, pruritus, etc. may resolve if the above methods are successful, particularly protein restriction and calcium and phosphate control. Others may need to await dialysis which almost invariably produces a notable improvement in general well-being.

Renal replacement therapy

The main place of renal replacement therapy is in ESRD patients whose GFR has fallen below 5–10 mL/min or in whom other complications are not responding to conservative therapy. Renal replacement therapy involves either the artificial techniques of dialysis or natural replacement with a transplant, but temporary dialysis may also be used in acute renal failure or poisoning.

Renal dialysis

Aim

Renal dialysis attempts to mimic the excretory and to a lesser extent the homeostatic roles of the kidney. Although dialysis cannot restore renal endocrine function, it ameliorates some of the secondary effects of endocrine dysfunction such as hypertension and hyperphosphataemia. Anaemia may also be improved. Many patients on dialysis lead near-normal lives and half of them return to work. There is a reduced quality of life compared with normal or after a transplant, but there are far fewer restrictions compared with conservative treatment in the later stages of CRF.

When the GFR falls below about 5 mL/min, toxic nitrogenous metabolites, potassium, acid and water start to accumulate to a life-threatening degree. Serum creatinine at this stage would be above 1000 micromol/L and blood urea more than 30 mmol/L. If there are persistent complications such as neuropathy, pericarditis or refractory hypertension, intervention is made even earlier.

Although there are few patients for whom transplantation is absolutely contraindicated, most will have to wait months or years for an organ to become available, and dialysis is essential to keep them alive until then. Many patients have been successfully maintained on dialysis for decades. Nevertheless, their poor general health results in a greater mortality than that of the general population.

Principles

Two general techniques are currently available, namely haemodialysis and peritoneal dialysis. Ideally these would perform the same functions as the natural kidney (reviewed on pp. 151–153) where ultrafiltration is followed by reabsorption. Filtration involves removal of water and dissolved small molecules via a size-selective semipermeable membrane (the glomerular basement membrane (GBM)) driven by hydrostatic pressure (arterial blood pressure). Reabsorption involves partially selective, sometimes active recouping of useful substances (in the tubules).

These processes cannot be mimicked exactly. Almost all artificial kidneys utilize a membrane that is analogous to the GBM, but with a different pore size. In haemodialysis (HD) the membrane is artificial, while in peritoneal dialysis (PD) the patient's own peritoneal membrane is used. In PD the dialysis almost reaches equilibrium before the dialysis fluid is changed, whereas in HD fast cycling of fresh dialysis fluid speeds diffusion by continually exposing the blood to maximal concentration gradients. Thus HD is more efficient.

In addition to its principal use in CRF, dialysis is also used in the oliguric phase of ARF and for drug overdose and poisoning. Some conservatively managed early CRF patients may need temporary dialysis during acute-on-chronic exacerbations, after which they may stabilize again.

Water removal

In both forms of dialysis, water removal is by **ultrafiltration**. In HD the driving force is hydrostatic, using negative pressure on the dialysate side; in PD, water is removed osmotically.

Removal of waste solutes

In its simplest form dialysis means solute transfer by diffusion through a membrane down a concentration gradient. It is therefore arranged that blood on one side of the membrane is exposed to a dialysis solution on the other, the dialysis solution having low concentrations of the substances that one is trying to remove (or they may be completely absent; Fig. 4.14). Haemodialysis can effect urea clearances of up to 100 mL/min. Yet because it relies on diffusion, clearance is inversely proportional to molecular weight, so that 'middle molecules' are less efficiently removed than small molecules such as urea and creatinine. With high transmembrane flow rates and especially with larger pores, larger solutes may also be drawn across by solvent drag – a process known as **convection**.

Conservation of useful substances

There is no equivalent in dialysis to the subtle processes of natural tubular reabsorption. However, in practice significant electrolyte and nutrient losses are uncommon. Two rather crude substitutes may be used. There can be replacement by dietary supplementation, e.g. of water-soluble vitamins or amino acids, or else the dialysis fluid can be loaded with the desired substances at normal plasma concentrations, thus inhibiting diffusion. The latter technique may be extended by adding substances to the dialysis fluid in excess, to promote net transfer to the patient's circulation, e.g. bicarbonate to combat acidosis, or insulin for diabetics on PD.

Haemodialysis

Unlike modern units the early artificial kidneys were cumbersome and inefficient. Resembling filter presses the size of large trunks, they had to be painstakingly disassembled and cleaned between treatments. Modern artificial kidneys

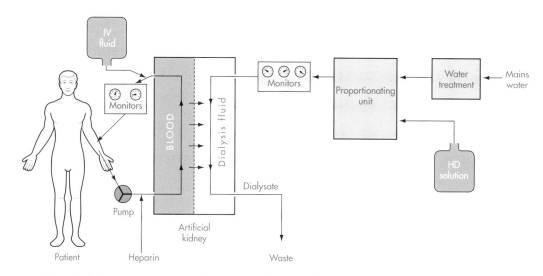

Figure 4.14 Block diagram of the essential elements in a haemodialysis circuit (not to scale). (Modified with permission from Greene R, Harris N (1985) *Chemist Drugg* **224**: 164.)

are disposable and little larger than the organ they replace, though they have about the same filtration area of $1\,m^2$. In some there are multiple thin cellophane films which separate alternate layers of blood and dialysis fluid; in others the blood is pumped through fine, hollow, coiled fibres that are surrounded by dialysis fluid.

Basic system and apparatus

A diagram of the basic HD system is given in Fig. 4.14 and the apparatus is shown in use in Fig. 4.15. The sequence is:

- Arterial blood is directed outside the body.
- The blood is anticoagulated (heparin) and circulated through the artificial kidney.
- A countercurrent of haemodialysis fluid runs against the blood.
- A small negative pressure is applied to the blood.
- Blood is returned to a vein and the dialysate is discarded.

Apart from the artificial kidney itself, the function of most of the HD apparatus is the maintenance of a safe extracorporeal blood circulation and the preparation of a suitably purified dialysis fluid. The blood circuit is *heparinized* using an infusion pump at a rate that prevents clotting within the apparatus. The heparin is inactivated naturally by the time blood is returned to the patient; rarely, *protamine* may be needed as an antidote, or *epoprostenol* may be used if the patient has bleeding problems. About $200\,mL/min$ of blood is removed from the patient and this must be returned free of air bubbles and clots and at the correct pressure and temperature. Physiological saline is flushed through the blood circuit beforehand to prime it, and afterwards to return as much blood as possible to the patient. This also facilitates a top-up infusion if an overshoot in ultrafiltration has caused fluid depletion.

Vascular access

The patient is usually connected to the HD apparatus via a subcutaneous arteriovenous fistula in the arm (Fig. 4.16(a)). After a few weeks, the fistula is mature and the vein becomes swollen ('arterialized'), facilitating repeated puncture for both access and return. For temporary dialysis, or during the few weeks while a fistula matures, either an external shunt (Fig. 4.16(b)) or a temporary intravenous line (jugular or subclavian vein) is used. Fistulae last for several years before

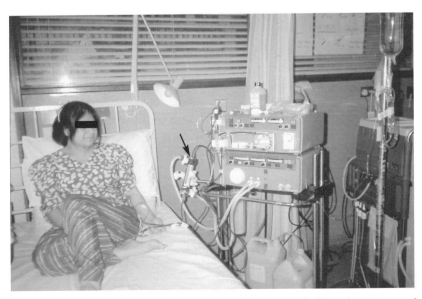

Figure 4.15   Patient on haemodialysis. The artificial kidney unit is the small cylinder in the centre, just below the lamp (arrow). The cabinet beside it is the monitoring and proportionating unit. (Reproduced by courtesy of Dr J R Curtis, Renal Unit, Charing Cross and Westminster Hospital, London.)

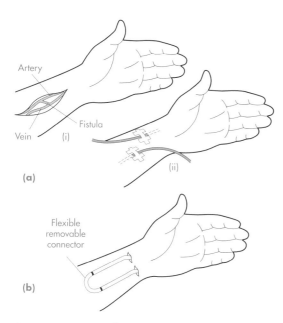

Figure 4.16 Types of vascular access used for haemodialysis. (a) Arteriovenous fistula showing (i) surgery involved and (ii) needles inserted for treatment. (b) Arteriovenous external shunt closed off between treatments. (Reproduced with permission from Greene R, Harris N (1985) *Chemist Drugg* **224**: 164.)

becoming unusable, when a different site needs to be fashioned. Shunts, although quick to set up, last less than a year and are very inconvenient.

Dialysis fluid

The 100–200 L of dialysis fluid needed for each treatment are prepared automatically in the proportioning unit using concentrated dialysis solution, diluted as required with mains water which has been cleared of potentially toxic ions by ion exchange or reverse osmosis. Aluminium and calcium are the main problems long term: the former causes encephalopathy ('dialysis dementia') and calcium causes acute neurological problems during dialysis.

Haemodialysis fluid need not be sterile because the membrane is bacteria-proof, but of course all tubing and apparatus carrying blood, including the artificial kidney, must be sterile. The ionic composition of the dialysis fluid is adjusted individually to normalize each patient's plasma, i.e. low in those ions to be removed, high in those to

be taken up. Usually it is equimolar in Na^+ and Mg^{++}, K^+ is at about 1.5 mmol/L, Ca^{++} is variable and alkali is supplied as lactate or acetate, bicarbonate being incompatible with Ca^{++} and Mg^{++}. For diabetics, glucose is sometimes added to prevent hypoglycaemia.

Routine therapy

Most patients need 3–6 h of HD two to three times each week, depending on their fluid and electrolyte retention between treatments, which partly depends on residual urine output. Dialysis requirement is often empirically monitored by weight gain, just as the progress of HD can be followed by using a weigh-bed. Ideally the patient should not gain more than 1500 g between treatments to avoid cardiovascular system and pulmonary problems. Moreover, removing more than this in 4–6 h can cause temporary fluid or electrolyte imbalance, the so-called 'disequilibrium syndrome'.

Dialysis may be carried out overnight, thus maximizing the utilization of hospital dialysis facilities, although in hospital it is more usually done during the day. Many patients continue full or part-time work. Patients can also make temporary arrangements with units in holiday areas. Once patients are stabilized, dialysis equipment may be set up in their homes. This depends on whether the patient can cope physically, intellectually and psychologically, and also on logistical factors, such as whether there is a spare room (some patients have Portakabins erected in their garden) and whether there is someone to help them cope with their problems.

Most CRF dietary restrictions regarding potassium, phosphate, etc. still need to be observed by patients on HD, and daily fluid intake must not exceed 500 mL plus urine output. Expert advice and encouragement from a dietician is important. Antihypertensive treatment is frequently continued, although the hypertension may improve. Vitamins B complex and C are required to compensate for losses of these water-soluble substances to the dialysate, as are iron and folate supplements to compensate for the blood losses incurred. Immediately after treatment some patients need an oral sodium supplement for cramps caused by electrolyte deficiency. Treatment for osteodystrophy needs to be continued.

Problems

Acute problems include fluid or electrolyte imbalance resulting from the rapid changes causing cramps, hypotension, headaches, etc. and ischaemia distal to the access site, e.g. in the hand. The main chronic problems are related to the vascular access and include thrombosis, local or systemic infection, haemorrhage, phlebitis, haemolysis, etc.

Patients do very well on HD and feel better than they did in the later stages of CRF before starting dialysis. The quality of life is reduced on account of regular disruption and dependence on machinery, but some patients still prefer this to the continuous commitment of PD.

Haemofiltration

Drawbacks to the conventional HD system include complex apparatus and poor clearance of 'middle molecules'. The intermittent nature of the treatment can impose high haemodynamic stresses, especially in ARF. Several alternatives have been developed which are particularly useful for short-term dialyses, e.g. in ARF or cases of poisoning.

In **continuous arteriovenous haemofiltration** (CAVH) no dialysis fluid is used. The system operates more like a plasma exchange, with large quantities of fluid (up to 20 L per day) being removed in an artificial kidney with a more permeable membrane. Crystalloids follow by convection, rather than diffusion as in haemodialysis. Fluid and electrolytes (without unwanted toxins) are replaced continuously via the return line, the volume replaced depending on how much net loss is required. Where urea levels are high, e.g. in the hypercatabolic states of severe ARF, a blood pump and negative pressure are used which also improves the removal of 'middle molecules'. Alternatively, there may be additional intermittent haemodialysis.

The newer technique of **continuous arteriovenous haemodiafiltration** (CAV-HD) represents a compromise. Dialysis fluid and a more porous dialyser unit are used but no pump is required. Fluid removal is controlled by the dialysis fluid flow rate, which is generally much slower than in normal HD. In **haemoperfusion** a sterile activated charcoal column is put in the blood circuit rather than an artificial kidney. This is sometimes useful in poisoning treatment. In **continuous venovenous haemofiltration** a single dual-lumen intravenous catheter is used.

Peritoneal dialysis

This process is far simpler mechanically. Two litres of sterile dialysis fluid are run directly into the patient's peritoneal cavity under gravity via an indwelling silastic catheter, over about 10 min (Fig. 4.17). Dialysis then takes place between the

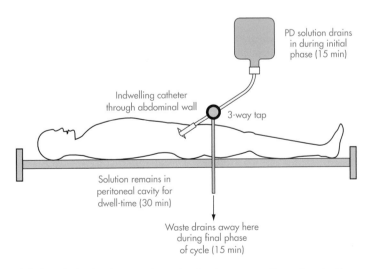

Figure 4.17 Peritoneal dialysis (PD). The diagram shows the simplest system. (Reproduced with permission from Greene R, Harris N (1985) *Chemist Drugg* **224**: 164.)

blood in peritoneal capillaries and the dialysis fluid in the peritoneum. The dialysing interface is composed of the vascular basement membranes and the peritoneal membranes, both of which are semi-permeable. The process is thus analogous to the formation of tissue fluid or ascites.

Sterile PD fluid comes ready-made, and is similar in composition to diluted HD fluid but with little potassium, the clearances being lower than in HD. Also, because hydrostatic pressure cannot be used for water removal different concentrations of glucose are added (1.5–4%) to effect different rates of osmotic removal. The system is relatively cheap to set up and maintain and requires far simpler equipment and fewer specialized staff when used in hospital.

There are several different ways of organizing and scheduling PD.

Intermittent peritoneal dialysis (IPD)

This method in its conventional hospital-based form involves multiple hourly fill–drain cycles with short dwell times, repeated 24–48 times over 1–2 days. The rate of diffusion of molecules (equivalent to their clearance) declines as their concentration in the peritoneal dialysate increases, so a 30-min contact time within the peritoneum is optimal. The entire fluid volume, including excess water and dialysed substances, is then drained out again under gravity, often by simply putting the empty dialysis fluid bag on the floor below the patient.

IPD is only about 20% as efficient as HD, with urea clearance at about 20 mL/min. The cycle must be repeated, two or three times weekly, using 50–100 L of PD fluid each time. Perhaps surprisingly, it is not overly uncomfortable for most patients, although they are physically restricted for long periods. However, IPD is rarely used nowadays except in patients awaiting some other management, in those for whom all other methods have failed, and in those with some residual renal function when the inefficiency of IPD is less of a problem.

Continuous ambulatory peritoneal dialysis (CAPD)

Originally devised to exploit the simplicity of PD but free the patient of its restrictions, CAPD yielded unexpected additional benefits and is now the most popular form of dialysis in the UK (about 40–50% of cases). Instead of the frequent fluid changes being made during several specified periods in the week, the patient carries the fluid in his or her abdomen continuously, day and night, while living an otherwise almost normal life. The solution is changed two to five times daily, the longest dwell being overnight.

PD fluid (2–2.5 L) is run in from a soft plastic bag, and the line is then closed. After 4–6 h the dialysate is drained out and fresh fluid run in. The changeover takes 30–40 min, and the patient needs training in aseptic technique. CAPD is not suitable for all: some cannot cope emotionally or intellectually, while others have manipulative difficulties, e.g. the aged or arthritic; others do not appreciate the need for strict asepsis. On the other hand, some patients are even able to judge the right glucose concentration to use each time.

In the original system the dialysis fluid bag, after being emptied into the peritoneum, was not disconnected but rolled up and secured around the waist (Fig. 4.18). The dialysate was subsequently drained back into the same bag, which was disconnected and discarded. A new bag was then aseptically connected and run in. The current 'disconnect-flush before fill' system reduces the chances of infection. The intraperitoneal catheter terminates externally as a Y-tube, both arms of which can be sealed. At changeover both an empty and the new bag are connected. The dialysate is first drained off, flushing away potential contamination from the connection procedure; the new fluid is then run in.

Successful patients achieve a continuous clearance of water, electrolytes and uraemic toxins with stable – if somewhat higher than normal – blood levels so that the process resembles normal renal function more closely than other forms of dialysis. There is little of the peaking and troughing of electrolyte levels characteristic of both HD and IPD. In addition, the use of a natural membrane and longer dwell time improves the removal of 'middle molecules'. Thus there is a more stable fluid and electrolyte balance and consistently lower levels of toxins, and consequently patients feel very much better.

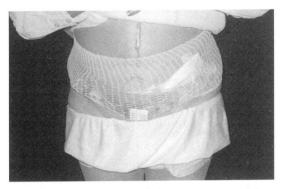

Figure 4.18 Continuous ambulatory peritoneal dialysis (CAPD) patient showing empty bag carried in waist pouch between changes. This shows the original system. More recently, patients completely disconnect during the dwell period. (Reproduced with permission from Henderson RG (1981) *Hosp Update* August: 834.)

Moreover, there are few dietary restrictions, the main remaining modification being an increased protein intake to compensate for losses across the peritoneum. Water-soluble vitamins are given as usual.

Automated peritoneal dialysis (APD)

This technique is increasingly used where CAPD has failed to provide control or where it produces unacceptable daytime restrictions for patients. The method involves automation of intermittent PD, with a machine to switch between bags and control the tap. It can be used easily at home, and when run overnight causes less discomfort because the patient is recumbent. The more rapid cycling compared with CAPD means that night-time exchanges may provide sufficient control and obviate the necessity for the patient to dialyse during the day, or else only require a few daytime cycles. Thus, APD is preferred by many patients and now is used by about one-quarter of PD patients in the UK.

Problems

Contraindications. Patients with respiratory or abdominal disease present difficulties. Diaphragm movement is impeded by the fluid-filled abdomen, and this possibly impairs respiration. Fistula formation might be encouraged in inflammatory bowel disease, with consequent peritonitis, and hernias may be aggravated. Gut surgery can leave fibrous adhesions which reduce the effective membrane area.

Peritonitis. Infections from contamination during bag switching are unfortunately common: a CAPD patient experiences one such episode every 2–3 years. It is less frequent in hospital-based PD. Usually, a commensal Gram-positive skin organism (*Staphylococcus epidermidis*) is implicated, but enterococcal infection (*Streptococcus faecalis*) that is suggestive of an intestinal fistula may occur and is far more serious. Infection may be painless and is usually detected when the dialysate becomes cloudy or takes much longer than usual to drain. CAPD patients must then report to the hospital immediately.

The dialysate should be sampled for culturing and sensitivity testing before antibiotics are given, but blind therapy must be started promptly to minimize the development of peritoneal fibrosis. Initial treatment is *vancomycin* plus an *aminoglycoside* in the dialysis fluid, with one or the other stopped according to sensitivity data. A loading dose, possibly IV, may be needed in severe cases: otherwise most episodes are managed with the patient at home or as an outpatient. Treatment should last 7–10 days, during which normal dialysis may be continued, although at an increased frequency because the inflamed membranes reduce urea clearance.

A less invasive and far cheaper recommendation for mild peritonitis is to perform three rapid exchanges at the first sign of infection and then simply to stop PD for 2 days and allow for natural resolution, though this requires careful supervision in hospital. It is claimed that dialysis fluid can inhibit healing.

Apart from the direct threat of a serious infection, each episode causes a reduction in the effective peritoneal surface area and ultrafiltration efficiency, owing to scarring and adhesions. The latter may be exacerbated by the continuous exposure of the peritoneum to an abnormal fluid volume, the long-term adverse consequences of which cannot yet be estimated.

Hyperglycaemia. The glucose in the dialysis fluid causes hyperglycaemia and obesity, especially in CAPD because there is significant absorption during the long dwell times. This is a particular problem with diabetics. The hyperlipidaemia which all renal patients suffer is exacerbated in PD patients, possibly due to the hyperglycaemia. Another consequence of glucose absorption is a gradual reduction in the osmolarity of the dialysis fluid, which reduces ultrafiltration as each exchange proceeds. Recent trials with glucose polymers (e.g. *icodextrin*) in the dialysis fluid, which exert a significant oncotic pressure but cannot be absorbed, have indicated a possible remedy.

Other problems include:

* Loss of protein and amino acids.
* Blockage of the catheter (usually they last many months, and are regularly cleared with a heparin flush).
* Local infection around catheter insertion site.
* Sclerosing peritonitis, a rare, potentially fatal complication, possibly associated with dialysis fluid contaminants or additives (e.g. chlorhexidine, acetate).

There is a high drop-out rate from CAPD, with up to half of patients switching to some other method within 3 years, and few lasting 10 years. In the UK many would regard CAPD as the treatment of second choice (after transplantation) for ESRD, and intensive efforts are being made into improving its success rate because of the quality of life it permits and its economic benefits. Up to 50% of dialysis patients are on CAPD and the rest on HD. However, the position is different in the rest of Europe; e.g. in Scandinavia, only 30–40% choose CAPD, the majority preferring HD. This may be because of a scarcity of physical and financial resources in the UK, which limits patient choice.

Drug therapy in PD

Many drugs can, like antibiotics, be given safely and effectively by the intraperitoneal route in CAPD fluid. The most notable example is insulin for diabetics with ESRD, and very smooth diabetic control can be achieved in this way. Further information on this subject may be obtained in the References and further reading.

Comparison of dialysis types

The 10-year survival rate for both methods is about 75%, with CAPD patients achieving a slightly better rate. Table 4.20 summarizes the other important features of the two main types of dialysis, and compares their relative advantages and disadvantages.

Transplantation

For the vast majority of ESRD patients a renal transplant is the best possible treatment. In Europe as a whole about 30% of patients receive replacement kidneys, but there are regional differences. The UK, with 30 kidney donations per million population annually, has the lowest rate.

The shortage of organs is still the major impediment to improving these figures, the situation having been adversely affected by seat-belt legislation which has reduced road traffic fatalities. However, as tissue matching and immunosuppressive regimens improve, surgical experience grows, and the survival rate of non-related or unmatched living grafts improves, so the admission criteria to transplant programmes have been relaxed.

Patients who formerly would not have been grafted owing to age or an underlying disease which predisposed them to renewed renal damage (e.g. diabetes, hypertension, arterial disease) are now considered. There remain few absolute contraindications; these include extensive neoplastic disease, serious infection, and the inability to withstand major surgery or immunosuppression (e.g. immunocompromised patients).

A successful graft is an almost complete cure: all fluid, electrolyte and toxaemic complications are reversed, and in time the anaemia and even the bone disease resolve. There may be some residual hypertension but the only significant disadvantage is the lifelong immunosuppression that is needed, with its attendant risks, and the (inconvenient) need for regular monitoring.

Organ donation

Using live donors is convenient and allows ample preoperative preparation. It also results in improved graft survival because of the reduced

Table 4.20   Comparison of haemodialysis and peritoneal dialysis

Haemodialysis	Peritoneal dialysis
Complex, expensive	Simple
Special staff (hospital dialysis)	No special staff needed, but patient needs training
Can be done at home, but detailed training and home modification involved	Can be done at home, but storage facilities needed
Needs another person	Complete independence possible; less social and employment disruption
	Patient motivation more critical
Patient tied to machine during treatment but free at other times	Patient must change 2–5 times every day (CAPD) but mobile
Fluctuating biochemical parameters	Stable biochemical parameters
Patient's condition varies between treatments and takes time to recover after each	Consistent well-being
Poor removal of 'middle molecules'	Good metabolic control and removal of 'middle molecules'
Vascular access complications	Can be used in patients with vascular problems
	Serious infective complications
Can be used for long periods (if vascular access maintained)	CAPD often only possible for a few years
	Difficult for diabetics
More effective in acute renal failure	
	Back-up fistula/shunt may be needed for CAPD failure
	Back-up support services required

CAPD, continuous ambulatory peritoneal dialysis.

time that the organ spends disconnected from a blood supply. Donors are carefully screened for renal disease or relevant risk factors, e.g. hypertension, and for general and psychological health. The loss of a kidney does not adversely affect an otherwise healthy person, and the operative risk is low (mortality about 1/3000). Their remaining kidney hypertrophies, giving an eventual GFR of about two-thirds the pre-donation level. Long-term follow-up of donors has shown no significantly increased risk of renal disease or hypertension.

Related donors are preferred. Obviously the ideal of an identical twin is rarely achieved; failing that, other siblings are preferred. However, genetically unrelated spouse donors are being increasingly used, with surprising success. Anonymous organ donation for profit is not permitted in most countries. In the future there may be transplants from other species such as pigs (**xenotransplantation**). One approach is genetically to modify the animals to make their tissues immunologically better tolerated by the human immune system. Increasingly, diabetic patients are being offered simultaneous renal and pancreatic transplantation (*see* Chapter 9).

About 70% of donations are cadaveric, mostly from brain-damaged patients taken off life-support systems. At 10%, the UK has a relatively low proportion of living donors to cadaveric, the highest being Norway with 45%. The criteria applied in this controversial area are affected by ethical, cultural, ethnic and religious considerations that are outside the scope of this book. However, it should be noted that rigorous criteria for determining brain death are now applied which effectively eliminate the risk of error.

All ESRD patients approaching end-stage are tissue-typed and registered centrally. When a kidney becomes available, several closely matched potential recipients are urgently called to their local renal unit and direct cross-matching is done. All other things being equal, the patient with the best match is then immediately prepared for surgery.

Graft matching

Histocompatibility

Two important immunological criteria affect the risk of rejection. Blood group (ABO) compatibility operates as in blood transfusion, i.e. group O is a universal donor, etc. More complex is HLA antigen compatibility (human leucocyte locus-A; *see* Chapter 2). Class II HLA-D antigens seem to be the more important in transplantation.

The intensity of an immune response and thus the likelihood of rejection depends on the degree of HLA similarity between donor and recipient; e.g. they may have the same HLA-A and HLA-B antigens (both Class I), but differ in HLA-DR. Children have a mixture of their parents' HLA genes. Identical (monozygotic) twins will have identical genes, as occasionally may two siblings by chance. The more distant the relationship, the less compatibility there is likely to be. Grafts from an identical twin (isografts) have a 95% chance of survival at 1 year. This figure gradually falls for more distant relatives (allografts), through non-identical siblings and then parents or children, down to about 75% for unrelated or cadaveric donors. The longer a graft survives the lower the incidence of rejection; at the best centres the 10-year graft survival rate with well-matched kidneys can reach 70%, although the average is about 50%.

Immunosuppressant drugs can keep rejection at bay at the cost of potential myelosuppression, infection and other chronic iatrogenic complications. Improvements here have brought about increased graft survival over the past decades. Better matching reduces not only the chance of rejection but also the immunosuppressant doses required.

Cross-matching

HLA-A, B, and C can be typed at any time using specific antisera and the patient's or donor's blood. For HLA-D, it is necessary to mix recipient lymphocytes and potential donor serum directly, from which donor lymphocytes must be deleted by a cytotoxic drug so that only the recipient's lymphocytes can respond to any incompatibility. Because typing takes 5 days, it is not practicable for cadaveric donors. The D subgroup called DR (D-related), currently the best predictor of graft tolerance, is detectable serologically, providing faster, more accurate matching.

Nevertheless, even completely HLA-mismatched grafts are sometimes successful and the significance of HLA matching is disputed. Blood group compatibility, general health, previous transfusions and effective immunosuppression seem to be equally important in determining graft survival. The survival rates of transplants from cadavers are fast approaching those from living donors.

The 'transfusion effect' is an immune tolerance which seems to be induced in ESRD patients. A wide variety of antigens are present in the pooled blood of the numerous transfusions usually received by ESRD patients during the course of their illness. Theoretically these would be expected to stimulate the production of multiple antibodies, some of which could – and sometimes do – reject a subsequent graft. However, a significant overall graft-sparing effect results, which has been attributed to transfusions given in the months before grafting, and pre-transplant transfusion is now routine in most units. Possibly the multiple foreign HLA antigens induce a hyporesponsive state.

A final direct cross-matching of recipient serum and donor lymphocytes is performed just before surgery to check if there are any pre-existing cytotoxic serum antibodies which would cause an immediate rejection. Such antibodies could have arisen from previous blood transfusions, transplants or pregnancy.

Surgical procedure

The operation is not complex surgically. The donor organ is placed extraperitoneally in an iliac fossa where it can easily be felt and biopsied after operation. This also preserves the peritoneum should further dialysis be necessary. The graft's renal artery and vein are connected to major local abdominal vessels and the ureter is implanted into the recipient's bladder. The bladder connection may occasionally cause subsequent problems, but the operation has few complications and a low risk.

The original kidneys are usually conserved even if the patient is anuric, unless there is strong evidence of renal hypertension, stones (a focus of infection) or a tumour. This utilizes any remaining function – especially important should the graft fail. Equally important, it helps maintain the haematocrit as some erythropoietic factor is still secreted even when the GFR is minimal. Bilateral nephrectomy introduces further operative risk for no improvement in graft or patient survival.

Kidneys are implanted as soon as possible after removal from the donor. This is easy to arrange with a living related donor using adjoining operating theatres, and this contributes to the success of this type of transplant. Cadaveric kidneys are perfused with physiological saline at 5°C immediately after removal to preserve their viability during transportation.

The ischaemic period after donor organ removal causes a variable degree of ATN, which manifests as ARF in the recipient for up to about 10 days after transplantation. During this time the patient may need to continue on dialysis, depending on their urine output and blood chemistry. The sooner the organ is implanted the less serious this episode is, and about half of recipients start producing urine within a few days.

Rejection

A kidney graft may be rejected at any time, although the longer it survives the less likely this becomes. Moreover, most rejection episodes can be controlled: a patient may undergo several episodes yet still ultimately retain the graft. However, if it cannot be saved it is removed and the patient returned to dialysis and the transplant waiting list. There are three main types of rejection:

- **Hyperacute** or **immediate rejection** is caused by either pre-existing plasma antibodies attaching to the graft and initiating an immune response or by ABO mismatch. This occurs within days or even hours, as soon as the organ becomes adequately perfused, and results in renal vascular thrombosis and loss of the graft. Fortunately rare, this condition is untreatable because the antibodies are already formed, although plasmapheresis has been tried.

- **Acute rejection** is the most common form. It can occur at any time, but usually in the first fortnight. It is a normal T cell-mediated response to HLA antigens involving primary sensitization, lymphocyte proliferation and subsequent attack. The resulting vascular and tubular damage initially causes non-specific symptoms such as fever and tenderness over the graft. If the organ has started functioning there will be a decline in renal function, with resultant oliguria and a rise in serum creatinine. There are problems in diagnosing acute rejection. If it occurs during the period of ATN which often follows cadaveric grafting, reduced renal function cannot be identified. Furthermore, a similar picture could be caused by a recurrence of the primary disease, by postoperative infection or obstruction, or by nephrotoxicity especially from ciclosporin (cyclosporine). Consequently, most such episodes are treated by default as if they were rejection while efforts are made to identify other causes.

- **Chronic rejection** may occur at any time after the first few months, and involves immune-complex deposition within the glomeruli and renal vessels resembling chronic glomerulonephritis. It is relentless and usually irreversible, and results in loss of the graft.

Prevention and treatment of rejection

Immunosuppressant therapy is started immediately before grafting, gradually reduced over 2–6 months, and except for isografts (HLA-identical) is continued lifelong. Treatment usually consists of combination therapy involving cytotoxic drugs, which depress bone marrow production of new immune cells, and non-specific and specific immunosuppressants, which reduce the activity of preformed immune cells. Common combinations in the UK use azathioprine, corticosteroids and ciclosporin (cyclosporine).

It is not known why the immune response to a permanently foreign transplant wanes over time, resulting in eventual partial tolerance under immunosuppression, but one theory is that donor cells carried over with the graft are in some way involved (microchimerism).

Prophylaxis

Treatment regimens vary between centres. There is no consensus as to whether combined therapy should be preferred, offering the prospect of lower individual doses, or eventual monotherapy, thus avoiding the toxicity of some drugs completely.

High-dose steroids (e.g. 60–100 mg or more of *methylprednisolone* IV daily) are almost always used initially, and then tailed off over 3 months to a maintenance level (10 mg *prednisolone* oral daily). Recently, the use of a lower oral steroid starting doses (30 mg prednisolone daily for 60 days) has resulted in fewer infective complications with no increase in rejection, and this is now favoured in the UK. Nevertheless, the main problems with this regimen remain the generalized depression of the immune response to infection and the typical adverse effects associated with long-term steroid use.

Cytotoxic drugs, e.g. *azathioprine* or *cyclophosphamide*, are initiated postoperatively at maintenance doses. *Mycophenolate mofetil* is a recent alternative to azathioprine. It acts similarly to azathioprine but is more effective; it is also more myelotoxic, causing more opportunistic infections and blood dyscrasias.

Ciclosporine (*cyclosporine*) and *tacrolimus* (calcineurin inhibitors) selectively inhibit the proliferation of immune cells, especially T helper cells sensitized during a rejection response, without depressing the bone marrow function. These drugs have greatly improved the success rates of renal transplantation, allowing the level of general immunosuppression and the steroid dose to be reduced. However, both have potentially serious long-term adverse effects, including hepatotoxicity, lymphoma and unfortunately nephrotoxicity (afferent glomerular arterial vasoconstriction) that results in hypertension. Toxicity is minimized by careful plasma level monitoring; concurrent vasodilator therapy with *nifedipine* may be used to reduce nephrotoxicity.

Triple therapy (steroids, azathioprine/mycophenolate mofetil, ciclosporin (cyclosporine)/tacrolimus) is a common regimen, although there are advocates of most possible combinations, all of which confer certain benefits. Maintenance monotherapy with ciclosporin is increasingly used, with the benefit of avoiding steroid toxicity.

A short course of ciclosporin (cyclosporine) plus steroids after grafting followed by continuous low-dose steroids plus cytotoxic drugs is an alternative. The best maintenance immunosuppressive regimen, and the role of newer drugs like tacrolimus and mycophenolate mofetil, remain to be determined.

Immunotherapy, when better developed, may prove to have a better risk/benefit balance. Currently its primary use is in steroid-resistant rejection episodes, but interleukin receptor monoclonal antibodies such as *basiliximab* and *daclizumab* are starting to be used in combination maintenance regimens.

Management of rejection

The standard response to suspected rejection is to increase the steroid dose substantially, e.g. *methylprednisolone* 1 g daily for 3 days. This will depress preformed and activated immune cells. There is no point in raising cytotoxic dosage as the cells doing the damage are already in the blood, so depressing the bone marrow function would be ineffective. The episode will usually be aborted within a few days and normal prophylactic doses can be resumed.

Should steroids fail, a number of other immunotherapeutic regimens, some still in the investigational stage, may be tried. Most involve more or less specific anti-lymphocyte therapy. Early work with *anti-lymphocytic serum* (ALS), raised in horses against a mixed lymphocyte inoculum, has given way to the purified globulin extract (anti-lymphocyte or *anti-thymocyte globulin*, ATG), but this is still non-specific. More recently there have been trials with *monoclonal antibodies* to proliferating lymphocytes (e.g. *Muromonab-CD3*), the object being to delete the entire clone.

Other post-transplant complications

Successfully transplanted patients are still not entirely problem-free, owing mainly to their immunosuppressant therapy. They need regular renal, liver and blood screening and are carefully monitored for infective or haematological complications.

Many patients still have **hypertension**: contributory factors may include iatrogenic disease (steroid-induced fluid retention, ciclosporin), an imperfectly functioning graft and the influence of the original, diseased kidneys. A slightly increased risk of **malignancy** (lymphoma and skin) is associated with long-term cytotoxic therapy. **Vascular** disease is common. Dyslipidaemia (steroids and ciclosporin) and hypertension lead to atherosclerotic complications, mainly ischaemic heart disease and stroke, that are a major cause of death. The increased incidence of **peptic ulcer** may be related to steroids, as may **osteoporosis** and **osteonecrosis**. Immunosuppression from cytotoxic drug-induced bone marrow suppression and steroids predispose to **infections**, especially cytomegalovirus, *Pneumocystis* and bacterial urinary tract infections. **Hepatic** disease may result from treatment with both azathioprine and ciclosporin.

Important renal diseases

In this final section we consider some of the more important renal diseases, many of which may be the underlying cause of ARF or CRF.

Obstructive uropathy

Obstruction can occur anywhere from the renal pelvis to the urethra and may be either unilateral or bilateral (Fig. 4.19). Certain forms produce acute symptoms; bilateral obstruction, if untreated, may lead to CRF. Drugs have little role in the management of this condition.

Pathology

The effect of obstruction depends on the site. Obstruction in the ureter or above (e.g. a stone or **calculus**) causes fluid accumulation in the renal pelvis (hydronephrosis) and a rise in tubular hydrostatic pressure. The increased tubular back pressure reduces the GFR but filtrate continues to be produced for some time, even following complete obstruction. The resulting increase in intrarenal pressure causes dilatation and gross damage owing to compression. The prolonged urinary stasis which follows

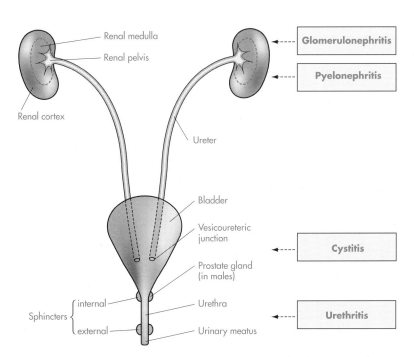

Figure 4.19   Urinary tract showing sites of major renal disease. (Reproduced with permission from Greene R, Harris N (1985) *Chemist Drugg* **223**: 853.)

can promote secondary effects such as urinary tract infection, because organisms are not regularly flushed out, in addition to stone formation.

If the obstruction is relieved promptly, there may be a complete restoration of renal function. There usually follows a massive and prolonged diuresis which can be fatally dehydrating: a urine output of up to 50 L in 24 h has been reported. Such losses suggest delayed tubular recovery (compare this with the polyuric phase of ARF; p. 180) in addition to the simple clearance of accumulated fluid. Because post-renal failure is potentially reversible, a patient presenting with sudden oliguria or anuria must always be investigated for possible obstruction. Although a comparatively rare cause of CRF, obstruction is one of the few causes that are preventable.

Chronic partial obstruction, which is often a result of congenital incompetence of the valve mechanism between the ureter and the bladder (the vesicoureteric junction; Fig. 4.19), leads to chronic renal inflammation, scarring and possible infection. **Vesicoureteric reflux** leading to **reflux nephropathy** usually starts in infancy, and may stabilize or progress slowly to CRF in adulthood.

In bladder outflow obstruction, e.g. prostatic hypertrophy, urinary retention may be accommodated by bladder distension, with little serious rise in intrarenal pressure.

Aetiology

The general causes of obstruction are listed in Table 4.21. In the West, the most common causes are gynaecological problems in women, prostatic hypertrophy in men, and stones in both.

Renal calculi

The causes of renal stone formation are poorly understood. **Calcium oxalate** stones, the most common type, may result from hypercalciuria (high urinary calcium) or excessive gastrointestinal absorption of oxalate. Stone formation is encouraged by an alkaline urine (e.g. from renal tubular acidosis) and hyperuricosuria (e.g. in hyperuricaemia or gout). Conversely, hyperuricaemia together with an acid urine predisposes to **urate** stones. In urinary infections caused by urease-producing organisms, especially *Proteus* spp., the urinary alkalinity and ammonium content cause co-precipitation of a mixed **phosphate** (calcium, magnesium and ammonium). In cystinuria, an inherited metabolic disorder, the reduced tubular reabsorption of cystine results in high urinary levels and **cystine** stone formation.

Clinical features and investigation

Symptoms depend on whether the lesion is above or below the bladder. In the latter case,

Table 4.21 Causes of renal obstruction

Cause	Example	
Renal calculi	Calcium oxalate	70%
	Calcium-magnesium-ammonium phosphate	20%
	Uric acid	5%
	Cystine	3%
Neuromuscular	Spasm, neurogenic bladder	
Structural	Congenital obstruction (e.g. pelvi-ureteric)	
	Urinary tract tumour	
	Stricture following infection	
	Prostatic enlargement	
	Abnormal mass (tumour, pregnancy)	
Iatrogenic	Anticholinergic drugs (spasm)	
	Sulphonamides (crystalluria)	
	Antineoplastic therapy (urate nephrolithiasis)	

dysuria, hesitancy, frequency, terminal dribbling or bladder distension and discomfort occur. Above-bladder obstruction usually causes renal colic (sudden severe and debilitating unilateral loin pain) often associated with haematuria and complete ureteric obstruction. Colic is also caused by the movement of stones in the ureter.

The urine flow pattern will also depend on the degree and site of obstruction and whether it is bilateral. Paradoxically, polyuria may occur as a result of tubular damage. Chronic reflux nephropathy may cause hypertension and recurrent renal infection (pyelonephritis).

Investigation ranges from simple examination and analysis of the urine to sophisticated imaging. A biopsy may be performed by percutaneous nephrostomy, in which a catheter is introduced directly into the renal pelvis, rather like a lumbar puncture.

Management

Whereas surgery used to be common in treating obstruction, conservative management is increasingly used, owing to the growing appreciation that renal function may be preserved or restored, and to the development of techniques of intrarenal manipulation. Surgical repair may be essential in some cases, e.g. congenital defect, but nephrectomy is now quite rare.

Small stones (especially cystine) may be passed in the urine if output is encouraged by ample *fluid* intake (more than 3 L daily), especially overnight. Antispasmodics such as *propantheline* (contraindicated in bladder outflow obstruction) or catheterization may also assist the passage of stones. *Penicillamine* will help to dissolve cystine stones. For oxalate stones, dietary calcium may be restricted and *thiazides* are used both to reduce urinary calcium and to increase urine flow. Reducing urinary urate levels with *allopurinol* may help. Alkalinization of the urine (e.g. with potassium citrate mixture) will also reduce hypercalciuria and in turn the formation of both urate and cystine stones. Urinary acidification, e.g. with *ammonium chloride*, will minimize phosphate stone production.

Nephrostomy may permit extraction of larger pelvic stones and drainage in hydronephrosis. Stones may be ultrasonically disrupted by extracorporeal shock-wave lithotripsy (ESWL) and the fragments passed out in the urine. Open surgery is rarely necessary.

In reflux nephropathy prompt treatment of infections and adequate control of hypertension are likely to prevent progression. Surgery is rarely indicated, except for reconstruction of a congenitally abnormal vesicoureteric junction.

Infection

As with obstruction, there is a significant difference between infections of the lower and upper renal systems. Lower **urinary tract infection** (UTI, e.g. urethritis, cystitis) causes discomfort, inconvenience and not a little pain, but is essentially benign if restricted to a single attack at that site. Conversely, infection of the kidney (upper urinary tract infection or **pyelonephritis**) is always serious and has systemic complications. It may even lead to CRF: indeed, chronic pyelonephritis accounts for at least 10% of all ESRD.

However, UTI and pyelonephritis are not completely distinct; both are related to obstructive disease. Most kidney infections are presumed to have ascended from asymptomatic, untreated or inadequately treated UTI, and this retrograde infection is encouraged by the urinary stasis which can result from obstruction. Repeated or serious UTI can itself lead to obstruction by causing fibrosis and stricture (narrowing). The pathological spectrum, from asymptomatic bacteriuria to what is still termed **chronic pyelonephritis**, is illustrated in Fig. 4.20.

Because pyelonephritis causes inflammatory damage there is also some pathological similarity to such conditions as nephrotoxicity, analgesic nephropathy, reflux nephropathy and the renal manifestations of connective tissue disorders, e.g. systemic lupus erythematosus (SLE). The overall term **interstitial nephritis** is often preferred.

Urinary tract infection

Because of the close pathogenetic links between UTI, reflux nephropathy, obstruction and pyelonephritis, some of the general features of UTI are discussed here so as to present a

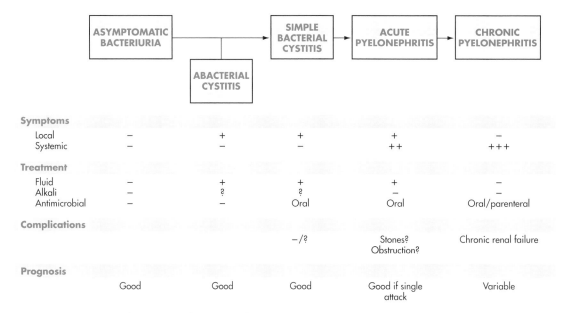

Figure 4.20   Spectrum of renal tract infection. −, absent (symptom) or useless (treatment), +, minor (symptom) or useful (treatment); ++, moderate; +++, substantial; ?, uncertain.

complete picture of renal system infections. Full details of UTI, especially the investigation and management, are given in Chapter 13.

Aetiology and pathology

Urine is normally sterile. The faecal commensal *Escherichia coli* is responsible for infection in 75% of those cases where a urinary organism is identified. Less common pathogens include staphylococci, faecal streptococci, *Proteus* and *Klebsiella*. **Non-specific urethritis** (i.e. non-gonococcal) is usually caused by *Chlamydia* spp.

Women.   Even with the strictest hygiene, contamination with skin commensals or faecal organisms is difficult to avoid in women. This is due to the anatomical proximity of the urethral and anal openings, and the relatively short urethra. Simple UTI is far more common among women than men.

The route of infection may be anus–vagina–vulva–urethra. Vaginal secretions, urine and the urinary tract all normally have protective antimicrobial properties, e.g. mucosal IgA, locally acidic pH, frequent flow. Thus, recurrent infection suggests a breakdown in these defence mechanisms (e.g. obstruction) or a protected

focus of infection (e.g. infected stones). Persisting vaginal organisms may be introduced into the urethra mechanically, especially during intercourse – hence the rather quaint but now anachronistic term 'honeymoon cystitis'.

Although bacteriuria is found in about 5% of adult women, few of these suffer symptoms. Such **asymptomatic** or **covert bacteriuria** generally does not require treatment except during pregnancy, where there is a 30% chance of progression to acute pyelonephritis. On the other hand, no organism can be found in up to 50% of women who do have symptoms of cystitis; this is known as **abacterial cystitis** (or 'urethral syndrome').

Men.   Infection in males is much more rare. Sexually transmitted non-specific urethritis is the most common cause in young men and chronic bacterial prostatitis in older men.

Both sexes.   In the elderly the prevalence of UTI may rise to 30% in both sexes; this is a particular problem in institutions. Catheterization alone carries a risk of infection variously estimated at between 2% and 20%. In diabetics, reduced host defence and glycosuria predispose to urinary bacterial growth.

Clinical features and course

The hallmark of acute urethritis/cystitis is an intense burning sensation on micturition, to which the simple term **dysuria** fails to do justice. The condition may be exacerbated by a more acid urine resulting from local bacterial metabolism. Urinary frequency is common and there may be suprapubic pain or discomfort. **Pyuria**, purulent discharge or even haematuria may also occur but, although alarming, none is necessarily sinister. There are no systemic signs. The elderly commonly present with fever, malaise or anorexia but few specific urinary symptoms, making it easy to miss during examination.

UTI is usually self-limiting within a few days and may have no complications in the absence of any other renal abnormality. However, recurrence is common owing either to infection with a different organism, or to relapse or re-infection with the same organism. The latter situation suggests the presence of a complicating factor that is preventing complete eradication.

Investigation

Two things must be determined: (i) which organism is responsible; and (ii) are there any underlying causes or correctable complications? The collection of urine samples and the indications for further investigation are discussed in Chapter 13.

Management

In the management of UTI the aims are:

- To reduce the risk of renal damage.
- To provide symptomatic relief.
- To render the urine sterile.
- Possibly, to provide prophylactic therapy.

The first of these aims is achieved by prompt attention and full investigation when appropriate. General measures include increasing the fluid intake substantially to promote urine flow, and providing advice on hygiene. For women, advice includes front-to-back wiping after defaecation, and micturition before and after coitus. Frequent recurrence or relapse in the absence of obstructive or other correctable complications may require prophylactic therapy. For details of treatment, *see* Chapter 13.

Acute pyelonephritis

Like lower UTI, most cases of acute pyelonephritis (APN) occur in women. *E. coli* is the usual organism, but *Proteus, Staphylococcus* and *Pseudomonas* are found more commonly than in simple UTI. Tubular inflammation causes polyuria and a dilute urine but severe cases may progress to acute oliguric renal failure.

Clinical features

An acute onset of severe loin pain is accompanied by systemic features such as fever, nausea and vomiting (Fig. 4.20). There may also be lower UTI symptoms of cystitis and urethritis. Rarely, if both kidneys are affected, tubular oedema and inflammatory exudate may cause intrarenal obstruction with acute postrenal failure.

Management

Prompt appropriate oral antimicrobial therapy and an increased fluid intake are always indicated. The same agents are used as in UTI. However, close attention to microbiological results is vital because of the likelihood of unusual or resistant organisms and the importance of characterizing recurrence as either relapse, i.e. the same organism, or re-infection possibly with another.

Most patients have a single attack of APN and recover completely, but recurrent attacks or persistent asymptomatic bacteriuria require further investigation. If the recurrence is a relapse with the same organism, either the antimicrobial therapy was inadequate or there may be obstructive/reflux abnormalities. Frequent re-infection with different organisms or strains suggests that the host defences are defective, and that prophylactic antimicrobial therapy should be considered. This can be continuous low-dose therapy, or intermittent 5-day full-dose courses at the onset of symptoms, which the patient can be instructed to initiate.

Chronic pyelonephritis (reflux nephropathy)

Definition

The term chronic pyelonephritis (CPN) has traditionally been used to describe a condition diagnosed radiologically where one or both kidneys appear irregular, shrunken and scarred. However, because evidence is accumulating of a strong association with reflux or infection, the term **reflux nephropathy** is now preferred. Although most cases do not progress to renal failure, CAPN can be extremely difficult to treat, and renal scarring is present in up to 20% of patients starting dialysis.

Pathogenesis

The relative contributions of chronic infection and sterile reflux (causing simple pressure damage) are still uncertain. Many patients have neither bacteriuria nor a history of UTI, and although UTI and APN are far more common in women, CPN shows equal sex distribution. One form may be from vesicoureteric reflux starting in the very young, and this has a poorer prognosis because initially it may be silent or undiagnosed. In adults, recurrent UTI or APN may be responsible.

Bacterial CPN commonly involves more virulent Gram-negative organisms, including *Pseudomonas*, and persistent infection with relapses is common. In contrast to the urinary tract the renal pelvis seems to have no natural antibacterial defences (presumably evolution never expected organisms there). There may even be factors which encourage the microbial persistence, and so complete eradication is difficult.

Clinical features and investigation

The condition may be asymptomatic or may present as proteinuria, hypertension or recurrent UTI. Rarely, the first indication may be symptoms of incipient renal failure such as polyuria or nocturia because the renal damage is primarily tubular. Early reflux damage may initiate the hypertension–renal failure vicious cycle, and sometimes a history of related childhood illnesses such as enuresis or cystitis may be traced. Diagnosis and investigation involve urography, urine microbiology and renal function tests.

Management

In the absence of renal impairment, all that may be required is regular monitoring of blood pressure, urine microbiology and renal function.

Infective episodes must be treated promptly as for APN, and antimicrobial prophylaxis may be indicated if bacteriuria cannot be eliminated. In children, surgery to correct reflux may be necessary.

Course and prognosis

Most patients have stable disease, especially if their BP and bacteriuria are managed successfully. Recurrent infective exacerbations carry a poorer prognosis, but only about 1% of patients progress to CRF.

Glomerular disease

Glomerular disease invariably affects both kidneys. Glomeruli seem especially sensitive to inflammatory immune damage, and most forms of glomerular disease involve immunological mechanisms. **Glomerulonephritis** (GN) is the single most important cause of CRF.

Classification

For such a small and apparently simple structure the glomerulus presents inordinate pathological complexity. Descriptions of glomerular disease have a long history in medicine, and understanding of the condition is confounded by the numerous methods of classification. Moreover, increasingly sophisticated microscopy and immunological techniques continue to identify new criteria and subgroups. Thus, in addition to simple clinical and aetiological classes there are histopathological and immunopathological groupings (Table 4.22).

There is no consistent correlation between these classes, and much overlap. No single classification provides an unequivocal guide to management, and usually each aspect needs to be specified when considering a particular patient. Thus, for example, diabetes is usually associated with chronically progressive glomerulosclerosis and a poor outcome. On the other hand, acute postinfective nephritis showing diffuse proliferative change has an excellent prognosis with minimal treatment.

Table 4.22   Classification of glomerular disease

Type of classification	Examples
Aetiological – describes cause	Primary (only the kidney affected) • idiopathic (i.e. unknown) • postinfective (e.g. post-streptococcal) • iatrogenic (e.g. gold, NSAID) • allergic (e.g. most iatrogenic causes) Secondary (systemic disease) • hypertension • connective tissue disease (e.g. SLE, PAN) • autoimmune (e.g. Goodpasture's disease) • diabetic nephropathy
Prognostic – describes course	Acute Rapidly progressive Chronic
Immunological – describes mechanism	Immune complex (type III hypersensitivity) Autoimmune (anti-GBM antibodies) IgA nephropathy
Histopathological – describes damage	Minimal change Membranous Proliferative Glomerulosclerosis

GBM, glomerular basement membrane; IgA, immunoglobulin A; PAN, polyarteritis nodosa; SLE, systemic lupus erythematosus.

Presenting syndromes

The histopathological classification is becoming the standard among nephrologists but glomerular disease remains perplexing for the non-specialist. It is best tackled by first understanding that there are four main ways in which it may present, ranging in severity from asymptomatic proteinuria through nephritic syndrome and nephrotic syndrome to irreversible renal failure. This is illustrated in Fig. 4.21, although this scheme must not be taken to imply an inevitable or direct progression.

Each syndrome can have various aetiologies and outcomes, so the likely cause should be identified if possible and the pathology described. It is then possible to decide treatment and judge prognosis.

The clinical features and management options for these syndromes will be summarized in general terms, including a brief description of the main varieties of nephritic syndrome as commonly classified by prognostic categories. The syndrome of chronic renal failure was described in detail on pp. 183–191.

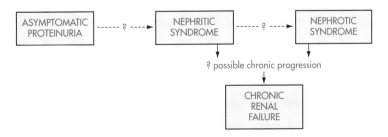

Figure 4.21   Spectrum of glomerular disease. Each syndrome can arise independently and progression is not inevitable.

Asymptomatic proteinuria

Normal urine contains only trace amounts of protein (usually less than 100 mg excreted over 24 h). Most plasma proteins are too large for filtration; smaller ones such as microglobulin are filtered to some extent, but most is reabsorbed in the tubules. **Proteinuria** means the presence of more than 500 mg protein in 24 h. If these are smaller proteins (a 'tubular pattern') it implies a tubular defect, i.e. a failure of reabsorption.

Albumin is larger, and its presence in significant amount suggests a 'glomerular pattern', i.e. a failure of filtration. Thus it is more correctly called **albuminuria**. Albumin is usually discovered as a chance finding during a general medical examination or during investigation of some other disease. Albumin loss below about 2 g/24 h may be benign, but such patients are always investigated and regularly monitored for the possible development of conditions such as glomerular nephritis, diabetes and hypertension. A medication history is also important. Intermittent proteinuria is quite a common normal finding after exercise or after prolonged standing or walking.

Microalbuminuria (<200 mg albumin per 24 h) is a prognostic marker of the possible development of nephropathy in diabetes. Urine dipsticks can currently detect this level of proteinuria. Microscopic **haematuria** may be benign. Even macroscopic haematuria need not be a sinister sign although it is obviously very alarming. Of course, both conditions also require thorough investigation.

Nephritic syndrome

Definition

The hallmarks of nephritis are renal impairment with oliguria, sodium and fluid retention, and peripheral oedema, mild to moderate proteinuria and possibly haematuria. Urinary red blood cell 'casts' are diagnostic; these are clumps of cells that have been shaped by the tubular lumen. Frequently there are no further complications but hypertension, hypertensive encephalopathy and pulmonary oedema may occur. Serum creatinine is moderately elevated, but only rarely does oliguric ARF supervene. The pathophysiological basis of these features is illustrated in Fig. 4.22.

Aetiology and pathogenesis

Acute nephritis following a non-renal streptococcal infection (e.g. streptococcal sore throat) is the most common form although other infections may be responsible, e.g. malaria, bacterial endocarditis. Drug reactions and connective tissue disorders are other possible causes.

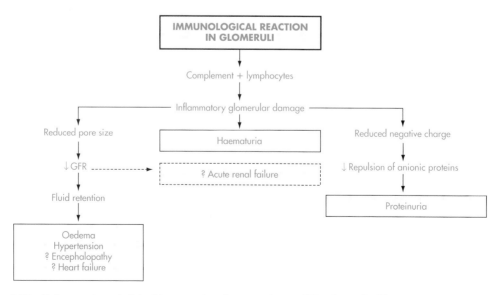

Figure 4.22   Pathogenesis and clinical features of nephritic syndrome. GFR, glomerular filtration rate.

Most cases are extra-renal in origin, involving immune complex (IC) deposition on the GBM. These complexes may be immunoglobulin plus, for example, streptoccocal antigen or a drug acting as a hapten. In connective tissue disorder, anti-nuclear antibodies may be involved. Why some patients react in this way, and why the ICs are deposited in the glomeruli rather than being cleared by the reticuloendothelial system as usual, is not known. Low plasma complement levels may be implicated, although this may be effect rather than cause (complement having been precipitated on the GBM).

Course and prognosis

Usually nephritis runs an acute florid course with excellent recovery, especially in children. Some older patients may have benign persistent or intermittent proteinuria for many months or years. A significant number progress slowly to CRF and a few follow a rapidly progressive decline.

Management

The aims of management are:

- To identify any specific cause (e.g. infection) and treat that.
- To institute simple symptomatic and supportive measures until the patient recovers.

The general approaches adopted and their rationales are summarized in Table 4.23.

Common presentations

Acute glomerulonephritis.   This is the classic post-streptococcal form usually seen in children or young adults. A very abrupt and severe renal inflammatory response might develop for example a few weeks after a severe throat infection. Disease severity usually correlates with the patient's titre of anti-streptolysin antibody (ASO). In children particularly, the prognosis is excellent with resolution in a week or less, and only supportive therapy is required. Anti-inflammatory therapy is usually ineffective.

Rapidly progressive glomerulonephritis. About 1% of patients who develop acute GN have a very aggressive, rapidly progressive form with a greater likelihood of acute oliguric failure. If this occurs the outlook is poor, with progression to ESRD within 2 years. Progressive GN may be associated with the presence of anti-GBM auto-antibodies (e.g. Goodpasture's disease), or arise in association with vasculitic connective tissue diseases (e.g. polyarteritis nodosa, PAN). The renal damage caused by malignant hypertension usually presents as a rapidly progressive GN; in this case the damage is not immunological.

Treatment and prognosis depend on the aetiology. For the connective tissue diseases early aggressive immunosuppressive therapy with *cytotoxic drugs* and *steroids* may induce a remission or retard progression. In idiopathic forms or in Goodpasture's disease this is rarely successful, but plasma exchange (plasmapheresis) may be

Table 4.23   Management of nephritic syndrome

Target symptom/feature	Management	Comment
Glomerular inflammation	*Steroids, cytotoxics*	Rarely indicated unless due to systemic disease, otherwise ineffective
Proteinuria	–	Protein supplementation not usually required
Fluid retention, oedema	Na/water restriction	As for acute renal failure (Table 4.14)
	Loop diuretic	Monitor fluid balance and blood pressure
	Dialysis	
Uraemia	Protein restriction	Rare
Hypertension	Hypotensive therapy	Avoid beta-blocker (heart failure)
Infection	*Antibiotics*	e.g. penicillin in post-streptococcal nephritis

helpful. The aim of this is to remove circulating auto-antibodies and ICs from the blood. Whole blood is removed and centrifuged: the supernatant plasma, containing the harmful immune products, is discarded and the cellular components are then re-injected. Fluid, electrolytes and albumin must also be administered to compensate for losses.

In the anti-GBM auto-antibody forms, plasmapheresis combined with immunosuppression has considerably improved the prognosis, either by inducing a remission or by reducing damage before a natural decline in disease activity. Nevertheless, eventual progression to CRF and renal replacement therapy is common. Following transplantation a recurrence of the disease is still possible, but the tendency nowadays is to transplant anyway.

Chronic glomerulonephritis. About 10% of GN patients, usually adults, progress to chronic illness. It is this slowly progressive, late-presenting form of GN which is the most common cause of CRF. Invariably there are co-existent hypertension and proteinuria. The cause of chronic GN is usually unknown. Diabetic nephropathy could be considered to be one form of the condition, although strictly speaking this is glomerular sclerosis rather than inflammation, and nephrotic syndrome is a more common presentation.

Specific treatment is rarely possible and the patient must enter a renal replacement programme. Certain forms of chronic GN with less glomerular damage ('membranous' and 'minimal change' GN) may respond to immunosuppressant therapy, but this is still controversial.

Nephrotic syndrome

The nephrotic syndrome is defined by the symptom triad:

- Heavy proteinuria.
- Hypoalbuminaemia.
- Gross pitting oedema.

The hallmark of nephrotic syndrome is hypoproteinaemia sufficient to cause severe generalized oedema associated with extensive urinary protein loss. The liver can synthesize albumin up to a maximum of about 15 g/24 h in an attempt to maintain plasma albumin levels, but paradoxically proteinuria no greater than 4–6 g/24 h may be sufficient to cause nephrotic syndrome. Thus there is probably another avenue of protein loss involved. This is likely to be an increase in the renal tubular catabolism of albumin, such that measurement of urinary protein loss underestimates the total deficit. These combined losses exceed hepatic capacity and lead to progressive hypoproteinaemia, regardless of dietary protein intake.

Aetiology
The nephrotic syndrome may be a complication or progression of GN, sometimes called the 'mixed nephritic-nephrotic' syndrome, or it may present *de novo*. Specific aetiologies include diabetes, drugs (e.g. penicillamine, captopril, heavy metals) and infections (e.g. malaria, endocarditis).

Pathophysiology
The apparently paradoxical combination of a reduced GFR with a 'leak' sufficient to pass albumin molecules of MW greater than 60 kDa may arise because the reduced plasma volume causes a mild pre-renal impairment of filtration while changes in the GBM electrostatic charge allow smaller proteins, that are normally repelled, to pass through (Fig. 4.22). In mixed nephritic-nephrotic syndromes there is also some glomerular obstruction. The phenomenon of proteinuria is still not understood.

The oedema forms by a quite different mechanism to that of simple nephritis. In the latter case there is redistribution of a raised total body water volume with increased volumes in all compartments, the hypervolaemia causing hypertension. By contrast, in nephrotic syndrome there is a reduced blood volume and often hypotension. The hypovolaemia results from the reduced plasma oncotic pressure brought about by the hypoproteinaemia, which permits a loss of plasma water to the extravascular compartment (Fig. 4.23).

The renin/angiotensin system acts to restore BP by increasing renal sodium and water reabsorption. However, blood volume cannot be expanded while plasma protein is low because renally retained fluid passes straight to the tissues,

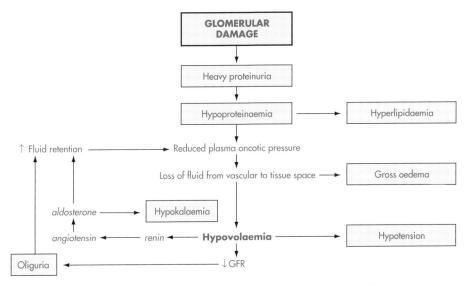

Figure 4.23 Pathogenesis and clinical features of nephrotic syndrome. GFR, glomerular filtration rate.

exacerbating the oedema and causing further fluid and electrolyte retention. This vicious cycle may result in gross oedema; indeed, the presence of over 20 L of oedema fluid has been reported. Nevertheless, many patients are not overtly hypotensive, possibly owing to the direct vasoconstrictor action of persistently raised angiotensin levels. Postural hypotension is usual, however. (This classical account of the pathophysiology of oedema in nephrotic syndrome has been challenged by recent research and is unlikely to represent the whole picture.)

Course and prognosis

The prognosis will depend on the age of the patient and the underlying lesion. In children the cause is usually acute GN and the outlook is good, with an 80% remission rate. In adults the underlying pathology is more likely to be a chronic progressive disease and the average remission rate nearer 20–30%.

Clinical features

The clinical picture is usually very distinctive. Nephrotic syndrome may have an acute or insidious onset and resembles acute GN, except that the oedema is usually greater, including pulmonary oedema and ascites, and the patient may be hypotensive. The patient is usually very ill, weak, anorexic and oliguric. A common

unexplained finding is hyperlipidaemia, possibly related to disordered protein metabolism (an attempt to synthesize new amino acids). High aldosterone levels often cause hypokalaemia.

Management

The aims of management are:

- To investigate and treat the cause (e.g. an underlying disease).
- To correct haemodynamic and metabolic abnormalities.
- To reduce glomerular inflammation.

Table 4.24 summarizes the treatment options. The effectiveness of immunosuppressant therapy, initially high-dose *steroids*, will depend on the cause, but in general steroid therapy is more beneficial than in simple GN. Patients who relapse after steroid withdrawal, i.e. are steroid-dependent, may benefit from cytotoxic drugs, e.g. *cyclophosphamide*.

Reversal of the hypoproteinaemia must usually await resolution of the glomerular damage, but high-protein diets are traditional. The principal clinical problems are oedema and sodium and fluid retention. Salt and water restriction and loop diuretics are used and high doses may be needed, e.g. 500 mg furosemide (frusemide). Care must be taken not to exacerbate hypovolaemia and precipitate pre-renal failure by too

Table 4.24   Management of nephrotic syndrome

Target symptom	Management	Comment
Glomerular inflammation	*Steroids, cytotoxics*, plasmapheresis	Often useful, especially in children
Proteinuria	Protein supplementation (>100 g/day)	Often given, efficiency unproven
Fluid retention, oedema	Na/water restriction	Care! Patient has hypovolaemia
	Diuretic: *spironolactone, thiazide, high-dose loop*	and hypokalaemia
Low plasma oncotic pressure	Albumin, mannitol infusion	Albumin effect short-lived
Hypokaleamia	*Spironolactone, amiloride*	

rapid a diuresis; thus the use of diuretics may be delayed until there is a recovery in urine output. This can be prevented by subsequent infusion of a plasma expander such as salt-free albumin. Hypokalaemia, which would be exacerbated by loop diuretics, can treated with high-dose spironolactone and potassium supplements.

Polycystic disease

Adult polycystic disease is the most common inherited renal disease. Both kidneys become enlarged up to two or three times normal size, owing to the development of many fluid-filled, inert cysts. These gradually crush adjacent renal structures.

The more common autosomal dominant form has a prevalence of 1/1000. The age of onset and progression are highly variable. Progression to end-stage renal failure usually occurs within 10–20 years of diagnosis, so patients who first present late in life may avoid this. Nevertheless, 10% of ESRD patients have polycystic disease. In a rarer recessive form, onset and rapid progression to renal failure occur in childhood.

Clinical features are similar to those of other forms of ARF. Hypertension is common; there may be loin or lumbar pain, and haematuria if a cyst ruptures. Diagnosis is based on ultrasound imaging.

There is no specific treatment beyond the standard procedures for CRF; control of BP will slow progress. Regular screening of siblings and offspring is important.

References and further reading

Ayers S, Magee P. *Beginner's Guide to Renal Pharmacy*. UK Renal Pharmacy Group.

Brady HR, Singer GG (1995) Acute renal failure. *Lancet* **346**: 1533–1540.

Gokal R, Mallick NP (1999) Peritoneal dialysis. *Lancet* **353**: 823–828.

Mallick NP, Gokal R (1999) Haemodialysis. *Lancet* **353**: 737–742.

Marshall WJ (1988) *Illustrated Textbook of Clinical Chemistry*. 3rd edn. London: Gower Medical.

Swanson P (1990) Drug treatment of chronic renal failure. *Pharm J* **244**: 365–367.

The Renal Association (1997) *Treatment of Adult Patients with Renal Failure*. 2nd edn. London: Royal College of Physicians.

Tomson CVR, Plant WD (1997) *Key Topics in Renal Medicine*. Oxford: Bios.

Vander AJ (1995) *Renal Physiology*. 5th edn. New York: McGraw-Hill.

Walker R (1997) General management of end stage renal disease. *Br Med J* **315**: 1429–1432.

5

Respiratory diseases

Respiratory diseases are major world-wide causes of morbidity and mortality, especially in Third World countries and those ravaged by war and natural disasters. The World Health Organization estimates that tuberculosis infects **one-third** of the world population, causing some three million deaths in 1998. This imposes great health burdens and large economic costs in terms of lost productivity, and comprises a major restraint on the growth of poorer economies. Developed Western societies are also affected. Increasing asthma is the most common chronic disease in the UK and affects about 12 million North Americans. Further, acute respiratory infections are still important causes of death in the elderly.

The respiratory tract is exposed to environmental hazards to a greater extent than any organ system except the skin. Lung tissue is extremely delicate and has limited protective mechanisms, so the high incidence of respiratory diseases is readily understandable. It is somewhat surprising that these are not more common, given the increasing airborne insults from expanding industrial activity and population growth.

Anatomy and clinical physiology of the respiratory system

Anatomy

The lungs are intimately connected with the heart in that they receive and process the entire cardiac output. To appreciate the effects of respiratory diseases it is essential to understand the cardiovascular system. This chapter outlines the anatomy and physiology of the respiratory system as an introduction to the aetiology, pathology and management of its important diseases.

The gross anatomy of the respiratory tract is illustrated in Fig. 5.1(a). The various parts have specialized functions, which are reflected in the types of tissue of which they are composed (Table 5.1). Most of the structures only serve to conduct gases between the air and the **acinus**, the smallest functional respiratory unit (Fig. 5.2). This comprises a **terminal bronchiole** which communicates with the **respiratory bronchioles**, **alveolar sacs** and **alveoli**. The majority of the exchange of oxygen and carbon dioxide between the inspired air and the capillary blood occurs across the walls of approximately 300 million alveoli, each about 250 microns in diameter, which together provide about $70\,m^2$ of membrane for gas exchange. The alveoli are not isolated units but are interconnected by pores.

Some of these structural and functional aspects (Table 5.1) are of interest here. Only those conducting airways which are not substantially supported by cartilage can be reduced considerably in bore by smooth muscle spasm, so it is these small airways which are involved in asthma and, to a lesser extent, in chronic bronchitis: supported airways can only constrict to a lesser extent. Thus, bronchodilators can be beneficial only if there is smooth muscle spasm causing bronchiolar constriction and **airways obstruction**. Further, because mucous glands and goblet cells occur primarily in the larger airways, their stimulation to produce excessive amounts of mucus, as in chronic bronchitis and

bronchiectasis, does not affect the smallest airways and the alveoli. In these diseases it is medium-sized airways obstruction, due to variable degrees and combinations of bronchoconstriction and mucus plugging, which causes the problems. Damage to the pulmonary blood vessels is also involved.

Ciliated epithelium provides an important defence mechanism. The cilia beat in organized waves, sweeping mucus, and microorganisms and other particles trapped in it, towards the larynx. The mucus and its trapped contents are usually swallowed and digested or, if large quantities are produced, coughed up.

Elastic tissue is present throughout the lungs and is especially important in the alveolar walls. The muscles of the airways and the thorax also have elastic properties. Although this elasticity produces a tendency for the expanded lungs to collapse, it accounts for only about one-third of the total recoil effect. The remainder is caused by interfacial tension within the film of fluid lining the alveoli, but this is counteracted by **surfactant lipoproteins** derived from dipalmitoyl lecithin, produced by specialized alveolar cells. These surfactants assist spreading of the fluid over the alveolar surfaces, keep the delicate tissues moist to provide for good gas exchange, and reduce both the tendency of the alveoli to collapse at low lung volumes and the work required to expand the lungs during inspiration. A brief increase in alveolar surface area increases the benefit of the surfactant. Hence the importance of the occasional deep breath or sigh during quiet breathing which expands any respiratory lobules (Fig. 5.2) that have collapsed under interfacial tension.

During the first 4 weeks of life of a small proportion of neonates, and especially in prematurity, a congenital deficiency of natural surfactant results in **hyaline membrane disease** and, if the deficiency is severe, the lungs collapse completely at the end of expiration and are difficult to re-expand. The infant may then exhibit **respiratory distress syndrome of the newborn (RDSN)**. If neonatal artificial ventilation is

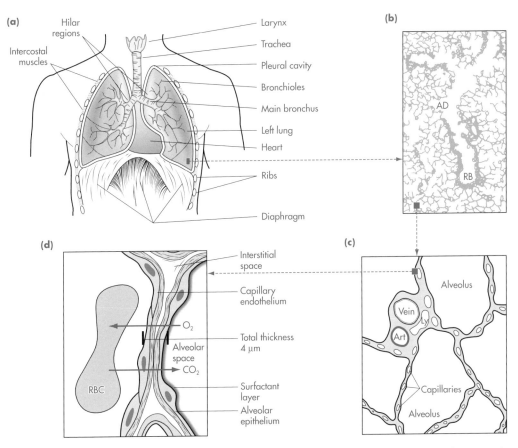

Figure 5.1   Anatomy and histology of the respiratory tract. (a) General view of the thoracic structures. (b) Section through the lung parenchyma. (c) Lung parenchyma at higher magnification. (d) Section through the alveolar wall. AD, alveolar duct; Art, arteriole; Ly, lymphatic vessel; RB, respiratory bronchiole; RBC, red blood cell.

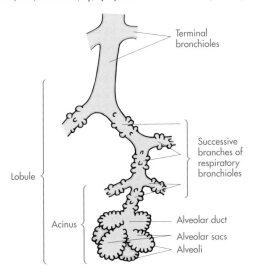

Figure 5.2   Respiratory lobule and acinus.

unsuccessful, the infant may die in the immediate postnatal period or, depending on the extent of the deficiency, in early infancy. Some 40–50% of the complications of RDSN may be prevented by giving the mother a short course of corticosteroids at least 24 h before a premature birth (<37 weeks' gestation). This is done preferably between the 24th and 34th week, e.g. 20–40 mg of *betamethasone* over 48 h. Artificial surfactants (e.g. *beractant, colfosceril palmitate, poractant alfa, pumactant*) are available for postnatal treatment, and a liposomal formulation of prostaglandin E is in clinical trial.

RDSN should not be confused with adult respiratory distress syndrome, which is usually due to trauma or inhalation of toxic material.

Table 5.1   Structure, histology and function in the respiratory tract

Organ or structure	Relative cross sectional area	Function[a]	Ciliate epithelium	Mucous and serous glands	Goblet cells	Lymphoid and phagocytic[b]	Muscle[c]	Elastic	Cartilage
Nose, etc.	1	C,O	+	+	–	A	V	–	+
Pharynx	1	C	+	+	+	T	V	+	+
Larynx	1	C	+	+	+	L	V	+	+
Trachea and bronchi	1	C	+	+	+	L	S	+	+
Bronchioles									
• larger	0.8	C	+	–	+	L	S	+	–
• terminal	1.3	C	–	–	+	(M)	S	+	–
• respiratory	3	C (E)	–	–	–	(M)	S	+	–
Alveolar									
• ducts	10	C,E	–	–	–	M	–	+	–
• sacs	2000	C,E	–	–	–	M	–	+	–

The "Type of tissue" spanning header covers: Ciliate epithelium, Mucous and serous glands, Goblet cells, Lymphoid and phagocytic[b], Muscle[c], Supportive (Elastic, Cartilage).

[a] C, conducting; E, gas exchange; O, olfactory; ( ), some function.

[b] A, adenoids; L, scattered lymphoid cells; M, macrophages; T, tonsils.

[c] S, smooth muscle; V, striated (voluntary) muscle.

Pleural membranes

Each lung is surrounded by a double membrane, the **pleura**, and is attached to the inner of these membranes. The outer membrane forms the lining of the thoracic wall and diaphragm. The **pleural cavity** between them is filled with a few millilitres of fluid, which is normally maintained at a negative pressure relative to the lung tissue. This negative pressure is essential for respiration because if air enters the pleural cavity (a **pneumothorax**, e.g. due to trauma or disease) the affected lung tends to collapse. The pleural fluid lubricates the membranes, permitting them to slip easily over each other during breathing. Inflammation or infection of these membranes (**pleurisy**) causes the cavity to fill with inflammatory exudate, resulting in adhesions (see p. 42) between the layers of membrane and a variable degree of inspiratory pain which enforces shallow, rapid respiration.

Mediastinum

The mediastinum is the space between the pleural sacs around each lung (Fig. 5.1(a)), and contains the heart and major blood vessels, the trachea and bronchial bifurcation, important nerves (vagus, cardiac, phrenic, splanchnic), the oesophagus, lymphatic vessels and tissues (thoracic duct, lymph nodes) and the thymus gland.

Although mediastinal diseases are outside the scope of this chapter, the course of the recurrent laryngeal nerves, especially the left (which loops under the aortic arch before ascending to the larynx) has important implications for the occurrence of certain respiratory tract symptoms. Notably, persistent hoarseness may be produced by any condition causing pressure on these nerves, e.g. tumours or an aortic aneurysm.

Clinically relevant aspects of respiratory physiology

Lung function has three interdependent components:

1. Conduction of inspired air to the alveoli and of expired gases to the trachea.
2. Maintenance of blood flow to and from the alveoli.
3. Exchange of oxygen and carbon dioxide between the alveolar spaces and the blood.

Regulation of respiration

Respiration consists of two phases: **inspiration** is the expansion of the lungs and the conduction of air to the alveoli (alveolar ventilation) and **expiration** is the relaxation of the expanded lungs and the expulsion of alveolar gas. A combination of chemical and nervous stimuli adjusts the alveolar ventilation almost exactly to the bodily requirements, so that the partial pressures of oxygen (P_aO_2) and of carbon dioxide (P_aCO_2) in the arterial blood are relatively constant over a wide range of systemic demands.

These stimuli are derived from sensors in various organs and tissues and the principal factors which influence respiration are summarized in Table 5.2.

Central nervous reflex signals arise primarily from chemoreceptors in the cerebral ventricles, carotid bodies and brainstem, which are primarily sensitive to carbon dioxide levels, and so also to pH, in the blood. The cerebral cortex and muscles also drive respiration (and heart rate) according to voluntary exercise demand. The signals from all of these are coordinated in the 'respiratory centre' in the brainstem (medulla and pons). Perhaps surprisingly for such an

Table 5.2   Some humoral and nervous factors influencing respiration

Origin of stimulus	Factors that affect respiration	
	Increase	Decrease
Cerebral cortex	Arousal/fear Desire to exercise Fever	Sleep Depressant drugs Trauma
Respiratory centre	pH[a] ↓ Salicylate poisoning Fever	pH[a] ↑ Severe hypoxaemia Sedatives
Cerebrospinal fluid	pH[a] ↓	pH[a] ↑
Carotid and aortic bodies	P_aO_2 ↓ pH[a] ↓ Blood pressure ↓	P_aO_2 ↑ (weak effects) pH[a] ↑ Blood pressure ↑
Lungs • parenchyma • bronchioles	Relaxation Pulmonary embolism/oedema Smoking/irritants	Stretching
Periphery	Muscle stretch ↑ Chronic pain	Acute pain
	------------ Proprioreceptors in chest wall and joints ------------	

[a] [H+] is the primary mechanism and reflects P_aCO_2 (see text).

important function, the respiratory centre is not well-defined, there being three widely separated groups of neurones located in the upper part of the brainstem which interact and send appropriate signals to the respiratory muscles.

These central mechanisms interact with peripheral ones to form a series of complex interrelationships and feedback mechanisms. The most important peripheral input is derived from chemoreceptors which respond to blood levels of carbon dioxide, pH and oxygen, in that order of importance under normal conditions. The P_aCO_2 exerts by far the greatest influence, there being an approximately eightfold increase in respiration rate from low to high values (Fig. 5.3(a)). Conversely, P_aO_2 has little influence because, as the shape of the haemoglobin dissociation curve shows, there is an almost complete saturation of oxygen-carrying capacity over the whole of the normal range of oxygen levels (Fig. 5.3(b)), and because a change in P_aO_2 increases the sensitivity of the respiratory centre to carbon dioxide. A change in blood pH has a similar sensitizing effect on the respiratory centre and influences the oxygen-carrying capacity of haemoglobin more than oxygen does in the normal range (Fig. 5.3(b)). Further, both the P_aCO_2 and pH mechanisms react to exert a braking effect on the response to oxygen. Although the effect of pH appears to be small, if all other parameters are controlled, the principal agent acting on the respiratory centre becomes the hydrogen ion, because changes in carbon dioxide levels immediately change the pH, since:

$$[H^+] = K \; \frac{[CO_2]}{[HCO_3^-]}$$

The hydrogen ions affect the respiratory centre primarily via the blood and to a lesser extent via the cerebrospinal fluid.

Although the carbon dioxide effect is large initially, if the hypercapnia (high P_aCO_2, also known as hypercarbia) is sustained, as in severe chronic bronchitis, the respiratory centre becomes desensitized to the level of carbon dioxide. The patient then depends on their P_aO_2 to provide their respiratory drive.

Respiratory muscles

Inspiration is an active process, the principal mechanism being contraction of the **phrenic** (diaphragm) muscles and to a lesser extent of the **external intercostal** (rib) muscles. However, during quiet breathing expiration is a passive process which depends on the elastic recoil of the stretched muscles and lung tissue and interfacial tension effects in the alveoli. The force of expiration during exercise is increased by the action of the **internal intercostal** muscles.

In severe respiratory deficit the muscles of the shoulders, chest wall and abdomen are used to increase the force applied for both inspiration and expiration, so these are known as the **accessory muscles of respiration**. Use of these can be recognized by excessive movements of the shoulders and abdomen: in very severe disability the patient will grasp the arms of a chair, or other surface, in an attempt to increase the applied force. However, these manoeuvres may be counter-productive, because excessive

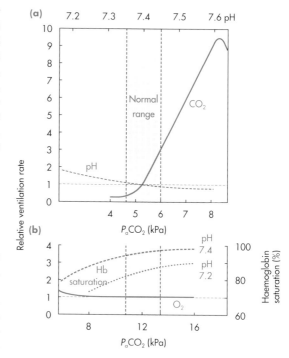

Figure 5.3   Influence of blood gases and pH on the ventilation rate. (a) Carbon dioxide and pH. (b) Oxygen and haemoglobin saturation.

respiratory force increases the intrathoracic pressure abnormally, so that the airways tend to collapse, especially if they are weakened by disease, thus increasing the resistance to expiratory flow (see below). Thus, difficulty in expiration may often be the first sign of respiratory obstruction.

Respiratory mechanics

Airways resistance

This is measured as the pressure difference between the mouth and the alveoli per litre of gas flow. It is the result of friction between the gas molecules themselves, and between them and the walls of the airways. Quiet breathing produces laminar gas flow but rapid breathing causes turbulence, so a greater pressure difference is then required to maintain the flow. Anything that causes airways narrowing, e.g. bronchoconstriction in asthma or mucus plugging in chronic bronchitis, will increase airways resistance markedly. In chronic bronchitis and emphysema there is a variable combination of airways inflammation and loss of both tissue supporting the airways and the elastic recoil pressure of the lungs. This makes the airways likely to collapse on expiration, when intrathoracic pressures increase, thus increasing resistance and making it difficult to exhale. Even small changes in airways bore make large differences to flow rate (Poiseuille's law: *see also* p. 52). However, bronchoconstriction may have some beneficial physiological effects, because it reduces the dead space (p. 221), and this improves the efficiency of ventilation when tidal volumes are low.

In normal respiration, airways resistance reduces gas flow almost to zero by the time the air reaches the entrances to the alveolar sacs, so diffusion is the final mechanism by which the gas molecules travel to and from the alveolar membranes.

Mechanical factors affecting gas flow

The lungs and respiratory muscles resist changes in size and shape because of tissue viscosity and elasticity.

Compliance is the term used to describe the ability of the lungs and thoracic wall to expand, and is a reflection of elasticity – the converse of stiffness. Compliance is reduced by any disease which increases lung stiffness, e.g. pulmonary fibrosis and oedema (pp. 273, 275), pneumonic consolidation and tuberculosis (p. 277). Compliance is **increased** in emphysema (p. 267), due to destruction of lung tissue, and in old age due to tissue weakening.

However, such factors account for only about 20% of the total pulmonary resistance and become a problem only if fibrosis or oedema are extensive. When this occurs, patients often breathe shallowly but rapidly. This is a normal physiological response which minimizes the effort required, but is very inefficient (see below).

Work of breathing

The energy expended during respiration is that required to overcome airways resistance and mechanical factors (e.g. compliance, muscular work). During normal quiet breathing this amounts to only about 2% of the total bodily energy requirement, and is negligible. However, disease may increase this so greatly that there is insufficient oxygen available for other purposes and patients become exercise-limited (e.g. in pulmonary fibrosis) or may be exhausted on admission to hospital (e.g. severe asthma).

Figure 5.4 shows the effect of lung volume on the change in pressure required to produce a unit change in that volume. Because air trapping occurs in obstructive lung disease (pp. 228, 266), increasing the lung volume, patients with severe asthma and chronic bronchitis have to exert a much greater effort to move air in and out of their lungs than do normal subjects, and this requires the expenditure of more energy.

Ventilation and perfusion

The composition of the alveolar gas varies markedly, depending on the respiration rate, blood flow, diffusion across the alveolar membrane, haemoglobin concentration, carbon dioxide production, etc. Further, the alveolar gas cannot be expelled completely from the lungs at expiration because about 150 mL of it is

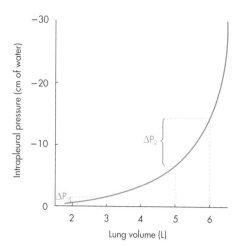

Figure 5.4 Relationship of intrapleural pressure to lung volume. ΔP_1, ΔP_2, the change in intrapleural pressure (negative, a measure of inspiratory effort) required to inspire 1 L of air at different lung volumes.

contained in the conducting airways (the **anatomical dead space**). This residual gas is the first to be washed into the alveoli during inspiration and is only removed by dilution with the inspired air. Hence shallow, rapid breathing may do little more than move this volume of gas in and out of the alveoli, and is a very inefficient mode of ventilation.

The **alveolar ventilation**, the total volume of gas exchanged in all the alveoli in unit time, is approximately 5 L/min during quiet breathing. The lungs receive the entire cardiac output, so in a normal resting adult the **pulmonary perfusion** is approximately 5 L/min. Thus, the overall resting **ventilation/perfusion ratio** (VPR) is about 1.0. However, this overall balance masks large differences which occur throughout the respiratory cycle and regional differences within the lungs. An imbalance between ventilation and perfusion is known as **mismatching**.

The resting value of VPR is not constant throughout the lung because blood flow decreases markedly from base to apex in an upright individual, whereas ventilation is less affected. Figure 5.5 shows that ventilation/perfusion mismatching is greatest in the upper lobes, so that oxygenation of the blood is relatively poor there. Ventilation is particularly unevenly distributed at low lung volumes (at the end of expiration or the beginning of inspiration) because the lungs are suspended in the chest only at the hilum, and so the weight of their upper part plus the weight and hydrostatic pressure of the blood contained in the lungs compresses the lower lobes. When we breathe in after a maximum expiration, air initially enters the upper lobes, which are less compressed, but when about 1 L has been inhaled the situation is reversed, the lower zone airways open and the lung bases are better ventilated.

The volume at which the lower airways close, due to intrathoracic pressure exceeding airways pressure, the **closing volume**, increases with increasing age until it encroaches on normal breathing. Consequently, elderly normal subjects often have poorly ventilated lungs with poor gas exchange and are exercise limited. An increased closing volume may be a sensitive

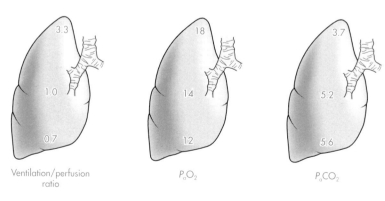

Figure 5.5 Variation of ventilation/perfusion ratios in the normal lung and its effect on arterial partial gas pressures.

early indicator of lung disease such as smoking damage or emphysema.

The value of VPR is crucial to oxygen delivery to the tissues. The arterial PO_2 (P_aO_2) results from a balance between the rates of oxygen delivery and its removal in the blood (i.e. the VPR). Thus high values of VPR lead to high values of P_aO_2, and vice versa. At the extreme limits, zero ventilation would give a P_aO_2 equal to that of venous blood and zero oxygen uptake, whereas minimal perfusion would give a P_aO_2 equal to that of the inspired gas, but no oxygen would be carried to the tissues. Such conditions can occur only locally, because neither of them is compatible with life if they were to occur widely. However, very high oxygen levels in the alveoli give only a limited increase in the oxygen-carrying capacity of the blood, because haemoglobin saturation is almost complete under normal conditions (Fig. 5.3), so a high VPR in one localized area of lung cannot compensate for low values elsewhere.

Although the alveolar–arterial deficit, i.e. the difference between the partial pressures of oxygen across the alveolar membrane, is negligible in the normal lung, it may be very severe in disease. The body attempts to compensate for this by vasoconstriction in hypoxic areas of lung, thus diverting blood from poorly ventilated or presumably damaged areas to those which are better ventilated, and this does give some improvement. However, if lung damage is widespread the pulmonary vasoconstriction produces pulmonary hypertension and this may lead to heart failure (**cor pulmonale**, p. 228; *see also* Chapter 3). Nevertheless, the VPR is the key factor controlling oxygenation of the blood, and no amount of increased ventilation or circulatory diversion can compensate for ventilation–perfusion mismatch in the diseased state: exercise limitation is inevitable.

The VPR is always grossly abnormal in **chronic obstructive pulmonary disease** (COPD, pp. 262–273), due to a combination of hypoventilation and a variable degree of diffusion limitation. Additionally, beta$_2$-bronchodilators tend to **reduce** the P_aO_2 by about 10% in some patients with COPD and asthma because they cause pulmonary vasodilatation and so increase blood flow to unventilated alveoli. However, the favourable action of bronchodilators in reducing airways resistance, and so increasing ventilation, outweighs this. Thus this adverse effect is negligible unless the patient is grossly hypoxaemic, when the additional oxygen deficit caused by the bronchodilator may be important.

Gas transfer

The transfer of gases across the alveolar membrane depends on the functional membrane area, the membrane thickness, the concentration gradient across the membrane, and the diffusion coefficient of the gas.

The **diffusion coefficient** of a gas is proportional to its solubility in extracellular fluid and inversely proportional to the square root of its molecular weight. Thus, carbon dioxide diffuses about 20 times as rapidly as oxygen, so its diffusion is not a limiting factor. Consequently, as ventilatory function deteriorates in COPD the P_aO_2 tends to fall before the P_aCO_2 rises.

The **functional membrane area** is the most important parameter controlling diffusion, and this is reduced in emphysema and by ventilation–perfusion abnormalities. The latter are also important in **concentration gradient** effects, because hypoventilation reduces the alveolar oxygen concentration. Diseases causing alveolar fibrosis or oedema produce a membrane which is up to five times thicker than normal and which interferes markedly with gas exchange, especially if the tissues become fibrosed.

The **transfer factor** is an overall measure of the effectiveness of diffusion, and is expressed as the rate of gas transfer per unit of partial pressure. The transfer factor is determined by taking a single breath of helium/air mixture containing a small amount of carbon monoxide, which is absent from normal blood, combines readily and completely with haemoglobin, and is easily measured: hence the term Tco (the old term, diffusing capacity, DLco, is now out of favour, because diffusion is only one aspect of gas transfer). The use of helium enables the alveolar volume to be determined. Tco is reduced in fibrosis, oedema, emphysema, pulmonary embolism, severe anaemia and in smokers, but is increased in polycythaemia, ventilation–perfusion remodelling and alveolar bleeding.

The overall effects of the ventilatory process

Table 5.3 Partial pressures of oxygen and carbon dioxide in the body

Partial pressures [a] Tissue	Oxygen	Carbon dioxide
Atmosphere	21.3	0.04
Alveoli	14.0	4.5
Blood capillaries		
Pulmonary		
• arteriolar	5.3	6.0
• venous		
Tissue	13.3	4.5
• arteriolar		
• venous		
Tissue cells	5.3	6.0

Transport mechanism	Oxygen (%)	Carbon dioxide (%)
Dissolved in plasma	3	7
HbO_2	97	–
HCO_3^-	–	70
HbNHCOOH	–	23

[a] kPa, approximate values only; 1 kPa = 7.5 mmHg.
HbO_2, oxygenated haemoglobin; HbNHCOOH, carbaminohaemoglobin.

are summarized in Table 5.3. There is a progressive fall in PO_2 from the alveoli to the tissue cells, and a converse increase in PCO_2. Under conditions of normal ventilation and blood flow, about 11 mmol/min of oxygen and 9 mmol/min of carbon dioxide are transported in and out of the body respectively, giving values for P_aO_2 of 10.6–13.3 kPa and for P_aCO_2 of 4.5–6.0 kPa.

Gas transport in blood

Table 5.3 also gives the relative proportions of oxygen and carbon dioxide which are transported by various mechanisms. Although most of the oxygen is carried by haemoglobin, that dissolved in the plasma may be important in patients in whom the oxygen-carrying capacity of the blood is significantly reduced, e.g. in

severe anaemia. Because haemoglobin is almost completely saturated under normal conditions, increasing the dissolved fraction may be the only way of increasing the oxygen content of the blood. This is one rationale for the use of hyperbaric (high-pressure) oxygen chambers.

The **oxygen saturation** of arterial blood (S_aO_2) is given by the expression:

$$S_aO_2 = \frac{O_2 \text{ combined with Hb}}{\text{Total } O_2 \text{ capacity of the blood}} \times 100\%$$

the denominator being the sum of the oxygen combined with Hb and the dissolved oxygen. This is an important parameter if a patient is anaemic. In this case **cyanosis**, due to the blue-purple colour of reduced haemoglobin, is an unreliable indicator of low oxygen saturation because its recognition varies with skin pigmentation, lighting, etc. and it is difficult to detect if the haemoglobin concentration is low. Hence the need to measure arterial blood gases, e.g. in a very severe asthma attack. Conversely, in the presence of polycythaemia cyanosis may be marked, resulting in the 'blue bloater' of COPD (p. 266).

Because of its high aqueous solubility, most of the carbon dioxide is carried in solution as bicarbonate, these two compounds forming an important pH buffering system. Haemoglobin is an important intermediary, picking up carbon dioxide in the tissues in exchange for oxygen.

Lung volumes and capacities

An idealized spirogram for a normal young adult male is shown in Fig. 5.6. This illustrates the trace obtained when the subject is initially breathing quietly at rest, and what happens when they then inhale and exhale maximally and as rapidly as possible. The **residual volume** cannot be used for ventilation but it plays an important part in buffering against the large swings that would occur in blood gas partial pressures if there were no gases in the lungs that could be exchanged with those in the blood at the end of expiration.

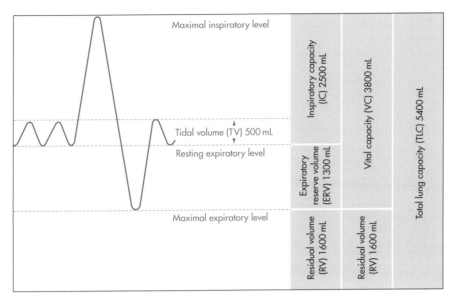

Figure 5.6   Lung volumes and capacities. Capacities are the sums of lung volumes. IC = TV + IRV; VC = TV + IRV + ERV; TLC = VC + RV.

Clinical aspects of respiratory disease

Classification

It will be obvious from the preceding discussion that the respiratory process can go wrong in numerous ways, and these are summarized in Table 5.4. There may be one of four basic problems:

1. Obstruction of gas flow in the airways.
2. Impaired alveolar diffusion.
3. A restricted thoracic capacity and expansibility.
4. Impaired ventilatory drive.

Obstructive defects (pp. 235–273) are the most common, and usually affect the smaller airways. They may be a consequence of bronchoconstriction, inflammation or excessive mucus production. However, **bronchiectasis** (chronic airways dilatation, usually resulting from infective damage, normally associated with massive sputum production: p. 272) affects the larger and medium-sized airways. Large airways may also be blocked by a foreign body: this may be inhaled food or, in children, almost any small toy or object, and is a medical emergency.

Chronic **diffusion defects**, in which there is impaired gas transfer across the alveolar membrane, usually result from a thickening of the respiratory membrane as a result of chronic inflammation leading to permanent fibrotic damage. However, in **pulmonary oedema**, e.g. following left ventricular failure, the accumulated fluid also acts as a physical barrier to prevent oxygen diffusion. An acute failure of pulmonary perfusion, or of the general circulation, e.g. due to myocardial infarction or shock, will also cause hypoxaemia similarly to a diffusion defect.

In **restrictive defects** (p. 273) there is an inability to expand the lungs adequately. Such defects may be caused by poor lung compliance, but are often due to problems outside the lungs. Thus pleural disease (fibrosis, effusion or adhesions) will limit expansion of the underlying lung. A similar effect results from a **pneumothorax**, because if gas leaks into the pleural space following rupture of peripheral lung tissue (e.g. due to emphysema, infection, trauma or surgery), a lung may collapse partially or completely. Provided that there is no serious underlying pathology the damaged area will heal, and fluid and gas will be reabsorbed fairly quickly by the pleural capillaries, thus restoring

Table 5.4   Types of respiratory disease

Type of defect	Pathological process	Some possible causes[a]
Obstructive	Obstruction or spasm of the airways	Asthma, chronic bronchitis, emphysema, bronchiectasis, carcinoma, cystic fibrosis, physical obstruction (e.g. food), severe chest trauma (e.g. crushing)
Diffusion	Alveolar damage	Hypersensitivity reactions (e.g. farmer's lung), emphysema, fibrosing alveolitis, iatrogenic (e.g. bleomycin, oxygen)
	Pulmonary oedema	Left ventricular failure, lymphatic obstruction, inhalation pneumonitis
	Acute circulatory failure	Pulmonary embolism, myocardial infarction, shock
Restrictive	Pulmonary fibrosis	Hypersensitivity reactions (e.g. farmer's lung), iatrogenic (e.g. bleomycin, chest radiotherapy), environmental (e.g. asbestosis, paraquat poisoning)
	Rigidity of chest wall or vertebral column	Obesity, ankylosing spondylitis, systemic sclerosis, sarcoidosis, congenital deformity, systemic lupus erythematosus, tuberculosis
	Inspiratory pain	Pleurisy, trauma
	Pneumothorax	Emphysema, pneumonia, trauma
Ventilatory	Nerve damage	Stroke, trauma or infection of brain or spinal cord, paralysis of respiratory muscles
	Depressed nervous transmission	Narcotics, psychotropic drugs

[a] A disease or condition may appear under more than one heading, e.g. emphysema causes both obstructive and diffusion defects, farmer's lung causes both diffusion and restrictive defects.

normality. Rib cage and spinal defects, e.g. due to congenital tuberculosis or ankylosing spondylitis (*see* Chapter 8, p. 503), also restrict lung expansion.

Ventilatory failure is the result of an inadequate ventilatory drive to the respiratory muscles or inability of these to respond. A primary loss of the central drive to breathe is rare except in:

- Head trauma.
- CNS disease and central depression by drugs, e.g. opioids, anaesthesia or trauma.
- Respiratory muscle damage due to disease, e.g. poliomyelitis, chest trauma.
- Neuromuscular damage, e.g. poliomyelitis, severe hypokalaemia.
- Severe airways obstruction causing cyanosis and carbon dioxide retention.
- Obesity, especially associated with rapid weight gain.

Clinical features

As in any other clinical situation an accurate history and examination are the essential first steps, and will often permit a reasonably confident diagnosis to be made before any investigations are carried out. The following symptoms and signs are characteristic of respiratory diseases.

Dyspnoea

This is a subjective, unpleasant sensation of breathlessness (**shortness of breath**, SOB) that probably results from an inappropriate effort of breathing. It does not correlate with blood P_aO_2. Objective signs, e.g. laboured breathing, rapid breathing (**tachypnoea**), breathing with pursed lips, hypoxaemia and hypercapnia, may also be present.

The time course for the development of breathlessness may help in diagnosis, e.g.

- Months to years: COPD, thyrotoxicosis.
- Weeks: anaemia, tumours.
- Hours to days: left ventricular failure (LVF), pneumonia.
- Minutes: acute severe asthma, major pulmonary embolism, pneumothorax.

Reduced exercise tolerance will initially present as **exertional dyspnoea** and should be defined quantitatively in terms of the patient's ability to walk on the flat or to climb stairs. However, there are many possible causes for dyspnoea apart from lung disease, e.g. cardiac disease, obesity, anaemia, anxiety and hyperthyroidism.

Orthopnoea is dyspnoea which occurs only when lying down, the symptom disappearing when the patient is erect. It may be of cardiac origin, and is consequent on the reduced gravitational load on the circulation when the patient lies down. The condition produces an increased venous return and **pulmonary congestion**, i.e. an excessive volume of blood in the lungs. Redistribution of fluid throughout the lungs also occurs. If there is severe airways obstruction, limitation of diaphragm movement when lying down will also produce dyspnoea, especially in the obese patient.

Pursed lip breathing occurs when lung compliance is increased by disease (e.g. emphysema) so that the airways have less support and an increased tendency to collapse on expiration. The patient then unwittingly breathes shallowly through partly closed lips to maintain a greater positive pressure than normal within the airways, thus keeping them open.

Breath sounds

Audible on examination
Wheezes (rhonchi) are sounds caused by gas flowing through airways narrowed by spasm or excessive secretions. This causes an obvious, more or less musical note which is usually **more marked on expiration** (see below). It is usually a symptom of obstruction but may be secondary to cardiovascular problems (so-called 'cardiac asthma').

Stridor is a harsher, **inspiratory** sound due to the obstruction of the larynx, trachea or other major airway.

Audible on auscultation
In the normal lung, respiration usually gives gentle, rustling sounds in the stethoscope. **Bronchial breathing** consists of higher-pitched sounds found on both inspiration and (more prolonged) expiration. **Crackles** (crepitations, 'creps'; râles) are fine crackling noises caused by the opening of blocked, small airways at the periphery of the lung. Coarse crackles are caused by gas bubbling through copious secretions in larger airways. A **friction rub** results from friction between inflamed pleural membranes or, similarly, to pericardial friction. Wheezes are also heard.

The complete absence of lung sounds is a very sinister sign that indicates an inability to move air in and out of the lung, e.g. in a very severe asthma attack or physical obstruction of a major airway.

Cough and sputum

Coughing is abnormal when it is persistent, or associated with pain or significant sputum production. It is usually due to minor infection. Although the nature of the cough may indicate the underlying pathology, e.g. the characteristic inspiratory 'whoop' of whooping cough or the softer, longer cough resulting from paralysis of the vocal chords, the associated features are usually more informative. A 'dry' cough (unproductive of sputum) may occur in asthma, early acute bronchitis or pneumonia. **Post-nasal drip**, the drainage of discharge from infected sinuses, etc. into the throat, also causes coughing.

A productive cough is one caused by the formation of sputum. **Mucoid sputum** (white or grey) is usually produced in chronic bronchitis, fibrosing alveolitis or asthma. **Purulent sputum** (green or yellow, containing pus) indicates infection that is often bacterial in nature.

Haemoptysis (coughing up of blood or blood streaked sputum) is an alarming symptom that is usually due to an acute lung infection, e.g. pneumonia or tuberculosis, or to an exacerbation of chronic bronchitis. It may also indicate the possibility of serious disease such as pulmonary oedema (producing pink, frothy sputum), bronchial carcinoma or pulmonary embolism.

Hyperinflation

Because expiration is more difficult than inspiration, severe obstructive airways disease leads to progressive **air trapping**, because not all of the inspired volume of gas in the lungs can be exhaled before the next inspiration occurs. The chest thus remains partially expanded at all times and, in extreme cases, this may eventually lead to a '**barrel chest**'. There will then often be abnormally large cavities (**bullae**) in the lung parenchyma which may be detectable by hyper-resonance on percussion. Hyperinflation tends to occur, together with pursed lip breathing.

Chest pain

Pain of respiratory origin may be due to **pleurisy** (pleural inflammation or infection), and a pneumothorax may give a similar sharp pain. Acute tracheitis or bronchitis and pulmonary emboli may also give pain, particularly if embolism causes infarction, but disease in the lung parenchyma is normally painless. Bronchial carcinoma may give only a vague, aching pain.

However, chest pain may also be due to trauma, cardiovascular or gastrointestinal conditions, bone tumours, herpes zoster, etc. Such pain may often be referred to the neck, back or abdomen because many major nerve tracts run in the mediastinum and may be affected secondarily. Thus, pain is a very non-specific diagnostic feature in most respiratory disease, even if linked to respiratory movements.

Finger clubbing

The cause of this sign (Fig. 5.7) is unknown, but it often indicates a serious chronic chest disease which produces chronic hypoxaemia, e.g. bronchial and other tumours, bronchiectasis, advanced tuberculosis, cystic fibrosis and lung abscesses. However, it may also be due to congenital heart disease or chronic gastrointestinal disease and may even occur as a familial trait.

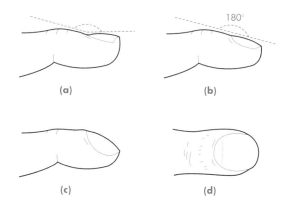

Figure 5.7   Finger clubbing. (a) Normal. (b) Early clubbing showing loss of the nail angle. (c) and (d) Late clubbing.

The early changes are subtle, there being the loss of the angle between the nail and the skin at its base. Eventually there is pronounced longitudinal curvature of the nail, softening of the nail bed and 'drum-stick' fingers.

Heart failure

Right ventricular failure (*see* Chapter 3, p. 75) secondary to lung disease is known as **cor pulmonale**. It is a consequence of **pulmonary hypertension** produced by:

- Alveolar and systemic hypoxia causing widespread pulmonary vasoconstriction and hypertrophy of pulmonary vascular smooth muscle.
- Distortion and fibrosis of the blood vessels.
- Destruction of blood vessels when alveoli are destroyed.
- Increased blood viscosity due to the polycythaemia resulting from chronic hypoxaemia.

The outstanding feature in these patients is fluid retention, with the usual symptoms of ankle oedema and progressive dyspnoea and exercise limitation. The increased afterload on the right ventricle, which has to work harder in order to perfuse the lungs, eventually leads to heart failure. However, in the early stages the heart may compensate for the failure by right ventricular dilatation (*see* Chapter 3, Fig. 3.12).

Investigation

Examination

From the above review of the clinical features the following are clearly relevant:

- Observation: pattern of respiration and cough, cyanosis, finger clubbing.
- Palpation: lymph nodes, diversion of the trachea (by a mass or pneumothorax), tenderness.
- Percussion: both sides are normally equally resonant. Hyper-resonance indicates a loss of tissue (a cavity) and dullness an area of consolidation (fluid).
- Auscultation (listening to breath sounds, etc.).
- Cardiovascular examination.

Imaging

A plain **chest X-ray** (CXR) is the most valuable adjunct to the history and examination. An erect postero-anterior (PA) view, i.e. the X-rays pass from front to back, is usually preferred. It shows the locations and sizes of the heart and other organs as well as lung tissue abnormalities. The lung fields should be evenly translucent and without shadowing, except in the hilar regions (where the main blood vessels and bronchi enter the lungs) and from the ribs (*see* Fig. 5.1). Excessive spacing between the ribs and a gap between the apex (bottom) of the heart and the left diaphragm indicate hyperinflation.

Complete collapse of a lung will cause a shift of the heart and other mediastinal structures into the area of collapse. Lesser degrees of collapse produce a well-defined shadow due to the increased density of the collapsed lung.

Ultrasound scanning has a limited role in investigating chest problems because currently it is possible only to visualize objects that are in contact with the chest wall with this technique. However, it is useful when guiding a needle biopsy for aspiration of an effusion.

Computed tomography (CT) and **magnetic resonance imaging** (MRI) are being used increasingly and provide valuable additional information. Both techniques permit accurate visualization of major organs and highlight the nature and extent of any abnormal or doubtful shadows in the CXR. Conventional CT scanning involves a high radiation dose, e.g. 40 to 250 times that of a normal CXR, but the advent of 'spiral' (rapid volumetric) scanning enables data to be obtained within seconds. This is less stressful to patients, reduces the X-ray dose and can provide dynamic information, e.g. visualization of pulmonary emboli by demonstrating obstruction to blood flow with injection of a venous contrast medium. MRI involves no radiation dose, and gives detailed images of the lung parenchyma; moreover, rapid acquisition scanning improves patient acceptability. Another technique, **magnetic resonance angiography** (MRA), may be used to visualize blood vessels, without having to inject contrast medium.

Fluoroscopy is an X-ray technique which is used to visualize dynamic events, e.g. the movements of organs, and is used only for specialized investigations. The use of image intensifiers and television-type display reduces the high radiation dose received formerly by radiologists, and has improved the utility of the technique.

Bronchoscopy and biopsy

Flexible **fibreoptic endoscopes** (*see* Chapter 6, Fig. 6.5) are indispensable for the direct observation of the airways and the biopsy of lesions located by imaging. Bronchial brushings and washings can also be taken for cytological and bacteriological examination. Modern bronchoscopes will reach nearly all parts of the lungs, especially in the upper lobes.

Most bronchoscopies are performed for the diagnosis of potential malignancy, infections and diffuse parenchymal disease, and to confirm uncertain diagnoses. Obstructing tumours may also be treated through the endoscope by diathermy or lasers if they are small enough. Older-type rigid bronchoscopes are still used for the removal of small inhaled foreign bodies from the trachea.

Superficial lesions and the pleura may be biopsied percutaneously using special needles, guided by X-ray or CT, and are less invasive. Open lung biopsy is done only when surgery is essential.

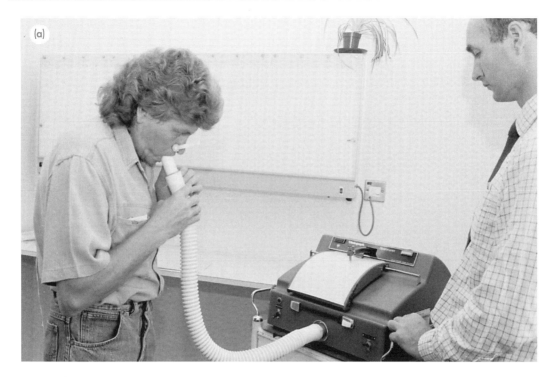

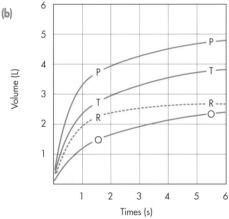

Figure 5.8   Pulmonary function testing with the Vitalograph respirometer. (a) Testing in progress, patient wearing a nose clip. (b) Traces obtained showing: O, typical obstructive pattern; T, improvement after a test dose of a beta$_2$-bronchodilator in an asthmatic patient (A), showing excellent reversibility; P, result after continuous bronchodilator prophylaxis in the same asthmatic patient; R, typical restrictive pattern (Patient B).

Patient[b]	Curve	FEV$_1$ (L)	FVC (L)	FEV$_1$/FVC (%)	Type of respiratory defect	Predicted normal values[a]		
						FEV$_1$ (L)	FVC (L)	FEV$_1$/FVC (%)
A	O	1.2	2.4	50	Obstructive,			
	T	2.3	3.8	61	becoming	4.2	5.2	81
	P	3.3	4.8	69	normal			
B	R	2.0	2.6	77	Restrictive	3.3	3.9	85

[a] FEV$_1$, forced expiratory volume in 1s; FVC, forced vital capacity; FEV$_1$/FVC, forced expiratory ratio.

[b] Patient A, asthma, male, 43 years of age, height 180 cm.

   Patient B, spinal deformity from childhood tuberculosis, female, 25 years of age, height 168 cm.

Lung function tests

These are used to determine the type of disease, its severity, and the response to therapy. **Ventilatory function** is assessed using a recording spirometer, such as the Vitalograph (Fig. 5.8(a)) or the Microflow, which both work on a simple bellows principle. The patient inspires maximally and then blows as hard and as fast as possible into the mouthpiece, producing a recording similar to that shown in Fig. 5.8(b). Several parameters can be derived from the curve, the most useful being the **forced vital capacity** (FVC), the maximum volume of gas which can be blown out, and the **forced expiratory volume**, usually recorded as the volume forced out in 1 second (FEV$_1$). The predicted values of these for a normal subject can be estimated from nomograms which relate them to age, height and sex. These parameters are relatively independent of the force applied during expiration.

Generally, a fit young adult will have an FVC of 4–5 L and the FEV$_1$ will be at least 75% of this, i.e. the **forced expiratory ratio** (FEV$_1$/FVC) exceeds 0.75, indicating efficient ventilation. Obstruction of the airways leads to a low FVC and to forced expiratory ratios of <0.65 (curve O, Fig. 5.8(b); in severe disease it may be as low as 0.3). Restrictive patterns of disease reduce both the FEV$_1$ and the FVC similarly, so that the ratio is normal (curve R, Fig. 5.8(b); Table 5.5). Forced expiratory ratios of about 0.6 lead to dyspnoea only on severe exertion, at 0.5 there will be significant exercise limitation, and below 0.3 there is likely to be chronic disability, orthopnoea, hypercapnia and frequent invalidism.

Figure 5.8(b) shows that the spirometer can also be used for a diagnostic trial of drugs and to monitor the benefits of therapy objectively. If an obstructive pattern is seen, the patient inhales a dose of a bronchodilator and repeats the test

Table 5.5 Changes in some common pulmonary function parameters and normal values[a] in respiratory diseases of moderate severity

Parameter	Values or changes[b]			
	Asthma	Chronic bronchitis	Emphysema	Restrictive lung disease
FVC	N/[↓]	N/[↓]	N/[↓]	50–60% of normal
FEV$_1$/FVC (%)	40–60	40–60	40–60	N/[↑]
Improvement with bronchodilator (%) (i.e. reversibility)	10–50	0–20	0–10	Nil
RV (% of normal)	150	150	150	75
PEF	↓/↓↓	↓/↓↓	↓/↓↓	N
TLC	N/↑	N/↑	↑	↓
Gas transfer	N	N/↓	50% of N	N/↓
P$_a$O$_2$	N/↓	↓/↓↓	[↓]	↓ (E)
P$_a$CO$_2$	N/[↑]	↑	N/[↑]	N
Lung compliance	N	N/↓	N/↑	N/↓
Dyspnoea	+/++	+/++	+/++	++

[a] Approximate normal values for adults aged 30 years; heights: males, 175 cm; females, 165 cm:

FVC (L): M, 4.8; F, 3.51;

FEV$_1$ (L): M, 4.0; F, 3.1;

FEV$_1$/FVC (%): M, 83; F, 89;

RV/TLC (%): M, 29.2; F, 26.2.

[b] Values determined at rest, unless otherwise stated: many asthma patients appear virtually normal (N) between attacks; (E), patient exercised; [ ], slight effect; +/++, present/strongly present; FVC, forced vital capacity; FEV$_1$ forced expiratory volume in 1 s; FEV/FVC, forced expiratory ratio; RV, residual volume; PEF peak expiratory flow; TLC, total lung capacity; P$_a$O$_2$, P$_a$CO$_2$, arterial partial pressures of oxygen and carbon dioxide.

after 20–30 min. Good to moderate **reversibility** (≥15% improvement) is observed in asthmatics (e.g. curve T) in whom there may be a return to a near-normal trace (curve P). There may be some reversibility in chronic bronchitics, but this rarely exceeds 5%.

The **flow–volume loop** is obtained by asking the patient to inspire maximally and to blow into the instrument as hard as possible to maximal expiration and then to inhale again to total lung capacity. This is a sensitive test which will discriminate between asthma and other types of airways obstruction (Fig. 5.9).

The **peak expiratory flow** (PEF), the maximum expiratory flow rate in L/min measured over the first 10 msec of expiration, may be determined directly from the flow–volume loop (Fig. 5.9) or calculated from the initial slope of the spirometer curve shown in Fig. 5.8(b). However, PEF is much more easily determined using a peak flow meter or gauge (Fig. 5.10), though this measures flow over only the first 2 msec of forced expiration. A nomogram, a simple 'slide rule' or a chart (Fig. 5.11) is used to predict normal values. The PEF is a simple and sensitive indicator of the presence and severity of airways obstruction, so the determination is popular in chest clinics as a simple, rapid, cheap diagnostic and monitoring tool. However, the accuracy of the test depends on the instrument used and on the patient making a maximal inspiration and applying maximal force during expiration, whereas the FEV_1 is less energy-dependent. The PEF is not diagnostically reliable because it will not distinguish between the different types of airways obstruction, unlike the flow–volume loop.

Peak flow gauges are particularly useful for observing rapid changes and monitoring the severity of disease and the effects of medication, especially in asthma. They are invaluable for the routine home self-monitoring of patients with significant asthma, when the absolute accuracy of the instrument is not important because it will still show changes in lung function. If a diary is kept, patients can detect the warning signs of an impending, possibly severe, attack and take appropriate therapeutic measures (p. 250). However, one study has shown that a high proportion of patient diaries are unreliable. Furthermore, PEF measurements are less useful in those with chronic asthma (p. 246) or **COPD** (p. 262) where there is significant fixed (irreversible) airways obstruction.

Other tests may be performed in specialist centres, e.g. determination of compliance, TCO, ventilation/perfusion estimates and lung volumes and capacities.

Blood gases

Measurements of P_aO_2, S_aO_2, P_aCO_2 and pH, done on a sample of arterial blood taken from the radial artery or the ear lobe, provide valuable information on the levels of hypoxaemia and hypercapnia, the response to oxygen and other therapy, the adequacy of ventilation, and the nature and severity of any metabolic disturbance. They are mandatory in hospital for the management of seriously ill patients.

Exercise testing

Preferably, a treadmill or cycle ergometer is used because performance can be related directly to predetermined levels of effort. The speed, slope or resistance is increased progressively until the patient stops, due to breathlessness, chest pain, etc., or reaches their predetermined safe heart rate. The ventilation rates, composition of the expired gas mixture and oxygen saturation of the blood are measured and an ECG is recorded (*see* Chapter 3, p. 72). These enable the severity of lung disease to be determined, abnormalities of ventilation or oxygen uptake to be assessed, and pulmonary or cardiac causes of disability to be distinguished.

However, simple walking tests are often done. The patient is asked to walk up and down a corridor for 2, 6 or 12 min, preferably with a pulse oximeter attached to a finger or earlobe. Oxygen saturation falls if there is ventilation–perfusion mismatch, e.g. in obstructive lung disease.

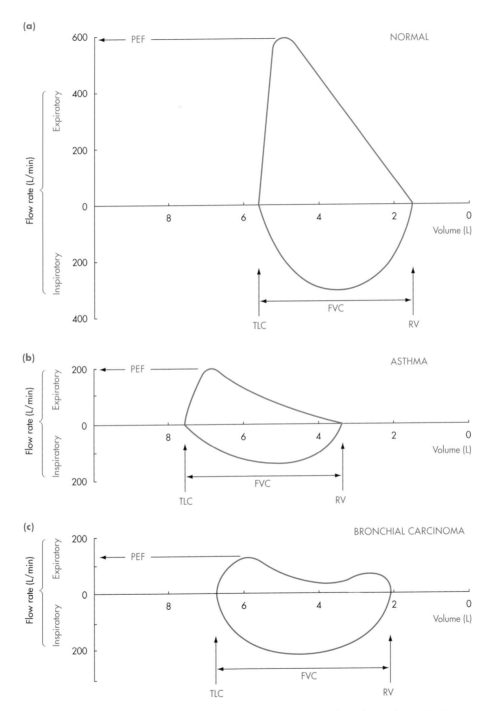

Figure 5.9   Flow–volume loops in obstructive respiratory diseases. (a) Normal. (b) Asthma. (c) Bronchial carcinoma. FVC, forced vital capacity; PEF, peak expiratory flow rate; RV, residual volume; TLC, total lung capacity.

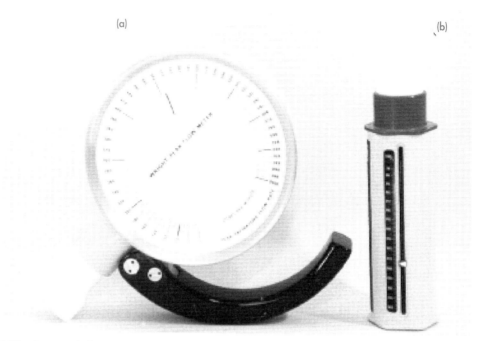

Figure 5.10   Some peak flow meters. (a) Type commonly used in hospitals. (b) Type suitable for patient self-monitoring (prescribable in the UK under the NHS).

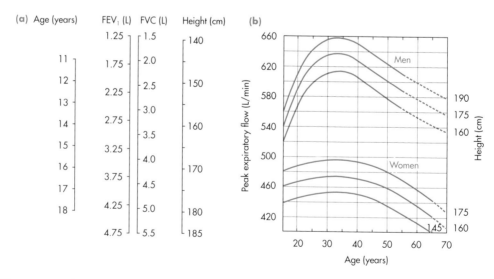

Figure 5.11   Some predictive charts for pulmonary function tests. (a) Nomogram for forced vital capacity (FVC) and forced expiratory volume in 1 sec (FEV$_1$); both sexes, 5–18 years. (b) Partial relationship for the prediction of normal peak expiratory flow in adults. Note that the PEF for adult males is higher than that for females of the same age and height and that ventilatory function peaks at 30–35 years, rather different from that for most physical attributes. (Reproduced with permission of Vitalograph Ltd.)

Obstructive pulmonary disease

Asthma

Definition

No entirely satisfactory definition exists, though the following covers most patients:

> Attacks of breathlessness, wheezing and chest tightness, usually reversible spontaneously or on treatment, characterized by wide variations in intrapulmonary airways resistance over short periods of time. The attacks are associated with airways inflammation and increased bronchial hyper-reactivity to a variety of stimuli.

This rather vague clinical definition reflects our lack of knowledge about the precise nature of the disease. This is 'bronchial asthma': the term 'cardiac asthma' has been used to denote pulmonary oedema consequent on left ventricular failure (*see* Chapter 3, p. 80) but this is now obsolete and so 'asthma' now invariably means 'bronchial asthma'.

Epidemiology and natural history

The overall prevalence of asthma in the West is about 5% and this has increased steadily in the past 20 years, with about 10–15% of the 10- to 20-year age group being affected. Indeed, the consulting rate for asthma doubled in the period 1971/2 to 1981/2. Some of this increase may be due to increased awareness of the disease and expectations of effective treatment and some to improved diagnosis, but it is considered to reflect a real change. Asthma is the most common chronic disease in the UK and the principal cause of childhood morbidity. The prevalence in some developing countries (e.g. South America, Fiji) appears to be similar, but is much less in some African and Indian countries.

The incidence peaks at age 10–12 years (some 15–25% of children wheeze annually), with a secondary peak at about 65 years (6%). These two peaks correspond to the two main clinical types of disease (Table 5.6). If triggered by iden-

tifiable external allergens in atopic individuals the condition is called **extrinsic** or **episodic asthma**. In other patients the agents, circumstances or conditions responsible for attacks are unknown or poorly defined. This latter form tends to be chronic, or becomes so after a time: this is **intrinsic** or **cryptogenic asthma**. Extrinsic asthma tends to occur in the younger age group and is usually relatively mild. In contrast, the intrinsic asthmatic is usually older, with more persistent disease. However, this distinction is of only limited value because about 30% of patients have mixed-type disease. On average, each doctor in the UK will have about 125 asthma patients, and a community pharmacy can expect to see about twice this number.

Table 5.6   The two clinical types of asthma

Feature	Episodic (extrinsic)	Chronic (intrinsic)
Proportion (%)[a]	20	50
Age of onset	Childhood	Usually adults
Atopic patient	Yes: family history common[b]	No
Known allergens or precipitating factors	Yes	None or URTI Often sensitive to aspirin
Skin tests	Positive	Negative
Severity	Usually episodic Often mild	Often chronic May be severe
Treatment	Effective	Moderately effective, oral corticosteroids may be required

[a] 30% have mixed type disease.
[b] There is often a personal or family history of eczema and allergic rhintis.
URTI, upper respiratory tract infection.

Up to 80% of children suffer episodic symptoms of wheezing, usually associated with respiratory infections, but most of these are not regarded as asthmatics. Asthma is the most common chronic childhood disease causing absence from school. Boys are more likely to develop asthma than girls, the relative prevalence before puberty being M : F ≥2 : 1). In many children, the frequency and severity of attacks declines from the age of 6–8 years, with at least 30% growing out of the condition by puberty, at which point the sex prevalence is about equal. However, a tendency to **bronchial hyper-reactivity** may persist throughout life, with a highly variable frequency of attacks or chronic wheeziness. Above the age of 20 years, more women are affected; the M : F ratio of incidence being about 1 : 1.5.

Interestingly, a high salt intake has been shown to increase bronchial hyper-responsiveness in men, but not in women. Further, a higher than normal dietary intake of magnesium has been shown to improve the FEV_1 and to reduce hyper-reactivity and wheezing. Clearly, the role of diet needs to be explored more fully.

The increasing prevalence of asthma points to the probable importance of environmental agents as triggers for the initiation of the disease in genetically predisposed individuals, but evidence for this is equivocal. In the UK, a recent study found little urban–rural or geographical variation in prevalence. The prevalence in the unpolluted Scottish highlands was found to be similar to that in nearby urbanized areas. However, studies in the USA have implicated outdoor, and especially indoor, air contaminants as important risk factors for the development of childhood asthma and as determinants of severity. One possible cause of this discrepancy may be the larger number of centrally heated, air-conditioned homes in the USA with limited fresh air exchange – conditions that favour the persistence of dust mite, animal and other airborne allergens and irritants.

The indicators of a poorer prognosis are:

- Severe or early onset.
- Persistent attacks.
- An atopic patient.
- A family history of atopy.
- Female sex.

Asthma accounts for about 1900 deaths annually in the UK, and many of these are the result of under-diagnosis and under-treatment. A 1998 study of 12- to 14-year-olds found that 4% had been diagnosed as asthmatic but were poorly controlled, and a further 1–3.4% had moderate to severe symptoms but were undiagnosed and untreated. Also patients may not appreciate the severity of an attack. The British Thoracic Society (BTS) surveyed 90 asthma deaths in North-West England some years ago and found that only 36 of the patients had been sufficiently alarmed to see their doctors, and of those only nine were then managed appropriately, though unsuccessfully. All of these factors are theoretically preventable. Although the situation has improved there is still some way to go before preventable deaths are reduced to an acceptable level.

Pathophysiology

The underlying problem is one of intense **airways inflammation**, leading to **bronchial hyper-reactivity**. Inflammation is present even when patients are asymptomatic. Everyone's airways will become constricted if exposed to a sufficient dose of a bronchoconstrictor, e.g. histamine or methacholine. Following viral respiratory tract infection the airways of non-asthmatics will be more sensitive than usual for up to 6 weeks as a result of mucosal damage and the exposure of receptors for pharmacological mediators (e.g. histamine, kinins, leukotrienes, platelet activating factor (PAF); *see* Chapter 2). Asthmatics may be up to 100 times more sensitive than normal subjects: atopic individuals suffering from hayfever but not asthma form an intermediate group.

The precise cause of this hyper-reactivity is unknown, though a number of putative pharmacological mediators have been identified and we know of many factors which may precipitate attacks (Tables 5.7 and 5.8; Fig. 5.12). Although some patients are sensitive to only a single trigger factor, most are sensitive to several, so attacks may be due to the combined effects of two or more of these. Inflammation is clearly the single most significant factor. In an acute attack, the epithelium is intensely infiltrated with eosinophils, causing eosinophil products (e.g.

Table 5.7   Some substances and conditions that may precipitate asthmatic attacks

Environmental and medical factors

Allergens	Pollens (especially grasses), mould spores, animal fur and dander, house dust mite (*Dermatophagoides pteronyssimus*), proteolytic enzymes (biological detergents)
Foods	Milk, eggs, nuts, alcoholic drinks, tartrazine colorant, sulphur dioxide preservative
Non-specific irritants	Dusts, cigarette smoke, atmospheric pollutants (especially sulphur dioxide)
Exercise	
Medical conditions	Pregnancy, menstruation, respiratory infections (especially viruses), thyrotoxicosis, levothyroxine (thyroxine) therapy, reflux oesophagitis
Medicines	*See* Table 5.8

Occupational causes[a]

Metal salts (platinum, chromium, nickel); laboratory animals and insects; plastics (epoxy resins, isocyanates, PVC); microorganisms (fermentation plants, humidifiers and air-conditioning plants, mushrooms); pharmaceuticals (antibiotics, acacia gum, ethylenediamine, formaldehyde, animal products); colophony fumes (soldering fluxes); proteolytic enzymes; dyes and hairdressing solutions; fabrics (silk); plant materials (pollens, coffee beans, tobacco, tea, wood, dust, cotton, flour and grain dusts)

[a] These may be legally recognized grounds for industrial injury compensation.

Table 5.8   Some drugs and medicines that may provoke asthmatic attacks

General drugs

Antimicrobials: cefaloridine, erythromycin, griseofulvin, nitrofurantoin, penicillins, streptomycin, tetracyclines
Beta-blockers, non-steroidal anti-inflammatory drugs, sulfasalazine, carbamazepine, iodine-based contrast media, dextrans, pituitary snuff, preservatives and dyes used in formulation

Drugs and devices used in asthma treatment

Ipratropium bromide, methylxanthines, hydrocortisone
Dry powder inhalers, aerosol propellants, nebulized hypotonic solutions

proteins, neurotoxins) to be released, and these damage the epithelium.

Other inflammatory cells (mast cells, basophils, etc.) also accumulate and release a large variety of inflammatory mediators, e.g. histamine, leukotrienes, prostaglandins, thromboxanes and PAF. These cause bronchiolar smooth muscle contraction and marked oedema of the bronchial mucosa, epithelial shedding and receptor exposure. The extent of the damage produced is reflected in the degree of airways hyper-responsiveness produced. Lymphocytes and macrophages are also abundant but less so than eosinophils. Goblet cell hyperplasia causes hypersecretion of mucus, which may be abnormally viscous and may plug the smallest airways.

The initial step in this inflammatory process is believed to be T cell activation. Lymphokines are produced which amplify the immune response, notably by the production of IgE antibodies and their induction of allergic reactions. Allergic mechanisms are especially important in episodic asthma.

Bronchoconstriction may also be mediated by cholinergic action via the vagus nerve. Although there is no adrenergic innervation of the airways, alpha- and beta-receptors are present and are targets for bronchodilating drugs.

About 80% of asthmatics suffer **nocturnal attacks**, described as 'morning dipping' (see below and Fig. 5.13), during which the peak flow

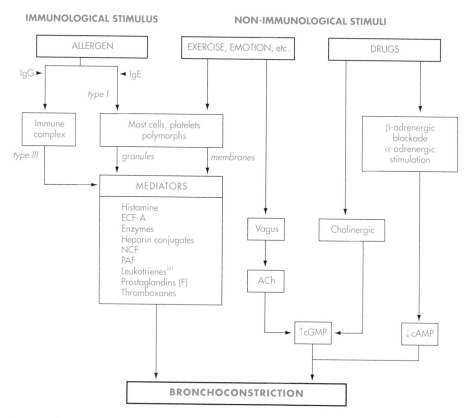

Figure 5.12 Some factors involved in producing bronchoconstriction. [a] Leukotrienes $C_4 + D_4 + E_4$ used to be known as 'slow reacting substance of anaphylaxis' (SRS-A). Reaction types I and III, Coombs and Gell classification (*see* Chapter 2, p. 29). ACh, acetylcholine; cAMP, cGMP, cyclic adenosine and guanosine monophosphates; ECF-A, eosinophil chemotactic factor A; NCF, neutrophil chemotactic factor; PAF, platelet activating factor; ↑, ↓, increased or decreased level.

may fall by as much as 50%. This marked diurnal variation in respiratory function is much greater than is seen in normal subjects, in whom nocturnal falls are about 8%. The tendency to nocturnal attacks is exacerbated by allergen exposure, especially following a severe attack, when patients are particularly vulnerable. It is tempting to associate this with the nadir of adrenal cortical activity, which occurs at a similar time, though evidence for this is lacking. The principal factor appears to be the physiological changes which occur during sleep, e.g. increased vagal (cholinergic) activity and reduced mucociliary clearance. Airways cooling during the night may also make a small, though significant, contribution, so it is reasonable to counsel patients not to sleep in cold rooms.

Although it has been suggested that a fish oil diet may be beneficial by promoting the forma-

tion of 5-series leukotrienes as opposed to the 4-series derived from arachidonic acid (*see* Chapter 8, Fig. 8.9), available data indicate that they are not clinically beneficial and may even be harmful.

Exercise-induced asthma occurs in many patients, especially the young. The attack comes on after a short bout of vigorous exercise or during a prolonged period, e.g. a football match, and may be the only symptom of asthma. The trigger seems to be the excessive cooling and drying of the airways epithelium by the air flow, because inhalation of cold, dry air can also provoke attacks, whereas swimming is the exercise least likely to do so.

The complexity of the mechanisms and mediators which appear to underlie asthma (*see* Fig. 5.12) may reflect our limited understanding of the pathological processes concerned. However, these uncertainties may be resolved within the

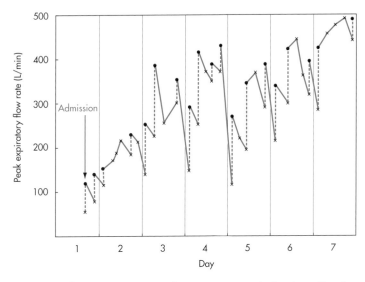

Figure 5.13 Peak flow chart of a patient recovering from a severe attack of asthma. The chart shows morning dipping and considerable variability imposed on a pattern of underlying improvement towards normality. ×, readings immediately before medication; •, readings 15 min after inhaling a beta$_2$-bronchodilator.

next 10 years by the application of new techniques from the rapidly expanding fields of genetics, immunology and molecular biology.

Occupational asthma is estimated to cause 5–10% of cases in adults (aged 20–44 years) in industrialized countries, notably cleaners, spray and other painters, and plastics workers. Agricultural workers also have a high risk but it is unclear how much of this is due to modern farm chemicals. A partial listing of possible agents is given in Table 5.7.

Clinical features

The classic symptoms of asthma following exposure to an identified trigger are attacks of breathlessness, wheezing and cough which commence within 15 min. Depending on the severity of the attack, peak flow may fall to 25–75% of those recorded between attacks, and usually recover over a period of 60–90 min without treatment (Fig. 5.14), but more promptly if a bronchodilator is used. Between attacks, patients may have an apparently normal respiratory function.

However, this pattern is shown in only about that 20% of patients showing an immediate allergic type (Type I) hypersensitivity reaction

(*see* Chapter 2). About 50% of asthmatics experience delayed attacks (see below) and a further 30% suffer both immediate and delayed attacks.

Dyspnoea in asthmatics is worse in the early hours of the morning, whether they experience acute severe nocturnal attacks or not, and most asthma deaths occur at night or in the early morning.

In a severe attack there will be hyperventilation and hyperinflation, to the extent that patients are incapable of speaking in complete sentences, with prolonged expiration and the use of the accessory muscles of respiration. Peak flow may fall below 100 L/min. Patients are very anxious, the heart rate may exceed 120 per min, and there may be palpable pulsus paradoxus (p. 240) and peripheral cyanosis. A 'quiet chest' on auscultation, indicating very poor air flow, also indicates a severe attack.

Many patients experience a variety of non-respiratory symptoms before an attack:

- Mild to moderate **chest pain** (about 75%), the severity being unrelated to asthma severity. The pain worsens on coughing, deep inspiration and most changes in position, but 65% obtain relief by sitting erect. This may result in abortive investigations for cardiac problems or pulmonary embolism (p. 274).

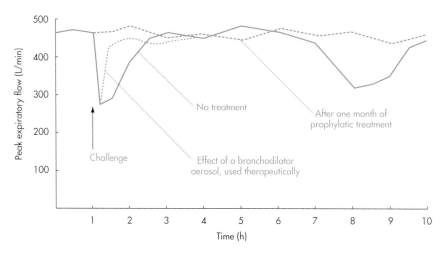

Figure 5.14 Peak flow chart of an asthmatic patient following an allergic challenge showing the effects of therapeutic and prophylactic treatment on the early and late reactions.

- Other symptoms are: nose or throat irritation, sleepiness, dry mouth, thirst, urinary frequency, flushing, irritability, depression.

Diagnosis

This is based on the history, examination and the investigations outlined below. It must be remembered that patients with episodic asthma may appear completely normal between attacks unless they have chronic symptoms or provocation testing is used.

Acute attacks

The following features may be found:

- Forced expiratory ratio <0.65. A spirogram has the general appearance of that in Fig. 5.15(b).
- PEF reduced to 80% of the predicted normal value or less.
- Flow–volume loop showing air trapping with increased TLC and RV (Fig. 5.9).
- Blood gases: P_aO_2 is reduced, but hypercapnia occurs only in severe attacks and is a serious sign.
- White blood cells: eosinophils $>0.5 \times 10^9$/L in blood in extrinsic asthma and they may also be present in sputum.

- Reversibility with an inhaled beta-agonist: a 15% increase (or more) in FEV_1 or PEF is conclusive; lesser degrees of reversibility do not distinguish between asthma and chronic bronchitis. In very severe attacks, or in chronic asthma, this reversibility may not be seen, because the airways become unresponsive.

Severe attacks

Retention of carbon dioxide in a very severe attack may be indicated by drowsiness, sweating and cyanosis, and a high-volume, bounding pulse. Central cyanosis is a serious sign but its absence does not preclude a severe attack.

Pulsus paradoxus is a sign of left ventricular failure and may be present in a severe attack. This is a pulse which decreases markedly in pressure during inspiration. It is not peculiar to asthma, because it also occurs in cardiovascular disease, e.g. constrictive pericarditis. A difference in pulse pressure between inspiration and expiration greater than 5–10 mmHg is abnormal. In severe asthma there may be a difference of 20–40 mmHg between weak and strong beats and, if present, the magnitude of the difference may be used to assess the severity of an attack and the patient's progress.

Other features have been described on pp. 246–248.

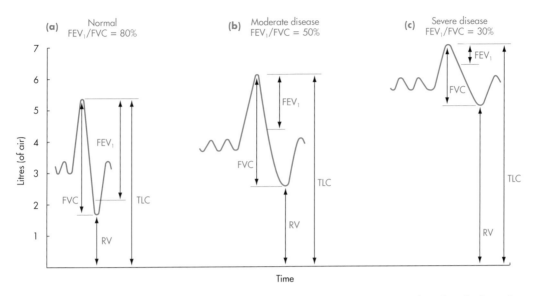

Figure 5.15 Spirograms in normal subjects and in obstructive lung disease. Expiration is slowed markedly in disease. The increase in TLC is due entirely to increased RV (unusable), the result of air trapping and, possibly, emphysema. FVC, forced vital capacity; FEV_1, forced expiratory volume in 1 sec; FEV_1/FVC, forced expiratory ratio; RV, residual volume; TLC, total lung capacity.

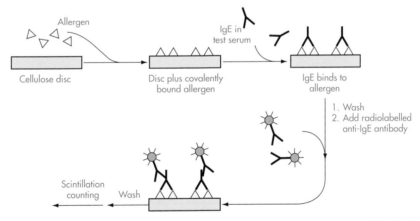

Figure 5.16 Radioallergosorbent test (RAST) procedure. IgE, immunoglobulin E (reaginic antibody). The final radioactivity on the disc is proportional to the amount of radiolabelled anti-IgE antibody which is bound to the disc by IgE bound from the test serum, i.e. the serum IgE level. The test is very sensitive because the disc carries large amounts of allergen.

Other investigations

IgE blood levels may be raised indicating atopic reactivity and are determined by the radioallergosorbent test (RAST) procedure (Fig. 5.16).

The aetiology may be ascertained by prick testing with allergens as a guide to allergen avoidance, though it may be impracticable to avoid allergens, especially if patients react to several simultaneously. However, negative skin tests may indicate an alternative diagnosis. **Bronchial challenge** by inhaling suspected allergen aerosols may be conclusive, but is hazardous and should not be attempted unless full resources for resuscitation are immediately available.

Exercise stress testing may also be helpful, especially in children, to assess the degree of exercise limitation and the role of exercise in inducing attacks.

Diagnostic problems

The following features may cause difficulties:

- Dry cough, sometimes with the production of small amounts of very viscid sputum. Cough, particularly troublesome at night, may be the only presenting symptom, especially in young children.
- Many infants have attacks of wheezing, possibly because they have rather small airways owing to maternal smoking during pregnancy, but only about one-third of these go on to develop asthma. Diagnosis in very young children is clearly difficult but relief following a trial of drugs (e.g. the inhalation of nebulized ipratropium or a beta-agonist bronchodilator, held near the nose, or an oral dose of a theophylline product) may be diagnostic. The likelihood of asthma is increased if wheezing is unrelated to respiratory infection or there is a family history of atopy (asthma, eczema, hayfever).
- Delayed attacks which occur some 6–8 h after provocation (Fig. 5.14) and recover slowly over a period of hours. These are associated with increased bronchial hyper-reactivity and are caused by an inflammatory (Type 3) hypersensitivity reaction (see Chapter 2).
- Recurrent 'chest colds' or 'wheezy bronchitis' in children, and sometimes adults, may be due to undiagnosed asthma. A proportion of patients eventually diagnosed as asthmatics have had repeated visits to their doctors with respiratory complaints (the 'wheezy baby' syndrome) for a year or more.
- Persistent airflow obstruction in an older patient with a limited degree of reversibility may be due to asthma, chronic bronchitis or emphysema. It may be impossible (and unnecessary) to distinguish between these because they may coexist: what counts is the extent to which treatment is effective.
- Paroxysmal nocturnal dyspnoea (PND; *see* Chapter 3, p. 81) may mimic nocturnal asthma, but is due to left ventricular failure ('cardiac asthma'). A therapeutic trial of a bronchodilator, with or without cortico-steroids, will distinguish between these conditions, because asthma will be relieved but not PND. Moreover, pulmonary oedema will usually show characteristic X-ray, ECG and clinical signs, e.g. a raised venous pressure and the presence of a third heart sound.
- Some undiagnosed asthmatics present for the first time with cor pulmonale (p. 228).
- Recurrent respiratory tract infections may cause difficulty. However, there will not be significant airflow obstruction or diurnal variation in PEF between infections.
- Large airways obstruction (outside the lungs) will usually be persistent, show inspiratory stridor rather than expiratory wheeze, and give a characteristic flow–volume loop (*see* Fig. 5.9).
- Delayed attacks (see above and p. 239), apparently unrelated to allergen exposure.

Management

Aims

The aims of management are:

- To control symptoms, minimize anxiety and permit as normal a life as possible.
- To educate the patient about the disease and its treatment.
- To identify triggers, thus minimizing morbidity and preventing death.

General measures

General management measures include:

- **Environmental control**, as far as is possible, by:
  - Removing pets, using non-allergenic bed clothing, etc. and minimizing house dust; these measures are particularly important in childhood asthma. However, it is not possible or practicable to eliminate all environmental allergens, e.g. normal vacuum cleaning does not significantly reduce the concentration of house dust mite allergens in the atmosphere, though cleaners with high-efficiency particulate air (HEPA) filtered output are now available and may help.

– **Stopping smoking** in both patients and their families.
* **Reduce stress** by effective treatment and educating patients about their disease.
* **Control infections** promptly.
* **Physiotherapy**, especially supervised swimming, may be helpful in developing respiratory function: the humid atmosphere of a swimming bath helps to avoid exercise-induced attacks.
* **Patient counselling** has a crucial role. There are repeated reports that patients are confused about their medication and its proper use. Patients (and their families, teachers, employers, etc.) need to understand the nature of the disease and how to prevent exacerbations and manage them effectively if they occur. Pharmacists can and should play an important part in this process: they understand the drugs and products and are readily accessible to patients. Active pharmacist counselling has been shown to reduce markedly both morbidity and the demands made on the community and hospital medical services. Additionally, there are the substantial benefits of increased patient well-being, less time off work or school and the satisfaction of patients being in control of their disease, rather than vice versa. Further, if patients are properly counselled and keep a diary, they can detect the first signs of deterioration in their condition (increasing dyspnoea, declining PEF, increasing medicines usage) and can adjust their medication to control the problem immediately, before seeing their doctor. Patients are reported as having a different perception of well-being from health professionals. Whereas patients see good disease control as freedom from constraints on activity, professionals use objective measures, e.g. absence of symptoms, low (or no) medicines usage. This gap can be closed by effective counselling, with improvement in patients' satisfaction with treatment.

Pharmacotherapy: general aspects

Drug treatment is often thought of in terms of either prophylaxis or the relief of symptoms. In asthma, both approaches are commonly used concurrently, and combination therapy is normal.

General strategy

A general approach to the control of the two cardinal features of asthma, airways inflammation and bronchoconstriction, is outlined in Table 5.9.

A stepwise addition of medication is used after diagnosis, starting with the occasional use of an inhaled, selective, short-acting beta$_2$-agonist bronchodilator for mild, infrequent attacks and often proceeding to this being used regularly in association with an inhaled steroid at appropriate dosage.

However, if attacks are frequent, or moderate to severe, it is preferable to gain control of symptoms promptly with greater initial intervention and to 'step down' treatment once this has been achieved. Control is usually gained with anti-inflammatory agents, usually low-dose or high-dose inhaled corticosteroids, plus a long-acting beta$_2$-agonist bronchodilator. A short-acting beta-agonist should also be available for rescue treatment (Tables 5.10 and 5.11). Other drugs may be introduced at any stage as the patient's condition and progress dictate.

All changes of treatment should be validated by careful monitoring of PEF and medicines usage, with ample time for prophylactic medication to take full effect (see below). Inhaled corticosteroids, bronchodilators and sodium cromoglicate (cromolyn sodium) (or nedocromil sodium for adults), used singly or in combination, will give excellent, safe control in most patients. Sedatives must never be used, because they may further depress an already compromised respiratory function.

The British Thoracic Society has published consensus guidelines for the management of adult and childhood asthma, and these are illustrated in part in Tables 5.10 and 5.11.

More detailed information on the drugs and their delivery systems are given below, but some general points are now discussed.

Treatment in an acute attack

This is designed to promote recovery and prevent deterioration to the point when hospital treatment becomes necessary.

Table 5.9　General approach to the treatment of target features in asthma

Target feature	Therapeutic aim	Drugs used	
		Class	Examples[a]
Inflammation and bronchial hyper-reactivity	Reduce • eosinophil recruitment and activation • lymphocyte activity • toxicity to epithelial cells	Corticosteroids	Beclometasone Budesonide Prednisolone
	• mast cell etc. degranulation	Inhibitors of mediator release	Sodium cromoglicate?[b] Nedocromil sodium? Theophylline? Selective beta$_2$-agonist
Broncho-constriction	Bronchodilatation: • increase sympathomimetic activity	Selective beta$_2$-agonist	Salbutamol, terbutaline, fenoterol, reproterol, tulobuterol Long-acting: bambuterol, eformoterol,[c] salmeterol
	• block parasympathetic activity • increase cAMP levels in bronchiolar muscle cells?	Antimuscarinic Phosphodiesterase inhibitor	Ipratropium Aminophylline? Theophylline? Sodium cromoglicate?[b]

[a] Some drugs fall into more than one class. Their precise modes of action may be unknown: ? = possible or secondary action.

[b] Cromolyn sodium.

[c] Formoterol.

cAMP, cyclic adenosine monophosphate.

Occasional attacks in an adult can be treated with an inhaled selective **beta$_2$-agonist bronchodilator** (p. 251). If a consistent trigger can be identified (e.g. sport, infection, drugs, visits to a home having a pet), prior use of a short-acting bronchodilator inhaler or regular use of a **corticosteroid** inhaler may prevent attacks (Table 5.10, Step 2). If there are **more frequent or severe episodes**, routine prophylactic treatment is indicated. This may start with a beta$_2$-bronchodilator when needed **plus** an inhaled **regular corticosteroid**, especially in adults.

In children, a **cromone** may be used as a regular prophylactic instead of a corticosteroid, especially *sodium cromoglicate (cromolyn sodium)* for exercise-induced asthma, but this may be ineffective in children aged under 4 years, in whom *ipratropium bromide* may be more useful. *Nedocromil sodium* is more appropriate for adults. It may take 3–4 weeks to establish the level of response to prophylactic inhalation therapy, so

persistence is required on the part of patient, doctor and carer. Older adults (aged >50 years) often do not respond well to beta$_2$-bronchodilators, probably because of a deficiency of bronchiolar beta$_2$-receptors, so the **antimuscarinic** agent *ipratropium bromide* may give better results in these patients.

High-dose inhaled corticosteroids are available for patients who do not respond adequately to normal doses, and may avoid the need for **oral steroids** completely or enable the dose of the latter to be reduced substantially. Alternatively, an inhaled long-acting beta-agonist, e.g. *eformoterol (formoterol)* or *salmeterol*, may be added to a low-dose corticosteroid. *Sodium cromoglicate* may also be helpful. Oral slow-release **methylxanthines** (e.g. *theophylline*) may also be introduced and, because they have a different mode of action from other bronchodilators, may augment the response to current bronchodilator treatment. Clearly, there will be no further benefit if the response to existing therapy is the

Table 5.10   Management of chronic asthma in adults and children 5 years and over

Start at step most appropriate to initial severity, use **'rescue course'** of prednisolone at **any time** or **any step**

Step 1: Occasional relief bronchodilators

Inhaled short-acting beta$_2$-agonist as required (up to once daily)

Note: Move to step 2 if needed more than once daily (or night-time symptoms)
Check compliance and inhaler technique

Step 2: Regular inhaled prophylactic therapy

Inhaled short-acting beta$_2$-agonist as required
PLUS EITHER regular standard-dose[a] inhaled corticosteroid
OR regular cromoglicate[b] or nedocromil (change to inhaled corticosteroid if control not achieved)

Note: Higher dose of inhaled corticosteroid may be required to gain initial control; some individuals benefit from
doubling for short period to cover exacerbation

**Step 3: High-dose inhaled corticosteroids or standard-dose inhaled corticosteroids plus long-acting inhaled
beta$_2$-agonist**

Inhaled short-acting beta$_2$-agonist as required
PLUS EITHER regular high-dose[c] inhaled corticosteroid
OR regular standard-dose[a] inhaled corticosteroid plus regular inhaled long-acting beta$_2$-agonist (salmeterol
50 micrograms twice daily or in those over 18 years, formoterol (eformoterol) 12 micrograms twice daily)

Note: In the few who have problems with high-dose inhaled corticosteroids use a standard-dose inhaled
corticosteroid with either an inhaled long-acting beta$_2$-stimulant option or regular modified-release oral
theophylline or try regular cromoglicate[b] or nedocromil

Step 4: High-dose inhaled corticosteroids plus regular bronchodilators

Inhaled short-acting beta$_2$-agonist as required
WITH regular high-dose[c] inhaled corticosteroid
PLUS sequential therapeutic trial of one or more of:
Inhaled long-acting beta$_2$-agonist
Modified-release oral theophylline
Inhaled ipratropium or, in adults, oxitropium
Modified-release oral beta$_2$-agonist
High-dose inhaled bronchodilators
Cromoglicate[b] or nedocromil

Step 5: Regular corticosteroid tablets

Inhaled short-acting beta$_2$-agonist as required
WITH regular high-dose[c] inhaled corticosteroid plus one or more long-acting bronchodilators (as step 4)
PLUS regular prednisolone tablets (as single daily dose)

Note: In addition to regular prednisolone, continue high-dose inhaled corticosteroid (may exceptionally exceed
licensed doses); these patients should normally be referred to an asthma clinic

continued overleaf

Table 5.10   (Continued)

Stepping down

Review treatment every 3–6 months

If control is achieved, stepwise reduction may be possible; if treatment was started recently at step 4 or 5 (or contained corticosteroid tablets) reduction may take place after a short interval; in other patients 1–3 months or longer period of stability is needed before stepwise reduction is undertaken

[a] Standard-dose inhaled corticosteroids are beclometasone dipropionate or budesonide 100–400 micrograms twice daily or fluticasone propionate 50–200 micrograms twice daily.

[b] Cromolyn.

[c] High-dose inhaled corticosteroids are beclometasone dipropionate or budesonide 0.8–2 mg daily in divided doses or fluticasone propionate 0.4–1 mg daily (in divided doses); use a large-volume spacer.

Desirable outcomes of treatment	
Steps 1–3: control of asthma	Steps 4–5: best possible result

• Minimal – chronic symptoms, including nocturnal ones
   – exacerbations (or infrequent ones)
   – need for relieving bronchodilators
   – adverse effects from medication (or none)
• Not activity or exercise limited
• PEF ≥80% of predicted or best
• Circadian variation in PEF <20%
	• Least possible – symptoms
	   – need for relieving bronchodilators
	   – limitation of activity
	   – variation in PEF
	• Best PEF
	• Least adverse effects from medication

Based on tables in British Thoracic Society et al. (1997) The British Guidelines on Asthma Management. *Thorax* **52**: Suppl. 1 and *British National Formulary* 38. (With permission of BMJ Specialist Journals and the Pharmaceutical Press.)

maximum that can be achieved in damaged lungs. They should be tried first when oral steroids are contemplated, the latter being a measure of last resort. However, severe acute exacerbations may require a short course of an oral steroid.

Morning dipping (*see* Fig. 5.13) was traditionally managed with an **oral** slow-release bronchodilator (beta$_2$-agonist or a methylxanthine) taken before retiring, but an inhaled long-acting beta$_2$-agonist is preferable nowadays. *Bambuterol* (an oral pro-drug of *terbutaline*) may also be useful.

Chronic adult asthma

Management of these patients is similar in principle to that just described, the basis being a high-dose inhaled corticosteroid (Table 5.10, Step 5), with a short-acting beta$_2$-agonist reliever for breakthrough attacks. Long-acting beta$_2$-agonists and a methylxanthine may be added later.

If necessary a further bronchodilator may be added, including an inhaled antimuscarinic (*ipratropium* or *oxitropium*) or an **oral** modified-release long-acting beta$_2$-agonist (*bambuterol* or

salmeterol). If there is an inadequate response to beta$_2$-agonists in these patients an antimuscarinic may enhance and prolong the effects of the adrenergic bronchodilator.

Steroids are always needed, often the high-dose inhaled form, but many patients will need oral prednisolone in addition. Even with oral steroid medication **the high-dose inhaled corticosteroid should always be continued** to minimize the oral dose required. In exceptional circumstances, **cytotoxic** drugs have been used to spare the oral corticosteroid dose.

Morning dipping is best managed with a bedtime dose of a long-acting inhaled beta$_2$-agonist, as described above.

Acute severe and life-threatening asthma

This comprises severe attacks which are not relieved by the patient's normal medication and is sometimes called **status asthmaticus**. Most such attacks do not develop very acutely but are preceded by warning signs which are indications for aggressive therapy to abort them. These signs are:

Table 5.11   Management of chronic asthma in children under 5 years

Start at step most appropriate to initial severity, use **'rescue course'** of prednisolone at **any time** or **any step**

Step 1: Occasional relief bronchodilators

Short-acting beta$_2$-agonist as required (not more than once daily)

Note: Whenever possible use inhalers (more side effects and less effective when given orally)
Check compliance, technique and that inhaler is appropriate

Step 2: Regular inhaled prophylactic therapy

Inhaled short-acting beta$_2$-agonist as required
PLUS EITHER regular inhaled cromoglicate[a] (powder or metered-dose inhaler via large-volume spacer)
OR regular inhaled standard paediatric dose corticosteroid[b]
CONSIDER (TO STABILIZE PATIENT) 5-day course of soluble prednisolone tablets[c] or temporary doubling of inhaled corticosteroid dose

Note: Try cromoglicate[a] for 4–6 weeks. For inhaled corticosteroids assess effect on symptoms after 1 month and adjust doses; if control not adequate consider doubling dose of inhaled corticosteroid for 1 month (alternatively give 5-day course of soluble prednisolone tablets or consider introducing other treatments before increasing dose of inhaled corticosteroid for long periods)

Step 3: Increased-dose inhaled corticosteroids

Inhaled short-acting beta$_2$-agonist as required
PLUS regular inhaled high paediatric dose corticosteroid[d]
CONSIDER: Short course of soluble prednisolone tablets[c]
Regular inhaled long-acting beta$_2$-agonist *OR* regular modified-release oral theophylline

Note: Long-acting beta$_2$-agonist should probably be reserved for supplementing treatment if child already receiving cromoglicate[a] or a corticosteroid; modified-release oral theophylline may be helpful (particularly for nocturnal symptoms) but has appreciable side effects in up to one-third of children (plasma- or salivary-concentration monitoring recommended)

Step 4: High-dose inhaled corticosteroid plus regular bronchodilators

Inhaled short-acting beta$_2$-agonist as required
WITH regular inhaled high paediatric dose corticosteroid[d]
CONSIDER: Short course of soluble prednisolone[c]
Regular inhaled long-acting beta$_2$-agonist
Regular modified-release oral theophylline
ALSO nebulized beta$_2$-agonist

Stepping down

Regularly review need for treatment according to disease severity and as child grows

[a] Cromolyn.
[b] Standard paediatric inhaled corticosteroid dose is beclometasone dipropionate or budesonide up to 400 micrograms daily (in divided doses) or fluticasone propionate up to 200 micrograms daily (in divided doses); initial dose according to age, weight and severity of asthma; use a large-volume spacer.
[c] Doses of prednisolone tablets are: child under 1 year, 1–2 mg/kg daily; 1–5 years, 20 mg daily; rescue courses usually for 1–3 days.
[d] High paediatric dose inhaled corticosteroid is beclometasone dipropionate or budesonide up to 800 micrograms daily (in divided doses) or fluticasone propionate up to 500 micrograms daily (in divided doses); use a large-volume spacer.
Based on tables in British Thoracic Society *et al.* (1997) The British Guidelines on Asthma Management. *Thorax* **52**: Suppl. 1 and *British National Formulary* 38. (With permission of BMJ Specialist Journals and the Pharmaceutical Press.)

- Decreasing exercise tolerance.
- Increasing respiration rate, dyspnoea and sleep disturbance.
- Increasing diurnal variation in PEF.
- Medication becoming less effective, with increased bronchodilator usage.

Acute severe asthma is characterized by:

- Pulse ≥ 110 beats/min in adults or ≥ 120/min in children under 5 years.
- Respiration rate ≥ 25 breaths/min at rest in adults, ≥ 40/min in children under 5 years.
- In young children, use of the accessory muscles of respiration (p. 220).
- Inability to speak in complete sentences or, in young children, inability to talk or feed.
- Decreasing PEF, which may drop below 100 L/min or 34–50% of the patient's predicted or best value in adults, and $\leq 50\%$ in children who can give reliable readings.
- Diurnal variation in PEF >25%.

In an **acute life-threatening attack** there may also be:

- A silent chest, i.e. no airflow in or out, or a feeble respiratory effort.
- Bradycardia.
- Exhaustion.
- Confusion or coma in adults, agitation or reduced consciousness in young children, who may not appear to be distressed.
- Cyanosis in adults.
- Peak flow $\leq 33\%$ of the patient's predicted or best value.

- If blood gases are measured, $P_aCO_2 \geq 6$ kPa, i.e. acidosis (pH <7.35); and severe hypoxia, $P_aO_2 <8$ kPa.

We have already noted that the severity of such attacks is often not appreciated by the patients or their doctors, so many patients arrive at hospital virtually moribund. Sometimes the severity of symptoms may be masked by over-enthusiastic use of beta$_2$-agonists, especially with a nebulizer (p. 285). It is better to recognize that a severe attack is impending and treat aggressively at the first signs to gain control and prevent deterioration, because it is more difficult to treat severe symptoms once they are established. Even large doses of beta$_2$-agonist bronchodilators and corticosteroids are safe in the short term. However, patients are often unresponsive to bronchodilators in severe attacks, so it may be dangerous to persist with these because they may aggravate hypoxia (p. 223). If a patient is unresponsive to a nebulized or parenteral beta$_2$-agonist, it may be better to use intravenous *aminophylline* (see below), which has a different mode of action.

The groups most at risk in an acute severe attack are patients who are aged between 12 and 25 years of age, who are immigrants, migrant workers and holidaymakers, and who:

- Were in hospital for asthma in the previous year.
- Have a history of severe attacks.
- Use regular or occasional oral or nebulized corticosteroids.
- Initiated an emergency call.

Figure 5.17 Flow chart for the management of acute severe asthma (status asthmaticus). Note that **severity** is often not appreciated by both the patient and the doctor: **peak flow rates should always be measured**. [a] This figure should be read in consultation with the text, particularly Tables 5.10 and 5.11, and with the BTS Guidelines on Asthma Management (*see* References and further reading), especially charts 2, 3, 4 and 8 of the latter. [b] If the GP is not available, patients should dial 999 or go to the nearest A & E Department. [c] High-flow oxygen (40–60% via face mask) does not depress respiration in asthmatics (pp. 219–220). It may not be available to GPs. [d] Soluble tablets are preferred: adults 30–60 mg per day; 1–15 years 1–2 mg/kg/day, maxima 1–5 years 20 mg/day, 5–15 years 40 mg/day. If very ill, oral prednisolone and IV hydrocortisone can be started together, with oral administration only used as soon as possible. Maximum daily IV dose at any age is 400 mg in 6-hourly divided doses. [e] An oxygen-driven nebulizer with a flow rate of 6–8 L/min should be used (p. 285). Some children will not tolerate a face mask, and similar doses can be give via a spacer. [f] Patients aged over 40 years may respond better to ipratropium, which is also used if there is a poor response to bronchodilators. [g] Bolus aminophylline must not be given to those already taking an oral theophylline. Blood level monitoring should be used where available, especially if treatment is continued for more than 24 h, and the dose given by slow, small volume IV infusion. Doses: adults 750–1500 mg/day; 1–15 years, loading dose 5 mg/kg over 20 min (omit if already receiving oral theophylline), then 1 mg/kg/h. [h] Treatment on admission will depend on prior GP/ambulance treatment. [i] See p. 293. [k] Percent of predicted or best value, provided that patients are not too ill or too young to give reliable results.

In addition, these patients may have:

- Progressive symptoms or signs (nocturnal, declining or increasingly labile PEF).
- Exposure to seasonal or occupational allergens.
- Psychosocial problems.

The general management strategy is outlined in Fig. 5.17, but this is empirical and needs to be considered in the light of the patient's current therapy. Thus if this already includes a nebulized beta$_2$-adrenergic bronchodilator and oral corticosteroids, it may be appropriate to give a slow IV bolus of aminophylline. If the patient is already

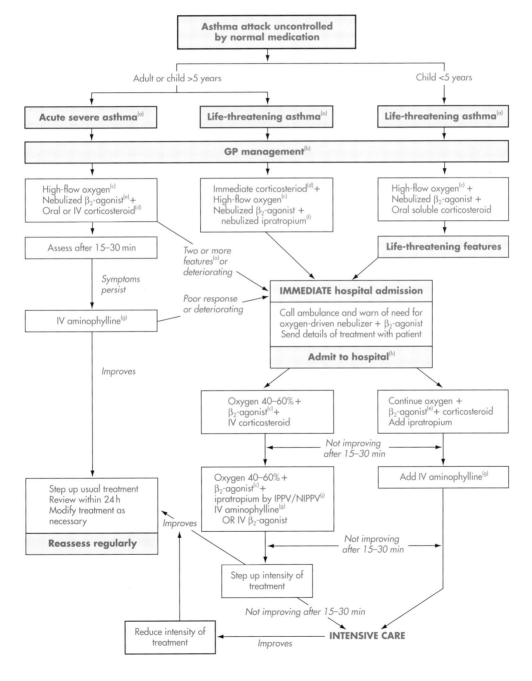

taking oral theophylline, the IV dose should be halved and the patient observed for cardiac arrhythmias. Lack of a satisfactory response then indicates the need for an IV steroid and oxygen as required, and the patient being admitted to hospital. Emergency self-admission ('open door') schemes may be life-saving.

Following admission, PEF, blood gases and serum electrolytes are monitored. The serum potassium level is particularly important, because there is a risk of serious hypokalaemia (see below and Chapter 4).

All patients should be educated to recognize any significant deterioration in their condition, e.g. with home monitoring of PEF, and about what action to take. These 'self-management plans' may involve:

- A protocol agreed with the patient's GP or consultant and instructions to see their doctor without delay.
- Increasing the dose of their inhaled corticosteroid.
- Reserve supplies of: (i) oral corticosteroids to take at the first signs of significant deterioration; and (ii) antibiotics, if severe attacks are known to be triggered by antibiotic-sensitive infection.

A few patients are '**brittle asthmatics**' and suffer severe attacks with very few or none of the warning signs described above. The peak flow charts of these patients will show a chaotic pattern. Provided that such patients are measuring and recording their PEF correctly, they need a reserve supply of oral corticosteroids and a nebulizer so that they can start intensive treatment immediately at the start of an attack. They must also obtain expert assistance without delay and often have special arrangements with their local hospital. Clearly, these patients will need to have been thoroughly assessed by a specialist respiratory physician and trained in the use of the equipment, i.e. peak flow meters, inhalers and nebulizers, and their medication.

Childhood asthma

Young children present special problems in diagnosis and treatment. The emotional response of the child (and parents) to the knowledge that they have a chronic disease, and the loss of time from school, are also important, so careful counselling of the child and its parents, siblings and teachers is essential.

Children cannot coordinate the relatively complex manoeuvres required to use an unmodified metered dose inhaler (MDIs, p. 281) before the age of about 7 years. A range of specially designed spacers and face masks for use with MDIs is available for young children. For older children, breath-actuated MDIs or dry powder inhalers are preferred. Nebulized drugs (p. 285) or oral medication may be used at any age, especially in infants and during severe attacks. However, children vary enormously in their rates of mental and physical development, so the route of administration has to be tailored to their abilities and tolerance of treatment. Regular monitoring is especially important because the requirements change rapidly with age.

Within these constraints, the management of childhood asthma (Table 5.11) is generally similar to that in adults. However, adrenergic bronchodilators are often ineffective in young children because only a small dose reaches the lungs; nebulized *ipratropium bromide* or oral **methylxanthines** may give better results. The latter tend to be more effective in children than in adults, but the dose must be monitored carefully to avoid toxicity. Careful consideration needs to be given to the use of methylxanthines in children because *theophylline* use has been associated with behavioural and learning difficulties.

It has recently been shown that a beta$_2$-agonist bronchodilator used with a large-volume spacer was more effective than a nebulizer in children aged over 3 years with acute asthma. This finding requires confirmation, but provides a less costly and simpler alternative to conventional nebulizer treatment.

Sodium cromoglicate (*cromolyn sodium*) or low-dose **corticosteroids** are recommended for first-line prophylaxis, and sodium cromoglicate or **long-acting beta$_2$-agonists** for exercise-induced bronchoconstriction. Higher doses of inhaled corticosteroids, administered via a spacer device (p. 282), are introduced as necessary. One study has shown that the early use of an inhaled corticosteroid may prevent the development of irreversible airways obstruction.

Oral corticosteroids must be avoided if at all possible, because they retard growth, even if given in alternate-day dosage, but it has been shown that *nebulized budesonide* may permit a dramatic reduction in oral corticosteroid usage. Although high-dose inhaled corticosteroids may also affect growth it should be remembered that growth retardation may also be a consequence of severe asthma. As usual with severe chronic diseases, effective control comprises a sometimes difficult balance between the harmful effects of the disease and the side effects of treatment.

Immunotherapy: hyposensitization

Many attempts have been made to 'desensitize' patients to allergens. Because episodic asthma is often associated with high levels of IgE, it is attractive to try to prevent IgE production and the resultant hypersensitivity reaction. This has been attempted by injecting a minute dose of an identified allergen and following this with regularly increasing doses, none of which must provoke a significant reaction. Theoretically, this should result in effective immunization with the production of sufficient IgG (so-called 'blocking antibody') to scavenge any allergen before it is able to elicit the formation of IgE.

However, it is rarely possible to achieve this effectively because, even if patients can be desensitized to a single allergen, they are usually sensitive to several allergens at first diagnosis and do not respond adequately. Further, being atopic they will later become sensitive to other allergens. Hyposensitization has largely been abandoned in the UK following a number of severe anaphylactic events and 11 deaths. The UK Committee on the Safety of Medicines has advised that desensitizing vaccines should not be used unless full cardiorespiratory resuscitation facilities are immediately available and patients can be observed for 2 h following each injection.

Current research in this field is directed towards the minimization of major reactions during immunization by using modified allergens or immunomodulatory agents. A more fundamental approach to immunotherapy involves the control of IgE production in atopic individuals. The role of immunotherapy, used in carefully selected patients under controlled conditions, requires reappraisal.

The term 'immunotherapy' may be stretched to include the blocking of the release or action of inflammatory eicosanoids and cytokines. The first agents with such properties, the leukotriene receptor antagonists, are now available (see below).

Drugs used in asthma

A summary of the treatment of target features was presented in Table 5.9 and the topic of inhalation therapy is dealt with separately on pp. 280–291.

Beta$_2$-agonist bronchodilators

Mode of action

These drugs interact with a membrane-bound receptor coupled to an intracellular protein with a sub-unit which regulates effector molecule activation in the cell, e.g. adenylcyclase, phospholipases, ion channels or transport proteins. Beta$_2$-receptors ultimately cause the opening of Ca^{++} channels and reduce both the phosphorylation of myosin light chains and calcium-dependent actin–myosin coupling, producing smooth muscle relaxation.

Secondary effects relevant to asthma are:

- Increased mucociliary clearance from the airways, reducing obstruction.
- The reduction of bronchial reactivity to a variety of stimuli, due to:
  - Decreased microvascular permeability, reducing the recruitment of inflammatory cells.
  - Inhibition of phospholipase A$_2$ activity.
- Inhibition of the liberation of leukotrienes and histamine from mast cells and other effector cells.

These secondary effects are probably less important acutely, but may contribute to the beneficial effect of the beta$_2$-agonists when they are used prophylactically.

Because the density of beta$_2$-receptors is greatest in the smaller airways, it is there (the site of the problem in asthma) that the beta$_2$-agonists exert their major effect.

Use

The short-acting selective beta$_2$-agonists are the drugs of first choice in the treatment of mild asthma and are used therapeutically as 'relievers' to control occasional acute attacks. However, anti-inflammatory agents and long-acting selective beta$_2$-agonists are now introduced into treatment much earlier than previously for the prophylaxis of more persistent moderate to severe symptoms.

Short-acting agents.   Most of the currently available drugs (*salbutamol*, *terbutaline*, *reproterol*) have very similar kinetic characteristics. The most widely used, *salbutamol*, has an intermediate duration of action of about 4 h and a peak effect about 60 min after inhalation. *Terbutaline* and *reproterol* seem to have a slightly longer duration of action, but this difference is not clinically relevant. These and similar short-acting drugs (e.g. *pirbuterol*) are therefore used up to three to four times daily.

Fenoterol may be less beta$_2$-selective than *salbutamol*, and doubts have been raised as to its safety. Until these are resolved it should be used cautiously.

Long-acting agents.   *Bambuterol* requires only once-daily oral dosing, while *formoterol* (*eformoterol*) and *salmeterol* are inhaled twice daily, giving enhanced convenience and patient compliance. It is important to note that these long-acting agents are not replacements for the shorter-acting drugs because they are suitable only for regular prophylaxis and not as relievers for 'rescue therapy': the shorter-acting drugs are still useful for treating the occasional acute attack. These long-acting agents are valuable in those patients who show significant morning dipping, or who continue to wheeze despite using low-dose inhaled steroids and short-acting bronchodilators. They now tend to be introduced at an earlier stage as adjuncts to low-dose inhaled steroids. With chronic use they may also have a significant anti-inflammatory action, though the clinical value of this is not yet clear: they must not be regarded as a replacement for inhaled corticosteroids.

Used regularly, the beta-agonists also have some additional prophylactic effects, possibly by providing a prolonged barrier to bronchoconstriction: even if a bronchoconstricting trigger is encountered, the result is unlikely to be a clinically significant reduction in ventilatory capacity. However, tolerance may develop, resulting particularly in a reduced duration of action. Thus the current trend is to use the short-acting beta$_2$-agonists on an 'as-required' basis.

Side effects.   It is clear from the distributions of the two types of beta-adrenoreceptors (Table 5.12) that the beta$_2$-selective agents are without significant adverse cardiac effects at normal dosage. This selectivity is enhanced because they can be delivered directly to their sites of action in the bronchioles where they are very effective at about one-tenth of the oral dose. They are thus very safe and have replaced the nonselective adrenergic agents (*adrenaline* (*epinephrine*), *isoprenaline* (*isoproterenol*), etc.), the CNS (restlessness, agitation) and cardiovascular side effects of which are particularly harmful in patients who are stressed by a severe asthma attack. Inhaled doses of terbutaline eight times the normally recommended maximum have been used to achieve greater bronchodilatation, with no increase in side effects.

The selective beta$_2$-agonists are not completely receptor-specific and so do have some predictable side effects (central stimulation and insomnia, headache, peripheral vasodilatation, tachycardia), especially if they are inhaled excessively or taken orally. Tremors, usually a fine hand tremor (due to direct stimulation of beta$_2$-receptors in skeletal muscle), are common and are a significant problem in a minority of patients. A very small proportion of patients may experience paradoxical bronchospasm with inhaled bronchodilators, possibly due to direct bronchial irritation. Although this is very rare, perhaps as low as one in 50 million doses, this possibility should be borne in mind. Because of the adverse cardiac effects of the **oral** use of these drugs, inhaled forms are preferred in the elderly or if there is evidence of cardiac insufficiency.

The beta$_2$-agonists, especially in high doses, are known to cause serious **hypokalaemia** by increasing cellular potassium uptake (*see* Chapter 4). This effect is potentiated by hypoxia and concomitant

Table 5.12 Beta-adrenergic receptor subtypes and some effects of their stimulation in certain tissues

Receptor type	Tissue in which present	Effect of stimulation
β_1	Heart	Increased rate, force, conduction velocity, automaticity
	Kidney	Renin secretion
	Fat tissue	Lipolysis
β_2	Smooth muscle	
	• bronchial	Bronchodilatation
	• vascular	Vasodilatation
	• intestinal	Reduced motility and tone
	• bladder	
	Skeletal muscle	Increased contractility, glycogenolysis, potassium uptake, tremor (overdose)
	Pancreas	Increased insulin secretion
	Liver	Glycogenolysis, gluconeogenesis
	Central nervous system	Nervous tension, headache, insomnia

treatment with **methylxanthines**, **steroids** and **diuretics**. Life-threatening hypokalaemia is fortunately rare, but the potential is clearly greatest during severe exacerbations of asthma when hypoxia and the use of drug combinations occur concurrently. Serum potassium levels must always be monitored during severe episodes.

Bronchodilators should be used with caution in patients with hyperthyroidism, who exhibit many of the symptoms just described, or with cardiovascular problems and in the elderly. As usual, they should be used with care in pregnancy, but the benefits of good asthma control outweigh any slightly detrimental cardiovascular effects on the mother or fetus; high doses of beta-agonists are used parenterally in obstetrics to control premature uterine contractions in the last trimester.

Antimuscarinic agents

Mode of action

Antimuscarinic drugs are competitive inhibitors of acetylcholine (ACh) at muscarinic receptors, of which there are several sub-types. M_1 receptors are present in ganglia in the airways walls and M_3 receptors in airways smooth muscle. *Ipratropium* and *oxitropium* block the uptake of ACh at both of these receptor types, reducing muscle tone and producing dilatation of both larger and small airways. They do not affect M_2 receptors, which are widespread elsewhere.

Use

Although anticholinergics were used widely in the past in the form of belladonna or hyoscyamus galenicals, and more recently as atropine, they were largely abandoned owing to the occurrence of widespread antimuscarinic adverse reactions. However, inhaled *ipratropium* and *oxitropium* bromides are useful because they appear to be fairly specific for lung tissue and are virtually without side effects. This results from their poor absorption, a consequence of their highly polar, quaternary ammonium structure. Because they do not penetrate mucous membranes they have no effect on reducing mucus secretion, though an antimuscarinic agent should theoretically do so, and there is no convincing evidence that any of these drugs, including atropine, affect sputum volume or viscosity. Further, they do not interfere with mucociliary clearance, so mucus is cleared normally.

The antimuscarinics show some synergism with beta$_2$-adrenergic bronchodilators, enhancing and prolonging their activity, though this has been disputed. This discrepancy seems to have been resolved by a recent survey of schoolchildren and adolescents, which found little support for using the combination routinely and for mild to moderate exacerbations of asthma. However, the addition of multiple doses of an antimuscarinic to beta$_2$-agonist inhalations improved lung function and reduced hospital admission in severe exacerbations. Antimuscarinics are particularly useful in older, chronic asthmatics in whom responsiveness to beta$_2$-agonists tends to decline progressively from age 40, probably owing to a reduction in the number of bronchiolar beta-receptors.

Ipratropium bromide has a slightly slower onset of action (30–60 min, peak effect at 90–120 min) and a slightly longer duration of action than the beta$_2$-agonists and so is normally used three times daily, for prophylaxis only.

Side effects

There are few significant problems. Nebulized ipratropium bromide occasionally causes paradoxical bronchospasm although isotonic, preservative-free formulations have been introduced to minimize this risk. Even so, this form of treatment should be initiated only in hospital with careful supervision for the first week. Although ipratropium is poorly absorbed topically, it sometimes causes dry mouth, rarely urinary retention or constipation. The use of nebulized solutions has been associated with acute angle closure glaucoma because of escape of drug aerosol and direct eye contact. Thus these should not be used in glaucoma patients and in the elderly and precautions should always be taken to prevent escape of aerosol from masks, which should fit closely. Mouthpieces are preferable. The occasional patient may be adversely sensitive to the bromide radical. A new longer-acting agent, *tiotropium*, is currently undergoing clinical trial.

Methylxanthine bronchodilators

Mode of action

Theophylline is the most potent of these agents. For many years it was thought to act solely as a cyclic nucleotide phosphodiesterase inhibitor (PDI), thus increasing the levels of cyclic 3′,5′-adenosine monophosphate (cAMP) in cells and causing airways relaxation. However, relaxation of the airways occurs *in vitro* at concentrations which have no effect on cellular cAMP levels. Also, several PDIs which are more potent than theophylline provide no significant benefit in asthma.

However, theophylline is now known to have other actions:

* Antagonization of receptor-mediated adenosine-induced bronchospasm.
* Direct effects on intracellular Ca^{++} concentration and indirect effects via cell membrane hyperpolarization.
* Uncoupling of intracellular Ca^{++} concentration from muscular contraction.

Thus, despite some 150 years of use the precise mode of action of the methylxanthines remains obscure. Other possible actions have been suggested, e.g. increased mucociliary clearance, inhibition of mediator release, central stimulation of ventilation and improved contractility of the respiratory muscles. However, it is doubtful whether these can contribute materially to the increases in FEV$_1$ or PEF which are observed. Recent evidence suggests that theophylline also has anti-inflammatory, immunomodulatory and bronchoprotective effects which may contribute to its usefulness as an asthma prophylactic.

There is evidence that cAMP modulation of intracellular calcium levels may be a common pathway for bronchodilatation, however caused, and it is interesting that beta$_2$-agonists share this effect. The action of theophylline to mobilize intracellular calcium as referred to above may prove to be its principal effect.

Use

Theophylline (1,3-dimethylxanthine) itself is relatively insoluble but is well absorbed from solutions, capsules and uncoated tablets, with peak concentrations occurring after 1–2 h. However, clearance is very variable (see below). Thus microfined, slow-release oral formulations have been introduced which, although they have poorer bioavailability, provide therapeutic blood levels which persist over approximately 12 h. Because peak blood levels tend to occur after about 8 h, the evening dose should be taken at about 8 p.m. to minimize morning dipping. These slow-release forms are taken once or twice daily. Methylxanthines should not be used unless the patient has failed to respond adequately to high-dose inhaled corticosteroids.

Theophylline, when combined with ethylenediamine, as *aminophylline*, is much more soluble and in this form is used parenterally, preferably as a low-volume IV infusion (see below).

Side effects

Theophylline can cause numerous side effects, e.g. central nervous (headache, irritability, insomnia) and gastrointestinal (nausea and vomiting), even when its serum levels are within the therapeutic range (10–20 mg/L). Above this level serious CNS reactions can occur, e.g. seizures, encephalopathy, coma, even death, and convulsions may occur without warning signs, especially if the patient is hypoxic, because cerebral hypoxia is exacerbated. Because the side effects of methylxanthines and beta$_2$-agonists are additive, and both cause hypoxaemia and are frequently used together, the risk of convulsions is increased.

Theophylline has been considered suitable for use in pregnancy. However, it needs especially careful therapeutic drug level monitoring because blood levels are affected by the stage of pregnancy and by delivery.

Aminophylline is more **irritant** than theophylline by any route. Even normal therapeutic oral doses may cause nausea and vomiting, though this is less likely with the modern modified-release products. Suppositories may cause proctitis. When aminophylline is given intravenously it is best given as a slow infusion (see below), because venous irritation may cause phlebitis and rapid bolus injections may cause cardiac arrhythmias, profound hypotension and hypokalaemia, resembling an acute overdose situation. A very few patients may be hypersensitive to the ethylenediamine component. In emergency situations in the community, it may be given as a slow bolus IV injection over 20 min.

Toxicity and therapeutic levels of theophylline and aminophylline. The therapeutic range of theophylline is rather narrow, and non-bronchodilatory side effects occur at concentrations below 10 mg/L. Thus, treatment should be instituted with blood level monitoring, especially if the patient has been taking an oral form and receives IV treatment in an emergency or if there is any evidence of theophylline toxicity (see below) or hepatic impairment. Blood samples must be taken at steady state: approximately 4–6 h after the start of an infusion and 8–12 h after a an oral dose of a modified-release product. Because only 10% of a dose is excreted renally, renal impairment should not affect blood levels significantly unless there is gross renal failure in a patient whose blood level is approaching toxicity. Regrettably, many patients in the community are given slow-release oral preparations on a standard dosage regimen and, because absorption may be erratic and metabolism variable, it is not known whether levels in the therapeutic range are achieved: an appreciable proportion have sub-therapeutic blood concentrations. A summary of the factors which influence theophylline serum levels is given in Table 5.13.

Because of the variations in patient response to the different formulations, modified-release forms from different manufacturers should not be changed without careful clinical and blood level monitoring. In emergency admissions, hospital A&E doctors must be informed if patients are taking an oral theophylline product, in which case the parenteral dose of aminophylline must be halved to avoid serious toxicity. In the absence of blood level monitoring, not more than four 250-mg doses should be given in 24 h. If therapeutic drug monitoring is available, an infusion rate of 500 microgram/kg/h is appropriate for maintenance in adults.

Despite their potential toxicity, methylxanthines have been widely used as the drugs of first choice in North America. However, they are used less frequently now and may be supplanted by the inhaled long-acting beta$_2$-agonists and corticosteroids over the next few years. Nevertheless, there is a subgroup of patients who seem to respond better to theophylline than to other drugs.

Other xanthine derivatives are used in the USA and continental Europe. *Enprofylline* (3-propylxanthine) is a soluble, well-absorbed, potent compound which does not yield theophylline on metabolism and does not have many of the side effects of the latter. Further, because it is excreted unchanged via the kidneys, it does not possess the complex pharmacokinetics and interactions of theophylline. However, it tends to cause

Table 5.13   Some drugs and conditions affecting theophylline plasma levels and activity

---

Increased plasma level or effect

Inhibition or reduction of liver microsomal enzyme activity
Cimetidine, ciprofloxacin, enoxacin, erythromycin, propranolol, combined oral contraceptives, viloxazine
Heart failure, hepatic diseases, age (neonates, old age), interferons and viral infections, immunization (possibly),
high-carbohydrate/low-protein diet (vegetarians)

Inhibition of xanthine metabolism[a]
Allopurinol

Decreased clearance (abnormal physiology)
Diltiazem, verapamil
Late pregnancy[b]

Reduced plasma level or effect

Induction of liver microsomal enzymes
Aminoglutethimide, barbiturates, phenytoin and other anticonvulsants, rifampicin
Cigarette and marijuana smoking, high-protein/low-carbohydrate diet

Increased clearance
Sulfinpyrazone, furosemide (frusemide)[c]
Pregnancy[b]

---

[a] Theophylline is 1,3-dimethylxanthine.

[b] The effect of pregnancy on blood levels is uncertain and varies with the stage of pregnancy, so careful therapeutic blood level monitoring is essential.
Parturition results in increased blood levels.

[c] The situation with furosemide (frusemide) is unclear. Plasma concentrations of theophylline may be increased with concurrent intravenous use of both
drugs; caution is necesssary.

---

headaches. *Diprophylline* (dyphylline, dihydroxypropyltheophylline) has similar kinetic and toxic properties to enprofylline and is better tolerated than theophylline or aminophylline.

Glucocorticosteroids

These are the most potent anti-inflammatory drugs available and thus are used extensively in the treatment of asthma and other respiratory diseases (Table 5.14). They are life-saving in severe asthma attacks and may modify disease progression in intractable, infiltrative lung diseases, e.g. rheumatoid lung disease, systemic lupus erythematosus (SLE) and polyarteritis nodosa (PAN) (*see* Chapter 8, p. 511 and p. 518).

Mode of action
These agents are presumed to diffuse passively into cells, bind to a specific receptor protein and finally stimulate the synthesis of **lipocortin**. The latter inhibits phospholipase A_2 and in turn the synthesis of prostaglandins and leukotriene mediators from macrophages, monocytes and mast cells. The formation and release of potent inflammatory cytokines (interleukin 1 (IL-1), IL-2, IL-3, IL-6, tumour necrosis factor (TNF) alpha, interferon (IFN) gamma) and the production of complement (C_3) acute phase reactants are also blocked.

Thus, steroids inhibit the production and release of a number of pro-inflammatory agents from a variety of immune and inflammatory cells, e.g. vasoactive and chemoattractive factors, lipolytic and proteolytic enzymes. Additionally, the extravasation of lymphocytes, fibrosis and production of PAF (an important inflammatory mediator) and immunoglobulin E (IgE) are also reduced. These actions combine to reduce inflammatory damage in the airways and **hyper-reactivity**.

Table 5.14 Some indications for the use of cortico-steroids in diseases with respiratory involvement

Primary lung disease
Asthma, prophylaxis and severe attacks
Allergic bronchopulmonary aspergillosis
Extrinsic allergic alveolitis
Interstitial lung disease

Secondary lung disease (*see* Chapter 8)
Granulomatous lung diseases, e.g. rheumatoid lung disease, sarcoidosis, histiocytosis X
Vasculitis, e.g. systemic lupus erythematosus, polyarteritis nodosa
Autoimmune, e.g. Goodpasture's syndrome

Table 5.15 The approximate relative potencies[a] of corticosteroids used for the treatment of respiratory diseases

Systemic use		By inhalation	
Hydrocortisone	0.2	Beclometasone	1
Deflazacort	0.8	Budesonide	1
Prednisolone	1	Fluticasone	2
Methylprednisolone	1.3		
Triamcinolone	1.3		
Dexamethasone	7		
Betamethasone	7		

[a] Relative to: prednisolone = 1 (systemic use); beclometasone = 1 (by inhalation).

N.B. The two columns cannot be compared as they have different baselines.

Use

Inhalation therapy. For the treatment of asthma, corticosteroids are preferably given by inhalation (*beclometasone, budesonide* or *fluticasone*). A single dose will not control an attack so they cannot be used for rescue. They must be used prophylactically, being particularly useful in controlling the delayed inflammatory response (*see* Fig. 5.14). It may take 7–14 days or more to obtain the maximal therapeutic response. Since the fundamentally inflammatory nature of asthma has been recognized, inhaled corticosteroids are introduced at an early stage, e.g. if there are significant nocturnal symptoms or more than three wheezy episodes per week or if short-acting bronchodilators are used more than two to three times daily. However, there is a reluctance on the part of many patients, and some doctors, to use these valuable agents because of unjustified fears of serious side effects, arising from experience with oral use. The relative potencies of these drugs are given in Table 5.15.

The dose requirement varies widely between patients and in any one patient over a long period. Although a high dose may be needed initially to control symptoms it may be possible to reduce the dose substantially (step down) once symptoms are well controlled. Once stabilized, temporary dose increases may be needed to treat acute exacerbations. A high-dose corticosteroid aerosol may be very useful in chronic asthma and may avoid the need for oral medication. A budesonide inhaler, used with a spacer and face mask, is reported to be particularly suitable for young children who are unable to use a MDI. Even if control is inadequate with inhaled steroids they should always be continued, so that the oral dose can be reduced to a minimum. MDIs deliver only about one-tenth of the oral dose required to give a comparable effect, so only minor side effects occur (see below).

Oral use: maintenance therapy. *Prednisolone* and comparable agents (e.g. *betamethasone, dexamethasone, methylprednisolone, triamcinolone*) may be taken orally as a last resort in chronic (intrinsic) asthma and may be the only practicable means of controlling symptoms adequately. However, as usual, dosage must be kept to a minimum to avoid their well-known long-term side effects as far as possible.

Oral use: rescue therapy. The prompt use of glucocorticosteroids may be invaluable in aborting a severe attack which occurs against a background of worsening symptoms and decreased response to bronchodilators, i.e. threatened acute severe asthma (p. 246). Doses equivalent to 30–40 mg or more of *prednisolone* daily (Table 5.15) may be required initially depending on the severity of symptoms. When the patient has been stabilized the dose may be reduced (*see* Tables 5.10 and 5.11). Whether the dose needs to be reduced gradually over 2–3 weeks to a suitable maintenance level, or reduced rapidly over a few days, will depend on the duration and intensity of rescue treatment: it is essential to continue treatment until it is clear that dose reduction does not lead to relapse. Peak flow monitoring should be maintained during and after rescue treatment to ensure adequate control and the absence of deterioration. There is evidence that some patients are relatively steroid-resistant and that this is a reflection of a generalized tissue resistance to steroids, and not confined to the lungs.

Alternate-day dosing, which is often used in other situations to minimize steroid side effects, is usually unsuitable in asthma because patients tend to deteriorate in the second 24-h period. As usual, dose reduction must always be gradual after any prolonged period of corticosteroid dosing to permit recovery from adrenal suppression and the resumption of adequate endogenous cortisol secretion. Further, patients on long-term corticosteroids may require temporary increases in dose to cover exceptionally stressful situations, e.g. severe illness, surgery or trauma.

Parenteral use. In acute severe asthma, *hydrocortisone* or *methylprednisolone* (up to 1 g daily) is given by slow IV infusion, with transfer to oral therapy as the patient improves (*see* Fig. 5.17). However, it has been suggested that oral dosage of 40 mg prednisolone may be equally effective. Oral steroids may also be useful in the occasional patient who bronchoconstricts in response to IV hydrocortisone.

Side effects

Too much emphasis has been placed on the harmful side effects of using steroids in asthma, leading to an aversion on the part of both doctors and patients, and subsequent under-use. As usual, the hazards of therapy need to be weighed against their undoubted benefits in the treatment of this potentially debilitating and life-threatening disease. It is clearly important to use minimal doses. This discussion deals primarily with the side effects of inhaled corticosteroids. Those occurring with oral administration are discussed in connection with rheumatoid disease (*see* Chapter 8, p. 495).

Inhaled steroids usually cause very few, minor adverse reactions, the most common being mild throat irritation and hoarseness (**dysphonia**). The oral deposition of drug may sometimes cause oral thrush. These effects are largely prevented by twice-daily administration, which is as effective as the same total dose given four times daily, by rinsing the mouth with water (or a mouthwash if preferred) after using the inhaler, and using a spacer device (p. 282). If thrush does occur, it is readily controlled with topical *amphotericin or nystatin*, an **imidazole**, e.g. *miconazole*, or a **triazole**, e.g. *fluconazole, itraconazole*, though *ketoconazole* and the triazoles should be reserved for resistant infections.

Although adverse systemic effects are unlikely unless the daily dose exceeds 1500–2000 microgram of inhaled steroid, osteoporosis, dermal thinning and, in children, growth retardation may occur. Toothbrushes have been reported to be reservoirs of *Candida* infection in patients using inhaled corticosteroids: patients should be advised to change their toothbrush if they develop hoarseness or a significant sore throat or mouth during treatment.

Recent long-term research in Scotland has shown that side effects on the height and weight of children are significant only in those on Step 4 of the British Thoracic Society's treatment scale (*see* Table 5.10). This effect was less than the effects of social deprivation, and independent of them. However, growth is also affected by the severity of asthma and the degree of control, so it may be necessary to accept some drug-related growth retardation to prevent that arising from severe disease.

Nebulized steroids given with a face mask may cause facial eczema and, if this treatment mode is used over a long period, then unacceptable skin damage may occur. This may be largely prevented by coating the skin under the mask with soft paraffin and washing the face thoroughly immediately after dosing. Masks should fit closely.

Rarely, a patient may be sensitive to the drug or propellant.

Chronic oral therapy may lead to the well-known side effects of these drugs (*see* Chapter 8), e.g. Cushing's syndrome, growth suppression in children, hypertension, electrolyte disturbances and immunosuppression, though these should be mild if the daily dose does not exceed 7.5 mg of prednisolone or its equivalent. A few patients may become steroid-dependent and rely on continuous therapy, relapsing whenever an attempt is made to reduce the dose.

Relative contraindications include hypertension, obesity, diabetes mellitus, peptic ulceration, psoriasis, pregnancy, childhood and intercurrent infection (especially tuberculosis).

Anti-allergic drugs: cromones

Considerable attention has been focused on drugs which prevent the release from leucocytes and mast cells of the pharmacological mediators of bronchospasm and bronchial inflammation. These include *sodium cromoglicate* (*cromolyn sodium*, SCG) and *nedocromil sodium* (NDCS).

Mode of action

The mode of action of these drugs is still uncertain, despite intensive research. SCG has been regarded as the classic drug which is alleged to stabilize mast cell membranes, preventing both immediate and delayed degranulation, and so the release of mediators of bronchoconstriction. This antagonism occurs whether the stimulus is immunological (IgE) or irritant (due to exercise, cold air or inhaled hypertonic saline). The development of bronchiolar hyper-responsiveness is also blocked by pretreatment with SCG. NDCS is a much more potent inhibitor of mediator release than is SCG, and also inhibits white blood cell, macrophage and platelet activation. However, doubts have been expressed about the importance of mast cell stabilization, and the true mode of action of these drugs in asthma remains to be elucidated.

Some stimuli, e.g. sulphur dioxide, are believed to produce bronchoconstriction via a neuronal mechanism, involving the release of the peptide neurotransmitter, **substance P**, at the endings of unmyelinated C-fibres. Substance P is a potent airways constrictor, the action of which in the lungs is also blocked by SCG and NDCS: it is also involved in the transmission of pain sensation (*see* Chapter 10). SCG also affects phosphodiesterase enzyme levels and calcium influx into cells, thus influencing smooth muscle contraction.

Use

The cromones are not absorbed orally and so must be administered by inhalation. SCG is particularly useful in exercise-induced asthma in children, but rarely in adults. It can only be used prophylactically and may take up to 3–4 weeks to achieve its full effect.

Nedocromil sodium has similar properties to SCG but is a more potent anti-inflammatory agent. It appears to have a wider spectrum of clinical activity and is more effective in adults, having a steroid-sparing effect. It may be useful in mild to moderate asthma and for those patients who are fearful of using corticosteroids. However, it should not be regarded as a replacement for the latter.

Side effects

SCG is a very safe drug, the most common adverse reaction being a transient bronchospasm from the dry powder inhaler form. A combination product with salbutamol is available to prevent this effect, but this is not recommended because some patients use this combined formulation primarily for its salbutamol reliever activity. This aspect needs to be tested: if a patient obtains relief only from the combination then SCG is ineffective.

NDCS tends to cause slightly more undesirable effects than SCG, e.g. headache, nausea and vomiting, dyspepsia and abdominal pain, though these do not normally cause discontinuation of treatment.

Ketotifen has similar properties to SCG but is taken orally. Because it is also an antihistamine (H_1-blocker) it may cause drowsiness. A 3- to 4-week trial may be necessary to establish its value, but it does not seem to be particularly effective in most patients, though it is sometimes used in young children.

Leukotriene antagonists

Mode of action

The **leukotrienes** are straight-chain eicosanoids derived from arachidonic acid, and are potent pro-inflammatory agents. They are mostly produced from arachidonic acid by phospholipase A_2 pathway (*see* Chapter 8, p. 491). The latter is activated by a specific protein, **5-lipoxygenase** activating protein (FLAP), which binds the enzyme to the cell membrane.

Leukotriene B4 (LTB$_4$) is derived from the labile intermediate LTA$_4$ and is mostly produced by neutrophils. It is a potent neutrophil chemotactic agent. However, the role of neutrophils in asthma is controversial because they are only found in the lungs in appreciable numbers in patients with some types of occupational asthma. Although eosinophils are present in increased numbers in the lungs of asthmatic patients, LTB$_4$ probably plays only a minor role in eosinophil recruitment. It has only a weak effect on eosinophils, with other chemoattractants, e.g. PAF, IL-2, IL-5, being much more potent.

LTA$_4$ is also converted into the cysteinyl leukotrienes LTC$_4$, LTE$_4$ and LTF$_4$, initially by conjugation with glutathione. All of these have been implicated in asthma because they are potent bronchoconstrictors and can be produced by a range of effector cells, e.g. granulocytes and monocytes, mast cells and macrophages. The leukotrienes have a long persistence in lung tissue and also stimulate mucus secretion, cause mucosal oedema and sensitize the airways to other spasmogens. The LTC$_4$/D$_4$/E$_4$ mixture used to be known as SRS-A (slow reacting substance of anaphylaxis).

Leukotrienes act via at least three distinct receptors, for LTB$_4$, LTC$_4$ and LTD$_4$/LTE$_4$, which are blocked by the leukotriene receptor antagonists. The CysLT$_1$ receptor is activated by LTC$_4$/LTD$_4$/LTE$_4$ and is also blocked by the leukotriene receptor antagonists (LTAs).

There are thus two routes by which leukotriene activity may be prevented in asthma: antagonism of an early step in their formation, by inhibiting phosphpolipase A$_2$, 5-lipoxygenase, FLAP or leukotriene synthase, or by blocking leukotriene receptors in the lung.

The first 5-lipoxygenase inhibitor, *zileuton*, is licensed in the USA for the prophylaxis and treatment of chronic asthma and two leukotriene receptor antagonists, *montelukast* and *zafirlukast* are marketed in the UK.

Use

These agents are useful adjuncts when existing treatment with inhaled beta-agonists or corticosteroids fails to provide adequate control. They are not substitutes for existing treatments, but may have advantages over corticosteroids because they inhibit bronchoconstriction induced by exercise and allergens, against which corticosteroids are relatively ineffective. Although promising and well tolerated, more experience is needed before their precise role in therapy can be determined. At present they probably fit into Step 4 of the British Thoracic Society guidelines (*see* Table 5.10), i.e. as an adjunct to an inhaled beta$_2$-agonist plus an inhaled high-dose corticosteroid.

Because they are oral products they may benefit patients who have compliance problems with inhaled therapy, e.g. the elderly and mentally or physically handicapped.

Side effects

These are mild and infrequent, but abdominal pain and headache have been reported. They thus avoid the principal disadvantage of corticosteroids.

Oxygen

Oxygen may be life-saving in very severe acute asthma and should be given in these circumstances, even if there is no overt cyanosis. Because the pure gas causes pulmonary damage and retinal fibrosis (**retrolental fibroplasia**) it is always mixed with air. Provided that there is no history of COPD (pp. 262–273), patients may be given 35% oxygen while being transferred to hospital, and up to 60% may be used for short periods after admission. The hazards associated with higher concentrations means that artificial ventilation by **intermittent positive pressure ventilation** (IPPV, p. 293) is preferable.

If alveolar ventilation is inadequate in a seriously ill patient both P_aO_2 and P_aCO_2 may be reduced initially and patients may be cyanosed even when breathing oxygen-enriched air. Later, the P_aO_2 may continue to fall while the P_aCO_2 rises, producing respiratory acidosis. This may occur very rapidly in children. Any increase in P_aCO_2 is a serious sign in an asthmatic patient. Blood gases should be determined initially and if the P_aO_2 is less than 8 kPa, serial determinations should be made to monitor therapy. The P_aO_2 may rise only slowly in these circumstances.

High-dose (50–60%) oxygen is normally

given with a suitable mask (*see* Table 5.23) but if patients are exhausted then IPPV may be used. The techniques of oxygen therapy are discussed on pp. 291–294.

Other drugs

A number of **fixed drug combinations** (e.g. a non-selective sympathomimetic agent plus a methylxanthine) were used before effective asthma treatments became available, and some of these are still marketed. Most are oral formulations which are not now prescribed in the UK, but if older patients who are already using them find that they give adequate relief there is no reason to interfere with that situation.

Non-selective bronchodilators are rarely prescribed for asthma treatment because of their undesirable cardiovascular effects. Bronchodilators combined with sedatives should be avoided because they may cause respiratory depression in patients whose ventilatory function is already compromised.

Respiratory stimulants (*doxapram*, *etamivan*, *nikethamide*) are generally of no value in asthma and may be harmful: they should be used only under expert supervision in hospital. In situations where they might be considered to be necessary artificial ventilation is preferred, but they may have a limited role in community practice to support a patient while awaiting transport to a remote hospital.

Antihistamines (H_1-blockers) are not useful in asthma and do not prevent histamine-induced bronchospasm in normal dosage. However, some of the newer H_1-blockers, e.g. *azelastine* and *cetirizine*, have interesting anti-inflammatory properties, including effects on kinin, leukotriene and prostaglandin production, and may be the precursors of new anti-asthma drugs.

Many **investigational drugs** are being explored, e.g. alpha-adrenergic receptor antagonists, inhibitors of lipocortin and prostaglandins (E series), and potassium channel activators (e.g. *cromakalim*). Intense research activity is also directed towards other methods of modifying LT activity (over 10 000 papers in 15 years). Inhibitors of 5-lipoxygenase prevent the conversion of arachidonic acid to LTB_4 and the cysteinyl LTs (C_4, D_4 and E_4). Thus, future progress is likely to be in the more specific control of bronchial inflammation and hyper-reactivity. For the present, the beta$_2$-agonists and corticosteroids have a central role in management.

Other allergic lung diseases

Bronchopulmonary aspergillosis

Spores of the mould *Aspergillus fumigatus* are ubiquitous and sometimes cause infections or allergy, resulting in asthmatic attacks, COPD, bronchiectasis and fibrosis. Other species of *Aspergillus* are occasionally involved.

Extrinsic allergic alveolitis

Although this is a restrictive disease (not obstructive, *see* p. 225), it is convenient to include it here. A variety of environmental or occupation allergens may cause Type III hypersensitivity reactions which affect the lung parenchyma (Table 5.16). Following an initial

Table 5.16   Some types of extrinsic allergic alveolitis

Disease	Allergen
Farmer's lung Mushroom worker's lung Bagassosis	Spores of thermophilic actinomycetes from mouldy hay, mushroom compost, etc.
Bird fancier's lung	Avian antigens from feathers, excreta, etc. of pigeons, parrots, budgerigars, chickens
Grain handler's disease	Dust derived from the grain
Malt worker's lung	Spores of *Aspergillus* spp. in mouldy barley or malt

exposure to these antigens subsequent exposure may produce a transient mild asthmatic type attack followed after 4–6 h by a 24-h episode of cough and dyspnoea with fever, chills, headache, etc. With repeated exposure, pulmonary fibrosis and a diffusion defect occur and pulmonary function tests then show marked respiratory restriction. Diagnosis is complicated by the interval between exposure and the onset of symptoms so that the connection between them is often not made.

Pulmonary eosinophilia

This term includes a number of conditions in which dyspnoea and radiologically identified lung changes occur, together with a very high blood eosinophil count. Asthmatic attacks may also occur. Cases may be due to aspergillosis, drugs (e.g. sulphonamides), intestinal or other parasites and, rarely, polyarteritis nodosa (*see* Chapter 8).

Management

This involves treatment of any infection, antigen avoidance and the use of corticosteroids to minimize inflammatory lung changes.

Chronic obstructive pulmonary disease (COPD)

Introduction

COPD (also known as chronic obstructive lung disease, COLD) is the collective term for a number of chronic, slowly progressive conditions, most of which are either caused by tobacco smoking or are aggravated by it. The conditions produce widespread, persistent airways obstruction which is fixed (largely irreversible) but somewhat amenable to inhaled bronchodilator and corticosteroid therapy. The conditions are the result of chronic inflammation and recurrent infection of the airways, and cause dyspnoea and abnormal blood gas levels. The underlying condition is usually chronic bronchitis or emphysema (or a combination of these) but chronic

asthma may also present similarly. Bronchiectasis and cystic fibrosis are less common causes.

Definitions

Members of this group of diseases may occur together. The British Thoracic Society defines COPD as follows:

> COPD is a chronic, slowly progressive disorder characterised by airways obstruction (FEV_1 <80% predicted and FEV_1/FVC ratio <70%) which does not change markedly over several months. The impairment of lung function is largely fixed but is partially reversible by bronchodilator (or other) therapy.

- **Bronchitis**, the principal disease concerned, is inflammation of the larger airways and may be acute or chronic.
- **Acute bronchitis** is occasionally caused by the inhalation of irritants but is usually due to viral infection accompanied by opportunist bacterial infections (*see* Chapter 13). The outstanding symptom is cough, initially dry, but becoming productive. Young children may have a very severe, harsh cough with inspiratory stridor, the condition known as **croup**. Inflammation of the lower airways (bronchiolitis) may also occur in infants, but this should settle in 3–4 days, though the cough may persist for 2–3 weeks. Acute respiratory distress in young children should always be taken very seriously.
- **Chronic bronchitis** (CB) is defined as a chronic cough with the production of sputum on most days for at least three consecutive months of the year in at least two successive years. This epidemiological, symptomatic definition enables patients to be classified for statistical purposes, but a lesser degree or duration of symptoms clearly indicates the early stages of the disease. It takes no account of airways obstruction, the principal problem for patients.
- **Emphysema** is permanent destructive enlargement of the airspaces distal to the terminal bronchioles, i.e. of the respiratory bronchioles, alveolar ducts and alveolar sacs and walls. This defines a pathological lesion,

not a clinical syndrome, which may occur as a separate entity but often accompanies chronic bronchitis.

Chronic bronchitis

Epidemiology and natural history

The overall prevalence of CB is much higher in the UK than in most other countries, being about 4% in men aged about 50 years, 9% at 60 years, 12% at 80 years, and 3% in women. It is known as the 'English disease' – a consequence of being the first intensively industrialized country at a time when the health hazards of environmental and occupational pollution were not appreciated.

The sex difference is wholly attributable to differences in smoking habits: in fact, it increases with advancing age because of the cumulative effects of long-term smoking in men. However, changes in smoking habits over the past 40 years, with an increasing proportion of girls and young women smoking cigarettes, may be expected to change this pattern. These prevalence rates are about three times that for angina pectoris.

CB is responsible for considerable morbidity and time off work, and causes about 20 000 deaths annually in the UK (male : female ratio about 5). Almost 30% of these deaths occur before retirement, though the death rate is declining with reduced smoking in men, less air pollution and better treatment.

The disease is characterized by an insidious onset starting with a 'smoker's cough' which is usually disregarded. Significant symptoms may not appear until after some 20 years or more of smoking, by which time there is appreciable irreversible lung damage. There is then a progressive decline over about 10–40 years with increasing dyspnoea, exercise limitation, difficulty in expectoration and an increased frequency of alarming, acute infectious exacerbations and hospital admissions. Occasionally, an acute respiratory infection is identified as the trigger for the initial onset of overt symptoms.

The prognosis is related to the degree of exercise limitation: about 40% of patients with significantly reduced walking ability on the flat die within 5 years, usually of heart failure.

Aetiology and histopathology

The disease is multifactorial in origin, but prolonged bronchial irritation and insult is the major contributor. The prime cause is **cigarette smoking**, and almost all clinical parameters, e.g. symptoms, work lost, hospital admissions and deaths, correlate with the extent of smoking. The death rate from COPD is increased about tenfold for each 15 cigarettes which have been smoked daily and regularly in the past. **Environmental pollution** and some occupations (e.g. coal mining) potentiate the effect of smoking, and the effects of urbanization are very marked in smokers. However, urban pollution has only very small effects in non-smokers unless it is extreme.

Climate plays a minor role, though morbidity is higher in the colder and wetter regions in the North and West of the UK, after allowing for the effects of urbanization. In Australia and New Zealand the age–mortality curve is displaced relative to that for the UK to higher age groups by about 10–15 years. This shift is due primarily to less urban pollution and differences in smoking habits. Also, the risk of severe respiratory infections is lower in the better climate.

A **low socioeconomic status** predisposes to both morbidity and mortality. The mortality in Class V (unskilled) is six times that in Class II (administrative). This is related to differences in smoking habits, hygiene, nutrition and attitudes towards achieving a healthy lifestyle. Educational and cultural differences lead to a lack of awareness in the lower socioeconomic groups of the importance of symptoms, the need for medical care and the facilities available.

There may be a slight familial tendency predisposing to bronchial mucus hypersecretion, but this is heavily outweighed by the effects of the risk factors outlined above. Respiratory infections have little or no role in causation, though they produce the severe exacerbations seen in the winter months and contribute significantly to the progressive lung damage.

The histological appearance of the lung tissues in COPD is illustrated in Figs. 5.18 and 5.19.

The outstanding features in chronic bronchitis leading to airways obstruction include the following:

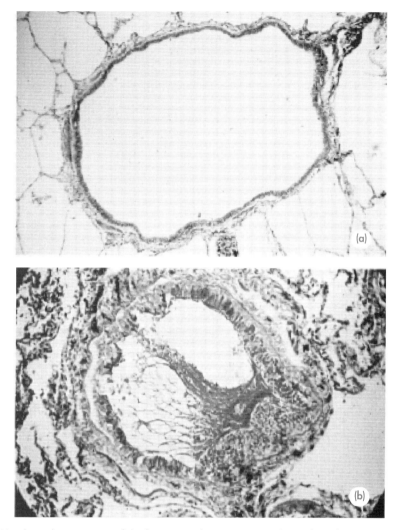

Figure 5.18   Histological appearance of the lung parenchyma in severe chronic bronchitis. (a) Normal: note the thin-walled, unobstructed bronchiole surrounded by well-defined, very thin-walled alveoli. Blood vessels, lymphatics, etc. are attached to the bronchiolar wall (top right and left side). (b) Chronic bronchitis, showing a thickened, inflamed mucosa, partial mucus plugging of the bronchiole, and distortion and destruction of the alveolar walls (emphysema). The mottled appearance of the tissues is largely from leucocytic (inflammatory cell) infiltration. (Reproduced with permission from Reid LM, p. 1253 in Fishman AP (1988) *Pulmonary Diseases and Disorders*, 2nd edn. New York: McGraw-Hill [Fig. 77-7 (c) and (e)]).

- Increased thickness of the bronchiolar lining from inflammation and hyperplasia of the mucous glands. The latter represent about two-thirds of the bulk of the increased tissue mass compared with the normal one-third (Fig. 5.19).
- Massive hypersecretion of mucus from the increased number of mucous glands and from irritated goblet cells.
- Impaired mucociliary clearance (chronic insult damages the cilia), so that mucus plugs the airways partially or completely.
- Numerous mucus-containing inflammatory cells (Fig. 5.18(b)) and trapped bacteria, the latter producing the infective exacerbations.
- A modest, variable degree of bronchoconstriction.

In late-stage disease there is extensive destruction of the lung parenchyma (i.e. emphysema).

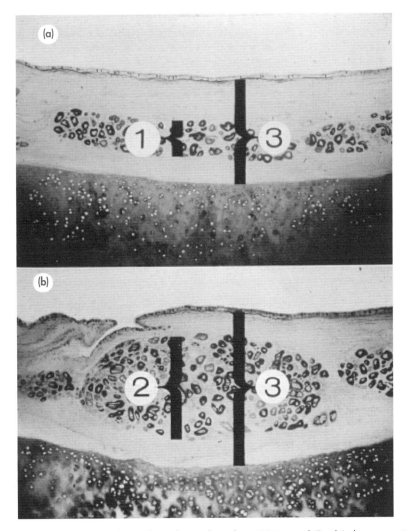

Figure 5.19 Histology of the bronchiolar wall in chronic bronchitis. (a) Normal (Reid Index approximately 0.3). (b) Chronic bronchitis (Reid Index approximately 0.7). Numbers in circles indicate one-third and two-thirds relationships. The Reid Index is the ratio of the thickness of the mucous gland layer to the total mucosal thickness. (Reproduced with permission of the editors of *Update*.)

Fibrosis contributes to obstruction, reduces lung compliance, increases the work of breathing and exacerbates dyspnoea, especially during passive expiration.

Clinical features

The **cardinal early symptoms** are as follows:

- *'Smoker's cough'*: initially present on winter mornings, but later throughout the year.
- *Sputum*: usually copious and tenacious (mucoid). It may be yellow, green or khaki-coloured during infective exacerbations (**mucopurulent**), but white or greyish between the infective episodes and occasionally streaked with blood.
- *Dyspnoea*: as with all obstructive airways diseases expiration is the difficult phase, the spirogram being similar to that shown in Fig. 5.15(b). Wheezing may occur, especially in the morning.
- *Fever* and the usual signs of infection during exacerbations.

In **mild disease** cough may be the only abnormality. Patients with **moderate disease** may also have sputum, breathlessness, with or without wheezing, and a general reduction in breath sounds on auscultation. In **late-stage disease** there is usually breathlessness at rest or on any exertion, together with a prominent wheeze and cough, plus the following features:

- *Cyanosis*: if the respiratory deficit is severe (frank cyanosis is discernible when there is about 5 g/dL of deoxygenated haemoglobin in the blood, i.e. about 30% of the total Hb, the P_aO_2 being about 6 kPa (normal = 12–13.3 kPa)).
- *Heart failure* (cor pulmonale, *see* p. 228) and *peripheral oedema*.
- *Plethoric complexion*: patients may have a high facial colour due to **polycythaemia** (erythrocytosis, a raised red cell count), a normal physiological response which increases the oxygen-carrying capacity of the blood. The resultant increased blood viscosity causes dilatation of the skin capillaries which are filled with blood containing excessive haemoglobin, thus causing the high colour.
- *Hyperinflation*: a consequence of air trapping.

At the extremes, two clinical patterns may be seen in patients. Type A ('**pink puffer**', the 'emphysemic type') is a thin, usually elderly patient with intense dyspnoea, pursed lip breathing, rapid shallow respiration and use of the accessory muscles of respiration. These patients produce little sputum but have severe airways obstruction with hyperinflation and evidence of emphysema. They have good respiratory drive and maintain near-normal blood gas levels at the expense of dyspnoea. Their thinness may reflect weight loss due to the energy required to maintain adequate ventilation.

At the other extreme, the Type B patient ('**blue bloater**', the 'bronchitic' type) is obese, has a plethoric complexion and moderate dyspnoea, lapsing readily into heart failure and presenting a picture of poor respiratory drive. Type B patients adjust to their abnormal blood gases at the expense of poor exercise tolerance, but do not experience dyspnoea at rest. There are considerable degrees of overlap between these patient groups, and their different appearances cannot be used diagnostically as most patients show elements of both types. The reasons for the occurrence of the two physical types are not clear, but may represent differences in ventilatory control.

Investigations

Pulmonary function tests.   These show the characteristic changes outlined in Table 5.5. If peak flow testing is used, serial recordings should be made over a week to show the absence of variability. The residual volume may be normal or, later on, somewhat increased by air trapping and destruction of lung tissue.

A trial of response to bronchodilator treatment is carried out using a nebulizer (p. 285) or an MDI with a large-volume spacer (p. 281 and pp. 283–284) to ensure that the dose is inhaled. The British Thoracic Society recommended protocol is to measure FEV_1 and FVC (PEF is less desirable) before:

- 2.5–5 mg salbutamol or 5–10 mg terbutaline by nebulizer and 15 min afterwards.
- 500 microgram ipratropium bromide and 30 min afterwards.
- Both in combination and 30 min afterwards.

The post-bronchodilator FEV_1 is an indicator of prognosis.

Breathlessness.   This is assessed by the ability to perform specific tasks, e.g. stair climbing, walking distance, or to manage the tasks of everyday living, e.g. shopping.

Blood gases.   These may be near-normal until the later stages of the disease. The P_aO_2 becomes reduced gradually and this effect becomes more severe during sleep, when patients may snore heavily and show 'sleep apnoea' (periods of failure to breathe during sleep). Although the P_aCO_2 is usually normal in the early stages, severely impaired respiratory drive may cause the P_aCO_2 to rise progressively later on, when patients may be in chronic respiratory failure (p. 279).

Chest X-ray.   This is usually normal, though in the later stages the heart may be enlarged and there may be evidence of emphysema and fibrosis.

Sputum microbiology.   This may be performed routinely in hospital. Most infections in chronic bronchitis are due to *Haemophilus influenzae*, *Streptococcus pneumoniae* and viruses, so community treatment is usually initiated on a 'best guess' basis. This may compromise subsequent sputum investigation even though the patient continues to produce purulent sputum. A sputum sample should always be taken **before** initiating antibiotic treatment, following usual good practice.

The management of CB will be discussed with that of emphysema on pp. 269–272.

Emphysema

When this occurs in association with CB (p. 263) it affects the alveoli closest to the respiratory bronchioles. Emphysema not associated with CB is uncommon and is more generalized: these patients usually show the clinical pattern of the 'pink puffer' group (p. 266).

Aetiology and pathology

The **aetiology** of emphysema is illustrated in Fig. 5.20. The principal underlying problem is reduced alpha$_1$-antitrypsin (AT) activity. This enzyme is a highly polymorphic glycoprotein produced by the liver and alveolar macrophages. In the lungs, the function of the enzyme is to protect the delicate alveolar tissue from autodigestion by elastase and other proteolytic enzymes that are produced to clear accumulated debris. Smoking produces both increased amounts of cell debris and reduced AT levels, and may also cause lung parenchymal damage by other mechanisms.

Hereditary AT deficiency is a rare autosomal recessive trait, which may be heterozygous or homozygous. AT is encoded for by the *Pi* gene on chromosome 14, of which more than 90 alleles are known. Disease is associated only with those mutations causing deficiency or greatly impaired function of the enzyme. These gene defects occur in between 1/2000–1/7000 European neonates and are the most common cause of liver disease in infancy and childhood. However, some further unknown genetic or environmental trigger is required because, although more than 50% of infants with total AT deficiency have abnormal liver function tests, only about 13% develop overt liver disease, usually by the age of 4 months. About 5% of these require liver transplantation by the age of 4 years, but the

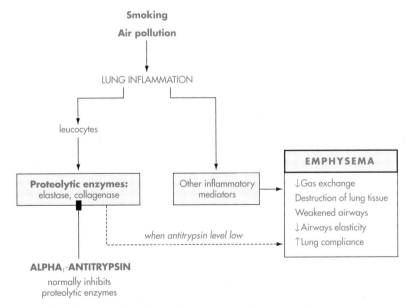

Figure 5.20   Aetiology of emphysema. The disease is characterized by proteolytic damage causing anatomical and physiological abnormalities. Normality gives normal alpha$_1$-antitrypsin levels and tissue and physiological integrity.

condition settles in the remainder, with a reasonable quality of life. Some 10% of the group suffer from malabsorption of vitamin K and the resultant **kernicterus** (bilirubin encephalopathy) causes permanent CNS damage if not treated early. A further 1–2% without any history of infantile jaundice present later in childhood or as adults with liver cirrhosis (*see* Chapter 6). Some develop emphysema as young adults. It seems likely that these various manifestations are associated with different alleles of the *Pi* gene. Symptoms are twice as common in males as in females.

The symptoms of emphysema are accelerated by environmental factors, especially smoking. Most emphysemics are smokers in whom the resultant chronic inflammation damages the alveoli rather than the airways, as in CB. However, there is considerable overlap between emphysema and CB.

Because there is destruction of lung tissue (Fig. 5.21) the TLC is increased, at the expense of an increased (unusable) RV, reducing the area available for gas exchange. The residual alveolar walls become thickened and fibrosed (Fig. 5.18(b)), thus limiting oxygen transfer.

Diagnosis

Correct diagnosis of emphysema rests on the evidence of obstructive lung disease associated with characteristic radiographical changes, though the latter are not always present. Obstruction results from weakened, narrowed, small (2-mm diameter) airways which tend to collapse on expiration (p. 221), owing both to inflammation and atrophy of their walls and the destruction of supporting alveolar tissue. Alveolar destruction also results in the loss of elastic tissue which provides an important proportion of the expiratory force. A definitive diagnosis may not be made during life and is often reached on inadequate evidence. Although a definitive diagnosis is possible by bronchoscopic biopsy, this is rarely done

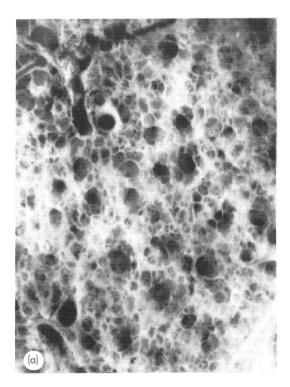 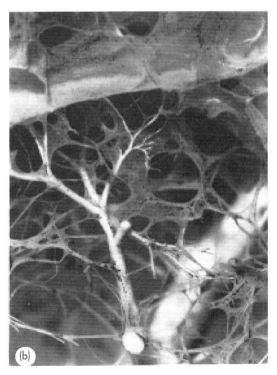

Figure 5.21   Low-power microscopic appearance of normal and emphysemic lungs. (a) Normal. (b) Emphysema showing tissue destruction and the production of enlarged air spaces, giving an increased total lung capacity. (Reproduced with permission from Heard BE (1958) *Thorax* **13**: 136.)

because it does not influence management. Because the damage is irreversible, treatment is symptomatic.

Management of COPD

Because most patients have a combination of emphysema and CB, their treatment is based on similar principles. There is unlikely to be a significant reversible element.

Aims

The aims of management of COPD are:

- To educate the patient about their disease and prognosis.
- To prevent deterioration.
- To minimize the frequency and severity of exacerbations and complications.
- To give the best possible symptomatic relief.
- To achieve a reasonable quality of life.

The ways in which these are achieved are discussed below, and summarized in Table 5.17.

General measures

General measures in the management of COPD include the following:

- *Education* is essential to any programme of rehabilitation. In a chronic condition such as COPD, patients need to understand the relevance of the general and pharmacotherapeutic measures and appreciate what is reasonable to expect from management.
- *Stop smoking*: this may reduce the risk of further deterioration substantially, and the patient may improve somewhat. In long-standing disease, significant improvement is not a realistic objective because irreversible damage may mean that the patient's lung function does not improve, merely that the decline is slowed or arrested.

Table 5.17   General approach to the management of target features in chronic bronchitis

Aim	Target feature	Management mode
Prevent deterioration	Bronchiolar irritation and inflammation	Stop smoking Avoid irritant and dusty environments Corticosteroids
Improve respiratory function	Poor ventilation Bronchoconstriction?	Physiotherapy Beta$_2$-agonist bronchodilator?[a] Antimuscarinic bronchodilator? Theophylline bronchodilator?
Symptomatic relief	Dyspnoea Excessive sputum Troublesome night cough	Oxygen Physiotherapy, inhalations Expectorants/mucolytics? Antitussives?
Treat exacerbations and complications	Infections Heart failure	Prompt antibiotics, influenza vaccination Reduce weight if obese Diuretics or vasodilators Digoxin if fibrillating Venesection
Improve quality of life	Poor mobility	Oxygen Occupational therapy Home improvements, social support

[a] These and any other potentially useful medicines (marked ?) should be tested objectively for benefit.

? = possible feature or potentially useful medication.

- *Avoid irritant and dusty environments.*
- *Weight loss* if obese to reduce the oxygen demand and the workload on the heart. **Healthy eating** should be encouraged and a planned **exercise** programme helps to improve cardiac and respiratory function.
- *Physiotherapy* to improve the use of what respiratory function remains and to teach **postural drainage**. For the latter the patient lies face down and on each side in turn, their chest wall, ribs and backs are percussed to help dislodge secretions. If secretions are very copious, a head-down position may help.
- *Occupational therapy* (aids in the home, etc.) and *social support*, e.g. more appropriate housing, transport to day care centres, may help severely exercise-limited patients to enjoy a reasonable quality of life.
- *Prophylactic influenza vaccination* annually in the autumn is recommended for all patients with chronic respiratory disease, regardless of age.

Pharmacotherapy

The British Thoracic Society guidelines (Table 5.18) set out the treatment of COPD according to the degree of impairment of respiratory function as assessed by FEV_1 (p. 231).

There may be an element of reversibility of airways obstruction, so *bronchodilators* are the cornerstone of therapy. However, the *antimuscarinic* and *corticosteroid* treatments used in asthma should be given a controlled trial. The drugs should be introduced singly at first, with respirometric or careful peak flow monitoring, to ensure that there is objective improvement (FEV_1 increased by 200 mL **and** 15% of baseline), and discontinued if ineffective. However, the patient's perception of their well-being

Table 5.18 Management of chronic obstructive pulmonary disease

Disease level	Symptoms and signs	Pharmacotherapy	Other considerations
Mild (FEV_1 60–80%)[a]	Currently asymptomatic 'Smoker's cough' Little or no breathlessness	Nil Beta$_2$-agonist as required OR antimuscarinic (depends on response)	Stop smoking Optimize inhaler technique
	Infective exacerbations	Antibiotics	All treatments subject to subjective ± objective benefit as guide
Moderate (FEV_1 40–59%)	Breathless on moderate exertion Wheeze Cough ± sputum Abnormal breath sounds	Beta$_2$-agonist as required (if responsive) Change to, or add, antimuscarinic bronchodilator if poor response	As above plus: Use large-volume spacer Long-acting beta$_2$-agonist only if clearly beneficial
	Infective exacerbations	Antibiotics	
Severe (FEV_1 <40%)	Breathless at rest or any exertion	Beta$_2$-agonist + antimuscarinic Assess for home nebulizer	Oral theophylline if tolerated and other bronchodilators not beneficial
	Prominent wheeze and cough Cyanosis Peripheral oedema and polycythaemia	Trial of corticosteroids Oxygen (if beneficial) Treat for heart failure: diuretics, etc. (see Chapter 3) Venesection	Objective proof of benefit
	Infective exacerbations	Antibiotics	

[a] FEV_1, percentage of predicted value.
Based on the British Thoracic Society (1997) BTS Guidelines for the management of chronic obstructive pulmonary disease. *Thorax* **52**: Suppl. 5.
Reproduced with permission of BMJ Specialist Journals.

should also be considered. Even a modest improvement in pulmonary function may give an apparently disproportionate symptomatic relief in a severely compromised patient, because a small increase in P_aO_2 greatly improves haemoglobin (Hb) saturation.

Some studies have shown that the antimuscarinic bronchodilators may be more effective than the beta-agonists in these patients.

A trial of *corticosteroids* is always warranted, especially in severe disease. Patients are assessed on the basis of a 15% (or 200 mL) improvement in baseline FEV_1 after a 14-day course of oral *prednisolone* (30 mg/day). If a positive response is obtained (about 20% of cases), an inhaled or oral steroid should be used: lack of such improvement requires discontinuation. Although it has been alleged that corticosteroids are grossly overused in COPD, in a careful study of nearly 1000 patients, inhaled *fluticasone* was found to reduce the decline in lung function (FEV_1) by 32% over the 3-year trial period and the exacerbation rate by 25%. Thus, the role of corticosteroid therapy in COPD has not yet been fully defined.

It is important to remember that in any trial of drugs for COPD – especially steroids – that a substantial response raises the possibility that some patients diagnosed as having COPD have either chronic asthma or asthma concurrent with COPD. Oral corticosteroids are also euphoriant in most patients, so they feel well despite the underlying disease state, and it may be difficult to wean them from the drug. However, a small proportion of patients feel anxious and depressed.

Although acute exacerbations of COPD are due to infections, the immunosuppressant action of steroids does not appear to compromise bronchitic patients.

Oxygen may be used for 15 h daily or more to improve mobility and relieve dyspnoea. In hospital, IPPV (p. 293) may be used to assist respiration. However, the oxygen concentration must be carefully controlled because patients become unresponsive to chronically raised carbon dioxide levels and depend on hypoxic drive to maintain ventilation. If the P_aO_2 is raised excessively the patient may then stop breathing: the aim is to improve the P_aO_2 somewhat, producing a significant increase in Hb saturation, without unduly increasing P_aCO_2 or exacerbating respiratory acidosis and without impairing respiratory drive. The patient's clinical condition and arterial blood gases must be monitored carefully, and the oxygen flow rate adjusted to give optimal oxygenation. However, such careful monitoring is not possible in a community setting, where the oxygen flow rate should not exceed 4 L/min, to give a maximum concentration of 28% in the inspired air with a suitable mask (p. 292). Even 24% oxygen may be excessive for some patients, so oxygen therapy should be initiated cautiously under careful supervision.

Evidence from two large trials indicates that continuous prophylactic oxygen used for at least 15 h/day in appropriately selected patients doubles the 5-year survival rate, so in the late stages of the disease, or if a patient has cor pulmonale or is in demonstrable respiratory failure, *long-term oxygen therapy* (>15 h/day) may be used. Oxygen therapy is discussed more fully on pp. 291–294.

Heart failure (cor pulmonale, p. 228) should be treated (*see also* Chapter 3). **Venesection** (removing 500–1000 mL of blood) may be used if polycythaemia causes such an increase in blood viscosity that cardiac function is compromised. *Oxygen* prevents progression of pulmonary hypertension and is the mainstay of therapy. A *diuretic* is indicated if there is peripheral oedema and a raised jugular venous pressure (JVP). Pulmonary vasodilatation with a *beta$_2$-agonist*, *calcium-channel blocker* or *alpha-adrenergic blocker* may also be helpful.

Respiratory acidosis consequent on hypercapnia must be treated promptly (*see* Chapter 4).

Steam inhalations may assist expectoration, but '**expectorants**' and **mucolytics** have not been demonstrated objectively to be useful, though some patients obtain subjective relief. There is no evidence that any drug can materially assist expectoration, so they are primarily placebos. *Cough suppressants* should not normally be used because, although effective, they may cause respiratory depression. However, a few patients have a troublesome unproductive night cough and this may need to be controlled.

Acute exacerbations

In such situations, either a bronchodilator may be added, or the dose may be increased after first checking the technique (*see* Table 5.22).

Infections should be treated aggressively at the first signs, but it is important to take a sputum sample for laboratory analysis before starting blind treatment because a significant proportion of the bacterial strains are antibiotic-resistant. However, antibiotics are effective only if two or all of the following are present:

- Increased sputum volume.
- Increasing breathlessness.
- Purulent sputum.

Broad-spectrum antibiotics for blind treatment, e.g. *ampicillin*, *trimethoprim*, *tetracyclines* or oral *cephalosporins*, are chosen on the basis of **local sensitivity data**. They are those usually active against the most likely bacterial pathogens (often pneumococci, *Haemophilus influenzae* or *Moraxella catarrhalis*). *Ciprofloxacin* is present in high concentrations in bronchial secretions, but the benefit of this is not clear. Ciprofloxacin has limited activity against pneumococci and numerous side effects and is not an appropriate first-line treatment.

Intelligent patients whose microbial status is well established can have a reserve supply of antibiotics available to start on their own initiative when they notice the first signs which trigger a deterioration in their condition. However, they should subsequently see their doctor as soon as possible. A few patients benefit from continuous antibiotic prophylaxis throughout the winter months, but the evidence for this is equivocal.

Oral corticosteroids, e.g. 30 mg/day *prednisolone* for 1 week, may be appropriate if the patient is known to respond to it or is already being maintained on lower doses, if there is no response to a bronchodilator or if this is the first presentation of increased airflow obstruction.

Oxygen therapy (pp. 291–294) may be required. **Respiratory failure** may need to be managed with IPPV or NIPPV (p. 293). **Respiratory stimulants** are used occasionally (e.g. *doxapram*, only in hospital) to tide patients over a bout of hypoventilation while other treatments are pursued.

When the patient has recovered sufficiently a full medication review should be undertaken. If hospital treatment was required there should also be detailed consideration of social and financial circumstances when planning for discharge.

Pure emphysema uncomplicated by an appreciable element of CB is uncommon, and patients primarily require *oxygen* because they are very breathless. *Oxygen therapy* will depend on the condition of the patient and the 'pink puffer' type, with relatively normal blood gases, will tolerate higher oxygen concentrations than those with a poor respiratory drive and hypercapnia ($P_a CO_2$ >9 kPa). Management is otherwise as for CB.

Rarely, surgical eradication of giant bullae (air spaces) in the lungs may relieve symptoms by relieving the compression of surrounding lung tissue.

Natural *alpha$_1$-antitrypsin* prepared from pooled plasma is available in the USA. Other experimental treatments for the replacement of AT are being explored, and gene therapy may become feasible in the future.

Bronchiectasis

Definition and epidemiology

This is abnormal dilatation of the bronchi, their walls becoming inflamed, thickened and irreversibly damaged. This may follow pneumonia or other severe bacterial lower respiratory tract infection, which may start in childhood as a sequel to measles or whooping cough. There is impaired mucociliary clearance, and chronic local inflammation and recurrent pyogenic infections cause massive mucus hypersecretion and airways obstruction.

Trapping of pus in the airways may also occur in **cystic fibrosis** and bronchial carcinoma and may cause similar damage. Bronchiectasis may also accompany chronic bronchitis and, occasionally, asthma.

The disease is much less common in developed countries, now that effective antibiotics are available, cystic fibrosis being the most common cause. Bronchiectasis persists in the Third World and in areas where natural disasters or wars disrupt social and political structures and medical services.

Clinical features

These vary greatly, depending on the severity of the disease, but the principal features include:

- Chronic cough, often productive of copious purulent sputum.
- A variable degree of haemoptysis.
- Breathlessness.
- Febrile episodes associated with infection, sometimes pneumonia.
- Anorexia and weight loss.
- Night sweats.
- Finger clubbing in the later stages if there is persistent infection.
- Immunodeficiency in about 10% of patients.

Investigation

Investigations of bronchiectasis include:

- Chest and sinus X-rays.
- High-resolution CT scanning.
- Sputum culture and antibiotic sensitivity testing.
- Serum immunoglobulins.

Occasionally bronchoscopy, sweat sodium levels (increased in cystic fibrosis) and a test for mucociliary clearance are also required.

Management

The aims of management are to improve respiratory function and prevent deterioration by eradicating infection, if possible. Treatment includes:

- **Postural drainage** of sputum (p. 270) and bronchodilators to improve airflow.
- **Corticosteroids** (inhaled or oral), to reduce inflammation and slow disease progression.
- **Antibiotics**: *cefaclor* or *ciprofloxacin* in mild cases, *flucloxacillin* if *Staphylococcus aureus* is isolated, other IV or inhaled drugs according to sensitivity, especially for *Pseudomonas aeruginosa*.
- **Heart/lung transplantation** in rare cases.

Restrictive lung disease (RLD)

In RLD the problem is an inability to expand the lungs normally, even though the airways are unobstructed. There are many diverse causes, some of which are given in Table 5.19.

Because of this diverse aetiology, treatment of RLD is often symptomatic rather than specific because by the time symptoms occur the pathological changes may be irreversible. Infections should be treated and any precipitating factors avoided as far as possible. There is clearly no effective way of treating thoracic cage deformity once it is established, though physiotherapy and surgery as soon as the problem is perceived may do much to help. Physiotherapy may also enable patients to make the best use of their limited ventilatory function.

However, some forms of RLD, e.g. Wegener's granulomatosis (WG) (*see* Chapter 8, p. 519 and Table 8.18), are eminently treatable, so it is important to reach a definitive diagnosis. Treatment of WG usually involves *corticosteroids* and *cytotoxic* drugs.

Diseases of the pulmonary circulation

Pulmonary embolism

Aetiology, epidemiology and pathology

This important, often preventable, condition has a 10% fatality rate. Pulmonary embolism usually results from thrombi in the systemic veins, usually the pelvic, abdominal and leg veins, but 10% of cases are cardiac in origin. The latter are due to right atrial fibrillation causing right atrial thrombosis or to right ventricular or septal infarction and resultant right ventricular thrombosis. Clot fragments break away and travel through the veins, which widen progressively, then through the heart and eventually become trapped in the pulmonary circulation where the vessels begin to narrow.

The factors predisposing to venous thrombosis are dealt with in Chapter 3.

Whenever there is a risk of a **deep vein thrombosis** (DVT), prophylactic measures should be taken. Thus low-dose heparin is appropriate after surgery and there should be passive exercising during a period of bed rest, with early mobilization. Low-molecular weight heparin is preferred and may be combined with rhythmic external compression applied to the legs. Elastic stockings are also used, but are less effective.

Table 5.19   Some causes of restrictive lung disease

Cause or disease	Examples, comments
Diseases causing diffuse pulmonary fibrosis	
Cryptogenic fibrosing alveolitis	Aetiology unknown. Occurs in late middle age with destruction of lung tissue
Rheumatoid and collagen-vascular diseases (*see* Chapter 8)	Rheumatoid arthritis, systemic sclerosis, systemic lupus erythematosus (SLE)
Iatrogenic[a]	Cytotoxic drugs: bleomycin, busulfan, cyclophosphamide, Ganglion-blocking agents: hexamethonium, mecamylamine, pentolinium Methysergide Nitrofurantoin Oxygen (>50%) Sulphonamides, sulfasalazine Radiotherapy Drugs inducing SLE (*see* Chapter 8, Table 8.22)
Occupational	Asbestosis, pneumoconiosis (miner's lung), silicosis, siderosis (iron, iron ores: also occurs if there is chronic alveolar bleeding)
Sarcoidosis	A Type IV (delayed) hypersensitivity reaction to an unidentified agent, causing granulomatous changes
Toxins	Paraquat weedkiller
Thoracic cage deformity	
Congenital	Severe kyphoscoliosis, tuberculosis
Rheumatoid	Ankylosing spondylitis
Pleural disease	
Fibrosis	Asbestos, methysergide
Effusion	Heart failure, infections (pneumonia, tuberculosis), malignancy, lymphatic disease

[a] This list of drugs is merely illustrative, not exhaustive. The effects may depend on dose level, accumulated dose, duration of treatment, etc. and may be reversible.

After embolism, lung tissue is ventilated but not perfused leading, after some hours, to failure of surfactant production and alveolar collapse. Lung tissue often does not infarct because it obtains sufficient oxygen by diffusion from the airways and the bronchial circulation.

Clinical features

The presentation will depend largely on the size and site of the embolus.

Small to medium emboli
These usually present with severe pleuritic chest pain, cough with bloody sputum and fever. Breath-lessness and hyperventilation are common but may be absent. Recurrence is unlikely, but any lung damage which may have occurred is irreversible.

Massive pulmonary embolus
This produces a precipitous fall in cardiac output so the patient will be shocked, pale and cyanosed, with marked tachypnoea and a raised JVP. Severe central chest pain occurs, due to cardiac ischaemia. There is a 30% fatality rate, sometimes immediate.

Repeated small emboli
These slowly produce progressive breathlessness and hyperventilation. Patients will become exercise-limited and may have angina pectoris (*see*

Chapter 3) owing to widespread restriction of pulmonary perfusion and consequent severe limitation of the coronary circulation. They may also faint on exercise in the later stages when they will also be chronically tired. Investigation will show the ECG changes associated with right ventricular hypertrophy and evidence of pulmonary hypertension. The condition is progressive.

Diagnosis

Small to medium emboli

The extent of obstruction of the pulmonary circulation may be determined using *Technetium* (*^{99m}Tc*) *Macrosalb Injection* (equivalents are Albumin Aggregated Injection [USP] and the Microspheres Injection [Eur. P]) for **radioisotope scanning**. The labelled particles lodge throughout the lung capillaries and so will show unperfused (non-radioactive) areas in which the circulation is blocked by an embolus when the chest is scanned with a gamma camera. This is preferably combined with a ^{133}Xe ventilation scintigram, the two investigations (**V/Q scan**) showing unperfused but ventilated areas.

CT angiography (spiral CT with venous contrast injection) or **MRI** have good specificity and sensitivity for medium-sized emboli. If **plasma D-dimer**, a breakdown product of fibrin, is not detected this positively excludes a pulmonary embolus. Raised erythrocyte sedimentation rate (ESR) and lactate dehydrogenase (LDH) levels indicate pulmonary infarction. The chest X-ray and ECG are usually normal. Ultrasound may be used to detect DVT.

Massive pulmonary embolus

The **ECG** exhibits characteristic changes. Ultrasound (**echocardiogram**) shows an actively contracting left ventricle (an attempt to restore adequate systemic circulation) and there may be a clot in the pulmonary trunk or a main pulmonary artery. Blood gas examination shows hypoxaemia and hypercapnia. **Pulmonary angiography** will locate emboli rapidly, but the technique is risky.

Repeated small emboli

Any of the tests described above may be done, especially CXR, ECG and V/Q scan, but may appear normal, so extensive investigations may be required.

Management

This includes:

- High-dose *oxygen*, unless the patients have COPD.
- *Analgesics* (opioids if necessary, taking care to avoid respiratory depression).
- Anticoagulants: *heparin*, to prevent further embolization, changing to *warfarin* after 48 h.

In the case of large emboli, management includes:

- Intensive care.
- Fibrinolytic therapy, e.g. *streptokinase* (by IV infusion over 24–72 h) or *alteplase* (bolus IV injection, then IV infusion over 90 min), may precede anticoagulation.
- **Surgical embolectomy** (clot removal, rarely) if cardiac function is severely impaired.

For repeated small emboli, management includes:

- *Anticoagulants;* these are continued for 3–6 months, but lifelong treatment may be necessary if there is a chronic thromboembolic disorder.
- *Antiplatelet drugs* (*see* Chapter 3, *aspirin, ticlopidine*; N.B. interactions with *warfarin*) may also be appropriate.

Pulmonary oedema

Clinical features and diagnosis

Pulmonary oedema can develop precipitately, e.g. as a sequel to myocardial infarction, and can be rapidly fatal. Acute pulmonary oedema is a medical emergency.

The condition is usually the result of increased pulmonary capillary pressure, due to left heart failure or mitral stenosis, which causes the accumulation of fluid in the normally minimal interstitial space of the lungs (*see* Fig. 5.1(d)). The increased vascular pressure compresses the bronchioles and reduces lung compliance, ventilation and perfusion. These changes are more marked

Table 5.20   Some precipitants of acute pulmonary oedema

Pulmonary	Large embolism
Cardiogenic[a]	Acute • arrhythmias • myocardial infarction • valvular regurgitation (aortic, mitral) • cardiac decompensation in chronic heart failure (non-compliance with medication)
Circulatory[a]	Hypervolaemia • pregnancy • excessive – infusion rate – sodium intake
Increased metabolic demand	Fever Excessive exercise Hyperthyroidism

[a] *See* Chapter 3.

initially in the lung bases because of the effect of gravity. If the condition persists, or occurs acutely, fluid eventually flows into the alveoli and the terminal bronchioles, producing severe dyspnoea. Some precipitants of acute pulmonary oedema are given in Table 5.20.

If the condition is of slow onset (pulmonary hypertension), the initial **symptoms and signs** are dyspnoea on exercise, then shortness of breath, cough, orthopnoea and paroxysmal nocturnal dyspnoea (PND) (*see* Chapter 3, p. 81 and p. 242). If symptoms are untreated, or if the onset is acute, these lead to extreme dyspnoea, tachypnoea, cyanosis, and coughing up of foamy, bloody sputum. Unsurprisingly, patients are extremely anxious and fearful.

Management

Pharmacotherapy of acute pulmonary oedema involves:

- An intravenous *loop diuretic* which sometimes produces a dramatic improvement (see below).
- High-concentration (60%), short-term *oxygen* to relieve dyspnoea.
- *Opioid analgesia* (*morphine* causes systemic venodilatation, reducing cardiac workload and tachypnoea, and is sedative and euphoric).

- *Vasodilators* to increase cardiac output.
- *Aminophylline*, given IV to control bronchospasm.
- Management of the underlying condition.

Diuretics have a dual action in this setting. In pulmonary oedema consequent on heart failure they reduce the blood volume and in turn the cardiac preload and cause vasodilatation, thus further reducing cardiac preload and also afterload. These combined actions improve cardiac function and reduce pulmonary venous pressure. If the condition is of renal origin, diuretics also reduce the hypervolaemia consequent on activation of the renin/aldosterone mechanism. Diuretics do not act directly to clear the oedema fluid which is cleared spontaneously when cardiac function improves and the pulmonary capillary pressure falls (*see* Chapter 3).

Treatment of pulmonary hypertension involves:

- Lowering pulmonary artery pressure, usually with a calcium channel antagonist, e.g. *nifedipine* or *diltiazem*.
- *Epoprostenol sodium*, by continuous IV infusion, as an antiplatelet agent and vasodilator.
- *Heparin* anticoagulation initially, followed by oral *warfarin*.
- Transplantation in otherwise suitable patients who fail to respond.

Respiratory infections

The general management of communicable diseases is discussed in Chapter 13 but some specific points are relevant here.

Pneumonia

Definition and aetiology

Pneumonia is a general term used to describe inflammation of the lung parenchyma. The disease is usually caused by any of a number of viruses and bacteria. In immunocompromised individuals tuberculosis, mycoplasmas, fungi and protozoa may also be implicated. However, inhalation of irritants (**inhalation pneumonitis**), including vomit, or severe allergic reactions can cause similar problems. Pneumonia is discussed more fully in Chapter 13.

Clinical features

These are very variable depending on the severity of the condition and the causative organism. There is an abrupt onset of malaise, fever and cough, often with some pleuritic pain. Tachypnoea and tachycardia are usually present, sometimes with dyspnoea and some cyanosis. Severe disease (respiratory rate 30/min, diastolic blood pressure 60 mmHg) may cause delirium, prostration and circulatory failure with oliguria and jaundice.

Management

Management of pneumonia involves:

- Sputum examination and culture (often negative).
- Prevention of dehydration.
- Analgesics, but opioids are contraindicated if there is concurrent COPD.
- Appropriate antibiotics.

In severe illness the following may also be indicated:

- Culture and serology of blood and endoscopic lung samples.
- Pleural and lung aspiration.
- Oxygen.
- IV fluids.
- Complete bed rest until the patient has been afebrile for 2–3 days.

Corticosteroids are sometimes used, though there is little evidence of their benefit.

Pneumonia must always be regarded seriously. Despite modern antibiotics the death rate varies from 4% to 25% in various European countries, with most deaths occurring in the first 5 days. Death can occur even in previously healthy subjects, and prolonged convalescence may be needed. Physiotherapy may aid recovery. Features associated with increased mortality risk are:

- Extensive lung involvement.
- Age 60 years or more.
- Respiratory rate 30/min or greater.
- Pre-existing disease state.
- Confusion or impaired consciousness.
- Diastolic blood pressure 60 mmHg or less.
- Atrial fibrillation.

Pneumocystis carinii pneumonia, a protozoal infection previously encountered only in some severely immunosuppressed cancer patients, is a significant problem in HIV/AIDS patients. It is treated with high-dose *co-trimoxazole* (sulfamethoxazole plus trimethoprim), or *pentamidine isethionate* if *co-trimoxazole* causes undesirable adverse reactions. *Trimetrexate*, *atovaquone* or *clindamycin plus primaquine* are used if other antimicrobials are not tolerated or are ineffective. *Trimetrexate* is a very potent dihydrofolate reductase inhibitor and must be used with *calcium folinate* rescue. There is a high mortality rate (about 20%) despite treatment, so at-risk patients should receive *co-trimoxazole* prophylaxis.

Tuberculosis

In the 19th century, tuberculosis (TB) was known as 'consumption', because of the body wasting caused, and was so devastating that it was described as 'The Captain of the Men of Death'. Tuberculosis is still the most common bacterial infection world-wide: the WHO estimates that one-third of the entire world population is infected. Easy and rapid travel, continued poverty, the mass movement of refugees and widespread HIV/AIDS infection make this a growing problem. The challenge for the affluent West is to control the disease before it again becomes a significant public health problem.

Pathology

This is an infection by the acid-fast bacteria, *Mycobacterium tuberculosis* and *M. bovis*, which cause necrosis and granuloma (tubercle) formation. It is usually a lung disease but may involve other organs or may be widespread (**miliary tuberculosis**).

Pulmonary disease produces a classical chronic inflammatory response with exudation into the alveoli and neutrophil infiltration. Subsequent macrophage activity leads to the development of cell-mediated immunity in 3–8 weeks and patients become tuberculin-positive, i.e. hypersensitive to the microbial proteins: this forms the basis of the Heaf and Mantoux tests for immunity to TB.

Clinical features

Primary infections are usually asymptomatic, but non-specific symptoms may occur, i.e. cough, malaise and wheezing. Occasionally pleural effusion, lung collapse, bronchiectasis or miliary disease ensue.

Post-primary lung infection usually arises from the breakdown of the tubercles with the release of infective bacteria, but it may also result from re-infection. Reactivation may occur in old age, neoplastic disease and following treatment with immunosuppressive drugs or high doses of corticosteroids, so prophylactic *isoniazid* is sometimes given before using corticosteroids.

There is a gradual onset of non-specific symptoms, commonly recurrent colds, malaise and anorexia. Later the full syndrome occurs with malaise, weight loss, persistent cough, haemoptysis and a resistant pneumonia. However, patients may be remarkably symptom-free even when there are extensive radiological changes. Patients, especially of Asian or African origin, may occasionally present with grossly enlarged lymph nodes ('glands') in the neck. The adrenal glands may also be involved, leading to **Addison's disease**.

Diagnosis

This is made on the basis of sputum examination (purulent sputum contains acid-fast bacilli), radiographic changes and clinical symptoms and signs. Night sweats are uncommon nowadays. It may be difficult to culture the organism and determine antibiotic sensitivities, but even if such information can be provided successfully it is not available for about 12 weeks. However, new DNA-based tests are becoming available which provide results in about 3 days.

Prophylaxis

As always, the production of active immunity is preferable to treatment of infection. Two types of **Bacillus Calmette–Guérin** (**BCG**) **Vaccine** are available, for either intradermal or percutaneous use. These must not be confused, because the latter is appropriate only for young infants in whom the normal intradermal route is difficult.

Vaccination is recommended for those who are unimmunized or are Heaf or Mantoux test-negative and who are:

* Contacts of those with active TB.
* Immigrants from endemic areas and long-stay travellers to such areas.
* Those who may be at risk, e.g. medical and paramedical staff, some veterinary staff, prison staff and workers with the homeless.
* Children aged 10–14 years.
* Neonates, children and adults for whom vaccination is requested.

Management

This is usually very effective and involves the use of an appropriate combination of antibiotics (*see* Chapter 13), to minimize resistance problems and because treatment has always had to be initiated on a best-guess basis immediately a provisional clinical diagnosis has been made and before the results of sensitivity tests are known.

This problem should be resolved with the advent of widespread rapid testing.

Patients improve rapidly, so the principal problem in most cases is one of compliance with therapy, especially because many patients have limited comprehension or understanding of the need for strict compliance and may have an unstable lifestyle. The response to this has been the initiation of **directly observed therapy** (DOT) to ensure compliance. However, this needs to be 'user friendly' and not authoritarian: one small study has shown that more patients who are well-counselled are more likely to comply if they are self-medicating than those in a DOT programme. The problem still remains of tracing dropouts who do not have a fixed address.

A new target for therapy is to stimulate dormant (antibiotic-resistant) organisms in the tubercles into growth, rendering them susceptible to antibiotics. This would enable elimination of post-primary infection. A small trial has identified a **resuscitation promotion factor** (Rpf) protein from *Micrococcus luteus* which may make this possible. Alternatively, a vaccine against Rpf could maintain organisms in the tubercles in permanent dormancy and so non-infective.

Respiratory failure

Respiratory failure is usually considered to be the occurrence of significant hypoxaemia (P_aO_2 < 8.5 kPa) with or without hypercapnia (P_aCO_2 > 6.5 kPa), and may be classified into two types (Table 5.21). Hypoxaemia is regarded as severe if the P_aO_2 is less than about 5 kPa. If sufficiently severe, hypercapnia causes acidosis (blood pH 7.3 or lower).

The **management** of Type I respiratory failure involves high-dose oxygen and treatment of the underlying disease state.

In Type II failure, high-dose oxygen is not used because patients either require mechanical ventilation or depend on a low P_aO_2 to provide their respiratory drive. These patients may develop severe respiratory acidosis which must be treated vigorously (*see* Chapter 4). In acute respiratory failure, extracorporeal oxygenation (in neonates) or carbon dioxide removal (in adults) are promising developments.

The best respiratory stimulant is vigorous physiotherapy, but drugs are used occasionally. *Doxapram* is a short-acting stimulant which is given by continuous IV infusion. It may be used to counter the depressant effect of oxygen in

---

Table 5.21 Types of respiratory failure

Type of failure, and the metabolic abnormalities observed		Some possible causes
Type I (P_aO_2 reduced or greatly reduced, P_aCO_2 normal or low)	Acute	Cardiovascular diseases Pneumonia Pulmonary oedema
	Chronic	Fibrosing alveolitis Interstitial lung disease
Type II (P_aO_2 reduced or greatly reduced, P_aCO_2 raised or greatly raised, acidosis)	Acute	Upper airways obstruction Sever acute asthma CNS damage COPD plus infection
	Chronic	COPD

COPD, chronic obstructive pulmonary disease; CNS, central nervous system.

Type II failure and to treat significant respiratory depression following anaesthesia. *Nikethamide*, an older agent best given by bolus IV injection, is sometimes used as a preliminary to artificial ventilation.

Inhalation therapy

Advantages

The development of inhalation therapy has produced considerable benefits for patients suffering from respiratory diseases, not only for asthma but also for chronic bronchitis, bronchiectasis and cystic fibrosis. Although simple devices had been used for many years, inhalation therapy was given a powerful impetus in 1969 with the introduction of the first selective beta$_2$-agonist bronchodilator (*salbutamol*) and the associated equipment to deliver precise doses direct to the lungs. The technique has subsequently been used successfully for the administration of corticosteroids, anticholinergics (*ipratropium*), anti-allergics (*sodium cromoglicate* (*cromolyn sodium*)), antibiotics (e.g. *bacitracin, aminoglycosides, cephalosporins, colistin, penicillins* and *polymyxin*, and the antifungal agent *amphotericin*). In terminal care it is used for administering mucolytics (e.g. normal and hypertonic saline, N-*acetylcysteine*), opioids (e.g. *morphine, diamorphine, fentanyl*) and local anaesthetics (*lidocaine* (*lignocaine*), *bupivacaine*).

Other applications include the administration of local anaesthetics before endotracheal intubation or endoscopy, water or saline for humidification, cytotoxic agents for regional cancer chemotherapy, vaccines for immunization and DNA for gene therapy in cystic fibrosis. It has also been proposed that many other drugs could be administered by this well-tolerated and non-invasive route which avoids first-pass hepatic metabolism, e.g. *insulin, heparin* and *vasopressin*.

In respiratory disease inhalation therapy is a simple, rapidly effective technique which delivers a small dose of drug directly to what is usually the desired site of action deep within the lungs. This gives a high local concentration and avoids (or minimizes, because some is absorbed from the lungs or swallowed) the side effects which occur when larger doses of drug are given systemically to achieve a similar effect. By avoiding first-pass metabolism, the bioavailability of drugs may be enhanced. The very high pulmonary blood flow and surface area, together with the very thin alveolar wall, may also serve to enhance activity.

Factors influencing pulmonary drug deposition

The principal factors are the particle size of the drug, the patient, the delivery system and the environment.

Particle size

The target area in the lungs depends on the site of the pathological changes, and may be the tracheobronchial region, the bronchioles or the respiratory bronchioles and alveoli. In adults, only some 8–12% of the inhaled dose reaches the distal lung, even with optimal delivery, and this may fall to below 1% in young children. The remainder is deposited in the oropharynx and is swallowed. This mechanism may also dispose of insoluble drugs deposited in the bronchi and escalated from there by mucociliary clearance.

Optimal particle size is crucial: particles need to be about 2 microns in diameter or less to reach the bronchioles and below 0.7 micron to reach the respiratory bronchioles. Below approximately 0.5 micron, particles will reach the alveolar sacs, but because this region does not possess any smooth muscle, bronchodilators will not have any effect there, though other drugs may do so, e.g. corticosteroids in extrinsic allergic alveolitis. Very small particles (<0.5 micron) may remain suspended in the alveolar gas and be exhaled (about 1% of the inhaled dose).

Larger particles (10 microns) are deposited in the mouth and oropharynx by **inertial impaction** (about 60% of the dose) and are swallowed, as is a large proportion of those in the 5- to 10-micron range. This gives rise to most of any systemic effects which occur. In the 2- to 5-micron range, particles are carried in the air stream until the velocity is slowed sufficiently by airways resistance to permit deposition in the bronchioles by **gravitational sedimentation**. Below approximately 2 microns, particles deposit on mucous surfaces, following accidental contact produced by random motion, partly Brownian. Thus, for most purposes we need the majority of particles to be in the range of 1–5 microns, with a median aerodynamic diameter of about 3 microns.

However, recent research with respirable polymer-coated insulin particles has shown that low-density particles ($<0.4\,g/cm^3$) greater than 5 microns in diameter can be aerosolized more easily than the conventional higher density, smaller diameter ones. Further, the light, large particles evade pulmonary phagocytosis, giving high bioavailability and more sustained drug release (96 h versus 4 h). If these findings can be replicated they will offer exciting possibilities for controlled drug administration to the lungs, and systemically via the lungs of drugs which currently are given only by injection.

Patient (physiological) factors

Although almost impossible to quantify, these are among the most important considerations. Modern equipment is well-designed and manufacturers take great care to produce aerosols of effective drugs having the appropriate particle size characteristics. Unfortunately, there is little control over what happens in use, especially if patients are counselled inadequately or if the devices are used without proper ongoing supervision by knowledgeable staff. The age of the patient, their ability to coordinate breathing with drug delivery, airways geometry, inspiratory and expiratory flow rates and times, tidal volumes, breath holding and the proportions of mouth and/or nose breathing may all influence the deposition of the drug in the lungs.

We can be certain only on some points, e.g. that pulmonary deposition is reduced in proportion to the severity of the ventilatory abnormality, with poor technique and in young children. It is clearly impossible to predict the response of an individual patient to a drug delivered from a particular piece of equipment. As in many other fields of therapy, there is no substitute for monitoring the actual clinical response and, if this is unsatisfactory, varying the conditions of use in a controlled way to determine whether this can be improved. If necessary, the drug and the delivery system itself may also be changed.

Drug delivery systems

There are four types available: the pressurized metered dose inhaler (MDI), dry powder inhalers (DPIs), gas driven nebulizers, and ultrasonic nebulizers.

Pressurized MDIs

This type of inhaler is the most widely used owing to its convenience. It consists (Fig. 5.22) of a metal canister filled with a suspension of a micronized drug in a propellant which is liquefied under pressure. The special metering valve gives doses that are reproducible within 5%.

Current propellants are CFC (chlorofluorocarbon, freon) compounds. Because of worries about the effects of CFCs on the ozone layer and the consequent environmental impact, these propellants are being replaced rapidly by hydrofluoroalkanes (HFAs). However, the latter still have some 'greenhouse' effect. The doses of propellant usually delivered are considered to be non-toxic, though they may cause small reductions in respiratory function. There do not appear to be any toxicity problems with these new inhalers.

In one new CFC-free formulation of *beclometasone* a change in its particle size has resulted in an increase from about 25% to 60% of the dose being in the respirable range, producing significant deposition in the small airways. There is evidence that inflammation in these small airways is an important component in both acute and chronic asthma. Thus the absolute loaded dose of beclometasone from this device is halved, with a reduction of about 30% in side effects at similar clinical effectiveness.

There may be additional features which may worry patients when they are changed to CFC-free inhalers:

- An altered sound made when the dose is released.
- A change in the taste of the spray.

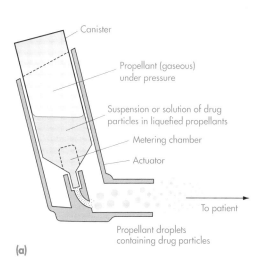

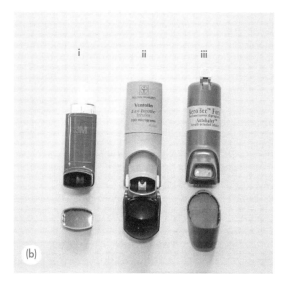

Figure 5.22   Metered dose inhalers. (a) General arrangement. (b) Some commercial inhalers. (i) Standard MDI, (ii) and (iii) breath-actuated inhalers: the dose is released when the patient seals their lips around the mouthpiece and starts to inhale. (ii) Easi-Breathe: the unit is set by opening the mouthpiece cover. (iii) Aerobec Forte Autohaler: the unit is shown in the set position with the top lever raised.

- Reduced pharyngeal impact.
- Incompatibility with their existing spacer device.

The European Commission has expressed concern about possible toxicity and has urged careful supervision of patients who are changed to CFC-free inhalers. Those with 'brittle' (difficult to manage) asthma will need especially close attention.

Patients using MDIs need careful counselling to ensure maximum benefit. Good coordination is essential for correct dose delivery and this is more difficult for the young, the elderly and the very anxious patient. It is essential to teach proper procedures and to check regularly that these are being maintained. A moderate inspiratory flow rate (about 30 L/min) gives the best lung deposition. Pharmacists, doctors and nurses need to acquire and maintain a good technique themselves (Table 5.22) and be able to teach this to patients: one survey showed that only 28% of adult patients and 48% of hospital pharmacists had a good inhaler technique.

If good coordination cannot be achieved, if patients dislike the sensation of the jet of cold aerosol impinging on the back of the mouth, or if it causes them to gag and involuntarily to stop inhaling momentarily, then several alternatives are available. These are the automatic (breath-actuated) inhalers, spacer devices and dry powder aerosols.

Breath-actuated inhalers

In these devices the inhaler cartridge has the same construction as in the normal MDI, but release of the dose is triggered automatically when the patient seals their lips around the mouthpiece and creates a sufficient pressure differential at the start of inhalation. However, some of these inhalers also have problems in use. Patients may dislike the sharp noise and the impact as the mechanism is activated in some inhalers. Further, a proportion of patients do not have sufficient inspiratory capacity at all times to trigger the mechanism or may not achieve a good enough seal around the mouthpiece. Recent designs have mitigated these problems. Once again, good counselling is essential for effective use.

Spacer devices

The object of these is to avoid the need for good coordination of dose release and inhalation for effective drug delivery, to maximize clinical

Table 5.22   Patient counselling points for the use of metered dose inhalers

Advice to the patient

- Keep the cap on the mouthpiece and keep the device clean. If necessary, wash with a warm, mild detergent solution and allow to dry thoroughly
- When using:
  - remove the cap and shake the inhaler (the drug is suspended in the propellant)
  - breathe out gently, but not fully, then immediately place the lips around the mouthpiece; start to breathe in slowly and deeply through the mouth, press down the inhaler cartridge to release the dose, and continue to breathe in steadily and deeply
  - hold the breath for about 10 s and breathe out slowly
- Good coordination to ensure release of the dose at the commencement of inhalation is essential to obtain the maximum benefit

Points for the pharmacist

- Demonstrate the correct method of use with a placebo inhaler, and ask the patient to show you how they use it. Never accept a patient's assurance that they know how to do so
- Most patients are on long-term therapy, and many develop bad habits. It is useful to ask them to demonstrate how they use their inhaler from time to time, and to reinforce correct usage
- Demonstration by a pharmacist, doctor or nurse is of limited value unless combined with supervised patient practice and testing
- The degree of benefit can be demonstrated to the patient by determining peak expiratory flow rates before dosing and 20–30 min afterwards, thus providing strong motivation
- Patients with anything other than mild, occasional attacks will derive considerable benefit from learning about their disease and how to manage it, especially in exacerbations. They should measure peak expiratory flow rates regularly and keep a diary of the results

Order of inhalation of drugs

- If an attack is not too severe, it may not matter which drug is inhaled first, so compound aerosols may aid patient compliance
- However, in a severe attack the airways may be too constricted to permit penetration of the drug, so the patient should proceed as follows to ensure that the airways are as dilated as possible:
  - inhale one puff of bronchodilator
  - wait 5 min and inhale a second puff of bronchodilator
  - wait 5 min and inhale other products as usual
- Unfortunately, this procedure may lead to non-compliance, owing to the waiting periods involved. If so, it is better to reduce wait between puffs to the maximum that the patient will tolerate

benefit, and to minimize adverse reactions. The dose is fired into a reservoir from which the patient then inhales, using several successive breaths if necessary. This gives comparable results to the use of an MDI with good coordination, so patients with good inhaler technique will derive little benefit in drug deposition in the lungs. However, another important function of the reservoir is to slow down the aerosol droplets so that there is more time for the propellant to evaporate before inhalation occurs; in this way particles are smaller and thus more likely to penetrate the bronchiolar tree. The reduced speed of the particles also reduces oropharyngeal impaction of drug. Thus the proportion of the dose swallowed and the incidence of hoarseness and oropharyngeal thrush with the corticosteroid aerosols is reduced.

Several commercial types of spacer are available (Fig. 5.23). The large volume (750 mL)

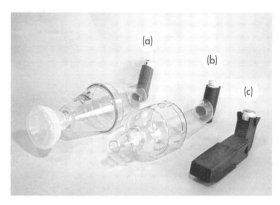

Figure 5.23 Some spacer devices. (a) Large volume (Volumatic) with paediatric mask. (b) Large volume (Nebuhaler). (c) Collapsible extended mouthpiece (Bricanyl).

larger doses. These types have a one-way valve through which only inspiration is possible, exhaled air passing out through side vents. Spacers increase the lung deposition from monodisperse aerosols, perhaps doubling the lung deposition from single doses (Fig. 5.24), with a significant increase in clinical response.

However, the larger spacers are too bulky for convenient use outside the home. Many manufacturers supply smaller tube spacers with their MDIs. Although almost any tube device will have a similar effect, extemporaneous devices give unpredictable results. Recently, spacers specially designed for young children have been introduced. These have a smaller volume and require less inspiratory effort in use.

A significant proportion of the aerosol dose is deposited on the walls of the spacers, largely due to electrostatic attraction. This can be reduced by washing the spacer with a detergent solution, as an antistatic. The inhaled dose is thereby increased, but it is not known whether this translates into clinical benefit.

devices (e.g. Fig. 5.23(b)) can be used flexibly: several breaths can be taken to achieve complete inhalation of the available drug and it is possible to discharge a number of puffs into the chamber, so a spacer may provide an effective alternative to the use of a nebulizer (*see* Fig. 5.27) for giving

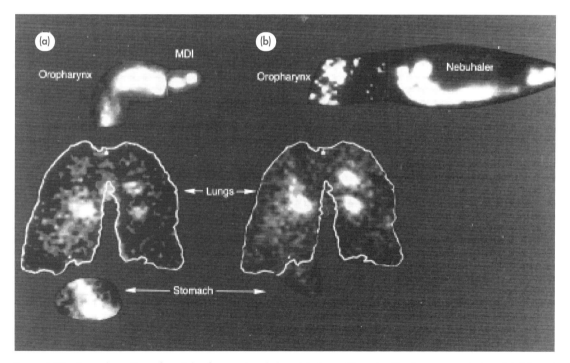

Figure 5.24 Lung deposition of particles from metered dose inhalers with and without a spacer device. (a) Bricanyl metered dose inhaler (MDI). (b) MDI with Nebuhaler large-volume spacer. Note the absence from the stomach of ingested aerosol and its relatively low deposition in the oropharynx. (Reproduced with permission from Newman SP (1984) *Thorax* **39**: 935–941.)

Dry powder inhalers

These devices are inherently breath-actuated and so also do not depend on good coordination for satisfactory performance. The dose is released into the inspired air when the patient inhales. There is no propellant, so these inhalers are more suitable for the occasional patient who is affected by the propellant or who is worried about its possible side effects. Several types of inhaler are available (Fig. 5.25), some of which use a lactose carrier for the drug, whereas others deliver pure drug. Although a number of innovative designs are in development these will have to demonstrate significant benefits in terms of clinical effectiveness or cost or both if they are to replace the Accuhaler and Turbohaler.

Some devices provide single doses from hard gelatin capsules, which have to be loaded into the device before each use. The newer ones provide a number of doses (up to 200) without recharging. They have either a dose counter or end-of-charge indicator so that the patient knows when a new device is required. If pure, carrier-free drug is used patients are scarcely aware that a powder is being inhaled.

Like the MDI, the DPIs are rather inefficient devices for the delivery of drug to the lungs. Many patients distrust the very idea of inhaling a powder, and some dislike the sensation produced. Patients with poor respiratory function may need to inhale several times to obtain the full dose.

High inspiration rates (approximately 60 L/min) are required to produce an adequate concentration of respirable particles to improve drug deposition within the lungs. Sustained breath holding does not seem to be necessary.

However, DPIs are simple to use and are generally more suitable for children. More importantly, the devices give a similar clinical benefit to that attainable with an MDI. If environmental pressures against aerosol propellants are maintained, then DPIs may become predominant.

Nebulizers

General principles

Nebulizers are devices for producing an aerosol from an aqueous solution of a drug. Two methods are generally used:

- **Jet nebulizers** use a jet of compressed gas (air or oxygen) to break a fine stream of

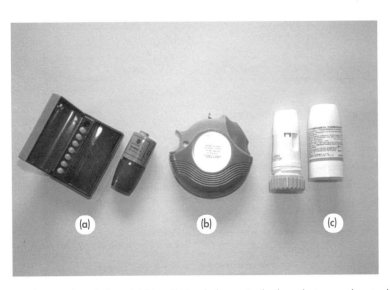

Figure 5.25   Some dry powder inhalers. (a) Ventolin Rotahaler; a single dose device, each capsule delivers one dose. (b) Becotide Accuhaler (refillable, 60-dose) opened ready for use, showing dose counter. The mouth piece is at 2 o'clock. A new dose is released by actuating the lever (at 10 o'clock). (c) Bricanyl Turbohaler (disposable, 100-dose) with protective cover. A new dose is released by twisting the knurled base. The small window below the mouthpiece shows a warning flag when the unit is becoming exhausted.

liquid into an aerosol, the smaller droplets emerging from the outlet as a fine mist.

• **Ultrasonic nebulizers** use electrically-induced ultrasonic vibrations to break the drug solution into an aerosol.

In the UK, nebulizers can be prescribed only via hospitals or must be purchased by patients. The following is a brief review of the topic: for more detailed information, readers are referred to the *Thorax* supplement listed in the References and further reading section.

Indications for nebulizer therapy

Nebulizers may be preferred for a number of reasons:

• Because young children, the elderly and very infirm patients may find it difficult to use MDIs and DPIs correctly or with sufficient benefit.

• Because some patients may require a higher dose than can be delivered by MDIs and DPIs and may be poorly controlled on these, notably some chronic asthmatics and those with COPD and cystic fibrosis.

• For self-medication at home, to give a larger dose of a drug when patients are inadequately controlled with an MDI, e.g. in severe or chronic asthma, exacerbations of COPD and chronic airflow obstruction.

• In acute severe asthma, either in hospital, in the doctor's surgery, or as an alternative to parenteral medication.

• When inhalation is desirable but drugs are not produced in a conveniently respirable form.

The latter point is especially applicable in the case of:

• *Antimicrobials* for cystic fibrosis, bronchiectasis and HIV infection or AIDS.

• *Dornase alfa* (recombinant human deoxyribonuclease, rhDNase) for reducing sputum viscosity in cystic fibrosis to aid expectoration.

• In palliative care, e.g. bronchodilators, *lidocaine* (*lignocaine*) or *bupivacaine* for relief of persistent dry cough and opioids for terminal dyspnoea.

The need for a nebulizer should be established by proof of additional benefit (Fig. 5.26). Patients must be carefully trained in the use and limitations of nebulizers because they may rely on them excessively and delay seeking effective treatment, with a consequently increased morbidity and mortality. Trials of therapy need to be continued for 3–4 weeks to assess benefit adequately and should normally give at least a 15% improvement over existing baseline to be considered worthwhile. However, due account should be taken of a patient's subjective perception of benefit, in addition to measurements of PEF or FEV_1.

Types of jet nebulizer

These work on the Venturi principle. High-pressure gas (air or oxygen) is forced through a very small aperture (venturi). As the gas escapes from the venturi it expands rapidly and gains velocity as it passes over the end of a feeding tube. The low pressure created sucks liquid up the feed tube and the liquid stream is broken into droplets which impinge onto a baffle. The largest droplets are trapped on the baffle and intermediate ones on the walls of the chamber. All of these drain back into the liquid reservoir. Only the smallest droplets are entrained in the gas stream and inhaled by the patient. The performance (dose delivery) depends on the precise sizes and designs of the feeding tube, venturi, baffles and chamber. The presence of a baffle distinguishes the nebulizer from a simple atomizer and its design is crucial to the droplet size produced.

Two forms of modern jet nebulizer are illustrated in Fig. 5.27.

Older, simple nebulizer designs which have been in use for many years are very inefficient because:

• They may produce <50% of particles in the 1–5 micron range.

• Some 95% of the primary droplets are trapped on internal baffles.

• About 65% remains in the chamber after nebulization and 65% of the inhaled aerosol is exhaled.

Thus only about 10% of the dose may reach the desired sites of action in the lungs. This situation can be improved in various ways.

Open vent nebulizers, e.g. the Sidestream, have an additional vent through which the low

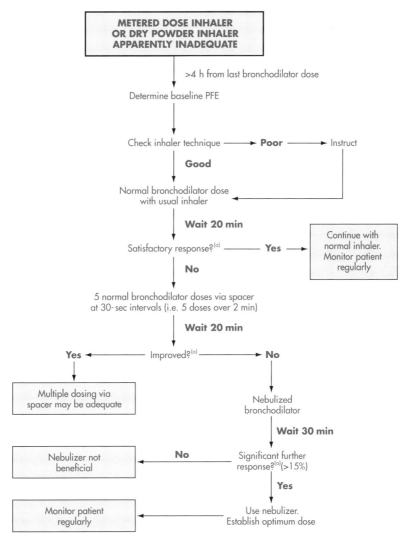

Figure 5.26 Protocol for establishing the need for nebulizer use. [a] Response or improvement is checked objectively at each stage by measuring peak expiratory flow (PEF): at least a 15% increase is required to justify a change of procedure. A trial of therapy or equipment needs 3–4 weeks to be confident of benefit or otherwise.

pressure in the chamber sucks additional air. The extra gas flow entrains more respirable particles, giving shorter nebulization times and possibly reducing particle size. Further, cheaper, low-output compressors can be used. However, patients with a low inspiratory flow, e.g. young children and the elderly infirm, may inspire less drug because more is carried to waste in the increased exhaust stream.

This drug loss may be overcome by the newer **breath-assisted open vent nebulizers** which

incorporate two valves, e.g. the Pari LC Plus (Fig. 5.27(b)) and Ventstream. An inlet valve opens only on inspiration, admitting ambient air as with the open vent design. On expiration the inlet valve closes and an outlet valve opens, so the aerosol loss is not increased by extra air flow through the inlet valve.

Aerosol loss when exhaling can also be reduced by using a holding chamber, e.g. the Mizer, with a conventional jet nebulizer, though this makes the set-up rather bulky.

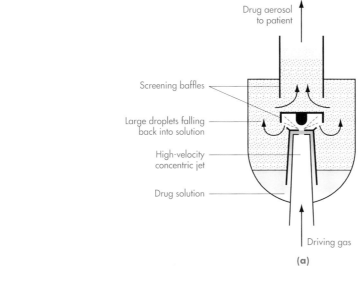

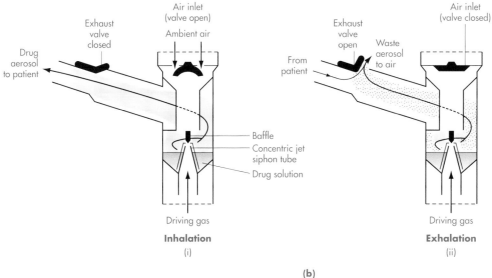

Figure 5.27   Some types of jet nebulizer. (a) A simple older type. (b) Breath-assisted, open vent type (Pari LC Plus).

Some factors affecting the performance of jet nebulizers

Gas flow rate.   This is the major determinant of output from a particular nebulizer, as particle size decreases markedly with increasing gas flow. The flow rate may be 6–8 L/min (high), 4–6 L/min (medium) or, occasionally, <4 L/min (low), but that required to yield the desired droplet size characteristics and dose output differs appreciably with different nebulizers. High

flow rates are needed to nebulize viscous solutions, e.g. antibiotics and rhDNase. Modern jet nebulizers have output rates comparable with those from ultrasonic devices.

Domiciliary oxygen equipment cannot deliver more than 4 L/min without a special controller and is unsuitable for use with most jet nebulizers. Electrically driven air compressors are preferred unless the patient needs oxygen (see below). However, if patients in the community need oxygen, a low-flow (<4 L/min) nebulizer, e.g. Cirrus, Pari LC Plus, can be used with an oxygen cylinder. Alternatively, a flow head capable of delivering up to 8 L/min from a gas cylinder should be used with a suitable nebulizer, e.g. Permaneb (4–6 L/min); or Micromist or Ventstream (6–8 L/min). If high flow rates are used, the normal size oxygen cylinder will have a very short life and the cost of supplying the oxygen will be very high. If oxygen is used, the patient must be capable of an adequate inhalation rate (see below). Oxygen concentrators (p. 292) are quite unsuitable for driving nebulizers.

The inhalation rate and pattern have only a small effect on particle size, but may be very important if oxygen is used as the driving gas and in determining pulmonary drug delivery.

Driving gas.   Under hospital conditions either piped oxygen or compressed air may be used. However, many patients, especially chronic bronchitics, are intolerant of oxygen. At the low inhalation rates which occur with exhausted and very infirm patients the oxygen concentration in the inspired air mixture may be very high (Fig. 5.28), so air is the preferred driving gas for hypoxic patients with carbon dioxide retention. However, some patients tolerate oxygen or may need it, e.g. in an acute severe asthma attack the patient may be severely hypoxaemic and this may be aggravated by the bronchodilator, so oxygen is then preferred.

Diluent, volume and formulation of solution. The preferred diluent for nebulizer solutions is sterile normal saline because hypotonic solutions may cause bronchoconstriction in some patients. Solutions diluted ready for use are preferable for domiciliary use because there is then no preservative to cause reactions and no possibility of a patient using a concentrated solution in error.

The fill volume of solution must be adjusted to suit the nebulizer being used, because some have an appreciable residual volume, and to give the desired delivery rate. The delivery rate of many nebulizers falls off markedly below approximately 2 mL. Tapping the chamber sharply and repeatedly throughout dosing to shake the solution to the bottom of the reservoir

improves maximum delivery somewhat. Because of evaporation, the residual volume underestimates the **residual mass** of drug at the end of nebulization, but there is little information on this because it is influenced by numerous factors, e.g. the humidity and temperature of the driving gas. Inhalation of the more concentrated drug solution may cause respiratory irritation in some patients towards the end of a treatment session.

The fill volume also controls the time over which the dose is delivered, this being one of the advantages of nebulizer therapy because there is then adequate time (10 min) for a physiological response (e.g. bronchodilatation) to occur and so better penetration of the latter part of the dose. Patients will not usually tolerate delivery times longer than 10 min.

Solutions of lower surface tension give greater volume deliveries because they adhere less to the walls and baffles of the nebulizers.

Hygiene.   Nebulizers must be kept clean to avoid microbial growth and consequent infection and are best washed out after each use, or at least daily. The manufacturer's instructions must be followed strictly to avoid damage to the precision plastic mouldings which are used.

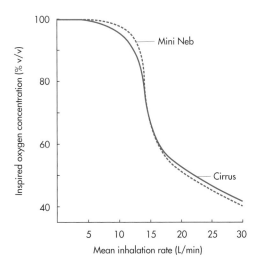

Figure 5.28 Influence of inhalation rate on the oxygen content of the inspired gas from two nebulizers (oxygen flow rate 8 L/min).

Drug solution delivery. This is the most significant attribute of a nebulizer, and solution outputs can vary in the range 0.01–0.75 mL/min, depending on the type of nebulizer and the gas flow rate. It is impossible to predict the actual delivery of drug from a particular nebulizer to a specific patient. We can only choose the device and adjust the conditions to get the best clinical response.

Nebulizer wear. Some nebulizers are durable, but should be replaced after about a year, e.g. Pari LC Plus, Sidestream Durable. However, most wear more rapidly and must be discarded after 3 months or if there is any sign of wear, e.g. increasing nebulization times, changed noise.

Ancillary equipment
A wide range of ancillary equipment is available from manufacturers. Either **mouthpieces** or **face masks** (p. 292) may be used, with similar clinical response. Young children and exhausted or very infirm patients usually do better with face masks because of their ease of use, but it is often a matter of patient preference. Very young children are often intolerant of masks, but reasonable results are sometimes achieved by merely holding the outlet tube or mask near the child's nose and allowing normal breathing. Although this reduces dose delivery substantially, it may accustom the child to the treatment and permit subsequent use of a more effective technique.

However, it is sometimes difficult to get a good fit with a mask and avoid leakage of aerosol, so mouthpieces may be preferred for use with corticosteroids, which may damage the facial skin, and antimuscarinic bronchodilators, which risk triggering or exacerbating glaucoma in the elderly.

There are concerns about the effects of drugs such as antibiotics on the environment and the possibility of spreading infections due to highly resistant microorganisms. For this sort of application **closed systems**, e.g. with exhaust **filters**, are used in hospitals to prevent cross-contamination. This is probably unnecessary for home use unless others in the family are at risk from respiratory infection, though nebulizers should be used in well-ventilated rooms.

Compressors must match the chosen nebulizer: many are supplied as complete outfits.

Ultrasonic nebulizers
Ultrasonic nebulization may be very fast, and output increases as the solution heats (whereas with jet nebulizers the output falls with time) due to the associated fall in viscosity. The output is usually adjustable by the user. Some patients find that the warm wet mist which they produce is unpleasant, especially if a face mask is fitted, and provokes coughing. Ultrasonic nebulizers are generally quieter than jet nebulizers and do not need a compressor or gas supply.

Improvements in nebulizers
The British Standard for jet nebulizers (BS7711, Part 3, 1994) requires them to be marked with maximum filling levels and recommended gas flows. Manufacturers must also supply details of:

- Intended use and any contraindications.
- Gas pressures, respirable outputs and residual volumes corresponding to the recommended, minimum and maximum flow rates.
- Aerosol particle size distribution at the recommended flow rates.
- Suitability for use with ventilators and anaesthetic systems.

However, BS7711 does not address many of the problems raised above.

Conclusion

Inhalation therapy has become a highly technical and sophisticated method of drug delivery which has brought tremendous advantages to sufferers from respiratory diseases. This is a research area of great interest and intense activity. Most difficult cases of asthma, in particular, can be controlled by the appropriate use of this technique, though occasionally oral medication may also be required.

Many new devices are likely to be introduced in the next few years, most of which are breath-actuated and provide more consistent dosing. For example, one new battery-powered DPI is claimed to deliver about 30% of the absolute loaded dose, i.e. some three times that from a conventional DPI. Another novel MDI delivers a high respirable fraction at lower velocity than current devices, similarly delivering some 30% of the absolute loaded dose. If these and similar devices perform to this level in daily clinical use they should permit significant reductions in loaded doses, and so also reduce both adverse reactions and drug costs. However, all new devices will have to demonstrate significant cost–benefit advantages.

The principal barrier to more effective control is largely a lack of appreciation of the potential benefits of inhalation therapy and inadequate understanding of the proper use of the equipment. The result is inadequate patient counselling and compliance, and sub-optimal control of the disease state. Although the situation has improved over recent years, more can, and should, be done to reduce morbidity and mortality. These comments apply to all health workers, including pharmacists.

Oxygen therapy

Aims

The aim of oxygen therapy is to increase the amount of oxygen carried by the blood in hypoxaemia by increasing either the haemoglobin saturation or the amount of oxygen carried in solution in the plasma (10 micromol O_2/L/kPa).

Increasing the oxygen concentration in poorly ventilated but well-perfused alveoli increases the P_aO_2 and also counteracts a reduced diffusing capacity. Patients with anaemia or heart failure may have good haemoglobin saturation but poor oxygen delivery to the tissues, due to low haemoglobin levels and low cardiac output respectively. These patients will also benefit from an increase in the dissolved oxygen concentration in the plasma.

Problems

It is important to remember that oxygen is a drug: **high concentrations of oxygen are toxic**.

They can cause blindness in premature infants and cause pulmonary oedema and irritation in adults, so concentrations greater than 60% are rarely used. If high-dose (60%) oxygen is required it should be given continuously and patients watched for any evidence of hypoventilation (i.e. respiratory depression), which may appear rapidly or develop gradually.

Patients who have had hypercapnia for some time (e.g. in COPD) rely on their P_aO_2 to provide their respiratory drive, so increasing the P_aO_2 artificially will inhibit this drive and may suppress respiration substantially. This aggravates the hypercapnia, and the raised carbon dioxide finally acts as a further respiratory depressant (CO_2 narcosis). Thus those patients who most need oxygen are often intolerant of it. Optimal delivery of oxygen to patients with prolonged hypercapnia can only be achieved by careful blood gas monitoring and clinical supervision.

Oxygen, unless from a concentrator, is supplied as a pure gas which must be diluted with air to a suitable concentration. If the concentration exceeds 40% the gas must be humidified with a nebulizer (preferably warmed), but masks delivering 35% oxygen or less carry sufficient moisture in the entrained air.

In the UK, domiciliary oxygen equipment supplied through the NHS will deliver up to 28% oxygen, depending on the type of mask used (p. 293). If concentrations other than this are required the appropriate equipment must be purchased or provided by a hospital. This long-term low concentration oxygen (p. 293) has been shown to improve survival in Type B patients ('blue bloaters', p. 266) with both dyspnoea and peripheral oedema, i.e. cor pulmonale, by up to 5 years. Although it does not arrest disease progression it does improve both exercise tolerance and the quality of life. In other forms of severe advanced respiratory disease it improves well-being, but does not prolong life.

Community pharmacists who provide domiciliary oxygen must ensure that a member of the family or helper is available and properly instructed in the use of the equipment. Oxygen is a fire hazard: it must not be used while smoking (if patients need oxygen they should not be smoking anyway!) or near naked flames.

Methods of administration

Types of supply

In hospital, oxygen is piped to bedside outlets. For UK **domiciliary use**, either cylinders (containing 1360 L) or **oxygen concentrators** may be supplied. The latter provide 95% oxygen plus 5% argon at 2 L/min, dropping to 85–90% oxygen at higher flow rates. Small lightweight portable cylinders can be supplied by the hospital or purchased by the patient and refilled from a liquid oxygen container, giving improved mobility to suitable patients.

Oxygen cylinders are suitable only for intermittent use, giving an 11-h supply at 2 L/min. When long-term oxygen therapy (LTOT) is required, oxygen concentrators are used. These are small portable machines for domiciliary use which can be set to deliver 24–28% oxygen via nasal cannulae at 1–2 L/min. They are cheaper and more convenient than cylinders, but cannot meet all types of requirement. Although the initial cost is high, this is justified when there is a need for sustained usage, i.e. 15 h or more per day over a long period.

In the USA about half a million patients use liquid oxygen, which is very flexible in use. A 30- to 40-L container lasts 8–10 days at 2 L/min output.

Cylinders with normal head units, oxygen concentrators and liquid oxygen containers are unsuitable for driving nebulizers.

Tents, masks and cannulae

For hospital patients who are severely ill or debilitated, or for whom minimal attachment of equipment is desirable, an **oxygen tent** or an 'oxygen hood' may be used, but this is uncommon. It is more usual to use **masks**, which cover the mouth and nose, or **nasal cannulae**. Fixed performance masks are preferable because the concentration delivered by variable performance masks varies with the breathing pattern.

These devices are illustrated in Fig. 5.29 and their characteristics are summarized in Table 5.23. Nasal cannulae have the advantage that there is no restriction on eating, drinking and talking, because the mouth is not obstructed. Further, patients in respiratory distress often do not tolerate masks. Although nasal cannulae give poor control of the oxygen concentration in the inspired air, they are generally preferred for the delivery of LTOT (see below). Endotracheal cannulae are sometimes used in hospital to achieve better control. Oxygen concentrators are designed to be used only with nasal cannulae.

Reservoir systems are available to reduce the wastage of oxygen in the expired air. They can reduce the oxygen requirement by about 50%. Pulse systems which deliver oxygen only on inspiration can reduce this to about 25%. The latter are unsuitable for use with concentrators. Neither of these arrangements are available on prescription in the UK.

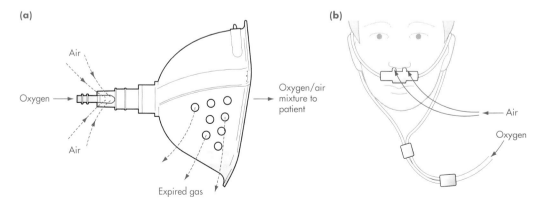

Figure 5.29 Typical oxygen mask and nasal cannula. (a) Ventimask 3 (Vickers). (b) Nasal cannula (Intersurgical).

Table 5.23   The types of oxygen masks and nasal cannulae, and their applications

Patient features	Types of performance[a]	Oxygen concentration delivered (% v/v)	Oxygen flow rate (L/min)[b]
Poor ventilatory drive, e.g. COPD	Constant	24 or 28[c]	2
Good ventilatory drive, e.g. asthma, pneumonia, pulmonary oedema	Constant Variable	31, 35, 40, 60 25–60[a]	[d] [e]

[a] Constant performance masks deliver a constant oxygen concentration over a wide range of flow rates. The output of variable performance masks depends on oxygen flow rate, the breathing pattern of the patient and other factors. Nasal connulae are the most commonly used form of variable performance device.

[b] Domicillary oxygen equipment provided in the UK under the NHS will deliver only 2 L/min at the 'Medium' setting and 4 L/min at the 'High' setting.

[c] The only type of mask which can be supplied in the UK through the NHS on prescription Form FP10 delivers 28% oxygen. It is unsuitable for use with oxygen concentrators with which nasal cannulae are usually preferred. If other concentrations are required the masks must be provided by a hospital or purchased.

[d] These are operable over a range of flow rates, as follows:

Oxygen concentration (% v/v)	24	28	31	35	40	60
Flow rates (L/min)	2–4	4–8	6–10	8–12	10–15	15–25

Oxygen flow rates must be sufficient to prevent inspiration of excess ambient air through the exhaust holes in the mask.

[e] See note (a); a nasal cannula operated at 2 L/min usually provides about 30% v/v of oxygen in the inspired air. These masks may be suitable for use with oxygen concentrators.

COPD, chronic obstructive pulmonary disease.

Intermittent positive pressure ventilation (IPPV)

These ventilators provide control of five parameters:

- Pressure of delivery of gas to the lungs.
- Duration of each pressure pulse.
- Degree of oxygen enrichment of the air.
- Inspiratory trigger pressure.
- End-expiratory pressure.

Initially, a low trigger pressure and a long, high-pressure oxygen pulse are used, forcing gas into the lungs. This removes the work of breathing from the patient but care is needed to avoid lung damage due to excessive pressures (**barotrauma**). As improvement occurs the trigger pressure is increased and the degree of assistance and oxygen enrichment reduced. A nebulizer is used to humidify the gas, so the equipment can also be used to deliver drugs.

However, if respiratory function is reasonable there is no evidence that the routine use of IPPV simply to deliver drugs is beneficial.

IPPV is instituted in hypoxaemic respiratory failure if the patient is in respiratory distress despite maximal treatment, e.g. exhaustion, inability to speak and a high respiration rate. IPPV requires endotracheal intubation, rarely tracheostomy, and also skilled initiation and supervision. A recent innovation is IPPV via a nasal mask (non-invasive IPPV, NIPPV), which is of particular value in **sleep apnoea**. Assisted ventilation has numerous hazards.

Guidelines for domiciliary oxygen therapy

Because of the cost of providing this service and the need to select patients and define objectives carefully, the following guidelines have been issued in the UK.

- Oxygen should be given only after a careful evaluation of the needs of the patient and never as a placebo.
- Patients should be supervised carefully, at least initially. A few patients may revert to an

adequate P_aO_2 (8 kPa) after several months of therapy, so oxygen may then be withdrawn.

- **Intermittent therapy**, using cylinders, is suitable for patients with:
  - Hypoxaemia of short duration, e.g. in asthma, pneumonia and pulmonary oedema.
  - Advanced irreversible respiratory disease to improve mobility and the quality of life, e.g. in chronic bronchitis, emphysema, pulmonary fibrosis, pulmonary thromboembolism and pulmonary hypertension.
- **Long-term therapy** implies the use of oxygen for a minimum of 15 h/day, including the night, so it is used for patients with chronic hypoxaemia and cor pulmonale. In these cases it is more economical to use a concentrator. The aim is to maintain the P_aO_2 at about 10.7 (9.3–12) kPa without producing hypercapnia, consequent on reducing the ventilatory drive. This can usually be achieved with a nasal cannula and a flow rate of 1.5–3 L/min. Because there are advantages for only a limited number of patients, clinical UK guidelines are published by the Department of Health which define the groups likely to benefit, i.e. those:
  - For whom there is an absolute indication with scientific evidence of benefit, e.g. patients with COPD (FEV$_1$ <1.5 L, FVC <2.0 L) associated with hypoxaemia (P_aO_2 <7.3 kPa) and hypercapnia (P_aCO_2 >6 kPa) who have had peripheral oedema. This improves both survival and quality of life.
  - Who would probably benefit but no scientific evidence exists for undisputed advantage, as occurs in COPD with hypoxaemia but no hypercapnia or oedema, e.g. patients with cystic fibrosis or chronic refractory asthma.
  - For whom oxygen would have a useful palliative effect, e.g. in severe kyphoscoliosis (spinal deformity), gross obesity, and terminally ill patients with persistent hypoxaemia, and neuropathies or myopathies which affect the respiratory muscles.
- Further criteria need to be satisfied before LTOT is prescribed:
  - Patients should be non-smokers and compliant, with optimal treatment.
  - Two measurements of blood gases should be made 3–4 weeks apart and repeated at 6–12 months and not less than 4 weeks after an acute exacerbation of the disease.
  - Regular home monitoring should be available.

The criteria for LTOT are liable to periodic revision and the BNF section 3.6 should be consulted for the latest information. Different criteria are used in other countries, e.g. the presence of cor pulmonale, oedema or polycythaemia (packed cell volume >56%). Oxygen may be prescribed much more loosely, possibly because of the emotive nature of the therapy, but this consideration lacks scientific support.

Almitrine dimesilate stimulates the carotid body and improves both ventilation and ventilation–perfusion mismatch. Given with oxygen, the drug further improves P_aO_2 levels.

References and further reading

Barnes PJ, Godfrey S (1999) *Asthma* (*Medical Pocket Books*). 2nd edn. London: Dunitz.

Brewis RAL (1998) *Lecture Notes on Respiratory Disease*. 5th edn. Oxford: Blackwell Science.

Brewis RAL, Corrin B, Geddes GM, Gibson GJ, eds (1995) *Respiratory Medicine*. 2nd edn. London: Bailliere Tindall.

The British Thoracic Society *et al.* (1997) The British Guidelines on Asthma Management: 1995 Review and Position Statement. *Thorax* **52**: Suppl. 1.

The British Thoracic Society (1997) BTS Guidelines for the Management of Chronic Obstructive Pulmonary Disease. *Thorax* **52**: Suppl. 5.

Clark TJH, Rees J (1997) *Practical Management of Asthma*. 3rd edn. London: Dunitz.

Cole RB, McKay D (1990) *Essentials of Respiratory Disease*. 3rd edn. Edinburgh: Churchill Livingstone.

Engels F, Nijkamp FP (1998) Pharmacological inhibition of leukotriene actions. *Pharm World Sci* **20**: 60–65.

Gross NJ, Skorodin MS (1984) Anticholinergic, antimuscarinic bronchodilators. *Am Rev Respir Dis* **129**: 856–870.

Johnson NMcI (1989) *Respiratory Medicine* (*Pocket Consultant*). 2nd edn. Oxford: Blackwell Science.

Muers MF, Corris PA, eds (1997) Current best practice for nebuliser treatment. *Thorax* **52**: Suppl. 2.

Rees J, Price J (1999) *ABC of Asthma*. 4th edn. London: BMJ Publishing.

Rees PJ, Dudley F (1998) ABC of oxygen: provision of oxygen at home. *BMJ* **317**: 935–938.

Royal College of Physicians (1999) Domicilliary oxygen therapy services: clinical guidelines and advice for prescribers.

Sugden L, Chamberlain J, eds (1997) Asthma: current topics and reviews. *J Pharm Pharmacol* **49**: Suppl. 3.

West JB (1995) *Respiratory Physiology – The essentials*. 5th edn. Baltimore: Williams & Wilkins.

West JB (1998) *Pulmonary Pathophysiology – The essentials*. 5th edn. Baltimore: Williams & Wilkins.

6

Gastrointestinal and liver diseases

Gastrointestinal problems are a frequent cause of GP consultations and comprise about 15–20% of the primary care workload. In the West, refined diets and food additives have been implicated in many gastrointestinal and systemic diseases, problems which are exacerbated by the increasing consumption of manufactured and convenience foods. Repeated health scares have led to a proliferation of diets that are often faddist and of dubious nutritional value, and there is a plethora of sometimes conflicting and confusing dietary advice. Intensive farming and increasing technology in the kitchen, e.g. frozen foods, refrigeration and microwave ovens, have combined with a generally poor understanding of basic food hygiene to produce an apparently inexorable rise in the incidence of 'food poisoning' in the UK.

Meanwhile in the Third World, poverty, population increase, crop failure, poor hygiene, political instability and wars have caused massive malnutrition and starvation and refugee problems. These factors have created the conditions for epidemics of gastrointestinal diseases. Underlying all of this are the endemic helminth, protozoal, bacterial and viral infections which are already responsible for intractable public health problems.

Gastrointestinal anatomy and physiology

Overall review

This chapter reviews briefly the anatomy of the digestive tract to assist in the association of symptoms with organs. This leads to a synopsis of gastrointestinal physiology as a basis for appreciating the pathophysiology underlying the principal diseases and disorders, and so their management. More detail about particular organs and their physiology is provided later in the sections dealing with the individual organs.

The gastrointestinal (GI) tract (alimentary tract, gut; Fig. 6.1) consists of an irregular tube some 6 m long, extending from the mouth to the anus. Accessory organs include the teeth, tongue, the salivary, gastric and intestinal glands, liver and gallbladder, and the pancreas.

For the purposes of this text, three groups of organs are distinguished:

- The **upper GI tract**, which includes the mouth, oesophagus, stomach and duodenum.
- The **lower GI tract**, which comprises the jejunum, ileum, colon, rectum and anus.
- The **liver and gallbladder**.

Upper GI tract

Food taken into the mouth is mixed with the saliva to form a plastic mass. The salivary glands secrete about 1 L of fluid daily; this contains a lubricant (mucin) and the polysaccharidase enzyme, salivary amylase.

The food bolus is then swallowed and transferred rapidly via the **oesophagus** into the **stomach**. The latter is joined to the oesophagus at the **gastro-oesophageal junction**, where there is a poorly defined **lower oesophageal sphincter** (LOS). The stomach is a highly distensible J-shaped organ that is enormously variable in size and shape depending on its food content. The stomach secretes a **gastric juice** containing hydrochloric acid and pepsinogen. The acid converts pepsinogen into the proteolytic enzyme **pepsin**, and also has a direct digestive function

by hydrolysing some foods. Infants, but not adults, also secrete the enzyme **rennin** (not to be confused with the renal enzyme, renin), which coagulates milk and so prevents too rapid a passage of liquid milk out of the stomach.

Gastric secretion is under complex nervous and hormonal control. There are three phases of acid secretion:

- **Cephalic**, arising centrally and mediated by vagal stimulation (appetite arousal).
- **Gastric**, which occurs when food both stretches the stomach and stimulates the parietal cells directly.
- **Intestinal**, initiated by the passage of food into the duodenum, which provokes intestinal (local) gastrin release.

The presence of food in the small intestine additionally provokes a nervous (enterogastric) reflex via the vagus nerve, which inhibits gastric secretion, and a further moderate inhibiting effect is produced by small bowel secretion of **secretin** and **cholecystokinin** (CCK). The purposes of these mechanisms are probably to delay further gastric emptying into an already full small intestine and to inhibit unnecessary gastric digestion, once digestion is focused on the intestinal phase.

Between meals, the stomach normally secretes only a few millilitres per hour of slightly alkaline mucus, though this is insufficient to neutralize residual gastric acid, so the basal pH remains acidic. Strong emotional stimuli may cause secretion of about 50 mL/h of acid and pepsin, via the cephalic mechanism.

Peristaltic waves ripple along the walls of the stomach every 15–30 sec, macerating the food and mixing it with the gastric juice, finally producing a fluid called **chyme**. Over some 2–6 h, the whole of the stomach contents is gradually emptied into the **duodenum** via the **pyloric sphincter**. The gastric residence time depends on a variety of factors, including the nature of the contents, being shortest for meals rich in carbohydrate and longest for those rich in fats. Gastric emptying depends on more powerful peristaltic waves which commence in the middle of the stomach and create a relatively high pressure, overcoming the resistance of the pyloric

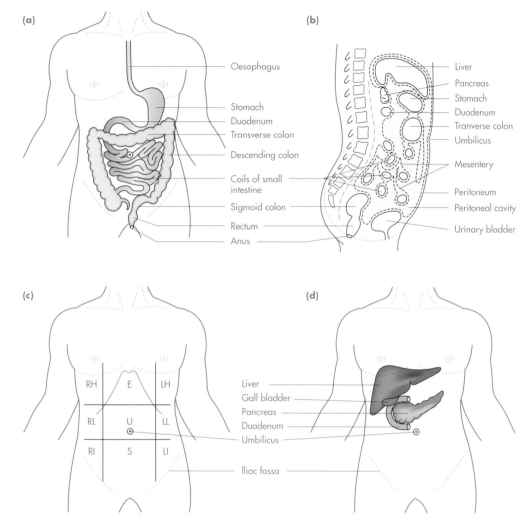

Figure 6.1 The human abdomen and alimentary tract. (a) General anatomy of the alimentary tract. (b) The abdomen in sagittal section. (c) Regions of the abdomen: E, epigastrium; RH, LH, right and left hypochondrium; RI, LI, right and left iliac; RL, LL, right and left lumbar (= lateral or loin); S, suprapubic (= hypogastric); U, umbilical. (d) Surface projections of the major associated organs.

sphincter and forcing out about 5 mL of chyme with each wave. Emptying is also controlled by feedback from the duodenum: in particular, fat in the duodenum delays gastric emptying. Little absorption occurs from the stomach, but salts, alcohol and some acidic drugs, being unionized in the acid environment and so lipophilic, may be absorbed there.

The chyme is discharged into the first part of the **small intestine**, the duodenum, a tube about 25 cm long which curves around the head of the pancreas to merge with the **jejunum**. The duodenal mucosa secretes an alkaline mucus which commences the neutralization of the acid chyme.

Lower GI tract

The jejunum is about 1.5 m long and merges with the final part of the small intestine, the **ileum** (3 m), which joins the **large intestine (colon)** (1.5 m) at the **ileocaecal 'valve'**, though it is unclear whether any histological structure or effective valve actually exists at this location. The walls of the small intestine are covered with **villi**; these are finger-like projections, each about 1 mm long, that enormously increase the small intestine surface area (Fig. 6.2(c)) and thus facilitate the absorption of nutrients and drugs.

Rhythmic contractions of the small intestine mix the chyme with the intestinal digestive secretions, and peristaltic waves gradually propel the mixture through the intestinal length.

Up to 3 L of intestinal juice is secreted daily. This contains mucus, digestive enzymes and bicarbonate, giving a pH of about 7.6. To this juice is added about 1.5 L daily of an alkaline, enzyme-laden, pancreatic juice which is discharged into the duodenum via the **pancreatic duct** (Fig. 6.3). The enzymes in the pancreatic juice convert proteins and protein fragments, fats, carbohydrate residues and nucleic acids into smaller, absorbable molecules.

The **large intestine** comprises the caecum and colon, and terminates with the rectum and anal canal. The **caecum** is a short (6-cm) blind-ended pouch located in the right iliac region (Fig. 6.1(c)), from which the **vermiform appendix** arises. The latter is a 10-cm blind tube for which no proven function exists, though it may have

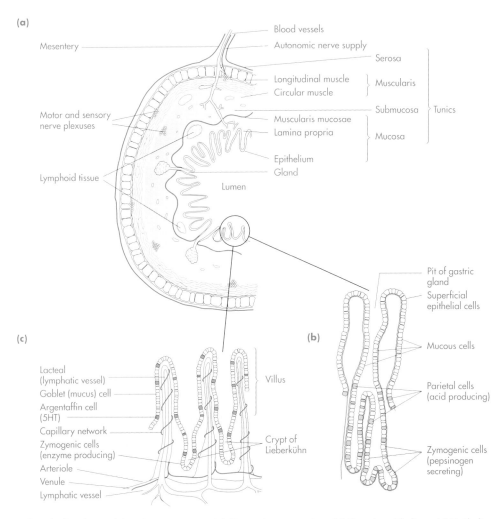

Figure 6.2 The histology of the alimentary tract. (a) General cross-section. (b) Gastric epithelium. (c) Epithelium of the jejunum and proximal ileum.

some protective lymphoid role. Infection of the appendix (**appendicitis**) is the most common surgical emergency. The caecum merges into the **ascending colon** (15 cm long), which turns sharply downwards and to the left, at the **right colic flexure**, to form the **transverse colon** (50 cm) which is concave upwards and ends at the **left colic (splenic) flexure** where it turns down sharply to form the **descending colon** (25 cm).

The final part of the colon consists of two S-shaped tubes, the **sigmoid colon**, which is a loop (40 cm) in the left iliac region, merging into the **rectum** (12 cm). The latter is curved, at first backwards and upwards and then finally downwards and forwards. At its end, the rectum narrows to join the **anal canal** (3.5 cm). The upper part of the latter has up to 10 longitudinal folds (the **anal columns**), and is surrounded by the muscles of the **internal anal sphincter** which holds the anal columns together very tightly in order to prevent faecal leakage. The terminal part of the anal canal, the **anus**, blends into normal skin. For greater security and control, the whole of the length of the anal canal is enclosed by the **external anal sphincter**; this consists of striated muscle which is under voluntary control, unlike the internal sphincter which is composed of involuntary circular smooth muscle.

Regions of the abdomen

The abdominal surface is thought of as being divided into nine regions, for ease of describing the location of organs or symptoms (Fig. 6.1(c)). A comparison of Figs 6.1(a), (c) and (d) indicates the regions under which the various organs lie, and these locations are further outlined in Table 6.1.

Table 6.1 Locations of the principal abdominal organs

Organ	Abdominal region[a]
Stomach	E (left side) and LH (right side)
Duodenum	E (lower right) and U (upper right)
Caecum, appendix	RI
Colon	
• ascending	RI and RL
• transverse	RL, U, LL
• descending	LL, LI
• sigmoid	LI and S (left side)
Liver	
• right lobe	RH and E (right upper)
• left lobe	E (left upper)
Gallbladder	RH (lower)
Pancreas	
• head	U (right upper)
• tail	U (left upper) and LH (right lower)
Kidneys	Around junctions of E, U, hypochondrial and lumbar regions
Spleen	LH

[a] Letters refer to Fig. 6.1(c).

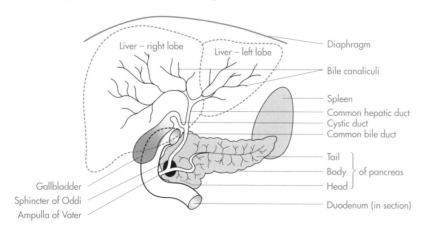

Figure 6.3 The anatomical relationships of the liver, gallbladder, pancreas, and related structures.

General histology of the alimentary tract

The whole of the alimentary tract, apart from the mouth, has a similar basic tissue arrangement. A generalized cross-section of the gut is illustrated in Fig. 6.2(a), which shows that there are four basic layers (**tunics**).

Tunics

The most important of these is the inner lining, the **mucosa**, which itself consists of three layers. The **epithelium** is in contact with the gut contents, has a protective function, and changes somewhat in character in the different areas of the gut. Although continuous with the epidermis (*see* Chapter 12), the epithelium is not keratinized, and permits a variable degree of absorption of foods and drugs to occur, depending on the precise site and local conditions. The **lamina propria** contains glandular epithelium which secretes digestive enzymes and adjuncts. It also contains the blood vessels and lymphatics, bound by loose connective tissue, by means of which absorbed substances enter the circulation and are distributed to the tissues. There are also lymph nodes which provide foci for protection against infective agents. The **muscularis mucosae** contains visceral smooth muscle, the tone of which throws the mucosa into small folds, providing for the considerable changes in volume that are required to respond to food intake while maintaining a large surface area for digestion and absorption.

The **submucosa** consists mostly of loose connective tissue, but has a rich blood supply and also contains glands and structures concerned with the autonomic nerve supply to the muscularis mucosae.

The **muscularis** throughout most of the gut consists of an inner circular layer of smooth muscle and an outer longitudinal layer. Contractions of these muscles tends to break down the food masses, and causes the food to mix with the digestive juices, after which it is propelled (by peristalsis) along the alimentary tract. The mouth, pharynx and oesophagus have a more complex, partly striated, musculature.

Within the abdomen, the gut is surrounded by the folds of the **peritoneum**, which form the outer layer of the gut, the **serosa**. These folds support the viscera, hold the organs in relation to each other and to the abdominal wall, and carry the blood, nerve and lymphatic supplies to the gut. Where these supplies enter the gut wall the tunics are structurally weakened, and this may result in pouches (**diverticula**, p. 346) being formed under pressure within the lumen. That part of the peritoneum which supports the small intestine is the **mesentery**, the **mesocolon** similarly supporting the large intestine. Other important peritoneal folds are the **falciform ligament** which attaches the liver to the abdominal wall and the diaphragm, the **lesser omentum** which suspends the stomach and duodenum from the liver, and the **greater omentum**, a large fold of tissue which hangs like an apron in front of the intestines. The greater omentum contains numerous lymph nodes and is the principal repository of abdominal fat. The large surface area and rich blood supply of the peritoneum make it valuable for **peritoneal dialysis** in renal failure (*see* Chapter 4). Peritoneal infection (**peritonitis**) is always extremely dangerous because the peritoneum is in contact with all the abdominal organs, which may be infected secondarily, and because it has a large surface area for the absorption of toxins.

Stomach

The mucosa of the stomach is highly specialized. It contains numerous minute openings which are the apertures of the gastric glands (Fig. 6.2(b)). These glands are lined with three types of secretory cells. The zymogenic (chief) cells secrete **pepsinogen**, which is converted into **pepsin** by the hydrochloric acid produced by the **parietal** cells. The parietal cells also secrete **intrinsic factor**, a glycoprotein which binds vitamin B_{12} (**extrinsic factor**) from the food and transports it to specific ileal mucosal receptors, where the vitamin B_{12} is liberated into the cells. The intrinsic factor remains in the gut lumen and is recycled. The mucous cells secrete an alkaline, bicarbonate-laden mucus which, together with other factors (*see* Fig. 6.9 and p. 323) protects the mucosa from the acid and pepsin and also further moistens and lubricates the food.

Small intestine

The mucosa of the small intestine (Fig. 6.2(c)) has many folds and numerous finger-like villi, which carry many more minute **microvilli** projecting from their surface. This arrangement produces an enormous surface area for the secretion of digestive enzymes and the absorption of food. The core of each villus contains specialized lymphatic vessels (**lacteals**) surrounded by a network of arterioles and venules. Between the bases of the villi are the **crypts of Lieberkühn**, which contain the zymogenic (enzyme-producing) cells. The epithelial cells are formed at the bases of the crypts and migrate upwards over a period of about 3–4 days, after which they are shed. Thus, the epithelium is being continuously regenerated, so that any acute pathological process is inherently self-limiting unless the damage is severe or becomes prolonged. This rapid cell turnover makes the gut highly sensitive to radiotherapy and cytotoxic chemotherapy, however, which may cause substantial damage.

In addition to the lymphatic vessels, the lamina propria of the small intestine contains numerous immunologically active cells, e.g. plasma cells, lymphocytes, macrophages, mast cells, etc., solitary lymph nodes and **Peyer's patches** (aggregates of lymph nodes). These are concerned with the immunological defence of the gut and are more numerous in the ileum than in other regions. Specialized **microfold cells (M cells)** above the Peyer's patches permit the ready localization of antigens which stimulate the local cloning of B cells (*see* Chapter 2). The latter secrete IgA (secretory immunoglobulin) into the gut lumen, providing surface protection against infective agents.

Large intestine

The colon has five principal functions:

1. To complete the digestion of residual foodstuff. Although the colon does not secrete enzymes, it harbours bacteria which ferment carbohydrate, convert amino acids to indole and skatole (which give faeces its characteristic odour) and bilirubin to urobilinogen. Bacterial action also produces some of our daily intake of B vitamins and vitamin K and breaks down some pro-drugs, e.g. sulfasalazine.
2. To secrete mucus, which lubricates faecal passage and protects the mucosa.
3. To convert the fluid ileal contents into faecal paste by mixing and the extraction of water.
4. To absorb electrolytes and vitamins.
5. To store the faeces until defecation is convenient.

Because colonic function is relatively simple, the mucosa is composed of only two cell types: columnar cells which primarily absorb water and electrolytes, and goblet cells which secrete mucus. There are isolated lymphatic nodules, which form part of the immune system.

Nutrient breakdown and absorption

Proteins

The digestion of protein commences in the stomach where pepsin (under acidic conditions) converts proteins into peptides; these then stimulate the pyloric antrum to secrete **gastrin**. The gastrin enhances the secretion of **histamine**, and so of acid, from the parietal cells and of bicarbonate-laden mucus from the superficial epithelial cells. Discharge of the acid chyme into the duodenum stimulates further **gastrin** release, which in turn promotes the production of bile and also stimulates the pancreas to secrete bicarbonate.

The presence of dietary fats in the small intestine triggers the secretion of CCK (pancreozymin), leading to pancreatic pro-enzyme release, e.g. trypsinogen, and bile ejection from the gallbladder. Vagally mediated acetylcholine release is also involved. The trypsinogen is converted into active **trypsin**, which in turn converts other pancreatic pro-enzymes into active proteolytic enzymes. These produce absorbable dipeptides and free amino acids, and longer-chain peptides. These longer peptides are finally converted into amino acids by specific peptidases in the cells of the microvilli or the epithelium, before their systemic absorption via specific transport mechanisms. Thus there is a complex, hormonal and neuronal positive feedback mechanism, which is responsive to the presence of food in the gut, and which controls the secretion and activation of appropriate enzymes (*see* Fig. 6.2).

Secretin and CCK are used clinically in tests of pancreatic function, their effects being measured in terms of total pancreatic secretion, enzyme or bicarbonate output. **Pentagastrin**, a synthetic gastrin analogue, is used in tests of gastric acid secretion: the 60-min basal acid output is compared with the maximal acid output after stimulation.

Carbohydrates

The digestion of carbohydrates starts in the mouth with **salivary amylase**, which continues to act until stopped by the low gastric pH. However, carbohydrates are mostly digested to monosaccharides in the upper small intestine, first by **pancreatic amylase** and finally by intestinal **saccharidases**. The resultant glucose, fructose and galactose are absorbed into the villi by sodium-dependent active transport systems. Deficiencies of maltase, sucrase and lactase enzymes cause accumulation of the corresponding disaccharides, which pass unabsorbed to the colon, producing an osmotic diarrhoea. Such deficiency may be congenital or may temporarily follow severe diarrhoea. Also, nucleic acids are converted into nucleotides by cleavage of their pentose-phosphate chain.

Fats

Dietary lipids consist principally of triglycerides, plus small amounts of cholesterol and its esters and phospholipids. Lipid digestion occurs predominantly in the small intestine after emulsification by **bile salts**. The resultant fat globules are hydrolysed, primarily by **pancreatic lipase** and, being insoluble, can be hydrolysed only at the globule surface: emulsification is essential to provide an adequate surface area for hydrolysis to proceed effectively. Thus bile salts are required for the absorption of fat-soluble vitamins (A, D) and enhance vitamin A uptake.

Pancreatic lipase hydrolyses triglycerides to monoglycerides plus fatty acids. All of these fatty materials are solubilized and emulsified by the bile salts before their absorption into the villi.

A lipase inhibitor, *orlistat*, is now available to reduce fat absorption and therefore obesity.

However, it must be used as part of a low-fat, weight-reducing diet because otherwise undigested fat will pool in the intestine causing wind (flatus), cramps, diarrhoea and, in the long term, deficiency of fat-soluble vitamins.

Following hydrolysis, the resultant monoglycerides and free fatty acids, which are solubilized in micelles, partition into the lipid membranes of the microvilli and are readily absorbed, the bile salts being recycled and reused. Cholesterol esters are similarly emulsified or solubilized, and are then hydrolysed by **cholesterol esterase**: without bile salt solubilization no cholesterol whatsoever is absorbed. Thus, diseases reducing gallbladder and pancreatic activity may result in only 30–50% of dietary fat being absorbed. The resultant fatty stools are pale, soft and particularly foul-smelling (**steatorrhoea**). Very short gut transit times can cause similar effects.

After absorption, the fatty acids are reconstituted into triglycerides. Globules of these, plus cholesterol and phospholipids, are coated with protein to yield **chylomicrons**, all but the smallest of which pass into the central lacteals of the villi (Figs 6.2(c) and 6.4) and into the general circulation via the thoracic duct.

Bile salts are highly conserved, with 95% being reabsorbed in the distal ileum; thus ileal diseases, e.g. Crohn's disease, may lead to a failure to reabsorb bile salts. When bile salts reach the colon they are highly irritant and are partly responsible for the severe diarrhoea of this condition. Indeed, bile salts used to be used as laxatives.

Fluid and electrolyte absorption and conservation

Sodium

Each day, about 25 g of sodium is secreted into the gut, and a further 5 g is ingested with food: this total of 30 g represents about 15% of the total body sodium. Active sodium resorption occurs in the upper jejunum, where it is associated with monosaccharide and amino acid absorption, and in the ileum and ascending colon. Sodium transport is always accompanied by water, so almost complete water resorption also occurs, especially in the distal ileum and in the colon (Table 6.2), such that only about 100 mL of water is lost daily in the faeces.

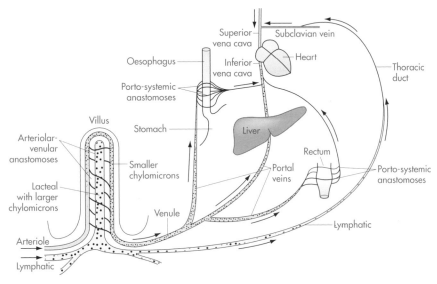

Figure 6.4   Portal and associated circulations (arrows indicate directions of flow).

Because the absorption of sodium from the small intestine must be accompanied by water, this mechanism is used to treat dehydration by oral rehydration. Sodium absorption is facilitated by glucose (facilitated active transport), so water absorption is enhanced. This is the rationale

behind the use of *oral rehydration salts* (containing glucose) and numerous similar proprietary products for the treatment of fluid loss due to severe diarrhoea and vomiting.

The ileal discharge is always fluid or semi-fluid (about 1 L/day), compared with the formed stools in the colon, and these differences have implications for the management of patients with stomas (p. 354).

Calcium

Absorption of calcium occurs in the small intestine, being intimately linked to the presence of the active form of vitamin D (*1,25-dihydroxycholecalciferol*, calcitriol) and a specific calcium-binding protein. Although described as a vitamin, it is clear that 1,25-dihydroxycholecalciferol (*see* Fig. 6.20) is a hormone which controls calcium homeostasis, primarily in association with parathyroid hormone (PTH). Vitamin D synthesis and calcium absorption are regulated principally by PTH, though other hormones (calcitonin, glucocorticoids, and sex, growth and thyroid hormones) are also involved.

Iron

In the UK, the average daily intake of iron is about 20 mg, only 2 mg of which is absorbed (in

Table 6.2   Fluid balance in the alimentary tract

Process		Approx. daily volume (L)	
Fluid intake from diet		1.5	
Excretion into the gut	Saliva	1.0	
	Gastric juice	2.5	
	Bile	0.5	
	Pancreatic juice	0.7	
	Small intestine	2.8	
	Total flow into the gut		9.0
Resorption from the gut	Small intestine	7.5	
	Colon	1.4	
	Total resorption from the gut		8.9
Excreted in the faeces			0.1

the duodenum and jejunum), although absorption increases in iron-deficiency states. The average daily requirement of iron for erythropoiesis is about 20 mg. Because there is a daily iron loss of about 750 microgram (plus about 2.5 mg/month in menstruation), it is clear that the iron content of the body is finely regulated, absorption being linked closely to needs. Most of the iron liberated by the breakdown of haemoglobin and other molecules is conserved. Some factors which influence iron absorption are given in Table 6.3.

Potassium
The average dietary intake of potassium is about 80 mmol/day, and a further 40 mmol is excreted into the small intestine in the succus entericus. As only about 10 mmol/day is lost in the faeces, about 110 mmol/day is absorbed in the ileum and colon. Diarrhoea and vomiting may produce substantial losses of potassium (and sodium), so fluid and electrolyte replacement is vital in severe or prolonged cases. Although some degree of potassium loss occurs with long-term diuretic use, especially with thiazide diuretics, oral potassium repletion is rarely indicated (*see* Chapter 3).

Absorption sites for nutrients and drugs

Some 90% of nutrients are absorbed in the small intestine, the remainder being absorbed in the stomach and large intestine. Absorption may be by processes of **active transport** (e.g. amino acids, sodium, potassium, calcium, iron) or of **diffusion** (e.g. water, chloride, fats). Fructose and some other nutrients are absorbed by the energy-independent process of **facilitated diffu-**

sion, which is faster than simple diffusion. The transport of amino acids, glucose and galactose is linked to that of sodium, the membrane transporter having binding sites for both sodium and the substance: this is **secondary active transport**. Water absorption always accompanies that of solutes, as a 'carrier', and water also moves freely, following osmotic gradients.

Whether substances (including drugs) are absorbed may depend crucially on their lipophilicity and, for some, also on their ionizability. Generally, lipophilic substances will dissolve in the lipoid villus membrane and then be released inside the cell, so the pKa of an ionizable substance and the local pH will decide whether that substance is absorbed or not.

Thus, for example, *aspirin* is unionized (lipophilic) in the acid gastric juice and so will be absorbed into the gastric mucosa. Once inside the cells it ionizes and is unable to diffuse out, and so is concentrated there. This property accounts in part for the ulcerogenic property of aspirin and related drugs.

Soluble substances and small chylomicrons enter the mucosal blood and then the portal vein and so are delivered direct to the liver (Fig. 6.4) where they are processed before discharge into the systemic circulation. This, together with any transformation which occurs during absorption, is **presystemic (first-pass) metabolism**. Although this occurs with many types of absorbed compounds, the term is usually applied to drugs and may be very important with some of them, to reduce or enhance their bioavailability. Thus with organic nitrates (e.g. glyceryl trinitrate, GTN) and propranolol, high oral doses must be given, while with levodopa the enzyme inhibitors benserazide or carbidopa are co-administered. Because presystemic metabolism is reduced in the elderly and in liver disease, doses of drugs that have a high 'first-pass extraction rate', i.e. are extensively metabolized in their first pass through the liver, may have to be reduced in such patients. For example, with propranolol the plasma concentration may be doubled in the elderly if the dose is not reduced. An alternative procedure is to avoid the portal circulation, and so bypass presystemic metabolism, by giving the drug buccally (GTN), transdermally (GTN, hyoscine (scopolamine), sex hormones) or

Table 6.3 Some factors influencing iron absorption from the gut

Increased by	Decreased by
Ferrous state	Ferric state
Reducing agents	Chelating agents (e.g. tetracyclines)
Gastric acid	Alkalis (antacids)
Inorganic state	Organic state
Iron deficiency	Iron overload
Erythropoiesis	Dietary phosphate
Alcohol	Dietary phytate (unmodified bran)

parenterally, if that is practicable or desirable. When drugs are formulated as pro-drugs to enhance absorption, we depend on metabolism to liberate the active form.

The larger chylomicrons are unable to enter the blood stream directly and are carried in the lymphatic circulation via the thoracic duct, discharging into the blood at the subclavian vein (Fig. 6.4).

Investigation

Only the common general investigations are described here. More specific tests are dealt with under the diseases to which they apply.

History

As usual, it is important to obtain a good history and to listen to patients and observe their appearance and behaviour carefully. Food and the GI tract are powerfully associated with emotional and social attitudes, and public misconceptions are common. Attention to these aspects may provide important clues to patient understanding, to social attitudes and to emotional state, all of which may have bearing on the interpretation of the information obtained.

It has been demonstrated that it takes only 5 min to obtain a good gastrointestinal history and, following this and an examination, a doctor will have about 80% of the information required for a probable diagnosis. The principal points to note are outlined in Table 6.4.

Table 6.4   The principal information to be obtained in a gastrointestinal history[a]

History of symptoms	
Duration	
	• intermittent, continuous, recurrent, progressive; if recurrent, are the symptoms the same or different from the last?
Severity	
Site and radiation	• initial, subsequent, now
Relationship to	• time of day
	• food intake
	• bowel motions
	• menstrual cycle
	• life events, e.g. bereavements, divorce, etc.
Relieving factors	• alkalis used
	• food and fluid intake
	• posture
	• local warmth, cold, etc.
Aggravating factors	• activity, work, stress (also as relieving factors)
	• appetite, taste, diet
Recent changes in	• weight, significant change without apparent cause
	• salivation
	• bowel action (frequency, consistency, colour, odour)
Pain	• site, type, severity, radiation, etc.
	• dysphagia (possibly serious), dyspepsia, heartburn or flatulence (wind)
Nausea and vomiting	

Other information
Recent travel (if so, where?)
Skin rashes, allergies, intercurrent diseases and medications
Previous treatments (especially abdominal or surgical)

[a] *See also* Chapter 1.

It is important for community pharmacists to be able to identify the signs and symptoms which may indicate the more serious gastrointestinal diseases, and to determine the urgency of treatment or referral, because they are often asked to advise on the treatment of conditions causing apparently minor symptoms. Specific symptoms and signs will be discussed under the various organs and diseases.

Imaging

Radiology

Plain X-rays of the abdomen are of little value in investigating most gastrointestinal diseases. However, they can be useful in investigating acute conditions, when they will show accumulation of air, toxic dilatation of the intestine and the presence of accumulated fluid (*see* Fig. 6.14).

Barium contrast studies
Using fine suspensions of radio-opaque barium sulphate, these were the mainstay of investigation for many years, including the following:

- Barium swallow to visualize the oesophagus or to demonstrate refluxing of gastric contents.
- Barium meal to examine the stomach and duodenum. This is often combined with a small-bowel follow-through, i.e. 'barium meal and follow-through', to visualize the gross anatomy of the small intestine, particularly the terminal ileum.
- Barium enemas. Barium is introduced into the empty large bowel rectally. This permits visualization of the whole of the colon and, usually, the terminal ileum, but not the rectum. A small-bowel enema uses a large volume of dilute barium suspension, introduced directly into the duodenum via an orally inserted tube. It provides more detailed information on areas of the small bowel which are suspicious on the follow-through.
- Double-contrast techniques are usually required for satisfactory visualization of the stomach and duodenum and the large bowel. A barium meal is followed by introducing a gas (carbon dioxide in the stomach, by giving bicarbonate, and air in the colon) to distend the organ and push the barium sulphate into and around lesions (*see* Figs 6.11 and 6.14).

Fluoroscopy
Direct continuous inspection of an X-ray image on a sensitive screen (nowadays a video monitor fed from an image intensifier to reduce the radiation dose to the radiologist) is especially useful for investigating disordered gut motility. The occurrence of gastro-oesophageal reflux (p. 310) can be observed directly.

Computed tomography (CT scanning)

This is a computer-enhanced X-ray technique which provides views of a succession of thin 'slices' of tissue, though in much greater detail and contrast than conventional radiography. Its principal use in gastroenterology is to examine organs outside the gut, e.g. the liver and pancreas. The radiation dose from CT is relatively high but is less with newer machines.

Nuclear magnetic resonance imaging (MRI)

The MRI scan is a newer technique than CT scanning and depends on atomic excitation by powerful magnets to produce images. It is capable of producing images of great detail and clarity, similar to CT though often superior to it. Both investigations are expensive, especially MRI, but have the advantage of being completely non-invasive. A problem with current MRI machines is the necessity for confinement of the patients in a small tunnel for some time, during which they must be absolutely still, and some find this intolerable: the newer machines are less claustrophobic.

Endoscopy

Endoscopes permit direct viewing of organs and structures within the body. The older type is a rigid tube containing a plastic 'light pipe' which connects the objective and eyepiece lenses. A channel is provided for powerful illumination of the object to be visualized. This type of instrument is now used only for proctoscopy and sigmoidoscopy (inspection of the rectum and terminal part of the sigmoid colon respectively) and for the removal of obstructions from the oesophagus, e.g. fish bones.

The **fibreoptic endoscope** (Fig. 6.5) is much more useful, and has revolutionized hospital gastroenterological practice. The light pipe and illumination channel consist of a **flexible** fibre-optic bundle which transmits light very efficiently and is completely steerable through the gut. **Gastroscopes** permit visualization of the oesophagus, stomach and duodenum, while **colonoscopes** provide views of the rectum, the whole of the colon, and the terminal ileum.

There is an increasing trend for **interventional endoscopy**, in which instruments are inserted through the tube and used to take biopsy samples and to carry out minor operations. These include the removal of foreign bodies, gallstones and colonic polyps, and cautery or injection of scle-rosant to arrest bleeding. Patients are first sedated with a benzodiazepine (*diazepam, lorazepam, midazolam* or *temazepam*), a procedure which has the advantage of producing amnesia, especially lorazepam, so patients have little recollection of an uncomfortable procedure. Temazepam has a rapid onset of action and gives rapid recovery, patients being reasonably alert after about 2 h. Local anaesthetic throat sprays (*see* Chapter 10) are used occasionally before gastroscopy.

Endoscopy is more invasive and uncomfortable than radiographic imaging and cannot be used for certain purposes, e.g. investigating refluxing. Which technique is used will depend on patient suitability and the availability of facilities and local expertise.

Ultrasound

This technique, which uses computer analysis of ultrasonic reflections from internal organs, is completely non-invasive and non-stressful. It can be used to visualize a variety of abdominal structures, especially the gallbladder and biliary tree and is being developed further.

Stool examination

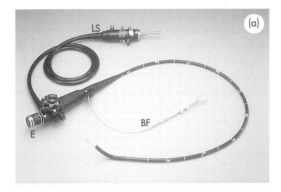

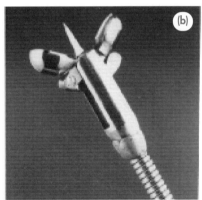

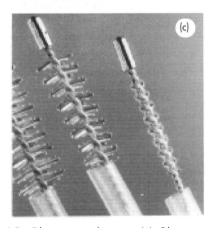

Figure 6.5   Fibreoptic endoscope. (a) Olympus gastro-scope and attached high-power light source conductor (LS) and biopsy forceps (BF) inserted. E, eyepiece. (b) Biopsy forceps. (c) Brushes for surface cytology. (b) and (c) are instruments for insertion through the endoscope. (Reproduced with permission from KeyMed-Medical and Industrial Equipment-Ltd, Southend-on-Sea, UK.)

Examination of the stool is used to look for:

- The passage of blood. Large amounts in the upper gut (>100 mL) are obvious as **melaena**, or on microscopy, while smaller amounts not apparent visually are detected by the **faecal occult blood** test, but this is of limited value because it yields a high proportion of false positives.

- Excessive fat (steatorrhoea) or undigested food in suspected malabsorption syndromes (p. 335).
- Pathogens by microscopy or stool culture.

Other investigations

The standard investigations provide valuable information about the possible origins of symptoms, as well as on the condition of patients and their progress. In cases of uncertainty the tests ordered should depend on the provisional diagnosis, because specialized tests are usually expensive and not readily available. Further, the best

yield of information comes from carefully targeted tests ordered on the basis of sound clinical evidence. Examples of a few specialized gastroenterological tests are given below.

In developed countries, nutritional deficiency is rare and vitamin assays are unusual. However, vitamin assays may be carried out for example in pregnancy (folate), strict vegans (vitamins B_{12}, D), anorexia (folate), liver and gallbladder disease (vitamins A, D), renal failure (vitamin D), alcoholism (B vitamins) and malabsorption syndromes.

Examples of other specialized tests in gastroenterology are oesophageal manometry in achalasia (p. 315), jejunal biopsy in malabsorption (Fig. 6.13), oral *sodium amidotrizoate* to locate fast gastrointestinal bleeds, and radiolabelled erythrocytes to locate slow bleeds.

Disorders of the upper gastrointestinal tract

Oesophageal disorders

Introduction

The principal oesophageal disorders are **gastro-oesophageal reflux disease**, **dysphagia** (difficulty in swallowing), **pain on swallowing** and **bleeding**. These may due to:

- Local problems within the oesophagus, e.g. infection, inflammation, ulceration, malignancy.
- A manifestation of generalized disease, e.g. oesophageal varices (consequent on hepatic disease, e.g. cirrhosis (p. 376), systemic sclerosis (*see* Chapter 8) and diabetes mellitus (*see* Chapter 9).
- Neuromuscular dysfunction, e.g. achalasia, spasm, myasthenia gravis.
- Pressure from neighbouring organs, e.g. goitre, left atrial enlargement due to hypertension.

- Pregnancy, causing refluxing of stomach contents into the oesophagus.

Gastro-oesophageal reflux disease (GORD)

Definition and aetiology

The most common symptom of GORD is **heartburn**, which occurs in about 75% of cases. Heartburn is a commonly occurring retrosternal burning pain of variable severity which accounts for about 30% of all cases of dyspepsia. It is usually due to **reflux oesophagitis**, i.e. the refluxing of gastric contents, occasionally with some bile, into the oesophagus, against which the oesophageal mucosa has little or no protection. A number of factors may reduce the competence of the LOS, and so predispose to refluxing. These include:

- Fatty foods, including chocolate, which lubricate the mucosa of the LOS.

- Excessive caffeine (coffee) consumption and anticholinergic drugs, which relax the smooth muscle of the LOS.

It is reported that the incidence of GORD (GERD in North America) is rising, and this is accompanied by a rapid, worrying rise in the incidence of oesophageal cancer. Up to 25% of duodenal ulcer patients from whom *Helicobacter pylori* has been eradicated (see below) may develop GORD.

About 50% of pregnant women suffer from heartburn, due to raised intra-abdominal pressure, reduced sphincter tone or to a temporary **hiatus hernia**. This is a protrusion of the stomach through the diaphragm (Fig. 6.6). Because the stomach is then subjected to abnormal pressure differentials, and the muscles of the diaphragm do not aid the sphincter action, this condition predisposes to refluxing, especially on bending forward. A **permanent hiatus hernia** may be congenital or occur in early infancy, but is more usual in the middle-aged and elderly. Although many patients with demonstrable hiatus hernia are asymptomatic, or show symptoms other than heartburn, the presence of a hiatus hernia may aggravate refluxing. Similar symptoms may also occur in normal subjects without demonstrable refluxing and with an undamaged oesophageal mucosa, resulting from an abnormality of oesophageal motility.

Other causes of oesophageal damage are excessive alcohol (spirits) consumption and candidiasis. Candidal infection may result from depressed immunity (e.g. by drugs, including inhaled corticosteroids, or malignancy) or from broad-spectrum antibiotic treatment, especially in debilitated or immunosuppressed patients. Taking tablets or capsules while lying down, or without adequate fluid, may result in the medication being retained in the oesophagus and release of the drug there, causing local irritation or ulceration. This is a particular problem with drugs such as *potassium*, *aspirin*, *indometacin* and other NSAIDs, some *antibiotics*, *alendronic acid*, and in elderly patients.

It is not known precisely why **smoking** aggravates symptoms, because it has numerous pharmacological effects, but increased gastric acid production, gastric and oesophageal stasis and local irritation may all be involved.

People with an abnormality which restricts the oesophageal lumen, e.g. oesophageal stricture, aortic aneurysm, bronchial carcinoma or an enlarged left atrium consequent on mitral valve disease, are also at risk. The left main bronchus, the heart and the aortic arch are in close proximity to the oesophagus and may indent it or cause its deviation. Disease of mediastinal organs may thus increase the risk of oesophageal restriction.

The relationship between oesophageal reflux, hiatus hernia and the occurrence of symptoms is illustrated diagrammatically in Fig. 6.7.

Clinical features and diagnosis

The pain often occurs after food, which induces the secretion of gastric acid. An alcoholic or other 'night-cap' often causes nocturnal symptoms because lying down promotes refluxing

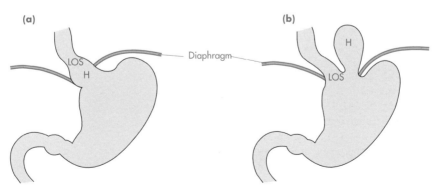

Figure 6.6   Types of hiatus hernia. (a) 'Sliding'. (b) Para-oesophageal ('rolling'). H, herniated portion of stomach projecting through the diaphragm; LOS, lower oesophageal sphincter.

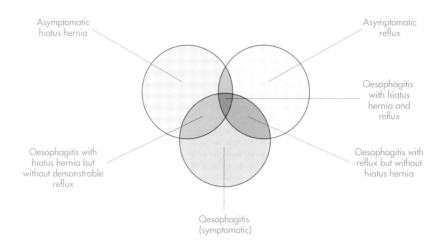

Figure 6.7   Relationships between oesophageal reflux, hiatus hernia and symptomatic oesophagitis.

from a consequently full, acid-laden stomach. However, refluxing does not usually disturb sleep. Exertion or bending forward may also produce refluxing. Occasionally the pain may be so severe as to mimic that of angina pectoris or myocardial infarction. There is an association between refluxing and asthma, because reflux causes vagally mediated bronchoconstriction in about 50% of asthmatics, making asthma diagnosis more difficult. The symptoms that may be associated with refluxing are outlined in Table 6.5.

Diagnosis is based on the clinical features and endoscopy, although there is a poor correlation between the severity of symptoms and endoscopy findings. GORD is the likely diagnosis if heartburn occurs on two days a week or more. It is also probable if upper abdominal or lower retrosternal symptoms are reliably relieved by antacids. Therapeutic trial with high-dose *proton pump inhibitors* (PPIs) is useful diagnostically.

However, other investigations which have been used widely in the past, e.g. fluoroscopic demonstration of reflux and production of symptoms on 24-h oesophageal acid exposure, are unreliable.

Table 6.5   Symptoms and conditions that may be associated with a hiatus hernia

Common conditions	Uncommon conditions[a]
Heartburn, especially postural (70%)	Dysphagia
Regurgitation of food, acid in throat (60%)	Gastric ulceration
Wind, bloating (45%)	Anaemia, haematemesis, melaena
Nausea (35%)	Severe upper abdominal pain
Sharp chest pain (35%)	
Stomach ache (25%)	
Breathing problems (20%)	
Aspiration pneumonitis	

[a] These require extensive investigation as they usually have some other cause. Severe pain may be due to strangulation, i.e. ischaemia of the hernia due to pressure from the muscles of the diaphragm and other organs.

Long-term complications

Although GORD usually occurs as a relatively brief acute attack of heartburn, repeated insult may cause oesophageal damage and chronic, persistent problems. Complications consequent on chronic mucosal damage include:

- Pain on swallowing.
- Ulceration.
- Haemorrhage.
- Oesophageal stricture causing dysphagia.
- Perforation or malignancy (rarely).

However, only about 5% of new patients with presumptive GORD are likely to experience significant local complications.

Management: general aspects

The **principal aim** is to prevent reflux occurring and so prevent damage to the oesophageal mucosa and the development of complications. Drugs may also be used secondarily to relieve symptoms by reducing the acidity and irritancy of the refluxed gastric contents, and to improve the competence of the LOS. Drug treatment is primarily with PPIs. Antacids, H_2-receptor antagonists and sphincter 'strengtheners' are also used. General measures involving lifestyle modification are of low efficacy, but may be useful as adjuncts to effective pharmacotherapy.

All treatments, especially the antisecretory agents, may mask the presence of gastric malignancy, so it is essential to exclude this possibility by gastroscopy before initiating treatment aimed at the reduction of significant pain or if a trial of therapy is unsuccessful.

General measures

These alone may be adequate in mild GORD, but good evidence for this approach is lacking. In view of this, patients should not attempt lifestyle modifications which impose excessive burdens. In the absence of good research-based evidence it seems sensible to avoid factors which precipitate symptoms, i.e.:

- Reduce weight if obese, to reduce intra-abdominal pressure.
- Take alcohol and caffeine-containing products only in moderation.

- Avoid:
  - Large meals, especially at night, acid foods.
  - A fatty diet and chocolate.
  - Tight clothing or belts.
  - Stooping and heavy lifting (bend the knees with the back straight).
  - Drugs which may reduce LOS pressure, e.g. *anticholinergics* (including tricyclic antidepressants), *diazepam*, *nifedipine* and *theophylline*.
- Stopping smoking may help some patients.

Management: pharmacotherapy

The properties of the drugs are described under 'peptic ulcer' (pp. 326–330), but aspects relevant to GORD are discussed below.

Antacids

Simple, infrequent, uncomplicated reflux oesophagitis should be treated symptomatically, using antacids as symptoms occur. Suspensions are more effective than tablets but, for convenience and prompt availability, the latter should be carried and sucked at the first sign of symptoms to minimize mucosal damage. They may also be sucked frequently between meals if symptoms tend to persist.

Alginate-antacid preparations.   These depend on the reaction between alginate, sodium bicarbonate and gastric acid to form a foam stabilized with viscous alginate gel. Thus an alkaline 'raft' of foamed alginate floats on top of the gastric contents and may tend to inhibit reflux. The raft will also be the first part of the gastric contents to be pushed into the oesophagus if reflux occurs, where it will form a protective alkaline coating. Most of the preparations in this class contain relatively large quantities of sodium, and so are likely to be unsuitable for patients with cardiovascular disease. Some preparations are now being marketed in which some of the sodium is replaced by potassium, but this may still cause a problem if patients are taking potassium-sparing diuretics.

If symptoms are not controlled in 6 weeks, the patient should be investigated by X-ray (barium swallow) or endoscopy.

The strength of the alginate gel is reduced by

aluminium and magnesium ions, so antacids containing these should not be used concurrently with alginates. Conversely, the addition of calcium ions is probably beneficial, because they react to produce a stronger calcium alginate gel, twice as much of which is retained in the stomach after 2 h. Anything which reduces the interfacial tension, e.g. liquid paraffin and *simethicone*, and so breaks the foam, is incompatible with alginate–antacid preparations.

Antisecretory agents

Confirmed refluxing or oesophageal damage is an indication for adding an inhibitor of acid secretion.

The drugs of choice, especially for resistant cases and if stricture or oesophageal erosion occur, are the **PPIs** (e.g. *omeprazole, lansoprazole, pantoprazole, rabeprazole sodium*) at double the normal dose. These are much more potent inhibitors of gastric acid secretion than the H_2-receptor antagonists. *Pantoprazole* may have fewer side effects than the others, but is a relatively new agent and is not recommended for long-term use (>8 weeks) at present. *Rabeprazole* is newer still and is currently licensed for 4–8 weeks' treatment for GORD. The other agents are licensed for maintenance use in refractory disease. Fears were originally expressed that prolonged suppression of acid secretion may predispose to malignancy, but sufficient experience has accumulated to discount this as a serious problem.

Patients who require **long-term maintenance** treatment should first be stabilized on a PPI. Those with severe oesophagitis will continue to need full PPI doses. Patients with **less serious disease** should be stepped down to the least expensive regimen which controls their symptoms effectively.

H_2-**receptor antagonists**, e.g. *ranitidine, cimetidine, famotidine* or *nizatidine*, are less effective than the PPIs and relieve symptoms in about 25% of patients, but higher than normal doses may be required. Greater benefit is achieved by using them in combination with *cisapride* (see below).

Sphincter 'strengtheners'

Metoclopramide is a dopamine antagonist which increases the tone of the LOS and may be added if symptoms persist. Once relief of symptoms has occurred, the regimen should be continued for at least 2 months, after which the dosages of individual medicines may be carefully reduced, titrating the dosage against symptoms for individual patients. Although not licensed for this indication in the UK, the anti-emetic agent *domperidone* is another dopamine antagonist which may be helpful (in the short term, because it is not recommended for chronic use). Because of their mode of action, both of these antagonize the effects of anti-Parkinson drugs, with an increased risk of extrapyramidal effects, and of some cardiac stimulants (*dopamine, dobutamine*). There is also an increased risk of extrapyramidal effects and neurotoxicity with *lithium*.

Motility stimulants

Metoclopramide and *domperidone*, referred to above, also help by hastening gastric emptying.

The prokinetic agent *cisapride* may also speed food transit by promoting acetylcholine release in the gut mucosa. It is probably suitable only for mild to moderate GORD, especially when associated with poor oesophageal or gastric motility. It may usefully be given to enhance the effect of H_2-receptor antagonists but may cause abdominal cramps, diarrhoea and mild CNS symptoms. However, it is **contraindicated** in pregnancy, breast feeding, or if gastrointestinal stimulation might be dangerous, e.g. if there is any possibility of gastrointestinal haemorrhage, perforation or obstruction. Moreover, there is a serious interaction with any drug that inhibits cytochrome P450 3A4, and hence its own metabolism, e.g. *clarithromycin, erythromycin* and any *imidazole* antimicrobial. There have been a number of fatalities due to cardiac arrhythmias caused by the increased blood levels. However, it may still be useful with expert supervision in premature infants and for 3 months after birth, despite unpredictable pharmacokinetics.

Other drugs

Mucosal protectants (*sucralfate, bismuth chelate*) have been used, but are only moderately successful. Sucralfate is most frequently used: the tablets are readily dispersed in water and for treating oesophageal reflux this mode of administration appears preferable to swallowing the tablets whole.

Carbenoxolone is a synthetic derivative of glycyrrhizinic acid. However, it is little used now, due to its limited effectiveness and side effects which arise because it is a steroid-like molecule.

Management: surgery

If symptoms persist despite an adequate trial of drugs, surgery may occasionally be indicated to repair a hernia or to refashion the cardia to minimize refluxing. Severe, prolonged oesophageal irritation may result in haemorrhage, with or without perforation. This is an emergency situation, the management of which is discussed below. It is now possible to repair oesophageal perforation by laparoscopic surgery, but results depend critically on the experience of the surgeon.

Dysphagia

Difficulty in swallowing food may have a large variety of causes, including motility and nerve disorders, local trauma and malignancy. It is an occasional symptom of diabetes mellitus, due to autonomic neuropathy, and of Crohn's disease (p. 338). Dysphagia is always a serious symptom that merits urgent investigation.

Globus syndrome is an apparent dysphagia, characterized by a 'lump in the throat', and is usually experienced by anxious or depressed patients who can nevertheless swallow food. Once investigations have ruled out significant pathology, the only treatment is reassurance, though extensive investigations may be needed to achieve this end.

Achalasia is caused by a failure of oesophageal peristalsis and/or of the LOS to open on swallowing. Oesophageal manometry will help to decide which of these is causative. The characteristic symptoms are a long history of central chest pain, progressive dysphagia and a tendency to regurgitate food, especially if the patient lies down after a meal. Achalasia often occurs in young patients, who sometimes experience severe pain due to ineffective oesophageal contractions. **Treatment** is usually by dilatation of the LOS, or occasionally surgery, but reflux oesophagitis tends to occur after both procedures. Injections of *botulinum A toxin–haemagglutinin complex*, which paralyses the neuromuscular junction and so relaxes the cardia, have also been used successfully.

Systemic sclerosis is characterized by widespread, diffuse tissue fibrosis, and is usually the province of the rheumatologist (*see* Chapter 8). In the oesophagus, systemic sclerosis causes a functional disability, with symptoms of dysphagia and heartburn. Treatment is symptomatic, because there is no adequate specific therapy.

Oesophageal bleeding

Aetiology

Bleeding usually occurs from **oesophageal varices**, which are distended anastomoses between the portal and systemic circulations. These occur around the lower part of the oesophagus (Fig. 6.6) and are a consequence of portal hypertension, which is usually caused by restriction of blood flow through the liver due to alcoholic cirrhosis (p. 376). Changes in pressure and local trauma may cause massive haemorrhage from the varices, with a 30–50% mortality rate. Any significant haemorrhage will cause haematemesis (vomiting of blood), while less serious bleeding will cause melaena (tarry, black, blood-laden stools). The risk of bleeding is related to the severity of the underlying liver disease (p. 375). In endemic areas of the tropics, **schistosomiasis** (bilharzia) is a common cause, because the parasites invade the liver and block the hepatic circulation.

Management

Bleeding varices are a medical emergency. Initially, treatment is with blood transfusions or plasma expanders. Applying direct pressure with a special balloon catheter in the oesophagus usually controls bleeding.

Terlipressin and *vasopressin*, which cause constriction of the splanchnic blood vessels and so reduce portal pressure, may be given as a temporary emergency measure. However, about 50% of patients fail to respond, even when these are combined with *GTN* to promote portal vein dilatation. *Terlipressin* is the better tolerated drug and has a longer half-life, but is considerably more expensive.

Once haemorrhage has been controlled (or occasionally as a first choice), **elastic band ligation** of the bleeding veins is preferred because it is probably more effective and leads to fewer complications. Alternatively, injecting a venous irritant (**sclerotherapy**, with *ethanolamine oleate, sodium tetradecyl sulphate* or *lauromacrogol 400 (laureth 9, polidocanol)* or *adrenaline (epinephrine)* via the endoscope either to obliterate the vein or to constrict it, is more than 90% effective. Both of these treatments may need to be repeated until all identifiable bleeding sites have been treated, but bleeds may still recur.

Octreotide, a long-acting octapeptide analogue of *somatostatin*, has also been used (presumably the recently introduced compound *lanreotide* also acts similarly), but this is an unlicensed indication. *Octreotide* appears superior to somatostatin and is safer and cheaper than terlipressin.

Very rarely, patients may require surgical intervention to fashion a portosystemic shunt, which diverts blood away from the varices. In severe cirrhosis, liver transplantation may be carried out on rare occasions.

In the longer term a negatively chronotropic antihypertensive, usually *propranolol* (*see* Chapter 3), may prevent recurrence.

Helicobacter infection as a cause of gastroduodenal disease

Organism and epidemiology

Helicobacter pylori was first identified in the early 1980s. It is implicated in chronic active **gastritis, non-ulcer dyspepsia, peptic ulcer, gastric cancer** and a rare low-grade lymphoma (MALT [mucosa-associated lymphoid tissue] lymphoma). It is a Gram-negative, multiflagellate, spiral, microaerophilic bacterium, which appears to be an obligate parasite of the gastric epithelium. *H. pylori* has been found only on gastric epithelium under the mucus layer and on areas of gastric-type epithelium in the duodenum. It has not been found elsewhere in the gut.

Two strains are distinguished on the basis of cytotoxin production, a virulence factor which determines duodenal ulcerogenicity: cagA+ (cytotoxic antigen positive) and cagA–. Both strains occur in Western countries, so typing for this may become a routine aid to determine whether eradication treatment is required or not. In developing countries, most isolates are cagA+, so typing is superfluous there.

H. pylori is potently urease-positive, i.e. breaks down urea to carbon dioxide and ammonia, and this property is used to demonstrate its presence. The patient drinks a solution of labelled urea, and the production of labelled carbon dioxide in the breath is detected. Endoscopic biopsy samples can also be examined for the organism microscopically and by culture: these samples are rapidly checked for urease by incubating on a medium containing urea, the production of ammonia being detected by the colour change of an indicator (CLO test). Both the isotopic and CLO tests have about a 95% specificity. PPIs and bismuth inhibit the bacterial urease and so should be stopped for at least 2 weeks before urease testing. Recent antibiotic use may also give false-negative results.

Serology is an unreliable indicator, due to the high carrier rate of *H. pylori* in the general population: 20% of people by the age of 30 years and 50% by 60 years are carriers. Much higher carrier rates occur in patients with active gastritis and duodenal ulcer (about 95%) and with gastric ulcer (75%). The high rate of gastric cancer in Peru is associated with a prevalence of *H. pylori* of 50% in infants from poor families, and 60% of children by age 10 years, whereas juvenile infection is uncommon in the UK and the gastric cancer rate is much lower.

Infection and epigastric symptoms

Although *Helicobacter* infection has not been proven unequivocally to be the prime cause of gastroduodenal ulceration, the circumstantial evidence is very strong:

- Gastritis developed in two research workers with previously normal gastric mucosa after deliberate self-infection.
- The presence of the organism in symptomatic patients.

- Resolution of symptoms when the organism is eradicated.
- Eradication of the organism results in longer remissions (up to 4 years in duodenal ulcer disease) than does simple suppression of acid production.
- The presence of mucosal changes in asymptomatic carriers, and association with a series of premalignant gastric changes.
- *H. pylori* causes:
  - Local cytokine release, e.g. IL-8, and so recruitment of inflammatory cells.
  - Suppression of somatostatin release and stimulation of histamine levels: both of these effects cause increased acid production, which produces gastric metaplasia in the duodenum, duodenal colonization with *H. pylori*, and duodenal ulcer (DU).

There appear to be two patterns of gastritis from *Helicobacter* infection: in the pyloric antrum and in the body of the stomach. Infection of the pyloric antrum seems to be associated with increased acid production and DU, but a low risk of gastric cancer. A minority of patients have infection of the body of the stomach and this is accompanied by reduced acid secretion and so protection against GORD: this may reflect colonization by the non-pathogenic (cagA–, commensal) strain or a genetic predisposition. Thus elimination of *Helicobacter* infection from the gastric body, which allows a variable recovery in gastric acid production, may be the cause of the observed increased incidence of GORD (see below).

Unfortunately, infection of the body of the stomach predisposes to gastric mucosal atrophy and, in some patients, to gastric cancer. This may possibly be due to suppression of ascorbic acid secretion into the stomach (ascorbic acid reacts with potentially carcinogenic nitroso-compounds and oxidizing free radicals) or to the prolonged inflammation of mucosal cells. There is limited evidence from Japan that elimination of *H. pylori* infection reduces the incidence of new gastric cancers in those who had undergone surgery for earlier gastric neoplasms. While it may be prudent to eradicate *H. pylori* in patients who need long-term acid suppression for peptic ulcer (PU), to prevent gastric cancer, this approach may exacerbate GORD.

Because chronic infection with *H. pylori* causes increased fibrinogen levels, it has been suggested that such infection may also be implicated in myocardial infarction.

The nature of the ulcerogenic interaction between *H. pylori* and non-steroidal anti-inflammatory drugs (NSAIDs) is unclear. NSAID-induced ulcers are more likely to bleed than are those caused by *H. pylori*, possibly because the organism stimulates the production of gastroprotective prostaglandin E_2 and this moderates the inhibition of prostaglandin production by NSAIDs (*see* Chapter 8).

Pharmacotherapy

Specific treatment should be used when *H. pylori* is found in association with peptic ulcer, especially duodenal ulcer. Some clinicians use such treatment prophylactically if *Helicobacter* is found, even in the absence of symptoms. However, if the preliminary observations reported above are substantiated, we may need to be much more selective in the treatment of patients with proven or suspected *Helicobacter* infection.

Eradication of *H. pylori*

This has been achieved using **triple therapy** with bismuth chelate, an H_2-receptor blocker or a PPI plus antibiotics. No single preferred regimen has been identified, but some which have been used successfully (about 90% eradication) are given in Table 6.6. There have also been reports of success with antibiotics alone. Dual therapy regimens comprising a PPI and a single antibiotic are not recommended.

One week of triple therapy is usually adequate, but 2 weeks' treatment has eliminated the bacteria in 91% of patients in one trial, with no relapse within a year. However, these longer regimens are often associated with more side effect and compliance problems. Other trials have demonstrated protection against relapse in DU for up to 4 years. It is not known whether this represents a 'cure'. Although re-infection is unusual, ulcer recurrence may be expected if recolonization occurs.

Amoxicillin, *imidazole* and *clarithromycin* resistance has been reported, and this is transmissible

Table 6.6   Triple drug regimens for *Helicobacter pylori* eradication

Treatment for 1 week with any of the combinations indicated below[a]		
Antisecretory		**Antibiotic combination**
Omeprazole		Clarithromycin + amoxicillin
OR		OR
Lansoprazole	PLUS	Clarithromycin + metronidazole
OR		OR
Ranitidine bismutrex		Amoxicillin + metronidazole

[a] i.e. any antisecretory plus any antibiotic combination. The combination of amoxicillin and metronidazole is slightly less effective than the others.

to other bacteria. Thus testing for resistance should preferably be done before treating: this requires endoscopy with biopsy and laboratory culture. Antibiotic-associated colitis is an uncommon side effect of triple therapy.

These regimens are recommended for patients with proven PU disease with *H. pylori* infection and where there is frequent relapse or a history of complications. They should be considered whenever long-term treatment with antisecretory agents is contemplated.

Treatment failure in confirmed cases of *H. pylori* infection is treated with quadruple therapy, i.e. a PPI + bismuth + two antibiotics.

Although successful triple therapy gives a high remission rate in MALT lymphoma, patients should be treated in specialist centres.

NSAID-induced ulceration and H. pylori infection

One study has shown that in patients with NSAID-induced symptomatic gastric ulcers, suppression of acid production with *omeprazole* (p. 326) is probably adequate. However, if there is a proven history of peptic ulceration and *H. pylori* infection, eradication before initiating essential NSAID treatment is preferable.

Dyspepsia

The general anatomy of the stomach and duodenum is illustrated in Fig. 6.8 and the physiology was outlined on pp. 302–307.

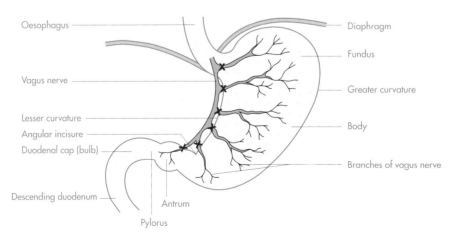

Figure 6.8   General anatomy of the stomach, duodenum and associated organs. X, points for highly selective vagotomy.

Aetiology

A self-diagnosis of 'indigestion' is one of the most common reasons for patients to consult a doctor or pharmacist. The term is used to describe upper abdominal discomfort, usually related to food intake.

Mistaken ideas about digestion are very common, but there is no evidence that any particular foods are 'indigestible', except for insoluble fibrous foods, the intake of which is beneficial. True dyspepsia, i.e. failure of digestion due to inadequate acid and pepsin production, is rare and a listing of the possible causes of symptoms is given in Table 6.7.

Clearly the range of possible pathologies is very large, so careful history taking, examination and investigation are necessary to exclude potentially serious disease. Only some of these diseases are dealt with here and the appropriate sections should be consulted. Many cases are described as 'functional non-ulcer dyspepsia', i.e. there is no demonstrable pathological basis for the symptoms and these are resistant to treatment.

Management

This depends on a proper diagnosis and treatment of any underlying disease(s) and reassurance. Over-enthusiastic medication or investigation may perpetuate false ideas of organic disease.

Pharmacotherapy

Antacids

Antacids are the mainstay of treatment. Self-medication with antacids is widespread and may be acceptable in patients under 40 years of age, provided that symptoms are not too severe and do not recur frequently.

The occurrence of drug-induced gastritis indicates a need to review whether this treatment should be continued. If it is essential, then an alternative formulation which is less irritant may be available. The concurrent administration of an H_2-receptor antagonist, prostaglandin, or sucralfate is probably appropriate.

Antacids are available in a large variety of preparations (Table 6.8). Soluble antacids (simple sodium, calcium and magnesium salts) are unsuitable for anything other than short-term use, because they may cause bowel upsets, aggravate fluid retention and heart failure, or produce metabolic disturbance. Patients who drink a lot of milk (from which they obtain relief) and take calcium concurrently are particularly liable to develop hypercalcaemia (the 'milk–alkali syndrome'). However, some patients like to take sodium bicarbonate, which aids eructation of wind and this may give relief. The side effects of antacids are summarized in Table 6.9.

The most desirable types of antacids are mixtures or complexes of aluminium and magnesium. Aluminium compounds alone tend to

---

Table 6.7 Some possible causes of dyspeptic symptoms

Oesophageal	Dysphagia, achalasia, reflux oesophagitis, hiatus hernia
Gastric	Gastritis, gastric ulcer, gastric carcinoma, gastric atrophy (elderly, pernicious anaemia), bile reflux, obstruction of gastric outflow, pyloric stenosis
Small bowel	Duodenitis, duodenal ulcer
Colonic	Crohn's disease, large-bowel disease, intestinal infections
Other organs	Pancreatitis, hepatitis, gallbladder disease, hypoglycaemia, diabetes mellitus, myocardial infarction, congestive heart failure
Other conditions	Stress, inappropriate diet, pregnancy, gastrectomy, dumping syndrome
Prescription and other drugs[a]	Aspirin, NSAIDs, oral corticosteroids, oral iron, antimuscarinics (see Table 6.11), cigarette smoking, excessive alcohol or caffeine consumption

[a] Almost any oral drug may cause gastrointestinal distress in some individuals and this may even be anticipatory, e.g. with placebos. NSAIDs are the most common cause of erosive gastritis in Europe and may cause chronic or acute gastric haemorrhage.

NSAID, non-steroidal anti-inflammatory drug.

Table 6.8   Some types of antacids in common use

Simple antacids

Soluble (more than about 10% of the dose is absorbed) | e.g. calcium carbonate, chalk; sodium bicarbonate

Insoluble (less than 5% of the dose is absorbed) | e.g. aluminium hydroxide, aluminium and magnesium mixtures (co-magaldrox), magnesium trisilicate, aluminium–magnesium complexes (e.g. almasilate, hydrotalcite), magnesium carbonate

Antacids with added ingredients

Alginates: for reflux oesophagitis; usually contain considerable amounts of sodium or potassium bicarbonate

Simethicone[a]: for wind; physicochemically incompatible with products containing alginates

Antispasmodics[b]: for griping or colicky pains; should be avoided in patients with reflux oesophagitis or paralytic ileus

Surface (mucosal) anaesthetics[a]: oxetacaine, for additional pain relief

[a] These are of doubtful benefit, but some patients appear to find them helpful.

[b] May be useful in a few patients.

---

cause constipation, and magnesium alone can cause diarrhoea. Thus, combinations of the two do not upset the bowel habit. Suspensions are more effective than tablets, though less convenient for patients with frequent symptoms. For unknown reasons, the pain relief is unrelated to neutralizing capacity, relief being obtained with doses (e.g. 10–20 mL of a commonly used suspension such as *co-magaldrox*) that do not markedly raise gastric pH. Antacids may have some mucosal protective effect by forming a coating on damaged tissue, and some may adsorb acid as well as neutralizing it. It is reasonable to start with a product of low to moderate neutralizing capacity and to change to one of higher capacity (Table 6.10) if relief is inadequate. However, patient preference is the best guide to antacid selection. Antacids should be taken regularly to be effective.

Very high doses of antacids (about 200 mL per day) are required to neutralize acid effectively: this abolishes peptic activity and assists ulcer healing. However, these high doses are usually unacceptable to patients, especially as they obtain satisfactory symptomatic relief with much lower doses. Further, the prolonged use of high doses of insoluble antacids is particularly likely to produce adverse reactions.

The basal (unstimulated) gastric acid output is about is about 3 mEq/h, and this is increased by about 30 mEq per main meal, plus smaller amounts for snacks. Accordingly, it has been suggested that doses sufficient to neutralize 200 mEq of HCl per day are effective in most patients. Further, buffering capacity is important, and that of *magaldrate* suspension has been reported to be high.

There is little evidence to suggest that products containing *simethicone* are of special benefit unless wind is a problem or patients find such products particularly useful. Equally, there does not appear to be a role for products containing alginates unless there is associated reflux oesophagitis. Despite this, these products are frequently prescribed as simple antacids. These latter two classes of product should not be used together because they are physicochemically incompatible.

Peptic ulcer disease

Definition

A peptic ulcer (PU) is an abnormal area of mucosa which has been damaged by the pepsin and hydrochloric acid of gastric juice, with consequent inflammation of the underlying and surrounding tissue. Erosion may subsequently occur

Table 6.9   Some side effects and interactions of antacid products[a]

Side effects	Examples
Constipation	Aluminium (obstruction with high doses), calcium
Acid rebound	Calcium, sodium bicarbonate
Diarrhoea or loose motions	Calcium, magnesium
Wind	Carbonates, bicarbonates
Nausea and vomiting	Aluminium
Electrolyte disturbances:	
• hypercalcaemia[b]	Calcium
• hypermagnesaemia	Magnesium
• hypophosphataemia[c]	Aluminium, magnesium, calcium
• impaired iron absorption	Any
Fluid retention	
Aggravation of hypertension	Sodium bicarbonate[b]
Metabolic alkalosis	
Renal calculi	Calcium
Encephalopathy	Bismuth[b] salicylate or subnitrate
Interference with diabetic control	
Dental caries	Sugar-containing antacids (some tablets)[b]
Antimuscarinic	See Table 6.11
Aggravation of coeliac disease	Tablets containing wheat gluten (p. 336)

Interactions Effect	Drug affected
Absorption reduced	Many basic drugs
	Antimicrobials: ciprofloxacin, pivampicillin, rifampicin, tetracyclines, itraconazole, ketoconazole
	Chloroquine, hydroxychloroquine
	Iron
	Penicillamine
	Phenothiazines
Renal excretion	
• reduced	Flecainide, mexiletine, quinidine
• increased	Aspirin, lithium
Effect reduced	Bismuth chelate, sucralfate
Physicochemical incompatibility	Simethicone with alginates

[a] Where a cation is given this refers to all compounds of it unless otherwise stated.

[b] Effects occur only with excessive intake or in renal impairment.

[c] With frequent, chronic use: osteomalacia has been reported in extreme situations.

into the lamina propria and submucosa to cause bleeding (*see* Fig. 6.2).

Most ulcers occur either in the duodenum or the stomach, where the pH is sufficiently low for peptic action, though ulcers may also occur in the lower oesophagus, as a result of refluxing of gastric contents, and rarely in certain areas of the small intestine.

Epidemiology

Dyspepsia (p. 318) is frequently thought of by patients as being due to ulceration, but it is benign and transient. Nevertheless, PUs are common: it has been estimated that up to 10% of the population has an ulcer at some time, though many of these are asymptomatic, the annual

Table 6.10   Some common liquid antacid preparations in approximately decreasing order of neutralizing capacity[a]

Aludrox, Asilone suspension, Mucaine
Aluminium Hydroxide Oral Suspension BP
Magnesium Hydroxide Mixture BP
Maalox
Magnesium Trisilicate Mixture BP
Magnesium Carbonate Mixture BPC
Asilone Gel
Kolanticon
Gelusil
Gaviscon

[a] The most active products have about eight times the neutralizing capacity of the least active.

the stomach, often near the angular incisure. These are usually benign, whereas an appreciable minority (5%) of those in the fundus and body of the stomach and the pyloric antrum are malignant. Most gastric carcinomas occur in the pyloric antrum, but it is rare for these to spread to the duodenum or for DUs to be malignant. Gastric malignancy is much more common in Japan, Chile, Finland and Iceland than in the UK, the difference probably being due to environmental factors, especially diet. The incidence of gastric carcinoma fortunately is declining fairly rapidly in the West, but it remains the third most common cause of death from malignancy in the UK and has a poor prognosis (10% survival rate at 5 years).

incidence of symptomatic PU being about 0.3%. **Duodenal ulcers** (DUs) are four times as common as **gastric ulcers** (GUs) and occur mainly in the duodenal cap (the first part of the duodenum; Fig. 6.8); among DUs, half occur on the anterior wall.

GUs occur mostly on the lesser curvature of

Aetiology

The aetiology of PU is multifactorial, the mechanisms normally operating to protect the mucosa from self-digestion by the acid and pepsin of gastric juice either failing or being overcome by a combination of injurious factors (Fig. 6.9). The

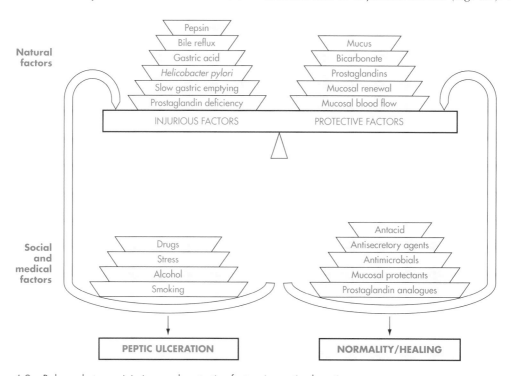

Figure 6.9   Balance between injurious and protective factors in peptic ulceration.

most common causes of PU in the UK are *H. pylori* infection and NSAID ingestion. The old hypothesis that ulceration is caused simply by hyperacidity is not tenable, because about 70% of GUs and 50% of DUs (i.e. about 55% of all ulcers) are not associated with abnormally high acid production. However, GUs occurring near the pylorus may be associated with *H. pylori* infection and high acid levels, as are most DUs (p. 316).

Heredity is also important: the development of DU at an early age tends to run in families. Ulcers are also more common in blood group O subjects and in those who do not secrete blood group antibodies into gastric secretions, but the reasons for this are obscure.

Added to these naturally occurring factors are a number of social and environmental ones, the most important being smoking. The ingestion of some drugs, especially NSAIDs and alcohol, also promotes acute ulceration. 'Stress ulcers' occur in seriously ill patients, and are common in those in intensive care. Whether sustained emotional stress leads to chronic ulceration is unclear, although it undoubtedly triggers gastrointestinal discomfort and may aggravate symptoms.

Balance between protective and erosive factors
Recently, much more attention has been focused on the factors responsible for the maintenance of mucosal integrity. These include the secretion of bicarbonate-laden mucus and the turnover of mucosal cells every 36–48 h – factors which depend on an adequate blood supply. These are opposed by several factors which either promote erosion or facilitate it, including bile reflux, chronic gastritis (from gastric stasis, diet or alcohol), local ischaemia and hyperacidity (40%). This balance is illustrated in Fig. 6.9. The damage caused to the mucosa by reflux of bile through an incompetent pyloric sphincter (Fig. 6.10) possibly accounts for the high incidence of ulcers in the pyloric antrum. Although the role of *H. pylori* has been discussed above, there has also been considerable recent interest in the role of prostaglandins, some of which (in small doses) have been shown, in animal studies, to inhibit acid secretion, promote the repair of damaged gastric mucosa, and to stimulate gastric blood flow. Prostaglandins have therefore been described as 'cytoprotective agents', though there is considerable debate as to whether this description is justified. This partly explains why NSAIDs, which inhibit prostaglandin synthesis, are ulcerogenic.

Clinical features

Pain is the outstanding feature, varying from 'discomfort' to 'severe'. It is usually felt in the epigastric region (Fig. 6.1(c)), though in long-standing, severe cases in which the ulcer penetrates into other organs, the patient may complain of backache or lower abdominal pain. The pain is often described as 'burning' or 'gnawing'. Sometimes a

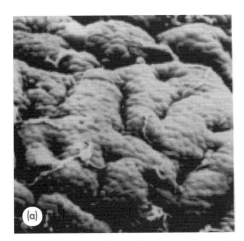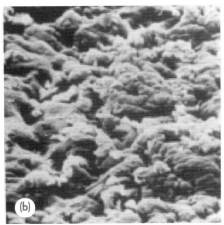

Figure 6.10 Effect of bile reflux on the gastric mucosa. (a) Normal antral mucosa. (b) After bile reflux from the duodenum. (Reproduced with permission from SmithKline Beecham plc.)

patient points with one finger to a spot in the epigastric region, the 'pointing sign', and this tends to indicate an ulcer rather than simple gastritis. The occurrence of pain in either the left or right hypochondrium is an unreliable guide to the site of ulceration.

Spontaneous night pain, which may be relieved by milk or antacid ingestion, may wake the patient regularly at about 2 a.m. and tends to be more common with DU, for unknown reasons. Generally, foods – or particular items of food – do not cause pain. Although it has been said that GU patients may complain of pain about 2 h after eating, whereas those with DU may find that food or milk relieves pain, this is fallacious.

None of these symptoms or signs is diagnostic, and GUs and PUs cannot be differentiated on clinical grounds. All PUs tend to give periodic symptoms, the recurrence having no obvious cause, and the symptom-free intervals decrease with time in the absence of effective treatment. The most important considerations are:

- Waking from sleep with epigastric pain.
- Periodicity of symptoms.
- A family history of PU.

Investigation and diagnosis

History

The discriminatory value of a history alone is poor, because it has been shown that symptoms such as postprandial pain and nausea occur with similar frequency (in about 40% of patients) in non-ulcer dyspepsia, peptic ulcer, irritable bowel syndrome, gallbladder disease and gastric carcinoma. However, **episodic pain** is very uncommon with the last two of these conditions. Nevertheless, history taking must not be omitted (*see* Table 6.4), especially because the information is quickly and easily obtained. Patients requiring special investigation are those with complications (haematemesis, gastrointestinal haemorrhage, suspected pyloric stenosis), those who fail to respond to treatment, and patients taking NSAIDs whose symptoms fail to remit when the drug is stopped.

Gastric secretion tests are of little value and are now used only in special circumstances.

Investigation

The principal concern when a patient presents with symptoms suggestive of PU is not to miss gastric cancer, but we have noted that the predictive value of the history is poor. The most significant factor for this disease is age, and any patient aged over 45 years with **new** persistent dyspeptic symptoms, which have no obvious cause, should be investigated urgently. Additional indicators of possible malignancy are:

- Male sex.
- Smoking.
- A family history of gastric cancer.
- Severe pain.
- Dysphagia, especially with vomiting.
- Unexplained weight loss.
- Microcytic, hypochromic anaemia (iron deficiency due to bleeding).
- Epigastric mass detected by palpation or ultrasound.
- Progressive symptoms.

In the UK, the average delay from the onset of symptoms to surgery for gastric cancer is about 7 months. This is far too long, because studies in Japan have shown that early diagnosis and treatment improves the prospects enormously. In Japan, the average overall 5-year survival rate is 25%, whereas it averages about 10% in the UK.

Fibreoptic endoscopy is the most accurate investigation for the diagnosis of PU and the differential diagnosis of gastric cancer, and also permits biopsies and brush cytology (removal of superficial cells for examination) to be carried out. If this technique is not readily available, or is contraindicated in a particular patient because of the possibility of oesophageal or gastric perforation, a barium meal radiograph (Fig. 6.11) gives good results. However, up to 20% of duodenal ulcers may be missed with this technique, especially if they are below the duodenal cap. The diagnostic yield from gastroscopy in most Western countries is poor and routine gastroscopy is not done, so early diagnosis is unusual, unlike the situation in Japan.

Complications

The most common of these is **haemorrhage**, which may vary from minor chronic blood loss

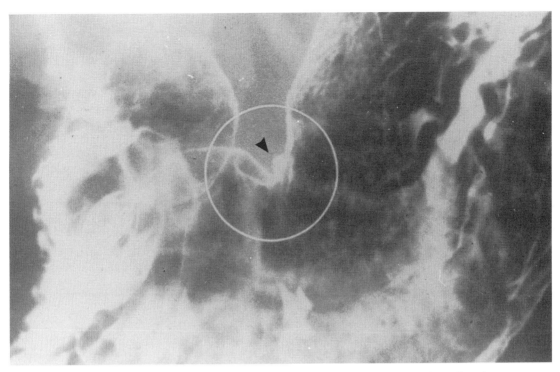

Figure 6.11   X-radiograph of peptic ulceration. The arrow indicates an irregularity in outline where barium contrast medium has filled an ulcer crater on the lesser curve of the stomach. (Reproduced with permission from SmithKline Beecham plc.)

that would eventually cause **anaemia**, to moderate bleeding causing melaena or haematemesis. The stomach is rather intolerant of blood: if the amount is small and the bleeding point is inactive, the blood may be partly digested and appear brownish in vomit (resembling coffee grounds). If bleeding is active and significant, then fresh blood will be vomited, and this is an alarming symptom.

A massive bleed, from the invasion of the arterial bed underlying an ulcer, may occasionally be life-threatening. Therapeutic endoscopy, using rubber band ligation, laser coagulation, electrocoagulation or injection therapy (*adrenaline* (*epinephrine*) or sclerotherapy), significantly reduces the need for emergency surgery.

Unobstructed **perforation** into the abdomen may occur and this is an emergency requiring surgery and broad-spectrum *antibiotics*. **Penetration** into adjacent organs (liver or pancreas) produces severe continuous pain, and **pancreatitis** may ensue.

Recurrent damage may result in scarring, the

consequent contraction causing **stricture** and obstruction, and this tends to be more common with DU. The symptoms of this are a feeling of fullness after modest meals, nausea and vomiting. A barium meal may show an 'hour-glass' stomach, or food trapping and gastric distension. Surgery is usually required.

If **gastric carcinoma** occurs it is usually present at the outset, but a benign chronic ulcer may undergo malignant change, though this is rare.

Management

The **objectives** of management are:

- To relieve pain and discomfort.
- To accelerate healing.
- To prevent recurrence and complications.

Approaches are usually based on patient age. Malignancy is rare below 45 years of age, so initially these patients may be treated conservatively. This may miss up to 3% of gastric cancers but gives a reasonable compromise between risk and workload. Those patients aged under 45y with neoplasms should be identified fairly quickly by their lack of response to treatment and/or early relapse.

General measures

Regular small meals are advisable, and strong coffee or tea should be taken only in moderation. Late snacks are best avoided, because they stimulate nocturnal gastric secretion. Apart from this there is no evidence that any special diet is beneficial, although it seems likely that some dietary factor is likely to be implicated in causation, though this may differ between patients. Clearly, patients will avoid any foods which they feel provoke or aggravate their symptoms. Rigorous dietary restriction is stressful and may be counterproductive, but smoking and alcohol should be strongly discouraged and patients should be warned against taking any medication, especially *aspirin* and *NSAIDs*, which are liable to cause gastrointestinal distress. Anxiety and stress should be reduced if possible, by the adoption of a more tranquil life style and the cultivation of hobbies, but this is difficult to achieve. Bedrest may be a useful adjunct in the short-term relief of severe symptoms, but has no advantage over modern drug treatment.

Pharmacotherapy

Aims

The aims of pharmacotherapy are:

- To relieve symptoms, by neutralizing acid or reducing acid secretion.
- To promote healing, by enhancing mucosal resistance, eliminating bacterial gastric infection and reducing acid secretion.

Ulcers are intrinsically self-healing if the imbalance between erosive and protective factors can be corrected. Healed ulcers are often found at post-mortem examination in individuals with no prior ulcer history. 'Ulcer-healing' drugs do not actually heal or stimulate repair, but correct the imbalance and so promote natural healing. About one-third of ulcers remit spontaneously.

Antacids

These are indicated as sole therapy in young patients (under 40 years of age) and those with chronic, stable, mild symptoms (*see* p. 330).

Antisecretory agents

These include the PPIs and H_2-receptor antagonists.

Proton pump inhibitors. *Omeprazole, pantoprazole* and the more recent agents *lansoprazole* and *rabeprazole*, powerfully inhibit H^+/K^+-ATPase, the final common pathway for hydrogen ion (proton) secretion. They are more effective antisecretory agents than the H_2-receptor antagonists, and are now often the drugs of first choice.

Omeprazole is a pro-drug which is concentrated selectively within the parietal cells. Following activation it binds irreversibly to H^+/K^+-ATPase to produce almost complete achlorhydria following a single dose. The drug has interesting kinetics: it is broken down by acid, leading to very variable absorption, but its effect in preventing acid secretion results in it enhancing its own bioavailability. It has a half-life of only 1 h, but because it produces irreversible enzyme inhibition its duration of action is at least 24 h. A single daily dose gives a peak effect after about 5 days of continuous dosing. After a single dose, or when treatment has ceased, inhibition of acid secretion persists until new enzyme synthesis occurs. The other agents are used similarly.

More rapid healing of duodenal ulcers is produced with PPIs than with H_2-receptor antagonists, but healing rates with gastric ulcers are similar. However, the relapse rates following cessation of treatment appear to be equivalent.

Side effects and interactions. Anti-secretory agents seem to cause only mild gastrointestinal and other side effects, e.g. diarrhoea or constipation, headache, rashes, pruritus and dizziness, nausea and vomiting, abdominal discomfort, bronchospasm, muscle and joint pain, depression, blurred vision and dry mouth.

Fears about possible carcinogenesis, which delayed licensing, are no longer believed to be significant. *Omeprazole* has been used for several years in some patients without untoward effects.

Unlike cimetidine, omeprazole does not have endocrine effects, e.g. gynaecomastia. However, it somewhat inhibits the hepatic microsomal metabolism of some drugs, whereas lansoprazole is a mild inducer. Caution is required with PPIs if patients have liver disease, are pregnant or are breast feeding.

H$_2$-receptor antagonists. These act by blocking histamine-mediated acid secretion from the parietal cells, and have gained wide acceptance as highly effective and safe drugs, having revolutionized the treatment of PU. There are now four drugs of this class available in the UK: *ranitidine, cimetidine* and the newer *famotidine* and *nizatidine*. Ranitidine and cimetidine have gained widespread acceptance, but all seem to be similarly effective at therapeutic dosage and are well tolerated. *Famotidine* is roughly equivalent to omeprazole in activity and is a potentially interesting introduction, as it may be useful in cases resistant to other H$_2$-receptor antagonists, but more experience with these newer agents is necessary before their place in therapy is clear. Famotidine and nizatidine do not appear to share the adverse reactions and interactions of cimetidine.

Ranitidine bismutrex (*ranitidine bismuth citrate*) is a compound of ranitidine with the mucosal protectant bismuth (see below). It is available for the treatment of benign GU and duodenal ulcers associated with *H. pylori*. The treatment period is 4–8 weeks for DU, but the longer period is always required for benign GU.

Dosing in acute attacks. *H. pylori*-negative patients normally use a dosage regimen consisting of a single night-time or twice-daily dose, though GU may need larger doses and more prolonged treatment than DU. There is some evidence that dosing after the evening meal gives superior results to bedtime dosage. Normal dosage regimens provide healing in about 70% of GU patients after 1 month and in about 80% after a further 2–4 weeks. Results for DU are somewhat better, and healing occurs in about 80% and 90% after 4 and 8 weeks, respectively. If patients are *H. pylori*-positive, then eradication therapy (see below) should be used.

Failure of therapy must always be investigated, to ensure that malignant change has not occurred and to exclude the unlikely possibility of **Zollinger–Ellison syndrome** (see below). Antacids may be needed additionally to obtain rapid symptomatic relief at the start of H$_2$-receptor antagonist therapy.

Side effects and interactions. There are gastrointestinal side effects, and occasional confusion also occurs, especially in the elderly. Very ill and older patients are also liable to suffer the rarer side effects of acute pancreatitis, bradycardia or AV block, depression and hallucinations. The doses of all of these drugs may need to be reduced in renal impairment.

Cimetidine, uniquely among the H$_2$-receptor antagonists, potentiates the actions of *warfarin, theophylline, phenytoin,* and *beta-blockers* and many other drugs, by inhibiting cytochrome P450-mediated liver metabolism. Cimetidine has oestrogenic (anti-androgenic) properties and may occasionally cause gynaecomastia (breast development in men) and loss of libido.

However, these drugs have proved very safe and *ranitidine, cimetidine* and *famotidine* are licensed for short-term OTC use in the UK. Although it may be reasonable to use these drugs to treat undiagnosed dyspepsia in patients under about 40 years of age, patients should always be investigated if there are prolonged (>14 days), severe symptoms, or associated systemic disturbance. A definitive diagnosis must always be made in older patients, to exclude the possibility of gastric malignancy.

Other indications. Ranitidine, cimetidine and famotidine are licensed in the UK for the treatment of patients with **Zollinger–Ellison syndrome**, a rare, slow-growing, gastrin-secreting pancreatic tumour which causes massive hypersecretion of acid and multiple large duodenal and ileal ulcers. These three agents are also used for reduction of gastric acid secretion, and so acid aspiration, during surgical and obstetric procedures.

H$_2$-receptor antagonists are also used for the prophylaxis of **stress ulcers** in intensive care. However, patients with nasogastric tubes may develop pneumonia, so *sucralfate* is usually used – provided that the patient does not have renal impairment and is not being fed enterally.

Cimetidine is used for reducing the breakdown

of pancreatic enzyme supplements (in cystic fibrosis) and in patients with **short bowel syndrome** after extensive bowel surgery.

Mucosal protectants

These form a protective sludge which binds to the ulcer crater, protecting it against further acid and pepsin attack. They are currently arousing considerable interest, as there is evidence that remissions are longer with these than are obtained with H_2-receptor antagonists.

Bismuth chelate (tripotassium dicitratobismuthate) is probably the preferred agent, because it has also been shown to be active against *H. pylori*, to increase mucosal prostaglandin levels, and to reduce pepsin secretion. If *H. pylori* is eradicated the relapse rate is reduced to about one-third of that which occurs if the organism persists (80%/year). The tablets are much more palatable than the liquid form, which is nauseating when ingested. The latter contains ammonia to maintain its colloidal nature and must therefore be diluted before use. Patients should be warned that the preparations cause blackening of the stools and, occasionally, of the tongue. The tablets should be swallowed with a glass of water, **not milk**, on an empty stomach: food, milk and antacids interfere with the coating of the ulcer by the drug, so none of these should be taken within 30 min before or after taking a dose. Bismuth chelate cannot currently be recommended for continuous maintenance therapy, as bismuth absorption and toxicity may conceivably occur. This has been disputed and is under investigation: reversible bismuth encephalopathy has been reported in patients taking normal doses of bismuth salts, notably in Australia and France. The current UK licence allows for two 28-day dosing periods, repeated if necessary after a gap of 1 month.

Other bismuth salts (e.g. carbonate, phosphate, salicylate, subnitrate) have been widely used as antacids and are used in some OTC products.

Sucralfate is also physicochemically protective and may additionally stimulate prostaglandin synthesis and the secretion of mucus. It is also used in intensive care (see H_2-receptor antagonists and stress ulcers above).

Although many patients take these products four times daily, there is evidence that twice-daily dosing is equally effective, and compliance is aided in this way.

Liquorice derivatives also have mucosal-protecting properties and were popular before the advent of the H_2-receptor antagonists; however, they are not now used for ulcer treatment in the UK. Deglycyrrhisinized liquorice products are of doubtful efficacy, but make useful placebos.

Other drugs

Antimuscarinics (antispasmodics, sometimes referred to less accurately as anticholinergics), which block the acid secretion produced by vagal activity, have a long history, starting with galenicals derived from belladonna and hyoscyamus. These still have a limited use today, but these and similar drugs (Table 6.11) are restricted in their use because they have a low therapeutic index and cause frequent and significant antimuscarinic side effects. They may occasionally be useful at night, when their side effects are less obtrusive, to reduce gastric motility and so retain antacids in the stomach. However, they are used primarily as adjuncts to antacids in the treatment of non-ulcer dyspepsia, if spasm is thought to be implicated. Because spasm is rarely, if ever, confirmed objectively, this application is questionable.

Pirenzepine binds selectively to gastric M_2-muscarinic receptors to reduce the secretion of both acid and pepsin. It has no advantages over the H_2-receptor blockers and has been discontinued in the UK.

Prostaglandins. Animal experiments have indicated that prostaglandins of the E series (PGE) have acid-inhibiting and cytoprotective properties. Among various PGE analogues, *misoprostol*, arbaprostil and enprostil have been tested fairly extensively, but to date only *misoprostol* has been marketed in the UK. The last two of these have been shown to inhibit both gastric secretion and gastrin release, whereas misoprostol does not have the latter effect. However, the prostaglandins appear to be less effective healing agents than the H_2-receptor antagonists and provide less pain relief. Prostaglandins tend to cause the side effects of diarrhoea and abdominal pain, which may be severe enough to require withdrawal.

The clinical value of prostaglandins thus

Table 6.11   Some antimuscarinics used for the treatment of dyspepsia and peptic ulcer, their side effects, interactions and contraindications

Drugs[a]

Atropine, ambutonium, dicycloverine (dicyclomine), glycopyrronium, hyoscine (scopolamine), mepenzolate, pipenzolate, piperidolate, poldine, propantheline

Side effects[b]

Dry mouth, thirst
Dilated pupils, photosensitivity, poor visual accomodation, glaucoma
Flushing, dry skin, rashes (occasionally)
Difficulties in micturition, urinary retention in the elderly
Tachycardia, arrhythmias
Confusion (in the elderly)

Interactions

Drug affected	Mechanism
Glyceryl trinitrate	Tablets may not dissolve sublingually
Metoclopramide	Antagonism of effect
Tricyclic antidepressants	Increased antimuscarinic side effects
Amantadine	
Ketoconazole, levodopa	Reduced absorption

Cautions and contraindications

Elderly patients
Breast feeding, infants under 6 months (especially dicycloverine (dicyclomine))
Urinary retention, prostatic enlargement
Cardiac problems
Oesophageal reflux (i.e. hiatus hernia, heartburn)
Paralytic ileus (obstruction due to a non-mobile bowel)
Ulcerative colitis

[a] Anions have been omitted.

[b] This list is not exhaustive and generalizations have been made for the sake of brevity. The *British National Formulary* and suitable texts should be consulted for full details.

remains to be assessed, though this is clearly an important research area. They are contraindicated in pregnancy, because they increase uterine tone.

Misoprostol reduces ulceration due to NSAIDs, but does not abolish it. It is probably more effective than H₂-receptor blockers for the **prophylaxis** of NSAID-induced GU, but has a similar activity against NSAID-induced DU. Misoprostol is marketed in the UK in combination with *diclofenac* and *naproxen*, to minimize the risk of ulceration from the NSAIDs. Its most appropriate use is in elderly and very frail patients in whom continued NSAID use is regarded as essential. However, it is probably less effective than an antisecretory agent once ulceration has occurred.

Eradication of H. pylori

Triple therapy (p. 317) is a proven effective treatment for duodenal and gastric ulceration. There is no good evidence for the benefit of a particular regimen, so choice depends primarily on the resistance of the organism to antibiotics in a particular patient or the known resistance pattern in the area: *metronidazole* resistance is most common and is increasing. Resistance is more likely in women, if there has been previous treatment with any of the antibiotics for any reason and in recent immigrants from countries where cagA+ strains of *H. pylori* are endemic. Except in severe cases there is ample time for sensitivity testing to be done. The second consideration is cost, as regimens using *clarithromycin* at full dosage are about twice as expensive as those not including this agent.

Treatment success should be confirmed after not less than 4 weeks by a negative urea-breath test, especially with GU. Careful counselling of patients about the rationale for treatment, the drugs, dosage regimen and possible side effects and the necessity for compliance reduces treatment failures, most of which are due to non-compliance.

Uncomplicated ulcers heal after eradication without further treatment. If there has been a haemorrhage or perforation, a PPI or H_2-receptor antagonist should be used for 4–12 weeks and healing then checked, preferably by endoscopy and biopsy, and followed up routinely. However, practice varies considerably between centres.

NSAID-associated ulcers are best managed with continuous antisecretory treatment as long as NSAID treatment continues.

Drug selection and maintenance therapy

Uncomplicated disease

The correct approach to maintenance in PU uncomplicated by *H. pylori* infection or bleeding is controversial, because treatment does not influence the course of the disease and relapse is common. The question is whether to stop when remission occurs, or to continue with prophylactic medication.

In younger patients who have infrequent recurrences (up to two per year), the usual approach is to use a PPI and discontinue this after 6–8 weeks and give further short courses when symptoms recur.

If relapse is more frequent, or attacks are severe, low-dose maintenance prophylaxis may be continued for long periods, though some patients may need to continue with full doses. Maintenance prophylaxis is also indicated in debilitated or elderly patients who are unfit for surgery.

It has been suggested that the prolonged hypochlorhydria produced by maintenance antisecretory therapy may be undesirable, because gastric digestion is reduced and bacterial overgrowth, resulting in nitrite-induced cancer, may conceivably result. However, there is no evidence that gastric malignancy occurs for this reason.

Complicated disease

PU accompanied by *H. pylori* infection, haemorrhage or perforation usually responds to one of the *H. pylori* eradication regimens described above. If symptoms persist or recur, despite confirmed eradication, retesting is indicated and a further eradication course prescribed, probably quadruple therapy. The re-infection rate is about 2% in Western adults.

It is important to realize that some PU patients may develop refluxing after eradication (p. 310) and the GORD symptoms may be misinterpreted as a recurrence of PU.

A flow chart for the management of dyspepsia and peptic ulcer is given in Fig. 6.12.

Surgery

Surgery is much less common now that effective medical management is available, but must be considered if:

- Patients fail to respond adequately to drugs.
- Malignancy is confirmed: all GUs should be reinvestigated to confirm complete healing and the absence of neoplastic change.
- Relapse and rebleeding occur frequently.
- Complications occur (p. 324).

The most common procedure is highly selective vagotomy (HSV), which is less invasive than partial or sub-total gastrectomy. HSV involves cutting selectively only those branches of the vagus nerve which supply the gastric body and fundus where acid secretion occurs (Fig. 6.8), so preserving motility in the antrum. Clearly, however, stricture or malignancy may dictate the removal of a variable mass of the stomach and the duodenum. HSV is a safe procedure with relatively few complications, but it gives a higher recurrence rate (10%) and incidence of diarrhoea (20%) than does partial gastrectomy (recurrence

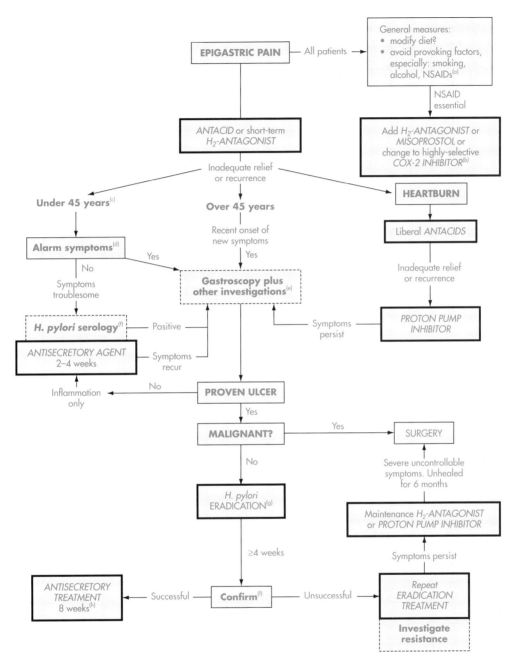

Figure 6.12 A general approach to the management of dyspepsia and suspected peptic ulceration. [a] Non-steroidal anti-inflammatory drug. [b] See Chapter 8, p. 491. [c] This cut-off age will miss less than 3% of gastric cancers. [d] Symptoms suggestive of malignancy; see p. 324. [e] Other investigations may include full blood count, abdominal X-ray or ultrasound (to confirm perforation) etc. [f] Serology is suitable for initial screening but cannot be used to confirm eradication (because antibodies persist). See p. 316. [g] Triple therapy (p. 317). [h] Improves rate of ulcer healing. The figure should be read together with text on Dyspepsia (p. 318) and Peptic ulcer disease (p. 320). **BOLD CAPITALS**, thin line boxes, indicate diseases or conditions; *ITALIC CAPITALS*, thick line boxes, indicate pharmacotherapy; **Bold normal text**, broken line boxes, indicate examinations and tests.

and diarrhoea, 3%). The more extensive operations leave some patients with distressing complications. These complications and their management are outlined in Table 6.12.

Nausea and vomiting

Definition and aetiology

Nausea is a prodromal symptom, i.e. it is the conscious recognition that the vomiting centre has been stimulated. **Vomiting** (emesis) is the forcible ejection of stomach contents through the mouth.

Vomiting is a common, usually benign, occasional, self-limiting condition, frequently with an obvious cause. When it occurs with diarrhoea, the cause is usually 'food poisoning', i.e. consequent on the ingestion of food or drink contaminated with bacteria, bacterial toxins, viruses or, occasionally, protozoa. Migraine, pregnancy and the indiscreet consumption of alcohol or food account for many other cases. If there are no associated symptoms, especially systemic ones, the origin may be psychogenic, e.g. bulimia nervosa or stress. However, vomiting may occasionally be due to more serious disease (Table 6.13).

Vertigo is an extreme, distressing form of dizziness in which the patient, or his or her surroundings, appear to be spinning. Unless of very brief duration, vertigo causes vomiting.

The vomiting centre in the brain consists of two areas, located symmetrically in the medulla, which coordinate the sequence of muscular contractions involved. Additionally, the **chemoreceptor trigger zone** (CTZ), which consists of twin areas in the floor of the fourth ventricle, detects noxious ingested chemical stimuli and may be stimulated directly by parenteral drugs.

Central and afferent signalling involves serotonin at $5HT_3$ receptors, dopamine at D_2 receptors, acetylcholine at muscarinic receptors and

Table 6.12 Some possible complications arising from partial gastrectomy for gastric ulcer or tumour and their management

Type of complication	Causes and comments	Management
Early after surgery		
Ulcer recurrence	Up to 10%	Avoid smoking and NSAIDs; antisecretory agents, sucralfate (mucosal protectant)
Diarrhoea	5%, mostly in the first month; due to short intestinal transit time	Small frequent meals, antidiarrhoeals, cholestyramine (for poor bile salt reabsorption), antibiotics (metronidazole?, for bacterial overgrowth due to low gastric acid)
Dumping	Faintness or giddiness up to 2 h after a meal. A 5HT-mediated component is involved	Eat dry meals (minimum fluid), lie down after eating Sugar if hypoglycaemic Methysergide (5HT antagonist)
Vomiting	Uncommon: • reduced gastric motility • emotional factors • obstruction	Anti-emetics, especially prokinetic agents, e.g. metoclopramide, domperidone, cisapride; surgery for obstruction
Late after surgery		
Malnutrition	May lead to anaemia, weight loss, hypocalcaemia	Symptomatic (vitamins, mineral supplements)
Malignancy	Incidence at about 20 years increased fourfold	Reoperation

5HT, 5-hydroxytryptamine, serotonin; NSAID, non-steroidal anti-inflammatory drug.

Table 6.13 Possible causes of nausea and vomiting

Dietary indiscretion, food 'poisoning', alcohol excess

Fever

Organic disease: e.g. renal failure (uraemia), diabetic ketoacidosis, hypercalcaemia, myocardial infarction, chronic bronchitis

Gastrointestinal disease: e.g. peptic ulcer, appendicitis, peritonitis, obstruction, gastric carcinoma, gastric surgery

Pregnancy

Central nervous system disease: e.g. migraine, meningitis, vestibular disease (Ménière's), abscesses and tumours, motion sickness

Psychogenic

Drugs: e.g. opioids, cytotoxic chemotherapy, digoxin overdose

histamine at H_1 receptors. Hence the benefits of the large range of anti-emetic drugs in use:

- Specific $5HT_3$ antagonists: e.g. *granisetron, ondansetron, tropisetron,* (*dolasetron,* not UK-licensed).
- D_2 antagonists: phenothiazines (e.g. *chlorpromazine, prochlorperazine, thiethylperazine*), butyrophenones (*droperidol, haloperidol*), benzimidazoles (*domperidone*), substituted benzamides (*trimethobenzamide,* not UK-licensed).
- $D_2/5HT_3$ antagonists: *metoclopramide,* cannabinoids (*dronabinol, nabilone*), corticosteroids? (*dexamethasone*).
- Antimuscarinics: *hyoscine* (*scopolamine*).
- Antihistamines: e.g. *cinnarizine, cyclizine, dimenhydrinate, meclozine, promethazine.*

Management

General considerations

The occasional episode requires no treatment except rest, abstinence from food or alcohol and frequent small amounts of carbonated drinks, as seems appropriate.

In persistent nausea and vomiting of unknown origin it is essential to find the underlying cause and to treat that appropriately. The use of anti-emetics in the absence of a definitive diagnosis may mask symptoms and result in a failure to recognize serious disease. However, many patients demand anti-emetics to avoid discomfort or social embarrassment.

It is always preferable to give medication in anticipation of symptoms, if that is possible, rather than to treat established vomiting. Anticipatory medication is especially important in the management of iatrogenic vomiting, notably in cancer treatment. Once vomiting has started, particularly if it is moderate or severe, the oral route clearly cannot be used, and rectal (suppositories), buccal or parenteral administration are needed. Doses adequate to control the vomiting are essential, otherwise the patient's confidence in their carers and their treatment will be undermined.

Acupuncture or **transcutaneous electrical stimulation** (TENS; *see* Chapter 10) of the P6 anti-emetic point may be a useful adjunct to pharmacotherapy.

Vestibular disorders

Motion sickness

This is best controlled with drugs which act at the vomiting centre, notably *hyoscine* (*scopolamine*). Hyoscine is available as tablets, slow-release tablets and a transdermal formulation. The latter two formulations may help to minimize the anticholinergic side effects of hyoscine, i.e. drowsiness, blurred vision, cardiovascular disease, dry mouth and urinary retention, and confusion in the elderly. Hyoscine is contraindicated in patients with closed-angle glaucoma.

In these patients, or if the side effects cannot be tolerated, **antihistamines** (H_1-antagonists, e.g. *cinnarizine*, *cyclizine*, *dimenhydrinate*, *promethazine*) are less likely to cause side effects, apart from drowsiness, but are less effective. The first dose should be taken 30 min before the journey commences (2 h for cinnarizine). Dimenhydrinate and promethazine are the more sedating and should not be used if this might create problems, e.g. if driving, though sedation may be useful in some cases, e.g. with children or at night. Other anti-emetics act selectively on the CTZ and are ineffective in motion sickness.

Ménière's disease

This is associated with idiopathic dilatation of the endolymph system of the inner ear. It causes recurrent attacks of vertigo, deafness and **tinnitus** (a subjective sensation of noise generated within the auditory system), associated with nausea and vomiting. Over a period of years the disease progresses to permanent deafness, and the vertigo remits. *Betahistine* reduces endolymph pressure in the inner ear and so is used in treatment, with variable benefit.

In an acute attack *cyclizine* and *prochlorperazine* (a phenothiazine), which can be given rectally or by IM injection, may be useful.

Other drugs, e.g. *cinnarizine*, *dimenhydrinate* and *hyoscine*, may also be beneficial. Salt restriction plus diuretics has been advocated, but is of doubtful value.

If the symptoms are distressing and refractory to treatment, surgical ablation of the auditory apparatus is sometimes done. This may relieve the vertigo, but it clearly causes deafness on the affected side and tinnitus often remains, sometimes severely.

Vomiting in pregnancy

Generally, nausea and vomiting in the first trimester can be tolerated and no drug treatment is indicated, because of the risk of teratogenicity. In common with other drugs, anti-emetics should be avoided in pregnancy, especially in the 3rd to 11th weeks, but in rare cases of severe vomiting *promethazine*, or occasionally *meclozine* or *thiethylperazine*, may be used in the short term (24–48 h), though they should be used only under specialist obstetric supervision.

Iatrogenic vomiting

This is most commonly associated with cancer chemotherapy and Parkinson's disease. Patients vary considerably in susceptibility to potentially emetic drugs. Emesis tends to increase with repeated exposure, though whether this is due to psychological factors, e.g. reinforcement of the unpleasant experience, or intrinsically increased sensitivity is unclear.

The *British National Formulary* (BNF) lists three classes of potentially emetogenic antineoplastic drugs and procedures but this depends on dosage (*see* Chapter 11):

- Highly emetogenic: *cisplatin*, *dacarbazine*, high-dose *cyclophosphamide*.
- Moderately emetogenic: *doxorubicin*, low to moderate doses of *cyclophosphamide*, high-dose *methotrexate*, *mitoxantrone* (*mitozantrone*).
- Mildly emetogenic: *etoposide*, *fluorouracil*, *methotrexate* ($<0.1 \, g/m^2$), *vinca alkaloids*, abdominal radiotherapy.

Anticipatory vomiting is best managed by prevention of **acute vomiting** during treatment, e.g. pre-treatment with a phenothiazine or *domperidone*, continued for up to 24 h afterwards. For more susceptible patients, *dexamethasone* and *lorazepam* can be added beforehand. The latter has an amnesic effect, so patients have no memory of the unpleasant treatment. High-risk patients will need a **$5HT_3$ antagonist**.

Delayed vomiting, occurring more than 24 h after treatment has ceased, is best managed with *dexamethasone*, with or without *metoclopramide* or *prochlorperazine*.

Nabilone may be used for intractable vomiting unresponsive to other anti-emetics.

The dopamine agonists used to treat Parkinson's disease (e.g. *levodopa*, *bromocriptine*) are very liable to cause vomiting. *Selegiline*, which increases the level of dopamine by inhibiting monoamine oxidase-B, has similar effects.

Metoclopramide has a wide spectrum of activity, and part of its usefulness derives from its enhancement of gastric motility, so hastening gastric emptying: an empty stomach reduces the volume of vomit, even if it does not abolish the reflex. High doses (maximum in 24 h 20 times normal) are used to prevent vomiting induced by cytotoxic chemotherapy. The side effects of metoclopramide resemble those of phenothiazines such as *prochlorperazine* (i.e. due to dopamine blockade), but are usually less severe. Prolonged administration is undesirable, as it may cause tardive dyskinesia and hyperprolactinaemia, the latter causing sterility.

Domperidone has similar uses but does not cross the blood–brain barrier and so is less likely than the phenothiazines to cause central effects, such as sedation. It is useful in treating nausea and vomiting caused by levodopa.

Nabilone is reported to be superior to prochlorperazine, but is more likely to cause side effects, and repeated or chronic use is contraindicated because it may be neurotoxic. The related compound *dronabinol* is used in the USA.

Granisetron, ondansetron and *tropisetron* (plus *dolasetron* in the USA) belong to the relatively new group of $5HT_3$ receptor-blocking drugs. They are used for the control of vomiting induced by cytotoxic chemotherapy and radiotherapy, and are more effective than metoclopramide and other anti-emetics for this purpose. Because of their specificity for $5HT_3$ receptors this group has a relatively good adverse effect profile, the principal side effects being headache, constipation and rashes, though hypersensitivity reactions have occurred. A combination of *ondansetron with dexamethasone* has been shown to be more than twice as effective as ondansetron alone in controlling severe vomiting induced by *cisplatin*. Nevertheless, single agents are preferred in moderate emesis.

It has been suggested that ondansetron may have other interesting properties, e.g. the improvement of memory in the elderly. All of these $5HT_3$ receptor blockers are considerably more expensive than other agents and are used as first-line drugs only in oncology and intractable vomiting.

Corticosteroids

Dexamethasone (see above) has also been reported to be as effective as *ondansetron* in controlling the acute emesis caused by moderately emetogenic cytotoxic chemotherapy, and is the drug of choice for preventing delayed vomiting. However, the basis for this, and the most effective dose and route, are unclear, though it may have actions at both D_2 and $5HT_3$ receptors. Moderately high IV doses are often used by infusion in cancer chemotherapy because an IV line is often already set up to ensure good hydration and renal drug clearance.

Anti-emetic adjuncts

Benzodiazepines, e.g. *lorazepam*, are useful for the management of cytotoxic drug-induced emesis, because they have sedative and amnesic effects. If benzodiazepines are administered before chemotherapy is given the patient has little recall of the procedure and its effects.

Problems of the small and large intestine

Malabsorption

Definition

This is a syndrome of numerous diverse origins resulting in failure to absorb dietary nutrients. The term is usually used to describe a global failure of absorption, and is not usually applied to a failure to absorb specific substances, e.g. vitamin B_{12}.

The most common causes are **gluten enteropathy** (see below), **Crohn's disease** (p. 338) and gastric or small-bowel surgery. Less commonly, pancreatic, hepatic or biliary disease, or chronic *Giardia lamblia* or other infections may be responsible. However, any condition causing chronic diarrhoea may lead to malabsorption.

Malabsorption may also be drug-induced. The lipid-regulating drugs *colestyramine* and *colestipol* bind bile salts and so may cause a failure to absorb dietary lipids. If these anion exchange resins are continued long term there may an associated failure to absorb fat-soluble vitamins, so supplements of vitamin A, D and K may be required. *Orlistat* also reduces lipid absorption, with similar consequences. Some broad-spectrum antibiotics, notably those which cause **antibiotic-associated colitis** (pseudomembranous colitis; *see* Chapter 13), may also be involved.

Clinical features

Generalized malabsorption commonly presents as **chronic diarrhoea**, often with **steatorrhoea**. Other gastrointestinal symptoms are abdominal cramps, borborygmi (bowel noises), flatulence, bloating and a swollen abdomen. However, nutritional symptoms may predominate (Table 6.14).

Gluten enteropathy (coeliac disease)

Epidemiology and aetiology

This is the most common cause of malabsorption in the UK (prevalence about 0.5–1/1000). It is more common in Ireland (up to 1/500), but very rare in Africa.

Patients are hypersensitive to the **alpha-gliadin** fraction of gluten, the protein in wheat and rye flour, which confers the physicochemical properties that make dough suitable for bread-making. Gluten enteropathy appears to be the result of an inherited hypersensitivity state, there being an association with hyperthyroidism, insulin-dependent diabetes mellitus and some other diseases. The jejunal plasma cells are IgA-deficient, there is an association with the MHC antigens HLA-B8, DR3 and DQW2, and splenic lymphoid tissue degeneration occurs.

Coeliac disease may mimic many other diseases, and a diagnosis may sometimes be reached only after a long period of unsuccessful treatment for other suspected conditions.

Clinical features and histopathology

Administration of gliadin or gluten to predisposed individuals results in shortening and eventually atrophy of the jejunal villi (Fig. 6.13). This effect commences about 4 h after ingestion, the mucosal damage being evident within 24 h. This time course and other factors point to a Type III hypersensitivity reaction.

In susceptible infants the disease usually appears as soon as cereals are introduced into the diet, causing abnormal stools, failure to thrive and occasionally vomiting. If the disease presents in later life, the diagnostic problems are considerable, e.g. adults may present with breathlessness and fatigue, consequent on anaemia. A definitive diagnosis can only be made by jejunal biopsy, remission of symptoms with gluten exclusion and relapse on challenge with its reintroduction.

Table 6.14 Some symptoms of malabsorption

Deficiency	Symptoms
Calorie, protein	Weakness, weight loss, oedema, hypotension
Iron, folate, vitamin B_{12}	Anaemia, glossitis (sore tongue)
Vitamin D, calcium	Rickets (children), osteomalacia (adults), tetanus (rarely)
Vitamin K	Bleeding tendency, haemorrhage
Vitamin B complex	Rashes, neuropsychiatric problems
Electrolytes	Widespread effects

Management

Management requires lifelong abstinence from gluten consumption. This is more difficult than may appear, because many processed foods contain gluten, or wheat or rye flour, as texture improvers. Gluten-free diets are prescribable in the UK through the NHS, and this is one of the rare indications for multivitamin therapy plus minerals. Following diagnosis, patients may need to persist with the diet for at least 3–6 months, though most respond more quickly.

Some 20% of patients fail to respond satisfactorily, being exquisitely sensitive to residual traces of gluten in the diet, or having poor compliance, very extensive small-bowel involvement, pancreatic disease or malignancy. Some of these problems may improve with corticosteroid therapy.

Complication: dermatitis herpetiformis

This is an infrequent, intensely itchy, burning, blistering sub-epidermal condition in which 70% of affected patients have associated gluten enteropathy. Malabsorption and the changes in the jejunal mucosa are usually less severe than in primary gluten enteropathy without skin involvement. The condition mostly affects adults in the 30- to 50-year age group, men more so than women, and follows a chronic, sometimes relapsing course.

Lifelong gluten avoidance is usually indicated, and this benefits both the skin condition and the malabsorption, though skin improvement may not be seen for 6 months or more. The rash is associated with the deposition of antigen–IgA complexes in the skin and responds to *dapsone*, which stimulates neutrophil and lymphocyte activity. *Sulfapyridine* is used occasionally but patients with glucose 6-phosphate dehydrogenase (G6PD) deficiency develop haemolytic anaemia with both this and dapsone. Other sulphonamides are ineffective. Gluten avoidance spares the dose of dapsone required. Topical steroids are of no benefit alone, but combinations with antimicrobial agents may be a useful adjunct to prevent secondary infection of

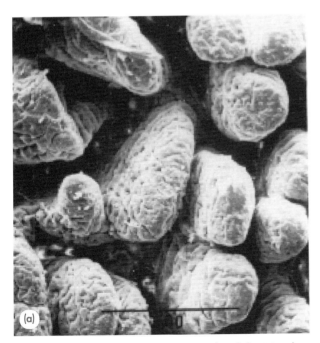
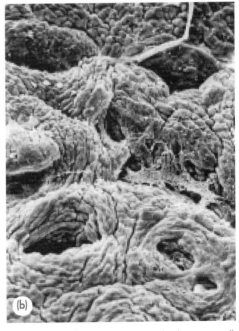

Figure 6.13 Scanning electron micrographs of the jejunal mucosa in coeliac disease. (a) Normal, showing well-developed villi. (b) After exposure to gluten: the mucosa is flat and has numerous pits and no villi. (Reproduced with permission from Dr MN Marsh, Hope Hospital, University of Manchester, UK.)

intensely itchy scratch sites. *Colestyramine* may also help, possibly by binding IgA in the gut.

Saccharide intolerance

Most patients in this group suffer from **disaccharidase deficiency**, so lactose (milk and milk products), sucrose, maltose or *iso*-maltose in the diet are not absorbed in the small bowel and high concentrations of these occur in the colon. This causes an osmotic diarrhoea (p. 351), with distension and flatulence. Treatment involves lifelong abstinence from contact with the disaccharides and the use of an appropriate monosaccharide.

Monosaccharide intolerance is rare and requires lifelong avoidance of glucose, galactose or fructose, and substances which yield these on digestion, as appropriate.

Nutritional deficiency

Vitamin D deficiency
Simple **vitamin D** nutritional deficiency is treated with *calciferol*. Because vitamin D is essential for the uptake and utilization of calcium, malabsorption may cause defective bone mineralization and deformity (**rickets** in children, **osteomalacia** if it occurs in adult life). The casual consumption of calcium supplements to correct this is inadvisable because hypercalcaemia may cause central nervous, cardiovascular, renal and abdominal symptoms and bone pain.

Iron deficiency
Iron deficiency in adults is normally treated with 200–600 mg/day of *ferrous sulphate*, and no other compound is significantly superior. This is better absorbed from an empty stomach, but tends to cause epigastric pain and so is often taken after food. The tablets may also cause constipation or diarrhoea. Treatment of iron deficiency is lengthy: it may take 3 months to restore normal haemoglobin levels and a further 3–6 months to replenish iron body stores. Injections (deep IM, *iron sorbitol* or *ferric hydroxide sucrose*) are used only if essential, e.g. failure

of oral therapy or severe side effects, persistent severe haemorrhage.

The use of compound iron preparations is rarely justified, except for prophylactic *iron and folic acid* in pregnancy.

Folic acid deficiency
Products containing about ten times the dose of folic acid used routinely in normal pregnancies are used for the prevention of neural tube defects, e.g. **spina bifida**, in mothers-to-be with known risk factors. However, compound iron and vitamins are appropriate in established severe nutritional deficiency.

Anaemia
In anaemia due to renal failure, *epoetin* (recombinant human erythropoietin, alpha or beta) may also be required (*see* Chapter 4). Epoetin may also be useful for treating the anaemia which accompanies most chronic diseases and is difficult to manage.

Inflammatory bowel disease

Inflammatory bowel disease (IBD) comprises two distinct diseases, **Crohn's disease** (CD) and **ulcerative colitis** (UC). Because the former can occur anywhere in localized sites in the gastrointestinal tract from the mouth to the anus, the term 'regional enteritis' has been used. UC is confined to the large bowel and may be difficult to distinguish from CD, which is restricted to the colon.

Although different, these conditions share many features and are considered together here, emphasizing important distinctions.

Aetiology

The causes of both CD and UC are unknown. Infective, immunological, dietary and psychosomatic causes have been suggested, but until recently there has been no evidence for any of these. However, an association has now been demonstrated with measles and mumps infections. Children who contract both in the same year appear to be up to seven times more likely to develop IBD some 20 years later. However, a causal link has not been demonstrated and these findings await confirmation. The research was related to natural infection with wild viruses and not to vaccination with measles/mumps/rubella vaccination, which is prepared from living attenuated measles and mumps viruses. Although most expert advice is that the vaccine is safe, this will inevitably cause parental alarm. It would seem prudent to change to well-spaced use of monovalent measles and mumps vaccines until the issue is resolved.

There may be an inherited predisposition to environmental agents, especially in CD, as there is familial clustering. The association between inflammatory bowel disease, ankylosing spondylitis and the histocompatibility antigen HLA-B27 suggests some autoimmune component.

Known associations in first-degree relatives are:

- About 50% concordance rate in monozygotic twins.
- An increased risk of occurrence (15%) and type of IBD.
- Clinical course.
- Sites of Crohn's disease in the gut.

Additional known associations are:

- Between CD and genes on chromosomes 7, 12 and 16.
- Between UC and HLA-DR1*103.
- In Japanese patients, between UC and HLA-DR2.
- Between antineutrophil cytoplasmic antibodies (cANCA) and 70% of patients with UC and granulomatous vasculitis in CD.

In addition, environmental factors which may be implicated are:

- Infection: viruses and bacteria (including bacterial L-forms). Apart from the measles and mumps viruses reported above, the most promising candidate is *Mycobacterium paratuberculosis* which causes Johne's disease in sheep and cattle, involving inflammation of the distal ileum. It is interesting that these animals only develop Johne's disease if they are infected by the mycobacteria as juveniles, though symptoms occur only in fully grown adults. This could account for the inability to isolate the organism from human CD patients. Further, some patients improve after antitubercular therapy.
- Consumption of refined sugar.
- Smoking: CD occurs more commonly in smokers, whereas UC, curiously, is often associated with smoking cessation and is twice as common in non-smokers.

The basic question to be answered is the mechanism by which initial infection is translated into a continuing autoimmune reaction after an interval of some 20 years. This problem relates to diseases other than IBD, e.g. rheumatoid arthritis.

Epidemiology

Both CD and UC occur throughout the world, and affect all races and both sexes. However, the incidence is generally higher in developed countries, especially in Northern Europe. Although we have noted an interaction between genetic and environmental influences, possibly diet, attempts to link IBD with a lack of dietary fibre have been disappointing. The true incidence in the tropics is unknown, because IBD may be difficult to distinguish from infective diarrhoeas. Jews of Central European origin seem to be about twice as liable as others to suffer from IBD, especially CD.

Crohn's disease has an annual incidence of about 6/100 000, with a prevalence of about 100/100 000, the figures for ulcerative colitis being about twice as high. There was a rapid increase in the incidence of CD between 1955 and 1975, but this appears to have stabilized. The reasons for this are unknown, but an increase in the consumption of manufactured foods may have been responsible. The 15-to 40-year age group is mainly affected and there is a second peak with UC at 55–70 years, but both diseases can occur at any age.

Pathology

Crohn's disease usually affects the terminal ileum and ascending colon (70% of cases). The inflammation is transmural and often involves even the mesentery and lymph nodes, causing adhesions between loops of bowel. Perforation and fistulae (a fistula is an abnormal connection between internal organs or between an internal organ and the skin surface) may occur, and peri-anal abscesses may precede the onset of more general symptoms by some years. Epithelial ulceration produces a 'cobblestone' appearance of the gut lining and is discontinuous, with apparently normal mucosa separating the affected areas, giving rise to what are known as 'skip lesions' (Fig. 6.14). The affected bowel is hard, rubbery and narrowed, with a small lumen (the 'string sign').

In UC, the rectum is involved in over 90% of cases, and inflammation may spread to involve the sigmoid and descending colon and, in severe cases, the whole of the colon (**pancolitis**). It may even affect the terminal few centimetres of ileum, though this is unusual. Only the mucosa and submucosa are affected, but continuously with no skips. Severe disease is usually chronic, rather than episodic, and may result in toxic dilatation of the colon and perforation.

Clinical features

These will clearly depend on the site, extent and severity of active disease. The outstanding symptoms of both diseases (Table 6.15) are diarrhoea (unless UC is confined to the rectum), fever, abdominal pain, malaise, lethargy and weight loss. In UC, the diarrhoea is bloody and contains mucus. Acute attacks may be triggered by infections, use of NSAIDs and severe stress.

Crohn's disease

Some patients may have only mild discomfort or may even present with general malaise, unaccompanied by gastrointestinal symptoms. Onset may be acute or insidious. Severe malabsorption, leading to hypoalbuminaemia and consequent

Table 6.15 Principal features of the inflammatory bowel diseases

Feature	Crohn's disease	Ulcerative colitis
Diarrhoea	Mild to severe	Mild to very severe
Stools	Steatorrhoea (small intestine affected), visible or occult blood (sigmoid colon or rectal disease)	Blood, mucus, pus
Usual site	Mostly terminal ileum and ascending colon but possible anywhere in the gut	Colon only, mostly distal
Sigmoid colon	Normal, or patchy ulceration	Always diffusely inflamed or ulcerated
Gut wall	Full thickness involvement	Mucosa and submucosa only
Extra-intestinal abdominal features	Yes; fatty liver, renal stones, adhesions	No
Fistulae	Common	No
Onset	Insidious or acute	Usually insidious, occasionally sudden and severe
Pain	Colicky, may mimic appendicitis	Discomfort
Oral aphthous ulceration	Common	Occasional
Peri-anal abscesses	Yes	No
ESR raised	Yes	Yes
Anaemia	Yes	Yes
Complications	Eyes, joints, skin, spine, liver disease, renal stones and gallstones	As for Crohn's disease, but no renal stones or gallstones

ESR, erythrocyte sedimentation rate.

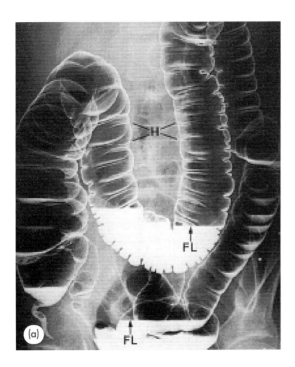

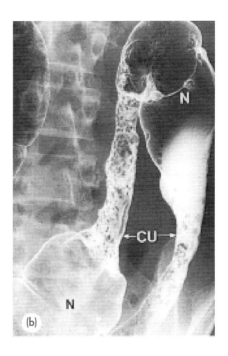

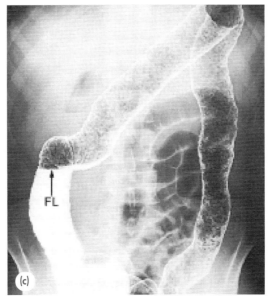

Figure 6.14 Radiological features in inflammatory bowel disease. (a) Normal double-contrast barium enema showing a distensible colon with well-marked haustrations (segmentations, H), and fluid levels of pools of contrast medium (FL). (b) Crohn's disease of the colon showing discontinuous ulceration, abrupt transition from normal areas (N) to diseased ones, good distensibility of normal (but not diseased) colon, 'cobblestone' ulceration and 'hosepipe' strictures (CU). (c) Advanced ulcerative colitis showing lack of distensibility, continuous ulceration of the whole colon (pancolitis) and loss of haustrations. There is a pool of contrast medium in the ascending colon, showing the fluid level. (Reproduced with permission from Pharmacia Ltd.)

peripheral oedema, may occur and cause growth retardation in children. Recurrences are common (50% in 10 years), though the relapse rate decreases the longer the disease-free interval.

Complications

A unique feature is the tendency to cause adhesions and fistulae. These are especially troublesome in small bowel and perianal disease. The occurrence of prodromal perianal abscesses has already been mentioned, and rectal and anal lesions cause considerable distress, as do also fistulae into the bladder or vagina. Failure of bile salt resorption may exacerbate diarrhoea and cause cholesterol gallstones and oxalate kidney stones. Mouth ulcers, rashes, finger clubbing, eye problems and arthritis are common. Rare complications include toxic megacolon, bowel perforation, renal and liver disease and amyloid disease (*see* Chapter 8). Obstruction may occur with ileocaecal disease.

Despite this long catalogue of possible symptoms patients sometimes present with unexplained weight loss as the sole symptom.

Ulcerative colitis

Diarrhoea in acute UC may be very severe, with 10–20 watery, bloody motions with mucus occurring throughout a 24-h period. However, disease confined to the rectum may cause severe constipation. The disease may present with mild symptoms, especially if restricted to the rectum and the sigmoid colon, though severe cases may be life-threatening.

Complications

Severe diarrhoea may cause dehydration, hypokalaemia, metabolic acidosis, anaemia, weight loss and hypoalbuminaemia and oedema. Biliary tract disease, including carcinoma, skin lesions, large joint arthritis and toxic megacolon may occur. Patients with long-standing disease (10 years), and those in whom a pancolitis has ever occurred, have a greatly increased risk of bowel perforation and carcinoma of the colon.

Diagnosis

This requires a careful history and examination. Investigations include a full blood count, ESR, electrolytes, barium meal and follow-through, double-contrast barium enema, sigmoidoscopy and/or colonoscopy and biopsy, and stool cultures.

Both diseases may be difficult to diagnose and distinguish from other causes of chronic diarrhoea, unless there is a high index of suspicion, or the patient's condition is severe and characteristic. Some diseases which may be confused with IBD are given in Table 6.16.

Management

Aims

The aims of management include:

- Rapid control of acute attacks.
- Correction of metabolic disturbances.
- Prevention of serious complications.

Table 6.16   Differential diagnosis of inflammatory bowel disease

Antibiotic-associated colitis (*see* Chapter 13)
Appendicitis
Bowel cancer
Coeliac disease (p. 336)
Diverticular disease (p. 346)
Irritable bowel syndrome (p. 353)
Ischaemic colitis
Lymphomas (*see* Chapter 11)
Infections: tuberculosis, *Campylobacter*, *Yersinia*, *Salmonella*, *Shigella*, sexually transmitted proctitis, giardiasis, amoebic dysentery, schistosomiasis

- For some patients, long-term immunosuppressive and/or anti-inflammatory therapy.
- Anticipation of the need for surgery and, if possible, avoidance of emergency procedures.

Both diseases are treated somewhat similarly. Because there is considerable variation in presentation and the severity of their symptoms, only very general guidelines can be given. The precise approach will depend entirely on the condition and response of each patient, and the likelihood of serious complications.

Acute attacks

General measures
These include:

- Bedrest.
- Correction of fluid and electrolyte imbalance.
- Correction of anaemia: oral or parenteral *iron*, or blood transfusion.
- A highly nutritious, low-residue ('elemental') diet, or total parenteral nutrition (TPN) if stricture is present and obstruction is possible. 'Bowel rest' does not seem to be beneficial and the concept does not appear to be valid.
- Vitamin supplementation as required, especially *vitamin B$_{12}$* and *folate* in CD.
- A low-fat diet if there is steatorrhoea in CD.
- Patient education about the nature of their disease and its treatment, and of the need for them to participate actively in therapeutic modifications to manage unpredictable variations in disease activity.

Pharmacotherapy
Anti-inflammatory and immunosuppressive drugs are used in the absence of precise knowledge of the aetiology of IBD. These include the following:

- **Corticosteroids**. These are the most effective agents and should be used to bring symptoms under control promptly. Patients with moderate to severe disease lose confidence in their physician if they have to suffer miserably during trials of less effective drugs. Oral *prednisolone* 30–60 mg daily, reducing over 6–8 weeks, is widely used. In severe cases IV *hydrocortisone* or *methylprednisolone* therapy is used, e.g. up to 100 mg *hydrocortisone* 6-hourly.
- Oral modified-release *budesonide* is also licensed for mild to moderate Crohn's disease, but is less effective than prednisolone if symptoms are severe. It undergoes rapid first-pass metabolism and so exerts its effect principally in the gut, with reduced systemic side effects.
- Corticosteroid retention enemas or rectal foams are routine for UC and spare the systemic corticosteroid dose, but are useful in CD only for rectal or distal colonic disease.
- **Immunosuppressants**. The use of these is controversial and their role in UC is unclear. *Azathioprine* may be used occasionally, especially in CD, and for its steroid-sparing effect. It is ineffective as sole therapy in active disease. Its metabolite, *mercaptopurine* is used in some centres. *Methotrexate* has been used experimentally.
- *Ciclosporin* (*cyclosporine*) is not useful in Crohn's disease. It is effective in severe, steroid-resistant UC, being used initially as an IV infusion, transferring to oral use when symptoms come under control. It may avoid the need for surgery or give time for surgery to be planned as an elective procedure, but this must be weighed against the risks of serious complications occurring due to delay. Experience in North America has been more favourable than in the UK, where *ciclosporin* use for UC is confined to specialist centres.
- **Antibiotics**. *Metronidazole* or *tinidazole* may be useful if there is bacterial overgrowth in the bowel or if septic complications occur, because anaerobes are often involved. Bowel perforation may lead to peritonitis and septicaemia, with an urgent need for surgery and parenteral antibiotics (and the identification of microbial sensitivities). *Co-trimoxazole* (trimethoprim plus sulfamethoxazole) has been used but is now appropriate only for infections of known sensitivity which are unresponsive to other agents.
- **Aminosalicylates**. These include *sulfasalazine* (*SSZ*), a salt formed between sulfapyridine (SP) and *5-aminosalicylic acid* (*5-ASA*), *olsalazine* (a dimer of 5-ASA), *mesalazine* (modified release 5-ASA) and *balsalazide* (5-ASA linked by a diazo bond to an inert carrier).

Among the aminosalicylates, SSZ is not absorbed in the small intestine, and the SP may act just as a carrier to deliver 5-ASA to the colon, where the SSZ is split by bacterial action, though the validity of this assumption has been questioned. The SP and some 5-ASA are subsequently absorbed, but about 50% of the 5-ASA remains in the colon to exert an anti-inflammatory effect.

Olsalazine is similarly split by colonic bacteria to yield only 5-ASA, and does not contain the SP, which is responsible for most of the side effects of SSZ (see below). *Mesalazine* is specially formulated for large bowel release, to avoid absorption of 5-ASA from the small intestine. However, both the time to reach the ileocaecal junction and the ileal residence time are very variable, both between individuals and in the same patient at different times, so the extent to which 5-ASA release is confined to the large bowel is unpredictable.

Balsalazide is a pro-drug of 5-ASA and resembles sulfasalazine, except that the carrier molecule is the non-toxic, inert 4-aminobenzoyl beta-alanine.

The aminosalicylates are used only to a limited extent to treat acute attacks. They are primarily used to maintain remission in UC (see below), and to a lesser degree in CD. SSZ may be adequate alone in mild attacks of UC, but moderate disease will also need corticosteroids, although the SSZ has a steroid-sparing effect. It has no place in the treatment of severe attacks, possibly because its hydrolysis to release 5-ASA is unpredictable in the diseased colon. SSZ may occasionally be used to treat CD confined to the distal colon. *Balsalazide* is licensed (in the UK) solely for the treatment of mild to moderate UC.

Topical rectal treatment. SSZ and *mesalazine* are available as retention enemas and suppositories. Some patients find the large volume (100 mL) of retention enemas difficult to use, but *mesalazine* is also available as a foam enema which is lighter and better tolerated. These products are useful for mild to moderate UC and for CD confined to the distal colon and rectum. They may spare the steroid dose.

Side effects. If the SP moiety in *SSZ* causes unacceptable side effects, and this is more likely in slow acetylators, *olsalazine, balsalazide* or *mesalazine* may prove more suitable. However, these also have side effects, e.g. nausea, headache, rash, and even diarrhoea and occasional exacerbation of colitis. SSZ causes a reversible oligospermia and so is unsuitable men wishing to raise a family. The monitoring of SSZ treatment is dealt with in Chapter 8.

There have also been occasional reports of nephrotoxicity with *mesalazine*. This is available as enteric-coated and modified-release tablets which release their contents in the small bowel and produce higher serum concentrations of 5-ASA than the azo-bonded products (SSZ, *olsalazine, balsalazide*). It is not clear whether this is due to *5-ASA* or to its acetyl metabolite, nor whether this can also occur with all aminosalicylates, but it seems prudent to reserve *mesalazine* for Crohn's disease affecting the small bowel.

All aminosalicylates may cause severe blood dyscrasias, e.g. agranulocytosis, aplastic anaemia, leucopenia, neutropenia and thrombocytopenia. Patients should be advised to report any unexplained bruising, bleeding, sore throat, fever or malaise. If any of these occur the drug should be stopped and a full blood count done.

Antidiarrhoeals. *Codeine* or *loperamide* may be used cautiously, to relieve discomfort. However, they are avoided as far as possible, because they tend to cause pooling of fluid in the bowel and may aggravate or prolong symptoms. In particular, they may induce obstruction in CD and toxic megacolon. They are not used in severe attacks: it is preferable to control diarrhoea by controlling the disease process with corticosteroids.

In CD, unabsorbed bile salts may contribute to the diarrhoea and *colestyramine* may then be indicated. Also, a milk-free diet is appropriate if lactase depletion is suspected.

Experimental agents. Antibody against TNF and infusion of IL-10 have been used as rescue therapy and help about 70% of patients with steroid-resistant disease. They are expensive and not generally available, but may point the way to potentially important developments in therapy.

Maintenance therapy

This is now the rule for both diseases, to reduce recurrence. Prophylaxis follows the general lines of the management of acute attacks, modified suitably according to disease activity and the severity of symptoms. In UC, the untreated recurrence rate of 80% at one year is reduced by about three-quarters. Because CD often follows an unpredictable relapsing-remitting course with symptom-free intervals of several years it has been common practice not to give maintenance therapy unless symptoms returned. However, high doses of the newer aminosalicylates, especially *mesalazine*, have changed this picture. The principal differences are outlined below.

Reduce stress. This advice is frequently given, but difficult to follow. It is not clear whether stress is a trigger factor for exacerbations of the disease or a consequence of the symptoms.

Diet. In contrast to the management of acute episodes, a high-residue diet is preferred unless there is a possibility of bowel obstruction, e.g. as the result of stricture formation. A high-carbohydrate, high-protein diet minimizes the possibility of nutritional deficiency due to chronic diarrhoea. Vitamin and mineral supplementation, especially iron, is often given. Avoidance of milk or milk products may occasionally be useful in some patients, especially those with UC.

Aminosalicylates. SSZ, or one of the alternatives mentioned above, is the mainstay of maintenance in UC. They reduce the relapse rate by about 75% and should be continued for life. Aminosalicylates (2 g/day or more, if tolerated) is beneficial in those with small-bowel or colonic CD. *Mesalazine* is preferred because it is released in the small bowel and should be started about 2 months after surgery or relapse, as soon as recovery permits. Enemas and suppositories are used for rectal and sigmoid disease and may spare the oral dose. Although SSZ frequently causes gastric distress, and enteric-coated tablets are available, it is doubtful whether these are beneficial.

Corticosteroids. Retention enemas and rectal foams, and sometimes suppositories, are used for rectal and colonic disease.

Chronic small-bowel involvement in CD is controlled with minimal oral doses, and intelligent patients should be counselled on judicious increases in dose to control exacerbations as soon as they occur: enemas spare the oral dose required. However, patients should seek medical advice for anything other than mild exacerbations. Oral corticosteroids do not influence the relapse rate in UC and should be stopped completely when symptoms remit, to minimize side effects. However, some patients are steroid-dependent and should be maintained on the minimal dose. *Budesonide* may be preferred in ileal and ascending colonic involvement. The addition of *azathioprine* (see below) spares the steroid dose.

Azathioprine. This cytotoxic immunosuppressant has a limited role in maintenance therapy for UC. However, it halves the relapse rate in Crohn's disease and may enable substantial withdrawal of corticosteroids. If tolerated it should be continued for at least 5 years.

Antibiotics. These should be used promptly for the treatment of any systemic infections, as there is evidence that infections may trigger exacerbations.

Surgery

Surgery is indicated if medical management fails, and also for the treatment of complications, e.g. toxic megacolon, perforation, obstruction, malignancy, and the repair of abscesses or fistulae. A further indication in children is retardation of growth and development despite intensive medical management.

In UC, colectomy is curative, ileoanal anastomosis with formation of a pouch being the preferred procedure. However, a permanent ileostomy (p. 354) may be necessary at some stage and is the procedure of choice in older patients. Colectomy is also carried out as an elective procedure in patients who have had extensive UC for more than 10 years, or if they have ever had a pancolitis, to pre-empt possible malignancy.

However, surgery is avoided as far as possible in CD, because relapse is common (30% in 5 years, 50% in 10 years) and repeated surgery is debilitating and carries a relatively high cumulative mortality. Thus only minimal surgery to deal with complications, e.g. fistula repair, is carried out unless there are frequent severe exacerbations. Patients with ileocaecal disease are more likely to need surgery than those with colonic or other involvement. However, about 80% of patients with CD have surgery at some time.

Prognosis

Virtually all CD patients have chronic or recurrent disease, with at least one serious relapse. The probability of recurrence is greater if there was extensive initial gut involvement, if perianal ulceration has occurred, or if an ileocolonic anastomosis has been formed at surgery. The mortality rate now approaches that for the population generally, with most deaths being associated with extensive severe small-bowel disease, onset in the third decade of life and emergency surgery.

In UC, some patients have only a single attack, but many have mild disease (proctitis only) and the outlook is correspondingly good, the overall mortality being near normal. About 10% of patients have chronic symptoms, and a further 10% have severe attacks requiring surgery. Although prompt surgery may be life-saving, severe attacks are associated with only about 1% mortality if managed in specialist centres (5% elsewhere).

Other colonic and rectal disorders

Diverticular disease

Definition

A **diverticulum** is a pouch in the wall of the gut. Diverticula can occur almost anywhere from the oesophagus to the rectum and may be congenital, e.g. Meckel's diverticulum in the ileum. Those in the small intestine tend to be either asymptomatic or cause only vague dyspeptic symptoms, and complications are unusual. However, diverticular disease of the colon (DDC) occurs frequently, often in the sigmoid colon where the wall is weakest.

Diverticulosis is the presence of diverticula, which may be asymptomatic or produce only mild, non-specific abdominal symptoms. **Diverticulitis** is the result of infection and inflammation of the diverticula.

Aetiology

DDC is believed to result from a lifelong lack of dietary fibre, because the disease is common in Western countries but is unusual in rural Africa. In the absence of adequate bulk, intense contractions of bowel segments produce high local intraluminal pressures and the mucosa and submucosa become ballooned out and herniate through the overlying muscle layers at points of weakness, usually where blood vessels and nerves pass through the intestinal wall.

The average age at diagnosis is 55 years and the incidence increases directly with age, being dependent on the loss of colonic muscle strength and the duration of the bowel insult. Consequently, diverticulosis is present in some 50% of people aged over 60 years.

Clinical features

Although diverticulosis is usually asymptomatic, it is so common that it may be blamed for symptoms due to other diseases. However, if the diverticula become filled with stagnant faecal residues, infection and inflammation may cause diverticulitis. The most prominent symptom is spasmodic or constant pain, usually in the lower abdomen, and especially in the left iliac fossa. Flatulence and constipation are common, though diarrhoea may also occur. Pain may follow meals and is relieved by defecation or passing wind (flatus). In severe cases, with numerous large infected diverticula, colonic obstruction or abscess formation may cause severe localized pain ('left-sided appendicitis'). Perforation of the bowel may cause peritonitis and septicaemia. Intermittent haemorrhage may cause rectal bleeding and a misdiagnosis of haemorrhoids.

Management

A **high-fibre diet**, possibly supplemented with a bulking agent (e.g. *bran, ispaghula*), is recommended to reduce intracolonic pressures and to prevent faecal stagnation and constipation which aggravates the condition due to straining. **Antispasmodics** (e.g. *alverine, dicycloverine (dicyclomine), mebeverine, propantheline* or *peppermint oil*) may be useful for colic and **antibiotics** (e.g. *cefoxitin with or without metronidazole, gentamicin plus metronidazole* if very severe) are used to control diverticular infection.

If pain is very severe, **analgesia** may be provided with *pethidine (meperidine)*. Morphine is contraindicated, because it reduces GI tract motility, and so aggravates constipation and increases intraluminal pressure. Related antimotility drugs, e.g. *codeine, loperamide*, may similarly aggravate symptoms and are also contraindicated.

Surgery is occasionally necessary to remove large, isolated diverticula or a badly affected section of bowel, or to deal with complications.

Constipation

Definition and aetiology

Constipation may be defined as a reduced frequency of defecation, i.e. less frequently than is normal for the individual concerned, accompanied by difficulty in passing hardened stools. There may also be sensations of incomplete defecation and that the rectum remains loaded with faeces.

Some possible causes are listed in Table 6.17. Defecation is a highly variable function and normality may range from three times per day to once in 3 days. One of the most common causes of constipation is a low-residue, low-fluid diet. This may be compounded by poor toilet facilities or a stressful busy life, resulting in an unwillingness to defecate or an inability to do so at adequate leisure.

In the elderly, poor muscle tone in the intestine and abdominal wall, perhaps associated with a lack of activity, depression and a low food and fluid intake, often leads to **faecal impaction**. The patient may then be aware of a hard mass in the left iliac region.

In young children, constipation may be due to inappropriate diet or to congenital defects, although it is to be hoped that the latter would be detected by the paediatrician or health visitor at an early age. However, it is more often the result of emotional conflict with (usually) the mother. If an attempt is made to toilet-train children before they are ready to accept it, or if the parent becomes anxious or obsessive about the problem, the child may see the withholding of defecation as a strategy for manipulating the parent. A 2-year-old often behaves negatively and a 4-year-old aggressively. Either behaviour pattern

Table 6.17	Some possible causes of constipation	
Simple	Diet: unusual (holidays), low fibre, low fluid intake	
	Lack of exercise, ignoring the call to stool	
Secondary	Inactive colon	especially in elderly
	Poor muscle tone	patients, after surgery
	Pregnancy	or febrile illness
	Irritable bowel syndrome (p. 353)	
	Disease causing painful defecation: proctitis, anal fissure or stricture, haemorrhoids	
	Metabolic disease (diabetes mellitus, hypothyroidism), obstruction (usually occurring acutely), Crohn's disease, carcinoma, sigmoid diverticular disease, volvulus, gallstones (occasionally), intussusception (usually in infants)	
	Spinal lesions: loss of transmission of sensation or sphincter control	
Iatrogenic	Most drugs can cause constipation. The following are commonly implicated: anticholinergics, amantadine, antacids (aluminium, calcium), antidiarrhoeals, benzodiazepines, codeine and opioids, diuretics, iron, phenothiazines, antidepressants, chronic laxative abuse	
Psychogenic	Anxiety, depression, disruption of routine (holidays)	

can result in a vicious cycle leading to the regular withholding of bowel motions and the start of chronic constipation, if the parent responds inappropriately.

Another common pattern is the reaction to a clinging, fearful child with over-permissiveness and over-indulgence. Moreover, if parents have incorrect ideas about what constitutes 'proper' bowel function, children may learn unsuitable behaviour, for example that 'tummyache' leads to illness and headache – symptoms which are rewarded with over-protectiveness, presents and time off school. All of these childhood behaviour patterns can persist into adult life.

Clearly, any condition which leads to pain on defecation, notably **haemorrhoids**, will lead to reluctance to evacuate the bowel and thus to constipation. Also, the passage of a large, hard stool may tear the anus, leading to further pain and reluctance to defecate, thus greatly aggravating the problem. It is perhaps surprising that such tears rarely become infected and usually heal well.

Occasionally, constipation may be a symptom of serious disease. Gallstones discharged into the duodenum may sometimes cause small-bowel obstruction, usually ileocaecal in nature, with an acute onset of symptoms, whereas colonic obstruction is more often insidious in onset. Obstruction may occasionally be due to **intussusception** (the bowel folding in on itself), which usually occurs in infants. In adults, it tends to be associated with a benign or malignant tumour. Acute obstruction may result from DDC (see above) or **volvulus**, i.e. twisting of the gut on itself. Fortunately, most of these organic or functional conditions are uncommon, though they must be considered, particularly in middle-aged or elderly patients or if there is no history of chronic or sporadic problems.

Psychogenic constipation, some aspects of which were discussed above, occurs frequently. Irrational beliefs about the optimal frequency for defecation, or the consistency and colour of faeces are widespread, and anxiety about the need to rid the body of 'unclean' wastes may develop in individuals with obsessional, perfectionist personality styles. Such ideas may result in laxative abuse, so that the bowel eventually fails to respond to normal stimuli: this is self-inflicted constipation.

Iatrogenic constipation is a common adverse reaction to medication and some of the drugs which produce this effect most frequently are listed in Table 6.17.

Finally, **drug abuse** with opioids (including codeine) must be considered as a possible cause, especially in teenagers and young adults; constipation may be the first indication of a drug abuse problem.

Clinical features

It is important to establish exactly what a patient means when they complain of constipation, as misconceptions and misdescriptions are common.

The usual symptoms are difficult and infrequent or irregular defecation, which may be accompanied by malaise, headache, tiredness and anorexia, possibly of emotional origin. Abdominal distension may also occur, with pain in the left iliac fossa or felt diffusely.

In elderly patients, faecal impaction may be accompanied by restlessness, confusion and **overflow**. The latter is a spurious diarrhoea resulting from the forcing of semi-fluid intestinal contents around the immobile mass, together with mucus, which may be secreted into the bowel as a lubricant. Impaction may also occur after prolonged bedrest and, rarely, in irritable bowel syndrome (p. 353).

Anal fissures (tears) are very painful, both at occurrence and at each subsequent motion until healing occurs; this aggravates the problem considerably because patients are understandably reluctant to defecate.

Management

Aims and strategy

Significant pathology must first be excluded. If constipation is of recent onset it is important to exclude secondary causes (Table 6.17), especially in patients over 40 years of age. The objectives are then to:

- Relieve any immediate distress.
- Remove any trigger factors and treat any underlying disease.
- Promote normal bowel function by: (i) re-educating the patient about correct bowel habits,

diet and exercise; and (ii) appropriate medication if the problem persists, i.e. faecal softeners, bulking agents, or osmotic or stimulant laxatives (Table 6.18).

General measures

In **simple constipation** the patient should be counselled on the value of a correct diet (wholemeal and bran products, fruit and vegetables are valuable), exercise, and an adequate fluid intake. Defecation with the thighs raised towards the abdomen assists by increasing intra-abdominal pressure, so a low toilet and/or a 'squat box' to raise the thighs may be useful. Regular, unhurried toilet habits should be encouraged.

The regular use of laxatives should be strongly discouraged. However, laxative avoidance may be very difficult in older patients who have been chronic laxative users. Advice to the elderly to abandon their accustomed laxative in favour of bulking agents and a high-fibre diet is unlikely to succeed. The best that can usually be achieved is some improvement in bulk intake and a reduction in laxative use.

Immediate relief

For the occasional simple constipation, e.g. in travellers whose normal diet and lifestyle are temporarily disrupted, **micro-enemas** (5 mL) based on *dioctyl sodium sulphosuccinate* (docusate) or *sodium citrate*, or **suppositories** (*glycerol* or *bisacodyl*) are useful as relatively fast-acting, single-dose products. Large-volume (100 mL)

hypertonic sodium phosphate enemas are also suitable.

In more severe cases, products containing oral **stimulant (irritant) laxatives**, e.g. *senna*, *bisacodyl* or *sodium picosulphate*, may be needed. If the faeces are very hard, especially if they are impacted or the patient has haemorrhoids or an anal tear, these may need supplementation with a **softening agent** such as oral liquid paraffin or an *arachis oil enema*.

Dantron was withdrawn from general use in the UK because of fears that it could cause bowel and liver tumours. However, it is an invaluable agent which has been reintroduced for the management of constipation produced by opioid analgesics in terminal care. It is sometimes used in combination with *dioctyl sodium sulphosuccinate* or *poloxamer 188* (known as *co-danthrusate* and *co-danthramer* respectively in the UK). It is also used in heart failure and myocardial infarction, in which straining must be avoided. Patients should be warned that it may colour the urine red; they may otherwise interpret this as bleeding. It is no longer licensed in the UK for the management of constipation in geriatric practice.

Oral **osmotic laxatives**, e.g. *magnesium sulphate* (Epsom salts) and *macrogols*, are also suitable for occasional use. An adequate fluid intake should be maintained. *Lactulose* and *lactitol* are semi-synthetic non-absorbable disaccharides which are hydrolysed by colonic bacteria to lactic acid, producing osmotic and mildly irritant

---

Table 6.18 Some drugs commonly used to treat constipation

Bulking agents	Ispaghula, psyllium, methylcellulose, sterculia, bran
Stimulants	Bisacodyl, sodium picosulphate, sennosides (standardized[a]), dantron[b]
Lubricants and softening agents	Arachis oil enemas, dioctyl sodium sulphosuccinate, sodium lauryl sulphate, liquid paraffin[c]
Osmotic agents	Lactulose, lactitol, magnesium salts[c], glycerol suppositories, sodium phosphate enemas
Motility stimulants[d]	Bethanechol, distigmine, neostigmine, pyridostigmine

[a] Unstandardized preparations of senna, and preparations of aloin, bile salts, cascara, colocynth, frangula, jalap, podophyllum and rhubarb, have unpredictable effects and are best avoided.

[b] Mutagenic in animals: for the management of opioid-induced constipation in the terminally ill only.

[c] Suitable for occasional use only.

[d] Exceptional use only.

effects. Although they take up to 48 h to act, they are useful agents with very wide applicability. Because they have a sweet taste they are useful in young children who might otherwise reject medication. Some patients may find lactitol less likely to cause cramps, wind and minor bowel disturbances. However, the regular use of these agents, or any other laxatives, should be discouraged, as the bowel comes to rely on them and becomes unresponsive, thus exacerbating the condition.

If there is an anal tear, topical *lidocaine* (lignocaine) is a useful local anaesthetic.

Prophylaxis

The most suitable measures are the general ones outlined above. However, patients often find it difficult to modify their lifestyle and **bulking agents**, e.g. *bran, ispaghula husk, psyllium, sterculia* or *methylcellulose*, may be needed. However, patients react very variably to these and any of them, including the 'natural' ones like bran, may cause discomfort, griping and flatus. Most bulking agents swell when added to water and must be taken with ample fluids. This may pose a problem with the frail elderly patient who cannot drink large volumes quickly or who has dentures. Bulking agents should not be used if faecal obstruction or impaction is suspected, because they add to bulk and may aggravate the situation. Nor should they be taken immediately before retiring at night. All of these take some time (days) to act.

Provided that a correct diagnosis has been made, bulking agents are also useful for modifying the consistency of bowel contents in:

- Stomatherapy (p. 354).
- Patients with chronic diarrhoea associated with DDC, irritable bowel syndrome (p. 353) and ulcerative colitis (p. 338).
- Haemorrhoids.

Motility stimulants

These agents are rarely used gastrointestinally but may help patients with colonic atony (non-motile bowel) in initial adaptation to new laxatives. They are given about 30 min before attempting defecation. Motility stimulants are either direct-acting parasympathomimetic compounds, e.g. *bethanechol*, or anticholinesterases, e.g. *distigmine, neostigmine* and *pyridostigmine*, so they can have widespread side effects such as sweating, salivation, intestinal cramps, diarrhoea, flushing, difficulty in breathing and hypotension. Thus they are generally contraindicated in elderly patients.

Although not currently licensed for this purpose, the prokinetic agent *cisapride* (p. 314) has been used to treat intractable constipation. However, this may have significant CNS and other side effects, especially ventricular arrhythmias in those with a prolonged QT interval.

Older laxatives and side effects

Products containing *liquid paraffin* may occasionally be useful to lubricate and soften a hard faecal mass, especially if defecation is painful due to haemorrhoids or anal tears. However, in the very young and elderly there is a risk of aspiration pneumonitis. If used long term, liquid paraffin reduces the absorption of oil-soluble vitamins and may cause anal leakage, especially in the elderly; thus it is unsuitable for use in children under 3 years of age, or for prolonged or repeated use, and should be employed only in exceptional circumstances. In **faecal impaction** an *arachis oil enema* produces softening and lubrication, and is preferable to liquid paraffin.

Although phenolphthalein has been very widely used in some proprietary medicines, it may cause skin rashes, albuminuria and haemoglobinuria. It may also cause colic and vomiting in young children and has been withdrawn in the UK.

The old vegetable cathartics, e.g. aloin, cascara, castor oil, colocynth and jalap, have a very drastic action and are likely to cause severe colic, so they have largely been superseded by less toxic agents.

Laxatives must not be used if there is a suspicion of appendicitis, as they increase the risk of perforation and peritonitis.

Bowel cleansing

'Bowel prep' is used with a low-residue diet to clear the bowel of solids in preparation for colonoscopy, radiology or surgery. The drugs used include high concentrations of salts, e.g. *magnesium citrate, sodium dihydrogen phosphate, macrogols plus salts, sodium picosulphate plus mag-*

nesium citrate and *oxyphenisatine*. None of these preparations is suitable as a routine laxative; oxyphenisatine may cause hepatitis in chronic use.

Diarrhoea

Definition, aetiology and pathology

Diarrhoea is an increased volume or frequency of bowel movement, relative to the normal for an individual, associated with greater fluidity of the motions. As with constipation, it is essential to establish just what a patient means by the term 'diarrhoea'.

Diarrhoea may be classified according to clinical criteria, i.e. **acute** or **chronic**, although there are many possible aetiologies (Table 6.19), some of which are dealt with in this chapter, for which the appropriate sections should be consulted. Alternatively, a **pathophysiological classification** can be made:

- **Malabsorptive**, owing to a failure to absorb nutrients, causing an osmotic diarrhoea, e.g. gluten enteropathy.
- **Osmotic**, in which hypertonic conditions prevent colonic water resorption, e.g. disaccharidase deficiency, saline purgatives.

- **Hypersecretory**, with massive secretion of water and electrolytes from the mucosa, e.g. cholera, verocytotoxin-producing *Escherichia coli* O157.
- **Exudative**, in which protein, blood and fluids leak from an inflamed or damaged mucosa, e.g. IBD, protozoal infection.
- **Neuromuscular**, leading to a shortened gut transit time and inadequate water and nutrient absorption, e.g. diabetic neuropathy, thyrotoxicosis.

The most common causes of acute diarrhoea are contaminated food or drinks (**gastroenteritis**), especially from recent travel abroad, and medicines.

Complications

Both chronic and severe acute diarrhoea may cause:

- Dehydration, with hypovolaemia, low blood pressure and tachycardia.
- Hypokalaemia and low bicarbonate, giving metabolic acidosis.
- Small-bowel lactase depletion.

Chronic diarrhoea may also cause anaemia (microcytic or macrocytic, low haemoglobin and folate).

Table 6.19   Some possible causes of diarrhoea

Acute	Gastroenteritis (food 'poisoning'): e.g. bacterial infections, especially *Salmonella typhimurium* and other *Salmonella* spp., *Campylobacter jejuni*, *Listeria monocytogenes*, enteropathogenic *Escherichia coli* (infants), typhoid and paratyphoid fevers, dysentery (*Shigella* spp.) Toxins: bacterial (staphylococcal, clostridial); plant (mushrooms, aflatoxins) Viral infections: rotavirus (infants), coxsackie, ECHO Protozoal infections: *Giardia lamblia*, *Entamoeba histolytica*
Chronic	Organic disease: Crohn's disease, ulcerative colitis, diverticular disease, irritable bowel syndrome, diabetes, biliary problems, malabsorption syndromes, pancreatic disease, cystic fibrosis, cancer Food-induced: food allergies, inappropriate diet Psychogenic: anxiety, depression
Iatrogenic	Almost all drugs can cause diarrhoea in some patients. The following are common causes: • antibiotics: clindamycin, lincomycin, tetracyclines, nalidixic acid, erythromycin, rifampicin • antacids: magnesium compounds (also 'health salts') • cardiac drugs: digoxin overdose Non-drug causes: intestinal radiotherapy

Management

Aims

The aims of management are:

- To relieve symptoms, without prolonging the condition.
- To prevent dehydration and electrolyte deficiencies, and to correct existing metabolic abnormality in severe disease.
- To treat any underlying disease or, if there is no effective treatment, give symptomatic relief.

Achievement of these aims is by:

- Removing any trigger substances, e.g. with adsorbents.
- Administering:
  - Glucose-electrolyte solutions.
  - Antidiarrhoeal drugs to reduce gastrointestinal motility.
  - Bulking agents, to improve faecal consistency.
- Investigating persistent symptoms (>2 weeks), and patients with severe constitutional upset.
- Using antibiotics (sometimes), if there is major systemic upset and a demonstrated pathogen of proven susceptibility.

General management

The treatment of **chronic diarrhoea** depends on controlling the underlying disease (Table 6.19).

Acute diarrhoea. Any medication which may be causing the condition (Table 6.19) or aggravating its metabolic consequences (e.g. diuretics) should be stopped and, if essential, a temporary or permanent alternative found.

Most cases of gastroenteritis are self-limiting, the most important aspect of treatment being the prevention of fluid and electrolyte depletion, or their adequate replacement, using *oral rehydration salts* (ORS) or a proprietary equivalent. The glucose, or other carbohydrate yielding it, is necessary as an energy source for electrolyte absorption. This is especially important in infants and young children, who can become dehydrated very rapidly, or in frail or elderly patients. Restlessness and fretfulness in an infant may be misinterpreted as a requirement for more food, and deaths have occurred from giving excessively concentrated feeds or feeds supplemented with glucose. If a baby is unwell, the safest course is to use fluid and electrolyte replacement at the recommended concentration until proper medical advice can be obtained. A properly nourished child will not come to harm if food is withheld for 24 h, but may do if fed excessively.

A short period of diarrhoea (<48 h) will not cause electrolyte depletion except in infants and the frail elderly, or unless the diarrhoea is very severe, so taking ample fluids such as water, fruit juices or commercial drinks containing glucose should be adequate. If diarrhoea is prolonged, the use of ORS or a proprietary equivalent is appropriate, but every effort should be made to identify a cause and treat the underlying condition.

It is difficult to identify dehydration clinically, but symptoms of diarrhoea, especially with vomiting, plus recent weight loss (especially in infants) or loss of skin turgor (in well-nourished teenagers and adults up to age 50 years) is significant. Skin turgor can be roughly assessed by lifting a skinfold on the back of the hand and releasing it; the skin should return briskly to normal. If it relaxes slowly, this may indicate fluid loss. This test is inapplicable in young children, because of their high fluid content, and in older patients (loss of subcutaneous and elastic tissue causes a normally slow relaxation).

Milk or milk products should be reintroduced cautiously after a prolonged period of diarrhoea, as the gut mucosa may be temporarily depleted of lactase, causing inadequate lactose absorption and a consequent **osmotic diarrhoea**.

Antimotility drugs. Examples are *loperamide* and *codeine*; these may be necessary in the short term for social reasons, or to permit the maintenance of some semblance of normality by a mother or a busy worker who can ill afford to take time off work. *Loperamide* is preferable, as it does not have central or addictive properties. These agents should be avoided if possible, because they are alleged to cause the retention of potentially inflammatory and toxic products in the bowel, thus prolonging symptoms. However, this is not an important consideration in most acute diarrhoeas, which are short, self-limiting conditions. Over-enthusiastic use may lead to constipation.

Antispasmodics. Examples are *alverine* and *mebeverine*, which do little to improve diarrhoea, but may help to relieve bowel cramps. They should not be used with antidiarrhoeals because the effects are additive.

Adsorbents and bulking agents. Examples are *kaolin* and *methylcellulose*; these serve primarily to modify stool consistency, but may aggravate symptoms by increasing stool weight. They may play a minor role if a known toxin is involved, but the ubiquitous Kaolin and Morphine Mixture is primarily a placebo.

Antibiotics. These are rarely indicated in uncomplicated infective diarrhoea. *Ciprofloxacin* is sometimes used for the prophylaxis of travellers' diarrhoea, but this is undesirable. The best prophylactic measures are awareness of potential sources of infection, sensible eating and drinking, and good food and personal hygiene. However, antibiotics may be required to treat properly diagnosed enteric infections, e.g. severe *Campolybacter* enteritis (*erythromycin* or *ciprofloxacin*) and *Salmomella typhimurium* infections (now often with multiple antibiotic resistance), typhoid fever, dysentery and antibiotic-associated colitis (*see* Chapter 13).

Irritable bowel syndrome

Definition and clinical features

This is one form of **functional bowel disease**, i.e. function is abnormal without any demonstrable specific abnormality and with a poor response to treatment. It is a diagnosis of exclusion, i.e. other possible causes of the symptoms are absent.

Clinical features
These include:

- Recurrent or chronic mild to moderate left-sided or more general abdominal pain or discomfort, commonly in the iliac fossa, often relieved by defecation or passing wind.
- Constipation with abnormal pellet-like or ribbon stools, or occasionally diarrhoea.

- Frequent small amounts of stool.
- A frequent feeling of bloating or incomplete evacuation.

Irritable bowel syndrome (IBS) accounts for more than half of all gastrointestinal consultations, and is a difficult problem for the gastroenterologist because extensive (negative) investigations may be needed.

Aetiology

The aetiology of IBS is obscure, but may include:

- A low-fibre diet.
- Sequel to severe bowel infection.
- Excessive colonic contractions, as part of a generalized disorder of smooth muscle function.
- Laxative abuse.

Although neurotic features are present in two-thirds of patients, they are not causative. However, they will determine how well the patient tolerates the symptoms, whether they seek medical advice and their presentation of symptoms to their GP.

Management

In the absence of organic disease and because the aetiology is obscure, treatment of IBS is symptomatic and empirical. It includes:

- Explanation and reassurance to allay fears of serious pathology.
- Treatment of any underlying depression or anxiety.
- A high-fibre diet or bulking agents to restore normal faecal bulk and consistency, though it is uncertain whether they produce significant improvement.
- Antidiarrhoeals (if indicated).
- Antispasmodics, e.g. *mebeverine* (a specific gastrointestinal musculotropic agent which reduces spasm without affecting colonic motility), *alverine*, *mepenzolate*, enteric coated peppermint oil capsules.
- *Activated charcoal* as an antiflatulant.

Stomatherapy

Stomas

These are artificial openings which are formed surgically between the internal organs and the skin. They are described according to the internal organ to which they are connected, e.g. **colostomy** (colon), **ileostomy** (ileum). Although **ureterostomy** is possible in some cases, an alternative procedure, a **urinary diversion**, is normally done (see below). Other types of stoma may be formed, e.g. tracheostomy for artificial ventilation, but these will not be considered here.

The indications for these operations are given in Table 6.20.

Location

It is important for the surgeon to site the stoma correctly in order to ensure that the patient can manage it properly and that it is in an area away from skin creases, which tend to cause leakage (Fig. 6.15(a)). The stoma is always formed separately from the main operative incision, because the scar causes skin irregularities and is particularly susceptible to damage by enzymes and irritants in bowel fluids leaking from the stoma. Other sites that should be avoided include old operation scars and areas where the skin surface is uneven or covered by breasts or skin folds, especially when seated.

Types of stoma

Colostomies

Although these are usually permanent, temporary ones may be formed to rest the distal section of bowel, following trauma or obstruction. This postoperative resting of damaged bowel should be distinguished from resting of inflamed, intact bowel in IBD, which is not helpful. Bowel continuity is restored after some 2–3 months. Thus temporary colostomies are mostly seen in the hospital setting. Other types of stoma are managed in the community, following surgery and initial hospital treatment.

Depending on the extent of disease, the colostomy may connect with the **ascending**, **transverse** or **descending** colon. The colon is turned back on itself to project about 1 cm above the skin surface to minimize skin soiling (Fig. 6.15(b)), and is stitched to the skin. The projecting stump of colon is moist and bright pink, like normal gastrointestinal mucosa. Although initially oedematous, the stump shrinks somewhat over the first few months, and this may cause leakage from an initially well-fitting appliance. Occasionally, retraction, prolapse or stenosis of the stoma may occur, or hernias may develop around it, necessitating surgical repair.

Temporary colostomies are usually 'loops', i.e. the colon is not completely divided and the partially separated surfaces are brought out through the skin, a plastic rod being used behind the loop of bowel to prevent retraction into the abdomen. There is thus an active and an inactive end of bowel (Fig. 6.16(c)), the former discharging faeces and the latter mucus.

Because the colon progressively absorbs residual water from the faeces, the consistency of the discharge will vary with the length of bowel removed: the less that is removed, the more normal the stools. However, the discharge is always fluid initially, due to inflammation, though this usually settles after a few months into a more formed stool, with a reasonably regular pattern of motions.

Table 6.20   Indications for stomatherapy

Colostomy	Ileostomy	Urinary diversion
Carcinoma of the rectum and colon	Extensive ulcerative colitis	Carcinoma of the bladder
Severe diverticulitis	Familial polyposis coli	Congenital or acquired
Uncontrolled ulcerative colitis or Crohn's colitis	Severe diverticulitis	neurological failure of
Traumatic abdominal injury	Uncontrolled Crohn's disease	bladder control

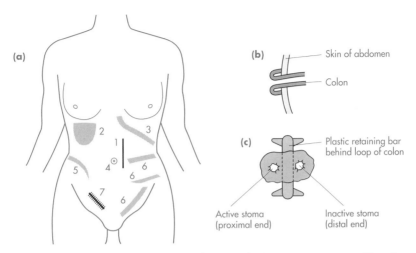

Figure 6.15 Location and formation of stomas. (a) Site of proposed main operative incision (1) and areas to avoid: 2, area under breasts; 3, margin of rib cage; 4, umbilicus; 5, iliac crest; 6, skin creases; 7, scars of old operations. (b) Formation (permanent colostomy): the cut end of colon is brought to the skin away from the main operative incision, reflexed and stitched down to form a 'spout'. (c) Temporary colostomy. (a) is modified from a drawing supplied by Convatec Ltd.

An interesting development is the 'continent colostomy plug', which is inserted into the stoma and then absorbs water and expands to fill the aperture, effectively blocking the passage of faeces. There is a built-in filter and valve, so that wind can usually be passed without noise or odour. The device is unobtrusive and overcomes many of the psychosocial problems of ostomists, but it is not suitable for all patients and its role is not yet clear.

Ileostomies

These are usually permanent, though occasionally the rectum and anus can be preserved and a subsequent ileorectal or ileoanal anastomosis (reconnection) performed.

The stoma is similar to that in colostomy, except that it is the ileum which is brought to the surface. As normal ileal contents are always fluid and rather irritant, owing to the presence of digestive enzymes, the stoma is usually formed to project further from the skin, to form a 'spout' and so minimize the possibility of skin soiling and damage immediately around the stoma.

A variant sometimes used is **Kock's continent ileostomy**, in which a reservoir is formed in the abdomen from the ileum. The stoma aperture is formed into a 'valve', to prevent leakage, and the reservoir emptied with a catheter several times a day.

Urinary diversions

These are usually formed as an **ileal conduit**. A segment of ileum is first removed with its blood supply, and the cut ends of the ileum are rejoined. The ureters are then transplanted into one end of the segment, the other end being used to form the urinary stoma. Because urinary output is continuous and liquid, the urinary stoma is always fashioned as a 2-cm 'spout' to carry urine away from the skin surface.

Management

Appliances

Unless a temporary stoma is formed, or a subsequent anal anastomosis is possible for colonic or ileal stomas, patients need to wear an appliance for the rest of their lives. There are many different types available. Initially, the choice will depend on the preference of the stoma care specialist, a drainable appliance being needed until the postoperative trauma to the tissues subsides.

However, modifications are necessary as recovery proceeds, and the final choice depends on the needs and preferences of the patient.

The general **criteria for selection** are:

- **Comfort.** There should be a reasonably close fit, without damaging the stoma. The gap around the stoma should be about 5 mm: if the clearance is significantly greater than this the skin may become damaged, creating considerable problems.
- **Security.** The patient should be able to have complete confidence that the appliance will not come off or be socially embarrassing.
- **Leak proof.** This is to avoid odour and skin damage.
- **Odour proof.** Deodorants are a poor substitute; fear of odour and social embarrassment is a major patient concern.
- **Convenience.** Light and unobtrusive, easy to

apply and change, easy to empty, or discard if disposable.

Most types of appliance in current use are disposable, though non-disposable types are still used occasionally. There is a trend towards two-piece appliances (Fig. 6.16), consisting of a self-adhesive base with an integral circular plastic gasket to which the bag is attached. The base remains on the skin for several days and enables easy, secure changing of the disposable bags. The advantages are that removal of the adhesive base is performed relatively infrequently, so skin trauma is minimized. Also, there is no fixed bag covering the stoma, so the skin immediately around the stoma is readily accessible and can easily be covered with protective pastes. With one-piece appliances, the adhesive gasket and the bag must be renewed more frequently as an integral unit and filler pastes applied first. In either case, the base must fit the stoma closely in

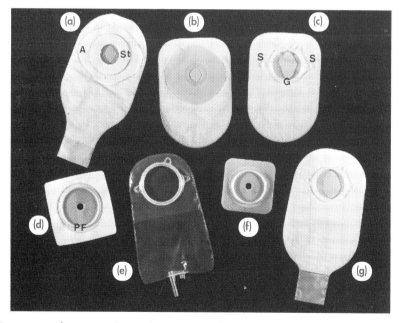

Figure 6.16 Some types of stoma appliance. (a) One-piece drainable ileostomy bag with Stomahesive seal (St) and adhesive patch (A). (b) Small one-piece non-drainable (closed) bag. This incorporates a flatus filter which is not seen in this view since it is on the underside, though the bulge it creates is just visible in the top left hand corner of the body. (c) Small two-piece closed bag with plastic gasket (G), incorporating belt supports (S). (d) Adhesive base for two-piece appliances with large plastic flange (PF) to suit bags (c) and (e). (e) Two-piece urostomy bag with large gasket and tap for drainage and attachment of night drainage bag (tap shown in open position). (f) Adhesive (Stomahesive) base with flange to suit bag (g). (g) Drainable two-piece ileostomy bag. The ends of bags (a) and (g) are sealed with a plastic clip in use. The apertures in the bases (d) and (f) are cut slightly larger than the stomas and, after application, the Stomahesive is moulded to fit closely around the stoma to protect the skin. (Reproduced with the permission of Convatec Ltd.)

order to minimize skin soiling, yet cause minimal trauma to the stoma itself. **Protective pastes**, e.g. Stomaseal, karaya paste, are essential to protect the skin and fill in awkward creases and scars, thus minimizing leakage.

Urostomy bags have an attachment for a **night drainage** tube and bag, to avoid wetting of the bed from accidental pressure on a full bag.

A high level of skin care and hygiene is essential. Cleansing routines must be gentle, and hair should be removed only with an electric razor. Barrier and other skin creams must not interfere with gasket adhesion. The key to skin care is a well-fitting appliance: it is more important to prevent skin damage than to treat it, however successfully.

Medicines and the ostomist

Because a variable length of bowel has been removed, previously suitable medicines may be unsuitable. Further, because the excreta are discharged into bags which display their appearances, or have to be emptied, patients are especially aware of changes in the colours of urine and faeces. Pharmacists should therefore avoid dispensing products which cause problems, if possible, and should counsel patients appropriately. A listing of drugs which may discolour urine and faeces is given in Table 6.21,

and of dosage forms which may cause problems in Table 6.22.

Diet

Diet is not usually a problem, and no specific restrictions whatever are required for urostomy patients. Colostomists have very individual requirements, but problems such as odour, fluidity and wind occur most often with salads, biscuits, tomatoes, onions, nuts and beer (Table 6.23). Odour is most frequently associated with baked beans, eggs, cabbage, cheeses, fish and beer. It is clearly a matter for each patient to learn to avoid those items that cause problems. If a major part of the colon is removed, *methylcellulose* may help to give firmer motions.

Ileostomy involves similar considerations, except that the discharge is always fluid and the larger volume of water lost with it must be replaced; thus patients need to drink up to 1 L extra daily, sometimes with added electrolytes.

Rehabilitation

Full physical and mental rehabilitation is the aim of stomatherapy, and many patients live remarkably full and normal lives. However, despite the enormous advances in the design of

Table 6.21 Some drugs which may discolour urine and faeces

Colour produced	Drug or drug class
Urine	
Blue or green	Amitriptyline, indometacin, sulphonamides, triamterene (in acid urine under fluorescent light)
Yellow or brownish	Chloroquine, metronidazole, nitrofurantoin, senna (acid urine)
Pink, red or reddish/brown	Cascara, dantron, levodopa, methyldopa, phenindione, phenothiazines, phenolphthalein, senna (alkaline urine), rifabutin, rifampicin
Darkening	Ferrous salts, senna (on standing)
Faeces	
Whitish or speckled	Insoluble antacids
Black	Bismuth salts, charcoal, iron salts
Pink or red to black[a]	Anticoagulants, aspirin and salicylates, non-steroidal anti-inflammatory drugs
Greenish or greyish	Antibiotics, indometacin

[a] May indicate gastrointestinal bleeding.

Table 6.22   Possible effects of dosage forms on ostomists

Drug or drug class	Type of patient[a]	Effects produced
Antibiotics	C, I	Diarrhoea, bacterial overgrowth
Antimuscarinics[b]	C, I	Constipation
Antacids	C, I, U	Constipation or diarrhoea
Beta-blockers	C, I, U	
Methyldopa	C, I, U	Diarrhoea
Opioid analgesics	C, I, U	Constipation
Sulphonamides	U	Crystalluria
Modified release preparations	C, I	May be ineffective due to impaired absorption
Diuretics	I	May cause impaired fluid and electrolyte balance
	U	Increased urine volumes in bags

[a] C, colostomy; I, ileostomy; U, urinary diversion. Ostomists are particularly susceptible to the side effects of drugs and react very variably. *See also* Table 6.21.

[b] Includes antihistamines, tricyclic antidepressants, phenothiazines.

Table 6.23   Dietary guidelines for colostomists and ileostomists[a]

General advice for achieving a consistent stoma output
- Eat regularly three times a day, in moderation
- Identify and avoid foods and drinks which give problems, or reduce their intake
- Eat wind-producing foods sparingly. Do not: eat too fast, talk while eating, or wash food down with drinks, especially fizzy drinks
- Balance intake of foods causing constipation and loose motions to produce a neutral effect

Some foods that may cause problems
- *Odour*: asparagus; beans, peas and other pulses; cabbage, brussels sprouts and other brassicas; coleslaw; cheese; eggs; fish; onions
- *Wind*: beans, peas and other pulses; cabbage, brussels sprouts and other brassicas; coleslaw; cucumber; fatty, rich foods; fizzy drinks; onions; radishes
- *Constipation*: bean sprouts; celery; chocolate; coleslaw; coconut and other nuts; eggs; fried foods; grapefruit; high fibre foods; nuts; macaroons; popcorn and sweetcorn; raisins and dried fruits; rice and tapioca; seeds; skins of fruits and vegetables
- *Diarrhoea*: alcoholic drinks, especially beer; green beans; broccoli and calabrese; fruit juices and raw fruit; mange tout; spinach; very spicy food

[a] The reactions of ostomists are highly individual.

appliances in recent years, and corresponding improvements in support systems for patient care, some patients (and/or their families) fail to come to terms with their stomas. The operations are major, emotionally traumatic, and are often performed at very short notice or as an emergency. When time allows, expert preoperative counselling of the patients and their families is essential, as is skilled and sympathetic postoperative support. Contact with one of the self-help groups is invaluable, and pharmacists can help greatly by dealing sympathetically with patients' problems and by ensuring the prompt supply of appliances and ancillary products. Good records ensure that the correct type of appliance is always supplied, because prescriptions are often incomplete. Most districts have a specialist stoma care nurse, and it is very helpful for community pharmacists to establish a working relationship with such personnel. Appliance manufacturers also employ nurse advisers who will provide technical advice by telephone and visit patients in their homes, though with a varying degree of commerciality.

Liver diseases

Because the liver is the largest single organ in the body and carries out vital metabolic functions (Table 6.24), liver diseases cause profound and widespread effects.

Many diverse pathological processes may cause liver dysfunction. This short section deals briefly with jaundice and some common liver diseases, notably those which may be caused by drugs. The reader is referred to the References and further reading section for further information.

Clinical physiology of the liver

Anatomy and histology

The liver is usually totally enclosed within the right lower rib cage (*see* Fig. 6.1(d)). The organ receives only 25% of its blood supply (but 50% of its oxygen) from the hepatic artery, the remainder being derived from the portal vein, which drains the gastrointestinal tract and the spleen (*see* Fig. 6.4). The liver has a modular

Table 6.24 Some functions of the liver

Type of function	Examples
Anabolic	Conversion of surplus glucose to glycogen and fat
	Manufacture of proteins, e.g. albumin, transferrin, lipoprotein (VLDLs, HDLs)
	Synthesis of coagulation factors, e.g. prothrombin; fibrinogen; factors V, VII, IX, X, XIII
	Production of heparin
	25-Hydroxylation of vitamin D_3
Storage	Energy (glycogen, fat)
	Vitamins A, D, E, K
	Minerals, e.g. Fe, Cu
	Non-metabolizable toxins, e.g. DDT
Catabolic	Breakdown of a wide range of compounds, e.g.
	• Hormones, e.g. insulin, glucagon, glucocorticoids, oestrogens, growth hormone
	• Conversion of:
	— nitrogen residues to urea
	— glycogen, fat and protein to glucose
	— haemoglobin to bilirubin with recirculation of iron
Detoxification	Bilirubin (to its glucuronide), drugs, alcohol, antigens
Scavenging and protective	Phagocytosis of blood-borne microorganisms and effete erythrocytes (by Kupffer cells)

structure, being divided into approximately polyhedral functional units, the **lobules** (Fig. 6.17), at the angles of which are branches of the portal vein and hepatic artery. The blood flows from these through irregularly shaped **sinusoids** into a **central vein**, and from there to the hepatic vein and the inferior vena cava. Between the sinusoids are cords of hepatic cells which carry out the crucial metabolic functions. Although most of the products of metabolism are secreted into the hepatic vein or are stored in the liver, the **bile** produced does not normally enter the blood. It is secreted into tiny capillaries (**canaliculi**) situated between the cells. These drain into small ducts and then into the **right** and **left hepatic ducts** which in turn unite to form the **common hepatic duct** that finally joins with the outflow from the gallbladder to form the **common bile duct**. The common bile duct is joined by the **pancreatic duct** just before it terminates at the duodenum, into which it discharges via the **sphincter of Oddi**. This sphincter closes the ducts when the duodenum is empty, at which point bile is diverted into the gallbladder where it is stored and concentrated until required.

Investigation

Imaging

Plain abdominal **X-rays** are of limited value, but do indicate the sizes of the liver and spleen and may show gas in the biliary tract, opaque gallstones, gallbladder and liver calcification, and ascites. An oral **cholecystogram** or IV **cholangiogram**, performed with an iodine contrast agent, visualizes both radiolucent and radioopaque gallstones. However, these traditional methods have largely been replaced by ultrasound, CT and MRI scanning and endoscopic retrograde cholangiopancreatography (ERCP) (see below).

Ultrasound scanning is now used routinely to define the size and shape of the liver and to detect intrahepatic lesions (e.g. cysts, tumours), ascites, abnormalities of the biliary tract and gallstones. This can be done during open surgery, with a sterile probe being used to guide the surgeon. **Doppler ultrasound** will measure blood flow. **Endoscopic ultrasonography** is being used increasingly in specialist centres to visualize the biliary tree, pancreas and portal vein, and also to obtain specific biopsy specimens.

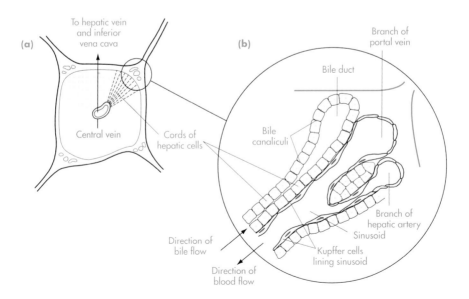

Figure 6.17   Liver histology (diagrammatic). (a) A lobule. (b) Arrangement of blood vessels and bile ducts.

CT scanning can also delineate organ size, and can detect internal lesions and the presence of fat and excess iron. The development of **spiral CT** scanning enables information on arterial and portal blood flow and hepatic lesions to be obtained rapidly. The use of contrast media enhances CT visualization of liver metastases and the biliary tree, but the agents used are rather toxic.

MRI is increasingly used because it can provide superior results to CT (with no radiation dose), and is less invasive than endoscopy.

Numerous compounds labelled with technetium-99m are used for **scintiscanning**. The procedure is more invasive, but can be used to define the shape and size of the liver and spleen, and to detect internal lesions. It also gives a direct semi-quantitative assessment of reticuloendothelial function, because the Kupffer cells preferentially take up the colloid. Radiopharmaceuticals can also be used to visualize the biliary tract and cystic duct and estimate biliary function. **Positron emission tomography** has been used for the detection of both primary and secondary tumours.

Visualization of the biliary tract may be done by X-ray following the injection of a radioopaque dye into an intrahepatic bile duct (**percutaneous transhepatic cholangiography**), with antibiotic cover. There is a small but significant risk to the patient, so ultrasound is being used increasingly.

ERCP (endoscopic retrograde cholangiopancreatography) can be used to visualize the common bile duct and biliary tract and the pancreatic duct. In this technique, the papilla of Vater is cannulated by endoscopy and contrast medium is injected to visualize gallstones. The pancreatic duct and other anatomical features can be examined simultaneously. The endoscope can also be used to remove stones which block the common bile duct. ERCP may also provide valuable further information on the aetiology of biliary obstruction, e.g. pancreatic carcinoma, or of its consequences, e.g. pancreatitis.

Blood (serum) and urine tests

Apart from the estimation of serum proteins (albumin, prothrombin), which are synthesized in the liver, the 'liver function tests' are only indirect indicators of hepatic function. Further, the finding of normal values does not exclude appreciable liver damage, because 20% of patients with stable, chronic cirrhosis have normal values.

Serum proteins

Because their synthesis occurs only in the liver, reduced levels of serum proteins, especially albumin, are a useful general indicator of hepatic disease.

Prothrombin (clotting factor II) is not measured directly but as **prothrombin time** (PT), i.e. the time taken for a fibrin clot to be produced in plasma under standard conditions. The test is always done in comparison with a normal sample of pooled plasma. In general, PT abnormalities are due to liver malfunction, indicating either defective prothrombin synthesis (liver disease) or vitamin K deficiency due to obstructive jaundice (see below). Inadequate bile function causes a failure to absorb fat-soluble vitamin K_1 (phytomenadione) from the diet. However, deficiency of vitamin K can also be due to malabsorption (p. 335) or oral anticoagulant therapy. These possibilities can be eliminated by repeating the PT test 24 h after a single IM injection of vitamin K. PT is probably the single most useful indicator for monitoring patient progress, being sensitive, specific to the liver (apart from vitamin K deficiency and anticoagulant therapy), and easily performed.

There are also unusually high immunoglobulin levels in alcoholic liver disease (IgA), chronic autoimmune hepatitis (IgG) and primary biliary cirrhosis (IgM), but these indicate possible causes of liver disease because they are not synthesized in the liver.

Other blood tests

Many others tests have been advocated, e.g. ammonia (p. 369), transaminases (ALT, AST), alkaline phosphatase (ALP), gamma-glutamyl transpeptidase (GT), bilirubin (p. 363) and LDH, but these may be useful only if targeted to carefully selected patients. The interpretations of the most common tests are outlined in Table 6.25.

Numerous other biochemical tests are carried out for the detection of specific abnormalities,

Table 6.25   Serum, blood and urine tests of liver function

Test and abbreviation	Notes and implications of results
Serum tests	
Bilirubin	>17 micromol/L (>1 mg/dL) + 80% unconjugated = haemolytic jaundice or congestive heart failure
	<80% unconjugated = hepatitic or metastatic liver disease
Alkaline phosphatase (ALP)	Non-specific. Raised levels = hepatic obstruction, or bone or pancreatic disease
Aminotransferases	For monitoring disease progression and the effects of therapy
• aspartate (AST, SGOT[a])	Levels normally parallel each other:
• alanine (ALT, SGPT[a])	• both very high = acute viral hepatitis
	• both high = myocardial infarction or shock
	• AST high, ALT normal = alcoholic liver disease
Albumin	Useful indicator of chronic liver disease ($t_{1/2}$ = 20 days)
Whole-blood tests	
Prothrombin time	2–3 s > normal = liver disease, vitamin K deficiency or anticoagulant therapy
Urine tests	
Bilirubin	Excess (dark urine = hepatic obstruction)
Urobilinogen	Total absence = cholestasis (also gives pale stools)
	High = haemolysis, chronic liver disease or portosystemic shunting of blood (e.g. due to alcoholic cirrhosis)

[a] SGOT and SGPT are former abbreviations that are no longer used.

e.g. serology for viral hepatitis (A, B, C) and autoantibodies (antimitochondrial, antimicrosomal), alpha-fetoprotein (a tumour marker; *see* Chapter 11), but the reader is referred to the References and further reading section for accounts of these.

Urine testing

This has been a conventional part of screening for liver disease, but is now less important with the introduction of improved serum biochemistry methods.

Dynamic tests

The blood and serum tests outlined above are static tests, i.e. they give a snapshot at the time of sampling, but little idea of liver function. The excretion of certain drugs, e.g. *sulphobromophthalein sodium* (*bromsulphthalein, BSP*) and *lidocaine* (*lignocaine*), is used in research and in specific cases to assess liver damage. These drugs have a high first-pass extraction, e.g. <5–7% of

BSP normally remains in the serum 45 min after injection, and their clearance is a measure of liver blood flow. However, these tests are done only infrequently nowadays.

The clearance of drugs with a low first-pass extraction, e.g. *phenazone* (*antipyrine*) and *aminophenazone* (*amidopyrine, aminopyrine*), is virtually independent of liver blood flow and is a better measure of liver function.

Other investigations

Invasive investigations, which may carry a significant risk, may also be undertaken. **Liver biopsy** may be needed to confirm a diagnosis, establish prognosis, monitor progress, and to diagnose certain systemic diseases, e.g. sarcoidosis, tuberculosis, brucellosis. Samples are taken percutaneously with a special biopsy needle, preferably under ultrasound or CT guidance. There should not be a significant clotting problem, but cross-matched blood or at least cross-matching facilities must be available, especially if the PT is prolonged. In skilled hands the procedure can be done as a day-case, but overnight observation may be required.

When occasionally the diagnosis is dubious, **laparoscopy** (examination of the abdominal organs with a fibreoptic instrument), or open **laparotomy** (surgical incision of the abdomen to permit examination of the organs) may be undertaken.

Clinical features of hepatic disease

General symptoms and signs

Many non-specific symptoms accompany early liver disease, e.g. malaise, anorexia, nausea and vomiting, and arthropathies. Fever is common, being mild to moderate in alcoholic hepatitis, though high fever with rigors may precede jaundice in acute viral hepatitis. **Steatorrhoea** (pale, bulky, fatty, abnormally foul-smelling stools) is a common feature in acute hepatitis, though less common in chronic disease, and may contribute to weight loss.

Dupuytren's contracture (tendon contraction causing permanent flexure of one or more fingers) and **parotid gland enlargement** tend to occur most commonly in alcoholic liver disease. Palmar tendon contracture may be the first sign of liver disease in people following sedentary occupations (it may be occupationally derived in manual workers).

Jaundice (icterus)

Definition

This most common symptom of liver disease is seen as a yellow coloration of the skin and sclera of the eyes, owing to the existence of **hyperbilirubinaemia**. Skin and scleral discoloration become visually evident at about two to three times the normal serum bilirubin levels (Normal = <20 micromol/L, <1.0 mg/dL). Although jaundice is always the result of a high bilirubin level, it will not occur if the bilirubin level is only slightly raised. A spurious jaundice may result from excessive ingestion of carotene (in 'health diets'), or drugs (e.g. *mepacrine*, *busulfan*), but in these cases only the skin is coloured, and not the eyes.

The formation and excretion of bilirubin is summarized schematically in Fig. 6.18, from which it is apparent that two forms of bilirubin exist. These appear differently in the urine and faeces in health and disease.

Excess **unconjugated bilirubin** is found in the serum when there is impaired hepatic removal and conjugation of bilirubin, e.g. in congenital glucuronidase deficiency (Gilbert's syndrome), or when excessive production of bilirubin overwhelms the capacity of the conjugation system, e.g. in haemolytic anaemias. Under these circumstances, bilirubin (water-insoluble) is absent from the urine, but urinary **urobilinogen** levels are raised to an extent which depends on the underlying cause and its severity. Although urobilinogen is colourless, the urine may darken on standing, as oxidation produces urobilin.

Excess **conjugated bilirubin** is present in the serum when there is **obstruction of the biliary tree**, e.g. due to gallstones or carcinoma. In this situation, bilirubin appears in the urine, because the conjugated form is water-soluble, but urinary levels of urobilinogen are reduced, or absent if obstruction is complete. If bilirubin is not discharged into the duodenum, urobilinogen and faecal bile pigments are not produced, so the faeces are pale and the urine is dark.

Classification

Jaundice may be classified according to its origin:

- **Prehepatic**, arising from the blood before it enters the liver, e.g. due to haemolysis (serum bilirubin 50–150 micromol/L).
- **Intrahepatic**, due to disease of the liver parenchyma, e.g. viral hepatitis or alcoholic cirrhosis (serum bilirubin 50–350 micromol/L).
- **Posthepatic**, the result of obstruction of the biliary tree outside the liver, e.g. by gallstones or carcinoma (serum bilirubin 100–750 micromol/L).

However, mixed types of jaundice are common, especially of the last two of these. Thus **cholestatic jaundice** (formerly called **obstructive**

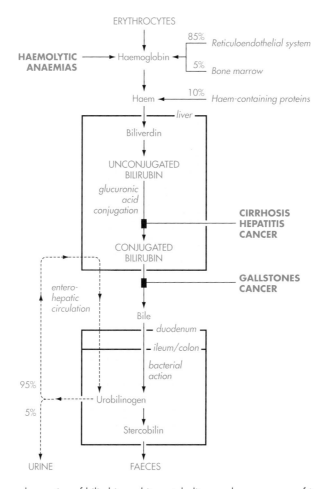

Figure 6.18   Formation and excretion of bilirubin and its metabolites, and some causes of jaundice. Causes of jaundice in bold capitals, sources of bilirubin and processes in italics (percentages are of bilirubin from the source indicated).

jaundice) may be due to inflammation of either the small bile canaliculi and ductules within the liver, or of the hepatic and common bile ducts outside it.

Obstruction of bile outflow causes a conjugated hyperbilirubinaemia and high concentrations of bile salts in the skin, often causing intense pruritus (itching). Pruritus may also be caused by increased endogenous opioid production (*see* Chapter 10) and consequent abnormal neurotransmission or neuromodulation of sensory nerves in the skin.

Aetiology

Jaundice is a symptom or sign and not a disease, so a cause must always be sought, especially because some are eminently treatable. The principal causes of jaundice are summarized in Table 6.26 and, in particular, the possibility of a drug aetiology must always be considered (Table 6.27).

Haemolytic anaemias may be inherited or acquired (Table 6.28), and may be due to intrinsic erythrocyte defects, or to extrinsic factors, such as immunological mechanisms, infection, drugs, or red cell damage, e.g. from prosthetic heart valves. Intrinsic defects, caused by abnormal membrane structure or biochemical abnormalities, may render the red cells more sensitive to extrinsic factors. Drugs may cause haemolysis directly, or trigger haemolysis in patients with an inherited tendency, e.g. G6PD deficiency (see below).

Table 6.26   Some causes of jaundice

Site of origin	Mechanism	Examples of causes
Prehepatic	Increased haem liberation	Haemolytic anaemias, malaria, reduced red cell lifespan
Intrahepatic	Defective liver metabolism	Congenital enzyme defects, iron storage disease, reduced hepatic bilirubin uptake
	Obstruction of small bile ducts	Alcoholic cirrhosis, autoimmune liver disease, drugs[a] and environmental chemicals, hepatic tumours, pregnancy, viral or other infections, gallstones (depends on diet), primary biliary cirrhosis
Posthepatic	Obstruction of large bile ducts	Infection or inflammation of the biliary tree; gallstones, carcinoma of the pancreas, gallbladder, bile ducts and ampulla of Vater; pancreatitis; drugs[a]

[a] See Table 6.27.

Table 6.27   Some drugs that may cause jaundice

Action	Examples[a]
Dose-dependent hepatocellular damage	Paracetamol (acetaminophen), salicylates, high-dose tetracyclines
Dose-independent hepatocellular damage	Halothane and methoxyflurane, dantrolene, ketoconazole, antidepressants, aminosalicylic acid, isoniazid, pyrazinamide, ethambutol
Haemolysis	Methyldopa, mefenamic acid
Cholestasis	Carbimazole, chlorpromazine, chlorpropamide, erythromycin estolate, oral contraceptives, sodium aurothiomalate, synthetic anabolic steroids

[a] This list is not comprehensive. Many drugs are capable of causing jaundice, but this is usually reversible on stopping the drug.

Table 6.28   Some causes of haemolytic anaemia

Inherited	Red cell defects Abnormalities of haemoglobin: thalassaemia (abnormal globin chains or haemoglobin), sickle cell disease Metabolic deficiencies: glucose-6-phosphate dehydrogenase, pyruvate kinase
Acquired	Immunological: autoimmune disease, isoimmunity (ABO and Rh blood group incompatibility), drugs (especially penicillins, methyldopa) Non-immune: red cell membrane defects, red cell damage (e.g. with mitral valve prostheses, in extensive burns), drugs (e.g. sulphonamides, aminosalicylates, hydroxycarbamide (hydroxyurea) or busulfan treatment for polycythaemia[a]) Infections: malaria (occasionally)

[a] Causes rapid breakdown of excess red cells.

Haemoglobinopathies also cause haemolytic anaemias, genetically abnormal haemoglobins being associated with abnormal red cell membranes. **Sickle cell anaemia** is common, especially in people of African descent, but also in the Middle East and the Indian subcontinent, and confers some protection against *Plasmodium falciparum* malaria. **Thalassaemia** affects people of Mediterranean origin and those living in a broad area from there across the Middle East into South-East Asia, there being several forms of the disease.

Management

Because jaundice is a symptom, management depends on treatment of the underlying disease.

There are no specific measures for the **anaemias**, which are treated supportively, e.g. blood transfusion, folic acid (or polyvitamin) supplements, removal of excess tissue iron with a chelating agent (e.g. *desferrioxamine*), stopping any drug which may precipitate haemolysis (*see* Tables 6.27–6.29), splenectomy.

Neonatal jaundice is common, and occurs in all preterm babies because liver glucuronyl transferase is poorly developed in neonates, especially if premature. The condition usually disappears spontaneously within 2 weeks, as liver function matures. However, moderate bilirubin levels (up to about 250 micromol/L) can be dealt with by exposure to blue light (phototherapy), which promotes bilirubin breakdown in the skin. Dangerously high bilirubin levels (>300 micromol/L) may require exchange blood transfusion to prevent **kernicterus** (deposition of bilirubin in the brain, the neonatal blood–brain barrier being permeable to bilirubin) and permanent brain damage.

Glucose-6-phosphate dehydrogenase (G6PD) deficiency. Inherited G6PD deficiency affects millions of people (mostly males) in the Mediterranean region, the Middle East, Africa and South-East Asia. G6PD is a crucial enzyme for maintaining adequate erythrocyte glutathione levels, and deficiency renders haemoglobin and red cell membranes liable to oxidation. The erythrocytes are then sensitive to a variety of minor insults, causing haemolysis. Thus lysis may be precipitated by drugs, especially oxidizing agents (Table 6.29) and acute illnesses, e.g. infections, diabetic ketoacidosis.

Skin signs

Generalized pruritus is itching of the skin. Patients with hepatic disease often present with severe, persistent itching of apparently normal skin, probably caused by the epidermal deposition of bile salts (see above). As the accumulation of bile salts and bilirubin are not necessarily related, pruritus can occur without jaundice, especially in early disease. Because itching may be due to many other causes (*see*

Table 6.29 Some drugs which may cause haemolysis in patients with glucose-6-phosphate dehydrogenase deficiency

Analgesics	Aspirin[a]
Antimalarials	Chloroquine[b], mepacrine[c], primaquine[c,d], pyrimethamine, quinine[c], quinidine[b]
Antimicrobials	Aminosalicylic acid, chloramphenicol, furazolidone, nitrofurantoin[c], nitrofurazone, 4-quinolones[c], sulphonamides[c,d], dapsone[c]
Others	Ascorbic acid, dimercaprol, diphenhydramine, methylthioninium chloride (methylene blue)[c], prilocaine, probenecid, sodium nitroprusside, vitamin K (water-soluble derivatives)

[a] Many other analgesics, e.g. acetanilide, amidopyrine, phenacetin, phenazone, which are no longer used in the UK, but are widely available in other countries, also cause haemolysis.

[b] Generally to be avoided but acceptable to manage acute malaria, the severity of which outweighs haemolytic problems.

[c] Drugs to be avoided in all cases.

[d] Primaquine and sulfasalazine do not cause haemolysis in some patients.

Chapter 12), the diagnosis of intractable pruritus in the absence of jaundice may require extensive investigation.

Spider naevi (spider telangiectases) is a frequent sign of liver disease, the naevi appearing as red spots on the upper trunk, above the nipple line. The naevi consist of a small central spiral arteriole with radiating small vessels. Central pressure with a finger or stylus causes blanching, showing that all the vessels are fed from the central arteriole. Naevi are probably caused by excessive oestrogen levels, a consequence of failing hepatic catabolism. Isolated spider naevi may occur in healthy individuals, especially in pregnant women or those on oestrogen therapy, but multiple spider naevi strongly suggest liver disease.

Raised oestrogen levels also cause body **hair loss** (including pubic and axillary), testicular atrophy and gynaecomastia (breast enlargement in men).

Palmar erythema occurs as a result of increased blood flow through the skin, caused by obstruction of the portal circulation. **Leuconychia** (white nails) is a reflection of impaired liver protein synthesis.

Abdominal signs

Pain

The liver parenchyma has no sensory nerve supply, so pain is not a marked feature of liver disease unless the **capsule** is damaged or stretched or other organs are involved. However, right hypochondrial pain is a common feature of acute **alcoholic** liver disease.

Ascites

Ascites is the accumulation of a large volume of fluid in the peritoneal cavity. In liver disease the causes are hypoproteinaemia, hepatic venous obstruction and failure of hepatic metabolism (Fig. 6.19). Ascites produces a tense, painfully

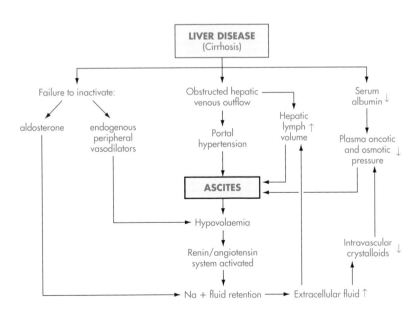

Figure 6.19 Mechanisms of ascites formation in hepatic disease (it may also have intestinal, renal and cardiac origins).

distended abdomen, though clinical signs are not apparent unless the volume exceeds about two litres, depending on the patient's stature. Peripheral (ankle) oedema may also occur in liver disease, though this is secondary to ascites, rather than being a primary event, as it is in heart or kidney failure (*see* Chapters 3 and 4). Ascites of hepatic origin is usually due to cirrhosis (see below), but there can also be non-hepatic causes, e.g. advanced congestive heart failure, nephrotic syndrome, malignancy, tuberculosis.

Similarly to the formation of oedema fluid (*see* Chapter 4), the principal initial event is that intravascular hydrostatic pressure (in this case in the portal vein) greatly exceeds the plasma oncotic pressure. This pressure difference is greater than usual in liver cirrhosis, because the portal pressure is increased owing to restricted flow through a fibrosed liver, while the oncotic pressure is reduced due to a failure of protein synthesis. These two causes combine to give increased outflow of fluid from the portal vein into the tissues.

Complications

Complications of ascites include:

- Consequences of the increased volume of intra-abdominal fluid, e.g. restricted mobility, respiratory distress.
- Spontaneous bacterial peritonitis (owing to the failure of the reticuloendothelial protection mechanisms of the liver.
- Hepatorenal syndrome (renal failure consequent on hepatic failure), which may be due to hypovolaemia causing pre-renal failure and an abnormality of tubular sodium handling. It may be precipitated by certain drugs, e.g. *diuretics*, *NSAIDs*, *ACEIs* and *aminoglycosides*.
- Encephalopathy (see below).
- Clotting defects.

Management

Management is primarily supportive and symptomatic. Bedrest improves hepatic blood flow and function.

Paracentesis and drainage, i.e. the removal of a limited volume of fluid (1–2 L) via a fine needle inserted through the abdominal wall provides fluid for diagnostic purposes and improves patient comfort. The drainage of large volumes of fluid by this means may prove fatal unless plasma expanders (low-salt albumin, polymerized gelatin) are given proportionately to the drained volume. If the plasma oncotic pressure is not increased the ascites volume is rapidly replaced, so the patient suffers further fluid and protein depletion, and the shift of further fluid from the blood into the abdomen causes hypovolaemia, hepatorenal syndrome and shock. However, up to 15 L (5 L/day) may be removed.

Salt and fluid restriction is a useful adjunctive therapy, but fluid restriction is only appropriate if the patient is hyponatraemic.

Potassium-sparing **diuretics** are used. *Spironolactone* is preferred initially, for several reasons: patients tend to be hypokalaemic, any hyperaldosteronism is counteracted, and its action is slow. Slow action is beneficial as the rapid mobilization of fluid and electrolytes causes harmful imbalances. Careful monitoring of serum electrolytes is essential to avoid hyperkalaemia and hyponatraemia. If gynaecomastia is a problem, *triamterene* or *amiloride* are suitable alternatives. If these give inadequate fluid loss, it is normal to add a low dose of a loop diuretic, e.g. *furosemide* (frusemide), rather than use high doses of potassium-sparing agents, but this increases the risk of hepatorenal syndrome.

Under certain circumstances, diuretics should be avoided:

- In hyponatraemia, to avoid further sodium depletion.
- If renal function is impaired; serum creatinine is the best guide, as liver failure results in failure of urea formation.
- If there is evidence of encephalopathy (see below). Diuretics may aggravate encephalopathy or precipitate it, by causing further disturbances of electrolyte and fluid distribution.

In refractory chronic ascites, fluid can be shunted from the peritoneal cavity into the internal jugular vein through a subcutaneously implanted catheter (transjugular intrahepatic portosystemic shunt). Alternatively, ascites fluid may be pumped from the abdomen, treated by ultrafiltration and the protein-enriched fluid returned to the circulation through a peripheral vein. Both techniques provide symptomatic relief, but carry the hazards of peritonitis, cardiovascular problems and infection.

Encephalopathy

This complex neuromuscular/neuropsychiatric syndrome occurs in severe liver disease, either late in chronic disease or as a presenting symptom of acute hepatic failure (see below). It is characterized by changes of mood and behaviour, confusion, disordered sleep rhythm, drowsiness and, eventually, delirium and coma. There is a strong similarity to senile dementia, and it is important to distinguish between them as encephalopathy is potentially correctable. **Liver flap (asterixis)** is an irregular, coarse, rapid, flapping movement of the hand(s), occurring when the arm is extended or the fist is clenched. It reflects metabolic disturbance, but the precise origin is unclear. It may occur in the absence of overt central nervous symptoms and is often the earliest sign.

The term **portosystemic encephalopathy** (PSE) describes the aetiology, i.e. it is triggered by substances which are shunted from the portal vein into the systemic circulation, escaping hepatic detoxification. The syndrome has been attributed to:

- The action of gamma-aminobutyric acid (GABA), benzodiazepine receptor agonists and a GABA-ergic neurosteroid. The levels of these are enhanced by ammonia produced by colonic bacteria.
- A changed branched-chain amino acid/aromatic amine ratio in the CNS, causing the production of false neurotransmitters, e.g. octopamine, phenylethanolamine, serotonin.
- Fatty acids, mercaptans and other substances which may also act as false neurotransmitters.

High blood levels of ammonia occur in 90% of patients, but this does not wholly account for the syndrome. Some potential precipitants of PSE are given in Table 6.30.

In acute liver failure, if there is a short interval between the appearance of jaundice and the onset of PSE, e.g. progression from mild to severe in 1–2 h, there is a high risk of potentially fatal cerebral oedema. In contrast, PSE complicating cirrhosis or a portosystemic shunt rarely causes cerebral oedema, so it is clearly important to distinguish these situations.

Management

Management of encephalopathy involves:

- Withdrawal of precipitants, e.g. alcohol and drugs.
- Control of infection, hypotension and renal impairment.
- Correction of metabolic abnormalities.
- A prophylactic antisecretory agent, to reduce the risk of haemorrhage from gastric erosions.

Table 6.30   Some precipitants of portosystemic encephalopathy

Mechanism	Examples of precipitants
Increased absorption of ammonia and other nitrogenous metabolites	GI bleeding (extra GI protein), especially from bleeding oesophageal varices (p. 315), excessive dietary protein, constipation (prolonged colonic residence times), uraemia
CNS depression	Sedatives, acidosis, uraemia
CNS excitation	Febrile infections, alkalosis
Decreased cerebral, renal and hepatic perfusion	Hyponatraemia, diuretics, heart failure, myocardial infarction, hypovolaemia, shock Drugs (see Table 6.35)
Liver damage	Diseases: e.g. viral hepatitis, Wilson's disease, malignancy

CNS, central nervous system; GI, gastrointestinal; MAOI, monoamine oxidase inhibitor.

- Suppression of colonic bacterial metabolism.
- Removal of toxic nitrogenous substances from the gut, including ammonia.

Pharmacotherapies used to achieve the last two of these objectives include the following:

- Purging with *phosphate enemas*. Magnesium enemas are sometimes recommended, but absorption may cause electrolyte disturbance.
- *Lactulose* or *lactitol* to maintain bowel evacuation, and to acidify the colon, so inhibiting bacterial metabolism and minimizing the absorption of ammonia and nitrogenous bases. This is sometimes used with antibiotics, the effects possibly being additive.
- An oral antibiotic (*neomycin*, occasionally *metronidazole* or *vancomycin*) is sometimes used to 'sterilize' the bowel. Because of toxicities with these, it is usual to rely on lactulose or lactitol.
- *Ornithine aspartate in fructose* IV increases ammonia excretion, but causes nausea and vomiting.
- *Flumazenil*, a benzodiazepine receptor antagonist, gives rapid improvement if encephalopathy was induced by benzodiazepines or other GABA-ergic drugs.

The restriction of dietary protein has been widely advocated, based on the ammonia–aromatic amine–amino acid theory of PSE aetiology. However, there is no evidence of clinical benefit for this. The 1997 guidelines of the European Society for Parenteral and Enteral Nutrition recommend a daily protein intake of 1–1.5 g/kg body weight for patients with liver disease, if tolerated. Those intolerant of this should have 0.5 g/kg/day of protein initially plus amino acids to make up the deficit, possibly as branched-chain amino acids, though this last point is unclear. The value of aggressive nutritional support has been demonstrated for patients with alcoholic liver disease and may apply to all those with severe hepatic disease. Expert dietetic involvement is clearly desirable.

Vitamin D deficiency

The functions of vitamin D are outlined on p. 305, and its formation is illustrated in Fig. 6.20, from which it is clear that either hepatic or renal failure can lead to vitamin D deficiency, in addition to poor nutrition and lack of sunlight.

Vitamin D deficiency due to malabsorption or hepatic failure is treated with *calciferol* (ergocalciferol, vitamin D_2) or *colecalciferol* (vitamin D_3) whereas *1-alpha-hydroxycholecalciferol* (alfacalcidol) or *1,25-dihydroxycholecalciferol* (calcitriol) is used in renal failure. Although expensive,

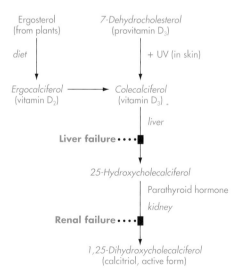

Figure 6.20   Formation of the active form of vitamin D.

alfacalcidol and calcitriol have a shorter duration of action than the older vitamin D derivatives and are less likely to cause **hypercalcaemia**, so they are safer in use. The most potent derivative is *1,25-dihydroxycholecalciferol*, which can be given either orally or intravenously.

Gallstones (cholelithiasis)

Epidemiology

Gallstones are common, with some 10–15% of adults in Western countries having stones that can be demonstrated by ultrasonography, though only about one-third of these are symptomatic. About 50 000 cholecystectomies (gallbladder removals) are carried out each year in the UK. Gallstones can occur at any age, though they are rare under the age of 10 years and most common at 50–60 years in both sexes. Women are more prone to develop gallstones than men, the M:F ratio rising from 1:2–4 at under 40 years of age to about 2:3 at over 80 years.

Relatively high prevalences occur in Italians and Swedes, Mexican women and North American Pima Indians. Black women are less likely to have stones than Caucasians, and Asians less than Europeans. These differences are real, having allowed for predisposing factors. The typical patient has been described (somewhat lightheartedly) as '5Fs', i.e. Female, Fair, Fat, Fertile and (approaching) Forty.

Aetiology and pathology

Most gallstones are composed of mixtures of cholesterol and bile pigments in varying proportions. They are usually calcified to some extent. It is not known why only a minority cause symptoms.

The pathology is uncertain, but several factors are implicated in producing bile supersaturated with cholesterol:

- Reduced low density lipoprotein uptake by the liver.
- Up-regulation of HMG CoA reductase, thus increasing cholesterol synthesis.

- Down-regulation of bile acid synthesis, causing reduced cholesterol solubilization.

It has also been suggested that a defect of **cholecystokinin** release, or of gallbladder response to it, causing delayed gallbladder emptying, is a precursor to gallstone formation.

Predisposing factors for **cholesterol stones** include:

- Obesity.
- Western diet (rich in saturated fats).
- Female sex, pregnancy and increased sex hormone levels (oral contraceptives increase cholesterol saturation of the bile).
- Diabetes mellitus.
- Iatrogenic: drugs (*clofibrate, octreotide*), parenteral nutrition (reduces gallbladder emptying) and ileal surgery (by reducing recycling of bile salts).

Pigment stones are brown/black in colour and relatively radio-opaque. They are associated with liver cirrhosis (p. 376) and haemolytic anaemia (p. 364), both of which cause increased bilirubin and calcium excretion. Distal ileal disease, causing reduced reabsorption and recycling of bile acids, is another risk factor because these acids are needed to solubilize bilirubin and calcium.

Clinical features and diagnosis

About 1% of individuals with asymptomatic, demonstrable stones in the gallbladder present annually with a gradual onset of non-specific symptoms, i.e. mild to severe right hypochondrial or epigastric pain, often referred to the right scapula, accompanied by a varying degree of anorexia and nausea. Symptoms are associated with impaction of stones in the cystic duct. Acute onset also occurs.

Diagnosis is by:

- Ultrasonography (this is sensitive, but cannot distinguish between types of stone).
- Radiography; plain X-rays detect only the calcified stones (20%), but oral radiocontrast medium enables the detection of radiolucent stones and gallbladder anatomy and contraction. Small stones are poorly visualized.

- CT scanning is better for detecting radiolucent stones.
- ERCP for complications, e.g. common bile duct stones. The technique also permits intervention for removal of small stones and stone fragments (see below).
- Liver function tests: serum conjugated bilirubin, ALP and ALT may be raised.

If the diagnosis is in doubt, serum amylase levels will indicate pancreatitis and exclude salivary gland disease and bowel perforation or infarction. High serum lipase levels are more specific for pancreatitis.

Patients' description of symptoms, such as 'biliousness', and the commonly held erroneous belief that symptoms are associated with fatty meals, are of no diagnostic value.

Complications

Common complications of gallstones include the following:

- Biliary colic (spasm of the inflamed gallbladder and/or bile duct) causes moderate to severe pain in the epigastrium or right hypochondrium, with excruciating exacerbations lasting for a few hours against a background of constant pain.
- Acute cholecystitis and cholangitis (inflammation of the gallbladder and common bile duct respectively), associated with the presence of stones or obstruction by a stone. These are usually followed by infection with intestinal bacteria that requires antibiotics and cholecystectomy (surgical removal of the gallbladder).
- Acute pancreatitis, caused by reflux of bile up the pancreatic duct, produces moderate to severe pain in the epigastrium. The pain penetrates to the back, usually causing vomiting. This is a potentially serious condition, occasionally causing acute respiratory or renal failure.
- Cholestatic jaundice (p. 363), usually fluctuating in character.

Other complications are uncommon. Upper abdominal pain with nausea, vomiting and wind has frequently been ascribed to cholecystitis, but there is no evidence that these symptoms represent a recognizable clinical entity.

Management

Treatment of gallstones may be either medical or surgical.

Pharmacotherapy

The drugs used are bile acids (*chenodeoxycholic acid* or *ursodeoxycholic acid*, or a mixture of the two because they have different modes of action). These drugs are taken for up to 2 years in order to dissolve radiolucent stones, as cholesterol is about 2×10^5 times more soluble in bile salts than in water. However, bile acid treatment may not be successful, or stones may recur, so this approach is usually reserved for patients who are unfit for surgery and as an adjunct to extracorporeal shock-wave lithotripsy (ESWL) (see below). Some patients find that symptoms are relieved very rapidly, well before stones could be dissolved, possibly because gallbladder and bile duct spasm are reduced.

Surgery and interventional endoscopy

Surgery nowadays is almost exclusively conducted by laparoscopic cholecystectomy (gallbladder removal via an endoscope inserted through the abdominal wall), because this technique is much less traumatic than conventional open surgery. Patients with a few noncalcified gallstones can have these dispersed ultrasonically (using ESWL), though endoscopic removal of residual fragments may be necessary. Other techniques include percutaneous lithotomy (removal of stones via a catheter inserted through the skin) and endoscopic laser fragmentation of stones, the endoscope being manoeuvred into the bile duct. The biliary system can also be intubated at operation and flushed with *monoctanoin*, a monoglyceride, to dissolve cholesterol stones in the bile duct, but this is effective in only 50% of cases.

Liver failure

Acute failure

Classification

There are three types of acute hepatic failure:

1. **Fulminant (hyperacute) hepatic failure** (FHF) is a syndrome of abrupt onset (fulminant = explosive), characterized by progressively severe encephalopathy occurring within 7–14 days of the onset of jaundice. FHF is the result of massive hepatocellular necrosis, i.e. death of the liver parenchyma, or other severe functional impairment.
2. In **acute hepatic failure** encephalopathy occurs within 28 days of the onset of jaundice.
3. **Subacute hepatic failure** is defined as acute failure occurring in patients without pre-existing liver disease, in whom the signs of encephalopathy develop more than 8 weeks after the onset of illness. These patients are generally older than those with FHF and tend not to have viral hepatitis. Survivors may have **autoimmune hepatitis** (p. 376).

Acute-on-chronic hepatocellular failure occurs owing to decompensation in a patient with chronic liver disease. This may result from protein overload (dietary, substantial gastrointestinal bleeding), sepsis, or intervention with drugs or surgery.

Aetiology of FHF

In the UK, *paracetamol (acetaminophen)* poisoning is the most common cause. Many other drugs may cause FHF (see below), anaesthesia with *halothane* or *methoxyflurane* being well-recognized, but monoamine oxidase inhibitors, anti-epileptics and antimicrobial agents may also be involved. FHF may also occur in Wilson's disease, Reye's syndrome (p. 382) and pregnancy and following solvent ingestion or 'glue sniffing'. About 1% of patients with viral hepatitis develop fulminant disease.

Clinical features

The symptoms and signs are similar for all types of acute hepatic failure. Because of the numerous functions of the liver, the initial signs are widespread and non-specific. Any of those outlined on pp. 363–371 may be present.

Jaundice may be absent, mild or obvious. Asterixis is virtually always present and **hepatic fetor** – an offensive breath odour of methyl mercaptan – is common. The liver size may be normal, enlarged, or small and hard. The presence of a small, hard liver, and the early onset of ascites, imply a very poor prognosis.

Management

Apart from general supportive measures, and the elimination of any precipitants, only limited treatments are available. A listing of some of the available measures is given in Table 6.31. Generally, everything depends on the severity of the failure and the regenerative ability of the liver.

In the case of FHF due to paracetamol (acetaminophen) overdose, gastric aspiration and absorption with activated charcoal is carried out if ingestion occurred within 2 h of hospital admission. *N-acetylcysteine* (NAC) given by IV infusion is the antidote of choice and is started immediately, but oral *methionine* is also used if appropriate facilities for infusion are not available, e.g. in remote areas. NAC should be given within 10–12 h of paracetamol (acetaminophen) ingestion to be optimally effective, but administration up to 36 h reduces mortality and limits the severity of symptoms.

The need for NAC treatment is assessed by nomogram, using the paracetamol (acetaminophen) plasma concentration determined on a sample taken not less than 4 h after ingestion, i.e. after complete absorption of the drug.

NAC protects the liver against the depletion of glutathione, thus detoxifying a reactive metabolic intermediate and preventing its binding to hepatocytes. NAC also acts as a cardiac inotrope, increasing peripheral blood flow and oxygen extraction, and may potentiate vasodilatation due to endothelium-derived relaxing factor (nitric oxide), thus increasing hepatic and cerebral blood flow.

Prophylactic parenteral H_2-receptor antagonists reduce the incidence of gastro-oesophageal bleeding, but regrettably have little influence on mortality.

Table 6.31   Management of hepatic failure

Problem	Aetiology or pathology	Treatment
Ascites	Malignancy, hypoproteinaemia, cirrhosis	*See* p. 367
Portosystemic encephalopathy	Ammonia?, other blood 'toxins'	*See* p. 369
Cerebral oedema	Unknown	Mannitol/glucose IV, dexamethasone?, *N*-acetylcysteine? Haemofiltration, surgical decompression
Hypoglycaemia	Inability to mobilize carbohydrate, control blood glucose	Glucose IV Potassium chloride IV + insulin Check blood glucose hourly
Electrolyte imbalance	Failure of regulation Fluid retention Vomiting/diarrhoea	Correct ion levels, restrict sodium, calcium gluconate IV, ion exchange resins
Respiratory failure	Fluid retention, restriction of diaphragm due to ascites	Ventilate; monitor blood gases
Infections	Impaired reticuloendothelial function Renal impairment causing uraemia[a]	Specific antibiotics
Anaemia, coagulation disorders	Haemorrhage Bone marrow depression Reduced prothrombin level	Blood, plasma or platelet transfusion, vitamin K, H_2-blocker IV (prophylactic)
Hepatocellular necrosis	Paracetamol (acetaminophen) overdose	*N*-acetylcysteine Charcoal + gastric lavage
General		Identify and treat any precipitating cause Low-protein, high-carbohydrate diet Barrier nursing Central venous line for TPN, manometry, blood sampling Purgation if constipated No sedatives or potentially hepatotoxic substances Transplantation

[a] Urea increases membrane permeability and facilitates microbial tissue invasion.

IV, intravenous; TPN, total parenteral nutrition.

It is usual to establish a central venous line to facilitate **total parenteral nutrition**, if required, and also to avoid repeated venepuncture for blood sampling in patients who often have coagulation defects.

Liver damage is maximal 3–4 days after ingestion, and reports exist of death occurring after ingestion of only 10–15 g of paracetamol (acetaminophen) (20–30 tablets). Over-dosage with the popular combination analgesic *co-proxamol* (acetaminophen + dextropropoxyphene [propoxyphene]) poses a greater risk than does plain acetaminophen because dextropropoxyphene causes CNS depression and inhibition of liver enzymes. *Naloxone* (additional to NAC) is required as an opioid antidote, and ventilatory support may also be needed.

Numerous attempts at more specific therapies have been tried, with variable, limited success. Corticosteroids are often used, though there is little rational basis for this. Many abortive attempts have been made to remove postulated blood toxins, e.g. by exchange transfusion. Haemodialysis, using a polyacrylonitrile membrane to remove small molecules (<5000 Da), is promising, but is unproven. **Liver transplantation** is rarely possible because a suitably matched donor organ is unlikely to be available at short notice. However, artificial livers have been developed and may offer support until a suitable donor organ becomes available, similarly to renal dialysis.

Chronic failure

Aetiology

Chronic liver failure may be the consequence of any chronic liver disease (Table 6.32). However, some patients show evidence of raised serum transaminases or persistent viral hepatitis (HBV), discovered by chance during investigations (e.g. when donating blood), without ever showing symptoms or progressing to liver failure.

Chronic progressive liver disease always leads to portal hypertension, resulting in ascites or bleeding oesophageal varices (p. 315), and encephalopathy. Cirrhosis (see below) frequently develops insidiously.

Management

Apart from the withdrawal of precipitants, which leads to recovery if the liver damage is not too severe (the liver has great powers of regeneration), management is again largely supportive and symptomatic.

However, there is some specific pharmacotherapy. *Penicillamine* is effective in Wilson's disease (hereditary abnormal copper metabolism) and *desferrioxamine* in iron overload. Immunosuppression with a combination of *corticosteroids* and *azathioprine* is beneficial in some forms of chronic hepatitis.

Table 6.32   Some causes of chronic liver disease

Aetiology	Examples
Alcohol abuse	
Drugs	*See* p. 379
Infection	Amoebic dysentery, helminths, tuberculosis, brucellosis
	Sequel to viral hepatitis (HBV, HCV)
	Secondary to biliary obstruction, diverticulitis, appendicitis or malignancy
Genetic	Abnormal copper metabolism (Wilson's disease) or iron metabolism
	Autoimmunity to hepatic nuclear, smooth muscle or microsomal antigens
	Inflammatory bowel disease
Iron overlaod	Repeated blood transfusion or excessive iron intake, abnormal iron metabolism, alcoholic liver disease

HBV, HCV, hepatitis B and C viruses.

Liver **transplantation** is the only satisfactory treatment for established severe failure, but the results depend on the aetiology of liver failure. The 5-year survival rate is currently about 85% in primary biliary cirrhosis, with most problems occurring in the first year. If the cause of cirrhosis is unknown, the 5-year survival rate falls to about 65%.

Autoimmune hepatitis

This is normally a chronic progressive disease of unknown aetiology, although it may also have an acute presentation resembling that of acute viral hepatitis. Because of the latter fact, the former description as 'chronic active hepatitis' has been abandoned.

Autoimmune hepatitis can affect both sexes at any age, the onset being most common in women aged 20–40 years. The condition is characterized by:

- Serum auto-antibodies.
- Hyperglobulinaemia.
- An association with other autoimmune diseases, e.g. sicca syndrome (*see* Chapter 8), renal tubular acidosis, Hashimoto's thyroiditis, ulcerative colitis (p. 338) and rheumatoid arthritis.

Prompt diagnosis of autoimmune hepatitis, to distinguish it from conditions such as chronic viral hepatitis (see below), Wilson's disease and other causes of liver cirrhosis, is essential to ensure appropriate treatment.

Pharmacotherapy is aggressive because severe disease has an untreated mortality rate of 30%. The mainstay of treatment is high-dose *prednisolone*, with or without *azathioprine*, depending on severity. For those intolerant of azathioprine, *ciclosporin* (*cyclosporine*) is used, and the latter may also be added to the prednisolone + azathioprine regimen for non-responders.

Liver **transplantation** is used for end-stage disease.

Cirrhosis

Cirrhosis is a chronic, irreversible degeneration of liver cells followed by scarring and infiltration

of the tissues with dense fibrotic strands. This leads to a progressive loss of liver function and circulatory obstruction, the latter causing portal hypertension (PH). The diagnosis can be made only on histological grounds.

Aetiology

Common causes include prolonged alcoholism and viral hepatitis (B, B+D, or C; see below). Less common causes include:

- Primary biliary cirrhosis (progressive idiopathic bile duct destruction), mostly in middle-aged females.
- Autoimmune hepatitis.
- Haemochromatosis, i.e. iron overload due to, e.g. repeated blood transfusions, genetic mutations, haemorrhagic conditions, impaired erythropoiesis, excessive oral iron intake.
- Wilson's disease.
- Schistosomiasis.
- Drugs and toxins.

Clinical features

The clinical features of cirrhosis are numerous and varied, consequent on liver failure and past history. The initial symptoms are non-specific and common to many liver diseases (see above). Generalized **pruritus** may precede jaundice by some years. **Ascites** and **encephalopathy** occur inevitably in the later stages.

Management

Management is similar to that for liver failure generally (*see* Table 6.31).

Viral and other infective hepatitis

Aetiology

Viral hepatitis is caused by one of several different viruses: hepatitis A virus (HAV), HBV, HCV, HDV, HEV, HGV and possibly other species.

Other viral infections may present with symptoms of liver disease, but these are not normally classified as viral hepatitis. The agents include the Epstein–Barr virus, which causes infectious mononucleosis (glandular fever), cytomegalovirus (usually in the immunocompromised), herpes virus, yellow fever, and such exotica as Lassa fever. Protozoa, helminths and to a lesser extent bacteria and fungi can also cause liver inflammation. Thus, Weil's disease, caused by *Leptospira icterohaemorrhagiae*, is a potentially severe infection that is contracted from infected rodents, usually after participating in inland water sports. The incidence of Weil's disease is increasing owing to the growing interest in such sports. In patients from tropical areas, amoebic dysentery, malaria, schistosomiasis and liver fluke infections may also be involved. The following account is confined to the hepatitis viruses.

Although these viruses are grouped together because they cause human hepatitis, they are structurally and taxonomically diverse:

- HAV, HEV and HGV are non-enveloped, single-stranded RNA viruses.
- HBV is an enveloped, polyhedral, double-stranded DNA virus.
- HCV is an enveloped, polyhedral, single-stranded RNA virus, related to the German measles virus.
- HDV is an unusual circular RNA, incomplete virus, requiring HBV for transmission and coated with the HBV surface antigen. Its genome resembles that of some plant viruses.

HAV and HEV cause **infective hepatitis**, the most common form, and this is responsible for some 40% of overt disease in the UK.

Clinical features

The diseases may be asymptomatic, for example about 50% of UK adults have antibodies against HAV, though there are relatively few identified cases. However, there is a complete spectrum of severity, from subclinical up to fulminant, life-threatening disease. The symptoms and signs are similar in all forms. There is initially a prodromal **anicteric** phase, i.e. no jaundice, with nausea, vomiting, headache, malaise, and a varying degree of fever. In moderate to severe disease this is followed by the **icteric phase**, with jaundice,

dark urine and pale faeces (produced by intrahepatic cholestasis), abdominal discomfort, liver (and sometimes spleen) enlargement and tenderness.

With HBV, the immunological response of the host causes a syndrome resembling serum sickness, sometimes with rashes and polyarthritis.

General prognosis

Nearly all patients with hepatitis A and E, about 95% with hepatitis B, and about 60% with hepatitis C have a self-limiting illness, followed by complete recovery. Fulminant hepatitis has a high mortality but is fortunately uncommon (1% of cases). Infection with HBV and HCV confers an increased risk of primary liver cancer. HGV is common in the USA and causes an apparently benign long-lasting viraemia.

There are no specific treatments, and full recovery may take several months. Infection due to HBV and HCV may cause chronic disease, a carrier state and cirrhosis (see below). Further, chronic HBV infection may cause hepatocellular carcinoma.

Hepatitis A and E

These RNA viruses have a faecal–oral route of transmission, causing infections which may be asymptomatic or acute. The incubation periods are prolonged, about 14–50 days, and symptoms start to resolve after about 3 weeks. There are no chronic carriers.

HAV infection occurs world-wide, often in autumnal epidemics spread by faecally contaminated food and water, and primarily under poor living conditions. HEV is responsible for most outbreaks in endemic regions (Africa, Asia, Central America, Middle East) but causes only about 1% of cases of acute hepatitis elsewhere.

The prognosis for HAV infection is usually excellent, though a few patients may have more severe disease. However, there is a fatality rate of about 2.5% in patients aged 50 or over. Although patients feel debilitated for many months, neither chronic disease nor a carrier state occurs.

HEV infection poses a special risk in pregnancy.

In the third trimester there is a high maternal mortality rate (20–25%) and a high fetal risk.

Treatment is symptomatic and supportive because neither diet nor drugs influence the course of the disease. Alcohol is best avoided, especially in the severe phase.

The most effective prophylactic measure is good **hygiene**, especially after defecation.

Passive immunoprophylaxis against HAV is conferred by *normal immunoglobulin* and lasts for 2–6 months, but a safe vaccine is now available which confers rapid, long-term active immunity. Booster doses of the vaccine are required after 12 months. A bivalent vaccine, against HAV and HBV, is produced. A vaccine against HEV is under trial.

Hepatitis B and D

Hepatitis B virus

HBV used to be called 'Australia antigen', because of its discovery in the blood of an Australian aboriginal. It occurs world-wide and is solely a human parasite, persisting in a human carrier reservoir. In Western countries the carrier rate is 0.1%, but some 12% may be carriers in Africa and the Far East. Spread is by infected blood, e.g. 'main-line' drug addicts, unhygienic tattooing and acupuncture, or by sexual contact, especially homosexual. In the Far East, mother-to-fetus transmission is common.

The course of chronic infection is very variable: there is an acute phase, followed by a slow elimination of virus, apparent recovery and then a second acute phase. About 5–10% of patients become chronic asymptomatic carriers, especially if they are male, immunosuppressed, are on long-term haemodialysis, or are long-term mental inpatients. Neonatal exposure also predisposes to chronic infection.

Some 3% of patients develop **autoimmune hepatitis** (p. 376), probably owing to a continuing immunological reaction.

HBV infection may be treated with:

- **Antivirals**, e.g. *famciclovir* and *lamivudine* (licensed in the UK; *adefovir* and *lobucavir* are under trial).
- **Cytokines**, e.g. interferons and *interleukin-2 + interferon-alpha* for 3 months being the

most successful, leading to eradication of the virus in about 40% of cases.

Prophylaxis is provided by an effective monovalent vaccine produced by recombinant DNA technology. The vaccine is used for those at special risk, e.g. doctors, nurses, pathology laboratory technicians, ward pharmacists and partners and spouses of patients. The initial course consists of three doses, usually given over 6 months, during which period effective protection should develop. The deltoid muscle is the preferred site: injection into the buttock reduces efficacy.

The divalent HAV + HBV vaccine is not recommended for accidental occupational exposure, e.g. needle-stick injuries and ocular contamination by aerosols, etc. In these circumstances, simultaneous use of monovalent HBV vaccine and specific HBV immunoglobulin is recommended.

For more rapid protection the initial course may be given over 2 months with a booster dose at 1 year. Some 10% of individuals respond poorly and need booster doses or revaccination. The duration of protection is uncertain, but a further booster dose is recommended after 5 years. Improved vaccines are under active investigation, and offer the hope of universal cheap immunization.

Hepatitis D virus

As noted above, delta virus depends on HBV for its replication. It may occur simultaneously with HBV infection, or as an opportunistic infection in HBV carriers.

HBV + HDV usually causes severe infections, being implicated in about 50% of patients with fulminant hepatitis, and is likely to cause hepatic cirrhosis (see below). Prophylaxis against HBV also protects against HDV.

Hepatitis C

Before characterization, this was described as Non-A Non-B hepatitis. HCV causes an acute infective hepatitis, with an incubation period of 6–12 weeks. Only about 25% of patients are jaundiced. Most chronic cases follow overt acute infection and the disease may last for several decades. Infection at an older age, concurrent infection and other illnesses may cause progressive cirrhosis and occasionally hepatocellular carcinoma.

It is believed to be responsible for up to 90% of cases occurring after unsafe blood transfusion. Organ transplantation patients and those receiving haemodialysis are also at risk. Intravenous drug abusers comprise 40% of patients, and high-risk sexual activity accounts for a further 10%.

There is no vaccine, but immunization with the **HAV + HBV vaccine** may prevent severe complications. A combination of *tribavirin (ribavirin) and interferon-alpha* holds some promise. Most other antivirals, etc. have not given a sustained benefit.

Drugs and the liver

The relationship between the liver and drugs is important for three reasons:

1. The liver is the principal site for drug metabolism. Consequently, while liver disease may impair hepatic drug-metabolizing activity, the drugs themselves may reduce or enhance these processes.
2. Liver failure has other physiological effects which affect drug handling and disposition.
3. Drugs may cause liver disease.

The bioavailability of drugs may be influenced by patient factors which are unconnected with liver disease: only those connected with the liver will be discussed here.

The liver and drug metabolism

A full discussion of this complex subject is out of place here, though some specific aspects are outlined below. A brief treatment of drugs to be used with caution in liver disease is given in Appendix 2 to the BNF and readers are referred to Chapter 1 and the References and further reading section of this chapter.

Biological (patient) factors influencing drug availability

Pharmacogenetic factors
Two points are relevant here:

1. Slow acetylators are more likely to experience toxic reactions with normal doses of drugs than fast acetylators.
2. Oxidative drug metabolism varies substantially (20-fold) between patients, so some patients fail to respond to doses of drugs which cause unacceptable side effects in others.

Disease state
Although diseases which compromise the blood supply to the liver may be expected to impair drug metabolism, the data are conflicting, and it is difficult to draw satisfactory conclusions. It is probable that liver function needs to be considerably impaired before significant effects are seen. The effects of liver disease are complex because several factors change simultaneously, e.g. metabolism, protein binding, volume of distribution and elimination in the bile. The greatest effects are seen when metabolism, especially first-pass metabolism, is high and protein binding is low, because the free plasma concentration is then markedly increased. Conversely, the plasma levels of drugs which undergo little first-pass metabolism and are highly protein-bound will be little changed. These effects are illustrated in Table 6.33.

Age
The decline in hepatic function with age leads to reduced levels of serum albumin and decreased hepatic metabolism, and these combine with other age-related changes to influence the availability of many drugs (*see* Chapter 1). Interacting factors and interindividual variation make it difficult to know what the effect will be in a particular patient.

Drugs and liver enzyme activity

The metabolism of many drugs may be either increased or decreased by the effects of other

Table 6.33   Some effects of liver disease on the availability of drugs with different pharmacokinetic properties

Drug		Effect of liver disease on availability	Examples
Hepatic extraction[a]	Protein binding		
Low	High	Nil	Diazepam, indometacin, phenytoin[b], rifampicin, theophylline, tolbutamide, warfarin
Moderate	Moderate	Increased	Chlorpromazine, isoniazid, pethidine (meperidine), metoprolol, nortriptyline, paracetamol (acetaminophen), quinidine
High	Moderate	Greatly increased	Labetalol, lidocaine (lignocaine), morphine, pentazocine, dextropropoxyphene (propoxyphene), propranolol, verapamil

[a] First-pass metabolism.
[b] Phenytoin clearance may be increased in the elderly.

drugs on microsomal mixed function oxidase, of which cytochrome P450 is the terminal enzyme. Table 6.34 lists the more important drugs that are known to induce or inhibit hepatic microsomal enzymes.

Generally, **enzyme induction** will reduce the biological availability of drugs and their activity. However, this is clinically significant only with drugs having a narrow therapeutic window and when loss of activity severely compromises the patient, e.g. *warfarin*, with which loss of activity may result in thrombosis, stroke or death, and the *oral contraceptive pill*, as enhanced metabolism of oestrogen may cause an unwanted pregnancy.

There are some drugs whose toxicity may be enhanced by metabolism, because the metabolite causes the damage, e.g. *paracetamol (acetaminophen)* and *isoniazid*.

Enzyme inhibition increases drug activity, if other factors do not change. Again, it is those drugs with a low therapeutic index that are important, e.g. *warfarin*, which may provoke severe spontaneous haemorrhage. *Phenytoin* has a non-linear dose–response curve, and small increases in plasma levels may give rise to acute toxic reactions, e.g. nausea, vomiting, dizziness, tremor, ataxia and blurred vision, if the steady-state level is near the top of the therapeutic range. With a hypnotic or sedative, enzyme induction only impairs the quality of sedation, but enzyme inhibition might result in over-sedation and confusion and serious falls in the elderly.

While inhibition occurs rapidly, enzyme induction depends on new synthesis, so the effects take some time to become apparent. Some of the drugs most likely to be affected by changes

Table 6.34   Some drugs which affect hepatic drug metabolism

Enzyme inducers
Alcohol, aminoglutethimide, barbiturates, carbamazepine, chlorpromazine, dichloralphenazone[a], griseofulvin, phenytoin, primidone, rifampicin

Enzyme inhibitors
Amiodarone, chloramphenicol, cimetidine, clofibrate, indometacin, omeprazole, sodium valproate, sulphonamides, tolbutamide

Drugs with which the clinical effects may be significant
Carbamazepine, clomethiazole, diazepam, phenytoin, theophylline, tolbutamide, warfarin, oral contraceptives

[a] Due to the phenazone component.

in liver enzyme activity are also listed in Table 6.34.

In addition, some drugs inhibit a specific enzyme, leading to higher levels of another drug which is metabolized by the same enzyme, e.g. *allopurinol* inhibits xanthine oxidase and may cause unacceptable toxicity with *azathioprine* and *mercaptopurine*.

Hepatotoxicity

As in other situations, side effects may be either **toxic** (Type A, predictable) or **idiosyncratic** (Type B, unpredictable). Table 6.35 lists some drugs which may produce these effects in the liver, though such adverse reactions are uncommon.

The principal risk factors for hepatic drug

Table 6.35 Some hepatotoxic drug effects

Type of reaction	Examples
Toxicity	
Hepatocellular necrosis	Paracetamol (acetaminophen)
Gallstone production	Clofibrate, oestrogens
Sensitivity (idiosyncrasy)	
Cholestasis	Chlorpromazine, co-amoxiclav[a], erythromycin estolate, fusidic acid, glibenclamide (glyburide), phenothiazines, sodium valproate
Hepatic dysfunction/failure	Methotrexate
Hepatitis	Amiodarone, azathioprine, dantrolene[b], halothane and methoxyflurane, isoniazid, monoamine oxidase inhibitors, methyldopa[b], nitrofurantoin[b], novobiocin, rifampicin, salicylates and sulfasalazine, sodium valproate
Granuloma formation (*see* Chapter 2)	Allopurinol, hydralazine, phenylbutazone[c], sulphonamides and sulfasalazine
Reye's syndrome	Aspirin, sodium valproate, high-dose tetracycline
Neoplastic disease	
Benign	Oral contraceptives, other steroids
Malignant[c]	Arsenic, thorotrast, plasticizers, benzene, toluene

[a] Amoxicillin plus clavulanic acid.
[b] May cause chronic hepatitis.
[c] Unusual, non-UK or discontinued drug. All these malignancies are due to environmental or industrial chemicals.

Table 6.36 Some risk factors for hepatic drug injury and side effects in liver disease

Risk factor	Mechanism involved
Liver disease (e.g. cirrhosis)	Reduced blood flow gives reduced oxidative metabolism Fluid retention causing changed volume of distribution Increased cerebral sensitivity
Age and sex	Females more susceptible Hepatotoxicity rare in children (except with sodium valproate)
Genetics	Impaired or absent enzyme activity, e.g. slow acetylators, glucose-6-phosphate dehydrogenase deficiency

injury are given in Table 6.36, together with the mechanisms involved.

Among these effects, *paracetamol* (*acetaminophen*) poisoning is the principal cause of acute hepatic failure in the UK (p. 373).

Halothane and *methoxyflurane* are generally very safe general anaesthetics. However, a small proportion of patients experience an unexplained fever, with mild signs of liver involvement. A second exposure to either anaesthetic should be avoided in such patients, as it may cause acute, often fatal liver failure – usually in obese, elderly females.

Reye's syndrome follows febrile illness in young children, though fortunately only rarely. Affected patients develop signs of liver disease with severe encephalopathy, and there is severe fatty degeneration of the liver. Because there is a high probability that the syndrome can be triggered by *aspirin*, this is contraindicated in children under 12 years of age. The mortality rate is about 50%, usually from cerebral oedema.

References and further reading

Aspinall R, Robinson ST (1997) *Gastroenterology: A Color Atlas and Text*. London: Mosby.

Dent J, Brun J, Fendrick AM, *et al.* (1999) An evidence-based appraisal of reflux disease management – the Genval Workshop Report. *Gut* **44** (Suppl. 2): S1–S16.

Farrell GC (1997) Drug induced hepatic injury. *J Gastroenterol Hepatol* **12**: S242–S250.

Farthing MJG, Ballinger A, eds (2000) *Drug Therapy for Gastrointestinal Disease*. London: Martin Dunitz.

Heuman DM, *et al.* (1997) *Gastroenterology*. Philadelphia: W B Saunders.

Morgan DJ, McLean AJ (1995) Clinical pharmacokinetic and pharmacodynamic considerations in patients with liver disease: an update. *Clin Pharmacokinet* **29**: 370–391.

Sherlock S, Dooley J (1997) *Disease of the Liver and Biliary System*. 10th edn. Oxford: Blackwell Science. (A substantial standard reference work.)

Sleisenger MA, Fordtran JS (1997) *Gastrointestinal and Liver Disease: Pathology, Diagnosis and Management*. Philadelphia: W B Saunders.

Travis SPL, Taylor RH, Misiewicz JJ (1998) *Gastroenterology: Pocket Consultant Series*. Oxford: Blackwell Science.

Zuckerman AJ, Thomas HC, eds (1998) *Viral Hepatitis. Scientific Basis and Clinical Management*. 2nd edn. Edinburgh: Churchill Livingstone. (A definitive and substantial reference work.)

7

Central nervous system

Mental illness is widespread in society but remains the object of considerable stigma and a great deal of misconception. Recurrent media scares about so-called 'maniacs' do not help the situation. Many people suffer from anxiety or depression at some stage and the lifetime prevalence of schizophrenia is about one in 100. In the UK, despite the admirable motives behind the campaign to depopulate the long-stay psychiatric hospitals, the *Care in the community* programme appears to have overwhelmed the community organizations who have to implement it. Increasingly, psychiatrically ill patients are seen in primary care.

Neurological disease is assuming greater importance in an ageing population, as the prevalence of conditions such as Parkinson's disease and dementia rises inexorably.

In almost all CNS conditions, although psychotherapy can help, drug therapy contributes enormously to making the problems manageable and relieving an enormous amount of suffering.

Physiological principles

To understand the mechanisms, symptoms and treatment of central nervous system (CNS) disorders it is necessary to review the functions of the more important brain centres, their interconnections and the transmitters which predominate in each. Only the most simplified outline can be attempted here. An overall view is presented in this section, but further specific information appears in later sections as appropriate. More detailed accounts may be found in the References and further reading.

Brain functions can be considered in three broad categories:

- **Input** or perceptual, i.e. handling the mass of sensory data passed up from receptors in the sense organs.
- **Processing** that data, i.e. the cognitive function, which involves integration, association with stored data (memory, experience) and, especially in man, the addition of an emotional component.

- **Output**, i.e. the action decided by the cognitive function in response to input: this will usually be either motor (mainly voluntary muscle) or homeostatic (mainly involuntary muscle and glands) (*see* Table 7.1 and Fig. 7.1).

Brain centres and their disorder

The brain is conventionally considered in six main anatomical and functional areas:

1. **Cerebrum** – two hemispheres of cerebral **cortex**, with **limbic system** and **basal ganglia**
2. **Diencephalon**, containing **hypothalamus** and **thalamus**
3. **Midbrain**
4. **Pons**
5. **Medulla oblongata**
6. **Cerebellum**

Alternatively, the brain may be sub-divided into distinct regions:

- The **forebrain**, which includes areas 1 and 2.

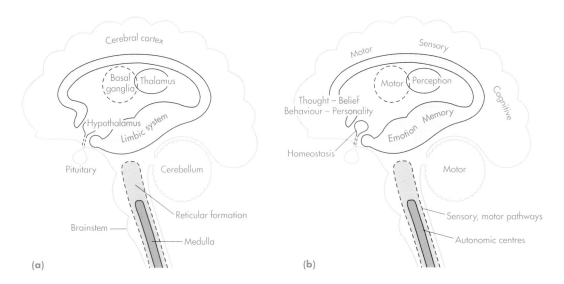

Figure 7.1   (a) Simplified schematic diagram of brain showing important anatomical areas. (b) Simplified representation of location of principal brain functions. Note: The locations of functions within the cortex are not intended to reflect specific cortical centres.

Table 7.1   Principal anatomical centres of brain function

	Function	Centre
Input	Perception	Sensory cortex, thalamus, reticular formation
Processing	Cognitive (intellectual)	Cerebral cortex
	Emotional	Limbic system
Output	Motor	Motor cortex, cerebellum, basal ganglia
	Homeostasis	Medulla, hypothalamus, pituitary

- The **hindbrain**, which includes areas 4, 5 and 6.
- The **brainstem**, which includes the midbrain, medulla and pons.

Interconnections between these areas are rich and complex, accounting for the richness and diversity of human activity, experience and achievement.

Cerebral cortex

The **cerebral cortex** is, in evolutionary terms, the youngest centre. It is the principal distinguishing feature of higher mammals. Notably developed in man, where it contains 90% of the total brain neurones, the cerebral cortex is the location of abstract thought, reasoning, judgement, creativity and also memory. It functions like a computer, providing a dispassionate, logical assessment of the environment as perceived via the senses, and then producing a plan for action in relation to experience and biological goals. Specific areas of the cortex are dedicated to subsidiary functions, such as the speech centre and the visual, auditory, and motor cortexes. Anatomically, the cerebral cortex is subdivided into various lobes, such as the frontal, temporal, parietal and occipital.

Cortical disorders usually have a profound effect on all CNS function. They are commonly manifested as disorders of intellect, e.g. mental handicap, dementia or Alzheimer's disease, or of movement, e.g. epilepsy. Strokes are caused by obstruction of blood flow usually to discrete cortical areas. The thought disorder characteristic of schizophrenia is partly cortical, but disordered limbic or thalamic influences on the cortex are probably more important.

Most proven and putative neurotransmitters are found in the cortex. Many of the more recently discovered mediators, such as the endorphins and peptides, have yet to be definitely linked with specific CNS functions, disorders or drug actions. They may modulate the action of the traditional transmitters.

Limbic system

This interesting evolutionary development of the higher mammals provides mental activity with an emotional dimension. The limbic system is responsible for feelings rather than objective reasoning and is perceived consciously as an emotional overlay, i.e. the **affect** or mood, which can modify the decisions taken by the cortex. The system may mediate rage, fear, pleasure and love and, by its influence on cortical function, is responsible for beliefs as opposed to rational thought. A materialist interpretation of one of the objectives of some Eastern philosophies, especially meditation, would be that it attempts to achieve control or even elimination of limbic influences ('the self', 'desire') on the cortex.

The contrast between limbic and cortical functions is illustrated by our response to being caught for a motoring offence. One part of us – our limbic system – is angry, fearful or ashamed (depending on our personality): at the same time, our cortex is calculating the effect on our insurance premium, the most effective way to appease the policeman, or perhaps even how to manage without a driving licence.

The limbic system has evolved from a structure in lower mammals concerned with olefaction (sense of smell), and indeed it retains this function in humans. Possibly this accounts for the emotional power of smells in humans. The limbic system is also involved in memory, and we are all familiar with how strongly smells can evoke memories. The system is structurally complex with many component nuclei and important connections with the frontal and temporal lobes of the cortex, with the reticular system and with the hypothalamus (all of which are sometimes considered partially within the limbic system). *Dopamine* is an important transmitter, as are *noradrenaline* (NA, norepinephrine) and *5-hydroxytryptamine* (5HT, serotonin). The action of benzodiazepines on emotion suggests that *gamma-aminobutyric acid* (GABA) is an inhibitory transmitter here (pp. 397–398).

Normally in a stable personality there is a balance between limbic and cortical influences on behaviour: one should be neither too emotional nor too unfeeling and cold. Of course, the relative contributions in any one person, which in effect defines their personality, will be determined by genetic, social and cultural factors, providing the diversity – and the unpredictability – of human behaviour. The affective dimension accounts for many of the differences between individuals, and also between man and most other animals. It is interesting to speculate on the biological advantage that the limbic system confers: possibly it is related to the social evolution of man.

Disorders of the limbic system are likely to cause inappropriate emotions, such as depression, mania or excessive anxiety. **Delusions** (inappropriate beliefs) may arise in the limbic system. Conversely, the now discredited **prefrontal lobotomy** (leucotomy), an operation to sever the links between the limbic system and the cortex in severe psychiatric disorders, resulted in the patient becoming emotionally flat. A similar phenomenon is sometimes seen in patients on long-term neuroleptics.

Basal ganglia

This group of interconnected nuclei lie deep within the cerebral hemispheres and are important coordinating centres for voluntary motor activity. If the cortex decides motor strategy and the cerebellum organizes the main muscular movements, then the basal ganglia look after the fine detail, especially of posture and tone.

The basal ganglia centres include the **corpus striatum** (putamen and caudate nucleus), the **globus pallidus** and the midbrain **substantia nigra**. There are important two-way connections with higher centres (especially motor cortex), the cerebellum and various motor nuclei of the brainstem. The basal ganglia are thus vital components in neural loops involved in the integrated control of muscular movement. They affect muscular activity indirectly by modulating motor cortex output and also directly by augmenting or suppressing motor neurones in the spinal cord via the descending **extrapyramidal** nerves tracts (see below). To assist them in this, the basal ganglia receive sensory information ascending from proprioceptor muscle spindles within voluntary muscle, via the **reticular** system (see below).

Disorders of the basal ganglia result in tremor or inappropriate muscular tone, e.g. Parkinson's disease. The three important transmitters here are *acetylcholine* (ACh), *dopamine* and *GABA*; the former two have opposing actions. Over 75% of brain dopamine is in the basal ganglia.

Thalamus

This important relay and preliminary processing centre for sensory data is situated in the main afferent pathway between the sense organs and the cortex. It may be involved, with other centres, in conditions where there is perceptual dysfunction, e.g. the hallucinations of schizophrenia. *Dopamine* is a likely transmitter in the thalamus, as are other *catecholamines* such as *adrenaline* (*epinephrine*) and *noradrenaline* (*norepinephrine*), and *ACh*. The thalamus is also involved in motor activity.

Brainstem

The brainstem comprises the 'lower', more primitive part of the brain (in effect the whole midbrain and hindbrain except the cerebellum). The midbrain houses visual and auditory sensory nuclei, as well as some motor centres. Throughout the brainstem is a more diffuse structure, the reticular formation (below).

Medulla

Here are located many vital homeostatic centres, notably the respiratory and cardiovascular centres but also controls for the gastrointestinal tract. These centres act via the autonomic nervous system. The medulla acts partly as an executive arm of the hypothalamus, which is the brain's principal integrating centre for homeostasis.

Hypothalamus

Through its connections with autonomic centres in the medulla, the hypothalamus has an important influence on the output of the sympathetic and parasympathetic nervous systems. The hypothalamus itself contains centres for satiety, sleep, thermoregulation, water balance and sexual appetite. It also controls a major part of the endocrine system through its connections with the pituitary gland. *Dopamine, 5-hydroxytryptamine* and *noradrenaline* (*norepinephrine*) are important transmitters in the hypothalamus. Drugs acting on dopaminergic receptors usually affect hypothalamic activity.

The reticular formation

This diffuse collection of tracts and nuclei permeating the brainstem monitors and modulates much of the brain's input and output. Before describing its two components it is necessary briefly to consider spinal pathways in general.

Efferent and afferent spinal pathways

Conventionally, neural pathways are classified according to whether they carry information to the brain or to a higher centre within it – the **ascending** or afferent pathways – or signals down from the brain to the periphery – the **descending** or efferent pathways. These subserve the input and output functions identified above.

Two main pathways carry the bulk of traffic. The afferent **spinothalamic** tract brings much of the sensory information from the periphery via the thalamus to the cortex (Fig. 7.2). The **corticospinal** tract (also called the **pyramidal tract** from the anatomical appearance in cross-section where left and right tracts cross in the medulla)

carries the signals to the muscles which execute the decisions taken by the brain. The corticospinal tract is routed via the cerebellum and it receives input from the basal ganglia (Fig. 7.3).

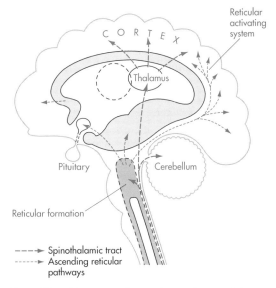

Figure 7.2 Main ascending pathways from periphery to brain.

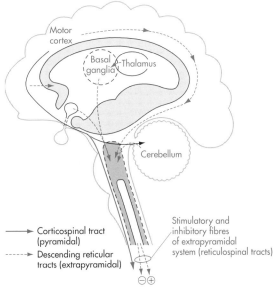

Figure 7.3 Main descending pathways from brain to muscles. Note: Only the main corticospinal efferent pathway is shown, there are several others; the positions of pathways within the spinal cord are not intended to be anatomically accurate.

Ascending reticular formation

Some fibres from the spinothalamic tract leave it as it ascends through the medulla, and run via the reticular formation directly to other centres. For example, the limbic system receives information directly from the sense organs, enabling an emotional colouring to our perceptions, e.g. the fear associated with pain. Fibres to the hypothalamus allow it to act very quickly if necessary to maintain homeostasis. Output from the reticular system also bypasses the thalamus and projects directly into the cortex: this is the so-called **reticular activating system**, which is concerned with alertness and sleep.

This system may also have an important role in focusing attention in that it allows unnecessary sensory 'noise' to be ignored. Clearly we are not conscious of all sensory input at all times. Just think about the messages from the various skin sensors in response to normal clothing: they are entirely ignored at the conscious level most of the time unless our attention is drawn to them. Conversely, recall how easily we are alerted, amid the noisy babble of a crowded room, the moment someone mentions our name. In a similar way the reticular formation may allow a mother to hear, when nobody else does, her baby crying in a distant room.

There has been speculation on the role of the ascending reticular formation in disordered perceptions, e.g. hallucinations. Although many psychotropic drugs act here (e.g. hypnotics, neuroleptics), it is difficult to link this with their clinical action.

Descending reticular formation

The descending reticular system, a vital component of overall motor function involved in the fine control and coordination, works in parallel to the corticospinal tract. The system passes signals from various brainstem reticular nuclei via **reticulospinal** tracts to synapses in the spinal cord with the motor neurones. These tracts run outside the main corticospinal tracts, hence the description **extrapyramidal**. There are both excitatory and inhibitory fibres, providing two net effects: smoothing of movement, and control of resting muscle tone that helps maintain posture.

This formation receives input from the basal ganglia (themselves connected to the motor cortex), the hypothalamus and cerebellum. The system obtains feedback via afferents originating in the muscle spindles (proprioceptors). Some of these synapse in the spinal cord with the motor neurones, while others run directly to the cerebellum.

Psychiatry and neurology

It is surprisingly difficult to make an unambiguous distinction between these traditionally separate specialities. Put simply, psychiatry concerns disorders of thought, belief, perception and mood, while neurology is concerned with disorders of movement, sensation and intellect (Table 7.2). Thus psychiatrists deal with disorders of the mind, e.g. depression and schizophrenia, while neurologists are concerned with brain disorders, e.g. parkinsonism and epilepsy. Unfortunately some conditions have both components. For example, mood changes may occur in epilepsy, and intellectual and motor deficits may occur in schizophrenia.

Looked at another way, neurological disease is generally felt to be caused by some **organic**

Table 7.2 Distinction between psychiatry and neurology

Psychiatric disorder	Neurological disorder
Disorders of mood, thought, behaviour and perception	Disorders of movement, intellect and sensation
Primarily 'functional' in origin	Primarily 'organic'
Psychological treatment may be suitable	Surgery sometimes effective
Drugs commonly used	Drug therapy usually essential
Examples: anxiety, depression, mania, schizophrenia	Examples: epilepsy, stroke, extrapyramidal disorder, brain tumour, migraine

(anatomical) lesion, whereas psychiatric disorder is **functional** – there is a problem with the way the mind functions but no identifiable structural defect. But epilepsy often has no obvious anatomical cause, and structural defects are sometimes found in the brains of schizophrenics. Changes in neurotransmitters, commonly found in CNS disorders, can be cited as evidence

for either model. Moreover, there is a school of thought which regards psychiatric illness also as organic.

Psychiatric disorders are generally treated by psychological means (psychotherapy, psychoanalysis) as well as with drugs, whereas surgery or drugs are usually appropriate for neurological disorders.

Psychiatric disorder

Clinical aspects of psychiatric disorder

Definition

In considering psychiatry it is impossible to omit reference to the philosophical and sociological controversies surrounding the human mind and its malfunction. Is the dichotomy between mind (spirit, soul, etc.) and brain (a collection of neurones and chemicals, essentially a machine and therefore ultimately predictable) just a subjective artefact? Just what is meant by 'mental illness'? Behaviour, beliefs, personality types and so on vary greatly from culture to culture and in different times in history. Mental disorder might simply be regarded as behaviour which is unusual or unacceptable to most people in the society in which the patient lives.

A more practical definition of mental illness, as opposed to just eccentric behaviour, needs to answer the question, when does a **person** becomes a potential **patient**? This is surely when they **cannot cope with everyday life**, or society cannot cope with them, because of their mental state.

Classification

There have been many attempts to classify mental illness and the situation changes constantly. The most widely accepted official classifications currently in use are the 10th edition of

the International Classification of Disease (ICD-10) and the 4th edition of the American Diagnostic and Statistical Manual of Mental Disorders (DSM-IV). The system adopted in this chapter broadly represents a consensus of these two, with conflation or simplification where this aids understanding.

At the most general level it is convenient to group psychiatric conditions into two broad types, **neurosis** and **psychosis**. As with most attempts to classify biological phenomena there is much overlap. Only a minority of patients exist entirely at either end of the spectrum, showing all the classical features. Nevertheless, this distinction remains useful (Table 7.3).

In general, patients with neurotic illness know they are ill and why others consider them so, and can see the effect it is having on themselves and those around them, i.e. they have insight. Although they are unable to control their symptoms, they retain a grasp of reality: they can reason and be reasoned with. They do not have **delusions** (fixed, false, irrational beliefs that they hold despite evidence to the contrary, after allowance for the context of their social or ethnic background) or **hallucinations** (false perceptions, that are not be perceived by anyone but them). Thus chronically anxious patients might agree that it is foolish to worry so much, but claim that they cannot help it. There may well be something happening to them which most people would consider distressing, but their reaction seems excessive. They are likely to have been an anxious, worrying type of person even

Table 7.3　Classes of psychiatric disorder

	Neurosis	Psychosis
Insight	Present	Absent
Grasp of reality	Present	Absent
Hallucinations, delusions	Absent	Present
Symptoms resemble normal personality	Yes	No
Plausible external cause or precipitant	Present	Absent
Treatment options	Non-invasive possible	Invasive often necessary
Examples	Anxiety, obsession, mild depression	Schizophrenia, mania, severe depression

before they became ill. Such patients often are difficult to treat; they generally respond poorly to drugs, but perhaps better to psychotherapy.

People with schizophrenia, by contrast, are psychotic. They have very poor insight into their illness. However, it would be untrue to suppose that they do not know they are ill. They suffer miserably, partly from the vague feeling that others find them or their reported experiences strange. Certainly, they do often have beliefs or perceptions which others find bizarre or frankly incredible. The onset of the illness may be linked to some life event, but this may bear no direct relationship to the specific symptoms. Nor will the patient's prior personality, although they, or their relationships with others, may have seemed a trifle strange. Ironically, the symptoms of psychosis are often easier to treat than those of neurosis, although it is unlikely that either type of disease can be fundamentally cured with current techniques.

Management

Treatment options

There are two broad categories of treatments:

- Invasive, such as drugs and electroconvulsive therapy (ECT).
- Non-invasive, including psychotherapy and conditioning methods.

These are compared in Table 7.4. The differences between these two approaches exemplify the principal differences between two fundamental concepts of the causation of mental illness.

The **functional** concept assumes there is a problem with the way a person thinks or feels; it is a matter of ideas and relationships. It follows that treatment methods should employ ideas, words, feelings and relationships; in short, psychotherapy.

Psychoanalysis is a form of psychotherapy in which the analyst explores the mental tensions or conflicts (complexes) that may underlie the psychiatric symptoms, especially anxiety. Causes are sought in experiences during infancy or childhood, or in family relationships. Psychoanalysis seeks to help the patient understand their problem on the assumption that resolution of the illness will follow. It is a lengthy, time-consuming and not always successful process. Simpler psychotherapeutic approaches often yield faster results, although some would argue that this represents a less fundamental solution.

Behaviour therapy takes a more pragmatic approach. A patient's illness behaviour is learned just like any other behaviour, i.e. it is conditioned. Being ill, and adopting the sick role, brings certain rewards, despite the suffering. Treatment should thus be aimed at modifying behaviour and reducing the benefits of it as perceived by the patient.

Conversely, the **materialistic** or **organic** concept of mental illness implies a distinct, and ultimately discoverable, anatomical or biochemical lesion; it is a matter of molecules. Thus drugs, physical traumas or manipulations, and even at one time the surgeon's knife, are seen to be appropriate.

As usual in the great schisms in science, probably the truth will ultimately be found to lie between the two extremes. Currently it seems that neuroses have a greater functional compo-

Table 7.4   Comparison of treatment options in mental illness

	Non-invasive methods	Invasive methods
Advantages	Represent a fundamental approach?	Rapid effect, cheap, relatively easy, predictable
Disadvantages	Slow effect, expensive and time-consuming, requires special skills, unpredictable, sometimes ineffective	Symptomatic relief only
Examples		
Neurosis	Anxiety management training Aversion therapy, desensitization Hypnosis, relaxation therapy Psychotherapy Counselling Group therapy, family therapy, cognitive therapy Psychoanalysis	Anxiolytics Tricyclics and SSRIs MAOIs
Psychosis	Skills training Simple counselling Rehabilitation Group therapy, family therapy	Neuroleptics Lithium Tricyclics and SSRIs ECT Psychosurgery

ECT, electroconvulsive therapy; MAOI, Monoamine oxidise inhibitor; SSRI, selective serotonin re-uptake inhibitor.

nent and respond better to non-invasive methods, while psychoses are often associated with biochemical defects and respond to invasive methods.

Nevertheless, either type of treatment can be appropriate and effective for either group of illnesses, depending on clinical factors. Most psychiatrists nowadays are eclectic. While non-invasive methods may be theoretically or humanely preferable, they may frequently be inadequate. For example, the first aim in treating severely depressed patients is to prevent them committing suicide, and psychotherapy is not rapid enough for this. Moreover, such patients may not have sufficient insight to allow this to be effective. Thus ECT has been found to be literally life-saving in such cases.

Diagnosis and management problems

The peculiar nature of disorders of the mind, and our incomplete knowledge of their causes, presents many problems in management (Table 7.5). Clearly, there is a difference between psychiatric diagnoses on the one hand and diagnosis of conditions such as asthma or diabetes mellitus on the other, because in the latter diseases there are agreed objective diagnostic criteria, and their pathology is relatively well understood. Further problems arise with pharmacotherapy, which are summarized in Table 7.6.

Anxiety

Definition

Anxiety is familiar to us all: dry mouth, 'butterflies in the stomach', heart pounding and the sense of fear, even panic or dread. It arises in **response to a threat** of some kind and prepares us to meet that threat. The physical symptoms are part of the sympathetic nervous system's

Table 7.5   Some problems in management of psychiatric disorders

Presentation	Often mixed, e.g. depression and restlessness
	May be masked, e.g. anxiety masked by depression
	Patient may deny illness, or compensate to mask it
Aetiology	Often unknown, so rational therapy difficult
Natural history	May be cyclic or self-limiting, so effect of treatment difficult to estimate
Diagnostic criteria	Subjective; international variation
Treatment modes	The most effective are often costly, risky or time-consuming
Compliance	Poor if patients often not fully aware of their illness

Table 7.6   Some problems with pharmacotherapy of psychiatric disorders

Mechanism	Mode of action of many psychotropic drugs not fully understood
Indications	Psychosis generally more responsive then neurosis
Biopharmacy/pharmacokinetics	Wide interpatient variation in drug handling
Efficacy	Often strong placebo effect
	Diagnostic uncertainties make assessment difficult
	No reliable animal models
Toxicity	Serious long-term side effects
	Some psychiatric side effects

'fight, fright or flight' response, and the subjective component (fright) is presumably a warning, rather like pain. All are mainly due to a rise in circulating adrenaline (epinephrine).

Anxiety then is a natural, healthy response of obvious biological value. Nowadays the kind of life-threatening dangers for which it was originally designed, like confronting wild animals, are rarely met. Instead, it has become adapted to modern life, helping us cope with less tangible stresses, like public speaking, examinations or athletic competition. Many of us find that a certain amount of anxiety, the feeling of being properly keyed up, can improve our overall performance.

However, above a certain degree of stress, performance levels off and then starts to decline rapidly. The point at which this happens varies from one individual to another – it is part of our personality. Some people have a low tolerance, worrying constantly and panicking easily: even quite a low stress level can impair their performance. Others, perhaps more laid back, seem to thrive on stress and can only work well under pressure, e.g. on the night before an examination (Fig. 7.4). We also know that some people,

with the so-called Type A personality, are exceptionally active and seem to thrive on stress.

Normally the threat, actual or anticipated, which is generating the stress is real and would be regarded by anyone as worrying or potentially harmful. It is important to distinguish between the normal physiological response to this **stress-related anxiety** and the characteristics of an **anxiety disorder**. Abnormal, counterproductive or pathological anxiety can be thought of as occurring when:

- The threat is only imagined by the patient (it may take the form of a vague but oppressive feeling of impending doom that the patient cannot explain but which makes them anxious, worried or tense).
- The threat is real but the response is out of proportion:
  - compared with the reaction of most people *or*
  - such that it interferes with normal functioning or everyday living.

Thus, a pragmatic definition of anxiety disorder would be: *a prolonged or exaggerated response*

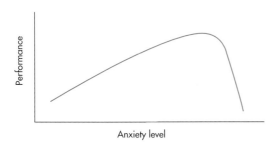

Figure 7.4 Hypothetical relationship between anxiety level and performance of tasks (arbitrary units).

to a real or imagined threat, which interferes with normal life.

The prevalence of anxiety disorder in the UK is estimated to be between 5% and 15% (depending on how it is defined) with approximately 15% of GP consultations arising from such disorder.

Pathogenesis

Pathophysiology

Figure 7.5 shows one way in which the mental and physical features of anxiety may be associated with the CNS structures discussed on pp. 384–388. The perceived threat, if real, reaches the cortex through both the normal sensory pathways (spinal cord–thalamus–cortex) and the ascending reticular system (which runs to the limbic system).

The former path causes appropriate voluntary muscular action (e.g. flight) via the motor cortex, and the endocrine and autonomic response (e.g. corticosteroid secretion and increased heart rate and blood pressure) via the hypothalamus and medulla. This would explain many of the symptoms associated with stress and anxiety. The limbic involvement accounts for the subjective feelings of fear or panic.

This may account for the low-tolerance type of anxiety, but how might the anxiety caused by an *imagined* threat be explained? Possibly it originates in the limbic system, perhaps as a misinterpretation of sensory input. Impulses would then pass up to the cortex, with all the consequences of a real threat, including what are then inappropriate autonomic responses.

This would provide a way of picturing how stress can be associated with increased heart disease or peptic ulceration: the drive to these organ systems becomes excessive, prolonged and unnecessary. It also agrees with the finding that anxiolytic drugs act on the limbic system.

Theories of anxiety

The **psychoanalytic** or functional view of anxiety disorder is that it results from internal mental conflicts. These may arise from man's socialization, which demands the repression of

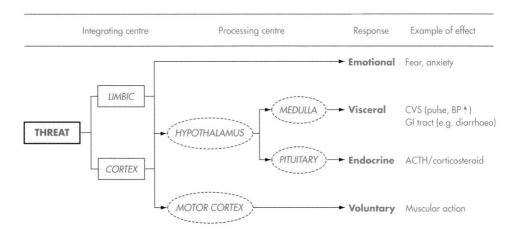

Figure 7.5 Possible pathways in pathophysiology of anxiety. BP, blood pressure; CVS, cardiovascular system.

primitive instincts, including the reproductive and sexual drives. This results in inappropriate ideas or feelings, which should be successfully modified by psychotherapy.

The **biological** theories, on the other hand, hold that the cause is biochemical, an imbalance of amines for example. One theory proposes a reduced **GABA-modulin** activity, which allows over-stimulation of the ascending reticular formation leading to **excessive arousal**. A former theory linked it to raised lactate levels secondary to sympathetically enhanced metabolic activity. It is also possible that **5HT** receptors are involved.

Although the success of drugs in controlling many of the symptoms of anxiety seems to support a biological model, the two theories are not necessarily incompatible. Functional mental events would have to alter brain activity in order to achieve anything, and neurochemical changes should result. Thus, chemical interference would be expected to bring about a symptomatic change but not to affect the underlying cause. This is in accord with the apparent effect of anxiolytics in suppressing symptoms, and argues for a combined, eclectic psychotherapeutic-pharmacotherapeutic approach to therapy.

Aetiology and classification

Both genetic and childhood developmental factors contribute to a predisposition to the illness, which usually starts in early adulthood. Environmental stressors and life events are frequently associated with its onset and persistence. An understanding of the aetiology and also of the management is helped by classifying it according to the nature of the perceived threat and the severity and course of the illness (Table 7.7).

Common forms of anxiety

Stress-related anxiety arises from a real external situation and is proportionate to that. It is usu-

Table 7.7   Classification[a] and aetiology of common anxiety disorders

Class	Course	Nature of threat	Features/examples	Severity
Stress-related	Acute	Real/plausible	Proportionate reaction to stressful life event, which will resolve itself, e.g. stage fright, examination nerves	Usually mild
	Chronic	Real/plausible	Proportionate **adjustment reaction**, e.g. unemployment, chronic illness	Mild/severe
Generalized anxiety disorder (GAD)	Acute, chronic or recurrent	Imagined, exaggerated or ill-defined	Response disproportionate to threat; related to patient's personality?	Severe
Panic disorder	Acute recurrent	Imagined, exaggerated or ill-defined	Sudden onset of severe disabling physical and psychiatric symptoms ('panic attack')	Very severe
Mild anxiety and depression	Chronic	Imagined, exaggerated or ill-defined	Mixture of anxiety and depression	Usually mild
Secondary anxiety	Acute or chronic	Underlying non-psychiatric cause	Physical illness, e.g. hyperthyroidism Iatrogenic, e.g. caffeine, adrenergic, substance abuse	Variable

[a] This classification broadly follows 10th edition of the *International Classification of Disease* (ICD-10).

ally acute and relatively benign, rarely needing treatment. The cause might reasonably be expected to resolve eventually, but the sufferer may require some treatment to help cope with symptoms temporarily. The more chronic forms are known as **adjustment reactions**.

Most patients fall into the category of **generalized anxiety disorder**. This is a disproportionate reaction to real or imagined adverse circumstances, related to a person's personality, and tends to be recurrent.

In **panic disorder** there are sudden onsets of florid autonomic symptoms, extreme distress and often a paralysis of action or decision, usually with no discernible cause. Patients may feel in imminent danger of death or insanity.

Possible causes of **secondary anxiety** must always be bone in mind when a patient first presents. Certain diseases (e.g. hyperthyroidism, phaeochromocytoma) can cause the physical symptoms of anxiety, as can certain drugs (e.g. excessive coffee consumption, alcohol or other drug abuse, adrenergic stimulants such as bronchodilators).

The commonly combined presentation of mild to moderate anxiety with depression is of particular importance to primary carers, including GPs and community pharmacists. Mixed anxiety and depression (mild or mixed affective disorder) presents a diagnostic difficulty: is the patient depressed in reaction to prolonged anxiety, or perhaps anxious over the problems caused by their depression? Interestingly, the distinction may not be that important because it does not influence management.

Insomnia, commonly associated with anxiety and other psychiatric illnesses, is a symptom rather than a discrete diagnosis. Nevertheless it may be a target for therapy, using **hypnotics**, which are largely the same range of drugs used for anxiety.

Less common chronic anxiety

A number of related neurotic syndromes with characteristic psychiatric symptoms are included in the wider definition of anxiety. They represent less common behavioural patterns with which the chronically anxious personality can present. They are summarized in Table 7.8 and a few will be briefly discussed here.

Obsessional and **compulsive** states usually occur together. Like many neuroses they are related to the patient's personality. Obsessions are commonly seen in the rigid, inflexible person, overly concerned with neatness and order. For example, a patient obsessed by the idea of cleanliness, and perhaps their own impurity, may be compelled to wash their hands 20 or 30 times a day. **Hypochondria** is a particular form of obsessional disorder with inappropriate or inaccurate thoughts or ideas about health and illness and a fear of disease. Such patients are constantly imagining themselves to be ill, consulting health professionals and self-medicating, when there is almost invariably no physical abnormality whatsoever. Hypochondriasis should not be confused with either psychosomatic illness or hysteria.

With **psychosomatic** illness there is a genuine physical dysfunction, usually autonomic, accounting for the symptoms, e.g. dyspepsia caused by gastric hypersecretion. The close relationship between the mind and the peripheral nervous system makes it easy to see how mental conflicts could alter physiological function in these cases. Indeed, psychosomatic symptoms may be the only indication that a patient is anxious: they may not complain of any mental stress.

Dissociative states usually start suddenly and dramatically, either as a neurological or neuromuscular deficit, e.g. blindness or paralysis, or an altered state of consciousness, e.g. the amnesic patient found wandering aimlessly. However, no physical cause can be found, e.g. no problem with the eye, optic nerve or visual cortex in hysterical blindness. Once again its origin seems to lie in mental conflict or instability, which is converted to a physical sign, hence the alternative term **conversion disorder**. The older term hysteria is now avoided to prevent confusion with lay concepts such as 'mass hysteria' and 'hysterical', which are quite different.

Phobias or morbid fears are easily understood to be expressions of underlying anxiety. Examples are agoraphobia (the fear of going out, of crowds or of open spaces) and arachnophobia (spiders). Recall that our definition of pathological anxiety involves the inability to cope. Thus simply being upset by spiders does not count:

Table 7.8   Less common classes[a] of chronic anxiety

Class	Features/examples
Obsession	Irresistible bizarre **thoughts** or preoccupations. Hypochondriasis is an obsession with and excessive concern for health in absence of physical disorder
Compulsion	Irresistible desire to perform meaningless or ritualistic **actions**
Psychosomatic illness (somatizaton disorder)	Genuine physical disorder, usually minor, brought about by mental conflicts, e.g. hyperacidity, palpitations, migraine, psychogenic pain
Dissociative disorder (conversion disorder, hysteria)	Serious physical expression of mental conflicts as physical or psychiatric symptoms, in absence of physiological or pathological basis (e.g. blindness or paralysis)
Phobia	Irrational, abnormal or excessive **fear** of an object or situation
Eating disorders	Anorexia nervosa (morbid fear of obesity, deliberate excessive weight loss, inappropriate body image) Bulimia nervosa (binge eating/vomiting; obsession with weight/shape)
Post-traumatic stress disorder	Response to overwhelming events outside normal human experience, characterized by delayed chronic anxiety, avoidance behaviour and intrusive recollections (flashbacks or nightmares)
Personality disorders	Enduring personal characteristics at extreme end of normal behavioural spectrum (e.g. obsessional, histrionic, schizoid, paranoid, dysthymic, cyclothymic)

[a] This classification broadly follows 10th edition of the *International Classification of Disease* (ICD-10).

but if the sight – or the unreasonable anticipation – of them disrupts everyday life, then there is a problem. However, the cultural and social context is also important: a fear of being eaten by a tiger might be phobic in Britain but a reasonable precaution in Bengal.

Clinical features

Anxiety is a neurotic disorder, in which insight and grasp of reality are preserved. Anxiety tends to be anticipatory, in that a future or current threat is perceived (compared to depression, which is generally retrospective).

As in all psychiatric illness we are concerned with intangible features such as the patient's demeanour, body language, facial expression or phraseology: precisely measurable physical signs may be absent although there will be variable physical features. Thus great skill is needed in eliciting a psychiatric history. The presentation is highly variable but usually includes many of the following:

- **Psychiatric features**:
  – Feelings of apprehension, tension, fear, panic or terror, being on edge.
  – Labile mood, outbursts of hostility.
  – Circling thoughts, inability to concentrate, easily distracted, lapses of memory.
- **Physical (somatic) features**:
  – Palpitations, bradycardia or tachycardia.
  – Elevated blood pressure.
  – Rapid shallow breathing (hyperventilation), possibly breathlessness (dyspnoea).
  – Gastrointestinal disturbances (e.g. diarrhoea, dyspepsia, dysphagia).
  – Agitation, restlessness, tremor.
  – Initial insomnia (difficulty in going to sleep).
  – Excessive sweating.
  – Flushing or pallor.
  – Elevated blood glucose and corticosteroids.

This is clearly a picture of sympathetic nervous system over-activity; even the mental features resemble the central actions of adrenaline (epinephrine). However, psychiatric presentations in general may frequently be mixed, masked or disguised. An anxious patient may present as depressed, or vice versa, or the patient may complain only of the physical symptoms and deny any mental problem.

Course and prognosis

Stress-related anxiety has a generally good outlook as long as the external stressor can be eliminated or the sufferer learns to cope with it. Most other forms of primary anxiety disorder tend to follow a chronic relapsing course, with the most serious cases requiring the intermittent refuge of acute psychiatric units. An unfortunate minority of patients suffer from chronic disabling anxiety.

Management

Aims and strategy

The aims in managing anxiety are:

- To discover any immediate cause and deal with that if possible.
- To assess the severity.
- To relieve the patient's suffering as soon as possible.
- In chronic anxiety, to institute long-term, potentially curative treatment.

Careful history taking and a full physical examination are important to eliminate any medical or iatrogenic causes. Any objective threat to the patient and its likely duration must be evaluated, as well as the patient's personality and the extent of their disability. It will often be necessary to address their social, economic or domestic situation.

If prompt symptomatic relief is felt necessary, short-term pharmacotherapy may be indicated. However, some psychiatrists believe that this only helps patients to avoid confronting their problems and may be counterproductive in the long term. Nevertheless, drugs may enable the patient to benefit from psychotherapy because mood is stabilized, concentration improved, and the patient becomes more receptive.

Drugs obviously cannot alter the reality of unemployment, bereavement or a disastrous marriage. However, it is vital to understand that they also do nothing to alter the underlying problem in chronic anxiety. Similarly, drugs cannot cure phobias or obsessive–compulsive disorder; they merely suppress symptoms. However, the relief of temporary stress-related anxiety, e.g. stage fright or examination nerves, with appropriate drugs (e.g. beta-blockers) is simple, harmless and usually effective.

Non-drug therapy

In most cases the problem lies within the patient, so any hope of overcoming the illness usually requires psychotherapy. Behavioural therapy is sometimes helpful, e.g. desensitization for phobias, aversion therapy for compulsions. Chronic anxiety may benefit from a combination of individual counselling (even a brief chat with a skilled counsellor can be very effective) and group therapy. Cognitive therapy and anger management help people to understand situations which precipitate symptoms and to deal with them. Hypnosis and relaxation therapies also have a place. Psychoanalysis is an option less commonly used in Europe than in North America. Psychiatric care requires a team approach, utilizing community nurses, social services, occupational therapists and clinical psychologists, to improve the patient's social, domestic or economic circumstances – often a difficult task.

Simple admission to a psychiatric unit may in itself sometimes be therapeutic, by removing the patient from a stressful domestic situation. However, some patients are regularly admitted this way. They partially recover and are returned after a few weeks to a life they cannot cope with, only to be re-admitted a few months later, and so on: the so-called revolving door phenomenon.

Drug therapy

Benzodiazepines

The initial enthusiasm for the benzodiazepines as universal panaceas, based with some justification on their great advantages over the barbiturates, has now cooled. Although they cause little generalized CNS depression and are remarkably safe in overdose, both dependence and withdrawal symptoms are now known to be quite common.

Action

The range of benzodiazepines available obscures the fact that there are few differences between them except in their pharmacokinetics. They all probably act at specific benzodiazepine receptors by enhancing the inhibitory activity of GABA at its receptors in many central and spinal sites, including the reticular activating system. Thus, they have a wide range of actions that makes them very useful drugs in the right circumstances. The anxiolytic action is quite selective for the limbic system at low doses, with only a small, but not insignificant, effect on cognition and coordination – hence the description 'minor tranquillizers' (the antipsychotic neuroleptic drugs being the major tranquillizers). At higher doses this selectivity is lost and they act as hypnotics (sleep inducers).

Benzodiazepines have several other actions. They are muscle-relaxant and anticonvulsant: rectal or IV *diazepam* is the drug of choice for status epilepticus. Parenteral use enables premedication and light general anaesthesia for minor procedures such as endoscopy, with the added benefit of short-term amnesia which covers the period of these disagreeable experiences. They are also useful adjuncts in anti-emetic regimens to cover cancer chemotherapy and are used in alcohol withdrawal therapy and for delirium tremens.

During use, **tolerance** develops owing to receptor down-regulation, although this should have little impact on use if prescribers adhere to the short courses that are currently recommended.

Pharmacokinetics

Benzodiazepines are lipophilic drugs that have good bioavailability, are widely distributed throughout the body and are avidly bound to plasma protein. Diazepam seems to have the most rapid onset of action, possibly because it is the most lipophilic and thus rapidly distributed to the CNS.

Benzodiazepines are cleared almost exclusively by the liver, the inactive glucuronide being eliminated renally. The principal difference between them is in their metabolism (Table 7.9). The shorter-acting agents, e.g. *temazepam*, are metabolized directly to an inactive form, and have half-lives of 3–15 h. The longer-acting drugs, e.g. *diazepam*, have one or more active intermediates thus may have effective biological half-lives of up to 100 h.

One result which is often overlooked is that the longer-acting benzodiazepines may take

Table 7.9 Comparison of some representative benzodiazepines

Half-life (h, approx.)[a]	Drug	Comment
Very short (<4)	Triazolam	
	Midazolam	Parenteral anaesthetic
Short (4–12)	Temazepam	
	Loprazolam	
	Alprazolam	
Medium (12–20)	Lorazepam	
	Oxazepam	
	Bromazepam	
Long (>20)	Chlordiazepoxide	The original *Librium*
	Nitrazepam	*Mogadon*
	Diazepam	*Valium*
	Flurazepam	
Very long (>50)	Clobazam	Anticonvulsant
	Clorazepate	Anticonvulsant

[a] Half-life likely to be much prolonged in the elderly.

several weeks to reach steady-state plasma levels. If the dose is increased too frequently during this period there will be accumulation, although the cumulative effect is to some extent offset by the development of tolerance (above). This can also occur with normal dosing in the elderly, in whom the half-lives given in Table 7.9 may be increased up to threefold. Similarly, the effects of the long-acting agents persist for many hours or days after discontinuation.

Advantages

Comparison of the benzodiazepines with their predecessors, the barbiturates, explains their initial appeal to prescribers (Table 7.10). They are selective, and largely avoid drowsiness at therapeutic doses. In addition, they are extremely safe in overdose because they do not cause depression of the respiratory or other medullary centres. Death from benzodiazepine over-dosage alone is extremely uncommon; the drugs rarely produce more than a light coma, from which the patient can be aroused. However, combination with other CNS depressant (e.g. opioids, alcohol – common components of deliberate overdose mixtures) or in otherwise compromised patients (the elderly, the very young, those with obstructive pulmonary disease) can be fatal. *Flumazenil*, a specific benzodiazepine competitive antagonist, is available for injection to reverse overdoses rapidly.

Habituation, dependence and withdrawal phenomena were initially thought to be rare. Benzodiazepines neither induce liver enzymes nor have their metabolism significantly affected by other drugs that induce or inhibit liver enzymes. They do not displace other drugs from plasma protein binding sites.

Disadvantages

The validity of many of these favourable initial impressions has been eroded. Benzodiazepines do cause unwanted CNS depression, especially a subtle impairment of motor coordination that is often unnoticed by the patient. This is thought to be implicated in a growing number of motoring accidents. In the elderly particularly, the longer-acting agents sometimes cause paradoxical excitement, giddiness, confusion or aggression (owing to disinhibition).

Dependence and drug-seeking behaviour and abuse, related to down-regulation of GABA receptors, are being increasingly recognized as major problems. Withdrawal symptoms seem to be more common with the short-acting benzodiazepines, especially if they are stopped abruptly, probably because of the subsequent rapid fall in plasma level. Dependence may occur after as little as 4–6 weeks, and up to half of patients may become dependent after 3 months of continuous treatment.

Weaning patients off benzodiazepines is not easy and inevitably takes a long time, if it can be done at all. One recommended procedure is to convert the patient to diazepam at an equipotent daily dose (see the *British National Formulary*, BNF), and then reduce the dose by one-eighth of this every fortnight.

Certain patients seem particularly prone to dependence, notably those with compliant, passive, dependent or anxious personalities, who tend to abuse prescription medication in low doses over long periods. Another group – impulsive, antisocial and more psychotic than neurotic – may abuse illicitly obtained benzodiazepines recreationally, in larger doses but with less likelihood of dependence. Pharmacists in the UK are

---

Table 7.10   Advantages and disadvantages of benzodiazepines

Advantages	Disadvantages and side effects
Effective as hypnotic/anxiolytic (symptomatic)	Tolerance, habituation, dependence
Specific anxiolytic effects	Subtle cognitive and psychomotor impairment
Safe in overdose	Withdrawal effects (especially long-acting agents)
Few interactions	May produce unnatural sleep pattern/sleep debt
	Paradoxical excitement
	Amnesia (may be beneficial – see text)

becoming actively involved in monitoring the use of benzodiazepines and countering their misuse.

When used as hypnotics, benzodiazepines produce abnormal sleep patterns and cause a rebound sleep debt on withdrawal. There is a hangover effect from all but the shortest-acting agents.

Indications and use

It is now strongly recommended that benzodiazepines are not used for more than 4–6 weeks at any one time. The longer-acting ones should be started cautiously with small dose increments. When stopping treatment, the dose should be reduced slowly, especially with the short-acting drugs.

A shorter-acting benzodiazepine is preferred for the elderly, for those with liver disease and for daytime use generally, even if this means more doses per day. Longer-acting drugs may be beneficial if compliance is doubtful, if the shorter-acting ones do not provide enough sleep, or if a combination of hypnotic effect and next-day sedation is desired.

It is necessary to tailor the choice of agent and dose carefully to the patient because of individual variations in clearance, response, residual effects and concurrent medication. If these precautions are observed, the value of benzodiazepines will be retained without incurring the potentially serious problems.

Other anxiolytic agents

If benzodiazepines are to be avoided, there are at present three alternatives for general anxiety: buspirone, beta-blockers, and tricyclic antidepressants. *Buspirone*, a partial 5HT agonist, is anxiolytic but not hypnotic. It probably has a lesser liability to habituation than benzodiazepines, but is expensive. Its main drawback is a slow onset of activity, up to 2 weeks, and this makes it unsuitable for treatment of acute anxiety. However, buspirone might be a suitable alternative where benzodiazepine-like activity is required beyond 1 month.

Beta-blockers are useful for some patients in stress-related anxiety with pronounced adrenergic physical symptoms, and they may also have direct a central anxiolytic effect. They may reduce the psychiatric symptoms by sparing patients further concern about the physical symptoms. However, beta-blockers are less useful in general anxiety or panic disorder. Their principal advantages are that they can be used for long periods if necessary and have no general sedative effect.

Antidepressants are useful and increasingly used for chronic anxiety, although just why they are effective is not clear. Some exert a non-specific sedative effect, e.g. older *tricyclics* like amitriptyline. Whether their specific antidepressant action is generally helpful is not clear, although clearly the combination of this with sedation is suitable for mixed affective disorder, when it obviates the necessity for precise differential diagnosis. Although not addictive like benzodiazepines, antidepressants do have common and distressing adverse effects. *Selective serotonin re-uptake inhibitors* (SSRIs) are also used. Antidepressants may occasionally exacerbate anxiety at first.

Dosage is similar to their use in depression (pp. 413–414), with low starting doses and gradual increments. Owing to the slow onset of action of antidepressants, and the initial increase in anxiety symptoms, patients with acute severe problems may need initial cover with a short course of benzodiazepines.

In addition, various antidepressants have specific indications in certain less common forms of anxiety (see Drug selection below).

Hypnotics

Alternatives to benzodiazepines as hypnotic drugs are the chemically distinct *zopiclone* and *zolpidem*, which also act on benzodiazepine receptors. They appear to offer little advantage and are costly. Other sedative drugs sometimes used include antihistamines (e.g. *promethazine*, *hydroxyzine*), chloral derivatives (e.g. *dichloralphenazone*) and *neuroleptics* in low doses. *Barbiturates* are now restricted to anaesthesia and continuing medication for epileptic patients long stabilized on phenobarbital; *meprobamate* is no longer used.

Drug selection

It must be emphasized that drug therapy has only a minor, strictly limited role in the management of anxiety. It should usually be restricted to short periods and have specific, agreed end points, e.g. to cover an acutely stressful temporary exacerbation of the patient's circumstances. Treatment must be monitored closely to ensure that the drug is withdrawn when the specific indications resolve. For most types of anxiety the preferred sequence is:

psychotherapy → short-term benzodiazepine → longer-term antidepressant

In some circumstances more specific recommendations can be made (see below), and the rapid effectiveness of benzodiazepines in the short term allows other therapies time to start working.

Stress-related anxiety

Short courses of *anxiolytics* can be very useful in acute conditions where the patient definitely needs support for a brief period before a specific stressful event. There is insufficient time for psychotherapy, and the duration of drug therapy is usually too short for dependence to develop, so that the *benzodiazepines* could be used. If the symptoms are mainly somatic (palpitations, gastrointestinal upset, tremor) *beta-blockers* are preferable, as they would be in situations when benzodiazepine adverse effects would be disadvantageous (e.g. musicians, actors, examination candidates). For chronic adjustment reactions, *antidepressants* are indicated.

Where the anxiety is **secondary** to an underlying medical condition, e.g. thyrotoxicosis, or drug use or misuse, obviously the aim is to diagnose and correct that.

Generalized anxiety disorder

This category perhaps presents the greatest dangers for inappropriate drug treatment. The temptation is strong to suppress the patient's unwelcome, distressing symptoms continuously with drugs – which seem so effective – rather than uncover the true cause of the patient's problems. This is particularly so if the problems stem from an adverse social environment, such as poverty or marital distress, when the clinician may feel frustrated by his or her inability to tackle the underlying difficulties. However, this temptation should be resisted. Short courses of anxiolytic drugs have a place in stabilizing the patient, but the only chance of a permanent

solution is to address these underlying problems. The alternative is the 'revolving door phenomenon' and anxiolytic dependence.

The idea of the 'pill for every ill' society is based mainly on the misguided drug treatment of this category of illness. The prevailing belief in the West (and perhaps especially in the USA) seems to be that all distress must be avoided, all stress reactions are pathological, and life must be perpetually serene. In his *Brave New World*, Aldous Huxley prophetically anticipated and ruthlessly satirised this idealistic philosophy. Modern-day critics also claim that too frequent recourse to drugs reduces people's capacity to confront stressful situations and may mask wider sociopolitical causes. There are Valium Anonymous groups in the USA and TRANX in the UK to counter this attitude and help those who are benzodiazepine-dependent.

With the growing recognition of the problems with the benzodiazepines, attention has turned to other forms of treatment. In the medium and long term, antidepressants or simple psychotherapy are far more effective than benzodiazepines. One exception is in serious organic illness and pain, especially cancer, where relief of symptoms becomes the prime objective.

Panic

For acute panic attacks a short course of anxiolytic therapy may be used. Longer-term prophylactic treatment requires antidepressants: *clomipramine*, *SSRIs* and *monoamine oxidase inhibitors* (MAOIs) are effective. However, psychotherapy or cognitive behaviour therapy may be useful at some stage, to try to discover the cause and tackle the problem.

Mixed anxiety and depression

Antidepressants with a sedative action are especially useful here. In some trials patients have been randomly assigned to either benzodiazepine or tricyclic treatment without reference to whether primary depression or anxiety was suspected: the *antidepressant* treated group had a better recovery rate.

Other neuroses

In certain syndromes drugs have been found to be particularly useful adjuncts to psychotherapy.

Tricyclic antidepressants (especially *clomipramine*, and the *SSRIs*) have a place in the treatment of **obsessive–compulsive** disorders, and both *MAOIs* and *tricyclics* are sometimes helpful in phobic states. All these have a low potential for producing dependence and so may be used for longer periods than benzodiazepines. For psychosomatic complaints, a short course of *anxiolytics* can aid psychotherapy.

Depression

Most people experience a depressed mood from time to time. Feelings of sadness are an appropriate response to a recent loss or disappointment, but they are expected to remit spontaneously sooner or later, depending on the personality of the subject and the cultural norms of their society.

As with all psychiatric conditions the normal response must be distinguished from an illness. One criterion is whether it is socially incapacitating or the patient can cope. Another is whether the sufferer's culture regards the apparent cause as meriting a period of depressed mood. Grieving for a close relative is a good example: almost all cultures recognize a period of mourning, although the acceptable duration varies greatly. In the UK, perhaps 6 months to a year is regarded as normal for a spouse. Much less would seem callous, but to dwell on it for much longer, remaining pessimistic, tearful and unable to function, would be regarded as abnormal.

On the other hand, someone who was depressed but whose life gave no apparent evidence of substantial adverse events would without doubt be regarded as suffering from a morbid depression. This distinction must be reflected in the classification of depression. It is also necessary to identify cases where there is an underlying primary medical or iatrogenic cause of which the depression is a secondary consequence.

Note that in psychiatry the term **affect** is an objective description of a person's transient emotional behaviour, whereas **mood** describes their prevailing subjective emotional state. Conventionally, **affective disorder** includes illnesses with abnormally high or low mood, i.e. mania and depression. Although it might seem logical to include anxiety too, the complexity of anxiety disorder has always meant it is considered as a separate major category of mental illness.

Classification and course

The difficulty with classifying depression is that it occurs in numerous forms, and different systems of classification use different criteria to distinguish between them. The range of criteria used by different classifications include:

- Severity.
- Presence or absence of physical (*somatic* or *biological*) features.
- Presence or absence of psychotic features.
- Course (duration and recurrence).
- Presence or absence of intervening manic phases.

The first three criteria are the characteristics of the single depressive episode, while the last two describe the pattern of occurrence (the course or natural history) and are the basis of the current ICD classification (Fig. 7.6).

A depressive episode usually lasts between 3 and 12 months. About half of patients only ever experience a **single episode** (which can then be differentiated on the basis of its severity; see below). Others experience a persistent mild depression for much of their adult lives, but this may be a feature of their personality. This is **dysthymia** or **chronic affective disorder**, and it may be interspersed with more severe exacerbations, when it is known as **double depression**; indeed, one-quarter of major depressive episodes occur against a background of dysthymia.

More commonly, depressive episodes – although naturally self-limiting – are prone to recurrence. A distinction is then made on the basis of whether the patient also suffers episodes of unnaturally elevated mood known as **mania**; this is known as **bipolar affective disorder** (pp. 418–422). A milder form, **cyclothymia**, is seen in persons who are subject to alternating periods of elevated or depressed mood outside what is considered as normal mood variation, yet the person is able to cope without resort to psychiatric support. Both cyclothymia and dysthymia are sometimes regarded as forms of personality disorder (*see* Table 7.8).

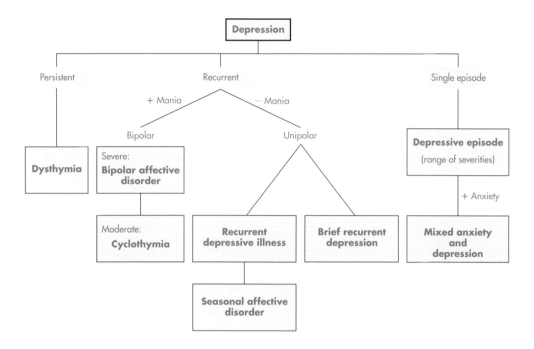

Figure 7.6   Course of affective disorders. This diagram is based the 10th edition of the *International Classification of Disease.*

In **unipolar affective disorder** there are recurrent episodes of depression (or far more rarely, mania) with periods of remission. With **recurrent depressive illness**, which is probably the largest single category, each episode is insidious in onset, developing over the course of months, and may last for months or even years. In some cases however there are **brief recurrent** depressive episodes, although each is severe. In **seasonal affective disorder** (SAD), depression recurs in the winter months, with either normal or hypomanic mood in the spring and summer.

A depressive episode, particularly the milder form, may coexist with anxiety, when the description **mixed anxiety and depression** is appropriate (p. 401).

Clinical features

Other classification criteria may be more helpful when summarizing the various clinical features of depression.

Psychiatric spectrum

Traditionally, depression was divided into two broad groups on the basis of the presence or absence of psychotic features (this roughly correlates with severity, see below). One group resembles an exaggerated response to an adverse life event that might be expected to depress anyone to a certain extent, such as a bereavement, but with which the patient is unable to cope. As such it is referred to as minor depression, or formerly as *neurotic* or *reactive* depression. The term *reactive* here can be taken to imply that the depression is a response to a life event, or that the patient still retains the ability to react emotionally to normal everyday events. However, the description *minor* should not be taken to imply that, for the patient, the depression is somehow more bearable.

This form resembles stress-related anxiety neurosis in that both are associated with real events and insight is preserved. However, depression is generally retrospective, whereas anxiety tends to be anticipatory.

At the other extreme are patients with no

obviously adverse events in the recent past, who become depressed for reasons they do not understand, and who have poor insight into their condition. This depression may involve psychotic symptoms such as delusions and is usually associated with a number of metabolic and physical (somatic) features. It is still sometimes referred to as *major*, *biological* or *endogenous* depression, although modern terminology has revived the poetic medieval description *melancholia*.

Figure 7.7 illustrates this distinction for some of the more important features of depressive illness. However, things are rarely as simple as this would imply and the distinctions are somewhat artificial. Biological variables within a population tend to occur as finely graded differences rather than clearly defined categories. The majority of patients appear somewhere on the continuum between the two extremes, and at different points for different features. Thus, a patient may have a strong family history and some delusions of guilt, but have an acute onset triggered by a bereavement.

Secondary depression can be caused by some antihypertensive drugs (methyldopa, clonidine, some beta-blockers), steroids (including oral contraceptives), and many CNS depressants such as benzodiazepines, opiates and alcohol. It also occurs secondary to dementia, stroke, Parkinson's disease, hypothyroidism, other psychiatric conditions (schizophrenia, alcoholism) and many serious chronic diseases, especially those involving pain, e.g. cancer, rheumatoid arthritis.

Severity

For a single depressive episode an alternative approach is to look at common presentations of the symptomatology at different degrees of severity (Fig. 7.8).

The core features of depression, present even in the mildest form, are:

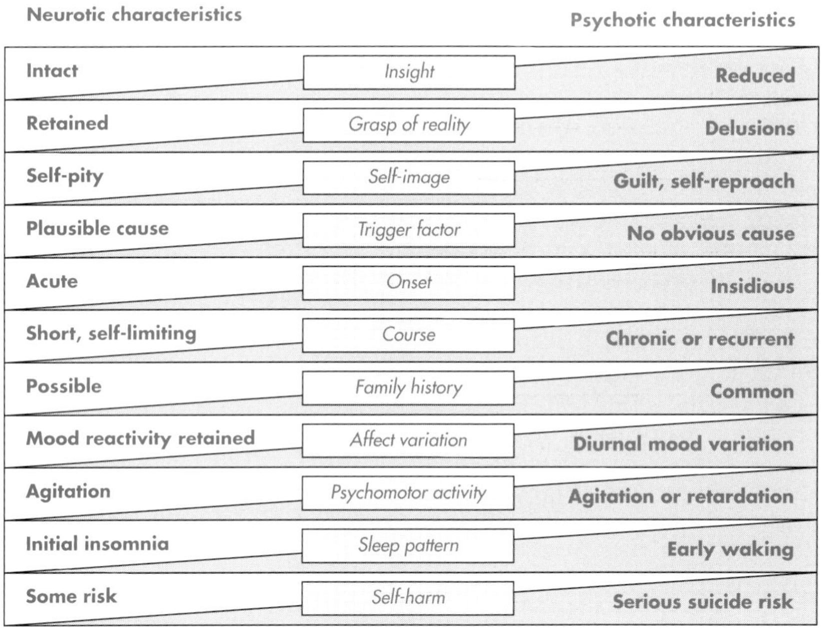

Neurotic characteristics		Psychotic characteristics
Intact	Insight	Reduced
Retained	Grasp of reality	Delusions
Self-pity	Self-image	Guilt, self-reproach
Plausible cause	Trigger factor	No obvious cause
Acute	Onset	Insidious
Short, self-limiting	Course	Chronic or recurrent
Possible	Family history	Common
Mood reactivity retained	Affect variation	Diurnal mood variation
Agitation	Psychomotor activity	Agitation or retardation
Initial insomnia	Sleep pattern	Early waking
Some risk	Self-harm	Serious suicide risk

Figure 7.7   Clinical spectrum of depression. This shows the range of psychiatric and physical features usually found in depression, and their presence, absence or quality for depressive episodes of different severity. For each feature the left-hand end represents the less serious form. An individual patient may be at different points along the spectrum for each feature. Few are wholly at one end or the other for all dimensions.

- **Depressed mood** (dysphoria) with **pessimism** (especially regarding the likelihood of recovering) and frequent tearfulness.
- **Loss of interest** and capacity for enjoyment (anhedonia).
- **Lethargy** and fatigue.

Patients may suffer a variety of additional neurotic symptoms (similar to those seen in anxiety). There are sleep and appetite disturbances and psychosomatic problems such as constipation or dyspepsia. Anorexia is common – per-

haps as an expression of general loss of interest in life's pleasures, but also possibly resulting from alterations in hypothalamic function. Patients tend to feel sorry for themselves but not guilty ('what have I done to deserve this?' rather than 'I deserve this as punishment').

The mood of patients with mild to moderate depression, although predominantly low, is labile, tending to fluctuate to some extent in reaction to the minor everyday joys and disappointments of life. They have difficulty getting off to sleep (i.e. initial insomnia or increased

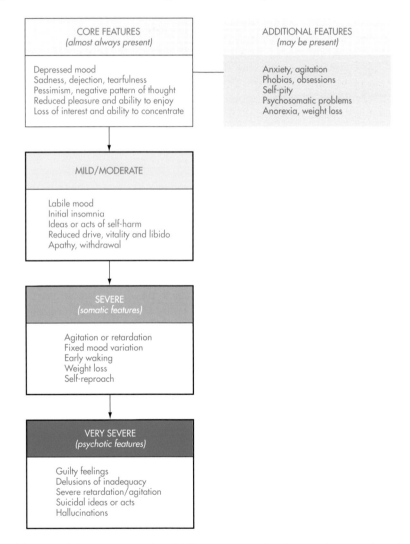

Figure 7.8   Clinical features of depressive episodes of different severity. This illustrates the general trend in episodes of depression of increasing severity. An individual patient may show a mix of features from different stages as represented here.

sleep latency), as in anxiety. They lose the capacity to initiate any action, and find making even quite trivial decisions difficult.

There is a marked loss of drive, vitality, ambition, libido and zest for life – a loss of appetite for more than just food. Patients have difficulty in concentrating and suffer selective memory impairment; past mistakes in particular are forgotten, or repressed. There is a persistently negative approach to everything.

In severe depression, more physical (somatic) features become evident. There may also be psychomotor impairment, either agitation, or conversely, mild retardation of thought, speech and action. Patients wake early, at 4 or 5 a.m. feeling at their worst; things improve slightly by evening. Mood variation tends to become fixed in this pattern, whatever the day brings. Rather than feeling sorry for themselves they somehow blame themselves for their plight: guilt, self-reproach and feelings of worthlessness are common. Because marital problems can follow the reduced libido, and impaired performance at work result from the loss of drive, the patient's low self-esteem is reinforced and justified – it becomes a self-fulfilling prophecy.

Very severe depression is accompanied by intensification of the biological features, with worsening of agitation or retardation. The psychotic dimension of depression also becomes apparent. For example, the general feeling of worthlessness and inadequacy becomes a firmly fixed, unrealistic false belief which no amount of appeals to reason can shift, i.e. a delusion. They believe themselves to be guilty, 'bad people', responsible for destroying their family and letting down their colleagues at work. These delusions may, rarely, be reinforced with another classic psychotic sign, hallucinations (false perceptions). They may hear voices chastising them for the evil or corrupt person they believe themselves to be.

Thus it is possible to get an inkling of how people may be driven to what is, in biological terms, the highly anomalous behaviour of intentional self-destruction. The perpetual misery, the firm conviction that you are causing serious problems for people around you, including loved ones, and the belief that things will not improve makes suicide for them an appealing, almost logical option.

Suicide and self-harm

There are some 5000 successful suicides a year in the UK. About 75% of these involve mental illness, mostly depression but also alcoholism, personality disorder and schizophrenia. Depressives are about 25 times more likely than others to attempt suicide, and 15% will eventually succeed. Prevention of suicide and attempts to change suicidal ideas are major targets of the management of depression.

In the UK, drug overdose is the usual means (up to 90% of cases) in both suicide and deliberate self-harm. Since barbiturates have become unavailable, the risk of serious consequences from drug overdose should have been reduced. However, the barbiturates have been superseded, and possibly exceeded in danger, by paracetamol (acetaminophen), which is freely available and hence widely believed to be safe. Yet as few as 20 paracetamol tablets can have the tragic unintended outcome of fatal liver failure. Overall, paracetamol and other analgesics are the most common choice, presumably because of ease of access (30%); sedatives are used in 15% of cases and antidepressants 10%. Alcohol use is also involved in over half of drug overdoses.

It is important to distinguish between suicide, which is intentional successful self-inflicted death, and deliberate self-harm, which is deliberate self-inflicted injury; the two are distinct entities presented by different types of patient. Those who decide to commit **suicide** are likely to be thorough: they will fail only through ignorance or bad luck. (When successful it is known as completed suicide.) They plan the suicide carefully for weeks so that it almost becomes an obsession. Although ostensibly keeping it secret, they may well give covert, even unconscious hints of their intention. More importantly, if asked directly they will usually admit to suicidal thoughts. Unfortunately, the topic is usually taboo among their family so they are driven to veiled hints which, tragically, are frequently only recognized in retrospect. Suicide is more often associated with major depression than minor, and patients frequently utilize means that are more likely to succeed and less likely to permit reversal; i.e. large overdoses, jumping in front of a train.

Patients with less severe depression may be driven to an ill-conceived, impulsive act of aggression directed at themselves. **Deliberate self-harm** (formerly parasuicide) is frequently preceded or immediately followed by a desperate phone call – the literal cry for help to complement the symbolic. Self-harm is not usually intended to be fatal: it rarely employs irreversible measures. Often it means ingestion of a few dozen hastily assembled tablets or some clumsy slashes at the wrist. Yet if someone is so disturbed that they demonstrate their hopelessness and their need to draw attention to their plight by self-harm, they surely merit help and sympathy, however manipulative they may appear.

The term 'attempted suicide' is no longer used because it does not convey whether or not there was an intention to die.

Epidemiology

Epidemiological statistics for depression are difficult to obtain because of the different definitions and the fact that most depression is encountered in primary care or is frequently unrecognized. About 20% of us develop a depressive episode at some stage in our life, and in a quarter of cases it becomes chronic. The prevalence of major depression is approximately 5%. About a quarter of all depression is bipolar.

Only one in 20 cases is referred to secondary care, the remainder being handled by GPs, one in 10 of whose consultations probably involve depression. Half these patients will only have a few minor depressive symptoms, which may well be missed, while one-quarter will have major depression. Depression is two to three times more common in women and its prevalence increases with age.

Diagnosis

A formal diagnosis of depression is made on symptomatic grounds. There must be low mood and at least four other symptoms from among:

- Pessimism.
- Negativism.
- Weight change.
- Sleep disorder.
- Psychomotor agitation or retardation.
- Fatigue.
- Feelings of inadequacy or guilt.
- Difficulty in concentrating.
- Suicidal thoughts or actions.

These must have persisted for at least 2 weeks, be inconsistent with the patient's prior personality and not be secondary to another medical condition or drug therapy.

The degree of depression may be rated by applying a standard scale based on a questionnaire, such as the Hamilton Depression Rating Scale or the Beck Depression Inventory. This can also be used to assess the efficacy and progress of any treatment. However, most depressive episodes remit and antidepressant drugs are slow to act, so any observed remission may be at least partially natural, although it may be tempting to ascribe it to the therapy.

In determining treatment, the finding that the depressive episode is associated with an adverse life event (and is therefore in some way understandable or 'reactive') is no reason to avoid drugs. The key criterion is severity.

Aetiology

As might be expected, there are both biochemical and psychological theories.

Biochemical theories

Most biochemical or organic theories of depression involve abnormalities in central monoamines or their receptors. However, the situation is still unclear and only a brief outline is given here.

The traditional model was deduced from two observations. First, the adverse effect of the now obsolete antihypertensive reserpine, a non-specific central amine depleter, which causes depression. Second, that the tricyclic antidepressants act by preventing amine re-uptake (following release at the nerve terminal) and hence could counteract such a depletion. The amines believed to be most involved are noradrenaline (norepinephrine) and serotonin (5HT).

Owing to its role in mood control, the limbic system is the most likely location of the lesion. Both transmitters are found there and the levels of both are affected by most, but not all, antidepressants. Moreover, 5HT is known to be involved in hypothalamic function, which could account for the sleep and appetite abnormalities of depression.

Recently this theory has been considerably modified. The tricyclics have been found to cause amine receptor subsensitivity (down-regulation) which takes about the same time to develop as the antidepressant effect, i.e. 2–4 weeks. MAOIs and ECT have a similar action. This provides a plausible explanation of the hitherto puzzling delay in the therapeutic action of antidepressants, because amine re-uptake block occurs within hours of entry of antidepressants into the CNS. On this newer model, depressed mood is associated with an initial increase in receptor sensitivity. Amine depletion could then be explained as a compensatory fall in amine release to reduce receptor stimulation. Alternatively, depression could represent the failure of a compensatory down-regulation mechanism which normally restores emotional stability.

It is likely that these various transmitters are interlinked along the polysynaptic neural pathways involved, so that action at one type could have secondary consequences on others. We are still a long way from understanding depression at the molecular level.

Metabolic markers

The diagnostic difficulties of depression have provoked a long search for a biochemical or metabolic marker so that the degree of depression could be measured simply and reliably, like blood glucose in diabetes mellitus. The identification of such a marker might also provide an insight into aetiology.

Thyroid function was an early candidate in view of the depression associated with hypothyroidism (which must always be a potential differential diagnosis in assessing affective disorder). There is some correlation between depression and thyroid-stimulating hormone release. There is a better, but still insufficiently consistent or specific, association between depression, raised serum cortisol and a **reduced suppression of corticosteroid** secretion by dexamethasone (the dexamethasone suppression test). However, this may be secondary to the feeding and sleep disturbances of depression. Neither of these measures is clinically useful.

At one time it was hoped that measuring the level of a metabolite of brain catechols, **3-methoxy-4-hydroxy-phenylethylene glycol** (MHPG) would yield specific information about central amine turnover. If the depression were associated with a catecholamine depletion, then urine or cerebrospinal fluid (CSF) levels of MHPG would be low: a 5HT deficit on the other hand would not affect the MHPG level. It is also possible, though less practicable, to measure CSF levels of 5HT, which are frequently found to be low in depression. These measurements could have an important bearing on drug treatment because some antidepressants selectively block noradrenaline (norepinephrine) re-uptake (e.g. protriptyline) while others block 5HT re-uptake (e.g. fluoxetine). They might also predict when *tryptophan* would be a logical replacement therapy. Unfortunately this approach too has proved inconsistent, and more pragmatic considerations still determine drug selection.

Mood disorders are frequently related to the season. Depression is usually more prevalent in the spring, but in SAD it occurs each winter. Lack of sunlight is an important aetiological factor in this. Abnormalities in melatonin metabolism may be involved because melatonin secretion is suppressed by light, and in manic depressive patients (p. 420) this response is augmented. However, the relationship between melatonin and mood is unknown.

Functional theories

An alternative to this reductionist biochemical approach is the functional or psychoanalytic one where unconscious mental conflicts are thought to be the cause of the disease (p. 390).

It is likely that a synthesis of these two approaches will eventually prevail, though at present the biochemical model probably provides a better explanation of major depression, while minor depression seems better accounted for in terms of mental conflicts and personality, or illness behaviour. A family history of depression tells us little, because the family environment is as likely as genes to influence personality development.

Genes versus environment

A family history is common in major depression but less so in the minor form. Environmental factors such as social class, unemployment, domestic pressures and childhood experiences are also important. The contribution of each factor varies from patient to patient.

Although a serious loss or disappointment does always precede major depression, an adverse or stressful event is frequently found in the patient's recent premorbid history. However, a careful history is necessary, including information from friends or relatives, to reduce the likelihood of confusing cause with effect. A depressed patient may first present with many problems in their life, any of which might plausibly have been the immediate cause of their depression. It is necessary to establish whether any did in fact predate their illness, or if they are all the consequences of depression. It may eventually become evident that there was no discernible trigger for the initial onset of symptoms.

Management

Aims and modes

The aims in managing depression are, in order of priority:

* To prevent suicide – consider custody and compulsory treatment if suicide is a risk.
* To identify possible primary causes, such as chronic illness.
* Symptomatic therapy to relieve the patient's misery.
* To investigate any adverse social, domestic or financial circumstances.
* To initiate long-term, potentially radical therapy.
* To prevent relapse or recurrence.

The three main modes of treatment are physical (invasive, with drugs, ECT, custody), social

and psychological therapy. The principal criteria for deciding between these for a particular patient are:

* Speed of onset/urgency.
* Effectiveness.
* Natural history/likelihood of recurrence.
* Presence of psychotic symptoms.
* Contraindications and adverse effects.
* Cost.

A multidisciplinary team approach involving clinicians, nurses, social workers and sometimes pharmacists is preferred. In severe depression, invasive methods are almost invariably indicated, if necessary including temporary custody and involuntary treatment to prevent patients harming themselves or making unwise decisions. Drugs and ECT are cheap and relatively rapidly effective, but in the long term, social or psychological therapies have a better chance of reducing recurrence. A distinction must be made between a depressive episode and recurrent depressive illness for which prophylaxis must be considered. If biological or psychotic features are prominent, the illness responds well to physical therapy. In mild depression drugs are generally ineffective.

Non-drug treatment

Psychotherapy
This is the preferred treatment for minor depression and frequently all that is needed: there is evidence that drug therapy is ineffective. Psychotherapy is also an important component in the management of major depression after the acute stage, when patients have improved insight, although the aim of some forms of psychotherapy is to further improve insight. At its simplest, psychotherapy may involve no more than giving the patient a sympathetic and concerned ear (*see also* p. 390).

Patients must be reassured that they are eventually going to get better – something which they find difficult to believe. In severe depression it is important to try to restore the patient's self-esteem. Patients should be advised against taking important decisions while depressed.

More specific treatments include group, marital and family therapy. **Cognitive behavioural** therapy has been used very successfully in numerous mental illnesses. In this approach, unhelpful ways of thinking are countered: the patient might be encouraged, for example, to think constructively about his or her illness, or to plan strategies to overcome specific symptoms. **Psychoanalysis** has a place in the management of neurotic depression. **Psychosocial** treatment involves improving the patient's social situation.

Although slow, often labour-intensive compared with drug therapy, and not always effective, psychotherapy does at least hold out hope of a recovery in that the patient becomes better able to cope and remains relatively symptom-free.

Electroconvulsive therapy (ECT)

While it may seem a bizarre and unlikely procedure, and thought inhumane by some, ECT is often rapidly effective compared with drug therapy in very severe and suicidal depression. It also helps patients who are resistant to other forms of therapy or intolerant of them, and there are surprisingly few proven harmful effects. It involves a brief electrical pulse being passed through the brain between two electrodes attached to the skull with electrode jelly (similar to that used in EEG and ECG techniques). The treatment induces electroencephalographic changes characteristic of a major tonic–clonic seizure (see p. 453). The patient is anaesthetized with a brief-acting intravenous anaesthetic and a muscle relaxant (e.g. suxamethonium) is used to prevent a physical seizure.

A course of ECT consists of treatments given about three times weekly, for 3 or 4 weeks. The procedure often produces a rapid elevation of mood in the severely depressed, minimizing the risk of suicide at the most vulnerable phase of depression and enabling the patient to start psychotherapy.

Psychiatry has often had recourse to what may be called trauma therapy. In less enlightened times, hydrotherapy involved drenching 'mad' patients in freezing water. Later, insulin was used to induce hypoglycaemic shock. ECT was partly an extension of this into the age of electricity. Presumably the rationale for these so-called treatments was akin to our predilection for

kicking a recalcitrant piece of machinery: and presumably they met with the same occasional success.

The original rationale for ECT was the observation, erroneous as it later turned out, that epileptic patients developing psychosis had fewer fits: it was reasoned that more fits in psychotic patients might reduce their psychosis. Subsequent research showed that only the cranial events of a seizure are important, so that the muscular seizure may safely be suppressed.

Double-blind placebo trials, using no actual current in controls, have subsequently demonstrated convincingly that the electric shock is essential. Previously, a variety of other factors had been suggested, including the anaesthetic, the muscle relaxant, the central hypoxia, the special care and attention the patient receives (because of the slight but real risks) or even the punitive element which a patient racked with guilt might welcome. ECT appears to produce changes in brain amines and receptor sensitivity similar to those produced by antidepressant drugs.

The common adverse mental effects are headache and confusion on recovering consciousness; similar symptoms occur after a major epileptic seizure. There is some loss of recent memory, which may reduce undue anxiety about subsequent ECT procedures. These side effects are minimized by passing the current through only the non-dominant hemisphere (unilateral ECT). Uncertainty over the possibility of long-term brain damage means that courses are kept to a maximum of about 12 treatments, although patients have had more without evident harm. ECT has none of the adverse effects or contraindications of antidepressant drugs. It can be used safely in pregnant women, the elderly and those in whom anticholinergic drugs are contraindicated. There is no long-term toxicity or suicide risk. However, ECT has no place in the treatment of mild or atypical depression.

Phototherapy

In SAD, 2 h of exposure each morning to full spectrum artificial light equivalent to bright sunlight seems to be effective but it must be continued as long as natural sunlight is unavailable.

Drug therapy

Antidepressant drugs

The antidepressant (thymoleptic or mood-elevating) drugs can be divided into several groups, mainly on the basis of clinical and adverse actions:

- *Tricyclics*, the original group.
- *2nd generation cyclics* ('heterocyclics').

Table 7.11   Comparison of cyclic antidepressants with selective serotonin re-uptake inhibitors (SSRIs)

	Tricyclic and related[a]	SSRI
Sedative potential	Sedative – most Less sedative[b] – *lofepramine, imipramine, trazodone, mianserin*	Less sedative/neutral[b]
Onset of activity	2–4 weeks	2–4 weeks
Side effects		
CNS	Drowsiness Weight gain	Stimulation – anxiety, agitation ? Weight loss 'Serotonin syndrome'
	Activation of acute mania Extrapyramidal symptoms (rare) Hyponatraemia[c]	Activation of acute mania Extrapyramidal symptoms (rare) Hyponatraemia[c]
Anticholinergic	Dry mouth, blurred vision, urinary retention	
Gastrointestinal	Constipation[d]	Nausea and vomiting Altered bowel function ($\uparrow\downarrow$)
Cardiovascular system	Tachycardia[d], hypotension	
Accident risk	Increased	? Less risk
Suicide risk	Significant	? Less risk
Discontinuation	General mild GI/CNS symptoms – withdraw slowly (after 8/52)	General mild GI/CNS symptoms – withdraw slowly (after 8/52)
Overdose	Convulsions; arrhythmias, heart block	Few problems
Treatment	Symptomatic; not specific	Few problems
Compliance/dropout	Common problems	? Few problems (few ADRs)
Dosage	Often can be given once daily Increment dose over 1–2 weeks	Often can be given once daily Usually full dose from start
Cost	Cheap	Relatively expensive
Efficacy	Very effective in adequate dosage	Equally effective

[a] Some newer cyclic drugs have fewer adverse effects – see also Table 7.12.

[b] *Protriptyline* (and to a lesser extent *fluoxetine*) tend to be stimulant.

[c] Dizziness, confusion, convulsions – central effect on antidiuretic hormone secretion.

[d] Anticholinergic effects.

ADR, adverse drug reaction; CNS, central nervous system; GI, gastrointestinal.

- *Selective re-uptake inhibitors*, especially for serotonin (SSRI).
- *Monoamine oxidase inhibitors* (MAOI).

The properties of the first two groups (referred to below generically as 'cyclics') and SSRIs are compared in Table 7.11.

Selectivity. The nomenclature of antidepressants has become somewhat confused owing to an informal classification by the principal neurotransmitter affected. The **original tricyclics** are non-selective. Most block both noradrenaline (norepinephrine) and 5HT re-uptake at central synapses to varying degrees and may also restore receptor sensitivity. They also block histamine-H_1 receptors, peripheral acetylcholine (muscarinic) and alpha-adrenergic receptors to a lesser extent; some also appear to interact weakly with dopaminergic systems. There is partial selectivity in that some (e.g. *protriptyline, desipramine*) have more effect on noradrenaline (norepinephrine) and others (esp. *amitriptyline*) on 5HT.

The **SSRIs** show high selectivity for 5HT re-uptake. Newer agents have noradrenaline (norepinephrine) selectivity (e.g. *reboxetine*) or noradrenaline (norepinephrine)/5HT selectivity (*venlafaxine*). *Nefazodone* has additional 5HT receptor block, while *mirtazapine* and *mianserin* appear not to affect any of the usual transmitters directly.

Certain anti-dopaminergic neuroleptic drugs, it has been claimed, also have moderate antidepressant action, particularly the thioxanthenes (e.g. *flupentixol*); *amoxapine* also affects dopamine. However, extrapyramidal and endocrine adverse effects (pp. 434–435) would limit their usefulness in depression without marked psychotic features. They are more useful in schizophrenia with associated depressive features.

No particular pharmacodynamic properties have been clearly shown to be of superior antidepressant efficacy. The most important clinical distinctions are the presence or absence of:

- Anticholinergic, anti-adrenergic and antihistaminic activity (conferring adverse effects).
- Non-specific sedative action (not linked exclusively to activity on any single transmitter).
- Cardiotoxic and convulsant action in overdose.

These properties governing the adverse affect and contraindication profile significantly affect drug selection. Thus antidepressant 'selectivity' means activity predominantly on the central transmitter(s) presumed to be involved in depression.

Tricyclics and related drugs
The traditional three-ring structure agents such as amitriptyline are effective and cheap, and their properties well known. However, they have significant adverse and toxic effects (Table 7.11). Second-generation drugs (e.g. *lofepramine, dosulepin (dothiepin)*), some not chemically tricyclic (e.g. *amoxapine, mianserin*) offer a number of advantages in that they have fewer adverse effects and are less toxic in overdose (Table 7.11).

Indications. *Amitriptyline* and many others have sedative as well as antidepressant action, and are particularly useful for **depression mixed with anxiety or agitation**. A single daily dose in the evening aids sleep but minimizes daytime sedation. The antidepressant effect, being unrelated to plasma level, is more prolonged.

Less sedative agents (e.g. *imipramine, lofepramine*) will be useful where neither anxiety nor retardation are problems. This will minimize daytime sedation which may otherwise restrict the patient's activity or occupation. By contrast, *protriptyline* has an alerting, mildly amphetamine-like action, suitable for depressed patients showing **retardation**.

Pharmacokinetics. Generally, tricyclics are rapidly and fairly well absorbed but are subject to considerable first-pass metabolism. The extent of hepatic clearance (by demethylation and hydroxylation) varies greatly, partly accounting for wide interpatient variation in response. Among the older drugs, tertiary amine derivatives (e.g. *imipramine*) are frequently demethylated to active secondary amines (e.g. *desipramine*) with a slightly different activity profile; this prolongs action.

The tricyclics are quite highly protein bound. However, they have a high volume of distribution with accumulation in extravascular sites so there are no significant displacement interactions. Plasma level monitoring is not a useful guide to dose titration or efficacy, but can be used to assess compliance. The overall pharmacokinetic effect is usually a long biological half-life, which may be further prolonged in over-dosage. Although therapeutic plasma levels are achieved within 24 h the clinical (antidepressant) effect is not seen for several weeks. Metabolism may be considerably reduced in the elderly, predisposing them to side effects.

Side effects.   Mild to moderate anticholinergic adverse effects, such as dry mouth, constipation, poor visual accommodation, tachycardia, etc. are common, as is drowsiness with many agents (Table 7.11). Although these effects are not serious and usually remit on continued use they may be troublesome at first and contribute to poor compliance. The visual problems may result in consultation with an optician, who should be informed about the drug therapy. If not evident as drowsiness, CNS depressive effects on cognition and coordination may be difficult to distinguish from the more retarded forms of the illness. Owing to this and postural hypotension (due to peripheral alpha-adrenergic blockade), antidepressants are believed to be implicated in a large number of falls and other accidents, especially among the elderly.

Weight gain is quite common. This may be in part the resolution of depressive anorexia, but a direct effect on appetite is also seen even in non-depressives (e.g. when used for migraine prophylaxis). In patients who are susceptible to bipolar mood swings, possible activation of mania must be watched for. A lowering of seizure threshold may destabilize epileptic patients and causes problems if a patient overdoses.

Hyponatraemia may occur owing to central stimulation of antidiuretic hormone (ADH) secretion, particularly in the elderly. This causes CNS depression (drowsiness, confusion) that may easily be attributed to other causes. Extrapyramidal symptoms occasionally occur. *Mianserin* has been implicated in bone marrow depression with leucopenia.

Toxic effects and overdose.   The acute toxicity of antidepressants is important because they are often involved in suicide attempts. For tricyclics there is no specific antidote; all complications must be managed symptomatically as they arise. The main problems are central (seizures and confusion) and cardiovascular (conduction defects giving heart block; vagal inhibition giving tachyarrhythmias; profound hypotension). Thus such overdoses are often fatal. A principal advantage of newer agents is a generally reduced likelihood of these complications, although *dosulepin* (*dothiepin*) is the most toxic of all in overdose.

Interactions.   Adrenergic over-stimulation occurs with *sympathomimetic* drugs (also included in some OTC decongestant preparations) and *MAOIs* causing potentially dangerous hypertension. *CNS depressants* (especially alcohol), which are frequently taken in association with an overdose, produce excessive sedation or coma. The effect of *anticonvulsant* drugs may be diminished. Arrhythmias may occur with *digoxin* or *quinidine*.

Contraindications and cautions.   Patients with heart disease (e.g. arrhythmias, previous MI), narrow-angle glaucoma, urinary retention (e.g. prostatism) or constipation, in whom anticholinergic effects could be harmful or dangerous, will need newer cyclic agents or SSRIs. Patients on antihypertensive medication should use *mianserin*, which does not interfere with amines. Care is needed in epilepsy. The elderly are prone to over-sedation because of the long half-lives and this problem can increase until steady-state concentrations are reached. The blood count of elderly patients on *mianserin* should be monitored (*see also* pp. 416–418).

Dosage and administration.   Drug treatment should be started as early as possible once major depression is diagnosed; this has beneficial effects on outcome and relapse. For optimal antidepressant effect, tricyclics must be used in adequate doses, for example, at least 125 mg daily of amitriptyline. However, this is achieved gradually over 2 weeks starting at 25 mg daily, unless adverse effects become unacceptable. The inconvenience of the initial side effects may be reduced by dividing doses unequally, e.g. two-thirds at night and one-third in the morning. If suicide is a likely or suspected risk, only small supplies should be given at any one time, although determined patients still accumulate them.

Patients must be forewarned that the antidepressant effect does not become apparent for several weeks, because most people expect all drugs to work very quickly. During this initial period they may only experience the adverse effects, which may be quite disabling. Combined with the as yet unrelieved depression this may lead to non-compliance.

Antidepressants should not be withdrawn too quickly to avoid a discontinuation syndrome with mild mixed gastrointestinal and central effects. After 8 weeks or more of therapy, dosage should be tailed off over at least 4 weeks. These effects do not indicate dependence, which does not occur, but are probably due to receptor sensitivity changes.

SSRIs

Indications. The main advantages of 5HT specificity are the absence of many of the troublesome adverse effects, toxicity and overdose problems associated with the older, less selective agents. Early hopes that they might be more effective or faster acting have not been realized. They are used for the same purposes as the tricyclics but at present are considerably more expensive. Their use is justified in several situations:

- Risk of suicide, because of their relative safety in over-dosage.
- Poor compliance owing to tricyclic adverse effects.
- In the elderly, who suffer more from tricyclic adverse effects.

Table 7.12 Advantages of second and third generation cyclic antidepressants and SSRIs compared with amitriptyline[a]

Drug	Less sedative	Less anti-cholinergic	Less cardiotoxic	Less convulsant	Less weight gain
Second and third generation cyclics					
Amoxapine	(+)	–	(+)	–	–
Dosulepin (dothiepin)	–	(+)	–	–	–
Doxepin	–	+	–	–	–
Lofepramine	+	(+)	+	–	–
Maprotilene	+	(+)	–	–	–
Mianserin	–	(+)	+	+	–
Mirtazepine	–	+	–	–	–
Nefazodone	+	+	–	–	–
Reboxetine	+	(+)	+	–	+
Trazodone	–	(+)	+	–	+
Venlafaxine	+	+	(+)	+	+
Viloxazine	+	+	+	+	+
Selective serotonin re-uptake inhibitors					
Citalopram	+	+	+	+	+
Fluoxetine	+	+	+	+	+
Fluvoxamine	(+)	(+)	+	+	+
Paroxetine[b]	+	+	+	+	–
Sertraline	+	+	+	+	–

[a] Sources differ on the extent of the effects cited. The evaluations are given for qualitative comparison only.

[b] More likely to cause extrapyramidal symptoms than other SSRIs.

SSRI, selective serotonin re-uptake inhibitor.

+, significant improvement; (+), moderate improvement; –, no improvement.

- When tricyclics are specifically contraindicated (see above).

However, even if an older tricyclic cannot be used, one of the newer cyclics may still be suitable (Table 7.12).

Pharmacokinetics. The SSRIs have broadly similar kinetic properties to the tricyclics, but are less likely to have active metabolites.

Side effects. SSRIs have a quite different profile from the tricyclics (Table 7.12). Most important is the almost complete absence of anticholinergic, cardiotoxic and convulsant properties; and there may be weight loss as opposed to weight gain. Psychomotor impairment is less. However, withdrawal phenomena, hyponatraemia, activation of mania and occasional extrapyramidal symptoms still occur.

The main problems are gastrointestinal and central. Nausea, diarrhoea and constipation are common and may be intolerable. Less common is CNS stimulation, occurring as anxiety, agitation, restlessness, headache or confusion. In general (i.e. apart from specific contraindications) the SSRIs are tolerated better than tricyclic antidepressants, as measured by dropout due to adverse effects; about one-third more patients cease tricyclic therapy.

Toxic effects and overdose. Another significant advantage of this group is the absence of serious cardiotoxic or convulsant actions in overdose. Thus they are much safer then tricyclics, although some newer cyclic antidepressants are also safer than original tricyclics (Table 7.12). It must also be remembered that SSRIs offer no greater protection from suicide by other means. Rarely, SSRIs may cause the 'serotonin syndrome', especially when interacting with other antidepressants. This is due to the liberation of excessive 5HT, causing CNS stimulation that results in restlessness and hyperthermia. The syndrome is usually mild, but may prove fatal; it usually responds to discontinuation of SSRIs if they are not tolerated, and in severe cases the 5HT blocker *cyproheptadine* can be used as an antidote.

Contraindications, cautions, interactions. Serotonin selectivity means these agents can be used in many situations when tricyclics are contraindicated. However, care is still needed in heart disease and epilepsy. Suitable washout periods (usually several weeks) must be observed when changing to other types of antidepressant, especially MAOIs, in order to avoid serious interactions.

Dosage and administration. Most SSRIs can be given once daily. The dose–response curve rapidly plateaus above the usual effective (and tolerable) dose. Therefore full doses can often be started at once (perhaps originally fostering the impression of more rapid onset of activity). However, withdrawal should still be staged over 2–4 weeks to avoid discontinuation symptoms.

Monoamine oxidase inhibitors (MAOI)

Indications. Frequent and hazardous dietary and drug interactions have always limited the use of MAOIs, especially in general practice. They may be of value in depression associated with atypical features characteristic of anxiety-neurosis (especially phobia or panic disorder), but they are not usually effective when used alone in severe depression. Their main role is as adjuncts or second- or third-line drugs in resistant disease. Their sometimes claimed superiority in mild depression is almost superfluous in the primary care environment where much of this disorder is treated, because their use should only be managed by clinicians experienced in their use. Moreover, dietary compliance is easier to ensure in hospital.

Side effects and toxicity. The range of mild to moderate adverse effects is very wide, and the potential toxic effects of MAOIs are serious. Many central, cardiovascular and gastrointestinal autonomic disturbances occur in normal use, especially anticholinergic and anti-adrenergic effects. Although interactions cause hypertension, adverse effects frequently involve postural hypotension. Peripheral oedema is also common. CNS stimulation and activation of mania can occur. Overdose with MAOIs (except *tranylcypromine*) is somewhat easier to manage than with tricyclics because specific alpha-adrenergic blockers (e.g. *phentolamine*) can be used.

Interactions. Normally, dietary tyramine is metabolized by MAO in the gut wall. Inhibition of MAO allows high levels of tyramine to be absorbed, causing widespread release of noradrenaline (norepinephrine) from nerve fibres, with predictable hypertensive cardiovascular consequences. Interacting prescription medication (e.g. cyclic antidepressants, CNS sedatives, opiate analgesics) can usually be avoided by professional vigilance. Greater potential problems arise with OTC preparations containing sympathomimetics (e.g. decongestants) and tyramine-containing foods (especially cheese, pickled meats or meat extracts, fava beans), which is why patient counselling and warning cards are so important. *Tranylcypromine*, the most stimulant MAOI, seems to be the worst offender (especially if combined with *clomipramine*); *phenelzine* is relatively sedating. Fatalities are still reported and MAOIs are likely to remain little used.

Because MAOIs cause irreversible enzyme inhibition, recovery of enzyme functions following cessation of therapy does not start for several days and may take several weeks to return to normal. Changing from an MAOI to a tricyclic requires at least a 2-week interval, but the reverse can be done safely after a week, though some SSRIs require longer.

Sometimes a tricyclic/MAOI combination is indicated, in which case a sedative tricyclic with a less stimulant MAOI (e.g. *amitriptyline* with *phenelzine*) is usually safe if managed by experienced psychiatrists. *Tranylcypromine* is the most dangerous in combination.

Other antidepressants

Moclobemide causes reversible inhibition of MAO type A (RIMA). This has two principal advantages: enzyme function is restored promptly following drug cessation, allowing quicker and safer switching to other antidepressants; and tyramine metabolism is little inhibited, so the patient is relatively free from dietary restrictions. It also has few of the autonomic adverse effects of the non-selective MAOIs and appears to be equally effective as the cyclics, particularly for retarded depression. However, it has not yet found its place in treatment protocols.

Tryptophan, a 5HT precursor, has proved disappointing considering the strong suspicion of a 5HT disturbance in some forms of depression. It is occasionally used as an adjuvant. Owing to an association with eosinophilia–myalgia syndrome, each case of its use has to be registered and monitored. *Lithium* and its use are discussed on pp. 421–422.

Treatment strategy and drug selection

The strategy for the drug treatment of depression involves the following stages (Fig. 7.9):

- Select the most **suitable** drug.
- Start **acute** treatment as **soon** as possible at **full recommended doses**.

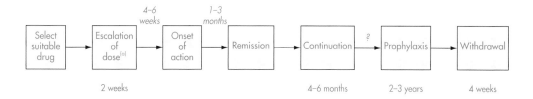

Figure 7.9 Phases in drug treatment of chronic depression. [a]Not needed with selective serotonin re-uptake inhibitor.

- **Continue** therapy and ensure **compliance** for 6 months after symptoms first respond.
- Consider up to 3 years **prophylaxis** if recurrent pattern.
- **Withdraw** slowly.

In deciding whether or not to treat an episode of primary depression, the criteria are the severity of depression and the patient's ability to cope. Whether or not the low mood is considered an appropriate reaction to an adverse event is not important. Moreover, prompt treatment reduces the length of the episode and the likelihood of recurrence. The use of full doses for 4–6 months after symptoms have subsided or remitted is essential to prevent relapse. Unfortunately, non-compliance is common once the patient has improved, especially if adverse effects are still troublesome.

Where there is a history of depressive episodes up to 3 years prophylactic therapy has been shown to limit recurrence. Although the best prophylactic dose level is not known, lower doses tend to be used than for acute therapy.

Drug selection depends on a variety of specific patient or disease factors, most of which are related to tolerance or contraindications (Table 7.13). Cyclic agents are usually first line unless non-drug therapy is indicated. For economic reasons older cyclics should be the first choice for all patients who can tolerate them and for whom they are not contraindicated. In many patients and situations the older agents are inappropriate, but even then it is not always necessary immediately to choose the more expensive SSRIs. The possibility of using a relatively cheap second-generation cyclic should always be considered, as one of these may be found that avoids the particular adverse effect or precaution limiting the use of the standard drugs in a given patient.

Mild/minor depression

Antidepressant medication is not always necessary for an isolated episode of mild depression associated with an adverse life event: psychotherapy is the first choice. If drugs are needed, treatment can be stopped when the patient

---

Table 7.13 First-line therapy in depression – special considerations

Situation/factor	Possible therapy[a]	Rationale
Mild symptoms	Consider psychotherapy	Drugs often ineffective
Mild – atypical symptoms	MAOI	
Severe – possibly suicidal	*Lofepramine, trazodone, mianserin,* SSRI	Less toxic in overdose
	ECT	ECT rapid
Severe – psychotic	Neuroleptic[b]; ECT	Antipsychotic and antidepressant
Elderly, CVS disease	*Lofepramine, venlafaxine,* SSRI	Less adverse effects, especially on CVS (arrhythmia, hypotension)
Cannot tolerate anti-cholinergic side effects	*Doxepin, mianserin,* SSRI	Less anti-cholinergic
Cannot tolerate sedation	*Lofepramine,* SSRI	Less sedative
Epilepsy	SSRI, *trazodone*	Less convulsant
Retarded	*Protriptyline*	Stimulant
Agitated, anxious, insomnia	*Amitriptyline, dosulepin* (*dothiepin*) Short-course *benzodiazepine*	Sedative
Recurrent bipolar	Initiate *lithium* therapy	*See* p. 421
Resistant	*See* Fig. 7.10	

[a] Only a few examples of possible drugs are cited in each case; see text and Fig. 7.15 for details.

[b] Caution needed combining neuroleptic (p. 430) with antidepressant and/or ECT.

CVS, cardiovascular system; ECT, electroconvulsive therapy; MAOI, monoamine oxidase inhibitor; SSRI, selective serotonin re-uptake inhibitor.

recovers; continuation and prophylactic therapy are not usually indicated. It is frequently claimed that MAOIs are more effective than cyclics, especially if there are atypical features such as anxiety, phobia, anger, hypochondria or increased appetite and sleep. However, their precautions limit their use and cyclics are most commonly tried first by non-psychiatrist clinicians.

For patients with anxiety, initial insomnia or mixed anxiety and depression short courses of anxiolytics or short-acting hypnotics are sometimes used. However, sedative antidepressants (e.g. *amitriptyline*) are preferable, given in the evening if needed for sleep problems.

Severe depression

Drug therapy is almost always necessary in severe, endogenous or psychotic depression, possibly preceded by a course of ECT. Cyclics or SSRIs seem to be the most effective, with MAOIs as second-line agents.

Patients suffering from psychotic symptoms, especially hallucinations, may benefit from a short course of a neuroleptic such as *haloperidol*. *Amoxapine* and thioxanthenes (e.g. *flupentixol*) have both been recommended because they have mixed antidepressant and sedative–antipsychotic–neuroleptic actions. In the case of the former, these effects are due to the metabolite *loxapine*. There is little evidence to support these uses.

Where suicide is a suspected risk, less toxic agents are preferable, including those with a lower convulsant potential, dispensed in small quantities. ECT is also used.

Contraindications or intolerance of adverse effects such as anticholinergic effects or sedation can usually be circumvented by judicious drug selection (*see* Table 7.13). If there evidence of a recurrent pattern, *lithium* therapy may be considered. If the pattern is recurrent unipolar, lithium may be as effective as tricyclics, but the need for plasma-level monitoring is inconvenient. However, lithium is the drug of choice in bipolar illness (with manic phases).

Resistant depression

For the minority of patients who do not improve after 6–8 weeks on optimal doses of a cyclic antidepressant, measuring the drug plasma level might first be considered to check for possible compliance problems or abnormal drug handling. Otherwise, changing to another antidepressant which acts in a different manner, such as from a noradrenaline (norepinephrine) to a serotonin re-uptake inhibitor, may help. A course of ECT could be considered. Thereafter, a variety of combinations are employed by psychiatrists, the only logical basis of which is that components have empirically different modes of action (Fig. 7.10). Adding *lithium* to other antidepressants (lithium augmentation) seems particularly successful. *Levothyroxine* (*thyroxine*) augmentation is also used, presumably on the basis that hypothyroidism is often associated with depression. Addition of a short course of steroids (e.g. *dexamethasone* 3 mg/day for 4 days) is sometimes used. Use of these combinations usually requires close monitoring and careful selection of agent and dose, and is too specialized to consider here.

Mania and manic-depressive disorder

Mania

Mania is a severe, usually recurrent, psychotic affective disorder that is almost the precise opposite of severe depression, although about one-tenth as common. There is an abnormally elevated mood – **euphoria** rather than dysphoria – unwarranted optimism, exuberance, overconfidence, inflated self-esteem, hyperactivity of thought and action, excessive libido, and little sleep. The patient has increased drive and is outgoing, but often socially tactless. The overconfidence is similar to that experienced by otherwise normal individuals during the usually pleasurable sensations of early alcoholic inebriation. In the same way, patients enjoy their episodes of mania, when they also often feel more creative, thus making compliance with treatment a problem.

A full-blown **manic** attack usually lasts no more than a few days, during which the patient sleeps little but appears to have boundless energy. **Hypomania** is more usual, where symptoms are less florid. Sufferers may require com-

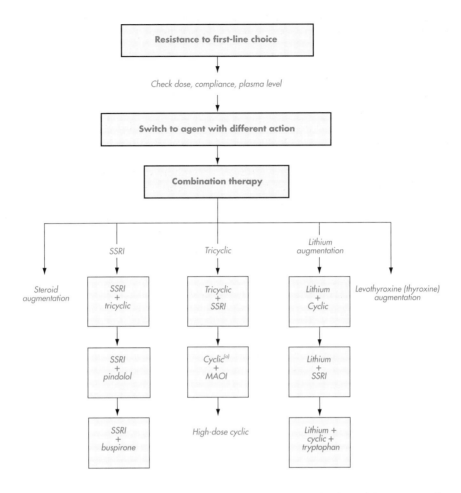

Figure 7.10   Some treatment options in resistant depression. MAOI, monoamine oxidase inhibitor; SSRI, selective serotonin re-uptake inhibitor. [a]Cyclic, tricyclic or second generation cyclic.

pulsory admission to hospital, although others manage to function adequately in the community. At the other end of the spectrum an even milder form is seen as a personality trait in some individuals. Such an individual retains insight, and may be thought of as simply a flamboyant character, a tireless and exuberant go-getter, even a 'Don Juan' or a 'nymphomaniac'.

Attacks are extremely disruptive socially, domestically and financially, because overconfidence causes patients to undertake wildly ambitious commitments. Patients discover when they finally 'come down' that they are hopelessly over-committed, double-booked and in serious debt.

The accelerated mental processes produce a short attention span, **flight of ideas** and **pressure of speech** as the patient jumps rapidly from subject to subject on apparently irrational grounds, such as a rhyme or puns (the 'clang association'). The mood too may suddenly change from euphoria to irritability and aggressiveness. The patient may thus appear quite incoherent, and the apparent thought disorder and delusions are not easily distinguished from acute schizophrenia. The differential diagnosis depends on whether mood disturbance or thought disorder predominates. An illness with elements of both is known as **schizoaffective disorder**. Clearly the lay term 'maniac' is related, but manic patients are no more criminal or violent than the general population.

Psychotic features such as lack of insight and delusions of grandeur, the counterpart of the depressive's delusions of worthlessness, are common during attacks, but the patient may seen quite normal and rational between them. Attacks rarely last more than a few weeks before the attention that patients draw to themselves means they are soon treated, although often involuntarily. Otherwise the patient would become exhausted. Mood returns to normal after a few months of therapy.

Manic-depressive disorder

Most patients experiencing mania also have episodes of severe depression, although the frequency, sequence and duration of mood swings vary enormously between patients. Depressive phases usually last longer than manic ones and are less obvious, and there are variable periods of normality between extreme swings. Mood swings can be quite abrupt, although manic phases tend to have a more rapid onset. 'Rapid cycling' is when there are four or more swings per year. Fluctuations become more frequent, and more frequently depressive rather than manic, as the patient ages.

Where the symptoms are serious or psychotic, the terms **manic-depressive** or **bipolar affective disorder** are used. An otherwise normal person with moderately exaggerated mood swings may be described as having a **cyclothymic** personality, which is not a psychotic illness.

Aetiology and pathology

Major depression, mania and manic-depressive disorder may have similar aetiologies. The underlying abnormality could be in the regulation of emotional responses by the limbic system, involving monoamine neurotransmitters. This hypothesis is supported by the prophylactic effectiveness of the single agent lithium in all three. In mania, however, cyclic antidepressants, SSRIs and MAOIs are not just ineffective but actually dangerous because they can trigger an exaggerated upswing from depression to mania.

As with severe recurrent depression, mania is a genetically linked, chronic but generally non-progressive disease. External triggers for attacks may sometimes be found in stressful life events but equally, as with some severe episodes of depression, there may be no apparent cause. There is usually a family history and the concordance rate in twins is over 70%.

Management

The aims of management are:

* To control acute manic or hypomanic attacks.
* To minimize recurrence and intensity of mood swings with prophylactic therapy.

The drug of choice in acute mania and in the prophylaxis of recurrent mania or bipolar disorder is *lithium*. However, in severe manic attacks initial sedation will be required to cover the 7–10 days while lithium takes effect. Either *neuroleptics* or *benzodiazepines* are indicated, depending on the presence or absence of psychotic features, e.g. loss of insight, grandiose delusions. Patients may need compulsory admission and treatment if they are a risk to themselves or others. ECT is an alternative to lithium in the acute phase.

If the patient is already taking lithium the plasma level must be checked: often patients will deliberately stop, either because of adverse effects or deliberately to induce mania. (This is an interesting inversion of recreational drug misuse, which more usually involves *taking* something to get high, rather than *avoiding* it.) Otherwise, lithium therapy is started.

If the patient demonstrates an alternating pattern (bipolar disorder) or a recurrent pattern, which is more common with mania than depression, they must be assessed for maintenance lithium therapy. This is a potentially lifelong commitment, and regular follow-up is essential to monitor both compliance and toxicity. As patients age, they will be more likely to start requiring drugs that potentially will interact with lithium (e.g. diuretics), so regular re-assessment is essential. Theoretically, long-term neuroleptics could be used, but they are usually avoided because of adverse effects. Once a patient is stabilized social and psychotherapeutic interventions should be introduced.

Not all patients respond to either of these traditional treatments, and a number of other approaches have become established as second-line alternatives (Table 7.14). The most promising are anticonvulsant drugs such as *carbamazepine* and *valproate*. These drugs may be more effective in rapid cyclers, or in those who fail to respond to lithium. More recently *gabapentin* and *lamotrigine* have been used; the calcium blockers *verapamil* and *nimodipine* also appear to have an anti-manic effect.

Lithium

Indications.   Lithium is an enigmatic drug. A monovalent cation seems an unlikely candidate for the stabilization of major affective disturbances, yet for single episodes its antidepressant action is similar to amitriptyline in potency and onset. However, the real value of lithium lies in the maintenance prophylaxis of recurrent unipolar or bipolar affective disorder. Here it is a safer and perhaps more effective proposition than the cyclics or SSRIs, and safer than neuroleptics or benzodiazepines, despite the need for regular plasma level monitoring.

Lithium treatment should be considered if there is evidence of recurrent episodes, either of severe depression or mania. Lithium will either abolish mood swings, or reduce their frequency, duration and intensity. A few patients complain that it produces a flattening of normal mood (blunting of affect), and manic patients may comply poorly because they value or enjoy some aspects of their attacks of (hypo)mania. Some believe themselves to be more creative in that state.

Dosage and side effects.   Lithium therapy is managed by monitoring the serum level. For acute attacks, up to 1.2–1.5 mmol/L may be needed initially. For prophylaxis, the goal is to maintain a plasma level within the narrow therapeutic window (0.4–1.0 mmol/L); in many patients control is obtained below 0.8 mmol/L.

Dosage should aim to maintain a stable plasma level throughout the day because **acute adverse effects**, such as nausea, polyuria, polydipsia and fine tremor, seem to be related to post-dose peak levels (Table 7.15). Thus, frequent daily doses or modified-release preparations are preferred. The formulation that a patient uses should not be changed needlessly. Many minor adverse effects remit on prolonged use.

Plasma levels of lithium above about 1.5 mmol/L produce **warning signs of toxicity** including diarrhoea and vomiting, coarsening of the tremor and CNS depression. Sustained **toxic** levels above 2.5 mmol/L cause hypotension, convulsions and coma; in such circumstances dialysis may be needed to bring about sufficiently rapid reversal. There are a number of lesser chronic effects, including hypothyroidism. The significance of long-term kidney changes remains controversial. Renal and thyroid function tests are recommended before commencing lithium therapy, and regularly thereafter.

Withdrawal of lithium, if it become necessary, needs to be gradual, staged over at least 2 weeks. Rebound hypomanic symptoms are sometimes noted.

Table 7.14   Alternatives to lithium in mania and manic-depressive disorder

Acute manic phase	Maintenance treatment of unipolar mania or bipolar disorder
Neuroleptics	Carbamazepine
Carbamazepine	Sodium valproate
Sodium valproate	Neuroleptic
Calcium channel blocker (e.g. *verapamil*)	

Table 7.15   Principal side effects and toxicity of lithium, in relation to steady-state plasma level

	Minor/reversible (therapeutic range: 0.4–1 mmol/L)	Early signs of toxicity (1.5–2.5 mmol/L)	Toxicity (>2.5 mmol/L)
Gastrointestinal	Dyspepsia	Anorexia Nausea and vomiting Diarrhoea	
CVS	Benign ECG changes	Hypotension, arrhythmia	Circulatory failure
Renal	Polyuria, polydipsia Oedema	Persistent polyuria	Acute: renal damage? Chronic: renal failure??
CNS and neuromuscular	Fine tremor, incoordination Muscle weakness	Coarse tremor, muscle weakness and twitch Lethargy, dysarthria Ataxia	Convulsions, coma Permanent neurological damage
Other	Non-myxoedemic goitre Neutrophilia Exacerbation of psoriasis	Hypothyroidism	Death

CNS, central nervous system; CVS, cardiovascular system.

Monitoring. Regular measurement of plasma lithium (12 h post dose) is essential, at first weekly until a stable level is obtained. Subsequently the interval may be increased up to 3- to 6-monthly in patients who understand the precautions. Extra measurement is indicated in suspected drug interaction or poor compliance, intercurrent illness, other circumstances which interfere with lithium level, or unexpected toxicity. Table 7.16 shows common circumstances which can interfere with lithium handling.

Pharmacokinetics and interactions. Lithium is distributed throughout body water, generally following the same pattern as sodium. This has lent support to body-water/electrolyte theories of affective disorder, but lithium has also been shown to affect monoamine levels and post-receptor intracellular signalling. It is cleared entirely by the kidney, which gives rise to many potential problems. Both fluid retention (e.g. dehydration, NSAIDs) and circumstances which cause increased renal sodium reabsorption (such as pyrexia, unaccustomed hot climate, electrolyte depletion, dehydration or diuretic therapy) tend to reduce lithium clearance and can cause dangerously high plasma levels. Patients must be warned about this, and those with renal or cardiovascular impairment need close attention. In pregnancy clearance is increased; however, lithium is moderately teratogenic and use in the first trimester will depend on the relative risks of withdrawal and continuation.

Despite these potential difficulties, lithium is a valuable drug. It has no anticholinergic or extrapyramidal effects, causes no amnesia, general CNS depression or psychomotor impairment, and has little effect on normal mood. Thus it has advantages over the other treatments available for depression or mania, although it is no less toxic in overdose than conventional antidepressants or neuroleptics. Diligent monitoring has enabled patients to take lithium for decades with little ill effect.

Schizophrenia

Schizophrenia is a much misunderstood disease. It has nothing to do with a so-called split personality. In schizophrenia, the split is between different components of the same personality – between mood and action, or behaviour and

Table 7.16   Circumstances enhancing lithium action or toxicity

Circumstances/concomitant drug therapy	Comment
Neuroleptics (especially *haloperidol*)	Accepted combination, but use caution
Cyclic *antidepressants* and *SSRIs*	Common combination. May trigger mania; enhanced toxicity (especially SSRIs)
ECT	
Increased renal **sodium** or **fluid** retention, caused by, e.g.: • renal impairment • dehydration • unusually hot climate • excessive perspiration • pyrexia • vomiting, diarrhoea • sodium depletion • low-salt diet • NSAID • *diuretic* (especially *thiazide*) • ACEIs	Reduced lithium clearance or increased lithium reabsorption → raised serum lithium level

Only the main interactions are shown; consult a formulary.

ACEI, angiotensin converting enzyme inhibitor; NSAID, non-steroidal anti-inflammatory drug.

belief, for example. The personality becomes fragmented or, literally, dis-integrated. (A very rare, genuine split personality disorder is known. More properly called dissociative disorder or multiple personality, in this extraordinary condition a person alternates between two or more usually completely integrated, rational personalities.) A more subtle solecism is the use of 'schizophrenic' as a synonym for ambivalent.

Although schizophrenia is generally what the lay public understands by madness, the popular idea that every 'mad axeman' has schizophrenia is wrong. Patients with schizophrenia are no more violent than the population as a whole. Violent criminals may be suffering from a 'psychopathic personality', a condition quite distinct from schizophrenia.

The experience of schizophrenia

It must not be assumed that people with schizophrenia, being psychotic and thus out of touch with reality and lacking insight, do not suffer from their disease: they do. There are lucid periods (possibly following treatment) during which they have sufficient insight to remember their experiences when acutely ill. Many patients give a strong impression of perplexity and bewilderment. They are convinced of the truth of their own reality and cannot reconcile this with the reaction this causes in others.

It is probably the most difficult mental illness to understand because the experience of sufferers is very remote from normal. It has been likened to that twilight world between sleep and waking, when the distinction between illusion and reality is blurred. Schizophrenic patients also have difficulty distinguishing between themselves and the outside world. While for most of us dreaming, thinking, saying and hearing are categorically distinct phenomena, in schizophrenia the distinctions are blurred. Consequently, patients may feel irrational external influences on their thoughts, or that their thoughts are available for all the world to read. This loss of the ultimate privacy – that of our thoughts – is possibly what makes schizophrenia so miserable and confusing for the sufferer.

Aetiology and pathology

Schizophrenia is a common condition: about 1% of the population are likely to have at least one episode during their life, although not all of these people will become permanently ill. Nevertheless, schizophrenia accounts for the majority of patients in continual psychiatric care. The condition has a uniform global prevalence. The apparent increased prevalence among lower socioeconomic groups is attributed to the 'downward social drift' of sufferers.

The causes of schizophrenia are unknown. Both genetic predisposition and environmental factors are important, as has been confirmed by studies on twins borne to schizophrenic parents. Among the **biological** causes suggested are autoimmune or viral encephalitis, abnormally large brain ventricles (i.e. reduced brain size), or imbalance between the right and left hemispheres. Recently, research has focused on neurodevelopmental abnormalities arising at a very early age. Another avenue utilizes new non-invasive imaging techniques, such as positron emission tomography (PET) and magnetic resonance imaging (MRI), which can be used to visualize the living brain and monitor changes in its activity with far greater precision than the relatively crude electroencephalogram (EEG). It is still unknown whether there are a structural abnormalities in various brain centres or defective interconnections between key centres.

Functional theories involve ideas of incomplete adjustment to society, especially the family. The 'antipsychiatrists' suggest, on the other hand, that schizophrenia is a response to an irrational, contradictory or hostile world.

The classical symptoms of inappropriate mood, delusions and hallucinations imply involvement of the limbic system, which is concerned with emotional responses and beliefs, and the ascending reticular system, concerned with monitoring and filtering of perceptions. On the other hand, the negative symptoms typical of chronic schizophrenia may involve lesions of frontal lobe cortical areas.

The predominant biochemical abnormality seems to be functional over-activity of dopaminergic pathways between midbrain and certain cortical areas (mesolimbic and mesocortical tracts). This is compatible with the known dopamine-blocking action of most antipsychotic drugs. Whether dopamine excess is a cause or an incidental consequence has not been established, and uncertainty remains about the relative roles of dopamine DA_1, DA_2 and DA_{3-6} receptors. Post-mortem studies on the brains of schizophrenic patients cannot distinguish the effects of chronic disease from those of many years of neuroleptic therapy.

Thus, the management of schizophrenia remains essentially symptomatic: relieve the patient's suffering, perhaps slow the progression, and help the patient to cope. As yet nothing can be done to reverse the disease process, nor is prevention possible.

Clinical features

Psychotic signs

The classification and symptomatology of schizophrenia are complex and have been endlessly debated among psychiatrists. Recently, WHO and the American Psychiatric Association have rationalized and harmonized diagnostic criteria. Table 7.17 describes the common signs in terms of normal brain functions. All are descriptive psychiatric signs; there are no objective physical, biochemical or metabolic signs.

The defining features of schizophrenia are thought disorder and delusions. Many patients have very strange ideas and make bizarre associations, sometimes inventing their own language (neologism) or using common words in an inappropriate way: "I'm in hospital because of my minarets". Some have elaborate paranoid delusions: everybody is spying on them or plotting against them, including relatives, neighbours, and governments East, West and even extraterrestrial. They may also hallucinate, hearing the voices of their tormentors talking about them, or they see their own name in newspapers or on television (ideas of reference). No wonder they are so miserable.

Patients may believe their actions are controlled by others – among patients from Western countries often by means of invisible rays, magnets or electric wires. They may hear on the radio

Table 7.17   Clinical features of schizophrenia[a]

Positive features (Type 1)	
Thought	**Distorted or irrational reasoning, reduced insight**
	Loosened associations, illogical cause–effect links
	Private language
Belief	Delusions
	• persecution (paranoia)
	• **external control (passivity)**
	• **thought broadcast**
	• **thought insertion**
	• grandeur
	Ideas of reference
	Delusional perception[b]
	Derealisation, depersonalization[c]
Perception	Hallucinations
	• **usually auditory**[d]
	• also visual
	• less common: tactile, gustatory, olfactory
Mood	Inappropriate emotional responses
Behaviour	Bizarre, irrational; occasionally aggressive, rarely violent

Negative features (Type 2)	
Mood	Blunting (flattening) of affect
Behaviour	Withdrawn, antisocial, apathetic, poor self-care
	Poverty of speech, anhedonia, avolition

[a] First rank symptoms (usually Type 1) are in bold.

[b] Special personal significance attributed to everyday phenomena ('primary delusion').

[c] Feeling of distancing from external world or from self, others or own emotions.

[d] First rank if voices heard referring to patient in third person, or echoing his/her thoughts.

an echo of what they have just thought, or feel that they have foreign ideas inserted into their brain. Often their emotional responses are fatuous or inappropriate (laughing or crying at the socially incorrect time); in others mood variation is generally reduced. The combination of all these features produces the markedly unusual behaviour popularly known as 'madness'.

There is often an almost tragic consistency about a patient's symptom complex. Their delusions reflect their hallucinations, or their hallucinations confirm their delusions; both appear to escape the logical censorship provided by fully functional insight. However bizarre, their behaviour may be consistent with their misreading of reality. Someone who believed that thoughts were constantly put into their head against their

will might well believe there was a plot against them, especially if they heard voices apparently confirming this. Their reaction might well be aggressive behaviour, or shouting out loud to tell the persons whose voices they heard to go away. The novels of Franz Kafka give us some inkling of the terror of paranoia.

Classification

Two broad syndromes are recognized (Table 7.17). Patients in the early acute stages have **Type 1** (classical or florid) schizophrenia with **positive** symptoms. Loosely, these resemble disinihibited exaggerations of normal activity. **Type 2** features, usually seen in chronic schizophrenia, are predominantly **negative**, such as flat mood, apathy, social withdrawal, lack of speech (alogia), pleasure (anhedonia) or initiative (avolition) are seen. These represent functions found in normal persons but absent in schizophrenia.

Type 2 features may represent long-term deterioration of chronic disease, ' burnt out' disease or possibly the consequence of long-term neuroleptic use. However, careful history taking will often reveal forerunners of these negative traits in early life, e.g. the withdrawn lonely child. At onset they are masked by the florid positive features but once the latter are under pharmacological control the former, less affected by drugs, emerge as the predominant signs of illness (Fig. 7.11).

Diagnosis

It is first necessary to eliminate any primary underlying cause such as iatrogenic psychosis (e.g. corticosteroids), drug misuse (e.g. amphetamines), brain tumour or infection, head injury, certain rare forms of epilepsy, hyperthyroidism, etc. The symptoms must have been continuously present for at least a month, and usually with evidence of deteriorating social functioning (work, family, friends, etc.).

Distinguishing between borderline schizophrenia and other psychoses (mania, depression) can sometimes be difficult. It is also important to recognize that delusions are defined as clearly ill founded but implacably held beliefs, not amenable to reasoned persuasion and completely at variance with the patient's religious, social or ethnic context. Traditionally the presence of at least two symptoms from the list given in Table 7.17, or just one first-rank symptom (positive symptoms, mostly specific forms of delusion) was needed to confirm schizophrenia. Type I patients usually show several florid positive symptoms and the diagnosis is clear.

In chronic schizophrenia, symptoms are predominantly negative and these are more difficult to diagnose and to treat. Moreover they must be distinguished from iatrogenic over-sedation or extrapyramidal effects, clinical depression or 'institutionalization' (i.e. the dependency and apathy which can result from long-term hospital care). The latest editions of both DSM-IV and ICD-10 also include negative symptoms as primary diagnostic criteria.

In different cultures and times the symptoms take different outward forms, but the overall pattern and prevalence are consistent. Nowadays the persecutors of paranoid patients are Martians or secret government spies, who control them with lasers or magnetism. In mediaeval Europe, and present day pre-industrial societies, devils or evil spirits using witchcraft or curses are to blame. This is one disease for which the stress of modern industrial society cannot be held responsible.

Course

The old medical Latin name for schizophrenia was *dementia praecox* (loosely, the madness of youth) because the most common time of onset is late adolescence or early adulthood. There may be a sudden deterioration (one form of 'nervous breakdown', the generic lay term for the acute onset of any psychiatric condition). However, this will usually have been preceded by a gradual reduction in social, academic or work-related functioning, loss of friends, deterioration in personal hygiene or other behaviour uncharacteristic of the patient's former personality.

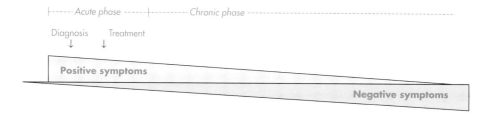

Figure 7.11   Typical course of chronic schizophrenia, showing change in type of symptoms.

About 25% of patients will suffer just a single episode, then recover and lead normal lives. Good prognostic signs are:

- The absence of a family history of schizophrenia.
- Stable premorbid personality.
- Acute onset.
- Preservation of emotional responses, initiative and coherent personality.
- Early recognition and treatment.

Conversely a poor outlook is indicated by:

- Positive family history.
- Disturbed, eccentric, antisocial or withdrawn premorbid personality.
- Difficulty in forming relationships.
- Disrupted domestic situation and poor social adjustment.
- Insidious onset.
- Loss of affect, initiative and drive.
- Delay in treatment.

About two-thirds of sufferers become chronically ill or suffer frequent relapses, and tend to develop Type 2 features. They have great difficulty forming relationships, do not marry, cannot keep jobs and drop out of education. Without treatment, follow-up and social or family support they drift down the social scale, becoming progressively more involved in vagrancy, petty crime, illicit drug use and alcoholism. Some 10% of all patients need long-term hospital care. The same proportion commit suicide.

Between these extremes are those who adjust to their disability and manage to cope in the community, while perhaps seeming just a trifle eccentric. The importance of social and family support is emphasized by the fact that the prognosis for patients in developing countries, with their extended families and perhaps greater tolerance of eccentricity and non-conformity, is better than in the developed world. Even in the UK, for example, many folk who are obviously quite 'mad', but harmless and able to look after themselves (after a fashion), are free to roam the streets.

Management

Drugs, psychotherapy and social interventions all have a place in the management of schizophrenia. Most patients are managed by a combination of family or community care with occasional hospital admission, supported by maintenance anti-psychotic drug therapy. Nowadays, few schizophrenic patients need permanent institutional care.

Before the discovery of chlorpromazine in the early 1950s, however, things were very different. Little could be done for persons with severe mental illness, if help was offered at all. There was only heavy sedation with barbiturates or, before them, bromides and straitjackets. Community care was unheard of: the idea was to keep 'maniacs' as far from 'normal' people as possible.

In the UK in the 19th century, the enlightened Victorians built asylums. Not then a pejorative term, asylum implied protection rather than imprisonment and neglect. In these enormous rambling institutions built at a safe distance outside the big cities, custodial care may have been the ethos but sedatives, locked doors, spiked walls and padded rooms were still the means (Fig. 7.12).

Aims

The aims in managing schizophrenia are:

- To control acute attacks and prevent self harm or harm to others.
- To attend to social and domestic factors.
- To rehabilitate the patient if possible.
- To start long-term support and maintenance therapy as appropriate.

Acute attack

An acutely psychotic patient is likely to be deluded, hallucinating, incomprehensible and quite without insight. The immediate objective is to control these features and to prevent the patient committing any mischief while his or her grasp of reality is impaired. In the UK, a section of the Mental Health Act allows compulsory admission to hospital for essential physical treatments in such circumstances, when the patient is likely to be a danger to him or herself or others (a process known colloquially as 'sectioning').

Day attendants must always have their keys attached to their person by the chain and belt provided...they are required to lock every door through which they pass.

...the patients are not to be permitted to sit or lie down on the floor or crouch in corners ...

...the patients must not be allowed to damage the shrubs and trees. Those having morbid appetites must be prevented from eating leaves, rubbish, etc.

...knives and forks must be counted and locked up in the proper box...under no circumstances must any patient be permitted to use the carving knife.

...all brooms, buckets, fire-irons, especially anything that may be used as a weapon of offence, must be kept clean, locked up, and placed in the cupboard set apart for the purpose.

Figure 7.12 Extracts from *Rules for the Guidance of the Attendants, Servants and all Persons Engaged in the Service of the Cornwall County Asylum at Bodmin*, 1900.

Prompt treatment at this stage improves the prognosis, and drug therapy is the only option. High doses of a sedating neuroleptic (antipsychotic) from one of the traditional or 'typical' groups is given, e.g. *chlorpromazine* 300 mg to 1 g daily or *haloperidol* up to 50 mg daily (lower doses if it is the first episode); a *benzodiazepine* may be added to a phenothiazine. At first, this may have to be administered parenterally to a reluctant patient, although the onset of action is hardly quicker and there is a much higher risk of serious acute extrapyramidal complications. In an aggressive patient *zuclopenthixol* (as acetate), in a relatively short-acting depot formulation, is effective once initial tranquillization is achieved.

Drug administration during this time is carefully supervised, and tranquillization and sedation are rapidly and reliably achieved. However, control of psychotic symptoms will not be evident for up to a month or so (Fig. 7.13) and full stabilization could take several months. If the patient does not respond in the first 1–2 months, some clinicians would advocate increasing the

dose; others would change to a different group for a further month. If extrapyramidal symptoms or other adverse effects are intolerable, or if there are specific contraindications, changing to an 'atypical' at this stage may be indicated; this would also be one of several possible strategies if the patient were treatment-resistant (p. 437).

Maintenance and prophylaxis

Patients who develop enduring disease need continuation therapy, either to suppress their symptoms (maintenance) or to prevent relapses (prophylaxis). The management of these patients has undergone a number of changes in recent decades.

The first was **changed social policy** which encouraged a reduction in the number of long-stay psychiatric hospital patients, many of them schizophrenic patients, and their return to the community. The inevitable lack of stimulation in long-stay hospitals is detrimental to recovery. Patients become institutionalized and incapable of independent existence, even if their disease eventually remits. Unfortunately, community services have not always been appropriately equipped or funded to care for this large increase in their dependent population. Only now is it realized that this process has been too thorough, as the discharged patients lose contact with the care services and become homeless, vagrant or imprisoned. In a very few cases – unfortunately those which attract most public attention – they have become dangerously violent. Second, the community care of these patients would not have been feasible without the development of long-acting depot forms of the antipsychotic drugs (p. 432).

However, recognition of the extent of tardive dyskinesia, a late-developing iatrogenic extrapyramidal syndrome (p. 436), is provoking a further re-assessment of the role of neuroleptic drugs in the long-term care of schizophrenia. The newer 'atypicals' have a lower propensity to cause this.

Duration of drug treatment

Once the acute phase of schizophrenia has been controlled, drug dosage can be gradually reduced. At least 12–24 months' maintenance

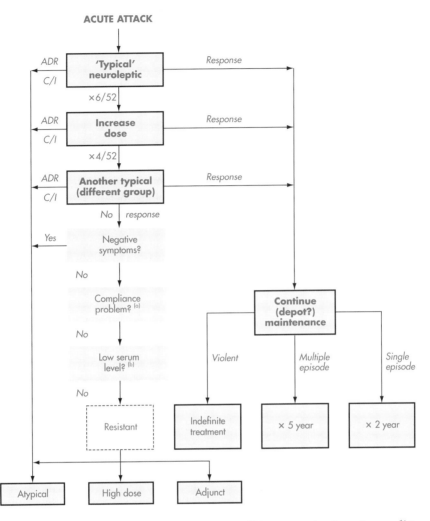

ACUTE ATTACK

Figure 7.13 A possible algorithm for treatment of schizophrenia. [a]If *yes*, consider depot therapy; [b]if *yes*, investigate possible drug interaction or other cause of abnormal kinetics. ADR, adverse drug reaction; C/I, contraindication.

treatment is needed after a single acute attack. Some 85% of patients will eventually relapse following a single attack, and how best to manage the patient prone to relapse is still debated. A patient who is a poor risk (violent, aggressive, never fully controlled) is still likely to be maintained on drugs indefinitely. For those who stay in remission for lengthy periods, attempts may be made to treat each acute attack aggressively, but gradually tail drugs off and stop them completely between attacks (targeted or intermittent therapy). Even so, an initial minimum 5-year maintenance period is recommended. There is a

relapse rate of about 15% per month on discontinuation, which is halved by prophylaxis, so a difficult judgement has to be made, in association with the patient and his or her carer.

Late initiation of treatment or continuation therapy for less than 3–5 years predisposes to more frequent, more severe, less easily treated relapses. However, the maintenance dose might be kept very low: oral doses as low as one-fifth the standard dose have been recommended, and depot injections might also allow reduced total drug doses. Drugs do little to alter the underlying disease process and may have insidious long-term effects on the brain; the spectre of tardive dyskinesia hangs over all maintenance neuroleptic therapy. Nevertheless, depot therapy has an invaluable place in the maintenance of many patients who would otherwise be unable to cope in the community.

Social and psychotherapy

Conventional psychotherapy is of little benefit in schizophrenia, and psychoanalysis even less so. Simple counselling however can help many patients to adjust to a chronic illness while remaining in the community. Coping-skills training, occupational therapy and hostel or 'halfway house' accommodation may be arranged. Family education and social therapy, where people in contact with the patient can be told what to expect and are encouraged to be supportive, can be very helpful in maintaining remission. Stormy home relationships and a lack of acceptance of the patient are the most common reasons for relapse, whereas a supportive home environment greatly reduces the chances of relapse.

Pharmacotherapy

Neuroleptic drugs

Pharmacodynamic action

The proprietary name *Largactil* was chosen for chlorpromazine, the original phenothiazine neuroleptic, rather prosaically because of its large number of actions. Its structural similarity to several natural neurotransmitter amines give it antagonist activity on cholinergic, histaminic, alpha-adrenergic, serotoninergic and dopaminergic receptors. Structural alterations during subsequent development have produced a number of groups of neuroleptics with varying receptor affinities, giving a range of adverse and therapeutic profiles (Tables 7.18 and 7.19).

Unfortunately, despite modern non-invasive imaging of the living brain, there is still much to learn about the relationship between receptor blockade, localization of CNS activity and antipsychotic action. One problem is that little is known of the inter-relationships and interdependencies between different receptor systems. For example, although most of the original antipsychotics are potent dopamine blockers, the newer ones preferentially target 5HT receptors. Could this be because one type of receptor is upstream or downstream of the other, with actions at either having a similar outcome? Again, the adrenergic alpha$_2$ activity shown by some agents could enhance dopaminergic transmission in the basal ganglia and thus moderate extrapyramidal adverse effects.

Among the original neuroleptics, antipsychotic action correlates well with blockade of the **dopamine** D$_2$ receptors assumed to be in the thalamus, limbic system and cortical projections of the ascending reticular formation. However, although the onset of antipsychotic action takes weeks, receptor blockade occurs within hours of starting therapy. A similar phenomenon is seen with antidepressants, and another similarity is that measurements of changes in the metabolite

---

Table 7.18 Pharmacodynamic actions of neuroleptic drugs

Receptor blocked	Therapeutic effect	Side effect
Dopamine	Antipsychotic, especially Type 1 (D$_2$)	Extrapyramidal symptoms (D$_{1,2}$?)
	Anti-emetic	Hypothalamic – ↑ prolactin (D$_5$?)
Acetylcholine (M$_1$)	Reduced extrapyramidal effects (sedative)	Antimuscarinic – various
Adrenaline	? Antipsychotic (α_2)	Sympatholytic (α_1) – hypotension
Histamine (H$_1$)	Antihistamine	
	Sedative	
Serotonin (5HT$_2$)	Antipsychotic	
	? ↓ Extrapyramidal symptoms	

Table 7.19 Comparison of therapeutic and side effects of main groups of neuroleptics in relation to principal receptor affinities

Chemical group	Example	Antipsychotic		Sedative	EPS	Side effects		
		DA_2[a]	$5HT_2$[a]	H_1	$DA_{1,2}$	Hypothalamic DA_1	Hypotensive α_1 Adr	Anticholinergic ACh
Simple phenothiazine[b]	Chlorpromazine	2	2	4	3	3	4	4
Piperidyl phenothiazine[b]	Thioridazine	3	2	3	1	4	3	4
Piperazinyl phenothiazine[b]	Trifluoperazine	4	1	3	4	3	2	2
Piperazinyl thioxanthene	Flupentixol	4	1	2	4	4	1	3
Butyrophenone	Haloperidol	4	1	4	4	4	1	2
Diphenylbutylpiperidine	Pimozide	4	0	0	3	4	2	0
Benzamide	Sulpiride	4	1	2	2	4	0	0
Dibenzazepine	Clozapine	4	4	4	0	2	2	4
Miscellaneous atypicals[c]	(Various)	1–3	4	0–3	0	2	0–3	1

Condensing inevitably entails considerable approximation, and the data are necessarily only for basic comparisons. Data compiled from various sources. Blocking potency: 0 none; 1 little; 2 moderate; 3 high; 4 very high.

[a] There may be up to five dopamine receptor subtypes, and many 5HT subtypes; both are simplified here.

[b] The three groups of phenothiazines are distinguished by different side chains on a common nucleus.

[c] Atypicals except the prototype, clozapine, are grouped together.

DA, dopamine; α_1 Adr, alpha-1 adrenergic; H_1, H_1 histamine; ACh, acetylcholine; $5HT_2$, 5-hydroxytryptamine$_2$; EPS, extrapyramidal symptoms.

of the presumed transmitter – homovanillic acid in the case of dopamine – do not correlate with clinical activity.

Dopamine blockade yields other useful actions (e.g. anti-emetic as with *prochlorperazine*) and many adverse ones, including extrapyramidal symptoms and endocrine (hypothalamic) actions. There are at least five subtypes of dopamine receptor, and research is attempting to differentiate these in terms of their anatomical location and clinical or adverse effect.

Actions at other receptors also have either therapeutic or adverse actions (*see* Table 7.18). **Anticholinergic** (antimuscarinic) action may reduce extrapyramidal symptoms (EPS); **antihistamine** action is sedative (exploited therapeutically as with *promethazine*); **adrenergic** blockade may cause postural hypotension; **serotonin** block has antipsychotic action.

Following the initial prolific development of the phenothiazines, other chemical structures have been developed (Table 7.19). These are usually more specific for dopamine D_2 receptors (e.g. *butyrophenones*) which appears to accentuate the antipsychotic clinical and extrapyramidal adverse actions, but reduces autonomic adverse effects. The *thioxanthene* and *benzamide* groups are claimed to have, in addition, stimulant and antidepressant activities. The *dibenzazepines* are forerunners of the so-called **atypical** neuroleptics, which have greater activity against resistant schizophrenia and negative symptoms combined with a significant reduction in extrapyramidal adverse effects. They mark a return to broad-spectrum receptor blockade, but with a greater relative affinity for 5HT receptors over D_2 receptors.

Psychotropic actions

These drugs have a wide spectrum of psychotropic actions (Table 7.20). Their ability to **sedate** without general impairment of consciousness, i.e. tranquillize, gives them an anxiolytic, tension-relieving effect. The **antipsychotic** action is a remarkable ability to banish hallucinations, diminish the power of delusions and straighten out distorted thought; this is the origin of their description as 'major tranquillizers'. **Psychomotor inhibition** is a specific depression of overactive thought and physical activity, again not at the expense of consciousness. Some antipsychotics have a stimulant or **alerting** effect on withdrawn patients, and others also a **mood elevating** or antidepressant action. These properties are shown to a different degree by different groups and their usefulness in treating the common target symptoms of various psychiatric illnesses is indicated in Table 7.20.

Pharmacokinetics and administration

No consistent predictions about neuroleptic effectiveness in a given patient can be made either from the dose used or from plasma level measurements. Most neuroleptics have a half-life greater than 24 h, so single daily doses are usually adequate in the maintenance phase; evening usually is the best time, especially if a sedating effect is required. There is often a first-pass effect, so parenteral doses are usually lower than oral ones. The apparent volume of distribution is high owing to the lipophilic nature and consequent accumulation in the CNS. Thus, although plasma binding is usually quite high (e.g. >95% for chlorpromazine) this does not present any potential interaction problems. Clearance is usually hepatic (an exception is the *benzamide* group), so the possibility exists for hepatic drug interactions. This is also important because hepatotoxicity occasionally occurs.

Recommended maximum doses are only guides: patient response is the principal criterion. Very high doses may be given if adverse effects are absent or tolerable, provided that a clinical effect is achieved. However, persistently high doses must be avoided, especially after the acute phase has been controlled. The Royal College of Psychiatrists has issued precautions about high dose therapy (*see* BNF).

Depot therapy

In depot formulations the neuroleptic is esterified and dissolved in an oily vehicle. The deep intramuscular dose is distributed throughout body fat during the first few days. Before exerting the clinical effect, the drug must be partitioned into the plasma from these lipid depots and then de-esterified by hydrolysis. Hence a single injection can maintain effective plasma levels for between 14 and 28 days. As would be expected, depot therapy, organized either via

Table 7.20   Psychotropic properties and target symptoms of the neuroleptic drugs

Psychotropic action	Target symptom	Psychiatric condition where symptom occurs	Drug group of choice
Tranquillize	Anxiety Tension	Anxiety neurosis	Simple *phenothiazine*
Psychomotor inhibition	Hyperactivity Agitation Racing thoughts Aggressive	Mania, schizophrenia	Simple *phenothiazine* *Piperidyl phenothiazine* *Zuclopenthixol*
Antipsychotic	Thought disorder Hallucination Delusion	Schizophrenia Schizophrenia, mania, severe depression	*Piperazinyl phenothiazine* *Butyrophenone* *Diphenylbutylpiperidine* *Benzamide*
Alerting	Apathy Withdrawal Negative symptoms	Schizophrenia (Type 2)	'Atypical', e.g. *dibenzazepine*
Mood elevation	Depressed mood	Schizophrenia; severe depression	*Benzamide; thioxanthene*

special outpatient clinics or community psychiatric nurses, has greatly facilitated the trend to community care for chronic schizophrenic patients.

If a patient is stabilized on neuroleptic therapy and seems to need medium- or long-term maintenance, there a number of advantages to transferring to depot therapy:

- Lower total dose.
- Facilitation of community care.
- Regular contact with the patient by carers.
- Supervised administration prevents defaulting.
- No accumulation or abuse of unused tablets.

There is at least one depot preparation available from each main group (except as yet the atypicals). Ideally, the patient is first titrated for a maintenance dose using the oral form of the selected neuroleptic. A test dose of the depot formulation is given to check for sensitivity to the vehicle. A formula may then be used to estimate the initial injected dose. For example, one method would convert a 10 mg daily dose of fluphenazine into an 25 mg fortnightly dose.

A cross-over phase follows, with the oral dose tapered off and the depot dose gradually increased. Subsequently, the depot dose must be titrated against effect, which is not as straightforward as with oral therapy because of the delayed onset, prolonged action and slow reversal of effect. Moreover there is no consistent relationship between oral and depot doses needed to achieve control in a given patient. Nevertheless, the final dose is usually lower than the previous total oral dose over the injection interval, partly because of improved bioavailability but also possibly due to the efficiency of a constant plasma level.

There are disadvantages to this approach. Injection site problems, including pain, are common. If adverse effects occur that were not identified in the preliminary oral dose ranging trial, the depot cannot be cleared quickly from the body. Although the lower total dose might be expected to reduce the incidence of adverse effects, including most EPS, this is not usually found; tardive dyskinesia may be more common. These may be incidental consequences of the imposed improved compliance, or related to the stable plasma level as opposed to the constantly varying levels of oral therapy.

Equally important is the fact that there is often considerable patient resistance to this form of therapy, which is seen as controlling, punitive or detrimental to autonomy. This is likely to be particularly the case with those patients who are poorly compliant with oral therapy and therefore one of the main target groups. Patient and family counselling and education are essential to explain the purpose and potential advantages of the technique.

Side effects

Many of the adverse effects of the neuroleptics derive from their various pharmacodynamic actions and so are, in principle, predictable. The widest spectrum of side effects is shown by the phenothiazines (Table 7.21), but the prominence of different adverse effects varies between groups (*see* Table 7.19). Generally, the greater the antipsychotic potency, the fewer the autonomic effects and the more likely the EPS, although this trend has been reversed with the newer agents, which are potent antipsychotics with greatly reduced EPS.

There also potentially serious **non-specific** or

idiosyncratic effects. Jaundice and photosensitivity are more common than agranulocytosis. *Clozapine* is particularly liable to depress the white cell count (incidence approx. 1% of patients per year) and it is mandatory that patients are regularly monitored. As with many psychotropic drugs, seizure threshold is lowered, a problem for epileptics at normal doses and for all patients in overdose. Retinopathy can occur, especially with *thioridazine*.

Autonomic blockade

The **anticholinergic** actions and consequent precautions are similar to those of the tricyclic antidepressants (Table 7.11). Peripheral alpha-**adrenergic blockade** can cause cardiovascular problems, particularly postural hypotension with reflex tachycardia. Autonomic symptoms tend to remit with chronic use.

Endocrine effects

Blocking dopamine in the hypothalamus inhibits some endocrine mechanisms. Most

Table 7.21 Side effects of phenothiazines and related agents

Pharmacological effect	System	Side effect
Dopamine blockade	Basal ganglia	Extrapyramidal symptoms
	Hypothalamus	Hyperprolactinaemia (gynaecomastia, impotence, galactorrhoea, etc.)
		Weight gain
	Hypothalamus?	Neuroleptic malignant syndrome
Adrenergic blockade	CVS	Hypotension, especially postural; tachycardia
Cholinergic blockade	GI tract	Dry mouth, constipation
	Eyes	Blurred vision, mydriasis, raised intraocular pressure
	Bladder	Urinary retention
	Heart	Tachycardia/palpitations
	CNS	Sedation, drowsiness, confusion
Membrane effects	Heart	Conduction defects, ECG changes
	CNS	Reduced seizure threshold, proconvulsant
Non-specific/unknown	Liver	Jaundice
	Skin	Rashes, photosensitivity (*chlorpromazine*)
	Eyes	Pigmented retinopathy (*thioridazine*)
	CNS	Impaired cognition: memory, attention, coordination
	Bone marrow	Agranulocytosis

CNS, central nervous system; CVS, cardiovascular system; GI, gastrointestinal.

important is the rare but potentially fatal **neuroleptic malignant syndrome**, which is probably hypothalamic in origin. The syndrome involves hyperthermia, muscle spasm, impaired consciousness and cardiovascular instability, and has a 10% mortality rate. Treatment is with dopaminergic agents (e.g. *bromocriptine*), muscle relaxants (e.g. *benzodiazepines*, *dantrolene*) and antimuscarinics (e.g. *procyclidine*), as well as cooling and rehydration. Hyperprolactinaemia is quite common and has many consequences that are very unacceptable to patients, such as galactorrhoea, amenorrhoea, gynaecomastia, loss of libido and impotence. Less serious, but equally likely to discourage compliance, is weight gain.

Extrapyramidal syndromes (EPS)

Movement disorders, although usually harmless, are a major cause of non-compliance among schizophrenia patients. A drawback of using dopamine blockers for antipsychotic action in the limbic and reticular systems is that dopamine is also a transmitter crucial to the motor-controlling functions of the basal ganglia. (For a fuller discussion, *see* pp. 384–389 and pp. 439–449.) Both systems seem to involve D_2 receptors, for which most neuroleptics have a high affinity. Thus, for a long time disturbance of fine motor control was believed to be almost inevitable with potent neuroleptics: the two effects seemed inextricable.

Three ways around the problem are currently known:

- Intrinsic anticholinergic activity.
- Specificity for dopamine receptors in the limbic system.
- Preferential affinity for 5HT receptors rather than D_2.

Normally, dopaminergic action in the basal ganglia is counterbalanced by cholinergic activity, whereas in the areas presumed to be disturbed in psychosis dopamine does not appear to have a natural antagonist. Thus it is possible to counteract the adverse effects of dopamine blockade with a centrally acting anticholinergic drug without significantly diminishing the antipsychotic action; this effect is used to treat some neuroleptic-induced EPS. (Note that, by contrast, using the anti-Parkinson drug *levodopa* would nullify the antipsychotic activity.) Some standard neuroleptics with high anticholinergic activity (especially *thioridazine*) have a lower incidence of EPS and so reduce the need for ancillary anticholinergic drugs.

Many newer drugs (e.g. *sulpiride*, *clozapine*) have a far lower incidence of EPS, perhaps because of a selective affinity for receptors in limbic and cortical areas, but not in the basal ganglia. In addition, the antipsychotic activity of most atypicals, especially *clozapine*, is more closely correlated with blockade of $5HT_2$ receptors, an action which has little direct effect on motor coordination but may indirectly prevent it being disturbed.

EPS can be classified into four groups (Table 7.22). Unfortunately, there are no predictors of which type will occur to which patient, or when.

Acute dystonia. Some patients react with an alarming acute muscle spasm on the first dose or within the first few days of neuroleptic

Table 7.22   Extrapyramidal side effects induced by neuroleptics

Class	Common symptoms
Acute dystonia	Neck or spine spasm Neck, jaw or larynx rigidity Oculogyric crisis
Pseudo-parkinsonism	Dyskinesia and dystonia: rigidity, tremor, bradykinesia
Akathisia	Psychomotor restlessness and agitation Inability to sit still
Tardive dyskinesia	Abnormal face, mouth or jaw movement, e.g. lipsmacking, grimacing, tongue protrusion Bodily writhing (choreo-athetoid movements)

therapy, especially if given in high doses or by injection. This usually occurs in the head and neck region: commonly it presents as an exaggerated and uncontrolled rolling upwards of the eyes (**oculogyric crisis**), a stiff jaw or a hyper-extended neck. Occasionally there may be a dangerous choking laryngospasm. Fortunately these reactions are easily treated by parenteral anticholinergics (e.g. *procyclidine*) but they can severely damage the patient's confidence in the therapy.

Pseudo-parkinsonism.   Early in therapy up to 50% of patients develop a motor incoordination syndrome very similar to idiopathic Parkinson's disease. (Note that Parkinson's disease involves dopamine deficit; pp. 439–449). Almost any parkinsonian symptom can occur, and though iatrogenic parkinsonism often remits spontaneously after a few months of treatment, this is of little comfort to the patient, who loses confidence and may become non-compliant.

The temptation to use oral *anticholinergic anti-Parkinson* drugs prophylactically is strong. In the past they have been given routinely. However, this is now uncommon because they may cause various psychotomimetic effects such as delirium; they have even been misused for such effects. In addition, their adverse anticholinergic effects would be additive to those of neuroleptics themselves. Their use is no longer thought to be associated with an increased incidence of tardive dyskinesia. Even so, strong efforts are made to encourage the patient to tolerate the symptoms without anti-Parkinson drugs until they eventually subside.

Akathisia.   Marked restlessness and anxiety seem to be the most disturbing effects for many patients. Akathisia follows a similar course to pseudo-parkinsonism but responds poorly to conventional anti-Parkinson therapy. Some patients develop a more persistent form which resembles tardive dyskinesia. Sometimes a short course of *benzodiazepines* may help, and lipophilic centrally acting *beta-blockers* have also been used.

Tardive dyskinesia (TD).   A form of orofacial dyskinesia, TD may develop after months or years of successful therapy, or even after drugs have been withdrawn. Its bizarre symptoms involve lip-smacking, chewing, grimacing facial expressions. Although not directly distressing for the patient, these provoke unsympathetic or hostile reactions in onlookers because they give the patient the appearance of the popular idea of 'craziness', when paradoxically the drugs responsible are in fact controlling the psychotic symptoms.

The pathology of TD is different from that of other EPS and is poorly understood, although dopamine receptor supersensitivity has been suggested. Prevalence rates of up to 50% and annual incidences of 5% have been reported, the elderly being particularly susceptible. TD is unpredictable, but seems to occur more commonly after long courses and high doses of neuroleptics. Intermittent therapy (e.g. drug holidays, depot therapy) and anticholinergic therapy seem to predispose patients to TD. Perversely, reducing the neuroleptic dose temporarily intensifies symptoms, while increasing the dose may alleviate them. Aside from a correlation with potency, generally no one drug is more likely to cause TD than another. However, clozapine and possibly olazapine appear to cause TD less often; it is not yet clear if this applies to all atypicals.

Currently the best strategy seems to be to reserve neuroleptics for serious psychosis and keep doses as low and courses as short as possible. If TD occurs, it may only be mild and, with the agreement of the patient and his or her family, may be ignored, especially if the patient would be expected to relapse without neuroleptics.

If neuroleptic treatment needs to be continued but symptoms are intolerable, then the current management approach is unsatisfactory. Various drugs have been used, including *vitamin E, clonazepam, nifedipine, sodium valproate, reserpine* and *choline*, with little success. *Clozapine* is sometimes effective. If it cannot be controlled, the neuroleptic must be gradually reduced until the dyskinesia remits. If psychotic symptoms then recur, re-starting neuroleptic therapy with a different agent (especially clozapine) may be possible without recurrence of TD. If not, both the patient and clinician are in a difficult position indeed.

Drug selection and treatment problems

The main considerations when selecting a neuroleptic, and related problems with neuroleptic therapy, are:

- History of the patient's response.
- Whether an *atypical* agent is indicated.
- Contraindications, adverse effects, toxicity.
- Treatment resistance.
- Negative symptoms.
- Compliance.
- Specific target symptoms.
- Cost.

Patient response

A patient's past clinical response is an important guide. So too is any previous adverse effect. Patient preferences or aversions may be strongly influenced by these, and taking them into consideration should encourage a positive attitude and promote compliance.

Atypical neuroleptics

The scope for rational selection among the many, broadly similar **typical** neuroleptics is limited; there is little to choose between different members within each group. However, the development of the **atypical** agents has meant that there is now a genuine basis for choice.

The advantages of this group as a whole are superior activity in treatment-resistant disease, significant activity against negative symptoms, and freedom from EPS. Generally, atypical neuroleptics are as effective on positive symptoms as the older agents and share the same autonomic adverse effects (cholinergic and adrenergic blockade). Weight gain is worse but hyperprolactinaemia less. Experience is not yet sufficient to be certain, but some have a lower incidence of TD and perhaps neuroleptic malignant syndrome. There may be a lower risk of suicide with clozapine. Nevertheless, this is not a completely homogeneous group: there are important differences in their adverse effects (Table 7.23; compare with Table 7.19). The current UK practice is for atypical drugs to be reserved for combating certain specific problems with conventional drugs:

- Contraindication to an adverse effect.
- Intolerable adverse effect (especially EPS).

- Treatment resistance.
- Significant negative symptoms.

Experience with *clozapine* is greatest, and it is now the benchmark against which others are measured. Unfortunately, because of its propensity to cause bone marrow suppression its use necessitates regular, costly and inconvenient blood monitoring. Mainly because of possible orthostatic hypotension, most atypical agents need careful initiation and subsequent dose titration.

Side effects

The autonomic effects of the less potent drug groups (e.g. simple phenothiazines) may be contraindicated in certain patients, notably those with cardiovascular disease, glaucoma, urinary retention, etc. Excessive sedation is unwanted in a disease characterized by depression or negative effects such as apathy and withdrawal. Many patients find weight gain and the consequences of hyperprolactinaemia unacceptable (*see also* Tables 7.19 and 7.23).

Treatment resistance

This is usually defined as failure with at least two drugs from different conventional groups at optimal doses (Fig. 7.13). It occurs in about one-third of patients, and about half of these are likely to respond to an atypical agent. This is a very significant advance because the tendency in the past has sometimes been to use excessively high doses of typical agents, which over-sedate the patient. This causes iatrogenic **secondary negative features** because the resultant inactivity, slowness and apparent dysphoria are easily confused with genuine idiopathic features of chronic disease.

A true treatment refractory state must be distinguished from poor compliance, drug interaction or possibly enhanced elimination by the patient's hepatic or renal systems

Three strategies are currently used to manage resistance to conventional agents at maximal recommended doses. **High-dose** therapy can be tried, but the guidelines of the Royal College of Psychiatrists (*see* BNF) mean that this is contraindicated for many at risk patients, rigorous precautions must be taken and close monitoring

Table 7.23 Properties of some newer atypical neuroleptics[a]

Neuroleptic agent	Efficacy		Side effects				Other comments
	For negative symptoms	In treatment resistance	EPS	Tardive dyskinesia	Sedation	Hypothalamic	
Clozapine	+	+	–	–	+	–	↓ Seizure threshold, bone marrow suppression
Risperidone	+	–	+	?	–	+	EPS only in higher doses; orthostatic hypotension
Sertindole[b]	+	?	–	?	–	–	ECG changes – monitor regularly
Olanzapine	+	(+)	(+)	–	+	(+)	EPS only in higher doses
Quetiapine	?	?	–	?	+	–	

The data assembled here illustrate some important properties of the atypical drugs, and also important differences between them. *Amisulpride* is sometimes included in this group, but is probably best classed with *sulpiride*.

[a] Currently insufficient data on *zotepine*, but it generally seems to resemble other atypicals.

[b] Withdrawn in the UK in December 1998, owing to cardiac side effects.

+ effect present; (+) minor effect; – effect absent or reduced compared to typical agents; ? no data. No evaluation of relative potency or incidence of any of the properties listed. EPS, extrapyramidal symptoms.

is required. An **adjunct drug** can be added, such as *lithium* (especially in schizoaffective states), *carbamazepine* (especially in aggression or mood swings) or a *benzodiazepine* (especially if extra sedation is indicated); experience with the lithium is greatest. Probably the treatment of choice now is to use an **atypical** agent; *clozapine* has been reliably shown to benefit a significant proportion of otherwise treatment-refractory patients.

Negative symptoms

The other significant advantage of the atypicals is the ability to manage patients who have chronic disease in which negative symptoms tend to predominate.

Compliance

Poor compliance is a perennial problem in psychotic patients. The basis is reduced insight, combined with often quite severe and frequently embarrassing adverse effects. Paranoid delusional states add to the difficulty when patients perceive carers as spies or tormentors. Apocryphal tales circulate of caches of medication found under floorboards or behind radiators when psychiatric hospitals are refurbished. In the community, once-daily dosing or depot therapy ameliorate the problem. In hospital, or in other situations allowing supervision of drug administration, nurses and carers become adept at ensuring that patients are not hiding tablets in their cheek pouch rather than swallowing them. Concentrated oral liquid forms help because they cannot be hidden from a search of the oral cavity, but syrup-based preparations are inconvenient, messy, and in the long term, cariogenic and obesity-inducing; moreover, doses are difficult to measure accurately.

Target symptoms

There is little evidence that particular neuroleptics have a preferential effect on specific target symptoms. The less potent agents are indicated where tranquillization or psychomotor inhibition is needed, e.g. in hypomania or acute panic attacks. However, neuroleptics should not be used for simple anxiety or agitation. Medium-potency agents are usually sufficient for the short-term treatment of the less intense psychotic features occasionally found in severe depression.

If there is an affective, especially depressive, component to schizophrenia then a *thioxanthene* may be indicated. However, fixed-dose combination preparations of tricyclic antidepressants and neuroleptics are almost never used by psychiatrists. *Zuclopenthixol* is reputed to be effective in diminishing aggressive symptoms.

Cost

Pharmacoeconomic analysis, in comparing the conventional agents with atypicals, weighs the far greater drug costs of the latter against the resulting savings in reduced hospital admissions for relapse or inability to achieve control. Less easily quantifiable factors such as improved quality of life and reduced drain on social services costs should also be taken into account. Looked at this way, the balance between risk and benefit definitely favours using an atypical agent as soon as possible. However, in the UK there is no agreement yet on whether the relatively costly atypicals should now replace the cheaper but potentially more poorly tolerated typical agents as first-line choices. In part this may be a consequence of the fragmented nature of social and medical budgeting.

Neurological disorder

Parkinson's disease and the extrapyramidal syndromes

The **basal ganglia** (BG) and the **extrapyramidal pathways** play an important role in modulating and smoothing voluntary muscular movement (p. 386 and p. 388; *see also* Fig. 7.3). An imbalance between excitatory and inhibitory influences in these structures can result in disorders of movement and tone, collectively termed extrapyramidal syndromes (EPS). Idiopathic Parkinson's disease (PD) is the most common form; other similar conditions are often described as parkinsonism. Many cerebral diseases or lesions can cause EPS (Table 7.24).

Some important structures in the BG, and interconnections with other brain centres, are shown in Fig. 7.14. Of the numerous stimulant and inhibitory transmitters involved, the best characterized are dopamine (mainly D_2), acetylcholine, GABA and glutamate. These complex circuits, which are still being unravelled, allow a high degree of fine adjustment of voluntary movement and are also responsible for the resting muscular tone, necessary for example for posture. An important input comes from the substantia nigra (strictly speaking, a midbrain structure) and output from this system descends via the corticospinal tract and the extrapyramidal pathways.

Extrapyramidal syndromes arise from lesions of the inhibitory dopaminergic **nigrostriatal pathway** (Fig. 7.14). The reduced dopaminergic inhibition which results allows a preponderance of unopposed cholinergic action in the nigrostriatum and increased GABA-ergic inhibitory tone downstream. These imbalances have a major destabilizing impact on the whole motor system.

In Parkinson's disease it is likely that abnormal corticospinal output causes the abnormalities in muscle tone (dystonias and dyskinesias) while extrapyramidal output defects cause abnormalities in posture and gait.

Aetiology and pathology

The underlying cause of **idiopathic Parkinson's disease** is unknown, so preventative measures cannot be taken. Parkinson's disease is a chronic progressive **neurodegenerative** disease involving destruction of, predominantly, the pigmented dopaminergic cells of the substantia nigra and their axonal connections to the striatum. This results in a fall in the nigrostriatal dopamine output and a consequent increase in the activity of inhibitory GABA-ergic neurones. It is not simply a case of cellular dopamine deficiency or reduced turnover: there is a reduced number of dopamine-secreting cells. Other neuronal structures and transmitter systems may also be involved but the clinical signs derive mainly from this lesion.

There seem to be no strong genetic links, but there are suggestions of inherited susceptibility. Neither auto-immunity nor infection are implicated. Many people developed PD as part of the *encephalitis lethargica* syndrome following an influenza epidemic in the 1920s, but although these are now dying out the prevalence of PD is unchanged.

The process by which nigrostriatal cells are destroyed is still not clear. A histological characteristic of affected cells is a build up of 'Lewy bodies' (dark-staining hyaline inclusions), but their specificity and direct pathological significance is unknown. Theories on the pathology include accelerated ageing with increased apoptosis (cellular autodestruction; *see* Chapter 11),

---

Table 7.24   Varieties of extrapyramidal syndrome and possible causes

Variety	Possible causes
Idiopathic Parkinson's disease (most common form)	Impaired dopamine metabolism
	Reactive free radical damage
	Neurotoxin (e.g. MPTP – see text)
Infective	Viral encephalitis, syphilis, etc.
Iatrogenic	Neuroleptics, metoclopramide
Traumatic	Head injury, tumour
Ischaemic	Arteriosclerosis, atherosclerosis
Toxic	Heavy metals, carbon monoxide, pyridines

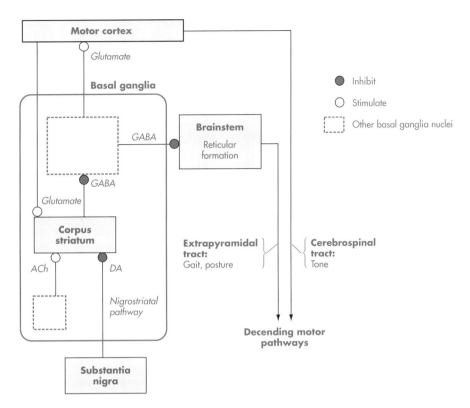

Figure 7.14   Simplified diagram showing transmitters and neural pathways within basal ganglia, and connections to other brain centres. ACh, acetylcholine; DA, dopamine; GABA, gamma-aminobutyric acid.

excessive build up of highly destructive oxidative free radical intermediates (which are normally neutralized), and impaired energy handling. Some investigators blame a free radical oxidized metabolite of dopamine itself.

A chance finding among drug misusers triggered a fruitful line of research. A contaminant in illicitly synthesized pethidine (meperidine) produced symptomatic and histological features very similar to idiopathic PD. This contaminant, MPTP (methyl-phenyl-tetrahydro-pyridine), is oxidized by monoamine oxidase B to MPP⁺. This is a toxic free radical which fatally interferes with mitochondrial energy pathways.

This discovery provided a primate model for studying the pathology and treatment of PD. However, its relevance to the naturally occurring disease in humans it still uncertain. MPTP is not common in the environment, although many herbicides and pesticides are pyridine-based and might be metabolized in a similar way. One pos-

sibility is a genetic defect in the ability to detoxify oxidative intermediates, leading to mitochondrial damage. It is unclear why only nigrostriatal cells should be affected by any of these effects.

Epidemiology and course

The overall prevalence of Parkinson's disease is 1–2 per 1000, but it is five to ten times more common among the elderly, the prevalence among people aged over 65 years being about 3%. Nevertheless, PD can affect people as young as 40. Men and women are affected equally and there seems to be little racial or social variation. This is not what would be expected if the cause were wholly environmental or toxic. However, the prevalence in Europe and North America is twice that of China and Japan.

PD has an insidious onset, with slowly

progressive non-specific signs such as vague muscle pain, stiffness, mild depression and general slowing down. A late onset may protect some patients from the worst ravages of advanced disease. Over 80% of nigrostriatal dopamine must be lost before symptoms become apparent, possibly because neurological and behavioural compensation mask symptoms before this stage. This prodromal phase may last for 5 years.

Parkinson's disease can be considered to proceed through five phases:

1. Prodromal phase – asymptomatic.
2. Early symptomatic phase – little disability; drugs may not be needed.
3. Main treatable phase (5–7 years) – levodopa effective.
4. Late phase – declining levodopa effectiveness.
5. Terminal phase – disease extremely difficult to control.

The early symptoms can easily be mistaken for simple ageing, although when the frank clinical features emerge the condition is unmistakable. Intellect is initially unimpaired, which may exacerbate the patient's distress. However, drug-resistant dyskinesias, intellectual degeneration, dementia and various psychiatric features can occur as the disease progresses. These may be due partly to the involvement of structures other than the nigrostriatum, within or outside the BG, becoming affected by the same degenerative process.

The rate of progression of PD is very variable and it is difficult to determine whether treatment retards the condition in any one individual. Untreated, the median survival is about 10 years from the onset of symptoms, and patients have three times the mortality of a matched normal population. Modern management with levodopa has improved the prognosis, partly by reducing the mortality and morbidity from the secondary complications of immobility. Optimal drug therapy has at least doubled the average survival time, and life expectancy now approaches normality. Death usually results from pneumonia.

Clinical features

The classical signs of parkinsonism are tremor, rigidity, slowness and abnormal posture. Most may be traced to disorders of muscle tone (**dystonias**) or muscle movement (**dyskinesias**). There are also signs of excess cholinergic parasympathetic activity. The clinical features are classified and described in Table 7.25. Clinical presentation is relatively uniform and diagnosis, which rarely causes diagnostic problems, is usually based on the following features:

- Flexed posture and shuffling gait.
- Expressionless face and reduced blinking.
- Distal tremor which relents during purposive movement.

It is necessary to consider possible primary causes, e.g. neuroleptic drug therapy, and to distinguish other conditions presenting similar features, e.g. stroke, hypothyroidism, dementia, etc. PD should be excluded when investigating falls, ankle oedema (possibly the result of immobility) and reduced mobility attributed to 'ageing'.

Management

Aims

The aims in the management of parkinsonism are:

- To provide general support.
- To reduce symptoms.
- To prevent further degeneration.
- To induce reversal or regeneration.

At present, most success has been obtained with the relief from troublesome symptoms and maintenance of the patient's independence and general health. Attempts at prevention and reversal are hampered by the lack of a clear understanding of the aetiology and pathogenesis, and so are still largely experimental.

Support
Exercise, physiotherapy, speech therapy and occupational therapy are essential to help the patient to cope with their progressive disability.

Table 7.25   Clinical features of Parkinson's disease

Dyskinesias	Example/comment
Bradykinesia/akinesia	General slowness
	Reduced voluntary movement, immobility
	'Stately' walk (straight arms swinging)
	Tiny writing (micrographia)
	Mask-like, expressionless face; drooling
Hypokinesia	Delays in initiating movement
Resting tremor	Disappears during activity, sleep
	Increases during stress
	'Pill rolling' hand movements

Dystonias	Example/comment
Limb rigidity	Lead pipe (plastic) or cog wheel (ratchet)
Stooped posture	
Stumbling, shuffling walk	(Festination)
Inarticulate speech	(Dysarthria)
Painful cramps	

Mood and cognition	
Flattening of affect	
Depressed	
Late dementia	

Other physical signs	
Dysphagia, constipation	
Reduced blink rate	
Greasy seborrhoeic skin	

It is important to maintain muscle and tendon strength in the face of reduced mobility. Psychiatric help may be needed for depression, which is common.

Symptomatic: drug therapy

The primary objective of drug therapy is to **enhance dopaminergic activity** within the damaged areas of the basal ganglia, and this is achieved various ways (Table 7.26). Parkinsonism has provided an exceptionally fertile field for rational drug design and formulation to specific clinical requirements. The two basic approaches are to augment dopaminergic activity, mainly with *levodopa* and similar compounds, or to use agents with effects on related receptor systems.

Residual dopaminergic activity can be enhanced by inhibiting neuronal re-uptake (*amantadine*) and the excessive cholinergic tone which dopamine deficiency causes can be countered (*anticholinergics*). However, anticholinergics exacerbate the psychiatric complications of Parkinson's disease and levodopa therapy, particularly in the elderly. They are helpful in tremor, but are little use for bradykinesia and have only limited effectiveness. Invariably some form of dopamine replacement becomes necessary.

Levodopa is currently the standard treatment. It is discussed in detail below. As levodopa inevitably becomes less effective over time its bioavailability can be enhanced with a monoamine oxidase B (MAO-B) inhibitor (*selegiline*) or

Table 7.26 Pharmacological rationales for enhancing dopaminergic transmission in the basal ganglia

Approach	Rationale	Example
Reduce cholinergic activity	Balance diminished dopaminergic activity	Anticholinergic, e.g. *trihexyphenidyl (benzhexol)*, *procyclidine*
Inhibit neuronal dopamine re-uptake	Maximize remaining dopaminergic activity	*Amantadine*
Supply dopamine precursor	Increase dopamine level in basal ganglia	*Levodopa*
Reduce peripheral destruction of precursor	Increase dopamine levels in brain	(i) Decarboxylase inhibitor, e.g. *carbidopa, benserazide* (ii) COMT-inhibitor, e.g. *entacapone*
	Reduce dopamine destruction in brain	MAO-B inhibitor, e.g. *selegiline*
	Use dopamine agonist	*Bromocriptine, pergolide, ropinirole*

MAO-B, monoamine oxidase B; COMT, catechol-O-methyl transferase.

a catechol-*O*-methyl transferase (COMT) inhibitor (e.g. *entacapone*). Where levodopa cannot be tolerated at all, direct-acting dopaminergic agents can be substituted. *Ropinirole, apomorphine* and the ergot-derived dopamine agonists (*bromocriptine, lisuride, cabergoline, pergolide*) do not require central activation by dopa-decarboxylase and have a longer duration of action than levodopa. However, they have worse dopaminergic adverse effects, especially peripherally; and although centrally they cause less dyskinesia, they cause more psychotic reactions. *Dopaminergic partial agonists* and drugs with affinity for *glutamate* receptors are still undergoing trials.

Although drugs are the mainstay of treatment, they do not relieve all symptoms in all patients, nor do they work indefinitely. In particular, the efficacy of levodopa tends to decline as the disease progresses.

Retard or prevent progression

With the discovery of the possible role of free radical damage in the pathogenesis of Parkinson's disease there was hope that antioxidants (e.g. *vitamin E*) or inhibitors of dopamine metabolism (e.g. *selegiline*) might prevent or retard the disease (as in the DATATOP trial). Unfortunately, these hopes have proved unfounded. Early observations on selegiline probably mis-attributed simple symptom control to disease retardation. On the other hand, the suggestion that

selegiline might actually increase mortality has also been refuted. A more recent theory that selegiline might after all retard progression, by inhibiting apoptosis, remains unconfirmed.

Although at present the progression of the disease seems inexorable, modern therapy, if started promptly, has undoubtedly improved survival.

Reversal or regeneration

Rarely, highly selective **surgery** to the thalamus (for intractable tremor) or globus pallidus (for all treatment-resistant symptoms and for levodopa-induced dyskinesias) has been used with some benefit in patients with advanced disease. This is designed to reduce or reverse the abnormal BG output. Trials of **implantation** of dopamine-secreting tissue into the brain have so far proved disappointing. Initially the patient's own adrenal tissue was used; more recently the transplantation of niagral tissue from aborted fetuses has been investigated.

Levodopa therapy

Rationale

Clearly, an ideal objective of Parkinson's disease treatment would be to replace the depleted dopamine in the BG. However, there is an important drug delivery problem because dopamine, being polar, is poorly absorbed orally and does not readily cross the blood–brain barrier (BBB). Further, dopamine has potent peripheral adverse effects.

Direct delivery of dopamine to the CNS is impractical; thus its natural amino acid precursor L-dopa (*levodopa*, L-dihydroxy-phenylalanine) is used (*see* Fig. 7.15). Levodopa is well absorbed from the gastrointestinal tract and, since it is the brain's natural source of neuronal dopamine, it is transported into the brain from the plasma across the BBB by an active uptake pump. Once in the brain, levodopa is decarboxylated intraneuronally to dopamine by dopa-decarboxylase. Decarboxylation is probably not confined to neurones of the nigrostriatum but also occurs in dopaminergic neurones elsewhere.

Levodopa is extremely effective for all symptoms of PD, and especially for bradykinesia; it is up to five times more effective than anticholin-ergics. Unfortunately levodopa is poorly tolerated, especially when given orally, when it produces severe side effects. Owing to peripheral decarboxylation, partly by dopa-decarboxylase in the gut wall during absorption, little of the administered dose actually reaches the CNS (Fig. 7.15). The free dopamine produced causes undesirable peripheral dopaminergic effects on the muscle of the gut, heart and blood vessels. Bioavailability is further compromised by a second pathway for peripheral metabolism, catalysed by COMT.

These problems are largely overcome by using a peripherally acting inhibitor of dopa-decarboxylase designed to be insufficiently lipophilic to cross the BBB, i.e. either *carbidopa* or *benserazide*. When one of these is combined with levodopa (as *co-careldopa* or *co-beneldopa*) the total levodopa dose may be cut by 75% and peripheral side effects are substantially reduced. The main

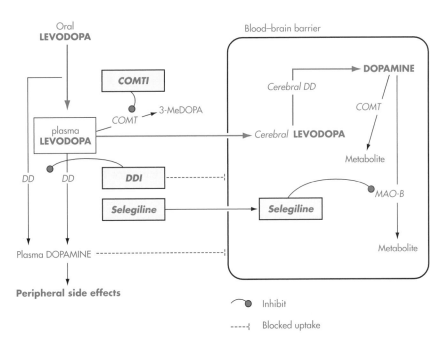

Figure 7.15 Dopamine metabolism and pharmacological intervention. Levodopa is partially decarboxylated and/or oxidized in the gut wall and plasma. From plasma, levodopa can enter the brain but dopamine cannot. Plasma dopamine causes peripheral adverse effects. Inhibiting the metabolism of levodopa in the gut or plasma increases its availability to the brain. Dopa decarboxylase inhibitors (DDIs) do not cross the blood–brain barrier, and so do not interfere with the central action of levodopa. See text for details. COMT, catechol-O-methyl transferase; COMTI, COMT inhibitor; DD, dopa-decarboxylase; MAO-B, monoamine oxidase B.

problem is a not unexpected increase in dopaminergic adverse effects in the CNS. The inhibitors themselves have few side effects.

About 90% of PD patients have a good to excellent initial response to levodopa; failure to respond to levodopa should prompt a re-evaluation of the diagnosis. However, some patients cannot tolerate levodopa at all, while others may have involvement of other neurotransmitter systems.

Unfortunately, even the combinations do not work indefinitely. A further means of enhancing dopamine activity in the CNS is to reduce its intraneuronal catabolism by MAO-B, the enzyme chiefly responsible for the termination its central action. *Selegiline* provides a moderate improvement in cases where levodopa effectiveness is waning. Because selegiline does not block MAO-A, the form of the enzyme affected by conventional antidepressant MAOIs such as phenelzine, it is not subject to the usual MAOI restrictions and dietary precautions. Selegiline may also inhibit neuronal re-uptake of dopamine and have glutamate antagonistic activity, both of which will also potentiate dopamine activity. Further increases in levodopa bioavailability can be obtained by using blockers of COMT (e.g. *entacapone*).

A number of unresolved problems remain. First, drug treatment is only really effective against dyskinetic symptoms. Other motor symptoms remain and indeed tend to deteriorate, especially dystonias causing gait and postural problems (*see* Table 7.25). These may be the patient's most disabling complaints despite otherwise good control; possibly they are mediated by defects in non-dopaminergic neuronal systems. Secondly, cholinergic features may still be troublesome. Finally, there is an inexorable, imperfectly understood decline in the effectiveness of levodopa after a number of years of satisfactory control.

Administration

All patients are routinely given combinations with a decarboxylase inhibitor. Low doses are used to establish tolerance and then gradually increased every 2 or 3 days until symptoms are controlled, the limit of tolerance is reached, or a compromise between these is achieved. The precise regimen, including the best ratio of levodopa to inhibitor, must be carefully individualized to balance tolerance, benefit and toxicity, and must remain continually under review. A variety of different combinations of absolute and relative strengths are available. Considerable ingenuity is exercised in tailoring levodopa drug regimens to extract maximum benefit as efficacy declines (see below).

Divided doses are necessary to minimize gastric intolerance, caused in part by dopamine generated in the gut wall, and to prevent swings in plasma levels which would be reflected in uneven clinical action. Levodopa is always taken with food; however, high-protein meals can reduce CNS penetration owing to competition for amino acid transport mechanisms.

Side effects

The side effects of levodopa are caused by the dopamine produced after decarboxylation, both peripherally and centrally, which acts on dopaminergic and adrenergic receptors (Table 7.27). Elderly patients are more prone to all side effects.

Gastrointestinal tract

Locally formed dopamine reduces gastrointestinal motility, slowing the absorption of further levodopa. Severe dyspepsia is minimized by taking small frequent doses with food. Nausea and vomiting are less common with the lower levodopa doses that decarboxylase inhibitors allow. However, if such doses remain troublesome, a peripherally acting dopamine blocker antinauseant such as *domperidone* may be used (metoclopramide and phenothiazines are unsuitable because they would antagonize the intended central therapeutic action of dopamine).

Cardiovascular system

Dopamine is active at both beta$_1$-adrenergic and dopaminergic receptors (it is used therapeutically as an inotrope and vasodilator; *see* Chapter 3). Most parkinsonian patients are in an age group that is prone to heart disease, and so care is needed in this respect. Elastic stockings are helpful to minimize the hypotension, but serious arrhythmias such as tachycardia and

Table 7.27   Important side effects of levodopa

System	Effects	Cause[a]
GI tract	Dyspepsia	Local irritation
	Reduced gastric motility	Inhibition of intestinal muscle
	Nausea, vomiting	Stimulation of chemoreceptor trigger zone
Cardiovascular system	Arrhythmias	Beta-adrenergic myocardial stimulation
	Hypotension	Peripheral vasodilatation
Central nervous system	Dyskinesias and dystonias	Action in extra-striatial basal ganglia centres?
	Psychiatric symptoms	Action in limbic or thalamic centres
Endocrine	(Rare)	Action in hyothalamus

[a] All except gastrointestinal (GI) irritation and arrhythmia are due to action at dopamine receptors.

premature ventricular beats may require anti-arrhythmic drugs, or the cessation of dopamine treatment. Fortunately, the cardiovascular effects seem to remit on continued therapy.

CNS

Dopamine is a transmitter in other areas of the BG besides the nigrostriatal pathway, and also in centres outside the BG, and actions in these areas may be intensified by decarboxylase inhibitors. Dopamine may, ironically, produce other **movement disorders**, chiefly writhing (choreoathetosis) or restless legs. These tend to occur in the later stages of treatment and are difficult to distinguish from late manifestations of the disease or declining disease control. The precise picture of these complex interactions is far from clear, and strategies for countering them, discussed below, are largely empirical.

Similarly, a variety of **psychotomimetic** effects can result from an excess of dopamine in, presumably, mesolimbic and mesocortical centres. (Recall that one theory of the pathogenesis of schizophrenia attributes it to excess dopamine here; p. 424.) Psychotic features such as hallucinations and paranoia may occur, as may delirium, depression or mania. These may be exacerbated by the use of anticholinergic drugs (anti-Parkinson or antidepressant). They may be confused with symptoms of advanced disease itself (dementia) or represent the unmasking of latent psychiatric illness (which is a relative contraindication to levodopa use).

For **psychosis**, traditional antipsychotic dopamine blockers such as the phenothiazines clearly cannot be used. Partly on the basis that the psychiatric symptoms may involve serotoninergic receptors, and also because they do not cause extrapyramidal symptoms, the atypical neuroleptics have been tried, and *clozapine* has been found helpful. The $5HT_3$ blocker *ondansetron* has also been tried.

Care is needed when treating **depression**. Conventional tricyclic antidepressants with anticholinergic effects must be avoided. There is a theoretical possibility of selective serotonin reuptake inhibitors worsening the parkinsonism (see above), and they also interact with selegiline (causing hypertension). Conventional nonselective MAO inhibitors interact with levodopa (causing hypertensive crisis) and with selegiline (causing hypotension). A sensible choice would appear to be an antidepressant with little anticholinergic activity, such as lofepramine.

Endocrine

There exists the theoretical possibility of mimicking dopamine's activity on hypothalamic releasing hormones. However, the potential results (e.g. hypoprolactinaemia) are not seen and are unlikely to be significant in the parkinsonian age group. (However, this effect is exploited therapeutically in the use of bromocriptine for hyperprolactinaemia.)

Long-term and late complications

Fortunately, no serious long-term haematological, renal or hepatic toxicity has yet been observed. However, the long-term dyskinetic and psychiatric side effects of levodopa are so varied and so difficult to distinguish from late complications of the underlying disease, that Parkinson's disease management has become almost a subspecialty in itself, with its own confusing taxonomy of complications. **Fluctuating therapeutic responses, dyskinesias** and **psychiatric symptoms** frequently become seriously disabling, with about half of patients experiencing problems after 5 years on levodopa and three-quarters after 15 years.

Numerous ingenious pharmacological, biopharmaceutical and formulation strategies are employed to optimize delivery of dopamine to the site of action and to minimize adverse systemic effects. This represents a tremendous clinical pharmacological challenge.

Early experience with levodopa had suggested that there was a limited window for effective levodopa treatment (phase 3, p. 442), after which these problems would arise. Thus, it was felt that levodopa therapy should be delayed as long as possible, conserving it for the later, more severe phases. However, many of the effects ascribed to long-term levodopa therapy are now considered to be probably related to disease progression.

Difficulties in interpreting irregular levodopa activity arise because of:

- Lack of correlation between plasma and brain levels, since CNS uptake of levodopa depends on an active pump, the activity of which may change.
- Lack of correlation between CNS levodopa levels and synaptic dopamine levels, because of reliance on neuronal uptake and dopa-decarboxylase action.
- Declining ability of reducing BG neurone population to decarboxylate levodopa and store dopamine, either within or outside the striatum.
- Normal dopamine activity in the BG varying smoothly, whereas treatment is pulsatile.
- Changes in post-synaptic receptor sensitivity.
- Involvement of dopaminergic systems outside the nigrostriatal system.
- Involvement of non-dopaminergic systems.

Management of levodopa complications

The motor problems of PD and levodopa therapy are classified in Table 7.28. It is unhelpful to attempt to specify a particular solution for each one, especially because many treatments are still experimental; moreover, when a particular problem is not responding, other methods are tried empirically. In general, three basic approaches are employed, depending on whether problems are related to reduced levodopa activity, excessive activity, or mixed intractable fluctuations.

For **reduced effectiveness**, e.g. 'end of dose' and other 'off' phenomena, the aim is to increase delivery of levodopa, modify its time

Table 7.28   Late motor control problems of Parkinson's disease and levodopa therapy

Origin	Description	Symptoms
Levodopa-related		
Reduced effect serum	End of dose wearing off	Declining effectiveness before next dose, related to trough level
	Delayed 'on'	Increasing time before onset of activity
Increased toxicity	Peak dose dyskinesia	Writhing (choreoathetosis) or akathisia related to peak serum level
	Diphasic dyskinesia	Choreoathetosis at onset and end of 'on' period
Disease-related		
	'On–off'	Unpredictable acute fluctuations in symptoms, unrelated to plasma level
? Treatment resistance	'On' period freezing	Transient immobility, especially of gait, in mid-dose period
? Disease progression	'Off' period dystonia	Writhing and spasm, especially of feet in morning

'On', desired therapeutic effect; 'Off', disease-related or iatrogenic motor symptoms.

course or smooth out variations in its plasma level. Increased frequency of lower doses (without allowing plasma levels to fall below the threshold of activity), liquid formulations or enteral systems (intraduodenal or intragastric) may help. The percutaneous, rectal and intranasal routes are being investigated. Modified-release oral preparations are often used, but these have reduced bioavailability and so require dosage adjustment. Continuous subcutaneous infusion of dopamine analogues such as *lisuride* and *apomorphine* is cumbersome but effective. Dopaminergic analogues generally have a longer half-life and may be added to levodopa. If a regimen can be developed with the right balance between levodopa precursor and direct-acting agonist, it may enable an acceptable compromise between prolonged activity and increased peripheral dopaminergic problems. The addition of *selegiline* or *entacapone* increases levodopa bioavailability. Delayed onset may be countered by avoiding simultaneous high-protein meals, using the motility-inducing agent *cisapride*, or enteral administration.

Increased toxicity, i.e. 'on' phenomena or dyskinesias, usually necessitates a reduction in dose, although spacing out doses or using modified-release preparations may help. Reducing the dose is likely to be at the expense of increased disease symptoms and decreased mobility. Again, an acceptable balance must be agreed with the patient.

A wide range of drugs have been tried for **intractable motor problems**, including atypical *neuroleptics*, adrenergic *beta-blockers*, and *SSRIs*. Painful dystonias may benefit from the antispastic agent *baclofen*. Still experimental are *partial dopamine agonists* and *glutamate* receptor blockers. 'Drug holidays', formerly recommended, are now thought unhelpful. Because no treatment definitely retards progression of the condition, it is to be expected that even a successfully managed patient will eventually go through increasing periods of instability.

Drug selection

Drug treatment is started when the degree of functional disability caused by the disease outweighs likely adverse effects. The principal con-

troversy concerns the stage at which levodopa therapy should be introduced. The arguments in favour of early initial therapy with levodopa are:

- It is the most effective drug.
- It is now widely agreed that levodopa does not have a strictly limited window of activity – it continues to benefit most patients to some degree.
- It is no longer believed that levodopa has long-term neurodegenerative effects which could accelerate disease progression.
- The elderly are very sensitive to the adverse effects of the possible alternatives (anticholinergics and dopamine agonists).
- It is no longer believed that selegiline retards disease progression.

On the other hand, the inevitable long-term adverse effects of levodopa, which usually start after 5–10 years of therapy, do mean that these are experienced earlier with earlier initiation of therapy, as would be the case with younger patients. Older patients should be started on levodopa as initial therapy (Fig. 7.16). This may also be the only effective therapy for younger patients with moderate or severe disease, but for younger patients with mild disease then other agents may be tried. Anticholinergics, and to a lesser extent amantadine, may help at first where tremor is the main symptom. There is a substantial minority of carers who would use dopamine agonists as initial therapy, even for moderate disease, but the evidence for their superiority over levodopa is lacking.

However patients commence treatment for PD, all will eventually need to take levodopa. Furthermore at some stage, when long-term complications supervene, this will fail to prove adequate. The numerous possibilities at this stage were discussed above. For a few patients it seems that, eventually, no drug combination will be satisfactory and surgical options may have to be considered.

Epilepsy

The word *'epilepsy'* is derived from the Greek, meaning *'to take hold of, seize'*. For centuries,

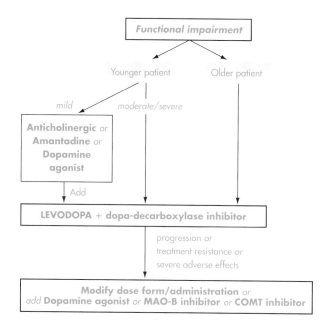

Figure 7.16   Drug selection in Parkinson's disease.

there has been the fear that the sufferer of epilepsy has been possessed, literally taken hold of, by some malign external force. The following ancient quotation describes many of the features of a major seizure in graphic terms.

> He begun to groan then like some terbel thing wer taking him and got inside him. He startit to fall and I easit him down I knowit he wer having a fit I seen that kynd of thing befor. I stuck the clof...be twean his teef so he wunt bite his tung. I wer on my knees in the mud and holding him wylst he twissit and groant...I cud feal how strong he wer tho he wernt putting out no strenth agenst me he wer sturgling with what ever wer inside him. I wunnert what wud happen it got pas him and out. It dint tho. It roalt him roun and shook him up it bent him like a bow but finely it pult back to where ever it come out of. When it gone he wunt do nothing only sleap nor I coulnt get him to walk 1 step.
>
> Russell Hoban, *Ridley Walker*
> (Reproduced with kind permission of the publishers)

For these reasons, epileptics have encountered as much prejudice as those suffering from psy-chiatric disorders. The lack of self-control that is evident during a seizure was feared, and the sufferer was therefore spurned. Yet only rarely does epilepsy directly cause psychiatric symptoms: it is predominantly a neurological condition involving disorders of movement or consciousness, and patients are asymptomatic for most of the time. There may however be secondary psychiatric morbidity in many long-term sufferers.

Epilepsy is a chronic recurrent disorder of intermittent disorganized electrical activity in the brain, which causes the seizure. Seizures are characterized most commonly by impairment of motor activity (convulsion), consciousness, perception or behaviour.

The term 'fit' is now avoided, as is 'epileptic' in reference to a patient. The term 'person with epilepsy' (PWE) is gaining currency.

Aetiology and classification

An isolated seizure can be precipitated in anyone if their brain is suitably provoked. Transient reversible triggers include drugs (e.g. tricyclic antidepressants), cerebral infection or inflammation, intracranial hypertension, head injury, stroboscopic lights and metabolic disturbances such as glycaemic, osmotic or pH imbalance. Fever can trigger seizures, especially in children. However, an isolated attack is not considered epilepsy, which is better defined as **a reduced seizure threshold with a continuing tendency to experience seizures**. Since it may have a variety of causes and triggers, epilepsy could be regarded as a syndrome rather than a discrete disease

In about 30–40% of epilepsy patients a structural abnormality can be located in a specific part of the brain (*see* Table 7.29). The origin may be a congenital or neurodevelopmental abnormality (especially in the hippocampus), ischaemia (arteriosclerosis, stroke, perinatal), trauma (post-infective, perinatal, postoperative or other head injury), tumour (5% overall; up to 40% of adult onset partial epilepsy) or alcoholic brain disease. Other cases are referred to variously as idiopathic (unknown cause) or cryptogenic (hidden cause).

Partial or generalized

Many seizures clearly originate in one particular area of one side of the brain, the epileptogenic focus (Table 7.30). The symptoms a patient displays in **partial** (focal or localization-related) epilepsy are usually readily identified as over-activity in this area (e.g. a particular sensory experience or abnormal muscular action, implicating an area in the sensory or motor cortex). Usually, a specific anatomical lesion will be found in the area predicted from the symptom. In other words most partial epilepsies are secondary, and even when no lesion can be traced, one is assumed to exist. There is little evidence of genetic links, and a family history is unusual.

In **primarily generalized** epilepsy the seizure involves the whole of the brain, on both sides, from the outset with symptoms involving impaired consciousness, major muscle groups, or both. This category includes the most familiar forms, **tonic–clonic** ('grand mal') and **absence** ('petit mal') epilepsy. There are strong genetic links in the generalized epilepsies, but no consistent environmental factors have been identified. Interestingly, even in cases where there is a clear cause, such as head injury, a family history may be found. This suggests that it is a tendency to lowered seizure thresholds which is inherited. Little is known of how the neuronal instability occurs or why it should be set off by particular triggers. One possibility could be that there is an increased tendency to allow random discharges, that are normally suppressed, to spread.

Although some partial seizures may be restricted to their area of origin, in other cases they spread rapidly to many other areas on both sides of the brain. This is known as **secondary generalization**. In such cases patients may experience, before the spread, a specific sensory or other warning symptom, the **aura**. The aura is characteristic of the epileptogenic focus, and in the restricted partial form would represent the entire seizure. In some cases the partial onset is masked or unrecognized because of very rapid generalization, but an attempt should be made

---

Table 7.29   Terminology of epilepsy

Term	Feature
Partial	Seizure arises from specific area of one side of brain
Primarily generalized	Arises simultaneously throughout all areas of both sides of brain
Secondarily generalized	Arises from specific area on one side, but rapidly spreads to all areas
Simple	Consciousness unimpaired
Complex	Consciousness impaired
Tonic	Muscular contraction
Clonic (myoclonic)	Alternate contraction and relaxation, jerking
Atonic	Relaxation, flaccid paralysis

to identify them because it affects prognosis and treatment.

Simple or complex

This diagnostic distinction among the partial epilepsies is based on whether or not consciousness is impaired during the seizure. Generalized seizures are almost invariably complex. The relationship between these different forms of seizure is illustrated schematically in Fig. 7.17.

Pathology

The ultimate defect in epilepsy may be a reduced threshold for neuronal membrane depolarization, for example, a reduced resting potential. This may result from a neurotransmitter imbalance, such as the reduced level of an inhibitory transmitter (e.g. gamma-amino-butyric acid [GABA], glutamate). Such inhibitors act physiologically by promoting chloride uptake into the neurone using the chloride ionophore membrane pump; this increases membrane potential and so stabilizes it. An imbalance theory is consistent with the apparent action of anti-epileptic drugs (AED), many of which facilitate the stabilizing action of inhibitory amines. However, although several specific mechanisms have been identified for the various AEDs, it is not certain that this is how they exert their anti-epileptic effect.

Epidemiology and course

About 1% of the population in the West and Asia have epilepsy, which is half the rate in Africa. There are about 250 000 patients taking AEDs in the UK. The onset is usually below the age of 30 years, with another peak in the elderly due to the presence of cerebrovascular disease.

In general, epilepsy does not deteriorate (i.e. it is not progressive) and children especially may grow out of it. Even in adults epilepsy can remit spontaneously but this can be extremely difficult to judge, and quite long seizure-free periods may – if medication is stopped – be followed by a seizure. Overall, the median period from diagnosis to being drug- and seizure-free (for at least 5 years) is 20 years. On the other hand, 30% of patients continue to have seizures despite optimal therapy.

Partial and secondarily generalized epilepsies account for up to two-thirds of cases, tonic–clonic about one-third, and absence seizures –

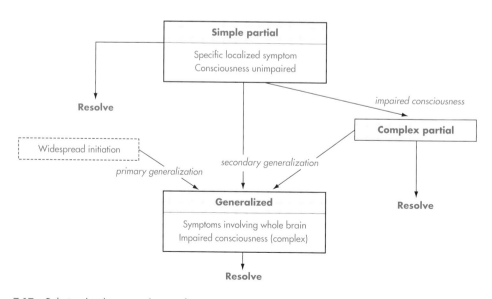

Figure 7.17   Relationship between classes of seizure.

which only occur in children – about 5%. The disease usually causes no intellectual impairment, although long-term AED therapy may do so. However, repeated uncontrolled convulsions can produce brain damage owing to cerebral hypoxia, and in some cases the seizure disorder is in fact the consequence of brain damage.

Clinical features

The features of different seizures are summarized in Table 7.30. Seizures are usually very short-lived, and although usually unpredictable are sometimes triggered in a characteristic way, e.g. flashing lights, altered mood, stress or relaxation. In all but simple partial seizures the patient is unaware of the seizure and may be unable to recall it afterwards.

If a patient presents with a fall, blackout or syncope (faint), or a transient absence, jerking, odd behavioural phenomenon or psychiatric symptom, this must be thoroughly investigated for a non-epileptic primary cause before epilepsy is diagnosed.

Partial seizures

The effects of these highly localized seizures are mostly self-explanatory once the focus is known; or more precisely, the features point to the focus.

Temporal lobe epilepsy is the most common form, representing about half of all cases. This condition can be manifested in a very wide variety of neurological, and occasionally psychiatric, symptoms, including aphasia (the inability to find words), mood disorder, hallucinations and fainting. This makes the differential diagnosis very difficult. There are many different types of partial seizures (*see* Table 7.30 and References and further reading), each of which usually lasts for a matter of minutes, but all are generally treated in a similar manner.

Tonic–clonic

The classic seizure, as described in the quotation on p. 450, is the type most widely associated with epilepsy, and goes through up to five phases:

1. In the **prodromal** phase, which is not experienced by all patients, the advent of a seizure is sensed subjectively, e.g. by a mood change.
2. Some patients then experience a more specific symptom, the **aura** – possibly sensory, sometimes epigastric – immediately before the attack. Auras are always the same for a given patient and suggest a primary partial seizure which subsequently becomes generalized.
3. Then follows the actual convulsion. In the **tonic** (contractile) phase there is a generalized contraction of many muscle groups, both

Table 7.30   Simplified classification of epilepsy, with features of different seizures

Type	Area affected	Function affected	Clinical features of seizure
Generalized (all parts of brain affected)			
Tonic–clonic[a]		Motor, consciousness	Tonic and clonic convulsions; loss of consciousness
Myoclonic[a]		Motor	Jerking of limbs
Absence		Attention; consciousness	Brief periods of reduced awareness
Partial (specific focus, unilateral)			
	Frontal lobe	Motor	Twitching, jerking (unilateral)
	Temporal lobe	Sensory	Smells, 'déjà vu', epigastric sensation, any other sensation
		Behaviour	Psychiatric
	Parietal lobe	Sensory	Tingling, etc.

[a] Other less common generalized motor seizures, usually associated with mental handicap, are purely tonic, clonic or atonic and are usually brief though equally debilitating.

somatic and visceral. Consequently, the patient loses balance and falls. The respiratory muscle spasm causes an initial brief involuntary cry, like being winded by a blow to the abdomen, followed by cyanosis.

4. After 30 sec or so the **tonic–clonic** phase starts. This series of alternating contractions and relaxations causes the jerking that is so alarming for the onlooker, although by this time the patient is usually unconscious. There may be frothing at the mouth, incontinence and tongue biting, and this is the most dangerous phase because of the risk of self harm. The tonic–clonic phase lasts a couple of minutes. The only first-aid practicable is, if possible, to get the patient into the semi-prone (recovery) position to prevent aspiration (inhalation) of vomitus or profuse saliva. The popular idea of putting a cloth in the patient's mouth is now strongly discouraged; any potential damage would usually have been done by the time this could be arranged, and the patient might choke on it. There is also a significant chance of damage to the helper's fingers.

5. In the **postictal** (after seizure) phase there is relaxation, with flaccid paralysis and continued stupor, gradually merging into sleep. After a few hours the patient wakes with a headache, confused, and often bruised, but with no recollection of the events. (A similar state follows ECT used to treat depression.)

Petit mal

In a typical **absence** seizure patients will seem briefly to lose concentration. There may be an obvious stare and fluttering of the eyelids. After a few seconds they continue with what they were doing, unaware of the hiatus. In more severe forms there may be a loss of consciousness for up to 30 sec, when the patient may fall; there may be muscular jerks (myoclonic seizure) but there will be no tonic–clonic convulsion. There are no prodromal signs and no postictal phenomena.

Such seizures usually occur in children and can easily be mistaken for 'daydreaming' or learning difficulty; or else they may be overlooked. Patients may have many attacks a day (sometimes hundreds), but the condition tends to remit as children grow up.

Status epilepticus

If a seizure does not terminate spontaneously, whether as a series of successive short fits or as one long one, it is defined as **status**. This may happen with any seizure type, but most commonly with the tonic–clonic form, and it is a medical emergency. Patients may cause themselves some physical injury, but the main problem is cerebral hypoxia owing to compromised respiration.

Complications

In addition to the seizures patients face considerable psychosocial difficulties. There is the general ignorance referred to in the introduction, as well as the associated stigma, causing difficulties with education, work, leisure and social relationships. The disease itself also imposes restrictions (e.g. driving). Thus depression is common and there is a fivefold risk of suicide. Temporal lobe epilepsy is associated with most psychiatric morbidity, including a schizophrenia-like psychosis. Unfortunately, most antidepressant and antipsychotic drugs lower seizure threshold and thus make treatment difficult. Examples of drugs with the lowest proconvulsant effects are *SSRIs* and *haloperidol*. The possibility of drug interactions then needs to be monitored.

Investigation and diagnosis

The first aim when a patient presents with an unaccountable fall, blackout, etc. is to ascertain if there is any identifiable underlying cause, e.g. medical or toxic (Fig. 7.18). A description of the seizure, from both the patient and especially a witness, is important. A seizure may be induced artificially under controlled conditions with EEG recording.

The EEG lacks specificity and selectivity. Some 15% of otherwise normal people will give an abnormal trace, while only 50% of patients with epilepsy will show abnormalities on random testing. An EEG is more useful in defining the

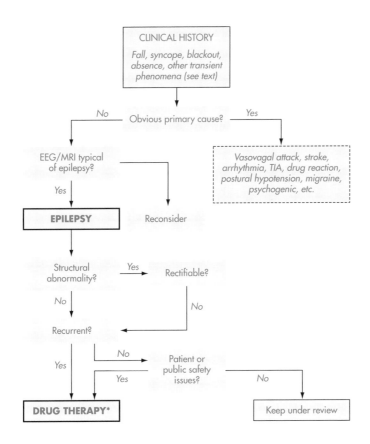

CLINICAL HISTORY

Fall, syncope, blackout, absence, other transient phenomena (see text)

Obvious primary cause? — No / Yes

No → EEG/MRI typical of epilepsy?

Yes → *Vasovagal attack, stroke, arrhythmia, TIA, drug reaction, postural hypotension, migraine, psychogenic, etc.*

Yes → **EPILEPSY**   Reconsider

Structural abnormality? — Yes → Rectifiable?

No / No

Recurrent?

Yes / No → Patient or public safety issues?

Yes / No → Keep under review

DRUG THERAPY*

Figure 7.18   Investigation of epilepsy. TIA, transient ischaemic attack. *See Fig. 7.19.

seizure type, since it is possible to distinguish generalized from partial or secondarily generalized seizures. MRI has replaced radiography as the procedure for the accurate identification of cranial lesions, which it can identify in over half of chronic cases. Surgery can sometimes rectify such problems, but often it cannot and drug treatment is usually required.

The decision to treat

There is disagreement about how frequent seizures must be before a confident diagnosis of epilepsy is made and treatment initiated. The diagnosis has serious legal and social implications (e.g. for driving, pregnancy, education, employment, leisure activities) and treatment involves the likelihood of adverse drug effects. Epidemiological evidence is ambiguous as to the probability of subsequent fits following a single episode, especially in childhood. Estimates of such probability range from 25% to 75%.

The circumstances of the first seizure are crucial to the decision. How likely is there to be a recurrence? Factors to consider are the cause (if known) and whether this is persistent, e.g. was it a manifestation of a transiently reduced threshold or a unique event, such as high fever (more than two-thirds of children who have a febrile convulsion have no further problems); is there objective evidence (EEG, MRI, etc.) or neurological abnormality? Certain types of seizure are more likely to recur, e.g. absences, juvenile myoclonic epilepsy.

Another factor is how serious would be the consequences of a further attack. Obviously if a patient drives a public service vehicle, for example, the risk cannot be taken. Even if treatment is delayed, avoiding driving for 1 year following a single seizure is advisable. The small but real risk of **sudden death in epilepsy** must also be considered if treatment is postponed.

The extent to which early treatment after the first seizure retards the subsequent development of the disease or reduces the likelihood of it becoming treatment resistant is unknown. Overall, about half of those suffering their first seizure will eventually experience recurrence. All decisions about starting drug treatment must involve informed discussion with the patient, and many prefer to await a second seizure before starting. Some patients who have fits no more than once every few years may prefer to risk these rather than long-term drug therapy and its associated problems.

Management

The aims of the management of epilepsy are:

- To investigate possible primary causes.
- To minimize social and psychological consequences and complications.
- To decide if active prophylaxis is necessary.
- To use drug therapy to prevent seizures *or* to keep seizures to minimum compatible with acceptable adverse reactions.

The over-riding consideration is to maximize the patient's quality of life by careful balancing of risks and benefits.

General measures

Careful, sensitive and thorough counselling is important, especially with children and their parents. Patients must be prevented as far as possible from being or feeling stigmatized. It must be emphasized that between attacks patients are perfectly normal, and that the disease causes no impairment of intelligence and no psychiatric disorder. It is helpful if not only the family but also a teacher, school friend or work colleague can be taught how to deal with a seizure.

Patients are encouraged to lead as normal a life as possible. There are certain legal constraints, notably driving. In the UK the current requirement for epilepsy patients to hold a driving licence is that the patient must have had no fits at all for a year, or no daytime fits for 3 years. Patients who are well controlled and seizure-free may have normal schooling, and even swim. The number of constraints is much reduced if the patient has recognizable prodromal signs or a consistent aura.

Principles of pharmacotherapy

Drug therapy does not alter the basic lesion, whatever it is, but can be very effective in preventing seizures. The limiting factor is the adverse effects, especially as treatment may be prolonged. Sometimes the doses needed for complete seizure suppression may be intolerable and it is preferable simply to aim for a reduced seizure frequency. In all cases the decision to initiate drug therapy should be based on a risk assessment. The risks of or from continued seizures in the absence of treatment must be weighed against the risks of adverse effects and the potential benefits of reduced seizure frequency with treatment.

A decision tree for managing drug therapy is given in Fig. 7.19. The following general principles should be observed.

Monotherapy
Monotherapy is now the accepted ideal. There are considerable benefits in avoiding polypharmacy in epilepsy in view of the many possible drug interactions. If the first drug proves inadequate or is not tolerated, another should be substituted, rather than adding another drug. Two first line agents appropriate for the patient and his or her seizure type should be tried singly before a combination is tried. Over two-thirds of patients are satisfactorily controlled on a single drug, and those who are not are likely to prove the most difficult to control.

Formerly, insufficient care was taken to achieve the optimal plasma level with the first drug chosen, so a second or even third drug was commonly added quite early. Some older patients may still be on polypharmacy (and

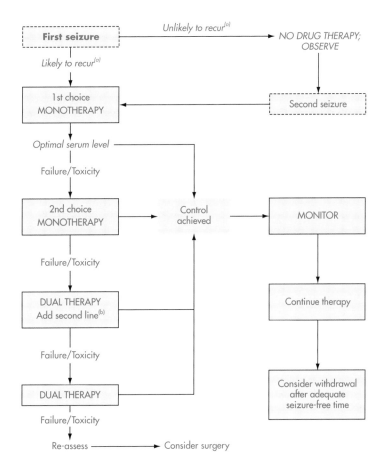

Figure 7.19   Treatment strategy for epilepsy. [a]Based on history, investigations, patient choice, etc. (*see* p. 454). [b]Prefer a drug with a different range of side effects. (Adapted with permission from Beghi *et al.* (1986) *Drugs* **31**: 249.)

should remain so), but this approach probably produces more problems than it solves and is now avoided.

Dual therapy

If two first-line agents used alone fail, a further 15% of patients may be controlled on a combination of two drugs. Selection of drugs to be used in combination involves consideration of minimal overlap in adverse effects, least chance of interaction and complementary modes of action. There are few evidence-based data on the relative effectiveness of different combinations.

The remaining patients can be difficult to control, but triple therapy should be avoided if possible. Failure to achieve control with a variety of drugs as monotherapy or dual therapy at optimal plasma levels suggests the need for further inves-

tigation and perhaps a revised diagnosis.

Gradual initiation

Low drug doses are used initially and gradually increased until control is achieved or unacceptable toxic effects occur, carefully adjusting doses according to individual patient response. This requires patience: a half-life of 36 h or more (e.g. phenytoin) means that a new steady state will not be reached until about 7–14 days after any change in dose.

Compliance

The importance of compliance must be stressed to the patient, and this must include a clear explanation about the range and likelihood of potential adverse effects. Seizure-free patients can easily decide that they are cured and stop taking medication: this is a common cause of 'failure' of therapy. This is especially true of younger patients. Abrupt withdrawal of drugs may precipitate a seizure.

Plasma level monitoring

It is no longer felt necessary to monitor patients' blood levels regularly. However, the non-toxic therapeutic ranges of most AEDs are known and therapeutic drug monitoring may be helpful in a number of circumstances to check for abnormalities in absorption, clearance, interaction and compliance:

- During initiation, if an expected response is not achieved.
- When previously stable control seems to become poor.
- In pregnancy.
- In suspected toxicity.
- When doses are changed or other drugs are taken.

Consistent formulation

Efforts should be made to ensure that patients continue taking the same proprietary form of AED. Unpredictable changes in bioavailability often follow changes in dose form or formulation, with loss of control or increased toxicity. Special vigilance is necessary when patients move between primary and secondary care, or between different prescribers or pharmacies, and for patients taking phenytoin.

Medication record

The patient should carry and maintain a complete medication record, including OTC drugs.

Antiepileptic drugs

It is possible to make some generalizations about AEDs where there are broad similarities, but the reader is referred to an official formulary for detailed information on each drug. Some of the more important features are given in Table 7.31 and discussed below.

Mode of action

Although most AEDs can be assigned a specific neuropharmacological mode of action, it is uncertain to what extent this correlates with their clinical action. Nevertheless, knowledge of the class to which a drug belongs facilitates rational combinations when these are necessary.

There are three main classes. Most AEDs interfere with voltage-dependent high-frequency **sodium channels** to limit the spread of the neuronal instability by inhibiting unnaturally rapid firing. This group includes the common agents used in generalized and partial seizures, such as *phenytoin, carbamazepine, lamotrigine* and perhaps *valproate*. Others facilitate the inhibitory transmitter **GABA**, which stabilizes neuronal membranes, especially the CNS sedative agents *phenobarbital* and the *benzodiazepines. Vigabatrin* irreversibly inhibits GABA catabolism. Although valproate also inhibits GABA-catabolic enzymes, other actions contribute to its wide spectrum of anti-epileptic activity. Some drugs active in absence seizures, especially *ethosuximide*, block voltage-dependent **calcium T-receptors**.

The modes of action of some of the newer AEDs have not yet been fully elucidated, e.g. *topiramate, gabapentin*. Approaches currently being explored include inhibition of excitatory transmitters such as glutamate.

Pharmacokinetics

The handling of AEDs is varied and complex. There may be great variation in plasma levels for a given dose, both between patients and even in the same patient at different times. For some drugs this may make plasma level monitoring advisable at certain times, but routinely it is usually sufficient to monitor clinically, by freedom from seizures and adverse effects.

Absorption

This may be highly formulation-dependent, especially with *phenytoin*, which makes it unwise to change brands or dosage forms. This does not preclude generic drugs *per se*, as is sometimes erroneously believed, provided that a particular formulation is used consistently. For drugs like phenytoin, with a narrow therapeutic index, bioavailability variation may permit seizure breakthrough on the one hand or excessive toxicity on the other; similar considerations apply to potential interactions. Absorption rate and

Table 7.31   Anti-epileptic drugs – notable features

Drug[a]	Action[b]	Pharmacokinetics	Side effects; other notes
Benzodiazepines	GABA	Rapid CNS penetration/action	Tolerance, sedation
Carbamazepine	Na	Auto-inducer; many active metabolites	Sedation, hyponatraemia
Ethosuximide	Ca	Hepatic clearance	Absence seizures only
Gabapentin	?	Renal clearance	Few interactions
Lamotrigine	Na	Inducible metabolism, long half-life; low binding; few interactions	Skin reactions Broad spectrum; several formulations
Phenobarbital	GABA	Active metabolites, enzyme induction	CNS depression
Phenytoin	Na	Variable absorption, high plasma protein binding, saturation kinetics, enzyme induction	Sedation, ataxia, etc. (see text) Many interactions; narrow therapeutic index
Tiagabine	GABA	Hepatic clearance, high plasma protein binding	Ophthalmological and psychotomimetic effects. Sedation
Topiramate	Na?	Renal clearance	CNS depression? Broad spectrum
Valproate	Na? GABA?	Twice-daily dosing	Hepatotoxicity (rare). Broad therapeutic spectrum
Vigabatrin	GABA	Once or twice-daily dosing; renal clearance	Visual field defects (monitor). Psychotomimetic effects

[a] For indications, see Table 7.32,

[b] Mode of action class:

Ca, calcium T-channel blocker; CNS, central nervous system; GABA, enhance GABA inhibitory activity; Na, voltage-dependent Na channels.

bioavailability may be reduced by food and antacids. Intramuscular phenytoin is very poorly absorbed, so the intravenous route is essential if parenteral therapy is necessary. The pro-drug *fosphenytoin* causes less local irritation.

Distribution

Clearly, all AEDs are sufficiently lipophilic to enter the brain but they do so at different rates. *Benzodiazepines* enter quickly to act most rapidly and so are the standard treatment for status epilepticus. They have the highest volumes of distribution due to central accumulation. Most AEDs are highly plasma protein bound; consequently, free drug levels may be sensitive to displacement owing to competition for binding by other drugs, including other AEDs.

Clearance

Most AEDs undergo extensive hepatic metabolism; exceptions are *vigabatrin, gabapentin* and *topiramate*, which are cleared renally. *Valproate, carbamazepine* and *phenobarbital* have active metabolites. Rates and extents of metabolism vary according to age, other disease, genetic factors and enzyme induction or inhibition by other drugs, usually in a predictable manner (*see* Chapter 1). A number of factors further complicate this.

Many AEDs are hepatic enzyme inducers, and some also cause auto-induction, producing subsequent difficulties in dosage adjustment. With *carbamazepine* and *valproate* the half-life can reduce from 50 h at the start of therapy to less than one-third of this later on. There is commonly a mutual interaction between AEDs, each enhancing the clearance of the other. AEDs will also enhance the clearance of other drugs; phenytoin and others reduce the efficacy of oral contraceptives in this way, which is especially important in view of the potential teratogenic action of many AEDs.

These enzyme systems are also saturable (especially with *phenytoin*). This may permit plasma levels easily to enter the toxic range inadvertently while treatment is being initialized or the dose changed: a dose increase similar to the previous one may produce an unexpectedly large effect (Fig. 7.20). Phenytoin dose changes must be gradual (allowing the usual five half-lives to

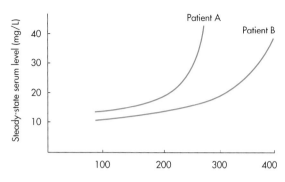

Figure 7.20   Graph illustrating effect of saturation kinetics on phenytoin steady-state plasma level. The dose/plasma level curve is linear up to about 300 mg daily (the exact threshold varies between patients). Above that the plasma level rises disproportionately for small increments in dose because the hepatic drug metabolizing system has become saturated.

attain steady state before alteration) and in small increments (25 mg) above about 200 mg/day.

Duration of action
Most AEDs have a sufficiently long half-life as to require only once-daily dosing. Notable exceptions are *valproate*, *carbamazepine* and *gabapentin*.

Side effects

Consideration of the adverse effects of the AEDs is important because they may have to be given

for long periods and compliance is sometimes a problem (*see* Table 7.31). This occurs in particular with adolescents on *phenytoin* because of the disagreeable though not dangerous cosmetic side effects. In addition, phenytoin causes dose-related toxic effects to occur at plasma levels that are only a little above the therapeutic range, and these are important markers of over-dosage (Fig. 7.21). Other AEDs do not have such a narrow therapeutic index.

CNS.   Most AEDs have some non-specific depressant or sedative action, but especially *phenytoin*, *phenobarbital* and its pro-drug, *primidone*. In the long term there may be cognitive and behavioural impairment with these older drugs, especially *phenobarbital*; nystagmus and ataxia may also occur. *Vigabatrin* can cause psychiatric disturbances. *Carbamazepine* and *valproate*, and many of the newer agents, are significantly less troublesome in these respects, which is one reason why they have replaced the former three as first choices.

Gastrointestinal tract.   Many AEDs cause gastrointestinal distress (especially *valproate*), but care is needed with the use of antacids as they may impair absorption of some AEDs. Enteric-coated preparations are preferred where available. Rarely, *valproate* causes hepatic or pancreatic injury (monitoring essential).

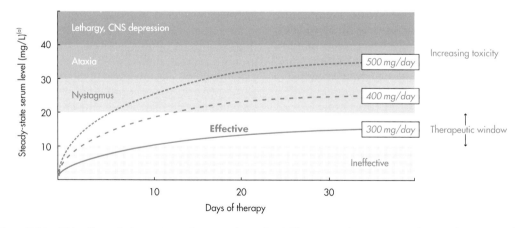

Figure 7.21   Side effects of phenytoin in relation to plasma level. The narrow therapeutic window can be seen, and also the long time required to achieve steady state. The effect of different doses is shown for illustrative purposes only; individuals vary widely in their responses. [a]For micromol/L multiply by 4. (Adapted with permission from Kutt H, McDowell F (1968) *J Am Med Assoc* **203**: 969.)

Skin. There are serious cutaneous reactions with *phenytoin*, including acne, hirsutism (excessive hair growth), coarsened looks and gingival hyperplasia (gum overgrowth). *Valproate* can cause hair loss. *Lamotrigine* and *carbamazepine* can cause rash that is severe enough to force discontinuation.

Metabolic. A number of AEDs, notably *phenytoin* and *carbamazepine*, lower vitamin D and folate levels, partly because enzyme induction accelerates the catabolism of these vitamins. Osteomalacia (rickets) or megaloblastic anaemia may follow. Folate supplementation is recommended in pregnancy to prevent neural tube defects

Systemic. Haematopoietic, hepatic or renal disturbances are rare. Nevertheless, blood and liver monitoring should be performed regularly. *Carbamazepine* occasionally causes hyponatraemia.

Teratogenic effects. Many AEDs present a serious dilemma in the therapy of young women. Many AEDs enhance the metabolism of oral contraceptives, possibly promoting failure and possible teratogenic effects before pregnancy is discovered. Since most teratogenic effects occur very early in pregnancy, possibly before it is realized, any damage would already have been done. AED therapy carries a small but definite risk (about two to three times normal) of fetal abnormality; particular offenders are unfortunately the most popular drugs: *carbamazepine, valproate* and *phenytoin*. Yet both fetus and mother may suffer, the former irreversibly from anoxia, if a pregnant woman has frequent major seizures.

Other toxic effects on the fetus include sedation, enzyme induction, and even neonatal withdrawal seizures. Neonatal bleeding may occur due to impaired vitamin K transplacental transport, and vitamin K is used immediately before delivery. In addition, the clearance of many AEDs increases during pregnancy, so plasma levels have to be monitored carefully. AEDs are secreted in small quantities in breast milk, but this does not seem to be a serious clinical problem.

Whether or not AED therapy should be continued depends on the risks of withdrawal. The current view is that treatment in women should be continued, but with careful monitoring to maintain control at the lowest possible dose, preferably with a single AED.

Drug selection

Despite determined efforts to produce a precise classification of epilepsy and frequently quoted recommendations for different types of seizure, a systematic rationale has not emerged for linking drug to seizure type. Few direct comparisons have been made and recommendations are still basically empirical.

Table 7.32 provides the currently agreed best choices. There seems to be no clear distinction between choices for generalized tonic–clonic seizures and those for partial seizures, but there is between these two seizures types and for absences. Patient factors such as tolerability, adverse effects and interactions are the main criteria once a decision on drug therapy has been made.

Epilepsy is the only remaining indication for phenobarbital which escapes the strict legal control of barbiturates in the UK, but its use is declining.

Interest continues in the use of high-fat *ketogenic diets* for resistant childhood epilepsy. This is based loosely on the apparent anti-epileptic effect of starvation, but it is not an established approach.

Withdrawal of drug therapy

After a suitable seizure-free period the possibility of gradual withdrawal should be discussed with the patient. The likelihood of a lengthy remission is increased in patients with childhood onset, epilepsy of short duration, previous good control, a normal EEG, and no evidence of a primary cause (head injury, mental retardation or an adverse MRI scan).

At present it is generally agreed that the patient must have at least two seizure-free years before stopping treatment can be considered, but the more cautious would wait for up to 5 years. It also depends on patient and clinician preference (e.g. does the patient need to drive?).

Table 7.32   First- and second-line drug selection in epilepsy

Primary generalized tonic–clonic	Absences	Partial	Juvenile myoclonic
First-line monotherapy			
Valproate	Valproate	Carbamazepine	Valproate
Carbamazepine	Ethosuximide	Valproate	Lamotrigine
Second-line monotherapy			
Lamotrigine	Lamotrigine	Lamotrigine	Clonazepam
Gabapentin		Gabapentin	
Phenytoin		Phenytoin	
Additional for dual therapy			
Topiramate		Topiramate	
		Tiagabine	

Withdrawal should be phased over at least 6 months, one drug at a time if on multiple therapy. Even if withdrawal is successful, the drug therapy itself cannot be considered to have brought about a cure: it is more likely that the disease has remitted spontaneously.

References and further reading

Agid Y (1991) Parkinson's disease: pathophysiology. *Lancet* **337**: 1321–1324.

Andreasen NC (1995) Symptoms, signs and diagnosis of schizophrenia. *Lancet* **346**: 477–481.

Angst J (1997) A regular review of the long term follow up of depression. *Br Med J* **315**: 1143–1146.

Anonymous (1995) Drug treatment of schizophrenia. *Drug Therap Bull* **33** (11): 81–85.

Anonymous (1995) Management of anxiety and insomnia. *MeReC Bulletin* **6** (10): 37–40.

Anonymous (1997) Atypical antipsychotics. *MeReC Bulletin* **8** (7): 25–28.

Bazil CW, Pedley TA (1998) Advances in the medical treatment of epilepsy. *Annu Rev Med* **49**: 135–162.

Bazire S (1999) *Psychotropic Drug Directory*. Salisbury: Quay Books.

Belmaker RH, *et al.* (1996) How does lithium work in manic depression? *Annu Rev Med* **47**: 47–56.

Daly I (1997) Mania. *Lancet* **349**: 1157–1160.

Fleischhacker VW, Hummer M (1997) Drug treatment of schizophrenia in the 1990s. *Drugs* **53**: 915–929.

Hale AS (1997) ABC of mental health. Anxiety. *Br Med J* **314**: 1186–1189.

Hale AS (1997) ABC of mental health. Depression. *Br Med J* **315**: 43–46.

Hughs AJ (1997) Drug treatment of Parkinson's disease in the 1990s. *Drugs* **53**: 195–206.

Kane JM, McGlashen TH (1995) Treatment of schizophrenia. *Lancet* **346**: 820–825.

Kantona C, Robertson M (1995) *Psychiatry at a Glance*. Oxford: Blackwell Science.

Lader M (1997) Treatment of anxiety. *Br Med J* **309**: 321–324.

Lang AE, Lonzano AM (1998) Parkinson's disease. *N Engl J Med* **339**: 1044–1052, 1130–1142.

Mir S, Taylor D (1998) Schizophrenia. *Pharm J* **261**: 55–58.

Paykel ES, Preist RG (1992) Recognition and management of depression in general practice: consensus statement. *Br Med J* **305**: 1198–1202.

Shorvon SD (1990) Epidemiology, classification, natural history and genetics of epilepsy. *Lancet* **336**: 936.

Taylor D, Kerwin R, Duncan D (1996) *Prescribing Guidelines*. 3rd edn. London: Bethlem and Maudsley NHS Trust.

Turner T (1997) ABC of mental health. Schizophrenia. *Br Med J* **315**: 108–111.

8

Rheumatology: musculoskeletal and connective tissue diseases

There are over 200 rheumatological disorders, producing about 25% of the average GP's workload. Some disorders are primary joint problems, but muscles, tendons and ligaments may also be affected. Systemic diseases may affect the joints and may trigger a rheumatological referral. Our progressively ageing population, with prolonged joint stresses and bad working practices may cause persistent problems, increasing the workload.

Many patients imagine that 'rheumatism' leads inexorably to chronic disability. This does not reflect current practice, but derives from times when life and work were much harder than now and good medical care was generally unavailable. Most patients are now treated effectively by their GP or paramedical staff and counselling can relieve inappropriate anxiety, but the drugs used can have serious side effects.

Introduction

This chapter describes the principal rheumatological conditions to aid an understanding of their treatment and to assist recognition of those signs (facial or other rashes, conjunctivitis, bowel problems etc.) indicating significant underlying disease and the need for prompt referral. The term 'rheumatism' is used loosely by patients to describe any form of pain or dysfunction associated with the joints or muscles. This covers a wide range of disease states (Table 8.1). None of the many attempts at classification is wholly satisfactory, because the aetiology of most of the diseases is obscure. Joint disease (arthropathy) and joint inflammation (arthritis) frequently accompany a variety of diseases whose principal effects are elsewhere than on the joints, e.g. diabetes mellitus, psoriasis and ulcerative colitis, so careful diagnosis is essential. Only the principal disease states in this group are discussed below. Table 8.1 also gives the disease abbreviations used most frequently throughout this chapter.

In this chapter, the terms 'rheumatoid' and 'arthritis' are used only for inflammatory joint conditions: 'rheumatic' and 'rheumatism' apply non-specifically to all types of pain or abnormality involving the joints, muscles, tendons and associated structures, e.g. in systemic lupus erythematosus (p. 511) or rheumatic fever (p. 520).

Specialization is especially important because of the large variety of diseases and drug toxicity: non-steroidal anti-inflammatory drugs are widely used and cause the largest proportion of adverse reaction reports of any drug group. Some of the other drugs used may also cause severe side effects. Unless the condition is severe, most patients are self-medicating when they seek advice, increasing the risk of drug interactions.

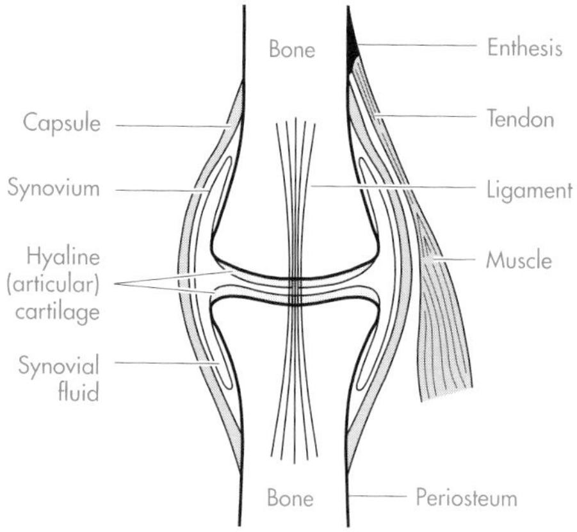

Figure 8.1 Generalized diagram of a synovial joint. The joint is stabilized by the ligaments and muscles (only one of each is shown). The **enthesis** is the point of attachment of the tendon to the bone. The **periosteum** is the specialized connective tissue, with bone-forming potential, which covers all bones.

Anatomy and physiological principles of the musculoskeletal system

Two types of joint are affected by rheumatic disease, namely **synovial** and **cartilaginous.** The former type allows a wide range of free movement and so includes all the hinge joints of the limbs. The latter type allows only limited movement and include primarily those joints of the vertebral column and the hip girdle, including the sacroiliac joints and the pubic symphysis (the anterior joint between the two pubic bones).

Disease of cartilaginous joints is primarily degenerative and traumatic, whereas problems in synovial joints tend to be inflammatory.

Synovial joints

This is the type of joint found in the legs, arms, hands and feet. From the generalized diagram given in Fig. 8.1 it can be seen that the ends of

Table 8.1   Some diseases and conditions that may give rise to rheumatic diseases and joint pain

Pathological class and examples	Abbreviation
Inflammatory arthritides	
Rheumatoid arthritis	RA
Juvenile chronic arthritis	JCA
Seronegative spondarthritides	
Ankylosing spondylitis	AS
Reiter's syndrome	
Psoriatic arthritis (*see* Chapter 12)	
Enteropathic arthritis (*see* Chapter 6)	
Degenerative joint disease	
Osteoarthritis, primary, secondary	OA
Crystal deposition arthropathies (metabolic disorders)	
Gout	
Pyrophosphate arthropathy (pseudogout)	
Systemic connective tissue diseases (collagen-vascular diseases)	
Systemic lupus erythematosus	SLE
Systemic sclerosis (scleroderma)	
Vasculitides:	
• polyarteritis nodosa	PAN
• giant cell arteritis	GCA
• polymyalgia rheumatica	PR
• Wegener's granulomatosis	WG
Reactive arthritis	
Rheumatic fever	
Secondary to systemic disease	
Amyloidosis	
Sarcoidosis	
See also Table 8.3	
Joint infections	
Septic arthritis	
Localized and traumatic	
Back and neck pain	
Carpal tunnel syndrome	
Tendinitis and tenosynovitis	
Fibrositis and fibromyalgia	
Enthesopathies and sports injuries	
Tennis elbow, golfer's elbow	
Iatrogenic	
Drug-induced: lupus-like syndromes, vaccines and sera, arthralgias	
Chronic haemodialysis (*see* Chapter 4)	

the two opposing bones are covered with a firmly attached layer of **hyaline** (articular) **cartilage**. This is about 6 mm thick in young adults but is only 1–3 mm thick in the elderly. The cartilage is radiolucent, giving the appearance of a joint space on X-ray (Fig. 8.2(a); *see also* Fig. 8.6(a)), though the two layers of cartilage are normally in close contact. The bearing surfaces of the cartilage are lubricated and supplied with nutrients by a small volume (less than 2 mL in a knee joint) of a viscous, pale yellow **synovial fluid** containing a hyaluronate–protein complex, albumin and some white cells, electrolytes, etc. The whole is surrounded and stabilized by a tough, **fibrous capsule** which may be thickened in places and by **ligaments**, which further strengthen the joint. However, joint stability depends largely on the strengths of the attached and surrounding muscles, and one of the objects of physiotherapy is to strengthen the muscles and so reinforce the joints. Some joints have additional structures, e.g. the tough, fibrous cartilage of the **menisci** in the knee joint (Fig. 8.2(a)) which helps to absorb stresses and further improve stability, and bursae (see below).

The synovial fluid is produced by the surrounding **synovial membrane** and contains phagocytic cells and those which secrete the fluid. This membrane is not flat and featureless: it has numerous folds, which allow for wide-ranging joint movement, and fat pads and inner projections which together fill much of the joint cavity. These internal projections ensure good distribution of the synovial fluid and provide some cushioning against mechanical shock to the joint. The synovial fluid does not normally clot but, if there is inflammation, fibrinogen enters the fluid, which is then able to clot like normal inflammatory exudate. The increased volume and pressure of fluid within the joint (due to inflammation), and any clotting, limit joint movement.

Joint pain derives primarily from the stretching and inflammation of the fibrous structures (capsule and ligaments) and the periosteum, the thin layer of tissue which covers all bones in the body: sensation in the synovial tissues is poor. Inflammation often results in joint deformity because the limb is unconsciously held in a position which provides the maximum joint volume,

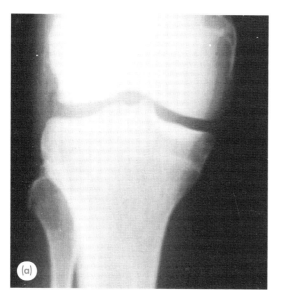
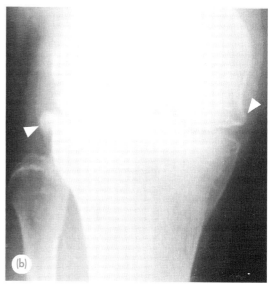

Figure 8.2 X-rays of normal and osteoarthritic knees. (a) Normal: note the smooth bone margins and the well-defined joint 'space', occupied by radiolucent cartilage. In the knee, this space is large being occupied by the cartilage covering the bone and two pads of cartilage (the **menisci**, one on either side) which absorb the shocks occurring during exercise. (b) Osteoarthritis: showing loss of joint space (owing to cartilage destruction and failure of cartilage repair), and osteophytes at the bone margins (arrows). (Reproduced with the permission of Dr AC Keat, Charing Cross and Westminster Medical School, London, UK.)

to accommodate the increased volume of synovial fluid and so reduce the pressure and pain.

Cartilaginous joints

The arrangement of the joints in the vertebral column is illustrated in Fig. 8.3. The vertebrae are covered with a thin layer of hyaline cartilage, similarly to synovial joints, but there is no capsule and associated synovium or synovial fluid. The vertebrae are separated by **intervertebral discs**, which consist of a strong fibrous capsule filled with a proteoglycan gel that provides an effective shock absorber.

Synovial sheaths and bursae

These occur where closely opposed structures move relative to each other, and especially where skin or tendons need to move freely over bony surfaces. **Bursae** are enclosed clefts of synovial membrane that are supported by dense connective tissue, the synovium sometimes being continuous with that of an adjacent joint. The central **potential** space is normally filled with a capillary film of synovial fluid which permits free movement to occur between the two layers of bursal synovium. Thus the **prepatellar bursa** lies between the skin and the lower half of the

patella (knee cap) and prevents damage to the skin and the tibial head when the knee is flexed. Similarly, the **olecranon bursa** prevents friction between the skin and the point of the elbow. Inflammation of these bursae (p. 522) causes the accumulation of synovial fluid, with swelling, tenderness, pain and restriction of movement and the conditions of 'housemaid's knee' and 'student's' or 'miner's, elbow'.

Synovial sheaths occur around tendons which pass under ligaments or through fibrous tunnels, e.g. the **carpal tunnel** (p. 521) in the wrist. The sheath consists of a closed, double-walled synovial cylinder enclosing a capillary film of synovial fluid. The inner wall is attached loosely to the tendon, and the outer wall to the bones, ligaments or other adjacent structures. This arrangement again permits free movement of the tendon through surrounding tissues, similarly to the bursae, and inflammation of the sheaths causes similar problems to bursitis.

'Ganglia' are synovial herniations (bulges) from a tendon sheath or joint and should not be confused with nerve ganglia.

Joint nutrition, maintenance and repair

The synovial membrane is supplied with blood and nutrients from the underlying vascular connective tissue. Nutrients for the **chondrocytes**,

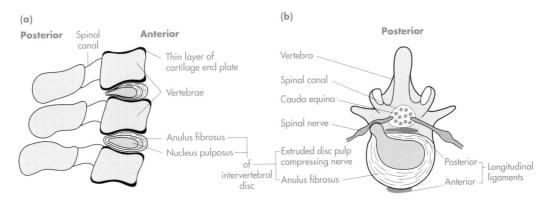

Figure 8.3 Diagram of cartilaginous joints in the lumbar region of the vertebral column and the result of disc prolapse ('slipped disc'). (a) General arrangement (saggital section). (b) Disc prolapse (transverse section): because the annulus fibrosus of the disc is thicker anteriorly and the rear of the disc is restrained by the posterior longitudinal ligament, the pulp (nucleus pulposus) tends to be extruded towards the back and side under pressure, compressing a spinal nerve on one side and causing unilateral symptoms.

which are responsible for synthesizing all of the components of the joint cartilage, diffuse from the blood supply of the synovium through the synovial fluid. The latter also returns waste products from the cartilage covering the bone, which is relatively poorly perfused, back to the circulation.

There is normally a slow continuous turnover of joint cartilage, which contains a unique type of collagen (Type II) plus highly hydrophilic proteoglycans. The latter bind the structurally important types IX and XI collagens, which are present in only small amounts but are crucial for cartilage stability. When collagen is compressed, the structural water (held by hydrogen bonding) is released from the proteoglycans and is regained when the force is removed. This mechanism temporarily increases the synovial fluid volume and makes it less viscous, thus cushioning stresses and facilitating movement. In adults the chondrocytes do not normally replicate, but repeated trauma reactivates their division. The resultant increased metabolism accelerates the dismantling and regeneration of damaged cartilage, but the effect is a **remodelling**, with an imbalance between cartilage degradation and synthesis, resulting in an inappropriate replacement.

In **osteoarthritis** (a degenerative joint disease; p. 474), the composition and size of the proteoglycan molecules is altered, with the Type II collagen fibrils being replaced with the more common, less suitable Type I collagen that is characteristic of skin and tendons. Changes also occur in the underlying bone.

The immune system and rheumatic diseases

Genetic aspects

There are clear associations between human leucocyte locus A (HLA) genes and rheumatic diseases, especially inflammatory ones. It will be recalled that the HLA system consists of a series of closely linked genetic loci located on the short arm of chromosome 6, and forms part of the major histocompatibility complex (MHC; *see* Chapter 2). Certain of the HLA antigens occur more frequently in patients with some rheumatic diseases than in general populations of the same ethnic origin (Table 8.2). For example, HLA-DR4 tends to be associated with severe rheumatoid arthritis (RA).

However, although associations between rheumatic diseases and HLA antigens are valuable pointers to pathogenesis, few of these are of diagnostic value and they do not currently influence management. The genetic status of an individual merely indicates an increased likelihood of suffering a rheumatic disease. Further, tissue typing is currently complex and expensive and does not help in prognosis, except in certain limited situations. The principal reason for pursuing these genetic relationships is the hope that better understanding of the fundamental mechanisms involved may lead to more effective, less toxic treatments and to better diagnostic and prognostic tests.

Table 8.2   Some associations between HLA antigens and rheumatic diseases

HLA antigen	Disease	Risk relative to normals[a]
DR4, Dw4	Rheumatoid arthritis (adult)	6
Dw14	Rheumatoid arthritis (adult)	5
DR2, DR3	Systemic lupus erythematosus	3
DR3	Sjögren's syndrome	6
DR4	Polyarticular juvenile arthritis	7
B27	Ankylosing spondylitis	90
	Reiter's syndrome	40
	Inflammatory bowel disease, psoriatic arthritis, and spondylitis	10

[a] Approximate values only.

Osteoarthritis

A mutation in the COL2A1 gene causes the production of a variant form of Type II collagen and is associated with the occurrence of premature osteoarthritis (OA). Further, the risk of needing a hip replacement for OA in siblings of a patient who has had the operation is three times that in the general population. **Aggrecan**, a protein–chondroitin–keratan sulphate macromolecule, is important in load dispersal in joints, and genetically determined variants are associated with hand OA in elderly men.

These and similar considerations have led to the estimate that about two-thirds of OA has a genetic basis.

Rheumatoid arthritis

The concordance rate for monozygotic (identical) twins, i.e. the risk of one contracting RA if the other has the disease, has been estimated as 12–30%. This is four to five times the risk in dizygotic (non-identical) twins. The general risk to other siblings is about eight times that in the general population.

Overall, about 40% of RA is linked to the possession of specific HLA antigens, especially DR4 and Dw4. This clearly points to RA being an autoimmune disease. The prevalence of HLA-DR4 is associated with the severity of RA and, in decreasing order of disease severity, is 90% in Felty's syndrome (p. 484), 70% in patients referred to rheumatologists, and 40% in general practice patients with RA.

Other HLA-DR antigens are implicated in the occurrence of RA in particular geographical and ethnic groups, e.g. DR1 in Southern Europe, DR10 in Spaniards, Indians and Jews, and DR14 in some North American Indians. Evidence for other genetic associations remains to be elucidated.

Interestingly, the likelihood of the occurrence of some side effects to gold or penicillamine (p. 489) is also genetically linked, e.g. nephrotic syndrome with HLA-DR3.

Ankylosing spondylitis

The association of ankylosing spondylitis (AS) with HLA-B27 is the strongest for any rheumatic disease and carries a 200 times increased risk. HLA-B60 carries only a threefold risk. Thus, the concordance rate for B27-positive monozygotic twins, one of whom has AS, is 75%. In a general group of dizygotic twins this risk falls to only 12%. Taking all genes into account, the chance of inheriting AS is about 90%, so inheritance far outweighs environmental factors as a risk factor for the condition.

The association is confirmed if we compare the prevalences of HLA-B27 and AS in different population groups: in some Native North Americans these are 50% and 8% respectively, in Northern Europeans these levels fall to 8% and 0.3%, and in Indigenous Australians to <0.5% and zero.

Environmental factors and other genes are also important for the disease to occur. It seems likely that the B27 gene requires additional genes, plus an environmental determinant, to cause rheumatic symptoms: no disease results if the additional gene is absent, even in the presence of the environmental trigger.

Tissue typing may be useful in prognosis in certain limited situations. Young patients with inconclusive symptoms and signs who are HLA-B27-positive need to be watched for the onset of significant disease, some of them being more likely to develop AS than typical juvenile chronic arthritis. Also, young male patients with low back pain who are HLA-B27-negative and do not have inflammatory bowel disease or psoriasis are unlikely to have AS.

Cytokines

Many of these small protein hormones have been implicated in rheumatic diseases, though their precise roles are uncertain. They may be **autocrines**, acting on the cell which secretes them, **paracrines**, acting on neighbouring cells, or they may have endocrine properties and act on remote tissues, e.g. *erythropoietin*.

One **tumour necrosis factor** (TNF-alpha) is released by macrophages, and induces **interleukin-1** (IL-1) production by T cells. IL-1 promotes the hepatic production of acute-phase proteins (p. 470), in association with IL-6, and is found in the synovial fluid associated with several types of arthritis. IL-1 has been implicated in stimulating the release of lysosomal enzymes, producing joint erosions in rheumatoid arthritis (RA, p. 479) and collagen degradation in OA (p. 474). Excess production of IL-1 may be responsible for maintaining a chronic inflammatory reaction in damaged joints.

Interleukin-2 (IL-2) is crucial in promoting antigen elimination, and a deficiency of it has been demonstrated in RA and systemic lupus erythematosus (SLE, p. 511). This deficiency may also contribute to the maintenance of joint inflammation, owing to a failure to clear antigens completely. **Interferons** (IFNs) are produced by several types of cell, and IFN-gamma may also be involved in joint pathology.

A deficiency of T helper cell production of erythropoietic interleukins (IL-3 and IL-5) may be implicated in causing the anaemia often seen in RA (p. 484). Finally, trials of IL-1 inhibitors, IFN-gamma and IL-2 for treating a variety of arthritides are in progress.

Examination, investigation and assessment

History and examination

Many diseases can give rise secondarily to muscular or joint pain (Table 8.3), and patient misconceptions may lead them to give misleading descriptions of pain which they ascribe to joint disease. It is therefore important for the rheumatologist to regard the patient as a whole and to decide whether there is actually an arthropathy or other related problem which falls within the speciality. The relevant details of the history and examination are given in Table 8.4.

Investigation

Although a wide range of investigations might be carried out, only those which are commonly performed are dealt with briefly below. They are discussed here only in general terms, the specific indications being dealt with under the various disease headings.

Haematology

Acute-phase proteins
These are a family of about 30 proteins that are produced by the liver in response to cytokines released from macrophages, etc. at the site of inflammation. Some of the proteins can be used as indicators of acute rheumatic disease activity; these include C-reactive protein, serum amyloid-A protein, serum ferritin and fibrinogen. The fibrinogen is not measured directly, its concentration being reflected in the erythrocyte sedimentation rate (ESR) and blood or serum viscosity.

ESR is a non-specific indicator of inflammation anywhere in the body. However, because

---

Table 8.3   Some non-rheumatic diseases which may give muscular or joint pain

Infections
Bacterial endocarditis, dysentery, gonorrhoea, hepatitis, meningitis, rubella, salmonellosis, streptococcal sore throat, tuberculosis. Fungal, protozoal

Metabolic and endocrine
Acromegaly, diabetes mellitus, hyperlipoproteinaemia, osteoporosis, osteomalacia, Paget's disease, parathyroid disease, thyroid diseases

Systemic diseases
Chronic renal failure, haemophilia, hypogammaglobulinaemia, inflammatory bowel disease, leukaemias, myelomas, neuropathy (loss of joint sensation), respiratory (e.g. bronchiectasis, fibrosing alveolitis)

Skin diseases
Erythema nodosum, psoriasis

Table 8.4   Aspects of the history and examination relevant to rheumatic diseases[a]

History

Age, sex, race
Occupation
Pain
- now: location, severity, duration
- pattern of onset, joint involvement, periodicity
- precipitating, aggravating and relieving factors
Associated symptoms
- stiffness, joint swelling
- skin, gastrointestinal, eye and respiratory
Presenting complaint (*see* Table 8.5)
Past medical history (*see* Table 8.6)
- medication history: drugs used, dose, period, effectiveness, side effects
Family history
Social history
- ability to cope; patient's attitudes, e.g. expectations of outcome and from the consultation and treatment, interpretation of symptoms and emotional response to them

---

Examination

Joints
- swelling, inflammation, pain or tenderness, deformity, symmetry of involvement
- surrounding abnormalities, muscle wasting
- movement: range, noises or grating
- stability
- functional capacity
The whole patient
- appearance, posture, gait
- nodules
- finger clubbing
- fever
- neuropathies (loss of sensation)
- review of all organ systems

---

[a] *See also* Chapter 1, Table 1.2. Items here are aspects of special relevance to rheumatic diseases.

the test is easily performed at the bedside, it is widely used as a rapid and simple screening test. The sedimentation rate increases owing to increased levels of fibrinogen and immunoglobulins which increase red blood cell (RBC) clumping, increasing in turn sedimentation, and so causing anaemia. Very high ESR values may be due to serious underlying disease, e.g. multisystem disorders (pp. 511–520), certain infections, or malignancy. Unfortunately, changes in RBC size or morphology that occur in some severe anaemias can also affect the ESR.

C-reactive protein (CRP) is another non-specific indicator of inflammation. The protein, so-called because it reacts with *Streptococcus pneumoniae* Type C polysaccharide, is synthesized in the liver and its concentration rises within 6 h of fever, inflammation, tissue damage or necrosis. This is a much more rapid response than the ESR, and CRP is the marker of choice in the diagnosis of inflammatory diseases. However, it is less useful than ESR and plasma viscosity for monitoring the progress of chronic inflammatory states.

Serum amyloid-A protein (SAA) is the probable precursor of **amyloid**, the fibrous protein which is characteristic of amyloidosis (p. 519). SAA levels are modestly raised in SLE, but are high in RA and Still's disease, though whether this predicts the development of amyloid disease is unknown.

Anaemia

Many chronic inflammatory diseases cause a mild, normocytic anaemia, related to reduced erythropoiesis. This may reflect the level of inflammatory disease activity, as also do ESR and CRP, and reduced levels of IL-3 and IL-5. Haemoglobin levels lower than about 10 g/dL in males and 9 g/dL in females may indicate other possible causes, e.g. iatrogenic gastrointestinal blood loss due to drugs used to treat rheumatic disease, such as NSAIDs. These irritate the gastrointestinal tract and also inhibit the production of gastroprotective prostaglandins.

Leucocytes

Leucocytosis (raised white cell count) may result from infection, severe exacerbations of RA, or treatment with corticosteroids. The condition may also be an indication of serious systemic inflammatory disease, notably polyarteritis nodosa (PAN). **Leucopenia** (depressed white cell count) may indicate the presence of SLE (p. 511), or Felty's syndrome (p. 484) in a patient with RA, but may also reflect drug-induced myelosuppression (bone marrow depression), e.g. due to *sodium aurothiomalate* (gold sodium thiomalate, sodium aurothiosuccinate), *penicillamine* or immunosuppressive drugs.

Platelets

The platelet count may be raised (**thrombocytosis**) in active inflammatory diseases or after an acute bleeding episode. The converse, **thrombocytopenia**, may indicate Felty's syndrome or drug toxicity. In the latter case, immediate drug withdrawal is essential because fatal bone marrow depression may sometimes follow.

Biochemistry

Serum phosphatases. Raised **serum alkaline phosphatase** (ALP) may be used to detect those patients whose bone pain is due to metabolic bone disease, e.g. Paget's disease and osteomalacia. High levels of **serum acid phosphatase** (ACP) in older men indicate the possibility of backache being due to metastatic deposits from prostatic carcinoma.

Creatine kinase (CK). CK is a useful screening test in patients who may have muscle damage in **polymyositis** or **dermatomyositis**. It is also a feature of heart muscle damage in myocardial infarction (*see* Chapter 3, pp. 139–140).

Serology

Rheumatoid factors (RFs). These are autoantibodies against the Fc portion of IgG (*see* Chapter 2). The tests routinely employed primarily detect IgMs, though some RFs are IgGs. Normally, the IgG molecule is folded and protected, but reaction with antigens exposes reaction sites so that flocculation can occur between RFs and immune complexes formed between IgGs and proteins from damaged tissues. Patients whose serum contains significant levels of RFs are described as 'seropositive', and the RF titre roughly reflects disease activity. Some laboratories use the **differential agglutinating test**, which gives a titratable measure of RFs in the serum.

Complement. Raised levels of complement components (*see* Chapter 2) occur in many of the significantly inflammatory rheumatic diseases.

Low levels of complement components, especially C3 and C4, reflect disease activity in SLE, because they indicate immune complex formation: decreasing levels imply a deterioration in the patient's condition.

Fluorescent antinuclear antibody test (ANA or ANF). This is used as a rapid preliminary, non-specific screening test for diseases in which autoantibodies to cell nuclei occur, e.g. SLE, mixed connective tissue disease.

DNA binding test. This radioimmunoassay detects antibodies against native (normal), double-stranded DNA. The level of DNA binding indicates disease activity in SLE, though the test is rather insensitive. It is usually used only in patients who are strongly positive in the ANA test.

Extractable antigens. A wide range of autoantibodies against soluble nuclear and cytoplasmic antigens detected by counter-immunoelectrophoresis are used to contribute to diagnosis in a variety of systemic connective tissue disorders, e.g. SLE, Sjögren's syndrome and systemic sclerosis.

Antistreptolysin 'O' titre (ASO). Levels of this antibody indicate recent streptococcal infection and may be used to confirm a diagnosis of rheumatic fever.

Tissue typing. Detection of the presence of the histocompatibility antigen HLA-B27 may occasionally help in the diagnosis or exclusion of seronegative arthropathies (p. 503).

Synovial fluid

This is normally present as a small volume of a clear, pale yellow, viscous fluid. It may be examined for the following:

- Protein (high in inflammatory arthritis).
- Leucocytes (high in RA, neutrophil counts are high in septic arthritis).
- Microorganisms (septic arthritis).
- Crystals of urate (gout) and pyrophosphate (pseudogout).

Urinalysis

This may give clues to the origin of symptoms, e.g.:

- Glycosuria: frozen shoulder (p. 522) and tendon contractures are associated with diabetes.
- Microscopic haematuria: Reiter's syndrome (p. 505), or metastatic bone pain caused by urinary tract carcinoma.
- Proteinuria: multiple myeloma as a cause of back pain.
- Sterile pyuria: tuberculosis causing bone and joint pain. *Mycobacterium tuberculosis* will not grow in the medium used for the normal bacteriological examination of urine.

Imaging

Radiology. X-rays are invaluable in revealing joint damage (Fig. 8.2(b); *see also* Fig. 8.6(b)) and for monitoring the progress of joint disease. Radiography is also useful in distinguishing between OA and RA, and as an aid in the diagnosis of AS and pseudogout. Occasionally, it may be necessary to use more specialized techniques, e.g. **computed tomography** (CT) scans, **nuclear magnetic resonance imaging** (MRI), arthrography (with radio-opaque contrast media injected into the joint) or **arthroscopy** (see below), and radionuclide bone scanning, when X-ray findings are negative or equivocal. CT and MRI scans can provide greater information on changes which are difficult to visualize using normal techniques, e.g. intervertebral disc prolapse (Fig. 8.3 and p. 523).

Arthroscopy. An endoscope (a thinner version of that shown in Chapter 6, Fig. 6.5) can be inserted into a joint to examine it, and this is a relatively safe and simple procedure. Arthroscopy is particularly valuable in the knee, where it permits complete examination of the cartilage, synovium and ligaments. Biopsies can be taken, synovial fluid aspirated and loose fragments or torn sections of cartilage can be removed with minimal trauma.

Scintiscanning. Technetium-99m-labelled *disodium etidronate* and similar agents are occasionally used to detect bone lesions.

Tissue biopsy

Biopsy is only occasionally helpful, as a confirmatory test, in some diseases associated with rheumatic symptoms, e.g. giant cell arteritis (temporal artery, p. 517), SLE (kidney, p. 511), and some myopathies.

Functional capacity

The principal components of a detailed assessment of functional capacity are listed in Table 8.5. However, a simpler approach is used for most clinical purposes, e.g.:

- Grade 1: completely independent.
- Grade 2: needs aids and appliances, but is still independent.
- Grade 3: needs help with daily tasks, e.g. bathing, dressing, cooking.

Table 8.5 Components contributing to the assessment of functional capacity

Duration of morning stiffness
Grip strength
Functional questionnaire: e.g. ability to dress, walk, open doors, turn taps, pick up small objects
Degree of joint movement: e.g. fingers, arms, hips, knees; chest expansion, spinal extension
Ability to perform activities of daily living: e.g. work-related tasks, maintaining the home, child care

- Grade 4: needs considerable and constant help; confined to a wheelchair or to bed.

Osteoarthritis (OA, osteoarthrosis)

Definition and epidemiology

As in all mechanical bearings, wear tends to occur in joints after a long period of use, and some degree of cartilage damage is almost universal in the elderly. This may affect the synovial joints (**osteoarthrosis**) or the cartilaginous joints of the vertebral column (**spondylosis**). Although inflammation is not the underlying pathology, a variable degree of secondary inflammation is very common and the term **osteoarthritis** may be used to indicate this, whereas osteoarthrosis may be used when inflammation is absent.

OA is often called degenerative joint disease, but this is inaccurate because symptoms are probably due to inappropriate repair (remodelling) secondary to joint damage. This remodelling process should be contrasted with the situation in rheumatoid arthritis (p. 479), where the underlying pathogenetic mechanism is a maladaptive immune response.

OA and soft tissue rheumatism (p. 521) together are responsible for most of the primary care rheumatological workload and of the prescriptions for non-steroidal anti-inflammatory drugs.

Classification

Osteoarthritis is classifiable into two groups:
- **Primary** (**idiopathic**): of unknown origin, that may be localized to a single joint or involve three or more groups of joints.

- **Secondary**: to other conditions. These are:
  - Consequent on trauma, overuse, joint misalignment, etc., or on bone disease, e.g. Paget's disease.
  - Congenital or developmental.
  - Inherited: e.g. metabolic disease, acromegaly, Gaucher's disease.
  - Neuropathic, e.g. Charcot's arthropathy.

Pathology and aetiology

Primary osteoarthritis

Important factors for primary OA are:

- **Age**: although OA is a very frequent condition in the elderly, it is not universal and so cannot be considered as a **normal** feature of the ageing process.
- **Wear and tear**: the subchondral bone (immediately underlying the cartilage) is known to undergo microfractures in normal use, and repeated fracture and healing results in bone changes that reduce its ability to absorb shocks. Further, muscle weakening with lack of exercise and advancing age results in loss of adequate joint support, thus allowing abnormal joint movement which causes further cartilage damage. However, excessive wear and tear does not, **by itself**, necessarily produce OA. Joint surgery, e.g. menisectomy (removal of the semilunar cartilage in the knee) predisposes to OA of the treated joint. The composition and size of the proteoglycan molecules of the joint cartilage is altered and the rate of repair no longer keeps pace with that of degradation. Further, the Type II collagen fibrils are replaced with the more common, less suitable Type I collagen which is characteristic

of skin and tendons. Changes also occur in the underlying bone, with new bone formation occurring at the margins of the articular cartilage to form osteophytes (bony outgrowths; Fig. 8.2(b)). Mutant genes (see below), producing abnormal collagen, may also be involved.

- **Obesity**: the persuasive argument that increased weight imposes additional stresses and wear on joints fails to explain why the ankle joint is usually spared.
- **Genetic predisposition**: e.g. **primary generalized OA (PGOA)**, in which there is widespread early joint involvement, is **sex-linked** in that it is 1.5 times more common in women and tends to run in families, as does the development of **Heberden's nodes**, i.e. bony enlargement of the distal interphalangeal (DIP; terminal finger) joints (Fig. 8.4). Less common are the similar **Bouchard's nodes** at the proximal interphalangeal (PIP; middle finger) joint. Involvement of the first metacarpophalangeal (MCP; thumb) joint gives the hand a squarish appearance. PGOA is unusual in Black populations, but is particularly common in people of British descent, with about 30% of white North American and Northern European adults having some osteoarthritic features. PGOA is not related to climatic or environmental factors, and there is no association with HLA antigens. Any genetic effect is likely to be polygenic.
- Local **biochemical factors** in individual joints.
- Acute exacerbations may be due to **calcium pyrophosphate deposition disease** (p. 511).

Secondary osteoarthritis

Accelerated wear due to joint damage or malfunction, e.g. obesity and sports injury, may lead to impaired or inappropriate repair mechanisms, as in osteophyte formation (e.g. Heberden's nodes: see above). A listing of some common causes is given in Table 8.6. The disease may develop insidiously over up to 60 years, and may be due to the production of an abnormal collagen structure that is less able to withstand the applied stresses.

Clinical features

The frequently used and weight-bearing joints (hands, hip, knee; Fig. 8.2(b)) are principally affected and contribute to disability. Unlike RA, there is no systemic (extra-articular) involvement (p. 484) in OA. The predominant features are:

- **Pain**. Onset is gradual, occurring initially after exercise but later also at night and at rest, with tenderness on pressure.
- **Stiffness**. This may be severe after a period of rest, but is transient, and although patients often complain of stiffness on rising ('morning stiffness') this usually lasts no more than 15 min. This should be compared with the situation in RA in which morning stiffness may be severe and prolonged.
- **Loss of function**. This is extremely variable and may occur early, even though the pain is slight. However, even gross joint changes may not be accompanied by significant functional

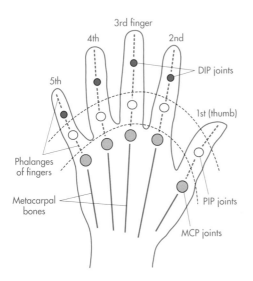

Figure 8.4 Joints and bones of the hand. DIP, distal interphalangeal; MCP, metacarpophalangeal; PIP, proximal interphalangeal. The joints of the foot corresponding to the MCP joints are the MTP (metatarsophalangeal) joints. The foot bones corresponding to the metacarpals are the metatarsals.

Table 8.6 Some conditions which commonly predispose to secondary osteoarthritis

Trauma
Obesity, fractures, dislocation, sports injuries, joint surgery

Genetic and congenital
Conditions affecting joint alignment, haemophilia, acromegaly, hyperparathyroidism, chondrocalcinosis, ochronosis

Postinflammatory
Rheumatoid arthritis, gout, pseudogout, septic arthritis

Bone disease
Paget's disease

impairment, though there may be limitation of movement.

- **Joint swellings**. These are hard (**Heberden's** and **Bouchard's** nodes) and due to **osteophytes** (outgrowths at the bone ends, Fig. 8.2(b)), or they may be softer and partly due to inflammation. The inflammation and tenderness may occur in the early stages and during the acute exacerbations, and last a few weeks. These conditions occur without apparent cause, notably if joints are over-used.

The **joints most commonly involved** are:

- DIP joints (Heberden's nodes, normally spared in RA).
- PIP joints (Bouchard's nodes, less common).
- The feet, especially the first metatarsophalangeal (MTP) joint (large toe), which takes the heaviest loading.

- The knees (Fig. 8.2(b)), hips, cervical and lumbar spine.

The **joints most commonly spared**, unless the damage results from repetitive occupational trauma, e.g. road drill operators, motor cycle despatch riders, are the shoulder, elbows, wrists, MCP joints (usually affected in RA) and ankle.

The course of OA is highly variable, and 25–30% of patients with established features may show no clinical or radiographic deterioration over long periods.

Investigation

X-radiography is an important aid in differential diagnosis and assessment of OA. Table 8.7 compares the principal radiographic features in OA and RA which are illustrated in Figs 8.2(b) and 8.6(b). There is a correlation between radiographic features and the reporting of pain, though not with pain severity.

All other tests are usually normal in OA, though there may occasionally be an increase in ESR during an acute inflammatory exacerbation.

Management

Aims

Because OA is not reversible, except by surgical interventions such as joint replacement, the aims of management are:

- To relieve pain.
- To maintain mobility and function.

Table 8.7 Comparison of the principal radiographic features in osteoarthritis and rheumatoid arthritis[a]

Feature	Osteoarthritis	Rheumatoid arthritis
Joint space	Reduced	Reduced
Erosions	No	Yes
Osteophytes	Yes	No
Bone density at joints	Increased (sclerosis)	Reduced (porosis)
Bone cysts	Yes[b]	No

[a] This table should be read in conjunction with Figs 8.2 and 8.6

[b] Although bone density is increased, cysts form under the cartilage, probably because some of the increased synovial fluid is forced into exposed bone.

- To prevent further joint damage.
- To improve the patient's mental health and quality of life.

The **modes** used in management include patient education and counselling, physiotherapy and occupational therapy, the correction of any exacerbating factors, drugs, and surgery.

Patient education and counselling

Many patients fear that they have crippling arthritis, so it is important to reassure them and to stress that disease progression is very gradual and that function is usually well maintained. Even if severe deterioration of major joints occurs, e.g. in the hips or knees, surgery is very effective.

Because the problem is basically one of joint wear, patients should understand that it is essential for them to follow proper physiotherapist guidance on exercises which are designed to maintain muscle strength without undue joint stress. Unwise exercise causes further damage to joints which are already compromised. However, rest is not advisable except during an acute exacerbation because it may lead to loss of muscle power and to excessive stiffness: patients need controlled exercise.

Attaining an ideal weight reduces joint stress in overweight patients.

Research has demonstrated that mental health improves with effective treatment and thus reflects disease activity.

Physical therapies

Physiotherapy (**PT**) and **occupational therapy** (**OT**) have an important role to play in maintaining muscle strength and so increasing joint stability, in giving the patient additional confidence to manage independently, and in maintaining mobility and independence as far as possible. The modes used involve the following. **Exercises** to maintain and restore muscle power and function are effective, especially after surgery. The power of the quadriceps muscles in the thigh must be sufficient to preserve general mobility, balance and the ability to rise from chairs, etc. Muscle power should be improved before a patient undergoes elective surgery as this greatly aids recovery: any period of bed rest causes a rapid loss of muscle mass and power. **Isometric exercises**, in which muscles are exercised against fixed resistance with minimal joint movement and change in muscle length, improve muscle power without joint wear. **Swimming** and **hydrotherapy** (exercising in a warm pool against water resistance) are also excellent forms of exercise, because the weight of the body is supported by the water, thus reducing joint stress.

Occupational assessment and training, i.e. advice on alternative methods of carrying out tasks at home and at work, or retraining, by occupational therapists to minimize joint trauma includes the following:

- Provision of **aids** and **appliances**, and modifications of the home to improve mobility and ease tasks, e.g. splints, easy-turning taps, specially adapted implements and, in exceptional circumstances, widening doors and providing ramps for wheelchair access.
- Local heat, diathermy, ultrasound, etc. are widely used, but provide only temporary relief.
- **Physiotherapists**, **osteopaths** and **chiropractors** can help by mobilizing and realigning joints and relieving associated muscle spasm.

Correction of exacerbating factors

The effects of OA may be exacerbated by a variety of conditions, some of which are potentially correctable, at least in part. Corrective measures include:

- Reduction of obesity to minimize stress on weight-bearing joints.
- Correction of any underlying or concurrent disease.
- Surgical or other orthopaedic correction of anatomical abnormalities which place abnormal stresses on other joints. For example, unequal leg length causes wear both to the leg joints and to those of the pelvis and vertebral column.
- Maintenance of physical activity and general fitness.
- Wearing of correct footwear and use of appropriate walking aids.
- Encouraging a positive outlook.

Pharmacotherapy

Medicines have only a limited role in the treatment of OA patients, the aims being the relief of:

- Pain and discomfort.
- Inflammatory exacerbations.
- Depression and anxiety.

Analgesics and non-steroidal anti-inflammatory drugs (NSAIDs)

Opinions differ as to which of these groups is most appropriate.

Simple analgesics (*see* Chapter 10) are widely used, but there is considerable variation in their tolerance and efficacy between patients. Most patients are maintained on a single product (*paracetamol (acetaminophen)*), normal analgesic doses (600–900 mg) of *aspirin*, occasionally *dextropropoxyphene (propoxyphene)*, *codeine* or *dihydrocodeine* (depending on pain severity), taken regularly. *Benorilate* (p. 496) combines the effects of both aspirin and paracetamol and is generally well tolerated. Combinations of paracetamol or aspirin with the other analgesics are widely used.

NSAIDs are discussed more fully under the treatment of RA (p. 489), but some points are relevant here. Although NSAIDs are popular, there are reports that some, e.g. *ibuprofen* and *naproxen*, may accelerate cartilage damage or prevent its repair. Although the clinical significance of this is unclear, it may be appropriate to use a drug which is alleged to promote cartilage repair, e.g. *aceclofenac* (or tenidap, experimental). Some prescribers prefer to reserve NSAIDs for the occasional painful exacerbation or when there is a significant inflammatory component. Several NSAIDs seem to be unsuitable in OA on grounds of toxicity, e.g. *azapropazone (apazone)*, *indometacin*, *ketoprofen* (and tolmetin, not licensed in the UK).

Meloxicam, the first 'second-generation' NSAID to be marketed as a relatively selective cyclooxygenase 2 (COX-2) inhibitor (Fig. 8.9), is licensed for the short-term treatment of exacerbations of OA, but may still cause severe gastrointestinal and skin reactions. However, existing NSAIDs, e.g. *diclofenac*, *etodolac*, *nabumetone*, *naproxen* and *piroxicam*, are also somewhat COX-2-selective and are licensed similarly.

'Third-generation' NSAIDs are highly selective COX-2 inhibitors, with no effect on COX-1 at therapeutic doses. *Rofecoxib* is the first of these to be licensed in the UK for symptomatic relief in OA treatment. *Celecoxib* is available in North America and is likely to be licensed soon in the UK. Although the risk of significant gastrointestinal side effects is much reduced with these drugs it has not been eliminated completely, though *rofecoxib* can be taken with or without food.

Rofecoxib is **contraindicated** in the presence of:

- Active peptic ulceration or gastrointestinal bleeding.
- Moderate to severe hepatic dysfunction.
- Significant renal failure.
- Hypersensitivity to aspirin or other NSAIDs.
- Pregnancy, or in women wishing to conceive, because:
  - The products of COX-2 activity are probably involved in ovulation, and implantation of the fertilized ovum and COX-2 inhibition may thus affect fertility.
  - Prostaglandin E1 (PGE_1) maintains patency of the ductus arteriosus. Inhibition of COX-2 may reduce fetal PGE_1 levels and cause premature closure of the duct (*indometacin* is used to close a persistent duct in young babies), thus damaging immature fetal lungs and causing undesirable fetal haemodynamic effects.

Other drugs

Disease-modifying antirheumatic drugs (DMARDs; Table 8.13 and p. 496) and *systemic corticosteroids* have no place in the treatment of OA. However, a severely affected joint which is inflamed or in which there is a fluid effusion may respond well to an intra-articular *corticosteroid injection*, though the benefit is usually only temporary. Because there is the possibility of long-term joint damage with repeated injections, owing to suppression of protein (cartilage) synthesis, this should only be done occasionally.

Intra-articular injections of *sodium hyaluronate*, given weekly on three to five occasions, is reported to be more beneficial than a steroid injection (unlicensed indication in the UK).

Levels of the pain transmitter, **substance P** (*see*

Chapter 10, p. 575), are raised in OA and this also increases synovial levels of prostaglandins and collagenase. Reduction of the substance P level is therefore desirable and this can be done using topical *capsaicin cream*. This product is thus a logical second-line agent after a simple analgesic, or as an adjunct to systemic treatment.

Antidepressants are used to alleviate the depression associated with chronic pain and may also improve the analgesic response.

Women receiving *hormone replacement therapy* (HRT) have been shown to be less likely to develop OA, especially of the knee, and HRT can also be mildly euphoriant. The benefit on the knee, which is lost if HRT is stopped, may be related to the prevention of osteoporosis and so to the maintenance of bone density adjacent to joints.

Surgery

Severe, uncontrolled pain or serious loss of function may necessitate surgery. **Arthroplasty** (joint replacement) is especially successful for the hip, the pain relief being excellent and mobility usually being returned close to normal, provided that the operation is carried out before joint damage is too severe and collateral damage, e.g. to the joints of the vertebral column, has not occurred. Knee and finger joint replacement are slightly less successful and that of other joints still less so, though techniques and results are improving continually.

Joint lavage with physiological saline benefits some patients, possibly by removing debris or inflammatory mediators from the joint space.

Other operations to fix joints permanently (**arthrodesis**) or to remove osteophytes (e.g. for bunions) may be undertaken occasionally for particular patients. In patients in whom arthroplasty is inappropriate, **osteotomy**, i.e. cutting the bone or removing a section of bone near a joint, with or without re-alignment, may be successful for pain relief in disease of the knee or hip joints. The reasons for this are poorly understood, but correction of misalignment of the limbs clearly relieves stresses on associated joints. Also, diversion of healing functions to the surgically produced wound may switch metabolic activity away from the neighbouring joint.

Rheumatoid arthritis (RA)

Introduction

Unlike OA, which is a local, generally non-inflammatory disease, RA is usually a chronic, progressive, inflammatory, **systemic** disease, that primarily affects synovial joints (cf. OA, pp. 474–478).

The most common extra-articular features are anaemia, soft tissue nodules (p. 484), vasculitis, sicca syndrome (p. 514) and fibrosing alveolitis.

Epidemiology and aetiology

In the UK, about 1.5% of the population is affected, with a 3:1 female:male premenopausal sex ratio, though among the elderly the incidence is equal in both sexes: this points to a strong hormonal influence. The peak period of onset of RA is between 35 and 55 years of age, though it can start at almost any age. Worldwide, only minor racial and geographical variations occur: the global prevalence is about 1%.

The concordance rate in monozygotic twins has been variously reported as between 12% and 30% (about 4% in dizygotics), so there is only a limited contribution from genetic factors, mostly HLA DR4 and DR1. However, these genes probably determine disease severity and persistence rather than causation.

The trigger factors and the basis of the prolonged, intense inflammatory process of RA are largely unknown: despite extensive research and our much greater understanding of immunopathology, current explanations are speculative. The concept of RA as an autoimmune disease is popular and there are large numbers of mature memory T cells (CD45RO) in rheumatoid joints, derived from CD4 cells. These promote immunoglobulin production by B cells, and there is no negative feedback, hence the production of **rheumatoid factors** (RFs, a class of antibodies, see below).

The presence of CD45RO cells implies prior exposure to antigen. It has been suggested that there is a persistent antigenic stimulation by Epstein–Barr virus, the cause of glandular fever.

Retroviruses have also been suspected in experimental animals, though as yet no virus has been implicated. Bacterial causes, e.g. *Proteus mirabilis*, are also disputed. There is a high incidence of HLA-DR1, DR4 and Dw4 genes in RA patients. DR4 carriers have a high reactivity to *M. tuberculosis* and, interestingly, T cells cloned from the synovial fluid of RA patients seem to react with tubercular antigens. There may also be an association between DR4 and T cell receptor genes.

It is possible that RA was introduced into Europe in the 18th century by contact with Native Americans, who have seven times the prevalence of most of the world. This would imply an infectious aetiology.

Course

The onset of classical RA is normally insidious, polyarticular (several joints are affected) and symmetrical. The small joints (PIP, MCP, MTP, wrists) are affected first, although a monoarticular onset, usually in the knee or the wrist, occurs in some 20% of patients. Fatigue and malaise may precede joint symptoms by several months.

Occasionally, there is an abrupt onset with marked systemic symptoms. This acute form has a better prognosis and, following recovery, many years may pass before another attack occurs. Even less common is a **palindromic** onset, with acute episodes affecting one joint for hours or days, followed by remissions and exacerbations affecting other joints at intervals of days to months. RA often remits in pregnancy (75% of women), a situation that may be related to the suppression of IL-2 production, a promoter of T cell proliferation and cytolytic killer cells. Susceptibility to RA, and changes in disease activity, may be related to sex hormone levels, which may modulate T cell responses.

Disease activity waxes and wanes unpredictably and spontaneously, so patients who experience a remission while taking or using some product will naturally – though often mistakenly – attribute their improvement to that use. This natural variation in disease activity is one of the principal problems in the evaluation of new anti-arthritic drugs: large numbers of patients have to be used in very well-designed trials over long periods in order to obtain statistically meaningful results.

Patients with severe disease have significant morbidity and mortality. Of those referred to hospital consultants only about 50% are likely to be working after 10 years of disease and after 20 years a similar proportion will probably have died or be severely disabled. However, these data are over 12 years old and the situation has since improved.

Pathology

Inflammation of the synovial membrane is the cardinal initial feature (Fig. 8.5). The cells lining

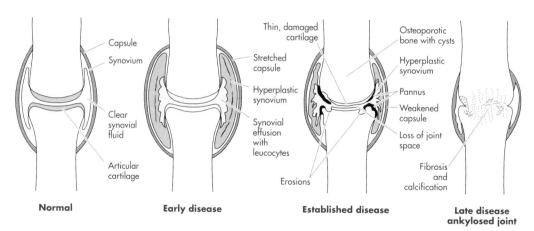

Figure 8.5 Progression of joint damage in rheumatoid arthritis. The end result in severe disease is an ankylosed (rigid), painless, non-functional joint.

the synovium multiply, the surface becomes thickened and covered with villi, and fibrin is deposited from the inflammatory exudate. In severe cases the synovium may be 1 cm thick (normally less than 1 mm).

The deeper layers become infiltrated with lymphocytes and plasma cells, the latter of which produce rheumatoid factors. Most patients become seropositive within a year of symptom onset and show high RF titres. However, there are few neutrophils in the synovium, though they are the most common cells in the synovial fluid. Phagocytosis of the immune complexes formed in the fluid results in an increase in oxidative metabolism, liberating damaging free radicals and lysosomal enzymes which attack tissues.

If the inflammation proceeds, the synovial margin develops outgrowths of metabolically active **pannus** which dissolves underlying cartilage and bone to produce the characteristic **erosions** (Figs 8.5 and 8.6(b)). With severe disease progression, the supporting ligaments and tendons are weakened and the joint will **sublux**

(become partially or completely dislocated; Fig. 8.6(b)), becoming deformed and eventually non-functional. Finally, the joint may become ankylosed, i.e. fibrosed and calcified and thus stiff and non-functional, but pain-free. This progression of changes is illustrated in Fig. 8.5. Tendons and tendon sheaths undergo changes similar to the synovial changes described above.

The mechanisms responsible for these changes are unknown but activation of T cells by macrophages and unidentified antigens cause cytokine release. Thus TNF-alpha and IL-1 are important in the initiation and maintenance of cartilage and bone damage and synovitis. It has also been suggested that deposition of iron in the synovial tissues, which does occur, promotes free radical damage. Hence chelating agents have been used to treat some patients with severe RA, and this approach is still being investigated.

Immunodeficient patients, e.g. those with AIDS and hypogammaglobulinaemia, are particularly susceptible to the complication of an episode of septic arthritis (joint infection).

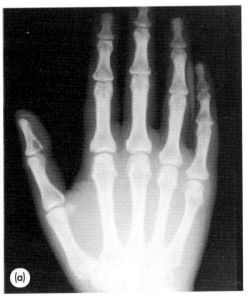 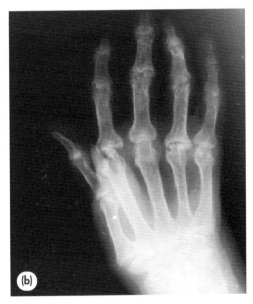

Figure 8.6 X-ray of the hand in rheumatoid arthritis. (a) Normal: note the clearly defined joint spaces in both the hand and the wrist. (b) Severe rheumatoid arthritis: note the loss of joint space owing to cartilage destruction and substantial erosions of the heads of the metacarpal bones (Fig. 8.5) and the carpal (wrist) bones. The first metacarpal (thumb) has subluxed under the second and there is slight ulnar deviation (Fig. 8.7). Most of the finger bones are osteoporotic (showing grey = radiolucent). (Reproduced with the permission of Dr AC Keat, Charing Cross and Westminster Medical School, London, UK.)

Clinical features

Articular features

These are outlined in Table 8.8. The most characteristic form of onset involves:

- **Symmetrical small joint polyarthritis** commencing in the MCP and PIP joints of the hands (Fig. 8.6(b)), the wrists and the corresponding joints in the feet.
- **Morning stiffness.**

With disease progression, morning stiffness becomes prolonged and disabling, and it may take a patient some 2 h to dress. Almost any joint may be affected, especially the wrists and the upper cervical spine. Wrist involvement (Fig. 8.6(b)) always suggests a diagnosis of RA, because the wrists are usually spared in OA.

Despite this catalogue of disability, it is important to appreciate that the majority of patients have only mild to moderate disease and are treated adequately by general practitioners: 25% recover completely. A minority, perhaps 10%, are referred to hospital consultants and about 50% of these, i.e. some 5% of the total, suffer serious disability. Thus, most GPs are likely to have such a patient.

More advanced disease may produce characteristic hand deformities, resulting in a progressive loss of function that manifests as:

- **Subluxation** of the MCP joints, so that the proximal phalangeal heads slip partly under the metacarpal heads.
- **Ulnar deviation** (Fig. 8.7(a)), in which the hand is tilted sideways towards the ulna (the large bone of the forearm), i.e. away from the thumb.
- **Boutonnière** and **swan neck** deformities of the fingers (Fig. 8.7(b)) due to damage to joint ligaments.

Changes in the upper cervical spine may cause serious instability, because ligament damage may allow subluxation of one or more vertebrae, producing kinking and compression of the spinal cord (Fig. 8.8), resulting in occipital, neck, shoulder and arm pain, and sensory loss. In particular, subluxation of the atlas on the axis may allow the dens to compress the upper cervical spine, and traumatic injury in this area, e.g. caused by a whiplash effect in a motor accident, may even cause death, though this is fortunately rare. Similarly, **manipulation of the cervical spine in RA may result in permanent disability**, even tetraparesis (partial or total paralysis of all four limbs), and so physiotherapy or other manipulation of this area is usually totally contraindicated in RA.

Periarticular features

These changes are those associated with the joints, but not arising from within the joint. Pain

---

Table 8.8 Principal articular and periarticular features of rheumatoid arthritis

Joints involved and frequency[a]	
Hands, 90; wrists, 85; knees, 80; feet, 70; shoulder, 60; hip, 10	

General features	
Inflammation	Any joint may be involved, but DIP[b] joints of the hands and feet tend to be spared
Muscle wasting	Associated with disuse of any joint
Joint deformity	Hands, especially MCP[c] joints; feet, especially MTP joints[c]; wrists[c], knees. The shoulder and hip joints are relatively spared
Joint erosions	At any joint actively affected
Other lesions	Hands, tendons; feet, bunions; wrists, carpal tunnel syndrome (p. 521); knees, Baker's cysts (p. 484), bursitis (p. 522)

[a] Numbers are the approximate percentages of patients affected.

[b] DIP, MCP, MTP, joints of the hands and feet (Fig. 8.4).

[c] Subluxation may occur (see above).

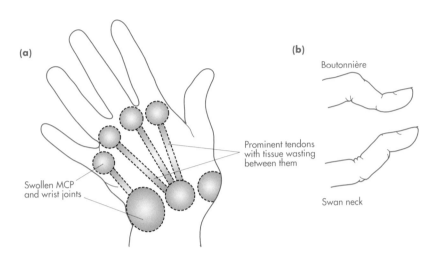

Figure 8.7   Hand in severe rheumatoid arthritis. (a) The hand shows ulnar deviation and the thumb is subluxed under the palm. (b) Types of finger deformity.

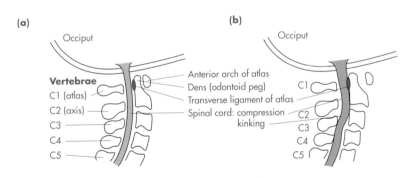

Figure 8.8   Cervical spine and the effects on it of severe rheumatoid arthritis. (a) Normal: the spinal cord and the vertebrae lie on a smooth curve, and the dens is held firmly by the transverse ligament of the atlas. The atlas is so-called because it carries the weight of the 'globe' (the head). The axis is the vertebra on which the head and atlas rotate. (b) Severe RA: weakening of the ligaments has allowed the vertebrae to sublux forwards so that they lie on a stepped curve causing kinking and compression of the spinal cord. The weakened transverse ligament of the atlas has allowed the dens to move away from the anterior arch of the atlas, compressing the spinal cord.

Table 8.9 Principal extra-articular (systemic) features and complications of rheumatoid arthritis

General	Malaise, tiredness, depression, fever
Skin	Nodules, sweaty palms, palmar erythema, nail fold infarcts
Blood and lymphoid	Anaemia, lymphadenopathy, splenomegaly, Felty's syndrome (see Table 8.10)
Cardiovascular	Raynaud's syndrome, pericarditis, myocarditis, heart nodules, vasculitis
Eye	Keratoconjunctivitis sicca, episcleritis, scleritis
Neurological	Nerve entrapment, peripheral neuropathies
Respiratory	Lung nodules, pleurisy, pulmonary fibrosis

and stiffness within a joint may result in wasting of the associated muscles. Because tendon sheaths resemble synovium, **tenosynovitis** (p. 522) may occur with pain and diminished joint movement. Tendons may be extensively damaged and may even rupture. Swelling of the tendon sheaths within the restricted confines of the carpal tunnel often causes **carpal tunnel syndrome** (p. 521). **Raynaud's syndrome** (p. 516) and carpal tunnel syndrome may appear before the joint symptoms.

Bursitis (p. 522) is also common, especially in the feet, with resultant **bunion** formation.

In the knees, high intra-articular pressure may cause the synovium to balloon out into the popliteal fossa to form a **Baker's cyst**. If this ruptures, due to increased pressure occurring in the joint during knee flexion, synovial fluid is forced into the calf, causing severe pain and mimicking a deep vein thrombosis (see Chapter 3).

Extra-articular features

These are sometimes described as **complications** of RA, but because RA is a systemic disease, signs and symptoms (often inflammatory) may occur almost anywhere in the body (Table 8.9). **Haematological** abnormalities are common. **Anaemia** is the most frequent of these, and is an almost invariable accompaniment to active diease. Iron-deficiency anaemia is common in patients being treated with aspirin and NSAIDs, and this may be superimposed on the normochromic, normocytic type associated with many chronic diseases, caused by bone marrow hypoplasia. **Splenomegaly** is common, occurring in some 5% of patients (see Table 8.10). Most of the other types of blood abnormality which

occur are associated with drug therapy and include leucopenia, thrombocytopenia and, infrequently, aplastic anaemia.

Involvement of the **lymphoid system** is common and **lymphadenopathy**, enlarged, rubbery non-tender glands, occurs in some 30% of patients, usually in association with active disease.

Felty's syndrome is an uncommon (1% of patients with severe RA), late feature of seropositive RA, and is characterized by splenomegaly and neutropenia, though widespread haematological and other signs may occur (Table 8.10). The syndrome runs an unpredictable course, with severe neutropenia predisposing to serious infections. In rare cases systemic corticosteroids and splenectomy are required.

Rheumatoid nodules are painless, often subcutaneous, granulomas (see Chapter 2) that are 0.5–3 cm in diameter. They usually occur near the elbow but may occur in bursae, tendons or tendon sheaths at any pressure site. They may also occur internally, e.g. in the lungs or heart or, fortunately rarely, in the eye. If the nodules occur in the lungs, then bronchoscopy with biopsy is indicated to distinguish them from bronchial carcinoma. If bronchoscopy is not available, the nodules are usually removed to

Table 8.10 Principal features of Felty's syndrome

Seropositive rheumatoid arthritis
Splenomegaly, causing pancytopenia, especially neutropenia (infections) and thrombocytopenia (bleeding)
Haemolytic anaemia
Skin pigmentation, leg ulcers

provide a certain diagnosis and protect the patient from the latter possibility, as far as possible. Although nodules usually occur in seropositive RA and are virtually diagnostic, they are also found in a few patients with SLE (p. 511).

Investigation and diagnosis

Classic criteria

A diagnosis of definite RA requires at least four of the following criteria, developed by the American Medical Association (AMA) and revised in 1988. To satisfy criteria 1 to 4, symptoms or signs must be present continuously for at least 6 weeks.

1. Morning stiffness for ≥ 1 h.
2. Arthritis of three or more joints.
3. Arthritis of hand joints (wrist, MCP or PIP joints).
4. Symmetric arthritis.
5. Rheumatoid nodules.
6. Serum rheumatoid factor (positive in <5% of normal control subjects).
7. Radiographical changes (hand X-ray changes

typical of RA must include erosions or unequivocal bony decalcification).

Strict formal application of these criteria is helpful in doubtful cases, but most doctors would make a provisional diagnosis on less rigid ones.

Investigation

Typical results of some common investigations in patients with RA are given in Table 8.11. The general picture is that of a chronic inflammatory disease, primarily affecting the joints, with an immunological component.

The **anaemia** is typical of that which accompanies many chronic diseases, and serum iron studies may be unhelpful in diagnosis. In particular, **serum ferritin** acts as an acute-phase reactant, and levels may be elevated in RA. Confirmation of the nature and extent of anaemia may therefore require bone marrow examination. Another common cause of anaemia in RA is drug-induced gastrointestinal bleeding, and this may complicate the interpretation of haematological data.

Table 8.11 Typical results of investigations in rheumatoid arthritis

Haematology			Serology	
ESR	↑		RFs	Present (75%)
CRP	↑		Complement	N/↑
Hb	↓		Immunoglobulins	↑ (often)
TIBC	↓/N		**Synovial fluid**	
Serum iron	↓			
Serum ferritin	N/↓		(Changes **not** specific)	
			Translucent or opaque	
	Usually N		Viscosity	↓
White cell count	↑ (severe episodes)		Protein	↑
	↑ (infection)		White cell count	↑
	↑ (steroid therapy)			
			Radiology	
	Usually N		Early disease: osteoporosis, marginal bone erosions	
Platelets	↑ (in active disease and acute bleeding)		Established disease: loss of joint space, bone erosions, subluxation or dislocation, ankylosis?	

↑, ↓, increased or decreased level; CRP, C-reactive protein; ESR, erythrocyte sedimentation rate; Hb, haemoglobin; N, normal; RFs, rheumatoid factors; TIBC, total iron binding capacity.

The white cell count is usually normal, but **leu-cocytosis** may be associated with severe exacerbations. **Neutropenia** may occur in Felty's syndrome, and also result from iatrogenic myelosuppression and predisposes to infections.

Platelet counts may be high in active disease, or as the result of bleeding from iatrogenic gastric ulceration. Once again, low counts may occur in Felty's syndrome and iatrogenic myelosuppression.

Plasma viscosity may be increased, due to increased levels of acute phase proteins, notably fibrinogen, complement, gamma globulins and RFs.

Diagnosis

Although full-blown RA is unmistakable, many patients show only certain features and, because there is no pathognomonic test, the diagnosis is sometimes revealed with certainty only after some time. The tetrad of early morning stiffness, symmetrical painful polyarthritis, high RF titre and joint erosions, i.e. AMA criteria 1, 2, 4, 6 and 7, is usually conclusive. The occurrence of certain features makes a diagnosis particularly difficult, i.e.:

- Mono-articular involvement.
- Lack of erosions after several years of disease.
- Seronegativity.
- High antinuclear antibody titre.
- Involvement of the lumbar spine, skin, kidneys or CNS.

Functional assessment

Regular functional assessment (Table 8.5) is essential in charting the progress of the disease and the effectiveness of treatment.

Complications

Complications of RA fall into four groups.

Inflammatory
Eye involvement is common:

- **Sjögren's syndrome** (pp. 514) may affect about 20% of patients, 85% of them female and mostly seropositive. The syndrome causes dry eyes and a dry mouth, resulting from lymphocytic infiltration of the lachrymal and salivary glands: other exocrine glands may also be affected. The syndrome may occur in association with related diseases, e.g. SLE, systemic sclerosis and polymyositis.
- **Episcleritis**, causing a localized or diffuse hyperaemia of the sclera (white of the eye) is less common.
- Severe **scleritis**, which involves the deeper layers of the sclera, is uncommon but more serious.

The principal **cardiovascular** problem is **arteritis** (vasculitis), which causes widespread obstructive lesions and is an indication of severe disease. Arteritis usually presents as **nail fold (periungual) infarcts**, i.e. small areas of black or brown dead tissue around the nail margins. The involvement of larger vessels may result in leg ulceration or peripheral neuropathies.

Respiratory complications reflect diffuse inflammation and include **fibrosing alveolitis** and, especially in men, **pleurisy** and pleural effusions ('rheumatoid lung').

Infective
Septic arthritis, due to joint infection by *Staphylococcus aureus* (in adults and children) or *Haemophilus influenzae* (mostly in children), is a rare but important complication, especially in debilitated or immunosuppressed patients.

Secondary to abnormal metabolism
Mild **anaemia** is very common. **Osteoporosis** may lead to bone fractures. **Amyloidosis** (p. 519), the widespread deposition in tissues of abnormal amyloid protein, may occasionally cause clinical problems, notably nephrotic syndrome (*see* Chapter 4).

Iatrogenic
Problems with medication are very common because the drugs used (see below) tend to cause a high incidence of adverse reactions. **Eye damage** may be caused by *corticosteroids*, which can cause or accelerate cataracts and glaucoma, and antimalarials may induce retinopathy or corneal opacity, though these are rare if *hydroxychloroquine* is used at the correct dose.

Management

Objectives and strategy

The aims are:

- To relieve pain and discomfort and ameliorate symptoms.
- To arrest or limit disease progression and, if possible, reverse pathological changes.
- To maintain mobility and function, and promote the best possible quality of life.

These are achieved by a **holistic approach**, considering the patient's functional, medical, social and economic problems. The **modes** used are:

- Patient **education and counselling.**
- **Physical**: physiotherapy, osteopathy, occupational therapy, appliances, etc.
- **Social**: domestic assistance, modification of the home environment, financial support.
- **Pharmacotherapy**: analgesics, anti-inflammatory agents (NSAIDs, corticosteroids), disease-modifying antirheumatic drugs (immunoregulators, cytotoxics).
- **Surgery**: synovectomy, arthroplasty and other joint surgery.
- Appropriate management of anaemia and other complications.

Patient education and counselling

Because of the wide range of symptoms and their severity, and because patients almost inevitably fear that they will be completely crippled, it is important for them to comprehend as fully as possible the nature of the disease and the various procedures which are being used for management. Useful information is given in the patient leaflets provided by the (UK) Arthritis and Rheumatism Council, but these can only supplement verbal information. Such patient education needs to be an ongoing process because of the need to respond to the development of new symptoms and because there is a large amount of information to assimilate, which is impossible to convey in one or two sessions.

Physical methods

Rest may be valuable in an acute episode. Complete bedrest is occasionally used for a minority of patients but if not properly supervised this may lead to permanent disability owing to joint disuse.

Physiotherapy is very valuable, and includes the use of splints or support bandaging to rest particular joints or to correct deformity. A carefully planned series of exercises (e.g. swimming, isometric exercises) is important in maintaining muscle power without over-stressing damaged joints. Other widely used methods, e.g. the application of heat, cold, wax baths, short wave therapy, etc., may provide some short-term relief of pain and stiffness.

Occupational therapy is an essential component of management.

Pharmacotherapy: introduction

An algorithm for the drug treatment of RA is given in Table 8.12. Early drug management for mild disease is similar to that used in OA (p. 478), though **anti-inflammatory drugs**, mostly NSAIDs or somewhat higher doses of aspirin than normal are used, with an increased risk of adverse reactions. Inadequate relief or control, more severe symptoms or a definite diagnosis of seropositive RA leads to the use of **disease-modifying antirheumatic drugs (DMARDs)**. Despite this terminology, the extent to which any of this group of drugs significantly modify disease progression in the long term is arguable.

Although the inflammation responds to current treatments, the destructive process due to the pannus (p. 481) are less amenable.

Anti-inflammatory drugs comprise:

- High-dose aspirin and salicylates.
- NSAIDs.
- Corticosteroids.

By comparison, the **DMARDs** (Table 8.13) include:

- Immunomodulators (immunosuppressants; e.g. methotrexate, ciclosporin, leflunomide).
- Sulfasalazine.
- Gold compounds, penicillamine and antimalarials.

Table 8.12   The management of confirmed rheumatoid arthritis[a]

Step	Criterion	Action[b]
1	All patients	Education Physiotherapy, controlled exercise
2	At any stage	2.1 Inadequate pain relief: 'top-up' simple analgesics, increase dose of NSAID 2.2 A few painful joints: rest, e.g. splinting; intra-articular corticosteroid 2.3 Surgery: e.g. synovectomy, arthroplasty, arthrodesis
3	Very mild symptoms	Simple analgesics
4	Mild to moderate disease	NSAIDs[c] 4.1 Ibuprofen or diclofenac 4.2 Change to naproxen or meloxicam or piroxicam 4.3 Morning stiffness >1 h: change to indometacin 4.4 Others
5	Severe presentation or exacerbation or elderly	Corticosteroid[d]
6	Severe or aggressive disease	DMARD[e] 6.1 SSZ or MTX or hydroxychloroquine 6.2 Azathioprine or ciclosporin (cyclosporine) 6.3 Gold or penicillamine 6.4 Cyclophosphamide 6.5 Experimental treatments
7	Significant functional impairment of a few joints	Surgery: e.g. synovectomy, arthroplasty, arthrodesis

[a] This is an example of common usage and does not represent a firm recommendation of one drug or course of action over another. Patients vary widely in disease presentation and response to treatment and prescribers have individual approaches.

[b] Numbers represent a possible sequence at each step.

[c] NSAIDs should be tried for 2 weeks at the minimum appropriate dose, unless contraindicated. If relief is inadequate, the dose should be increased for a further 2 weeks. If still ineffective, a change should be made to a different chemical class (Table 8.14). All patients aged over 65 years and younger patients who develop epigastric discomfort should also take an H_2-antagonist or proton pump inhibitor.

[d] A severe presentation or exacerbation should be treated promptly with prednisolone. Corticosteroids provide prompt relief, but the dose should be reduced to the minimum required to control symptoms, preferably nil, once control has been gained. Low doses may be needed until DMARDs take effect. Patients aged over 65 years tolerate NSAIDs poorly and may be better off with prednisolone, despite the adverse effects.

[e] With moderate to severe or progressive disease, a DMARD should be introduced as soon as a definite diagnosis of RA has been made because joint damage may commence early. All take some time before their full effect is obtained.

DMARD, disease-modifying anti-inflammatory drug; MTX, methotrexate; NSAID, non-steroidal anti-inflammatory drug; SSZ, sulfasalazine.

Monitoring

The American College of Rheumatology has recommended the following criteria for defining improvement. There should be demonstrable improvement in:

• The number of swollen and tender joints.

Table 8.13 Disease-modifying antirheumatic drugs

Drug	Cautions, contraindications and side effects		Monitoring procedures
All	CCI:	Increase dose slowly to minimize adverse reactions (except antimalarials) Elderly Pregnancy Hepatic or renal disease	Generally[a]: careful examination of the patient and inquiry for adverse reactions (especially bleeding or bruising tendency, fever, sore throat or mouth[b]; also kidney and liver damage, rashes); regular full blood counts[b]
	SEs:	Gastrointestinal disturbance (oral forms[c]) Blood dyscrasias[b]	
Sulfasalazine	CCI:	G6PD deficiency Porphyria	Regular liver function tests for first 3 months
	SEs:	Hypersensitivity to salicylates or sulphonamides	
Gold (auranofin and Na aurothiomalate)	SEs:	Pruritus (may herald severe skin disease) Breathing problems[d] Kidney damage	Annual chest X-ray
Penicillamine	SEs:	SLE, hypersensitivity reactions	
Hydroxychloroquine	CCI:	Psoriasis[e]	Regular eye checks (see text, retinopathy very unlikely at low doses)
	SEs:	Headache, myopathy retinopathy	

[a] These are additional to the specific requirements listed for individual drugs.

[b] Indicators of possible blood dyscrasias (rare with antimalarials).

[c] All are orally administered, except sodium aurothiomalate (IM).

[d] Pulmonary fibrosis.

[e] May severely exacerbate existing psoriasis. There are numerous other contraindications (see *British National Formulary*).

CCI, cautions and contraindications; G6PD, glucose 6-phosphate dehydrogenase; SEs, side effects; SLE, systemic lupus erythematosus (p. 511).

- At least **three** of the following measures of disease activity:
  - Patient assessment.
  - Physician assessment.
  - Pain score.
  - Disability score.
  - Serum levels of acute-phase reactants (e.g. CRP, ESR, plasma viscosity).

An appropriate goal for treatment is a better than 50% improvement in these criteria.

Pharmacotherapy: anti-inflammatory drugs and analgesics

Non-steroidal anti-inflammatory drugs

NSAIDs have been the drugs of first choice for the treatment of mild RA for many years because they possess both analgesic and anti-inflammatory properties. A large and increasing number is available (Table 8.14). They are also used as an adjunct to DMARDs if symptomatic support is required.

Table 8.14 Chemical classification of non-selective[a] non-steroidal anti-inflammatory drugs

Anthranilic acids	Mefenamic acid, flufenamic acid[b], meclofenamate sodium[b]
Arylalkanoic acids	Arylacetic acids: aceclofenac[c], diclofenac, tolmetin Arylbutyric acids: fenbufen Arylpropionic acids[c]: ibuprofen, fenoprofen, flurbiprofen, ketoprofen, naproxen
Alkanes	Nabumetone
Enolic acids (oxicams)	Piroxicam, meloxicam, tenoxicam
Indole and indene acetic acids	Etodolac, indometacin, acemetacin, sulindac
Pyrazolidines	Azapropazone (apazone)[c], phenylbutazone
Salicylates	Aspirin, diflunisal[c]

[a] Agents with relatively greater COX selectivity have recently been introduced (see text).

[b] Not licensed in the UK.

[c] Azapropazone, aceclofenac, diclofenac and diflunisal have similar properties to the arylpropionic acids.

Patient response to NSAIDs and tolerance of them is very variable, so it may be necessary to try several products to determine which has the best combination of efficacy and tolerability. The basis for this inter-patient variability is unclear, but it is likely to be more related to disease activity than to drug pharmacokinetics or anti-prostaglandin activity. These drugs have a rapid onset of action but the full analgesic and anti-inflammatory effect may not be apparent for a week or so, largely dependent on dose frequency and the consequent time to reach steady state. If adequate relief is not obtained within 2–3 weeks at full dosage, a change to another product is indicated. However, relief of pain and early morning stiffness is often incomplete at tolerable doses.

Mode of action

The activity of NSAIDs is ascribed to their inhibition of **cyclooxygenase** (COX) activity and thus of prostaglandin (PG) synthesis. Recent research has shown that COX exists in two isoforms which are expressed constitutively in only a limited range of tissues.

COX-1 is constitutive in the stomach, kidneys, intestines and platelets, while COX-2 is found in the brain, kidney and reproductive tract. Activation of COX-1 leads to the formation of autacoids, e.g. protective prostacyclins in the gastric mucosa and vascular endothelium, prostaglandin E_2 (PGE_2)

in the kidney and thromboxane in the platelets. COX-2 activity is involved in fever, the central modulation of pain and the initiation of uterine contractions and fetal expulsion in childbirth, but its physiological roles are not fully defined. *Nimesulide*, a selective COX-2 inhibitor (not UK licensed), is being investigated for delaying premature labour.

Although COX-2 may play a role in ulcer healing in animals and occurs around human gastric ulcers, the clinical significance of this is unknown. COX-2 is also **inducible** by cytokines and other pro-inflammatory stimuli, causing an inflammatory response **localized** to the site of production, e.g. in joints (Fig. 8.9).

COX-2 differs from COX-1 only by the substitution of isoleucine by valine in the active site; this leads to a larger NSAID binding site which is the basis for the development of COX-2-selective NSAIDs.

Aspirin and most of the older NSAIDs inhibit both COX isozymes but the relative effects differ considerably between drugs, and most of the older NSAIDs inhibit COX-1 more than COX-2. This may be clinically significant because preferential inhibition of leukotrienes produced by COX-2 induction should therefore spare distant, uninflamed sites, e.g. the stomach. Also, COX-1 constitutive actions in the stomach and kidney will still produce the eicosanoids necessary for normal gastrointestinal and renal functions.

Differing potencies and selectivity against

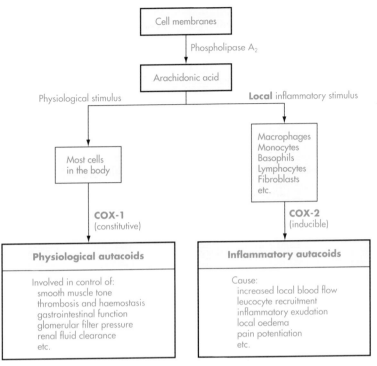

Figure 8.9   Simplified scheme for physiological and inflammatory autacoid formation by cyclooxygenase (COX) isozymes. Non-selective non-steroidal anti-inflammatory drugs inhibit COX-1 and COX-2: selective NSAIDs inhibit COX-2 preferentially.

COX-1/COX-2 are alleged to account for the differences between NSAIDs. It has been suggested that inhibition of COX-1 causes most of the side effects of NSAIDs, while that of COX-2 is responsible for the anti-inflammatory action. If these results are confirmed, and the clinical benefit of highly selective COX-2 inhibition is proven in prolonged use, it is clear that the highly selective COX-2 inhibitors represent a valuable new generation of NSAIDs.

Side effects

NSAIDs are responsible for the largest number of 'yellow card' reports to the UK Committee on the Safety of Medicines of any drug group, reflecting both their numerous side effects and interactions (Table 8.15) and their frequency of use. Most adverse drug reactions (ADRs) are minor, but the principal adverse reaction – **gastric ulceration** – may lead to significant bleeding and severe anaemia, even perforation. Taking NSAIDs increases the risk of these reactions in RA patients about three times, with a sixfold increase in the risk of perforation of the gut. Patients do not become tolerant to this effect and the incidence of hospital admission due to gastrointestinal haemorrhage is increasing.

Factors which increase the risk of serious gastrointestinal side effects by at least 50% include the following:

- Age >65 years.
- History of gastrointestinal problems, e.g. recent upper abdominal pain, regular or recurrent use of antacids or antisecretory drugs, and peptic ulcer.
- Previous NSAID intolerance or cessation of treatment due to gastrointestinal disturbance.
- Cigarette smoking.
- Alcohol consumption.
- Any concurrent chronic disease and associated medications.

Antisecretory agents, e.g. *H₂-receptor antagonists* and *proton pump inhibitors*, help to protect against NSAID-induced gastric ulceration. Also, *misoprostol*, a 'cytoprotective' prostaglandin (PG)

Table 8.15   Possible side effects, interactions, cautions and contraindications

Side effects[a]

Gastrointestinal	Gastric discomfort, nausea, diarrhoea, bleeding (occasionally severe), peptic ulceration, rectal irritation (suppositories)
Neurological	Headache, dizziness or confusion, vertigo, tinnitus, psychiatric disturbance, eye problems
Dermatological	Rashes, photosensitivity
Hypersensitivity reactions	Asthma, angioedema
Haematological	Purpura
Fluid retention	May precipitate heart failure or exacerbate hypertension, renal failure (rare)

Some important interactions[b]

Warfarin[c]	Enhanced anticoagulant effect (especially azapropazone and phenylbutazone; other NSAIDs may also interact)
Diuretics	Antagonism of diuretic effect, increased risk of hyperkalaemia with potassium-sparing diuretics
ACEIs	Antagonism of hypotensive effect, increased risk of hyperkalaemia and renal failure
Digoxin	Increased serum concentration of digoxin, antagonism of effect on heart failure (due to fluid retention)
Ciclosporin (cyclosporine)	Increased risk of nephrotoxicity
Methotrexate	Increased risk of toxicity
Lithium	Increased serum concentration of lithium, possible toxicity
Probenecid	Reduced excretion of indometacin, ketoprofen and naproxen
Quinolone antibiotics	Risk of convulsions

Cautions

Elderly, respiratory disease, asthma, allergic disorders, peptic ulceration, renal, cardiac or hepatic impairment, pregnancy, breast feeding, dehydration, diuretic therapy, haemorrhoids (suppositories)

Contraindications

Gout, children under 12 years, anticoagulant therapy (especially with aspirin), hypersensitivity to aspririn or any NSAID

[a] Side effects vary in severity and frequency between drugs and, especially, between patients.

[b] Only the most important interactions are listed: phenylbutazone, azapropazone and indometacin are the most likely to interact with other drugs.

[c] Potentially life-threatening interaction.

ACEI, angiotensin converting enzyme inhibitor; NSAID, non-steroidal anti-inflammatory drug.

analogue, is marketed for co-administration with NSAIDs to minimize gastric damage, and fixed combinations with *diclofenac* and *naproxen* are available. Misoprostol may be slightly more effective than the H_2-receptor antagonists in preventing gastric ulcers, but both types of drug are equivalent in protecting against duodenal ulceration. However, misoprostol may cause severe diarrhoea and other gastrointestinal, central nervous and gynaecological side effects, and these may necessitate withdrawal.

These agents are intended to overcome the damaging effects of NSAIDS on the gastric mucosa while permitting the anti-inflammatory benefits to continue. With the older acidic NSAIDs, gastric side effects are due to a combination of local irritation and systemic mechanisms, but the selective COX-2 agents described above may make it possible to maintain the systemic benefits without the side effects. They will at least minimize the need for antisecretory and other drugs.

Selective COX-2 inhibitors should be less likely to cause renal effects, especially papillary necrosis. However, they may still cause deterioration in renal function, with fluid retention and oedema, particularly in the elderly and in patients in whom this is already compromised, e.g. creatinine clearance <30 mL/min. All NSAIDs tend to cause fluid retention, and this may cause acute cardiac decompensation in patients with heart failure and limited cardiac reserve. There is one Australian report suggesting that 29% of the hypertension cases found among in the elderly Australian population are due to NSAIDs.

Although rofecoxib (and presumably other selective COX-2 inhibitors) does not affect the antiplatelet effect of low-dose aspirin it is not known whether long-term co-administration enhances gastrotoxicity.

Other side effects are **rashes**, notably with *diclofenac*, *fenbufen* and *sulindac*.

All NSAIDs cause premature closure of the ductus arteriosus if used regularly during pregnancy, delay childbirth and increase the duration of labour.

Effects on cartilage repair.   It has been alleged that NSAIDs increase cartilage damage in the long term. They are known to suppress bone formation, and have been used to prevent undesirable ossification following total hip replacement. The clinical significance of this in treating RA is unclear.

There is a continuous turnover of articular cartilage throughout life, and the glycosaminoglycan (GAG) matrix turns over considerably more rapidly than the fibrillar collagen. This remodelling has been reflected in the regression of joint pathology in some arthritic patients. Changes in chondrocyte activity affect this process and may be the pathological basis of OA and some other arthritides. Local cytokine release, notably IL-1, may interfere with natural repair mechanisms and we know that human cartilage is more sensitive than animal tissue: this emphasizes the need for caution when interpreting the results of experiments with animal models of rheumatic diseases. Further, it is known that some NSAIDs modulate IL-1 activity, e.g. indometacin increases it seven times.

One short-term in-vitro study with human osteoarthritic and normal cartilage has shown that NSAIDs probably fall into three groups on the basis of their effects on GAG synthesis: i.e.:

- Stimulatory, e.g. aceclofenac.
- No effect, e.g. aspirin, diclofenac, tiaprofenic acid (the effects of aspirin and diclofenac appear to depend on individual cartilage metabolism, ketoprofen and piroxicam may stimulate GAG synthesis in young cartilage but not in adults).
- Inhibitory, e.g. ibuprofen, indometacin, naproxen.

This result with indometacin may reflect its known effect on IL-1 activity.

Although these laboratory results were obtained at NSAID concentrations similar to the plasma levels achieved with normal dosing, it is notoriously difficult to extrapolate from short-term in-vitro studies to the clinical situation. Thus, these findings provide some rational basis for NSAID selection, at least in OA. These considerations may be unimportant if, for example, indometacin is used for the short-term treatment of acute gout, but may be significant if long-term use is contemplated in patients with demonstrable cartilage damage. The effects are quite distinct from the analgesic properties of this drug group.

It must be concluded that, despite the advantages and wide use of NSAIDs, there is an obvious need to develop safer alternatives to the present generation of NSAIDs.

Selection

NSAIDs are often classified on the basis of their chemical structures (*see* Table 8.14), but this is generally unhelpful in choosing a product for a patient except to select a chemically unrelated drug if an adverse reaction, e.g. hypersensitivity, dictates a change of medication. The main differences between the approximately 20 available NSAIDs are their potency and incidence of side effects. However, these criteria do not assure clinical effectiveness and patient acceptability which, together with disease severity, are the basis for selection:

- *Ibuprofen* has a low incidence of side effects and so is a common first choice for patients with mild symptoms, but it has relatively weak anti-inflammatory properties.
- *Naproxen* is more potent, has a reasonable effectiveness/toxicity balance and is conveniently taken twice daily: it is probably the first-line drug for those with moderate symptoms.

- Modified-release forms of *diclofenac* and *ketoprofen* are widely used alternatives.
- *Nabumetone* has been shown to produce less endoscopically proven gastric lesions than many other NSAIDs.

The selective COX-2 inhibitor *meloxicam* is licensed for the treatment of pain and inflammation in rheumatic diseases generally, though the *British National Formulary* (BNF) does not currently suggest a lower incidence or smaller range of side effects. The highly selective compounds, *celecoxib* and *rofecoxib*, may be somewhat safer, especially as far as gastrointestinal ulceration is concerned. Rofecoxib is currently licensed only for the treatment of OA, but use in RA awaits further evaluation. It is too soon to be clear about the benefits of any of the highly selective COX-2 inhibitors, but they seem likely to emerge as first-line drugs for rheumatic diseases generally. They also appear to be useful analgesics. COX-2-selective NSAIDs which do not affect cartilage repair adversely (see above) would be of great interest.

Because of its toxicity, *azapropazone* is subject to special safety restrictions in the UK. It may be used only when other NSAIDs have failed and special care must be taken in the elderly and in those with a history of inflammatory bowel disease (*see* Chapter 6), or any blood disorders. Azapropazone may also cause severe photosensitivity and is specifically **contraindicated** if there is any history of peptic ulceration. *Meloxicam*, may cause serious skin and gastrointestinal reactions. *Tiaprofenic acid* may cause severe bladder irritation.

Table 8.16 gives the approximate rankings of some older NSAIDs on the basis of their potency and likelihood of causing gastrointestinal side effects. Unfortunately, effectiveness and toxicity seem to be associated with the current range of drugs.

Because the products will be taken for long periods, compliance is aided by the use of drugs or products with convenient dosing patterns (once or twice daily). However, the differences in the pharmacokinetic properties of the drugs has been blurred by the introduction of modified-release versions of those with a short half-life.

A procedure used by some rheumatologists is to give a patient a 14- or 21-day supply of each of three products, to be taken consecutively, and allow the patient to choose the most acceptable. The initial choice may be made on the basis of the criteria outlined above. If none of the first group chosen is acceptable, a further selection is tried. Some 50% of patients are likely to respond to the first agent tried, and a further 30% to the second. Approximately 5% fail to derive satisfactory benefit from any of this group of drugs.

However, NSAIDs are probably over-prescribed. They are the principal cause of drug-related problems in the elderly and are often used when there is no evidence of inflammation and a simple analgesic would suffice.

Topical NSAIDs

These are popular, partly because when patients rub in the product they feel that they are contributing to their own treatment and because the massage also stimulates local blood supply, so contributing to healing. Penetration into joints has been demonstrated and a meta-analysis found that *ketoprofen*, *felbinac*, *ibuprofen* and *piroxicam* gave at least 50% pain reduction in

---

Table 8.16 Relative effectiveness and toxicity of some non-steroidal anti-inflammatory drugs[a]

Effectiveness

Phenylbutazone > indometacin > flurbiprofen > naproxen ≈ azapropazone ≈ diclofenac ≈ fenoprofen ≈ nabumetone ≈ piroxicam ≈ tenoxicam ≈ tiaprofenic acid > ketoprofen > ibuprofen ≈ tolmetin ≈ mefenamic acid

Likelihood of causing gastrointestinal side effects

Phenylbutazone > azapropazone > piroxicam > indometacin ≈ meclofenamate[b] > ketoprofen > diclofenac ≈ fenoprofen ≈ flurbiprofen ≈ naproxen ≈ sulindac ≈ tenoxicam ≈ tiaprofenic acid > ibuprofen

[a] Rankings are very approximate owing to considerable differences in reported data and wide interpatient variation: clinical effectiveness also depends on the dose and the disease state.
[b] Not licensed in the UK.

acute soft tissue trauma, sprains and strains. Similar benefits were seen in chronic conditions (tendinitis, osteoarthritis). However, the BNF states that these products provide only limited pain relief.

Although they avoid the gastrointestinal side effects associated with oral dosing, the use of large amounts of topical products and occlusive bandaging may cause excessive penetration and systemic effects, e.g. renal impairment, especially in older patients, and/or skin problems.

Corticosteroids

These are the most potent anti-inflammatory agents available and also have immunosuppressive properties. They produce a dramatic response. Some studies have suggested the prevalence of use of corticosteroids in RA to be as high as 80%, accounting for about 25% of all steroid usage. Although it used to be generally accepted that corticosteroids have little effect on the underlying disease process, they may limit the extent of joint damage if used in early RA (see below), and during a severe inflammatory episode.

Because they are associated with numerous, well known **side effects**, the corticosteroids have a strictly limited role in the treatment of RA. Even patients given relatively low doses (as low as 5 mg *prednisolone* daily) over long periods may show:

- Fluid retention and hypertension.
- Weight gain (additional to fluid retention).
- Loss of bone density (osteoporosis) and increased risk of fracture.
- Increased susceptibility to infections, e.g. chickenpox may be fatal, shingles.
- Reduced glucose tolerance.
- Cataract formation and glaucoma.
- Impaired wound healing.
- Loss of subcutaneous tissue.
- Proximal myopathy.

Corticosteroids down-regulate the production of leukotrienes, prostaglandins, complement components, interferons, other cytokines and histamine. However, they are not myelosuppressive because they act on mature immune cells to prevent B cell and T cell clone proliferation. In contrast, the cytotoxic immunomodulators (see below) act on immune cell precursors in the bone marrow, and incidentally on all other haematopoietic cells.

Corticosteroids reduce blood levels of salicylates. Thus, the introduction of steroids in a patient taking aspirin as an analgesic is illogical. Further, if a patient is taking an effective dose of aspirin plus a steroid, withdrawal of the steroid may precipitate aspirin toxicity.

Uses

Corticosteroids are invaluable when serious complications occur, e.g. intolerable pain, uncontrolled loss of function and especially vasculitis. High doses (up to 100 mg of *prednisolone* daily PO, or an equivalent intravenous or intramuscular injection of *methylprednisolone*) may be used in severe uncontrolled disease or for serious systemic complications, e.g. vasculitis. Pulsed high doses, e.g. up to 1 g of *methylprednisolone* IV on three consecutive days, are sometimes used to avoid the corticosteroid dependence that occurs with gradual progressive or prolonged regimens. Corticosteroids also have a place in the prompt, **short-term** relief of severe exacerbations, and possibly as an adjunct to early DMARD treatment, to give rapid relief and to prevent early joint damage, until the DMARD effects are manifest. A few RA patients derive adequate benefit from low-dose (5 mg/day) oral *prednisolone*.

Recent evidence has shown that the early introduction of 7.5 mg/day of *prednisolone*, in addition to other treatments, retards joint erosion over a 2- to 4-year period. Withdrawal of the steroid in the third year may result in the initiation of joint damage in some patients and its resumption in those with joint damage at the start of corticosteroid use. This anti-erosive dose should be reduced gradually after 2–4 years, in order to avoid long-term ADRs.

In very elderly patients, corticosteroids may be used for the maintenance of already limited mobility and function, when their advantages, including an increased sense of well-being, may outweigh their long-term disadvantages.

Local treatment. Water-insoluble corticosteroids, e.g. *triamcinolone hexacetonide* or *methylprednisolone acetate*, may be injected into a particular joint, with aspiration of excessive synovial exudate, to control a flare-up in that joint. Provided that the injection is placed correctly in the joint, and leakage does not occur, peri-articular subcutaneous atrophy should not be a problem. This procedure provides periods of relief that vary from a few days to months, but such injections should not be done more than three times annually, in order to avoid joint damage. If greater frequency is indicated, an alternative treatment should be sought. Corticosteroid joint injections must always be carried out with scrupulous aseptic technique to avoid the possibility of infection. Joints must not be injected if infection is suspected as the steroid is likely to exacerbate the problem.

Tendons and bursae may also be injected. However, it is essential to inject the tendon sheath and not the tendon itself, otherwise tendon rupture is likely. Because the **Achilles tendon** (in the heel) does not have a proper sheath it **should not be injected**: tendon rupture may occur.

Corticosteroid eye drops are essential for the control of serious eye complications (p. 486).

Salicylates

These have largely been replaced by the NSAIDs. Until the advent of the latter, *aspirin* (up to 5 g/day, depending on body weight: normal anti-inflammatory dose about 3.6 g/day) was the first-line drug for the treatment of RA. Aspirin is very effective, but because of the high incidence of gastrointestinal disturbance it should be given as a product formulated for release in the small intestine. Buffered forms are also used but these tend to be less effective in preventing gastric distress. However, gastric and small bowel bleeding may still occur with any dosage form because gastric bleeding results from both local irritation and the inhibition of prostaglandin release, which is a systemic effect.

Benorilate is an aspirin–paracetamol ester pro-drug, being hydrolysed to its two constituents after absorption. It thus combines the anti-inflammatory properties of aspirin and the analgesic and antipyretic properties of both drugs, and their side effects and limitations. Overall tolerance is good, but benorylate should not be used in patients with a history of peptic ulceration, or in children aged under 12 years (because of the risk of Reye's syndrome; *see* Chapter 6). Benorilate should be used with care in the elderly and in those with renal or hepatic impairment. There is also a risk of inadvertent overdosing:

patients must be warned not to self-medicate with OTC analgesics.

Patients vary considerably in the dosage at which side effects occur, especially older patients. One approach is to increase the dose slowly (weekly, possibly fortnightly in older patients), until the maximum tolerable dose which does not produce tinnitus is achieved.

Although *diflunisal* is a fluorinated, aryl-substituted salicylic acid, its clinical action more closely resembles that of propionic acid NSAIDs (ibuprofen, naproxen, etc., see below).

The principal **side effects**, **interactions** and **contraindications** of this drug group are given in Table 8.17.

Analgesics

Simple and compound analgesics, e.g. paracetamol (acetaminophen), co-proxamol (in the UK, *see* Chapter 10), are used at any stage as 'top up' therapy if additional pain control is required. However, because inflammation is central to RA, analgesics are inappropriate as monotherapy.

Pharmacotherapy: disease-modifying antirheumatic drugs (DMARDs)

Introduction

Patients with mild disease are treated satisfactorily with NSAIDs. Those with moderate to severe disease, or if there is a progression from mild to moderate symptoms or signs, need a DMARD (*see* Table 8.13). If a DMARD is effective and tolerated in a particular patient, any of these second-line agents will improve both the joint problems and any extra-articular symptoms and will abolish the need for corticosteroids, or spare the steroid dose. Patients usually require an NSAID in the early stages, if they are not already taking one, to provide symptom relief until the DMARD is fully effective. If there is no objective evidence of benefit with a DMARD after 6 months, then it should be discontinued and an alternative sought.

Irreversible joint damage and impairment of function tend to occur early in the course of the disease, especially in the 2 years following diagnosis, so DMARDs should be used immediately a

Table 8.17 Principal side effects and interactions of salicylates[a] and their cautions and contraindications

Side effects[b]

Gastrointestinal	Dyspepsia, nausea and vomiting, peptic ulceration, blood loss (70% of patients; may cause anaemia), Reye's syndrome (in children, affects liver)
Neurological	Tinnitus, deafness, Reye's syndrome (liver, children)
Haematological	Increased bleeding tendency (inhibition of platelet aggregation)
Hypersensitivity[c]	Severe asthma, urticaria, anaphylaxis

Interactions

Oral anticoagulants	Potentiation[d], potentially life-threatening
Oral hypoglycaemics	Potentiation[e]
Uricosuric agents	Effect inhibited[f] (low-dose aspirin)
Alcohol	Increased (additive) gastric irritation
Antacids[g]	Reduced serum salicylate levels
Corticosteroids[h]	

Cautions

Asthma, impaired renal or hepatic functions, dehydration, pregnancy

Contraindications

Gastrointestinal ulceration, anticoagulant therapy, bleeding disorders, age under 12 years

[a] Includes benorilate.
[b] Side effects may vary between compounds and patients.
[c] Especially in patients who have both asthma and nasal polyps.
[d] Owing to displacement of warfarin from protein binding and the antiplatelet effect of aspirin.
[e] Owing to the hypoglycaemic action of the high-dose aspirin and salicylates, and displacement from protein binding.
[f] Tubular secretion of urate reduced.
[g] Increased urinary pH causes increased salicylate excretion.
[h] Owing to cation retention, causing increased salicylate clearance: withdrawal of the steroid can cause salicylate toxicity.

firm diagnosis of moderate to severe RA has been made, i.e. much earlier than previously recommended and certainly within the first 2 years, to achieve improved benefit. Careful monitoring for both effectiveness and toxicity is essential, especially in the early stages. It may be important to try to identify those patients in the subset who are likely to suffer more aggressive disease.

Some patients may benefit from combination DMARD therapy, especially if they have responded partially to monotherapy, but the response is very variable. One small North American study found that *methotrexate–sulfasalazine–hydroxychloroquine* triple therapy gave at least a 50% improvement in symptoms over single agents, with no evidence of excessive toxicity. In a Dutch trial, an intensive regimen with *methotrexate–sulfasalazine–prednisolone* gave significant improvement over sulfasalazine alone, but this benefit disappeared when the prednisolone was withdrawn. Patients who respond well but incompletely to *methotrexate* (MTX) may benefit from the addition of *ciclosporin*.

The modes of action of most of these agents in RA are unknown or uncertain.

Cytotoxic immunomodulators

These are arguably the most effective of the second-line agents, but they have a relatively high incidence of adverse reactions (*see also* Chapter 11, p. 656) and there are hazards associated with long-term immunosuppression.

They are therefore used only for patients with proven, moderate to severe or progressive disease which is not adequately controlled by NSAIDs, or who cannot tolerate other products. This is especially important with RA because, although distressing, it is rarely fatal and requires prolonged treatment. Use is usually restricted to specialized units with adequate monitoring facilities, particularly for myelosuppression caused by damage to bone marrow stem cells generally (undesirable) in order to damage immune stem cells (desirable) and produce immunosuppression. In contrast, corticosteroids act on mature immune cells and so do not cause myelosuppression.

All cytotoxic drugs are teratogenic and may have side effects on spematogenesis. They are therefore avoided, used with great care, or may be absolutely contraindicated, in women of child-bearing age and those who are breast feeding. Exceptionally, they may be considered for the control of a severe exacerbation in a woman who is already pregnant: this is a matter for discussion and cooperation between rheumatologist and gynaecologist, and possibly a specialist in cytotoxic chemotherapy.

Methotrexate (MTX)

This is a dihydrofolate reductase inhibitor, its mode of action being to block folate synthesis. MTX is unsuitable for the treatment of RA in pregnant women (it has been used as an abortifacient), and contraceptive precautions must be taken both during and for 6–12 months after therapy. MTX also damages spermatozoa, and there should not be any attempt made at conception within 6 months of its use. Similar considerations apply to other cytotoxic drugs. MTX is licensed for the treatment of severe active RA that is unresponsive to 'conventional' therapy, and is relatively well tolerated at the lower doses (5–25 mg weekly) used in rheumatology. MTX is currently the first choice of many rheumatologists and is increasing in popularity because it has a simple once-weekly dosage regimen; moreover, its drop-out rate after 1–2 years is only about 40–50% of that found with other DMARDs. However, MTX must be used with great care if there is any evidence of renal or hepatic impairment or of the pulmonary complications of RA. The CSM advises a full blood count, and also that renal and liver function tests be made initially and weekly until patients are stabilized, and then at 2- to 3-month intervals thereafter. Patients should promptly report any occurrence of sore throat or fever, and also any signs of infection.

Azathioprine

This agent is a pro-drug, being metabolized slowly to 6-mercaptopurine, a purine antagonist. Like MTX, azathioprine is widely used, but it has a slower onset of action. In addition to their use in treating RA, these two drugs are used to treat severe, progressive **psoriatic arthropathy** (*see* Chapter 12, p. 694). In this setting, azathioprine seems to be the more effective for the arthritic symptoms, and methotrexate for the skin lesions.

Cyclophosphamide

This nitrogen mustard is an effective DNA alkylating agent, with a rapid onset of action, though it causes a very high incidence of side effects (in 90% of patients). *Chlorambucil* is chemically related to cyclophosphamide, but tends to produce less short-term side effects.

Azathioprine, *cyclophosphamide* and *chlorambucil* are used as reserve agents.

Other immunomodulators

One promising development is the use of low-dose *ciclosporin* (*cyclosporine*) (*see* Chapter 4, p. 202), which can improve all clinical parameters in severe RA. Ciclosporin inhibits T cell activation and cytokine production, and so is immunosuppressive but not myelosuppressive. Because long-term treatment is required, careful determinations of drug blood levels and serum creatinine are essential to avoid nephrotoxicity. This does not appear to be as significant a problem with the low-dose regimens which have been used in RA as in those used for immunosuppression in organ transplantation. However, ciclosporin is usually reserved for non-responders or those intolerant to other drugs. Two formulations with very different oral bioavailabilities are available, so extra care is needed in prescribing and dispensing.

Leflunomide (to be introduced in 2000) is a reversible inhibitor of dihydro-orotate dehydrogenase, an enzyme believed to be involved in the autoimmune processes leading to RA. Leflunomide significantly reduced the symptoms and signs of RA and retarded joint damage in Phase III clinical trials, and appears to be well tolerated.

Sulfasalazine (SSZ)

This has been used mostly for the treatment of inflammatory bowel disease (IBD; *see* Chapter 6). In RA, SSZ is as effective as penicillamine, and slightly less so than gold, but has significant advantages over both of these. It has a faster onset of action than the older agents and is less toxic and so is emerging as a drug of first choice, together with methotrexate, if NSAIDs are ineffective or are not tolerated, or symptoms are moderate to severe.

Side effects (*see* Table 8.13) are more likely to occur in older patients, those who have previously used other disease-modifying agents and in slow acetylators. The most serious side effects are due to myelosuppression, e.g. occasional leucopenia, neutropenia and thrombocytopenia, rarely agranulocytosis and aplastic anaemia, and hypersensitivity reactions, e.g. anaphylaxis, Stevens–Johnson syndrome and exfoliative dermatitis. Thus full blood counts, including differential white cell and platelet counts, should be performed before starting treatment and at monthly intervals for the first 3 months. Hepatic function tests should be carried out at the same time. The UK Committee on the Safety of Medicines advises that patients taking sulfasalazine should be advised to report any unexplained bleeding, bruising, purpura, sore throat, fever or malaise. Those with glucose 6-phosphate dehydrogenase deficiency may develop haemolytic anaemia.

The UK product licence in RA is only for the enteric-coated tablets, because trials were carried out with that dosage form. It was felt that patients who had been taking NSAIDs for some time might be more susceptible to gastrointestinal disturbance, though this has not been established, and the benefits of enteric coating have been challenged for patients with inflammatory bowel disease. Though these points require confirmation, it is reasonable to proceed more cautiously in patients who have experienced gastrointestinal problems or have been taking other DMARDs and to increase the dose at 14-day intervals, rather than the recommended 7 days, up to the normal maximum of 2–3 g daily. However, as many patients may withdraw from SSZ treatment as from gold and penicillamine, mostly in the first few months.

Patients should be warned that the urine may be coloured orange-yellow and that extended-wear contact lenses may also be stained.

Perhaps surprisingly, the activity of SSZ in RA (and its side effects) appears to be related to the sulfapyridine moiety and not to the salicylate component, which provides the benefit in inflammatory bowel disease. This latter finding has prompted a re-investigation of the possibility of a bacterial aetiology for RA. As antimicrobials, the sulphonamides are competitive antagonists of *p*-aminobenzoic acid, thus inhibiting folate synthesis. However, human cells are unable to synthesize folate, so this cannot be its mode of action as an anti-inflammatory agent. Thus the basis for its activity is unknown.

Older DMARDs

Like most other DMARDs, these agents (*gold, penicillamine* and *antimalarials*) have a slow onset of action, unlike the NSAIDs, and some 3–6 months may be required before their effectiveness is apparent. Consequently, they have also been described as 'slow-acting anti-rheumatic drugs (SAARD)'.

Modes of action. These are mostly unknown and several different mechanisms are likely. *Gold salts* may inhibit the activation and maturation of mononuclear and T cells, but their anti-inflammatory activity in conditions other than RA is minimal. The only certain activity of *penicillamine* is as a chelating agent for heavy metals. In RA it causes a marked reduction in the levels of RFs (IgMs), by unknown mechanisms. *Antimalarials* are known to have mild cytotoxic activity.

Clinical activity. Up to 70% of patients may show improvement in both symptoms and the objective indicators of disease activity (e.g. ESR,

CRP, RFs, anaemia), though the extent of such improvement is very variable. Older DMARDs are usually reserved for patients who are unresponsive to methotrexate, sulfasalazine or ciclosporin, or who are intolerant of these. Because DMARDs are not curative, drug administration is necessary for as long as active disease persists and side effects are tolerated.

Toxicity. DMARDs are significantly more toxic than NSAIDs, and so are used only in moderate to severe and progressive disease. They require careful monitoring with full haematological and other tests as appropriate (*see* Table 8.13). It is thus essential that patients are counselled carefully to ensure that they appreciate fully the possible advantages and disadvantages of treatment with these drugs, and that they are prepared to cooperate in the regular monitoring procedures required.

Gold salts

These are available as both oral and intramuscular formulations. The most common **side effect** with the oral form is diarrhoea, but the range of toxicities of the oral and IM agents is otherwise similar, though the injectables are more troublesome.

Auranofin is the orally active agent. The initial twice daily dose is increased by 50% (three daily doses) after 6 months if the response is inadequate. The bioavailability is about 25%, but when steady-state serum concentrations are reached after about 10 weeks, less than 1% of the ingested dose is retained in the body. However, serum levels do not correlate with the activity or with side effects. Patients can be transferred from parenteral gold to auranofin directly, without overlap or washout.

Sodium aurothiomalate (gold sodium thiomalate) is the only injectable gold salt available in the UK and is equivalent to others which are available elsewhere, e.g. aurothioglucose. It is given by deep IM injection, followed by gentle massage at the injection site. Therapy is initiated with one or more small test doses to minimize the possibility of a major idiosyncratic adverse reaction. Aurothiomalate is continued with weekly doses until clinical improvement is apparent, usually at 2–4 months (about

300–500 mg total dose), or significant side effects (rashes, blood dyscrasias, renal or hepatic toxicity) occur. If a favourable response is seen, maintenance is continued with a lower 2- to 4-weekly dose, as long as the drug is tolerated, for up to 5 years after complete remission. If relapse occurs treatment is stepped up until control is regained. Complete relapse must be avoided if possible because second courses of gold are usually ineffective. Treatment is stopped if no benefit occurs when a total dose of 1 g is reached (about 6 months).

Because of this toxicity, careful monitoring is mandatory, especially with *sodium aurothiomalate* (*see* Table 8.13).

It has been suggested, on anecdotal evidence, that wearing gold rings limits damage in the adjacent joint.

Penicillamine

This orally active agent is slightly less active than gold and has a similar spectrum of side effects, though it is somewhat better tolerated. The daily dose is increased every 4–8 weeks until clinical improvement occurs, and the maintenance dose is then held at that level. Administration is usually stopped if it has not produced benefit in 6 months or if unacceptable side effects or toxicity occur.

Side effects may occur in up to 50% of patients, but often respond to dose reduction or to temporary withdrawal of the drug.

Hydroxychloroquine

Chloroquine and *hydroxychloroquine* are relatively weak antirheumatic agents which are used at about five times the dose used for malaria prophylaxis. Although they are often taken as antimalarials for prolonged periods without problems occurring, the combination of the increased dose, possible greater susceptibility of rheumatoid patients and the fact that antirheumatic treatment is likely to be very prolonged, greatly enhances the possibility of significant side effects, notably rashes, myopathy and retinopathy.

Although the last of these side effects is rare in patients with normal renal function, fear of blindness has limited the use of these drugs. Chloroquine, which is significantly the more toxic to the retina, should no longer be used to treat RA. The BNF advises that retinal toxicity is very unlikely with doses of *hydroxychloroquine sulphate* up to 6.5 mg/kg daily, calculated on the basis of lean body weight in obese patients. Early retinopathy appears to be reversible: this places a premium on patient counselling to ensure that they appreciate the importance of stopping treatment immediately they are aware of any visual impairment, and of seeing the prescriber promptly.

The Royal College of Ophthalmologists gives the following advice (modified from Jones SK (1999) *Br J Dermatol* **140**: 3–7, with permission):

- Baseline assessment should include:
  - Establishment of normal renal and hepatic function.
  - Enquiry for visual impairment not corrected by glasses.
  - A recording of near visual acuity (with glasses if used) by a reading test.
  - A check by an optician if there is any visual impairment.
- If no abnormality is detected, commence treatment with *hydroxychloroquine sulphate:*
  - Annual evaluation should comprise a simple enquiry about vision and repetition of the reading test.
- Patients should:
  - Be referred to an ophthalmologist if any visual impairment or eye disease is detected at baseline assessment.
  - Stop treatment and see the prescriber immediately if any change in visual acuity or blurred vision develops.

These drugs have rather complex **pharmacokinetics**, with a wide variation in elimination half-life. The route of excretion is mainly renal. The drugs are widely distributed in the body and are very strongly bound in the melanin-containing tissues of the skin and the eye. They are very persistent; indeed, chloroquine has been reported to be detectable in the retina of a patient 16 years after stopping treatment!

There are anecdotal reports of benefit from normal antimalarial doses when patients with RA travel to malarious areas and some patients with mild disease may benefit from such doses, with their preferable safety profile.

Other drugs and treatments

Many other approaches, mostly immunomodulatory, have been used in an attempt to control RA, but all of these procedures remain experimental.

Intra-articular injection of *osmium tetroxide* (osmic acid, preceded by a local anaesthetic plus methylprednisolone) has been used for synovial ablation, as an alternative to surgical synovectomy. About 70% of patients with severe refractory joint problems may benefit, but pain may recur. Complete regeneration of both synovial membranes and nerve endings occurs after a variable period.

Thalidomide has marked anti-inflammatory and immunomodulatory properties, suppressing superoxide and hydroxyl free radical formation. It has shown good results in RA within a few weeks, and remission may last for years in some patients, though others may relapse 2 months after stopping the drug. Some patients may remain symptom-free with low-dose maintenance treatment. The most common side effects are drowsiness, constipation and leg oedema, with no evidence of neuropathy. The well-known teratogenicity of thalidomide restricts its use to males and post-menopausal females and to fertile females taking effective contraceptive measures.

Epoietin may correct the resistant anaemia of active disease and in addition to haematological improvement also reduces the ESR and improves well-being.

Monoclonal antibodies (anti-CD4+), combined with a TNF-alpha receptor antagonist, have helped some patients with refractory RA. There seems to be a possibility of long-lasting improvement after a single course. Anti-CD5 and anti-T cell vaccines have also been used, as has the removal of lymphocytes and immune complexes from the lymph and serum (lymphopheresis and plasmapheresis). *Tumour necrosis factor* (TNF-alpha) has been implicated as a pro-inflammatory agent in RA and *monoclonal anti-TNF-alpha antibody* and *TNF-receptor-Fc fusion protein* have been used with some success in small trials in patients with severe disease.

As in asthma (*see* Chapter 5, pp. 259–260), *leukotriene antagonists* are under investigation for use in the arthritides. *Tenidap* appears to have multiple actions: it blocks COX and 5-lipoxygenase and also IL-1 formation and action. Injection of IL-1 receptor antagonist protein (*IRAP*, IL-1ra) has improved symptom scores in patients with active severe RA, with minimal side effects. A liposome formulation of the latter has been proposed for injection into joints, but as yet no products have been marketed.

It is becoming likely that synovial macrophages and fibroblasts may be more important than T cells, and this is an active research area. One problem with the biological agents is that they are themselves immunogenic, so they need to produce long-lasting results with a single short course of treatment: repeat courses are unlikely to succeed.

Levamisole, an immunostimulant, and *dapsone*, which has both immunosuppressive and pro-inflammatory properties, have also been used.

Yttrium-90 radiocolloid has been injected into inflamed joints as an immunosuppressive agent, with variable success.

Tetracycline antibiotics (e.g. *minocycline*) have been used on the hypothesis that RA is caused by mycoplasma infections, or is associated with them. Although some success has been achieved it is unclear whether this is due to the antimicrobial or immunomodulatory properties or to inhibition of phospholipase A2 and collagenases.

It has also been suggested, but unproven, that *selenium* supplementation is beneficial. Selenium is an essential trace element (it is a component of glutathione reductase), but the recommended daily allowance should not be exceeded because it is very toxic in overdose. This is difficult to manage because the selenium content of drinking water varies widely with the locality.

Fish oil supplements may help some patients with RA, but not OA.

Surgery

Orthopaedic surgery has a great deal to offer in the management of local problems when medical management has failed to give adequate control. However, it is important to carry out surgery before joint damage is so far advanced that good function cannot be restored. The most successful procedures are:

- Arthroplasty (overall probability about 20–25%).
  - Total hip replacement (success rate >95%).
  - Total knee replacement (success rate >90%).
- Removal of metatarsal heads (for eroded, subluxed MTP joints).
- Elbow synovectomy and removal of the radial head.

Other procedures include hand and wrist surgery, especially for tendon release, and fusion of the cervical spine if instability causes spinal cord compression. Arthroplasty of the PIP joints has successfully restored hand function. Operations on other joints are less common.

Juvenile chronic arthritis (JCA)

Definition

JCA is not a single condition, but includes several diseases, the true nature of which may become apparent only some time after the first appearance of symptoms. It is usually defined as arthritis starting before age 16 years and affecting four or more joints for at least 3 months, or a lesser number of joints confirmed by a biopsy, other diseases being excluded. Systemic JCA is sometimes referred to in the UK as **Still's disease** and in the USA as **juvenile rheumatoid arthritis**. It is not known to what extent the childhood arthropathies are simply early-onset adult disease, although there are certain similarities. Some children clearly have true juvenile RA, which may be severe in up to 50% of cases.

The disease states are currently classified according to the pattern of clinical presentation, but the boundaries between the various groups are difficult to define. The diagnosis and management of juvenile arthritis is normally carried out in specialist centres.

Diagnosis, management and prognosis

As indicated, the diagnosis of systemic JCA may initially be difficult because of the variety of systemic diseases which can cause joint symptoms (*see* Table 8.3), so these diseases need to be excluded.

Generally, the outlook is better than in adult RA of comparable joint involvement, and about 75% of patients have no significant residual disability. Occasionally, amyloid disease (p. 519) and eye involvement may be severe.

The principal **aim of management** is to ensure that there is a minimum of physical, educational and social disability when the disease eventually becomes inactive.

Pharmacotherapy resembles that in adult RA, with appropriate allowance for the fact that chil- dren are particularly vulnerable to blood dyscrasias and developmental abnormalities. *Aspirin* and *benorylate* must not be used in young children because of the risk of Reye's syndrome until an unequivocal diagnosis has been made. However, aspirin is sometimes used as an antipyretic, though paracetamol (acetaminophen) is preferred. NSAIDs (usually *diclofenac*, *ibuprofen*, *naproxen* or *piroxicam*) are the basis of treatment. Corticosteroids, MTX and hydroxychloroquine are used as a last resort in severe systemic disease.

Seronegative spondarthritides

This group of diseases have two features in common, as the name implies: they affect the spine and rheumatoid factors are absent. They include:

- Ankylosing spondylitis (see below).
- Reiter's syndrome (p. 505).
- Psoriatic arthritis (*see* Chapter 12).
- Inflammatory bowel disease (IBD, *see* Chapter 6).

Ankylosing spondylitis (AS)

Definition, epidemiology and aetiology

AS is a seronegative, chronic, spondarthritis (spondylarthritis), i.e. it primarily involves inflammation of the spine, leading to fusion of the vertebrae. Young adult males are most likely to have significant symptoms.

The disease affects about 1% of Caucasian populations with a male : female ratio of about 4 : 1 for moderate to severe disease, though mild disease is more common in women, the overall M : F ratio being about 2 : 1. The principal age of onset is 17–25 years. Some 5% of first-degree relatives also have AS, and there is a familial association with the other diseases mentioned above via HLA-B27 (*see* Table 8.2).

Aetiology

This is unknown, but HLA-B27 occurs in more than 90% of patients with uncomplicated AS showing no other symptoms (the prevalence in the general population is about 6%). HLA-B27 occurs infrequently in Black races and Japanese, who rarely suffer from AS, and the frequency of this gene in patients suffering from both AS and psoriasis or IBD is reduced to 60%. The possession of HLA-B27 clearly confers a predisposition to develop these diseases, though there is an environmental component, possibly an (unknown) infective agent. HLA-B27 has an important role in antigen presentation to T cells. One small trial has indeed shown the presence of cytotoxic (CD8) T cells which recognize arthritogenic bacteria (*Salmonella*, *Yersinia*) and possibly also auto-antigens in arthritic joints, and kill infected cell lines. A suggestion that *Klebsiella pneumoniae* is implicated has been disputed.

Pathology

The hallmark of AS is bilateral inflammation of the sacroiliac joints (non-synovial) at the base of the spine. The **synovitis** which occurs at other joints is similar to that in RA, but **enthe- sopathy** – inflammation of the points of attachment of the ligaments to the bone – is a prominent feature. There is a high tendency for anky-losis and calcification. This usually results in an ascending spinal ankylosis, and the spine may eventually become rigid in patients with advanced disease.

Clinical features, complications and diagnosis

Onset is usually insidious, initially with episodic low back pain and stiffness, especially in the morning. Much of this arises from pelvic joint inflammation, especially the sacroiliac joint, causing moderate to severe pain and stiffness in the buttocks. Systemic malaise, tiredness, anorexia and weight loss also occur but are less severe than in RA. Some 20% of patients, usually the younger ones, present with peripheral joint problems. **Plantar fasciitis**, i.e. inflammation at the heel of the entheses of the ligaments in the sole of the foot, is common. If spinal rigidity occurs, this compromises posture and movement, and respiration becomes wholly diaphragmatic if the rib articulations in the thoracic spine are severely affected.

Iritis (anterior uveitis) may occur in 25% of patients, the severity being unrelated to that of the arthropathy. Serious spinal fractures can occur in patients with rigid spines.

Diagnosis is based primarily on the clinical features and X-rays.

Management

The **aims** of management are the relief of pain (with drugs) and the minimization of stiffness and deformity (by physiotherapy).

Early diagnosis and forceful education about the value of a programme of morning exercises, to prevent bridging between vertebrae, are the basis of successful management.

Without good pain management it may be impossible to maintain an effective exercise reg-imen. *NSAIDs* are the mainstay of symptomatic treatment and are very effective if used in full dosage. *Indometacin*, one of the most potent, is often the drug of first choice, though any NSAID which is tolerated will usually be satisfactory. Once improvement has occurred, the dose is stepped down to the minimum necessary to give reasonable control of symptoms, and this level should be maintained as a permanent pro-phylactic dose, regardless of apparent disease activity, provided that side effects are not too obtrusive.

Azapropazone is a potent drug, but its toxicity – especially in the elderly – has led to its use being restricted only to situations when other NSAIDs have failed to provide adequate relief. *Phenylbutazone*, a highly effective drug is restric-ted to hospital use only (in the UK) because of its toxicity, and is the NSAID of last resort in severe cases. Careful patient monitoring, espe-cially haematological, is essential with both of these agents.

DMARDs (*gold, penicillamine*) are not gener-ally useful. *Sulfasalazine* or *methotrexate* may help to control any associated peripheral arthropathy, but have little effect on spinal inflammation.

Local corticosteroid injections may also be help-ful for peripheral joint problems or enthe-sopathies, e.g. plantar fasciitis.

Active physiotherapy, with a planned daily (morning) exercise programme, is invaluable for the minimization of spinal rigidity, the mainte-nance of function and to prevent spinal defor-mity. Swimming is especially recommended because the increased body buoyancy permits exercise but minimizes joint stress. Rest and immobility (e.g. splinting) increase the risk of deformity.

Surgery (arthroplasty) may be necessary for severe hip involvement (total hip replacement), and to manage the vertebral fractures that occur in a rigid and osteoporotic spine. Other spinal procedures are hazardous.

A single course of spinal radiotherapy is used occasionally, and is anti-inflammatory within the radiation target area. Repeat courses are contraindicated because they produce a high incidence of leukaemia and soft tissue tumours.

Reiter's syndrome

Definition

This multi-system disorder is usually characterized by:

- Urethritis.
- Seronegative spondarthritis.
- Conjunctivitis.
- Skin lesions.

These may follow sexually transmitted diseases, e.g. non-specific urethritis or cervicitis. The acronym 'SARA' (Sexually Acquired Reactive Arthritis) has been coined for this condition, about 50% of cases being associated with *Chlamydia trachomatis* or *Ureaplasma* urethritis. Gut infections, e.g. bacillary dysentery, may also be involved.

This is almost exclusively a male problem (80–95%), with most patients aged 16–35 years. There is a strong association with HLA-B27 (between 60% and 95% in various reports) that suggests the existence of a genetic susceptibility to an infection-triggered, immune-mediated disease.

Clinical features

Typically, there is a low-grade fever, conjunctivitis, arthritis and urinary tract symptoms. The arthritis tends to affect a few joints asymmetrically, primarily in the lower limbs, and usually remits after a few weeks or months. Back pain is associated with severe disease. About 50% of patients experience a single episode, but recurrences occur in the remainder over a period of years, probably as a result of repeated gastrointestinal or urinogenital infections, and sacroiliitis and spondylitis can occur at any stage. Repeated attacks lead to joint damage which is sometimes severe.

Management

Management of Reiter's syndrome involves:

- Rest, except in the mildest cases.
- Treatment of any infection (*tetracyclines* for most urinogenital infections, including *Chlamydia*).
- NSAIDs.
- Corticosteroids for severe systemic complications, or for injection into isolated affected joints.
- Aspiration of badly swollen joints.

Crystal deposition arthropathies

Common features and pathology

The diseases in this group share the feature of deposition of crystals of metabolites in the joints, with consequent inflammation and joint damage. Their principal characteristics are given in Table 8.18.

It is not known what factors promote the deposition of crystals in the synovial fluid. Once there, the positively charged crystals become coated with negatively charged proteins, especially IgG and phospholipids, thus enhancing phagocytosis by macrophages. This results in the liberation of lysosomal and cytoplasmic enzymes, which attack the synovial membrane, and promotes the release from neutrophils of a specific pro-inflammatory

Table 8.18   Some features of crystal deposition

Disease	Metabolite deposited	Crystal shape	Joints involved	Prevalence[a]
Gout	Monosodium urate	Needle	Peripheral Small	1%, mostly males 40–50 years of age
Pyrophosphate arthropathy	Calcium pyrophosphate	Rhomboidal	Large (knee)	0.4%, M : F = 3 : 2, 60–80 years of age

[a] Approximate international prevalence.

glycoprotein. Injection of this glycoprotein into joints produces symptoms that are indistinguishable from those of gout. Chemotactic factors are also released and promote leucocyte recruitment, thus multiplying the effect.

Similar effects can be produced by a variety of crystals or other substances introduced into the joint space, e.g. corticosteroid suspensions injected to relieve joint inflammation, glove powder (avoided nowadays) and cholesterol. Exacerbations of osteoarthritis may be due to microcrystals of hydroxyapatite released from the bone causing a similar effect.

Gout

Gout is an arthropathy resulting from the deposition of crystals of monosodium urate in the joints and surrounding tissues.

Aetiology and epidemiology

Gout is the result of **hyperuricaemia**, though it is difficult to define the latter satisfactorily because there is a continuous normal distribution of serum urate levels. The solubility of uric acid in serum is about 0.38 mmol/L (6.3 mg/dL). The 95% population limits are 0.18–0.42 mmol/L (3.0–7.0 mg/dL) for men and 0.13–0.34 mmol/L (2.2–5.7 mg/dL) for women, so it follows that the serum is supersaturated with urate in about 3% of UK men and that gout is overwhelmingly a male problem (90–95% of cases). Fortunately, only a minority of men with high serum urate levels show clinical symptoms, but

it is not clear why this is so. Further, some patients with gout have relatively low urate levels. However, clinical symptoms are overwhelmingly associated with hyperuricaemia.

A simplified outline of uric acid metabolism is given in Fig. 8.10, from which it may be deduced that hyperuricaemia could result either from excessive production of uric acid or from reduced renal elimination, the latter being the most common cause. In **primary gout** there are numerous factors operating on a background of genetic predisposition to produce clinical symptoms. The causes of **secondary gout** are given in Table 8.19. Treatment with thiazide diuretics often causes some degree of hyperuricaemia, but fortunately does not often cause an attack of gout. However, diuretics are a relatively common cause of gout in elderly women.

The prevalence of gout varies widely, being about 0.3% in the UK and about 2% in France. In Maoris, who have a strong genetic predisposition, it is about 10%.

Pathology

If hyperuricaemia results in the crystallization of monosodium urate in synovial fluid, small, needle-shaped crystals can also be seen within the leucocytes, causing the release of lysosomal enzymes.

If untreated, gout leads initially to the deposition of urate crystals on the surface of the cartilage, with subsequent cartilage damage and finally to the deposition of masses of urate crystals within and around the joints, producing extensive joint destruction. Nodular accretions of monosodium urate (**tophi**) may occur. A

Table 8.19   The aetiology of secondary hyperuricaemia

| | Factors causing uric acid | |
	Under-excretion	Overproduction
Iatrogenic	Diuretics, especially thiazides[a] Low-dose aspirin or fructose administration Ciclosporin (cyclosporine) (due to renal toxicity)	Cytotoxic drugs, radiotherapy (increased cell destruction)
Self-inflicted	–	Obesity Excessive consumption of alcohol or purines (meat)
Renal	Renal failure Hypertensive nephropathy Sarcoidosis Lead poisoning	–
Cardiovascular	Heart failure	–
Metabolic	Ketosis Starvation Myxoedema	Inherited enzyme defects
Other conditions	Hypercalcaemia	High cell turnover (neoplastic diseases, psoriasis)

[a] Probably the most common cause of secondary gout.

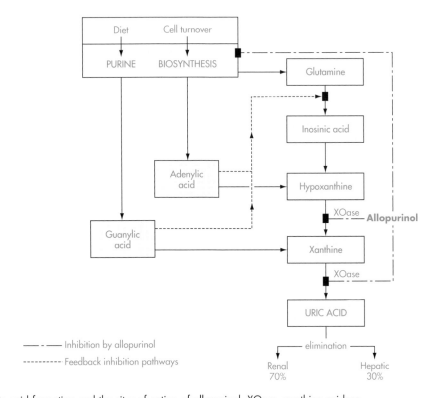

Figure 8.10   Uric acid formation and the sites of action of allopurinol. XOase, xanthine oxidase.

characteristic site for these is the cartilaginous margin (**helix**) of the pinna of the ear, but they occur also on tendons and in bursae associated with the affected joints. They are granulomatous structures containing the urate crystals in a protein–lipid–polysaccharide matrix and eventually become calcified. In long-standing chronic gout, joint erosions occur which contain calcified deposits. Urate deposition tends to occur in sites where the temperature is lower than the core body temperature, resulting in reduced urate solubility: cartilage is avascular and the affected joints are environmentally exposed.

The precipitation of monosodium urate from urine within the kidney, or of uric acid under acid conditions, may result in the formation of renal stones, possibly causing urinary tract infection and obstruction and renal failure (*see* Chapter 4, p. 204).

Clinical features and diagnosis

Acute gout

In some 75% of cases a first attack affects the big toe, and this form is called **podagra**. Other common sites are the ankles, knees, elbows, wrists and fingers. An attack often starts overnight or a few hours after an acutely stressful episode, e.g. myocardial infarction or surgery. The joint becomes exquisitely painful and inflamed and the overlying skin may flake over the next few hours: this sign plus the symptoms is almost conclusive. The attack subsides spontaneously over a few days or weeks, though most sufferers seek treatment. There may be no recurrence, or a second attack may follow after a variable period ranging from days to years.

Attacks tend to be more severe in younger patients (aged <30 years).

Chronic gout

This is uncommon, except in non-compliant patients or those with a metabolic abnormality. Acute episodes occur with increasing frequency, leading to tophus formation and permanent joint damage. Renal impairment increases with time and this is aggravated in about one-third of

patients by associated hypertension, though the latter probably reflects the kidney damage.

Diagnosis

This is on the basis of the symptoms and signs outlined above, and the finding of a high serum urate level. However, the association of the latter with joint pain does not necessarily imply a diagnosis of gout: there may be a coincidental association of hyperuricaemia with arthritic problems. The principal diagnostic confusion is with septic arthritis. The diagnosis can be confirmed unequivocally only by the demonstration of urate crystals microscopically in the synovial fluid of the affected joint, but this is necessary only in doubtful cases. Aspiration of small joints is impossibly painful during an attack.

Management

Aims

The aims of management of gout are:

- The prompt relief of pain in an acute attack.
- To eliminate secondary causes, if possible.
- The prevention of recurrence and complications in chronic sufferers by correction of hyperuricaemia.

General measures

Acute attacks
The approach is to:

- Rest the affected joint, splinting may help in the severe acute stage.
- Maintain a high fluid intake to reduce hyperuricaemia and prevent renal urate stone formation.

Chronic gout
The approach is to:

- Maintain high fluid intake.
- Lose weight if obese, to reduce tissue mass and so urate production and to reduce loading on joints.
- Provide dietary advice:

- Avoid alcohol (reduces urate solubility), especially beer (high in purines).
- Reduce carbohydrate intake (protein-sparing).
- Avoid foods rich in purines, e.g. offal, shellfish, spinach.
- Endoscopic shock wave lithotripsy (*see* Chapter 4, p. 205) for urate kidney stones.

However, even a strict low-purine diet has only a small effect, reducing the serum urate level by about 10–15%.

Pharmacotherapy

Acute attacks

Immediate initiation of treatment is important, and NSAIDs are given as early as possible. High-dose *indometacin* is the drug of choice, e.g. 75 mg immediately, 50 mg 6- to 8-hourly on the first and second days, 100 mg on the third day, then slowly tapering to zero over 10–14 days. In the elderly, or if this regimen is contraindicated or is not well tolerated, a choice may be made from *naproxen*, *diclofenac*, *ketoprofen*, *piroxicam* and *sulindac* at comparable dosage, depending on acceptability to the patient.

Exceptionally, if none of these drugs provides adequate relief, *azapropazone* (*apazone*) may be used, provided that there is no history of peptic ulceration. However, the dose should be reduced in the elderly or if there is any suspicion of moderate to severe renal impairment. Azapropazone is very liable to cause photosensitivity, so high-factor sunblocks are required if it is used. In addition to having analgesic and anti-inflammatory properties, azapropazone is also a potent uricosuric agent (see below) and may thus be particularly useful for the treatment of gout.

Occasionally, moderately potent opioids may need to be added to control intolerable pain.

If NSAIDs are not tolerated, or if there is a history of peptic ulceration, hypertension or heart failure, or if the patient is taking warfarin (possibly potentiated by NSAIDs, especially by azapropazone and phenylbutazone), then *colchicine* is indicated. This is very effective: it suppresses macrophage recruitment and multiplication and specifically inhibits production of the pro-inflammatory glycoprotein. The pain normally starts to remit in 12–24 h and is completely controlled in 2–3 days. However, colchicine is more toxic than NSAIDs and tends to cause diarrhoea and vomiting: these side effects are often used as an index of adequate dosage. Colchicine has been used at the outset as an aid to diagnosis, but a prompt response to it is not specific. Pseudogout (less common, see below), tendon calcification and other conditions with symptoms similar to gout, which may cause diagnostic difficulty, also respond.

In resistant cases, systemic injections of *corticotrophin* or a *corticosteroid* may be used. Steroids may also be injected into an affected large joint in the course of aspiration for diagnostic purposes.

Paradoxically, *allopurinol* or *uricosuric agents* (see below) must not be started during an acute attack because they will often worsen and prolong symptoms (except *azapropazone*, see below). It is known that sudden changes in serum urate levels tend to precipitate attacks. These exacerbations probably result from mobilization of urate from the joints. Allopurinol also interferes with uric acid excretion. If an acute attack occurs during existing urate-lowering treatment, the treatment should be maintained, and the acute attack treated normally.

Interval control

This is management of the patient in the intervals between attacks. It includes:

- Control of precipitating and aggravating factors, e.g. diet, alcohol intake, obesity and drugs (especially thiazide diuretics): these must be dealt with regardless of possible pharmacotherapy.
- Evaluation of the need for pharmacotherapy, e.g. management of hyperuricaemia, other antigout drugs.

An isolated attack is not an indication for prophylactic pharmacotherapy unless the serum urate level is consistently very high (it is usually high, >0.60 mmol/L [10 mg/dL] in an acute attack), there is evidence of urate nephropathy or there are tophi. The disadvantages of long-term prophylaxis need to be weighed carefully before lifelong treatment is initiated.

Infrequent attacks. These are best managed by general measures and high-dose *NSAIDs*, as in an acute attack, because otherwise therapy needs to be lifelong. Continuous *low-dose colchicine* is used occasionally, though it is contraindicated in pregnancy (it is an antimitotic agent) and if a mother is breast feeding. Colchicine must be used cautiously in the elderly and if there is any suspicion or evidence of gastrointestinal, cardiac, hepatic or renal impairment.

Management of hyperuricaemia. If there are specific indications (more than two attacks in a year, tophi, joint or renal damage) or if the patient insists on treatment, then lifelong prophylactic pharmacotherapy is considered at least 3 weeks after an initial attack has subsided. Urate-lowering drugs are used, two methods being available: either by reducing urate production or by increasing renal urate excretion.

The target serum urate level is about 0.25 mmol/L (4.2 mg/dL), maintained over long periods to achieve regression of tophi. Because rapid reduction of serum urate levels tends to provoke attacks of gout, *prophylactic colchicine or NSAID* cover should be given for the first 3–6 months of either treatment mode, continued if necessary until urate levels are normalized.

Allopurinol is the drug of choice for **reducing urate production**. It is a **xanthine oxidase inhibitor** (Fig. 8.10) which also inhibits purine biosynthesis. Treatment should be initiated at a low dose, increasing gradually until urate levels are normalized. An adequate fluid intake (2–3 L/day) should be maintained to minimize the possibility of kidney stone formation.

Increased renal excretion is achieved with **uricosuric agents** (*probenecid* or *sulfinpyrazone*). These inhibit renal tubular reabsorption of uric acid, and so are ineffective if renal function is impaired. Although these drugs are less used nowadays because they are more toxic than allopurinol, they retain a place for patients intolerant of the latter. Initiation of treatment is undertaken with the same precautions as for allopurinol. They may also be used in addition to allopurinol if the latter provides inadequate control of serum urate levels.

Azapropazone, which has uricosuric properties, is an exception to the rule that uricosuric agents should not be used in an acute attack,

because it also provides effective simultaneous analgesic and anti-inflammatory cover. A high fluid intake should be maintained.

Side effects and interactions
Allopurinol is usually well tolerated, the most common side effects being rashes, sometimes with fever. The dosage should be reduced in renal or hepatic impairment. In the former case an active metabolite, oxypurinol, may accumulate and precipitate the potentially life-threatening **allopurinol hypersensitivity syndrome**. Thus if rashes occur, treatment must be stopped immediately, because they may indicate a potentially severe reaction. Treatment may be restarted cautiously following a mild skin reaction, but recurrence is an absolute contraindication to further use, as is an initially severe reaction. Gastrointestinal discomfort may be reduced by taking allopurinol after meals. Because the metabolism of xanthine is suppressed, high concentrations of the latter may be excreted and may crystallize in the urinary tract, hence the need for an adequate fluid intake, especially in the early stages of treatment.

The activity of the cytotoxic purines *azathioprine* and *mercaptopurine* is potentiated by the use of allopurinol, which also inhibits their metabolism, so if these drugs are used in neoplastic disease their dose should be reduced to one-quarter if allopurinol is also indicated. Treatment with allopurinol should be commenced before cytotoxic treatment is initiated, if possible, because cytotoxics or radiotherapy may cause rapid tissue and leucocyte breakdown, leading to increased urate production.

The action of oral anticoagulants may also be potentiated, so particular attention needs to be paid to prothrombin time/INR measurements. However, the clinical significance of this interaction is doubtful.

Probenecid and *sulfinpyrazone* are generally well tolerated, but should be used carefully if patients have peptic ulceration (they may cause gastrointestinal distress) or renal impairment (their action depends on adequate renal function). They must not be given with aspirin or salicylates, which antagonize their action in the renal tubules. The urine should be alkalinized (e.g. with citrates) if the uric acid level is high, to give the maximum solubility of uric acid and prevent urate stone formation. A night-time dose of *acetazolamide*, a carbonic anhydrase inhibitor and weak diuretic, has also been used to alkalinize the urine (unlicensed indication). Gastrointestinal disorders occur most commonly, but hypersensitivity reactions and blood dyscrasias may also occur: regular blood counts are advisable with sulfinpyrazone.

Pyrophosphate arthropathy

Pyrophosphate arthropathy (also known as calcium pyrophosphate deposition disease, CPPD, **pseudogout** or **chondrocalcinosis**) results from the excessive deposition of calcium pyrophosphate in joints: minor deposits are common and are usually asymptomatic. The aetiology is usu-

ally not identified, but genetic and predisposing factors, e.g. age and hyperparathyroidism, are known. CPPD is about one-third as common as gout.

The calcium pyrophosphate crystals probably form initially in cartilage and are shed into the synovial fluid. Thus microscopic examination of the latter gives a clear diagnosis. It is probable that acute exacerbations of osteoarthritis are due to calcium pyrophosphate shedding from damaged cartilage.

The disease may present acutely, resembling acute gout, or as a degenerative chronic arthritis, sometimes with intermittent acute episodes. *Colchicine* is as effective in CPPD as it is in gout. Otherwise there is no specific treatment: NSAIDs are effective in acute attacks and intra-articular injections of corticosteroids are highly beneficial. Otherwise, management resembles that of osteoarthritis.

Multisystem disorders and associated diseases

There is currently no satisfactory classification for this group of chronic, progressive inflammatory diseases, formerly called 'collagen-vascular diseases'. A possible grouping is given in Table 8.20. They share the following features:

- Widespread inflammation of organs and systems throughout the body, notably causing vasculitis and arthritis.
- Autoimmune features, with circulating autoantibodies and immune complex deposition.
- Unknown aetiology.

Two types of antineutrophil cytoplasmic antibodies (ANCA) are seen in the systemic vasculitides: cytoplasmic (cANCA) and perinuclear (pANCA). Both are anti-enzyme antibodies. One current hypothesis is that there is a defect in T-suppressor cell regulation, leading to excessive T-helper cell activity, so causing an autoimmune

state: there is a possible association with chronic viral infection.

Patients often show features of more than one of these diseases. The syndrome described as **'mixed connective tissue disease'** may be a distinct entity, but is possibly a variant of scleroderma.

Because fever and arthralgias are common presenting symptoms, patients are usually referred to rheumatologists.

Systemic lupus erythematosus (SLE)

Definition and epidemiology

This non-organ-specific, multisystem, autoimmune disease primarily affects young women. The female:male ratio is about 10:1, the onset

Table 8.20   The multisystem disorders and associated diseases

Disease grouping	Examples
Chronic autoimmune diseases	Systemic lupus erythematosus (SLE)
	Sjögren's syndrome
	Scleroderma and systemic sclerosis
	Raynaud's syndrome
Systemic vasculitides	
Large vessel vasculitis (aorta and main branches)	Giant cell arteritis (GCA)
	Polymyalgia rheumatica (PMR)
Medium vessel vasculitis (main visceral arteries, e.g. renal, hepatic, coronary, mesenteric)	Polyarteritis nodosa (PAN, small arteries also involved, but less so)
Small vessel vasculitis (distal vessels connecting with arterioles	Wegener's granulomatosis
Other multisystem disorders	Amyloidosis
	Sarcoidosis

being in the age range 20–35 years, notably in the early twenties. There is a profound immunological disturbance characterized by autoantibodies directed against normal double-stranded DNA.

SLE occurs world-wide, and may affect up to 0.5% of females in the West Indies and the Far East, there being a possible association with sunny climates. There are over 30 000 diagnosed patients in the UK.

Aetiology

There is an **inherited tendency** for SLE, the concordance rate for monozygotic twins being about twice that for dizygotic twins. There is about a 3% risk among first-degree relatives. In Caucasians, this is linked to an increased frequency of HLA-B8 and DR3, and in Japanese with DR2.

Inherited deficiencies of a number of components of the complement system occur, e.g. of C4a, C4b and C2 in 83% of patients, these being linked to the HLA changes.

The sex hormone status may also be involved because oophorectomy (ovary removal) or treatment with *androgens* has relieved lupus-like symptoms in experimental animals.

Pathology and diagnosis

SLE causes damage to a wide range of tissues. Damage to cells is known to release DNA, and this may provoke the formation of anti-DNA antibody. DNA has a high affinity for the collagen in the glomerular basement membrane, so binding of DNA in this region may be expected to lead to the formation of immune complexes (ICs), triggering local inflammation. These observations provide an explanation for two of the features of SLE: the presence of antinuclear antibodies (see below) and renal involvement. A further reason for glomerular involvement is local glomerular hypertension, which promotes extravasation from the circulation of cells and nuclei which can then attach to the basement membrane.

Fluorescent antibody studies show widespread IC deposition in cellular basement membranes. This probably accounts for most of the manifestations of the disease, especially the vasculitis in the arterioles and capillaries. Although the ICs may be formed in all individuals, SLE sufferers may be unable to clear them because of complement deficiencies referred to above.

The standard screening test is the **fluorescent antibody antinuclear test** (ANA; ANF, antinuclear factor) which detects antinuclear antibodies and is positive in virtually all patients with SLE. However, the ANA test is not specific (some 3% of the population is ANF-positive, but only about 3% of these have SLE) and so is used only as a routine screening test. More confidence can be placed in **dsDNA binding tests**, though some 15% of patients are falsely negative in these, especially in early or mild disease. Because this test is applied only to patients who are strongly positive in the ANA test this type of result does not give rise to ambiguities.

Despite the inflammation, the CRP is not raised, though the ESR is raised in concordance with disease activity. The criteria for diagnosis are given in Table 8.21.

Drug-induced SLE

Many drugs are capable of producing a lupus-like syndrome (Table 8.22), but this is usually relatively mild, rarely provoking renal involvement, and tends to remit when the drug is withdrawn. It is doubtful whether this is related to true SLE.

Drugs may trigger attacks only in susceptible subjects, and all pharmacotherapy in SLE patients needs careful supervision. A history of drug allergies is common in patients with drug-induced SLE.

Clinical features

SLE may affect almost any organ, though the liver is rarely involved. The approximate percentage frequencies of the principal organs involved are: joints, 95%; skin, 80%; CNS, 60%; kidneys, 50%; lungs, 40%; heart, 40%. Fever and arthralgias are common, accompanied by headaches, depression, malaise and tiredness.

There is often a symmetrical malar (facial) 'butterfly'-shaped rash, giving a wolf-like pattern: hence the name 'lupus'. The occurrence of the rash may be triggered by sunlight, with or without photosensitizing drugs. If rash is the principal presenting symptom, patients may be referred initially to a dermatologist.

Table 8.21 Criteria for the diagnosis of systemic lupus erythematosus (SLE)

For a diagnosis of SLE, at least four of the following criteria need to be present simultaneously, or serially, during a period of observation:
- Malar (facial) rash
- Discoid rash (see p. 514)
- Photosensitivity
- Oral or nasopharyngeal ulcers
- Serositis
- Non-erosive arthritis involving two or more peripheral joints
- Pleuritis *or* pericarditis
- Renal disease (persistent heavy proteinuria)
- Fits *or* psychotic features
- Haemolytic anaemia *or* thrombocytopenia *or* leukopenia
- Antinuclear and other auto-antibodies

Table 8.22 Some drugs which may cause a lupus-like syndrome

Cardiovascular drugs
Beta-blockers, hydralazine, methyldopa, procainamide, quinidine

Antimicrobial agents
Griseofulvin, isoniazid

Anti-epileptics
Ethosuximide, phenytoin, primidone
Antipsychotics: chlorpromazine, lithium carbonate

Others
Oral contraceptives, penicillamine, propylthiouracil

Although an episodic course is usual, some patients have chronic disease. Exacerbations and complete remissions may occur over a very variable time period. The disease used to be represented as a relentlessly progressive, fatal condition, but the 10-year survival rate is now about 90%. Severe problems are unlikely if they have not developed within this time: most patients now do reasonably well.

Management

General

Because of the potential widespread and diverse nature of symptoms, patients need to be counselled carefully and told to report any new symptoms as they occur. Reassurance is appropriate for most. They should be warned of the need to protect themselves from bright sunshine, because of photosensitivity, and of the potential for drug allergies.

Pregnancy is not contraindicated, except in severe disease, but specialist gynaecological care is essential.

Pharmacotherapy

Corticosteroids are the mainstay of treatment, using high doses in acute severe episodes and low-dose maintenance therapy in most patients. Their well-known side effects make it important to step down the dose to about 7.5 mg/day of *prednisolone*, or less if possible, once symptoms are controlled. However, not all patients need continuous maintenance therapy.

Mild disease confined to the joints can usually be controlled with *NSAIDs*. *Hydroxychloroquine* is useful if these are inadequate and for the control of skin lesions. *Immunosuppressants*, usually *azathioprine* or *cyclophosphamide*, are often used for their steroid-sparing effect and to control renal involvement or severe symptoms. Other treatment is supportive and symptomatic, e.g. renal dialysis.

Chronic discoid lupus erythematosus (CDLE)

Clinical features and pathology

CDLE is a benign, chronic, episodic, erythematous skin disorder which mostly affects the face, although the scalp, hands and feet may also be affected. The rash may be symmetrical (like SLE) or asymmetrical. The lesions are sharply defined, slightly scaly, erythematous discs about 5–10 mm in diameter, sometimes slightly larger. If a scale is removed, the underside will show a 'hairy' appearance due to the adherent pilosebaceous plugs which filled the hair follicles: this is pathognomonic. Older lesions tend to heal with scarring and hair loss. Pigmentation may occur in white skin and depigmentation is common in coloured skin. Usually, there are no systemic features with CDLE, but about 5% of patients eventually develop SLE.

Similarly to SLE, the lesions are caused by the deposition of ICs, in this case in the basal layer of the skin, causing cell destruction. There may be a high ESR and cells usually associated with SLE or similar diseases (LE cells) occur in the serum.

Pharmacotherapy

High-protection factor *sunblock preparations* are used for photosensitivity. CDLE is one of the few indications for the use on the face of potent or moderately potent *corticosteroids*, e.g. *clobetasol;* **even** intralesional injections are sometimes used.

If this does not achieve control, *antimalarials* may be helpful (as in SLE). Also, antimycobacterial drugs are sometimes used because they have anti-inflammatory properties. The antileprotic drug *clofazimine* is preferred to *rifampicin*, so as not to prejudice the use of the latter for tuberculosis.

Sjögren's syndrome (keratoconjunctivitis sicca)

Definition

Classically, Sjögren's syndrome is defined as a triad of:

- **Xerophthalmia** (dry eyes).
- **Xerostomia** (dry mouth).
- A connective tissue or rheumatoid disease, usually RA.

If only the first two of these symptoms occur, this is described as the '**primary**' form, sometimes called '**sicca syndrome**'. It is not known whether this represents a complication of occult connective tissue disease or whether the two conditions are triggered by a common agent. There is an association of sicca syndrome with lymphoid hyperplasia and high levels of circulating antibody, suggesting the presence of a distinct autoimmune disease.

However, Sjögren's syndrome is usually **secondary**, occurring in about 20% of those with other autoimmune and connective tissue diseases, e.g. RA, SLE or systemic sclerosis (see below).

Overall, about 0.5% of adult females are affected, the female : male ratio being 9 : 1.

Pathology

This is a chronic autoimmune disease causing destruction of the exocrine glands due to lymphocytic infiltration. The aetiology is unknown, but there is an association with an HLA-DR3 allele.

There is also hyperactivity of B cells, shown by auto-antibodies, e.g. RFs and antibodies to small RNA–protein complexes.

Clinical features

The general drying up of exocrine secretions may cause effects on many organ systems, though in most patients the disease remains a minor mouth and eye problem. These effects include:

- **Eyes**: grittiness, irritation, morning lid stickiness, conjunctivitis.
- **Mouth**: difficulty in chewing and swallowing food; inability to speak continuously; tongue smooth, erythematous and sensitive; greatly increased dental caries; parotid gland enlargement; candidal infection common.
- **Respiratory tract**: predisposition to infection.
- **Genital tract**: atrophic vaginitis and **dyspareunia** (difficult or painful coitus) in premenopausal women.
- **Kidneys**: some patients develop nephritis, but major renal pathology is rare.
- **Raynaud's syndrome** (in 25% of patients; see below).
- Non-erosive **arthritis** (33%).
- **Vasculitis** causing purpura and sometimes glomerulonephritis.

Other features may be seen, e.g. leg ulceration and an increased tendency to hypersensitivity reactions. Patients with persistent parotid gland enlargement may develop non-Hodgkin's B cell **lymphoma**, but this can be predicted by the presence of circulating cryoglobulins (IgMs precipitated at low temperatures).

Management

In **secondary disease** this consists of management of the underlying condition, plus symptomatic relief, as in the primary syndrome.

Treatment of **primary Sjögren's syndrome** is solely symptomatic, and focuses on replacement of secretions, thus minimizing discomfort and any damaging effects. They include:

- **Eye drops**: frequent use of preparations containing *hypromellose, polyvinyl alcohol* or *acetylcysteine* ('artificial tears').
- **Mouth problems**:
  - Scrupulous attention to dental hygiene to minimize premature, gross dental caries.
  - *Compound thymol glycerin* or more potent antiseptic mouthwashes, e.g. *chlorhexidine gluconate* if toothbrushing is painful.
  - Commercial '*artificial saliva*' preparations, and **sugar-free** demulcent pastilles, to alleviate dryness; *pilocarpine* may also help.
  - *Fluconazole* or *itraconazole* for oropharyngeal candidiasis.
- *Hydroxychloroquine* for joint problems.
- *Corticosteroids* or cytotoxic immunosuppressants (*cyclophosphamide*) for severe systemic problems, e.g. vasculitis.
- **Lymphoma**, normal treatment (Chapter 11).

Diuretics and anticholinergic drugs aggravate the lack of secretions and should be avoided.

Scleroderma and systemic sclerosis

Definition

Scleroderma is characterized superficially by a dense hardening of skin collagen, especially of the hands and face, giving a tense, shiny appearance to the affected skin and puckering around the mouth.

If the internal organs are affected, the term **systemic sclerosis** is more appropriate, but the terms tend to be used interchangeably. **Systemic sclerosis** may lead to renal, pulmonary or cardiac failure.

Clinical features and pathology

The disease is uncommon (UK annual incidence 18 per million, USA slightly higher) and occurs principally in women aged 30–50 years (overall female : male ratio about 3 : 1).

The symptoms described above are the result of three features:

- **Vascular damage**: Raynaud's syndrome (see below) occurs in nearly all patients, often months or years before other symptoms. This, and finger joint arthropathy, are common presenting features.
- **Fibrosis**: from the deposition of collagen and adhesive proteins (e.g. fibronectin) etc., produced by fibroblasts.
- An **activated immune system**: the active fibroblasts are associated with T_H lymphocytes (CD4+), macrophages and degranulation of mast cells.

A genetic susceptibility has been mapped to HLA genes. Intriguingly, similarity between the target of some antiscleroderma auto-antibodies, DNA topoisomerase-1, and some mammalian retroviruses raises the possibility that scleroderma is triggered by viral infection.

The disease follows a chronic, highly variable course.

Management

Management of scleroderma is primarily symptomatic. *Corticosteroids* may be used to suppress synovitis. *Cytotoxic immunosuppressives* and *antithymocyte globulin*, if given early enough, may be helpful. *ACEIs* have vastly improved the morbidity and mortality from renal involvement, and the principal cause of death is pulmonary fibrosis. *Penicillamine* and *IFN-gamma* have been used experimentally to stem fibrosis.

The survival rate at 5 years after diagnosis is about 50%, but in some patients the disease stabilizes or regresses at about this time.

Raynaud's syndrome

The nomenclature of this condition is confused. The primary (idiopathic) form, which occurs without any underlying rheumatoid or connective tissue disorder, has been called 'Raynaud's disease', that secondary to such disease being called 'Raynaud's phenomenon'. This division seems artificial, not least because Raynaud's disease may precede the onset of symptoms of the underlying disease by many years and is then seen to be a prodrome of that disease. In this text the neutral term 'Raynaud's syndrome' is preferred.

Primary Raynaud's syndrome, which especially affects young women, is due to spasm of the arterioles and small arteries, especially in the fingers and toes, resulting in intermittent blanching of the overlying skin. Occasionally other extremities, e.g. the nose, tongue and ears, may be affected.

The secondary form (Table 8.23) may reflect local nerve damage, similarly causing vasospasm, or the use of vasospastic drugs, but may be due to inflammation, e.g. vasculitis.

Table 8.23   Some causes and associations of Raynaud's syndrome

Cause	Examples
Idiopathic	Genetic, mostly young women
Trauma	Pneumatic drill workers, motor cycle dispatch riders
Secondary	Arteritis, mixed connective tissue disease, myxoedema, progressive systemic sclerosis, rheumatoid arthritis, Sjögren's syndrome, systemic lupus erythematosus
Drug-induced	Beta-blockers, ergotamine, methysergide

Clinical features

The primary form causes intermittent, reversible attacks, precipitated by exposure to cold or emotional upset. The hands are most often affected, but attacks rarely involve the thumb. The affected fingers go white and may even become cyanosed and finally red as rewarming occurs. Paraesthesias, e.g. numbness, tingling or burning are common, and pain may be severe during rewarming.

The primary disease is a common condition which affects 5% of the population. It usually causes bilateral symptoms whereas secondary disease may produce unilateral, irreversible symptoms, the affected area being permanently sensitive to adverse conditions, especially cold.

Diagnosis

The symptoms described above are pathognomonic. However, attacks of secondary Raynaud's syndrome may precede the onset of symptoms due to the underlying disease, e.g. RA or scleroderma, by months or years. It is thus essential to look carefully for the markers of any underlying disease.

Management

General measures

In secondary Raynaud's syndrome, treatment is that of the underlying disease. The most useful basic approaches, whether or not the condition is primary are:

- To avoid:
  - Cold; keep warm locally and generally.
  - Peripherally vasoconstricting drugs, e.g. ergotamine, beta-blockers.
  - Smoking.
- To be scrupulous about hand hygiene, cuts, etc. and skin care.
- Physiotherapy needs to be started at the onset and performed regularly to promote good circulation.

Pharmacotherapy

Drugs are widely used, but most drug use is empirical. The following may help:

- **Vasodilators:**
  - Calcium-channel blockers (*see* Chapter 3) are sometimes effective. *Nifedipine* is the only one licensed for this purpose in the UK, but *nicardipine*, and possibly *amlodipine* and *felodipine*, may also be useful. They tend to cause headache, flushing and dizziness.
  - Other vasodilators (*see* Chapter 3) may help, e.g. *prazosin*, ACE inhibitors (e.g. *captopril*, *enalapril*) and *thymoxamine*, but may cause postural hypotension and the side effects described for calcium-channel blockers.
  - *Epoprostenol*, an anti-platelet drug, is also a potent vasodilator and has been used if there are seriously compromised ischaemic areas. It must be given by continuous IV infusion because of its very short half-life. Epoprostenol may cause severe flushing, headache and hypotension and so its use must be closely supervised. It is unsuitable for patients with ischaemic heart disease because it diverts blood from ischaemic areas and aggravates the problem. Its more stable analogue *iloprost* (not licensed in the UK) may be preferred if epoprostenol is not tolerated.
- **Other agents:** *gamolenic acid* and *halibut liver oil* have been reported to be helpful.
- Nitric oxide, generated topically by mixing sodium nitrite and ascorbic acid gels, has recently been reported to improve the microcirculation.

Surgery

This may help, e.g. to relieve median nerve compression in associated carpal tunnel syndrome (p. 521). Sympathectomy has been used if there is a risk of digital gangrene, but the long-term outcome is uncertain.

Vasculitides

Large-vessel vasculitis

Giant cell arteritis (GCA)

Clinical features

This disease usually involves only the carotid arterial tree. Patients present with fever, severe malaise, weight loss and jaw pain on chewing. **Polymyalgia rheumatica** (see below) is a commonly associated condition. Most patients are over 50 years of age, and women are affected more than men. Severe, localized headache is common, usually unilateral (temporal), with marked tenderness of the temple or scalp, hence the alternative names **temporal** (or **cranial**) **arteritis**. The ESR is high, 50–120 mm/h (Normal <20 mm/h), as is the CRP level. One important complication is sudden, reversible or irreversible, unilateral or bilateral **blindness** (25% risk).

Pharmacotherapy

High-dose corticosteroids, e.g. 60–100 mg *prednisolone* daily, are essential to prevent blindness. The dose may be reduced after one month, depending on the condition of the patient and the reduction in ESR. Some consultants favour lower starting doses of 40 mg. The headache remits within hours of the first dose, and this feature is sometimes helpful diagnostically.

The disease remits within 24–36 months' treatment in about 75% of patients, but the remainder require maintenance low-dose steroids. Recurrence of symptoms at any stage dictates a return to full steroid dosage.

Patients need to be taught to manage their disease and to increase the corticosteroid dose immediately according to an agreed protocol if their condition deteriorates. They should then see their doctor. A prompt reaction to deterioration may pre-empt the need for more aggressive treatment later.

Polymyalgia rheumatica (PMR)

Aetiology and epidemiology

PMR is defined by its clinical features. Some cases are associated with GCA, though most show quite distinct features and more widespread arteritis. PMR occurs mainly in the elderly, with two-thirds of patients being aged over 60 years, and is uncommon before the age of 50 or after 80 years. The female : male ratio is 2 : 1.

PMR is more common in Northern Europe. There are marked seasonal variations in incidence (about 70 per 100 000 in the over-60s),

and these have prompted a search for infective causes, albeit without success. Because PMR is unusual in patients' partners, environmental factors are unlikely to be implicated.

Clinical features

The principal **symptoms** are stiffness and aching, principally in the shoulder and pelvic girdles (neck, shoulders, upper arm, buttocks and thighs). There is prolonged (>1 h) and severe early morning stiffness, malaise, depression and weight loss. **Onset** may be sudden and dramatic (overnight), but in most cases occurs gradually over about 2 weeks. In the latter case it may all too easily be dismissed as part of 'ageing'.

Pharmacotherapy

Symptoms respond rapidly to moderate doses of *prednisolone*, e.g. 15–25 mg daily. If there is any evidence of vasculitis, the higher doses used for GCA should be used because of the risk of sudden blindness. The dose is gradually reduced to the minimum required to control symptoms and normalize the ESR. It is possible to withdraw steroids completely in about 75% of patients within 2–3 years. In the remainder, disease duration may be 7–10 years and the risks of prolonged corticosteroid treatment have to be weighed against those associated with the disease, notably blindness.

The same considerations apply to patient self management as in GCA.

Medium- and small-vessel vasculitis

Polyarteritis nodosa (PAN)

This intense inflammation of the small and medium arteries commonly occurs at the junctions of vessels. The widespread distribution of the lesions leads to correspondingly extensive and severe symptoms.

PAN is a rare disease that affects men more than women (male : female ratio, 3 : 1). In about 20% of patients PAN is associated with hepatitis B infection. A small number of cases appear to be associated with hypersensitivity reactions to penicillins and sulphonamides. However, the aetiology is generally unknown.

There is infiltration of all of the layers of the affected arteries, leading to degeneration of the arterial walls, and to obstruction and ischaemia. Inflammation and thrombosis may lead to tissue infarction in almost any organ.

The **clinical features** are the result of widespread organ damage (skin, cardiovascular, renal, pulmonary, nervous) associated with non-specific symptoms, e.g. fever, weight loss and malaise. Such extensive symptoms clearly indicate a severe and alarming disease. Joint involvement is common, but is rarely serious. The disease runs a very variable course from a mild cutaneous vasculitis to severe, life-threatening involvement of major organs.

Management is with high-dose *corticosteroids*, immunomodulators (*azathioprine, cyclophosphamide*) and appropriate symptomatic support.

Wegener's granulomatosis

This rare disease mostly affects adults over 40 years of age, causing widespread small vessel arteritis. Pulmonary, renal and sometimes eye lesions occur. The initial **symptoms** may be severe rhinorrhoea, cough and pleuritic pain, so patients usually present to chest clinics. Some 85% of patients have nephritis (*see* Chapter 4) which is rapidly progressive without prompt diagnosis and treatment. The aetiology is unknown, but it has been suggested that drugs may be involved, though no consistent associations have been demonstrated.

Pharmacotherapy
The condition, once uniformly fatal, responds well to *high-dose prednisolone plus cyclophosphamide*.

Other multisystem diseases

Amyloidosis

This is the deposition of abnormal fibrous protein in various tissues throughout the body. The proteins include immunoglobulin fragments and precursors of normal serum proteins and are resistant to proteolysis *in vitro*. The deposits may be localized or widely distributed. Several different forms are distinguished.

Because many organs may be involved, patients may present with any of a diverse range of symptoms, e.g. heart failure, nephrotic syndrome, purpura, peripheral neuropathy and weight loss. **Dialysis arthropathy**, **Alzheimer's disease** (senile dementia) and **Creutzfeldt–Jakob disease** are all associated with amyloid deposits.

Amyloidosis may be hereditary or an acquired complication of RA, JCA and any of the systemic connective tissue diseases. It usually presents with renal syndromes (proteinuria) or heart failure.

Once regarded as relentlessly progressive, many patients can now be managed effectively, e.g. with *cytotoxic chemotherapy* (*see* Chapter 11), *colchicine* (for familial Mediterranean fever, triggered by rickettsial infection) or transplantation of almost any organ, as is practicable. Patients who respond to treatment show gradual regression of amyloid deposits. Transplant patients do little worse than others without amyloid, but surgery may be complicated by haemorrhagic problems and poor wound healing.

Sarcoidosis

Epidemiology and clinical features

This is a relatively common (UK prevalence about 20 per 100 000) granulomatous disorder mostly affecting young adults (aged 20–40 years), with widespread organ involvement. It usually presents with respiratory symptoms (bilateral hilar lymphadenopathy, often detected on routine X-ray), eye lesions (25% of cases), or skin lesions (10%; *see* erythema nodosum, Chapter 12, p. 716). Afro-Caribbeans usually have a more severe form of sarcoidosis, but it is less common in Asians.

The presenting symptoms may be small joint, tendon and associated soft tissue swelling, occurring in about 5% of patients. The picture may strongly resemble RA, but this frank arthritis is usually associated with lung problems or erythema nodosum. Cardiac symptoms may also occur in isolation.

The underlying abnormality appears to be the sequestration of T lymphocytes in the lungs, causing depression of both T cell function and cell-mediated immunity (*see* Chapter 2).

Löfgren's syndrome is characterized by the abrupt onset of malaise, fever, large joint arthritis, erythema nodosum and lung symptoms.

Management and pharmacotherapy

About 65% of patients do well simply with *NSAIDs*. Those with Löfgren's syndrome usually respond similarly, though symptoms may take up to 3 months to resolve, and lung lesions up to 18 months.

Corticosteroids are the mainstay of treatment for lung, cardiac, CNS, liver and spleen involvement and for hypercalcaemia. Severe disease may necessitate the use of **second-line drugs**, e.g. *methotrexate* or *hydroxychloroquine*, as in RA. *Ciclosporin* (*cyclosporine*) has been used experimentally but its value has been disputed. It is usually reserved for non-responders to conventional treatment.

Eye problems (**uveitis**) are usually treated with topical corticosteroids, e.g. *dexamethasone* or *clobetasone* (lower risk of glaucoma), but also require **mydriatics**, e.g. *cyclopentolate*. They may be severe enough to require *systemic corticosteroids*.

Combined heart–lung and kidney **transplantation** has been used in end-stage non-responders, but the disease is likely to affect the transplanted organs subsequently.

Other rheumatic diseases

Reactive arthritis

This is an ill-defined entity, but it is usually used to describe arthritis which follows an identifiable infection, often rheumatic fever or enteric infections, e.g. *Campylobacter* infection, dysentery, antibiotic-associated colitis. Reiter's syndrome (p. 505) may also be classified in this group.

Rheumatic fever

Aetiology and clinical features

Rheumatic fever is an inflammatory arthropathy consequent on infection with group A beta-haemolytic streptococci, especially certain sub-types. There appears to be some antigenic cross-reactivity between streptococcal antigens and cardiac tissue, resulting in **carditis** in some 50% of cases, followed by progressive damage to the mitral and aortic valves. One graphic description is that it 'licks the joints but grips the heart'.

Attacks may last for a few weeks or months, and are characterized by a mild to severe sore throat, followed after 1–5 weeks by fever (38–40°C) and a painful, migratory, large-joint arthritis. Abdominal pain, **epistaxis** (nosebleeds) and **chorea** (writhing, e.g. Sydenham's chorea, St. Vitus' dance) may occur.

The joint disease is usually fully reversible, but the permanent mitral and aortic valve damage may produce cardiac symptoms several decades later.

Because the infection is associated with poor living conditions, it is uncommon nowadays in developed countries (0.01% of children, 5–15 years of age). In Third World countries it is common and affects about 2% of children with streptococcal infections.

Management

Acute attacks
Treatment involves the following:

- **Anti-inflammatories:**
  - *High-dose aspirin* (60–100 mg/kg/day), to give a blood level of 25 mg/dL, once the diagnosis is clear and there is no risk of Reye's syndrome (not in children under 12 years of age).

 – In severe cases with carditis, prednisolone 2 mg/kg/day, though its value is disputed.
* **Antibiotics**: *benzylpenicillin potassium* does not affect the course of an attack, but it is commonly used to eradicate the streptococci.
* Strict bedrest for 3 weeks is traditional, though of unproven value, and may be psychologically undesirable.

Treatment is continued for 4 weeks and, if the patient's condition is satisfactory, is gradually reduced over a further 2 weeks.

Prophylaxis

It is essential to prevent subsequent infections in order to protect the heart valves and endocardium from further damage, so antibiotics are normally continued for at least 5 years after the last attack or until age 25 years, whichever is the longer. Oral *phenoxymethylpenicillin* twice daily is normally used. *Sulfadiazine* is suitable if the patient is penicillin-sensitive.

Patients with consequent heart disease should have lifelong prophylactic antibiotic 'cover' for any dental procedures or surgery, however minor, in order to prevent endocarditis. Streptococcal infections should be treated promptly and aggressively. In high-risk patients, *ampicillin plus gentamicin* (*vancomycin plus gentamicin* if penicillin sensitive) have been used.

Soft tissue rheumatism

This section describes briefly the most common minor non-arthritic soft tissue lesions. They are relatively common and treatable. Topical therapy with creams and liniments is popular (p. 494, Topical NSAIDs). Physical treatments (physiotherapy, osteopathy, chiropractic) and acupuncture are widely used, and help to relieve pain and associated muscle spasm.

Carpal tunnel syndrome (CTS)

Definition

This entrapment neuropathy is the result of compression of the median nerve at the wrist, where it passes between the tendons and the transverse ligament (Fig. 8.11).

Aetiology and epidemiology

CTS may be idiopathic or occur in association with many diseases or conditions: e.g. rheumatoid arthritis, Raynaud's syndrome, fluid accumulation (e.g. pregnancy, premenstrual, postmenopausal), tenosynovitis (e.g. sports injury, overuse of the wrist, repetitive strain injury), local trauma, obesity, diabetes mellitus, hypothyroidism, amyloidosis, acromegaly.

The condition may occur at any age, mostly in women.

Clinical features

These include:

* **Paraesthesias** (tingling, sensory loss and numbness in the first three-and-a-half digits of the hand; Fig. 8.11(a)), although symptoms may be rather diffuse. The patient often wakes at night and hangs the arm over the bedside or wrings the hand to obtain relief.
* **Pain** in the hand, wrist or forearm.
* **Weakness** of the hand and wasting of the ball of the thumb.

Management

This comprises:

* Management of any underlying disease or predisposing condition.
* Local injection of corticosteroids.
* Splinting.
* Nerve decompression by surgical division of the transverse ligament of the wrist. However, a precise diagnosis is an essential prerequisite; this procedure may give no benefit if the root of the problem lies elsewhere, e.g. nerve compression at the neck or shoulder.

Tendinitis and tenosynovitis

Tendinitis

Tendon inflammation is rarely diagnosed precisely in general practice, and many syndromes

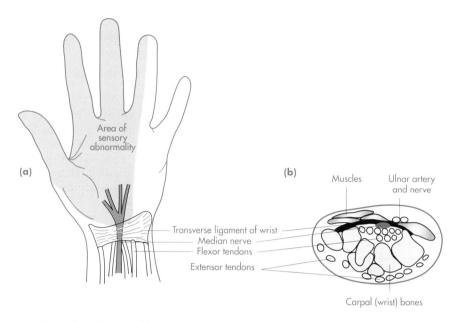

Figure 8.11 Carpal tunnel syndrome and the associated anatomy of the hand and wrist. (a) Left palm showing the usual area of sensory abnormality in carpal tunnel syndrome, i.e. the area served by the median nerve. (b) Section through the wrist showing the median nerve lying immediately under the transverse ligament, in the 'carpal tunnel' formed by the ligament and the carpal (wrist) bones.

are **enthesopathies**. The aetiology is uncertain but may be associated with an inflammatory arthropathy or minor repetitive trauma. The most common lesions include:

- **Supraspinous tendinitis**, characterized by pain on straight arm raising.
- **Frozen shoulder**, a more serious condition, occurring at any age in adult life, but mostly in older patients; it may cause restriction of shoulder movement and severe pain, especially at night.
- **Tennis elbow**, with pain occurring over the lateral (outer) aspect of one elbow joint.
- **Golfer's elbow** causes pain on the medial (inner) side of an elbow.
- **Achilles tendinitis**.
- **Plantar fasciitis** gives pain in the sole of the foot.

Tenosynovitis

Inflammation and swelling of the tendon sheaths is commonly caused by trauma and overuse injury, but it is also a frequent accompaniment to RA and other inflammatory

arthropathies. Type II hyperlipoproteinaemia (*see* Chapter 3, p. 120) is a predisposing factor.

The use of *fluoroquinolone antibiotics*, e.g. *ciprofloxacin, cinoxacin, norfloxacin* and *ofloxacin*, has been associated with **tendon rupture**, especially in the Achilles tendon, but also in the shoulder and hand.

Management

Rest and the application of heat or cold, as the patient finds most effective, and NSAIDs are used. Local injection of corticosteroids is used in resistant cases, but it is important not to inject the tendon itself because tendon rupture may ensue. Physical therapies are used progressively as the condition improves, and are helpful in preventing adhesions. Surgery to divide tendon sheaths or remove calcified deposits may be needed in persistent cases, and may be curative.

Bursitis

This is inflammation of a bursa, the most common sites being the large toe (bunion), shoulder, lower pelvis ('tailor's bottom'), knee ('house-maid's knee'), and elbow ('miner's or 'student's elbow').

The **aetiology** is often unknown but may be the result of trauma, inflammatory arthritides, gout or infection.

There is pain and local tenderness, and swelling is a feature of the last two conditions mentioned above. Occasionally, chronic bursitis may follow repeated trauma, e.g. from shoes (bunions), unresolved infection or gout.

Management includes rest, with or without splinting, and high-dose *NSAIDs* **plus** local injection of *corticosteroids* in severe or persistent cases: NSAIDs alone are of limited value. Physical therapies are used progressively as the pain and inflammation subside.

Fibrositis and fibromyalgia

This is a group of non-specific conditions presenting with diffuse pain, tenderness and stiffness of muscles and their connective tissues, with local tender points. Pain is felt most frequently in the back, neck, shoulders, chest and buttocks.

There is no specific disease entity. It is assumed to be due to trauma, exposure to cold, viral infection or stress. **Management** is purely symptomatic with analgesics, and topical and physical treatments.

Low back pain

Definition

This is pain in the lower lumbar, lumbosacral and sacroiliac regions. It is sometimes accompanied by **sciatica**, which is neurological pain occurring in the distribution of the sciatic nerve, i.e. in the buttocks and the lateral (outer) aspect of the leg and the foot. It can be very severe and incapacitating.

Aetiology

The pain is mostly the result of degenerative joint disease (OA) and so is very common in the elderly (50% of the 60+ age group). However, buttock pain in younger patients may be due to ankylosing spondylitis (p. 503).

A common cause is a **prolapsed intervertebral disc** (PID, 'slipped disc'), when the capsule of an intervertebral disc ruptures or herniates under strain (lifting, bending stress, sports trauma, sneezing) and the **nucleus pulposus** (pulpy centre) is extruded into the spinal canal to press on the nerve root. A strong longitudinal vertebral ligament usually prevents the extruded pulp pressing directly on the spinal cord, so pressure is normally directed to one side to give unilateral symptoms (*see* Fig. 8.3(b)). There is associated muscle spasm, which exacerbates the condition. PID is uncommon in the elderly.

One iatrogenic cause is prolonged systemic corticosteroid therapy, leading to osteoporosis and collapse of one or more vertebrae (**crush fractures**), often causing bilateral nerve root compression and severe pain.

Pregnancy or obesity may also cause strain and low back pain.

Diagnosis

Frequently, no abnormality can be demonstrated with X-rays, so it may be difficult to make a precise diagnosis, unless there is a fracture, dislocation or PID. CT scanning and MRI may be useful, and justified if symptoms are severe.

More invasive investigations are rarely justified. However, a **myelogram** (X-ray following injection of a radio-opaque dye to visualize the spinal cord) may be done in difficult cases to determine the extent of spinal cord damage, though MRI will usually show this. This is important if there is evidence of neurological deficit (leg paraesthesias, loss of control of bladder or bowels), or to direct surgery.

Management

Acute back pain
Management is conservative because most patients recover completely in 6–8 weeks of partial rest with warmth, plus analgesic support. However, excessive rest is undesirable, causing muscle wasting and delaying recovery. If pain is

severe, recovery is prolonged or there are neurological signs, active treatment is indicated, including:

- Local injections of *pethidine (meperidine)*, *local anaesthetics* or a long-acting *corticosteroid*, if there is severe pain. Oral pethidine is ineffective (*see* Chapter 10).
- Muscle relaxants, e.g. *diazepam* or *meprobamate*, to relieve muscle spasm.
- Manipulation, provided that it is certain that there is no PID or fracture, otherwise serious neurological damage may be caused.
- Traction and surgery may occasionally be indicated for persistent motor weakness, as a matter of urgency if there is loss of control of bladder or bowel function.
- *NSAIDs* are often used in the community but are seldom indicated.

Chronic back pain

No generally satisfactory treatment is available. Orthodox management includes:

- Weight reduction.
- Treatment of any underlying disease.
- Analgesics.
- Counselling on the avoidance of back strain and poor posture, including advice on working conditions and suitable seating.
- Carefully graded exercises and physiotherapy to strengthen the back muscles and so improve joint stability.
- Spinal supports (corsets, belts) in an acute exacerbation, but prolonged use is undesirable because muscle tone, and therefore support, is lost.
- Occasionally, surgical removal of the disc (**discectomy**, usually percutaneously) or a vertebral arch (**laminectomy**). Enzyme injections are sometimes used to dissolve the disc pulp (**chemonucleolysis**, e.g. with *chymopapain* from the papaya plant), but are less satisfactory because of allergic reactions.
- Spinal fusion is undertaken rarely.

Other physical modalities (osteopathy, chiropractic) are of undoubted benefit to many sufferers, who tend to seek a variety of 'alternative' medical treatments, sometimes in desperation at the unsatisfactory outcomes of orthodox medical treatment.

References and further reading

Abdel-Nasser AM, Rasker JJ, Valkenburg HA (1997) Epidemiological and clinical aspects relating to the variability of rheumatoid arthritis. *Semin Arthritis Rheum* **27**: 123–140.

Anonymous (1998) Modifying disease in rheumatoid arthritis. *Drug Ther Bull* **36**: 3–6.

Arthritis and Rheumatism Council (UK): Patient leaflets and booklets, Practical Problems series, Student Handbook, Topical Reviews Series.

Clarke AK, Hart FD (1993) *Clinical Problems in Rheumatology*. London: Martin Dunitz.

Creamer P, Hochberg MC (1997) Osteoarthritis. *Lancet* **350**: 503–509.

Dingle JT (1996) The effect of NSAIDs on human articular cartilage glycosaminoglycan synthesis. *Eur J Rheum Inflamm* **16**: 47–52.

Hunder GG (1997) *Current Review of Rheumatology*. 9th edn. Rapid Science Publishers.

Klippel JH, Dieppe PA (1995) *Practical Rheumatology*. London: Mosby International.

National Prescribing Centre (1996) Second line drugs in rheumatoid arthritis. *MeReC Bull* **7**: 9–12.

National Prescribing Centre (1997) Topical non-steroidal anti-inflammatory drugs: an update. *MeReC Bull* **8**: 29–32.

Pincus T (1995) Long term outcomes in rheumatoid arthritis. *Br J Rheumatol* **34** (Suppl. 2): 59–73.

Rains CP, Noble S, Faulds D (1995) Sulfasalazine: A review of its pharmacological properties and therapeutic efficacy in the treatment of rheumatoid arthritis. *Drugs* **50**: 137–156.

Smith WL (1992) Prostanoid biosynthesis and mechanism of action. *Am J Physiol* **268**: F181–F191.

Snaith ML, ed. (1995) *ABC of Rheumatology*. London: BMJ Publishing Group.

Van Ryn J, Pairet M (1997) Selective cyclooxygenase-2 inhibitors: pharmacology, clinical effects and therapeutic potential. *Expert Opin Invest Drugs* **6**: 609–614.

9

Diabetes mellitus

Diabetes mellitus is one of the most serious and probably the most common of multisystem diseases. In this text the term 'diabetes' refers exclusively to diabetes mellitus, which is primarily a disorder of carbohydrate metabolism. The metabolic problems in treated diabetics are not usually troublesome and are relatively easy to control. It is the long-term complications of diabetes which are the main causes of morbidity and mortality. Diabetics suffer far more from cardiovascular and renal disease than other people, and diabetes is the principal cause of acquired blindness in the West. Most diabetics do not die from metabolic crises such as ketoacidosis but from stroke, myocardial infarction or chronic renal failure.

The hallmark of diabetes is hyperglycaemia, owing to abnormalities in insulin secretion or action. Consequently glucose can be neither adequately assimilated into cells nor utilized within them; energy must be derived from the breakdown of fats and possibly protein. There are two primary causes of diabetes and a variety of minor secondary ones. In **Type 1** diabetes (insulin-dependent diabetes mellitus, IDDM) there is usually gross destruction of the pancreatic beta-cells. In **Type 2** diabetes (non-insulin-dependent, NIDDM), insulin is secreted but is either insufficient or insufficiently effective to meet metabolic needs.

Epidemiology and classification

Definition

The current World Health Organization (WHO) definition of diabetes is based on standardized measurements of blood glucose concentrations. It defines two classes, diabetes and **impaired glucose tolerance** (Table 9.1). Patients in the latter category, which encompasses conditions that used to be termed 'latent diabetes', 'pre-diabetes', etc., must be carefully followed up because up to 5% per year develop frank diabetes. Often, a single random blood glucose reading of 10 mmol/L (plasma glucose 11.1 mmol/L) is sufficient for diagnosis in a patient with classic symptoms, although this should be confirmed with a fasting blood glucose greater than 6.7 mmol/L. (Note that laboratories may report *plasma* glucose levels, as specified by the American Diabetic Association diagnostic criteria, whereas finger prick test sticks measure *blood* levels.) In borderline cases the oral glucose tolerance test (OGTT) may be performed: the patient's blood glucose is measured before and at 2 h after a standardized 75 g glucose load, given orally following an overnight fast; however, this is becoming obsolete.

Epidemiology

Diabetes is known to affect greater than 2% of the UK population, and probably as many again would probably be discovered to have impaired glucose tolerance or even frank diabetes if screened. The incidence varies considerably between populations. For example, Europeans are prone to IDDM, especially in northern Europe, whereas the incidence in Japan is less than 10% of that in Finland.

NIDDM seems to be related partly to the affluence of a population, possibly through the prevalence of obesity and/or inactivity, which are major risk factors. However, genetic factors are also important. In some ethnic groups the prevalence is very high, e.g. in some Pacific islanders and the North American Pima Indians it reaches 50%. Among Indian immigrants to the UK it is five times that in the host population, suggesting a possible genetic susceptibility to changed environmental factors

Natural history

Onset

About 80% of patients have Type 2 diabetes, which tends to occur late in life, hence the obsolete description 'maturity onset'. Its onset is usually insidious and gradual, patients tolerating mild polyuric symptoms perhaps for many years. Diagnosis is often a chance finding, e.g. following urinalysis during routine medical screening or investigation of a complaint which turns out to be the consequence of one of the complications, such as recurrent boils, a non-healing foot lesion or a persistent urinary tract infection.

The other 20% who require insulin at the outset are almost invariably dependent from an early age: the peak onset of Type 1 diabetes is around puberty, starting most commonly in the winter months. Although the disease may be present sub-clinically for some considerable time (months, or possibly years; *see* p. 533) clinical onset is invariably abrupt. This is usually associated with some metabolic stress (e.g. infection) and presents with florid urinary symptoms, fluid imbalance, weight loss and possibly acute metabolic decompensation (ketoacidosis). There may follow some months of apparent remission with a reduced or absent insulin requirement, the so-called 'honeymoon period', but these patients then rapidly deteriorate. Before the isolation and therapeutic use of insulin in the 1920s they inevitably died shortly thereafter.

Progression

Insulin secretion in Type 2 diabetes declines relatively slowly, but up to one-third of patients

Table 9.1   WHO definitions of diabetes mellitus

Class	Blood glucose (mmol/L)		
	Fasting		OGTT at 2 h
Diabetes mellitus	>6.7	and/or	>10
Impaired glucose tolerance	<6.7	and	6.7–10
Normal	<6.7	and	<6.7

Usually venous whole blood is used. These figures would be approx. 10% higher (7.8 and 11.1 mmol/L) if either capillary blood or venous plasma is used.

The apparently non-uniform thresholds derive from conversion from old mg/100 ml units, as still used in North America.

A new fasting blood level of 6 mmol/L has recently been proposed but not yet agreed; this would introduce a new category of *impaired fasting glucose* between 5.5–6 mmol/L.

OGTT, oral glucose tolerance test.

may eventually need exogenous insulin ('insulin-requiring' as opposed to insulin-dependent diabetics). For most Type 1 diabetics, pancreatic beta-cell destruction is already almost complete at diagnosis, and routine insulin requirements do not generally increase. However, in both types the multisystem complications progress throughout life at rates which vary considerably between patients and will very likely be the eventual cause of death. Diabetics have a reduced life expectancy, although the prognosis has greatly improved with advances in treatment. Younger patients have mortality rates of up to five times that of the general population, while for older ones it is about twice normal. The precise prognosis for any given patient will depend on many factors, but particularly the overall consistency of control of blood glucose.

Classification

Primary diabetes

In the vast majority of cases there is direct damage to the pancreatic islet cells. Different attempts to classify diabetes comprehensively have been confounded by using criteria which are not mutually exclusive (e.g. age at onset, need for insulin). For example, some 'maturity onset' patients eventually require insulin, some older patients need it from the start (latent autoimmune diabetes in the adult, LADA) and a few younger patients may not ('maturity onset diabetes of the young'). The most practical distinction is whether the patient needs insulin.

However, a classification based on the pathogenesis of the pancreatic damage is now accepted to be the most meaningful (*see also* pp. 533–534). This distinguishes the two broad types referred to above and does correspond roughly with insulin dependency (Table 9.2).

Secondary diabetes

A minority of cases with identifiable primary causes (e.g. severe pancreatitis, steroid-induced diabetes) do not fit readily into either of the conventional categories. They may or may not be insulin-dependent (p. 534).

Physiological principles of glucose and insulin metabolism

Insulin action

Insulin is the major **anabolic** hormone. It expands energy stores during times of adequate nutrition against times of food shortage. Opposing this action are several **catabolic** 'counter-regulatory' or 'stress' hormones which mobilize glucose for use when increased energy expenditure is necessary. The most important of these are *adrenaline* (*epinephrine*), *corticosteroids*, *glucagon* and *growth hormone*. These two opposing systems work in harmony to maintain glucose homeostasis. Insulin also enhances amino acid utilization and protein synthesis, the latter action being shared with growth hormone.

Table 9.2   Comparison of the main types of idiopathic diabetes mellitus

	Type 1	Type 2
Therapeutic class	Insulin-dependent (IDDM)	Non-insulin-dependent (NIDDM)
Endogenous insulin	Absent	Present
Insulin deficiency	Absolute	Relative or partial Insulin receptor defect?
Insulin resistance	Usually absent	May be present
Pancreatic islet damage	Severe (destruction)	Slight/moderate
Immunology	Auto-immune; islet cell antibodies	No antibodies demonstrated
Usual age of onset	<30 years	>40 years
Build of patient	Thin	Obese (usually)
Genetics	Weak family history; HLA-linked	Strong family history
Ketoacidosis prone?	Yes	No

Insulin action has three main components (Fig. 9.1):

- **Rapid**: in certain tissues only, insulin facilitates the active transport of glucose and amino acids across cell membranes enhancing uptake from the blood.
- **Intermediate**: within all cells, insulin promotes the action of enzymes which convert glucose, fatty acids and amino acids into more complex, more stable storage forms.
- **Long-term**: because of increased protein synthesis, growth is promoted.

One important consequence is the prompt clearance of glucose from the blood after meals.

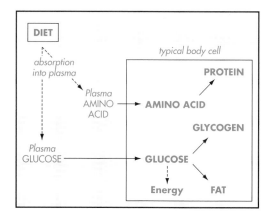

Figure 9.1 Simplified scheme showing the anabolic actions of insulin. Insulin aids the uptake of metabolites into body cells and enhances the action of enzymes which utilize them as precursors to synthesize more complex molecules. Note: not all actions occur in all body cells.

Some would otherwise be lost in the urine because of the kidney's limited capacity for re-absorbing glucose filtered at the glomerulus.

Glucose transport

Glucose uptake into cells across the cell membrane is dependent on the concentration gradient between the extracellular medium (e.g. blood plasma, gastrointestinal contents) and the cell interior. However, because glucose is such an important metabolite, there exist a number of membrane transport pumps or facilitators in different tissues (Table 9.3). Certain tissues, notably muscle and adipose, depend on an insulin-requiring active pump for glucose uptake, so insulin deficiency deprives them of glucose. Other cells, particularly in the liver and gastrointestinal tract, do not require insulin for glucose uptake, but diffusion is nevertheless facilitated. In the liver, enhanced phosphorylation of glucose drives intracellular concentrations down, encouraging uptake. Insulin lack does not deprive tissues such as these of glucose; on the contrary, the hyperglycaemia associated with diabetes can produce intracellular glucose overload, and this may be responsible for some diabetic complications (pp. 536–546). This is particularly relevant to tissues such as nerves, which are freely permeable to glucose.

Insulin also facilitates the uptake of amino acids into liver and muscle, and of potassium into most cells. This latter effect is exploited therapeutically for the rapid reduction of hyperkalaemia (*see* Chapter 4).

Metabolic effects

By facilitating certain enzymes and inhibiting others, insulin has wide-ranging effects on intermediary metabolism in most tissues (Table 9.4; Fig. 9.1). The synthesis of the energy stores (glycogen in liver and skeletal muscle, fat in liver and adipose tissue) is facilitated, and their breakdown is inhibited. Tissue growth and cell division are also promoted by enhanced nucleic acid synthesis (DNA, RNA) synthesis, amino acid assimilation and protein synthesis.

Overall effect

Only a general appreciation of how insulin and the catabolic hormones control everyday metabolic variations is given here (*see also* References and further reading).

Table 9.3   Insulin requirement for glucose transport in different tissues

Tissues not requiring insulin	Tissues requiring insulin
Liver	Adipose
Gastrointestinal endothelium	Muscle – skeletal, cardiac, smooth
Nerves, brain	
Kidney tubules	
Eye – retinal vessels, lens	
Leucocytes	
Blood vessel endothelium	

Table 9.4   Metabolic effects of insulin

Metabolite	Process	Tissue		
		Liver	Muscle	Adipose
Carbohydrate				
Increased	• glycogen synthesis (glycogenesis)	✓	✓	↔
	• glucose oxidation (glycolysis)	✓	✓	✓
Decreased	• glycogen breakdown (glycogenolysis)	✓	✓	↔
	• glucose synthesis (gluconeogenesis)	✓	↔	↔
Lipid				
Increased	• fat synthesis (lipogenesis)	✓	↔	✓
	• utilization of dietary fat	✓	↔	✓
Decreased	• fat breakdown (lipolysis)	↔	↔	✓
	• fatty acid oxidation (ketogenesis)	✓	✓	✓
Protein				
Increased	• protein synthesis	✓	✓	✓
Decreased	• protein breakdown (proteolysis)	✓	✓	↔
Nucleic acid				
Increased	• DNA and RNA synthesis	↔	✓	↔
	• cell growth	↔	✓	↔
	• cell division	↔	✓	↔

✓, insulin has important effect (increase or decrease) on process in that tissue; ↔, no effect.

Anabolic actions of insulin

Following a meal, glucose is absorbed from the gastrointestinal tract into the blood and rapidly transported into the cells, to be converted into forms suitable for storage and later use.

In the **liver** some glucose is converted into glycogen and stored but most is converted into lipid (free fatty acid, FFA, and triglyceride). Lipid is released into the blood as very low-density lipoprotein (VLDL), to be taken up and stored in adipose tissue; however, the release of glucose into the blood is inhibited. Hepatic regulation of glucose is an important mechanism for limiting the uptake of glucose into tissues where transport is independent of insulin.

In **adipose** tissue, fat breakdown is inhibited and glucose uptake promoted. The glucose provides glycerol for esterification with FFAs, and the resulting fat is stored. Adipose tissue also takes up the fat-containing chylomicrons obtained by digestion (*see* Chapter 6, p. 304 and p. 306). In **muscle**, glycogen is synthesized and fat metabolism is inhibited; this increases glucose availability for immediate energy needs. Amino acid uptake is promoted so that growth can be continued.

Catabolic actions of counter-regulatory hormones

During stresses such as 'fight or flight', infection or any major trauma, catabolic hormones reverse these processes. Blood glucose is rapidly raised to supply energy for the muscles and if this is insufficient fats can also be mobilized. Peripheral oxidation of FFAs produces large amounts of energy, but in the liver excess acetyl-CoA is produced. This is condensed to produce high-energy ketoacids such as acetoacetate, which many tissues can utilize in small amounts. In insulin insufficiency these 'ketone bodies' may accumulate in the plasma, causing **ketoacidosis**.

Insulin deficiency

The consequences of insulin deficiency, and thus many of the clinical features of diabetes, can be deduced from these considerations (Fig. 9.2). It will be explained below that obese Type 2 patients may not at first have an absolute defi-

ciency of insulin; rather, there is a degree of insulin resistance. This may be described as a relative lack because the result is the same; moreover, eventually their insulin levels do fall. There are important differences between the physiological effects of partial (or relative) and total insulin deficiency.

Partial deficiency (Type 2)

Even small amounts of insulin will prevent severe metabolic disruption, especially accelerated fat metabolism, i.e. ketosis. Thus, the main problems only arise after meals, as a result of impaired glucose transport and cellular uptake. Adipose and muscle tissue cannot take up glucose efficiently, causing it to remain in the blood, and glucose deficiency in muscle may cause weakness. As other tissues cannot compensate sufficiently to assimilate the whole postprandial glucose load, the blood glucose level rises causing **hyperglycaemia** (>11 mmol/L). When the concentration exceeds the renal threshold (*see* Chapter 4, p. 156) glucose is lost in the urine (**glycosuria**). Urinary glucose acts as an osmotic diuretic carrying with it large volumes of water (**polyuria**), resulting in excessive thirst and fluid intake (**polydipsia**). Because of reduced fat uptake by adipose tissue, plasma

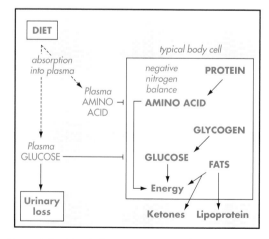

Figure 9.2 Metabolic consequences of insulin lack. Cellular uptake of glucose is prevented so that after exhausting their glycogen supplies, cells need to use fats and even protein for their energy needs. Compare with Fig. 9.1. Note: not all actions occur in all body cells.

lipid levels rise, especially those of triglycerides and lipoprotein. Although protein synthesis may be reduced, patients will generally still be obese, and if they do lose weight in the weeks before first diagnosis, this is partly due to dehydration.

Total deficiency (Type 1)

With no insulin at all there is severe hyperglycaemia at most times. This may raise the blood osmotic pressure sufficiently to cause neurological complications; diabetic coma is discussed on pp. 537–539. Cellular metabolism is profoundly disturbed. No glucose is available for energy metabolism, and the first result is a depletion of liver and muscle glycogen stores. Subsequently fat is mobilized, mainly from adipose tissue, so that plasma triglyceride, FFA and lipoprotein (an atherosclerosis risk factor) levels rise. This supplies energy needs for a little longer while the patient loses yet more weight. The brain switches to metabolizing the hepatically produced ketoacids. Fat stores are not replenished, and eventually may be exhausted. Finally, protein has to be broken down into amino acids which can be converted to glucose in the liver (**gluconeogenesis**), at the expense of lean muscle mass. Other than in uncontrolled diabetes, this process normally only occurs in times of prolonged starvation and is a desperate remedy that is akin to burning the house down to keep warm. Further, without insulin, glucose so produced cannot be utilized effectively anyway and this situation is inevitably fatal within months.

Thus many of the clinical problems in Type 2 diabetes are a direct consequence of hyperglycaemia, while in Type 1 diabetes there is also disrupted intracellular metabolism. In addition, chronic complications occur in both types, related to both hyperglycaemia and hyperlipidaemia.

Insulin physiology

Insulin (MW about 5800 Da) is composed of 51 amino acids in two chains of 21 (A chain) and 30 (B chain) amino acids that are connected by two disulphide bridges. It is synthesized in the pancreatic islet beta-cells. Other cells in the islets – which altogether comprise less than 3% of the pancreatic mass – are the alpha-cells (producing glucagon) and the delta-cells (producing somatostatin). Insulin is stored in granules in combination with **C-peptide** as proinsulin (MW 9000 Da), which is split before release into the portal vein. Insulin has a plasma half-life of only about 5 min. Approximately 50% of insulin is extracted by the liver – its main site of action – and after utilization it is subsequently degraded. Eventually, kidney peptidase also metabolizes some insulin. C-peptide is less rapidly cleared and is thus a useful index of beta-cell function. The main stimulus to insulin release is plasma glucose, which also stimulates insulin synthesis. Amino acids and possibly fats also promote release.

A wide variety of neuronal, hormonal and local influences have been identified, but their physiological or pathological significance is not established (Fig. 9.3). Adrenergic beta-receptors

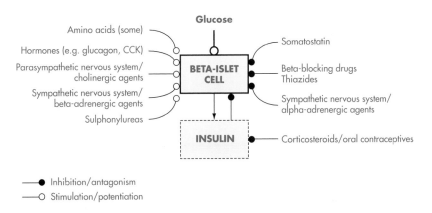

Figure 9.3 Factors affecting the release or action of insulin. CCK, cholecystokinin.

mediate release, so beta-blockers can theoretically inhibit this, though stimulation of inhibitory adrenergic alpha-receptors, magnified during the hyperglycaemic stress response, usually predominates.

Interestingly, glucose is a more powerful stimulant orally than parenterally, and various gut hormones have been implicated in this. Glucagon also promotes insulin release, possibly to facilitate cellular uptake of the glucose which it causes to be released into the plasma. In non-diabetics, the normal daily secretion of insulin is probably rather less than the average daily requirement in Type 1 diabetics of 50 units of exogenous insulin. Following a meal there is a biphasic secretory response. Within 1 min of blood glucose levels rising, preformed insulin is released from granules in beta-cells into the blood. This release is stimulated by oral hypoglycaemic agents and it is the first component to be compromised in early diabetes. Should hyperglycaemia persist, further insulin synthesis is stimulated and there is a delayed second phase of secretion after about 45 min.

Thus, normally the plasma insulin curve closely parallels the plasma glucose curve throughout the day, reflecting every small change in nutrient supply or demand (Fig. 9.4). It is important to note also that there is a continuous basal level of insulin secretion through-out the 24 hours, independent of food intake, which contributes to the regulation of metabolism and promotes glucose uptake into cells. Considering these subtle and sometimes rapid adaptations, it can be appreciated how far current therapeutic methods fall short of mimicking the physiological ideal.

Amylin

It has recently been found that the 37-amino acid peptide amylin is co-secreted with insulin from beta-cells. This appears to contribute to glucose regulation by a local (paracrine) action on islet cells, by moderating intestinal glucose uptake (thereby reducing the load presented to the pancreas) or by suppressing glucagon secretion. In diabetes, amylin deficiency parallels that of insulin and it is believed that patients whose postprandial hyperglycaemia is not adequately controlled by conventional therapy may benefit from amylin agonists.

Insulin receptors

These are present on the cell surfaces of all insulin-sensitive tissues and are normally down-regulated by insulin, especially if it is present at continuously high levels, e.g. the hyperinsulinaemia of over-eating, obesity or obesity-related Type 2 diabetes. This may account for the

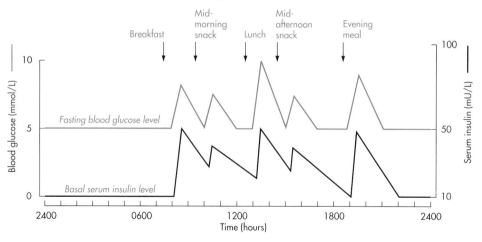

Figure 9.4 Schematic representation of normal diurnal variations in blood glucose and insulin levels. As the blood glucose level rapidly rises after a meal, it is closely followed by an increase in insulin level to prevent too great a rise. The insulin returns towards the basal level as blood glucose reaches the normal fasting level once more. Note how the two substances follow almost parallel curves. The small but positive basal insulin level serves to emphasise that insulin has functions other than just dealing with dietary glucose.

reduced insulin sensitivity (insulin resistance) found in some patients and the beneficial effect of weight reduction on glucose tolerance: there is a vicious cycle whereby hyperglycaemia and reduced insulin action reinforce one another. Long-term insulin treatment also often gradually reduces the insulin requirement, perhaps for related reasons. However, there is still much to be learned about the interactions between insulin, insulin receptors and carbohydrate metabolism.

Aetiology and pathogenesis

Primary diabetes

Despite having similar clinical pictures and complications, Types 1 and 2 primary diabetes have very different causes (Table 9.5).

Type 1 diabetes

In Type 1 diabetes the islet beta-cells are almost completely destroyed by an autoimmune process. Antibodies against all islet cells, and beta-cells specifically, are found in 80% of patients and the islets are invaded by inflammatory cells (insulitis). Insulin autoantibodies may also be found. As is usual with autoimmune disease, there is rarely a strong family history: siblings or children of Type 1 diabetics have about a 5% chance of developing the disease. However, there is a correlation with the patient's HLA tissue type and in a minority of patients an associ-

ation with other autoimmune diseases, especially of endocrine tissues, e.g. thyroiditis, pernicious anaemia.

Overt diabetes may follow many years of subclinical pancreatic damage, and when it occurs there is usually less than 10% of functional islet cell mass remaining. Clinical onset is usually abrupt (over a few weeks) and often associated with, or precipitated by, a metabolic stress such as viral infection which acutely increases insulin demand beyond capacity. This might account for the winter seasonal peak in incidence and also the brief temporary remission which follows (when the infection is reversed and the marginal insulin levels once again just compensate) before full-blown disease irreversibly takes hold. As with other autoimmune diseases, viral infection may be causing the expression of a normally suppressed HLA receptor, which subsequently activates lymphocytes (*see* Chapter 2). Other environmental triggers such as toxins or certain foods (including milk protein) may also be involved.

Autoantibodies are often found in patients up to 15 years before the onset of acute disease. This could eventually provide a means of early identification of prediabetics, so that they may be treated prophylactically, possibly by immunotherapy. However, such markers are also often found in close relatives who never develop the disease, and the chance of the identical twin of a diabetic patient subsequently developing diabetes is less than 50%.

Thus it seems that in Type 1 diabetes there is a genetically determined, HLA-dependent susceptibility which requires an environmental trigger

Table 9.5 Aetiology and pathology of primary diabetes

	Type 1	Type 2
Risk factors	HLA antigens (DR3, DR4)	Family history Over-eating Toxin? (Amyloid?)
Trigger factors	Viral infection Metabolic stress/excessive demand Environmental toxin?	Obesity Metabolic stress/excessive demand
Pathogenesis	Autoimmmune destruction of islet cells	Islet cell depletion? Peripheral insulin receptor defect?

for full expression. Following contact with this trigger, which may never be encountered, swift deterioration and complete insulin dependence are inevitable. There is still considerable ignorance of the relative contributions of genes and environment and of specific environmental factors.

Type 2 diabetes

Type 2 diabetes patients have one or more of the following fundamental abnormalities, and in established disease all three commonly coexist:

- Absolute insulin deficiency, i.e. reduced insulin secretion.
- Relative insulin deficiency: not enough insulin is secreted for metabolic increased needs (e.g. in obesity).
- Insulin resistance and hyperinsulinaemia: a peripheral insulin utilization defect.

There are at least two main sub-groups (Table 9.6). Non-obese patients may have a primary pancreatic defect with low insulin levels and a reduced insulin secretory response to hyperglycaemia. Post-mortem examination may reveal up to 50% destruction of islet cells; the nature and cause of the damage are still being elucidated. One form of this type of diabetes occurs in younger patients (maturity onset diabetes of the young, MODY).

In most cases (75%), Type 2 diabetes is associated with obesity on first presentation, and in a quarter of all diabetics simple weight reduction reverses the hyperglycaemia. This form is commonly associated with peripheral insulin resistance owing to receptor-binding or post-receptor defects. Obesity and reduced exercise also contribute to insulin resistance and are modifiable risk factors for Type 2 diabetes. The resultant hyperglycaemia induces insulin hypersecretion, hyperinsulinaemia and insulin receptor down-regulation, i.e. further insulin resistance. Hyperglycaemia itself is known to damage beta-cells. The vicious cycle eventually depletes ('exhausts') the beta-cells; insulin levels fall and some patients come to require insulin therapy. Thus, Type 2 diabetes is usually a progressive disease, although the late onset usually means that many patients die before requiring insulin.

There is still much debate as to the primary defect of Type 2 diabetes. Certainly insulin resistance usually precedes impaired glucose tolerance, but this may not be causal. Recently, the possibility has been investigated that inadequate fetal nourishment and low birth weight may impair pancreatic development and lead to the development of diabetes in later life.

It has also been proposed that the **amyloid** deposits (insoluble protein) long known to be found in the pancreas of Type 2 patients are related to abnormalities in amylin secretion (p. 532) and contribute to the pancreatic defect. Thus therapeutic manipulation of amylin in order to reduce disease progression is being investigated.

Genetics

The genetic component in Type 2 diabetes is much greater than in Type 1. A family history is common, often involving several relatives. Identical twins almost always both develop the disease, and offspring with both parents diabetic have a 50% chance of developing the disease. The 'thrifty gene' hypothesis proposes that the ability to store fat efficiently – and hence develop obesity – conferred a survival advantage in more primitive societies where famine was a regular phenomenon, hence its persistence in the genome. This may explain why some pre-industrial groups (e.g. Pacific islanders) readily develop diabetes when exposed to the industrialized lifestyle.

Secondary diabetes

Most diabetes results from primary defects of the pancreatic islet cells. Occasionally however, there are other causes of ineffective insulin action, impaired glucose tolerance and hyperglycaemia (Table 9.7).

Table 9.6 Sub-groups of Type 2 diabetes

Patient weight	Insulin level	Pathology
Non-obese	Low	Degenerative pancreatic damage
Obese	High	Peripheral insulin receptor defect

Table 9.7   Some causes of secondary diabetes

General mechanism	Aetiology	Example
Hepatic glucose metabolism defect	Liver failure	Viral hepatitis, drugs
Pancreatic destruction	Cirrhosis Pancreatitis	Alcoholism
Anti-insulin hormones	Corticosteroids	Cushing's disease Steroid therapy Pregnancy ('gestational diabetes') Major trauma/stress
	Growth hormone	Acromegaly
	Adrenaline (epinephrine), etc.	Phaeochromocytoma Major trauma/stress Adrenergic drugs
	Glucagon	Glucagonoma
	Thyroid hormones	Hyperthyroidism
Hyperglycaemic/anti-insulin drugs		Thiazide diuretics, diazoxide Oral contraceptives
Insulin antibodies	Autoimmune disease	
Abnormal insulin receptors	Congenital lipodystrophy	

Clinical features

Presentation

Diabetes is usually first diagnosed following one of four common presentations. For Type 2 diabetes these are:

- A chance finding of glycosuria at a routine medical examination.
- An incidental finding of glycosuria when the patient complains of symptoms subsequently found to be secondary to diabetes.
- The patient complains of increasing polyuria and/or polydipsia.

Type 1 patients often have an acute severe onset associated with metabolic decompensation:

- Severe acute hyperglycaemia, hyperosmolar coma and possibly ketoacidosis.

Type 2 patients may be asymptomatic or may have been only mildly symptomatic for several years, and their diabetes is only detected when they undergo a medical examination for insur-

ance purposes or a new job. More commonly, they present with hyperglycaemia-related symptoms such as tiredness, weight loss, visual problems or persistent urinary tract infection. Alternatively, as the complications proceed insidiously even during this early period, the primary reason for consultation may be vascular disease, retinopathy, neuropathy or impotence. One common manifestation is the 'diabetic foot', where the patient has a possibly gangrenous foot lesion, probably following a recent injury and subsequently infection. Sometimes the Type 2 patient does actually complain of the classical polyuria and thirst symptoms of diabetes. These are usually associated with tiredness, visual problems and recent weight loss, even though the patient may still be relatively obese. Often a strong family history is then discovered.

Only very rarely will a Type 2 patient first present with metabolically decompensated disease (ketoacidosis). These patients will have had impaired glucose tolerance for some time and then have undergone some major stress such as myocardial infarction or serious infection. Such stresses may also uncover latent disease in a less dramatic manner.

Unfortunately, acute presentation is more common at the onset of Type 1 disease. After a variable period of ostensibly normal life these patients deteriorate very rapidly, with the classic symptoms of rapid weight loss, weakness, extreme thirst, severe polyuria, urinary frequency and multiple nocturia. If this is not attended to, or if it develops very rapidly, the patient will become ketoacidotic and even comatose, and may be practically moribund on hospital admission.

Symptoms

The symptoms of diabetes as summarized in Table 9.8 are best understood in relation to their pathogenesis.

Symptoms due to hyperglycaemia

The classic symptoms which give diabetes mellitus its name ('sweet fountain') are easily explained by the osmotic effect of the elevated blood glucose levels that occur when glucose is denied entry to cells. They are more pronounced when the blood glucose level rises rapidly, e.g. in decompensation or acute onset. The osmotic effect of chronic hyperglycaemia will to some extent be compensated by hyponatraemia and an increased intracellular osmolarity.

When the blood glucose level exceeds the renal threshold (about 10 mmol/L), glucose appears in the urine in large quantities. The traditional method of distinguishing diabetes mellitus from diabetes insipidus – almost the only two idiopathic causes of chronic polyuria – was simply to taste the urine: in the former case it is sweet, and in the latter literally insipid (tasteless). Glycosuria predisposes to urinary tract infection partly because of the favourable growth medium presented to perineal organisms and partly because diabetic patients are generally more susceptible to infection (see below). Diabetic urine dries to leave a white glucose deposit, a clue which sometimes leads to diagnosis: there may be underwear stains or white specks on the shoes of elderly males (from careless micturition). Severe hyperosmolarity may reduce the intraocular pressure, causing eyeball and lens deformity and so blurred vision. This is sometimes a prodromal sign (early warning) of hyperglycaemic crisis.

Impaired metabolism and complications

The metabolic consequences of insulin lack were discussed in detail on pp. 527–533. The pathophysiology of hyperglycaemia and ketoacidosis is considered below.

Complications

Most complications of diabetes are due to either acute metabolic disturbances or chronic tissue damage.

Table 9.8   Clinical features of diabetes

Direct consequences of high blood glucose levels
Polyuria, frequency, nocturia, polydipsia (osmotic diuresis)
Visual disturbance (osmotic changes to intra-ocular pressure)
Urethritis, pruritis vulvae, balanitis (urinogenital infection)

Metabolic consequences of impaired glucose utilization
Lethargy, weakness, weight loss (intracellular glucose deficit)
Ketoacidosis (increased fat metabolism)

Long-term complications of hyperglycaemia and hyperlipidaemia
Vascular disease, heart disease, renal disease, neuropathy, eye disease, infections, arthropathy (stiffness)

Table 9.9 Causes of acute disturbances in diabetic control

Hypoglycaemia	Hyperglycaemia/ketoacidosis
Excess (mis-measured?) dose	Missed dose
Potentiation of oral hypoglycaemic (interaction)	Hyperglycaemic drugs, e.g. thiazides, steroids
Missed meal	Excess dietary intake
Unexpected activity	Metabolic stress, e.g. infection, surgery, pregnancy
Alcohol	

Acute complications

The most common acute complications are disturbances in glycaemic control. Optimal management of diabetes aims for a delicate balance, namely to prevent excessive glucose levels but not to force glucose levels too low. A variety of circumstances can drive the glucose level outside these narrow limits, and if treatment is not adjusted accordingly the result is either excess or insufficient glucose in the blood (Table 9.9).

Hyperglycaemia/ketoacidosis

Causes, pathogenesis and symptoms
Hyperglycaemia in treated diabetics usually arises because normal medication is somehow omitted or becomes insufficient to meet an increased insulin requirement. Drugs which raise blood glucose levels can also interfere with control. When diabetic control is lost, blood glucose rises and the symptoms develop gradually over a number of hours. Above a blood glucose level of approximately 15–20 mmol/L, both hyperosmolar and metabolic problems develop (Fig. 9.5; Table 9.10).

Blood glucose levels can exceed 50 mmol/L and this high osmotic load, which is also in the extracellular fluid, cannot be matched within most cells because glucose is excluded. Thus, water is drawn from the intracellular compartment and this causes tissue dehydration. This particularly affects the brain where the resultant reduced intracranial pressure leads to CNS depression. The skin is also dehydrated, and loses its elasticity (reduced skin turgor).

The high load of glucose in the glomerular filtrate, all of which cannot be reabsorbed, pro-

Table 9.10 Clinical features of hyperglycaemia and ketoacidosis

Glycosuria, ketonuria
Polyuria, nocturia
Thirst, polydipsia
Hypotension
Rapid (bounding) pulse and respiration
Dry mouth, reduced skin turgor
Visual disturbance
Hyperkalaemia, acidosis, ketonaemia
Sweet smell of ketones on breath
Weakness, drowsiness, eventually coma

duces an osmotic diuresis. This results in a reduction in circulating fluid volume, leading to hypotension and reflex tachycardia. The high urine volumes also cause a loss of electrolytes, especially sodium and potassium. However, the plasma potassium level may be paradoxically high because the acidosis inhibits the Na/K pump throughout the body, preventing intracellular potassium uptake. Osmoreceptors and baroreceptors detect the electrolyte and fluid losses, causing thirst, but as CNS depression and confusion develop the patient cannot respond by drinking.

In the absence of glucose, many cells start to metabolize fat instead. Adipose tissue releases fatty acids, and the liver converts some of these to acid ketones that can be readily utilized as an alternative energy source by many tissues. The resulting metabolic acidosis, which is misinterpreted by the respiratory centre as carbon

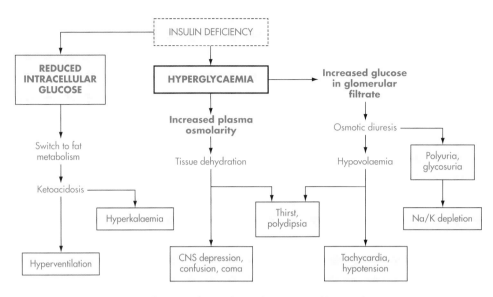

Figure 9.5   Pathogenesis and clinical features of acute hyperglycaemia and ketoacidosis.

dioxide retention, results in an increased respiratory drive and hyperventilation. Acidosis impairs oxygen dissociation from haemoglobin, exacerbating the gasping ('air hunger'), and also causes peripheral vasodilatation, exacerbating the hypotension. Both respiratory rate and blood oxygen level fall as coma supervenes.

Type 2 diabetics usually secrete sufficient insulin to prevent them developing ketoacidosis (except during severe stress), but they may still suffer hyperosmolar hyperglycaemic coma. Ketoacidosis is more likely to develop in Type 1 patients, although fortunately it is uncommon.

Management
Ketoacidosis is a medical emergency with about a 15% mortality rate. Close monitoring and very careful attention to the patient's fluid and electrolyte balance and blood biochemistry are essential (Table 9.11). Immediate attention is life-saving, but the patient may take several days to stabilize.

Intravenous *soluble insulin* is essential. An initial bolus of about 6 units is followed by continuous infusion (6 units/h). Fluid replacement needs are estimated from measurements of the central venous pressure and plasma sodium level. Hyponatraemia ('appropriate hyponatraemia', glucose having osmotically displaced sodium in the plasma) and/or sodium depletion require 0.9% saline administration. However, if the dehydration has caused hypernatraemia, especially in the non-ketotic patient, hypotonic saline (e.g. 0.45%) is indicated. Severe hypoten-

Table 9.11   Principles of the management of ketoacidosis

Problem	Treatment
Underlying cause	Discover and treat
Hyperglycaemia and hyperosmolarity	Insulin (soluble): small bolus plus continuous infusion
Dehydration	IV infusion: saline/dextran/plasma
Hyperkalaemia/potassium deficiency	Careful potassium repletion
Acidosis	Bicarbonate?
Hypoxaemia	Oxygen; up to 60% initially

sion or shock require plasma replacement (*see* Chapter 4, pp. 166–170). Potassium replacement is difficult to manage because the initial hyperkalaemia masks a total body potassium deficit. Once insulin is started, however, and potassium moves intracellularly, closely monitored intravenous potassium replacement is required. Acidosis will often resolve spontaneously with conservative therapy as ketone production falls and existing ketones are metabolized. Many clinicians would not use bicarbonate unless blood pH was below 7.00 for fear of overcompensating.

Hypoglycaemia

Causes

In all forms of diabetes, hypoglycaemia (blood glucose <3 mmol/L) is much more common than symptomatic hyperglycaemia, and it develops very rapidly, sometimes within minutes. Usually, either an excessive insulin dose is accidentally injected (many patients have eyesight problems) or else the normal dose of insulin or oral hypoglycaemic agent is not matched by an adequate dietary intake (Table 9.9). Insulin-induced hypoglycaemia is usually associated with injections of short-acting insulin. Deliberate overdosing is not unknown.

Hypoglycaemia induced by sulphonylurea oral hypoglycaemic drugs is rarer but more prolonged, more severe and more difficult to treat than insulin-induced hypoglycaemia. The elderly are especially prone, partly because the drugs are cleared more slowly and partly because of impaired homeostasis. Drug interactions which might potentiate oral antidiabetic drugs are considered on p. 557. Alcohol not only causes hypoglycaemia (by inhibiting hepatic gluconeogenesis) but also impairs the patients' perception of it, reducing their ability to respond.

Pathogenesis and symptoms

Hypoglycaemic symptoms fall into two main groups (Table 9.12). At glucose levels below about 4 mmol/L insulin release is inhibited and the counter-regulatory hormones such as glucagon and adrenaline are released in an effort to raise blood glucose. At a glucose level below 3.5 mmol/L the body responds by activating the

Table 9.12 Clinical features of hypoglycaemia

Adrenergic (autonomic) – enhanced sympathetic activity
- tremor, pallor
- sweating, shivering, palpitations
- anxiety

Neuroglycopenic – reduced CNS glucose delivery
- drowsiness, disorientation, confusion
- aggression, inappropriate behaviour
- apparent drunkenness
- convulsions, coma, brain damage; death

Other effects – multiple or indirect pathogenesis
- hunger, salivation, weakness, blurred vision

sympathetic nervous system and adrenal medulla (the 'fight or flight' response). The consequent **sympathetic/adrenal** symptoms (Table 9.12) provide the patient with a preliminary warning.

Below a glucose level of 3 mmol/L, neurological signs develop owing to the deficiency of glucose in the brain. These **neuroglycopenic** features may be noticed more by others than by patients themselves, although many patients do report an awareness of subjective prodroma. Sometimes the signs are subtle changes in mood or visual disturbances, but eventually there is almost always erratic behaviour resembling alcoholic inebriation. This has sometimes led to police arrest and delayed treatment, occasionally with fatal results. Frequent hypoglycaemic attacks may have a cumulative deleterious effect on higher brain function (cognition), especially in the elderly. All diabetics should carry, in addition to a readily available sugar source such as dextrose tablets, a card or bracelet stating that they are diabetics and should be given sugar if found acting strangely.

A patient's ability to recognize 'hypos' (**hypoglycaemic awareness**) should be checked regularly because it tends to diminish. Long-term diabetics become less sensitive to the warning signs and thus more vulnerable. This may result partly from autonomic neuropathy and partly from reduced counter-regulatory hormone response. It is also possible that frequent attacks may reduce the patient's ability to recognize them. There were reports when human insulin was first introduced that switching to it might also reduce hypoglycaemic awareness; this is no longer thought likely (p. 563).

Most of the adrenergic symptoms are mediated by beta-receptors, and so may be antagonized by concurrent beta-blocker therapy. Although this rarely presents a serious problem, such drugs should be avoided in diabetics; if they are essential, a cardioselective beta-blocker is preferred. Theoretically, beta-blockers might help by preventing beta-mediated insulin release (Fig. 9.3), but this is swamped by the symptom-masking effect.

Management

Although both hypoglycaemia and hyperglycaemia can result in coma, there is rarely any problem distinguishing them, especially as rapid blood glucose test stick methods are readily available. A test dose of glucose would clinch matters because hypoglycaemia will be very rapidly reversed but there would be no significant effect – either helpful or harmful – in hyperglycaemia. In contrast, insulin given blindly would severely exacerbate hypoglycaemia.

The conscious patient must take sugar, chocolate, sweet tea, dextrose tablets, etc. Semiconscious or comatose patients require intravenous glucose 50% or intramuscular glucagon (1 mg). The response is usually satisfyingly prompt, occurring within minutes. Glucagon injection can usually be managed easily by patients' relatives, who should be fully informed on how to recognize and deal with hypoglycaemic episodes. Unless patients or their relatives are taught to recognize the early signs, the patient may become comatose before being able to correct it. Newly diagnosed diabetics are usually given a controlled experience of hypoglycaemia.

Persistent hypoglycaemic attacks require reassessment of therapy. Dietary modification may be required, e.g. increased carbohydrate (although this might compromise weight reduction efforts). Modern intensive insulin therapy regimens aimed at producing 'tight' glycaemic control have increased the likelihood of hypoglycaemia, and a judgement of risk and benefit has to be made when such regimens are considered (pp. 559–560).

Brittle diabetes

A small proportion of Type 1 diabetics prove exceptionally difficult to control, experiencing frequent episodes of hypoglycaemia, hyperglycaemia or both. They are variously termed **brittle**, **unstable** or **labile**. It is unlikely that this condition is inherent to their disease, and specific causes are always sought. Poor compliance through error, ignorance or disability (e.g. visual problems measuring insulin doses), unrecognized intercurrent illness and drug interaction must first be eliminated. In older patients with recurrent hypoglycaemia the possibility of reduced hypoglycaemic awareness must be investigated.

Recurrent hyperglycaemia/ketoacidosis is more common in young patients and may sometimes be associated with psychological or psychopathological factors such as teenage rebellion or illness denial, self-destructive impulses or other emotional instability. A particular subgroup has been identified of slightly obese females aged 15–25 years who may be covertly manipulating their therapy adversely. Supervised intravenous therapy in some of these patients seems to resolve the problem temporarily.

Chronic complications

In many patients, even before diagnosis, widespread damage occurs in the kidney, nerves, eyes or vascular tree (Fig. 9.6). These long-term complications are to different degrees common to both types of diabetes, and their prevention or treatment are the real challenge for diabetes management and research.

Pathogenesis

It is important to know if these chronic problems are a direct consequence of hyperglycaemia. If so, then optimal control (normoglycaemia) would be expected to minimize them. Evidence has accumulated that this is broadly true for the so-called microvascular complications (mainly kidney, eye, nerves). The fact that similar complications arise in most types of diabetes, despite their very different aetiologies, supports the

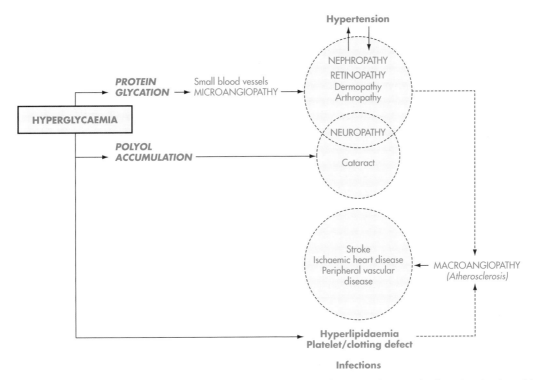

Figure 9.6   Possible pathogenetic mechanisms of chronic diabetic complications. The central column lists the clinical features. Also shown is possible interlinking of pathogenetic mechanisms.

hyperglycaemia hypothesis. The extensive Diabetes Control and Complications Trial (DCCT; 1992) confirmed that better control is associated with less severe complications in Type 1 diabetics. The UK Prospective Diabetes Study (UKPDS; 1998) also generally supported the hypothesis in Type 2 patients (p. 545).

Other hypotheses have been proposed. It could be that an as yet unidentified primary lesion in diabetes is responsible independently for both the hyperglycaemia and the complications: thus, correcting one would not necessarily improve the other. Some complications may be secondary to the abnormal pattern or amount of insulin secretion, which is not completely rectified by conventional treatment. For example, the hyperinsulinaemia seen in many Type 2 patients may contribute to blood vessel disease (macrovascular complications) or hypertension (p. 543). Alternatively, the abnormally high levels of counter-regulatory hormones usually found in diabetes may be deleterious. The involvement of growth hormone and insulin-like growth factor in angiopathy have also been

investigated. Finally, there seems to be a genetic variation in the susceptibility to different complications, regardless of the degree of glycaemic control.

Thus there is unlikely to be a simple answer. Currently three general mechanisms are proposed for the pathological basis of the complications: protein glycation (glycosylation); abnormal polyol metabolism; and atheromatous arterial changes. Glycation is probably mainly responsible for **microangiopathy** (small blood vessel disease), which affects many organ systems; accelerated atherosclerosis causes diabetic **macroangiopathy** (large vessel disease).

Glycation

Normally, almost all body protein is glycated to some extent, i.e. glucose molecules derived from body fluids are covalently bonded to free amine groups on side chains. The degree of glycation is directly proportional to the average blood glucose level. An accessible marker for this is haemoglobin glycation, particularly the HbA$_{1c}$ fraction. Other proteins throughout the body are similarly affected. Excessive glycation in chronic hyperglycaemia results in **advanced glycaemic end-products** which subsequently form abnormal cross-links between different parts of the protein chain. Protein configuration will thus be changed, disrupting secondary and tertiary structure and hence function. Basement membrane proteins seem particularly susceptible to glycation, the result being thickening and increased permeability (i.e. reduced selective barrier function). As basement membranes are present in most tissues, and especially in blood vessels, this could account for the widespread, multisystem distribution of diabetic complications.

Basement membrane damage in capillaries and smaller arterioles causes microangiopathy and subsequent ischaemia in any organ. **Retinopathy** is undoubtedly caused in part by this mechanism. **Neuropathy** may result from a combination of this and direct glycation of the sheaths of small nerves, e.g. sensory nerves. Similarly, glycation of the glomerular basement membrane probably causes the characteristic glomerular sclerosis of diabetic **nephropathy**, although renal arterial disease probably also contributes. Glycation of tendon sheaths and joint capsules may be responsible for the **joint** problems – particularly the stiffness in hands and feet – that some patients suffer; glycation of collagen in **skin** sometimes gives it a thickened, waxy appearance. The myocardium may also be affected, as may immune cells such as macrophages and leucocytes.

Polyol metabolism

Some tissues do not require insulin for glucose transport into their cells (Table 9.3), relying instead simply on diffusion down a concentration gradient. Thus, while other tissues are glucose-depleted in diabetes, these tissues will accumulate excess glucose in the presence of hyperglycaemia. Being surplus to energy needs, some of the glucose so accumulated is reduced to polyols such as sorbitol by the enzyme aldose reductase via an otherwise little used pathway (Fig. 9.7).

The resulting polyols are not readily eliminated from the cells, possibly because they are more polar than glucose and of greater molecular weight. Furthermore, low dehydrogenase activity, particularly in the eye lens and nerve sheaths, means that they are not metabolized efficiently. The resultant accumulation of osmotically active molecules draws water into the cells, causing them to expand and severely disrupting their function and possibly killing them. Retinal blood vessels, the eye lens and the glomeruli may be damaged in this way, contributing to retinopathy, cataract and nephropathy respectively. It has long been known that an analogous intracellular accumulation of galactitol in the lens is linked to the high prevalence of cataract in the inherited metabolic disorder galactosaemia.

A further abnormality may also contribute. Myoinositol, another polyol and an important intermediate in energy handling, may instead become deficient. By a poorly understood series

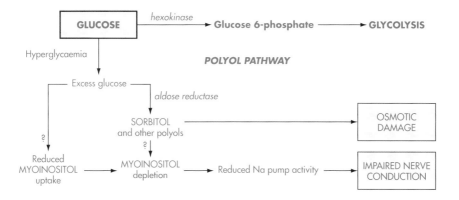

Figure 9.7   Polyol pathway and effects of polyol accumulation.

of steps this deficiency may impair nerve conduction (Fig. 9.7).

Macroangiopathy

Diabetics usually suffer from obstructive vascular diseases owing to a greatly increased predisposition to atherosclerosis. Several factors contribute to this. Because of their more active lipid metabolism, diabetics have raised plasma levels of triglycerides and total cholesterol, and lowered high-density lipoprotein (HDL), producing an unfavourable, atherogenic lipoprotein ratio (see Chapter 3, Fig. 3.25). Platelet aggregating ability is also usually raised, and hypertension is common. Furthermore, many Type 2 patients are initially hyperinsulinaemic and insulin may itself be a growth factor for atheromas. Thus major risk factors for atherosclerosis are intensified and cerebrovascular disease, stroke, ischaemic heart disease and peripheral vascular disease are common. Macroangiopathy also contributes to kidney disease.

Other mechanisms

As illustrated in Fig. 9.6, other complications of diabetes occur, the pathogenesis of which remains obscure. Moreover, different complications may be inter-related or coexistent. Neuropathy may result partly from direct neuronal damage and partly from impaired blood supply to the nerve sheath. Microangiopathy may result partly from glycation, partly from polyol accumulation and partly from hyperinsulinaemia. Once nephropathy is established, it promotes hypertension and vascular disease.

Diabetes and hypertension. There is evidence of an association between obesity, hyperinsulinaemia, insulin resistance, hyperlipidaemia, diabetes (especially Type 2) and hypertension, a condition sometimes termed 'syndrome X'. The precise cause and effect relationships have not yet been elucidated. Many hypertensives have insulin resistance, hyperinsulinaemia and impaired glucose tolerance, and insulin may have several hypertensive actions including promoting renal sodium retention, increasing sympathetic vasoconstrictor activity and directly increasing vascular reactivity (via an effect on sodium handling). In some cases hypertension may be secondary to diabetic kidney disease, although the converse may also be true (see Chapter 3, pp. 98–100). Alternatively, it may be that a third, as yet unknown, independent factor first causes insulin resistance which then leads to both Type 2 diabetes and hypertension. Hyperinsulinaemia could then be a common link in the vascular complications of both diabetes and hypertension. On the other hand, prolonged therapy with the two most common antihypertensive agents – thiazide diuretics and beta-blockers – while lowering blood pressure can also lead to glucose intolerance or even overt diabetes.

Clinical consequences

Almost any system in the body may be affected by diabetic complications, which is why diabetes is regarded as a multisystem disease (Table 9.13).

Table 9.13 Clinical consequences of diabetic complications

System	Clinical features
Eyes	Retinopathy, blindness; glaucoma; cataract
Nerves	Sensory, autonomic and motor defects
Renal	Glomerulosclerosis; chronic renal failure
Cardiovascular	Ischaemic heart disease (angina, MI), peripheral vascular disease, stroke; cardiomyopathy; congestive heart failure
Locomotor	Slow-healing peripheral lesions; 'the diabetic foot'; amputations; joint stiffness
Immune	Increased susceptibility to infection

MI, myocardial infarction.

Eyes. Diabetes is the most common causes of acquired blindness in developed countries. After 30 years of diabetes, about 50% of patients have some degree of retinopathy, and up to 10% become blind. The blindness is due to small-vessel damage in the retina, with dilatation, haemorrhage, infarction and ultimately excessive proliferation of new vessels that project into the vitreous humour. Retinopathy is frequently associated with nephropathy. Diabetics also have an increased incidence of glaucoma and cataract.

Nervous system. Diabetic neuropathy may affect any part of the peripheral nervous system, but most commonly starts with the peripheral *sensory* nerves, causing tingling and numbness (paraesthesias), loss of vibration sense or the sense of balance and limb position. It may also be quite painful. *Autonomic* neuropathy is potentially devastating because it can seriously disturb cardiovascular, gastrointestinal or genitourinary function, causing multifarious symptoms; postural hypotension and impotence are common. Voluntary *motor* nerves are less commonly affected.

Renal. Diabetic nephropathy is the cause of death in about 25% of Type 1 diabetics. Predominantly a form of sclerosis of the glomerular basement membrane, it develops very slowly and so most commonly occurs in Type 1 patients, up to 40% of whom may be affected. The increased glomerular filtration rate ('hyperfiltration') in early diabetes, which is due to hypertension and to the osmotic loading of hyperglycaemia, may overload renal capillaries. Nephropathy is heralded by microalbuminuria, with increasing proteinuria frequently progressing to worsening hypertension and end-stage renal failure. Progression varies between ethnic groups. Diabetics comprise about 15% of the caseload of UK renal replacement therapy centres. Renal decline is hastened by inadequate or tardy treatment of associated hypertension.

Cardiovascular. About half of diabetic deaths are from the consequences of large-vessel disease (macroangiopathy). Diabetics have a twofold risk of stroke and a fivefold risk of myocardial infarction compared with matched non-diabetic subjects. Peripheral vascular disease is also common, with a 50-fold risk of peripheral gangrene. Some patients undergo progressively extensive amputation; usually the lower limbs (especially the feet; see below) are affected, but fingers are also at risk.

As noted above, small vessel disease (microangiopathy) is also common, with serious consequences in other systems, particularly the eyes, nerves and kidneys.

Hypertension is often associated with diabetes. In Type 1 patients, the hypertension is probably secondary to nephropathy; in Type 2 patients the aetiology is uncertain ('syndrome X', p. 543), but obesity and hyperinsulinaemia each contribute. A rare complication is diffuse cardiac fibrosis (cardiomyopathy) which may lead to heart failure.

Locomotor. The 'diabetic foot' is a common problem. In normal people minor foot injuries such as a corn, blister or ingrown toenail usually heal before being noticed. In diabetics however, these often develop into non-healing painless ulcers which become gangrenous, with irreversible damage sometimes occurring before medical attention is sought. This results from a combination of poor peripheral sensation (neuropathy, so that the wound is not felt), poor peripheral circulation (angiopathy, so that healing is impaired) and reduced resistance to infection. All diabetics should see a chiropodist regularly. Correctly fitting footwear is essential. No pharmacist should attempt to treat any foot problem in a diabetic, or sell them 'corn plasters' or similar products. Any foot problem, however minor, should be referred to their chiropodist or doctor.

Diabetes can also cause soft tissue damage resulting in limited joint mobility (stiffness), and a characteristic osteoarthropathy (Charcot joints), usually in the feet, also owing to angiopathy and sensory neuropathy.

Systemic. Diabetics are very prone to infections owing to an impaired immune response caused by defects in immune and inflammatory cells. Recurrent bladder infection is common, which can ascend to cause pyelonephritis; autonomic neuropathy causing urinary retention and stasis exacerbates this. Skin infections are also frequent, and contribute to foot problems.

Management of complications

General strategy

The overall approach to preventing diabetic complications, minimizing them or delaying their onset combines control of blood glucose, risk factor reduction and regular monitoring.

Optimal glycaemic control. Although the aetiology and pathogenesis of the complications are still uncertain and likely to be multiple, the main clinical approach has been to aim for scrupulous control of blood glucose levels within the normal range, in an attempt to mimic physiological normality. This is based on the assumption that complications are due to hyperglycaemia (p. 540). This seems to be particularly likely for the microvascular (and possibly polyol-related) complications in nerves, eyes and kidney. Evidence derives from clinical trials including those using the more 'physiological' treatments such as continuous subcutaneous insulin infusion (p. 568) or other methods of achieving 'tight' glycaemic control. This means keeping fasting blood glucose levels below 7 mmol/L and never exceeding 11 mmol/L, and may mean conversion to insulin therapy in poorly controlled Type 2 patients.

Good control has been shown to reduce the incidence of complications. The most convincing evidence in Type 1 diabetes was the DCCT trial, which reported significant slowing of deterioration in retinopathy, microalbuminuria and, to a lesser extent, neuropathy. The UKPDS trial found broadly similar benefits in Type 2 patients and also strongly demonstrated the synergistic role of hypertension in exacerbating complications and the importance of achieving normotension as well as normoglycaemia. Unfortunately, this study failed to identify clearly the treatment mode which offered the best protection, although this had been one of its aims.

An unwanted side effect of tight control is that by keeping the average blood glucose low the incidence of hypoglycaemia is increased, espe-

cially among elderly and 'brittle' (unstable) diabetics. In the DCCT trial there was a threefold increase in the incidence of hypoglycaemia. This means that in some circumstances a compromise is necessary, because of the acute and the long-term complications of frequent hypoglycaemic attacks. Thus, older patients in whom the diabetes onset occurred quite late (i.e. Type 2) are usually allowed to run higher average levels. The long delay in onset of complications will mean that life expectancy may be little reduced, whereas quality of life would be markedly reduced by frequent hypoglycaemia.

An additional, unexpected effect is for established retinopathy to deteriorate rather than improve. This 'normoglycaemic re-entry phenomenon' is being investigated, but currently is not seen as a contraindication for good control, rather a caution for closer monitoring of susceptible patients.

For the macrovascular complications (cardiovascular, cerebrovascular and peripheral atherosclerosis) this approach is less successful, perhaps because insulin and related endocrine abnormalities and hypertension may contribute directly. It is still unknown whether the generally higher insulin levels associated with tight control regimens can actually exacerbate some macrovascular problems.

A recent experimental approach to reversing hyperglycaemia-related damage has been to attempt to cleave the protein cross-links that develop after glycation by the use of novel deglycation enzymes.

Minimize risk factors. It is important to control any additional risk factors which could exacerbate organ damage, especially via atherosclerosis. These include smoking, hypertension, obesity, hyperlipidaemia and hyperuricaemia.

Monitoring. This essential component in minimizing complications is discussed on pp. 568–569 (*see also* Table 9.20).

Reduce polyol accumulation. Based on the polyol theory of certain of the complications, it should be possible to impede this process by interfering with the metabolism of polyols. Unfortunately, **aldose reductase inhibitors**

(e.g. *sorbinil*), although they do minimize sorbitol accumulation and prevent myoinositol depletion, have not proven clinically successful in reversing or even retarding neuropathy, cataract, nephropathy or retinopathy. Dietary myoinositol supplementation has also been unsuccessful.

Specific complications

Nephropathy. There are currently four methods which have been shown to slow the rate of deterioration in renal function:

* Careful glycaemic control.
* Control of hypertension.
* Use of angiotensin converting enzyme inhibitors (ACEIs).
* Moderate protein restriction (in more advanced nephropathy).

It is essential that diabetics are monitored annually for the onset of hypertension and microalbuminuria. In treating hypertension, ACEIs seem to have an additional direct beneficial effect in diabetes, dilating intrarenal (efferent glomerular) vessels and thus minimizing glomerular hypertension. There is a growing tendency to use ACEIs increasingly early (unless contraindicated e.g. by bilateral renal artery stenosis). ACEIs should always be used when there is hypertension with proteinuria or microalbuminuria; some recommend their use in microalbuminuria even with normotension. At present, there is no evidence that ACEIs benefit normotensive diabetics with no evidence of nephropathy. It is also as yet unclear if other antihypertensives offer similar benefit

Once established, renal failure is managed in the normal way, except that haemodialysis is more difficult because of vascular and thrombotic complications. Continuous ambulatory peritoneal dialysis is particularly suitable in diabetes because insulin may be administered intraperitoneally (thus directly entering the portal circulation which is more physiological). However, there may be a problem with the glucose which is usually added to dialysis fluid to promote water removal. Diabetics are nowadays unlikely to be given low priority for renal transplantation, as they tended to be in the past, and this is sometimes combined with pancreatic transplantation (p. 547). There are however some problems: the poor general health of these patients and multiple organ damage increase operative risk, and there is an increased likelihood of post-transplant infection owing to the immunosuppression required. Nevertheless, graft survival is only about 10–15% poorer than the average for renal transplants.

Angiopathy. The usual dietary constraints on saturated fat and cholesterol are important. Monounsaturated fats (nuts, fish) are recommended. Although their benefits have not been specifically proven in trials on diabetics, lipid-lowering drugs such as the *statins* may be indicated. Other conventional atheroma risk factors such as smoking and hypertension must also be addressed (*see* Chapter 3, pp. 120–122).

Neuropathy. All treatment for neuropathy is symptomatic. Drug therapy may be of help in the sometimes excruciating pain of peripheral neuropathy. Conventional analgesic or anti-inflammatory drugs are generally ineffective. A variety of other drugs have been tried and the first-generation tricyclic antidepressants, e.g. *amitriptyline*, are standard first-line therapy. Second-line agents include *phenytoin* and *carbamazepine*. There have been some indications that ACEIs may benefit neuropathy as well as nephropathy.

Retinopathy. Retinal disease is conventionally treated by laser photocoagulation.

Management

Aims and strategy

Preventative methods for diabetes are as yet poorly developed. More progress has been made with potentially curative surgery. However, at present the vast majority of diabetics require long-term management of established disease.

The cardinal aim of management in diabetes is to keep blood glucose levels within the normal range, and to produce patterns of glucose and insulin levels in the blood similar to those that follow normal changes in diet and activity (*see* Fig. 9.4). Blood glucose levels should remain below the maxima in the WHO definition for impaired glucose tolerance (Table 9.1). Ideally, this would require a continuous basal level of insulin to maintain metabolism, supplemented by rapid pulses following meals and reduced during exercise.

Optimal management should attain three important interlinked aims:

- To prevent symptoms.
- To maintain biochemical stability.
- To prevent long-term complications.

At present, this ideal is not achievable. Even if pancreatic transplantation were to be perfected there might still remain insulin receptor defects. Current therapy is limited to artificially manipulating diet and insulin (endogenous or exogenous) in order to mimic normal patterns as closely as is practicable.

The older style directive, paternalistic medical model for such manipulation is now rarely practised, clinics preferring to negotiate a 'therapeutic contract' with the patient. The aim is to agree a desired level of control – optimal, prophylactic or perhaps merely symptomatic – based on the severity of the disease and the patient's age, understanding, likely compliance and normal way of life.

Sometimes it is inadvisable to strive too zealously to approach the ideal. For the elderly, where long-term complications are of less concern, keeping symptoms at a tolerable level without excessive disruptions to normal life patterns may be adequate. For this, the target need only be to achieve random blood glucose levels below 12 mmol/L. In some patients the incidence of hypoglycaemic attacks is unacceptably high if control is too tight. The advent of the 'insulin pen' (p. 565) has made such flexibility feasible.

Prevention

Because Type 1 disease involves immune destruction of the pancreas, immunotherapy has been attempted experimentally, as early as possible after initial diagnosis or even in the presymptomatic stage in at-risk individuals (e.g. where there is a strong family history). In animal models anti-T cell antibodies, bone marrow transplantation, thymectomy, azathioprine, nicotinamide and ciclosporin (cyclosporine) have been tried. Early introduction of insulin therapy has also been recommended (to 'spare' the beta cells and perhaps to reduce their expression of auto-antigens). In human studies, only high-dose *ciclosporin* has so far shown any promise. Even then, only prolongation of the honeymoon period has been achieved, with relapse occurring on stopping therapy.

However, considerable pancreatic damage has usually already occurred by the time symptoms are noticed. Only about 10% of functional islet cells then remain, so no great improvement can be expected. Research is now concentrating on discovering reliable early prognostic markers, such as islet cell antibodies (p. 533). Patients at risk could then be identified by screening.

No specific aetiological agents have been identified for Type 2 diabetes, but risk factors are known. These correspond with many of the well-established cardiovascular risk factors associated with the lifestyle of industrialized countries, i.e. diets high in sugar and fats and low in fibre, and slowly absorbable complex carbohydrates, lack of exercise, obesity.

Cure: organ replacement

Around 10 000 **pancreatic transplants** have so far been performed world-wide. Many of the early surgical problems, e.g. leakage of destructive digestive enzymes from non-islet cells, have now been resolved, and the current 1-year graft survival rate exceeds 75% using *tacrolimus* immunosuppression. In addition to the risks of surgery, successfully transplanted patients still have to contend with lifelong immunosuppression, possibly in the presence of multiple organ damage from established complications.

However, dual renal plus pancreatic transplantations are increasingly being performed on diabetics with end-stage nephropathy who qualify for a renal transplant, because such patients are going to have to undergo immunosuppression anyway. In the best centres the renal prognosis approaches that of kidney transplantation alone, although patient survival is currently poorer.

The implantation of pure beta-islet cells,

possibly from fetal sources, is under investigation. One approach to reducing rejection is to encapsulate the islet cells in a semi-permeable membrane which permits glucose and insulin diffusion but blocks access to immunoglobulin macromolecules.

Transplantation does not appear to reverse complications, nor is there firm evidence yet on whether it can prevent them. Currently transplantation is rarely considered in the absence of advanced nephropathy unless the patient has severe uncontrollable or brittle disease.

A number of **artificial pancreas** devices have been tested, although none is yet available for routine use (p. 565).

Therapeutic strategy

Using conventional methods (diet, drugs, insulin), the only way to allow relatively normal eating and activity in a diabetic (i.e. unpredictable, unplanned and uncontrolled) would be to give frequent, precisely calculated injections of soluble insulin or appropriate doses of a rapidly acting oral hypoglycaemic drug. The dose would be based on blood glucose measurement or guided by experience and recent diet and activity level: thus insulin is supplied on demand in a manner emulating normal physiol-

ogy (*see* Fig. 9.4). With the introduction of insulin pens, such an 'insulin demand-driven' strategy is becoming practicable, although dosage adjustment is still imprecise. The artificial pancreas, if perfected, may prove a better option.

'Insulin supply drive'

The alternative, which is still used for many older patients, is to turn physiology on its head and to accept a model driven by insulin supply. Instead of matching insulin supply to instantaneous changes in demand, demand in the form of diet and activity is adjusted and controlled to conform to available insulin (either endogenous or administered exogenously). Because both drugs and insulin must be given prospectively this is in effect 'feeding the insulin', as opposed to the normal situation where insulin follows feeding. Meals and activity must be regular and of predictable composition: explicit adjustments in drug or insulin dose must be made to allow for deviations (Fig. 9.8).

This places considerable constraints on patients, particularly children. Education and counselling are extremely important and the British Diabetic Association (BDA) performs a valuable role here. Generally speaking, diabetics are good compliers in the strict sense that the severe metabolic upset precipitated by drug

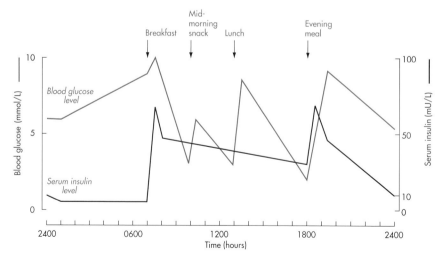

Figure 9.8 Matching food intake to available insulin. In the insulin supply-driven model, insulin levels are maintained artificially by either direct injection or by augmentation using oral hypoglycaemic agents. To prevent hypoglycaemia, sufficient glucose must be provided by the diet at regular intervals. Note what would be the effect of missing the mid-afternoon snack: blood glucose would start to fall dangerously low just before the evening meal. Unusual activity would complicate this picture.

defaulting is a powerful motivator. Nevertheless, good compliance with diet, and the very tight control of blood glucose which avoidance of long-term complications demands, are less common.

Treatment modes

Dietary management is the bedrock of treatment. All diabetics, irrespective of other treatments, require some control of their eating and exercise patterns, both in terms of total caloric intake, types of nutrients and eating schedule. Indeed, about half of patients will need no more than this, especially those who lose weight. A further 25% will need to augment their natural insulin with drugs. The remainder will need insulin.

The initial choice is usually related to how the patient first presents (pp. 535–536; Fig. 9.9). Younger patients, who are frequently non-obese, usually present unambiguously as Type 1 insulin-dependent diabetics, although a variable insulin-independent ('honeymoon') period may occur following diagnosis.

Older patients, who are often obese, will almost always be Type 2 and must be tried first on diet alone. Should this fail, drug therapy will be added. Although all drugs used in diabetes therapy are sometimes for convenience described as oral hypoglycaemics, only the sulphonylureas directly lower blood glucose level. Other oral agents are more correctly referred to as anti-hyperglycaemics. The generic term *antidiabetic drug*, while slightly inaccurate in implying a preventative or curative action, is nevertheless preferable.

Usually, a *sulphonylurea* is selected first, but a *biguanide* may be preferable for the obese, and increasingly an *alpha-glucosidase inhibitor* is being seen as a first-line agent, especially in the elderly. Sometimes a synergistic combination of the two types will be required. In the few for whom these measures are ineffective, and especially if ketoacidosis occurs, insulin treatment is needed, as it will be eventually in those whose disease progresses faster. Type 2 patients may also need insulin temporarily during periods of increased requirement such as major infection, surgery or pregnancy. Combining antidiabetic drugs with insulin therapy offers no advantages; once insulin is required for regular control it is usually better to convert fully to it.

At any point in this sequence an adjunctive drug which reduces intestinal glucose absorption or reduce insulin resistance may be added.

Initiation of treatment

On first diagnosis, all patients will be fully examined and investigated to establish baseline measures for the presence and progression of any complications. This will include ophthalmological, renal, cardiovascular, neurological, lipid and foot assessment (pp. 568–569).

Some patients will be treated first in hospital, especially Type 1 patients first presenting with ketoacidosis. Blood glucose levels will be measured 4-hourly during this period, to establish the diet and possibly the drug or insulin dosage necessary to achieve the agreed level of control. A test

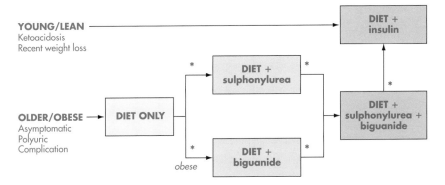

Figure 9.9 Treatment strategy for diabetes related to presentation. *Add or substitute *thiazolidinedione* or *glucosidase inhibitor* at any stage to attempt to improve control before moving to next stage. The role of *meglitinides* (e.g. *repaglinide*) is not yet established. See text, p. 559.

exposure to hypoglycaemia will be arranged to familiarize patients with the symptoms and the dietary constraints fully explained.

After discharge some will continue to attend as outpatients. Others will be managed by their general practitioner, although regular diabetic clinic visits are desirable. Some Type 1 and most Type 2 patients without acute complications may be treated by their GP from the outset.

Diet

All Type 2 patients must first be encouraged to try to control their disease on diet alone, and no patient taking antidiabetic drugs or insulin should believe that these obviate the necessity to control their diet. Recommendations about diet have evolved in several important ways. Fats are now discouraged, while complex carbohydrate and fibre are encouraged, and the overall approach is far less restrictive than formerly. The recommended diabetic diet, save in a few respects, now closely resembles the normal healthy diet that everyone should eat: regular meals low in fats, simple sugars and sodium and high in complex carbohydrate (starch) and fibre.

Formerly, inflexible, unrealistic or impractical prescriptions and restrictions (diet sheets,

'exchanges') took little or no account of the psychological importance of individual dietary habits, dietary preferences and ethnic variations. The result was poor compliance complicated by guilt and anxiety. The modern approach recognizes that:

- Dietary records or recall are an imprecise basis for future modification.
- Nutrient uptake varies even from precisely regulated and measured portions (owing to the interactions between foodstuffs, variations in temperature, physical form, degree of chewing, etc.).
- Compromise is needed to obtain a regimen with which the patient can reasonably be expected to comply.

Thus, a perfect diabetic diet is difficult to achieve in practice and although the pursuit of it is worthwhile, in some patients this could be counter-productive. Rather, efforts are made to ensure that patients understand, in their own fashion, what the aims are. Counselling and education are then used to maximize motivation. Advice from a dietician with experience in modifying diabetic diets to suit individual lifestyles can help achieve good compliance.

Four aspects of diet need to be considered (Fig. 9.10):

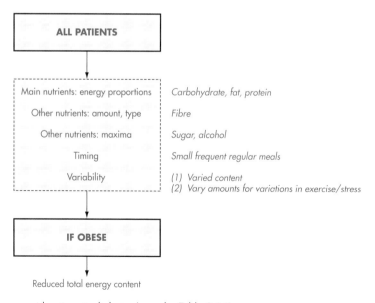

Figure 9.10   Dietary considerations in diabetes (*see also* Table 9.14).

- Total energy intake.
- Constituents.
- Timing.
- Variation.

Energy intake

All patients need to adjust their caloric intake to achieve and maintain the desired bodyweight for their size, aiming for a body mass index (BMI) of about $22 \, \text{kg/m}^2$. For most Type 2 diabetics, who are frequently obese, this implies a weight-reducing diet. Reliable tables are now available to predict the required energy intake according to age, gender, activity level and lifestyle.

Constituents

Macronutrients

The unselective restriction on **carbohydrate** which used to characterize diabetic diets is now considered misconceived. Carbohydrate is not harmful if taken mainly as slowly absorbed complex polysaccharides, i.e. starch. Such carbohydrates allow Type 2 diabetics to make best use of their limited endogenous insulin secretory capacity by not raising postprandial blood glucose too rapidly. Foods can be classified according to their **glycaemic index**, which represents the ratio of the total glucose absorption they produce compared with that from a standard test meal of wholemeal bread and cottage cheese. The lower the index the better, and representative values are rice 80%, potatoes 77%, pasta 60%, and lentils 45%. Foods acceptable to various ethnic minorities, such as chappatis, kidney beans, chickpeas, etc. are also now encouraged.

The relatively high **fat** content of early diabetic diets which was needed in a carbohydrate-reduced diet to provide calories more cheaply than with protein, is now seen to be dangerously atherogenic. A reduced fat intake, low in saturated fats and comprising about one-third polyunsaturated and one-third mono-unsaturated fat (e.g. nuts, fish, olive oil) is now encouraged. (Cholesterol is usually reduced inherently along with saturated fats.) There are no particular constraints on **protein** except for patients with suspected nephropathy, when restriction is indicated.

Other nutrients

A small amount of simple **sugar** (sucrose) is now considered acceptable, provided that the caloric content is accounted for. This is usually consumed as a constituent, e.g. of baked products. Artificial non-nutritive sweeteners are still preferred and patients must be advised to monitor intake of 'hidden' sugar in processed foods. So-called 'diabetic foods' often contain sorbitol or fructose and, while they may not raise blood glucose as much as sucrose, have a high energy content. They are also expensive, offer nothing that a well-balanced diabetic diet cannot offer, and are not recommended by the BDA.

Alcohol is not prohibited if its high caloric content is accounted for and its hypoglycaemic effect is appreciated, i.e. it should be taken with some carbohydrate. Recent evidence of its protective effect against heart disease suggests that once again similar recommendations should apply to diabetics as to the population as a whole. There should be little added **salt**, to minimize rises in blood pressure.

Fibre is extremely important. Although fibre is primarily carbohydrate, the terminology is somewhat inconsistent; however, the distinctions are relevant (Fig. 9.11). Starch, in staple foods like bread, potatoes and rice, is the main digestible carbohydrate energy source. Older classifications grouped all other indigestible matter together as 'dietary fibre', but there are important and distinct components. The **non-starch polysaccharides** (NSP) are now known to be particularly important in diabetes. They provide no energy but further delay absorption of glucose from starch digestion (see above), and by forming intestinal bulk promote a feeling of satiety that may reduce appetite and therefore help weight reduction.

The (**semi)soluble** or **viscous** fibres and gums found in fruit, vegetables and pulses (Fig. 9.11) in addition produce a modest reduction in blood cholesterol, possibly by binding bile salts thereby preventing enterohepatic recirculation. The **insoluble** NSP fibres, as in bran and unmilled cereals and grains, have little effect on cholesterol, but contribute to stool bulk along with other fibrous 'roughage' (e.g. lignin).

Although undigested in the ileum, some of

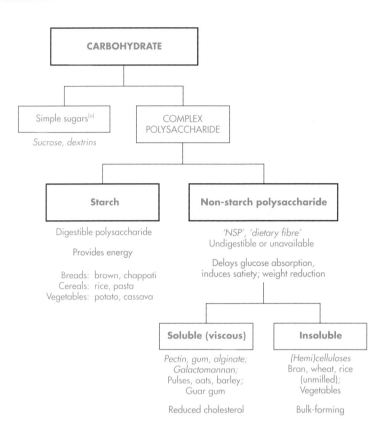

Figure 9.11   Different forms of dietary carbohydrate, including fibre; with functions and examples of foodstuffs. [a]Avoid as far as possible.

this material is hydrolysed by colonic flora to release absorbable and metabolizable carboxylic acids.

Proportions.   The recommended proportions of macronutrient energy intake are approximately 55:30:15 (Table 9.14; traditional diabetic diets used to be nearer 25:65:10). How the patient implements this has also changed. Clinics no longer issue rigid menus, kitchen scales and detailed tables of what can be exchanged for what. More generalized recommendations with much wider variability are found to be more successful.

One such approach simply visualizes a meal plate divided into segments: about one-fifth contains protein and fat sources such as meat or fish; the rest is divided equally between staple carbohydrate sources such as rice, pasta or potatoes and fibre such as fruit or vegetables. The patient is advised to construct each meal in these proportions (Fig. 9.12).

Timing

Small regular frequent meals are important. This means similar caloric intake at all main meals and regular snacks in between. For Type 2 patients this minimizes the load put on the pancreas at any one time. For both types it helps to keep blood glucose levels within closer limits, minimizing the risk of hypoglycaemia between drug or insulin doses and the risk of postprandial hyperglycaemia. There is some evidence that this too is a pattern that might benefit the general population. Nibbling or 'grazing' appears to produce lower average plasma lipid and blood glucose levels and less obesity compared with a similar caloric intake obtained from intermittent, larger meals.

Variation

Diabetics need to understand that these constraints do not prevent them having a varied,

Table 9.14   Nutrients in diets recommended for diabetic and general population

	British Diabetic Association Nutrition subcommittee[a]	National Advisory Committee on Nutrition Education (UK)[a]
Carbohydrate	50–60%	50%
Fat	30–35%	30–35%
Protein	10–15%	10%
Simple sugars	<25 g	10%
Cholesterol[b]	300 mg	
Soluble fibre[c]	>15 g	15–18 g
Alcohol	2 units (female)	2 units (female)
	3 units (male)	3 units (male)

[a] Percentages given as proportion of total energy intake. Amounts are per day.

[b] Cholesterol intake usually automatically reduced sufficiently if saturated fat intake less than 10%.

[c] 15 g soluble fibre equivalent to 18 g non-starch polysaccharides (NSP) or 30 g total dietary fibre.

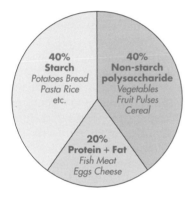

Figure 9.12   The 'plate model' of meal planning recommended by British Diabetic Association. Each meal should be constructed roughly of the types of foods and in the proportions shown, visualizing them as making up the complete plate of food. (Adapted from Nutrition subcommittee of the British Diabetic Association. Dietary recommendations for people with diabetes: an update for the 1990s (1992) *Diabetic Med* **9**: 198–202.)

appetising and nutritious diet. They should also understand how to augment their diet to match any unplanned or unusual exercise or stress so as to avoid hypoglycaemia. Temporary changes in a patient's metabolic requirements (such as in serious illness) or oral absorptive capacity (e.g. enteritis) require appropriate adjustment, which may involve temporary insulin therapy in a Type 2 patient.

Type 1 patients using the 'insulin pen' will generally be even more flexible (see below). In mildly diabetic elderly patients the diet will also be far less rigid, for reasons already discussed. On the other hand, the diets of growing children need constant reassessment. The availability of nutrients and the habits and constraints of different ethnic groups also need to be taken into account. Dieticians are an essential part of the diabetic team.

Diet as sole management may fail in up to two-thirds of Type 2 patients. Primary failure is usually due to poor compliance, poor motivation or inadequate counselling. Secondary failure usually results from disease progression, with falling insulin production. The next stage is to introduce oral antidiabetic drugs.

Oral antidiabetic drugs

Aim and role

Oral antidiabetic drugs (OADs) are used as the next step for Type 2 patients in whom diet has failed to control their condition adequately. The majority may then be controlled by a combination of diet and drugs for a number of years, but some Type 2 patients may eventually require insulin treatment.

There are four main therapeutic targets for OADs (Table 9.15). Doubts over the safety of some of these drugs have now been resolved. The results the 1970s' University Group Diabetes

Table 9.15   Oral antidiabetic drugs

Therapeutic target	Site of action	Group	Examples
Reduce or retard glucose uptake	Intestine	Alpha-glycosidase inhibitors	*Acarbose*
		Fibre	*Guar gum*
Enhance insulin secretion	Pancreas	Sulphonylureas	*Tolbutamide, glibenclamide (glyburide)*
Enhance insulin secretion	Pancreas	Meglitinides	*Repaglinide*
Enhance insulin action	Peripheral receptors	Biguanides	*Metformin*
Reduce gluconeogenesis	Liver	Biguanides	*Metformin*
Reduce insulin resistance	Peripheral receptors	Thiazolidinediones	*Troglitazone*[a]

[a] Licensed and then withdrawn in UK, 1997.

Programme (UGDP) trial, which suggested significant toxicity in the *sulphonylureas*, are now discredited. *Phenformin*, an early biguanide, caused numerous deaths from lactic acidosis and was withdrawn. Newer biguanides are much safer: only *metformin* is currently available in the UK; elsewhere *buformin* is used.

All OAD strategies depend on endogenous insulin secretion and are therefore effective only in patients with Type 2 disease who retain appreciable beta-cell function. Ketosis-prone patients, brittle diabetics or those whose fasting blood glucose exceeds 15–20 mmol/L, whether Type 1 or Type 2, almost invariably need exogenous insulin.

Action

These drugs have different, albeit complementary and sometimes overlapping, actions on the underlying abnormalities in Type 2 diabetes, so combination therapy is indicated if monotherapy fails.

Alpha-glucosidase inhibitors (*acarbose*) inhibit the final stage of the digestion of starch within the intestine by blocking the enzyme disaccharidase. This reduces the rate of glucose absorption and thus the postprandial glucose load presented to the islet cells. Thus, a pancreas with a limited insulin secretory rate might be better able to handle this load with less hyperglycaemia. They are generally only used as adjuncts to other therapy, but may be added at any stage to improve control. **Guar gum** pro-

duces a similar effect non-specifically, probably by binding glucose in the gut.

Both these groups can be regarded as oral *antihyperglycaemic* rather than oral hypoglycaemic agents.

Sulphonylureas enhance the release of preformed insulin in response to circulating glucose, partly by increasing beta-cell sensitivity to blood glucose. This mimics the acute phase of the normal response to hyperglycaemia. However, sulphonylureas do not directly stimulate subsequent insulin synthesis. Because sulphonylureas can produce hypoglycaemia it is believed that they also cause insulin release, even in the absence of the stimulus of blood glucose.

After prolonged sulphonylurea therapy insulin levels fall somewhat, but appreciable clinical benefit remains, suggesting additional extrapancreatic actions. They may up-regulate insulin receptors, both in the liver and peripherally, increasing sensitivity to lower insulin levels; inhibition of glucagon has also been suggested. However, sulphonylureas only work in the presence of functional beta-cells, so these extrapancreatic actions may be of limited significance. They could in part be secondary to reduced hyperglycaemia, preventing the 'glucose toxicity' known to inhibit both insulin release and receptor sensitivity.

The sulphonylureas are commonly divided into first- and second-generation groups. There are important pharmacokinetic differences, but pharmacodynamically they differ only in relative potency.

Meglitinides (benzoic acid derivatives) are a novel group which also stimulate insulin release. They are claimed to do so more specifically in response to the blood glucose level and thus to mealtime glucose load. This would make them more glucose sensitive and may reduce the likelihood of between-meals hypoglycaemia, but this remains to be confirmed by wider use. The first to be licensed in the UK is *repaglinide*.

Biguanides do not stimulate or mimic insulin. They appear to increase peripheral insulin receptor sensitivity and glucose utilization. The underlying effect is probably via a general inhibitory action on membrane transport. Intracellularly, this would prevent glucose entering mitochondria, thus promoting anaerobic glycolysis in the cytosol. Because this is a less efficient process, cellular glucose uptake and utilization are increased. This may also account for a tendency to cause lactic acidosis. In the intestine, reduced membrane transport may be useful in slowing and reducing glucose absorption; there may also be intestinal lactate production. Biguanides also reduce hepatic gluconeogenesis and release of glucose from the liver into the blood. They have an apparent anti-obesity action

Thiazolidinediones appear to switch metabolism from fatty acid to glucose by activating a transcription regulator for an insulin-responsive gene. The effect is to reduce insulin resistance and insulin levels and also alter blood lipids favourably (lowered triglycerides and raised HDL). There is hope that this group may reduce complications, both macrovascular (by reducing insulin and lipid levels) and microvascular (by reducing hyperglycaemia). However, *troglitazone*, the only drug in this group to be licensed in the UK, was withdrawn soon after release owing to liver toxicity.

Biopharmacy and pharmacokinetics

Sulphonylureas are generally well absorbed although potential bioavailability differences mean that patients should not change formulation. Most sulphonylureas are more than 90% protein bound (except *tolazamide*, 75%), and so are liable to competitive displacement interactions.

Important differences exist in clearance, half-life and duration of action which determine frequency of administration, precautions and contraindications. With one important exception, clearance is hepatic with subsequent renal excretion of inactive or less active metabolites (Table 9.16; Fig. 9.13). Those with inactive metabolites (e.g. *tolbutamide*) generally have the shortest half-lives. The older *chlorpropamide* is largely cleared renally which accounts for its long half-life. Some sulphonylureas have metabolites that are chiefly excreted in the bile, which makes them safer in renal disease but more reliant on hepatic function.

The duration of action, or biological half-life, is related to but often longer than the plasma half-life, owing partly to the activity of metabolites. *Chlorpropamide* has too long a duration of action and frequently produces between-meals hypoglycaemia; it has little if any role now and is contraindicated in the elderly. The other popular first-generation sulphonylurea, *tolbutamide*, fell from favour because its action was felt to be too short, requiring frequent dosing. However, it may for this reason be useful in the elderly, to minimize hypoglycaemia. Most newer second-generation drugs avoid these problems, but there are wide interpatient variations in the handling of all sulphonylureas and dose regimens must be individualized. *Glibenclamide* is a special case; being concentrated within beta-cells

---

Table 9.16   Duration of action of sulphonylureas

Relative duration of action[a]	Very short	Short	Medium	Long	Very long
Daily dose frequency	2–3	2–3	1(–2)	1	1
Examples	Gliquidone	Tolbutamide	Tolazamide, glipizide, glimepride	Glibenclamide (glyburide), gliclazide	Chlorpropamide

[a] Approximate descriptive indication of relative durations: precise time will vary from patient to patient.

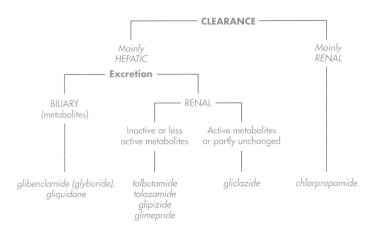

Figure 9.13   Clearance and excretion of the sulphonylureas.

its biological half-life is considerably longer than its plasma half-life.

Biguanides differ substantially from the sulphonylureas, being poorly absorbed, little protein-bound and cleared predominantly by renal excretion (with about 30% cleared by hepatic metabolism). *Metformin* has a short half-life, but higher doses may be given at longer intervals (i.e. 850 mg 12-hourly rather than 500 mg 8-hourly); *buformin* is longer acting. Renal clearance may exceed glomerular filtration rate, implying some tubular secretion. Thus minor renal impairment, unnoticed because of a normal serum creatinine level, might still permit significant accumulation, and renal function monitoring is essential with their use.

Troglitazone is well absorbed orally, highly bound to plasma albumin, cleared hepatically by conjugation and excreted into the bile, with a half-life of up to approximately 24 h. Once-daily dosing is usually possible. **Repaglinide** is rapidly absorbed, reaching a peak within 1 h; it has a very short half-life, being cleared and eliminated hepatically. This means that it may be useful in controlling blood glucose in close association with meals (p. 559). **Alpha-glucosidase inhibitors** are not absorbed, acting slowly in the gut.

Adverse reactions

Sulphonylureas are well tolerated and free from serious long-term adverse effects. The principal problem is hypoglycaemia, which may be pro-tracted and even fatal. A related drawback is the tendency to produce or maintain obesity. Both effects can be linked to increased insulin levels, which also are giving concern over a possible exacerbation of macrovascular complications (insulin being a possible growth factor in arterial walls).

Hypoglycaemia may be caused by an overdose, an interaction, a missed meal or unexpected activity and occurs more commonly with the longer-acting drugs (*glibenclamide* and *chlorpropamide*), especially in the elderly, who must avoid them. (The possible compliance advantage is far outweighed by the likelihood that a meal will be forgotten while plasma drug levels are still significant.) With the newer, shorter-acting drugs any hypoglycaemia that does occur is brief and more easily rectified.

Chlorpropamide can occasionally cause a mild disulfiram-like flush with alcohol (due to acetaldehyde dehydrogenase inhibition), and occasionally hyponatraemia and a syndrome of inappropriate secretion of antidiuretic hormone (ADH). These effects, as well as minor idiosyncratic reactions, are uncommon with second-generation sulphonylureas.

Biguanides (with the exception of phenformin) cause a few minor adverse effects, being somewhat less well tolerated than sulphonylureas. The nausea, diarrhoea, muscle discomfort and occasional malabsorption may be due to the membrane effects inherent in their mode of action. Biguanides are best taken with food, the dose being increased gradually to improve tolerance. Iatrogenic lactic acidosis, which has a high mortality, occurs rarely with *metformin* and its risk can be further reduced by careful monitoring of renal and hepatic function and ensuring that it is avoided in patients with hypoxaemic conditions such as cardiopulmonary insufficiency. Because biguanides do not release insulin, they cannot cause hypoglycaemia.

Alpha-glucosidase inhibitors frequently cause uncomfortable and sometimes unacceptable or intolerable gastrointestinal problems owing to the increased carbohydrate load delivered to the large bowel. Subsequent bacterial fermentation causes distension, pain, flatulence and diarrhoea.

Troglitazone causes mild generalized adverse effects, e.g. gastrointestinal upsets, headache. However, serious hepatic problems forced its withdrawal soon after release, although it may be re-introduced. **Repaglinide** is also well tolerated, with toxicity comparable with that of the sulphonylureas.

Interactions

Interactions with OADs are potentially serious because the patient's delicate biochemical balance is maintained by a specific dose. Potentiation can rapidly cause hypoglycaemia, whereas antagonism could lead to a loss of glycaemic control and a return of polyuric symptoms. Pharmacokinetic interference with absorption, binding or clearance occurs almost entirely with the sulphonylureas; the temporary introduction of an interacting drug can alter the free OAD plasma level, with potentially dangerous consequences. A number of drugs cause a pharmacodynamic interaction by a direct effect on glucose tolerance (Table 9.17). Fortunately, clinically significant problems are relatively rare – and certainly far fewer than the theoretical possibilities. Moreover, different drugs, especially among the sulphonylureas, have different tendencies to show a given interaction.

Pharmacokinetic potentiation
Drugs that increase stomach pH may enhance absorption of sulphonylureas. Highly plasma protein-bound drugs can theoretically displace sulphonylureas; however, following redistribution and alterations in clearance there may be little overall change in free drug levels. Moreover, the newer sulphonylureas bind to different plasma protein sites and are less prone to this effect. The hepatic clearance of sulphonylureas can be reduced by severe liver disease and by enzyme-inhibiting drugs and enhanced by enzyme inducers; similar considerations apply to the meglitinides (*repaglinide*). The thiazolidinedione *troglitazone* is an hepatic enzyme inducer and so care is needed if it is combined with a sulphonylurea. The renal clearance of unchanged drug or active metabolites of any of these drugs can be reduced by renal impairment and by certain drugs.

Pharmacodynamic potentiation
Alcohol is directly hypoglycaemic in fasting conditions, and it may also potentiate biguanide-induced lactic acidosis. Both monoamine oxidase inhibitors and beta-blockers tend to cause hypoglycaemia; the former probably stimulate insulin secretion and the latter inhibit hepatic glycogenolysis. Beta-blockers can 'mask' the effects of hypoglycaemia as perceived by the patient. Beta-blocker interactions are seen if at all mainly with non-cardioselective agents, but aside from those with *propranolol* are rare and usually insignificant. ACEIs enhance glucose uptake and utilization by cells, although the effect may diminish with continued therapy, and is of uncertain significance.

Antagonism
Drugs which induce liver enzymes can increase the clearance of hepatically metabolized sulphonylureas. Various drugs tend to raise blood glucose, either directly or via the suppression of insulin release. Paradoxically, given the masking effect referred to above, beta-blockers can block insulin release.

As a consequence of the inhibited disaccharide digestion, oral treatment of hypoglycaemia in patients taking glucosidase inhibitors should preferably be with glucose/dextrose rather than sucrose preparations.

Contraindications and cautions

The main precautions may be summarized thus:

- Diabetics need to take particular care when

Table 9.17 Important interactions and precautions with antidiabetic therapy

Potentiation → hypoglycaemia	Antagonism → hyperglycaemia
Interference with antidiabetic therapy generally[a]	
Beta-blockers – mask/may cause hypoglycaemia	(Beta-blockers, calcium channel blockers)[b]
ACEIs – increase glucose uptake	Corticosteroids
Alcohol – potentiates hypoglycaemia	Thiazide (and loop) diuretics
Fibrates	
Monoamine oxidase inhibitors	
Interactions with sulphonylureas[c][d]	
Absorption	
(Antacids, H$_2$-receptor antagonists)	
Binding displacement	
Salicylates – high doses	
Hepatic clearance	
Sulphonamides, chloramphenicol	Rifampicin ⎫
Warfarin	Anticonvulsants ⎬ enzyme inducers
Antifungals: imidazoles	Excess alcohol ⎭
Liver failure (enzyme inhibitors)	
Renal clearance	
Phenylbutazone (other NSAIDs)	
Sulfinpyrazone	
Renal impairment	
Interactions with biguanides	
Renal/hepatic impairment	
Alcohol – potentiates lactic acidosis	

[a] Problems here possible with either oral or insulin therapy.

[b] Entries in parentheses are known to be rare or minor.

[c] There are wide variations in the significance of specific interactions with individual oral antidiabetic drugs, and not all possible interactions are indicated. This table is merely to show possible effects and mechanisms. A detailed text is recommended to ascertain clinical significance of an interaction.

[d] Meglitinides (repaglinide) have similar pharmacokinetic properties to the sulphonylureas.

ACEIs, angiotensin converting enzyme inhibitors; NSAIDs, non-steroidal anti-inflammatory drugs.

changing dose, brand or type of antidiabetic medication.

- Medication records should be monitored to identify the introduction of potentially interacting drugs.
- The elderly are particularly prone to hypoglycaemia with the longer-acting OADs; these patients may be forgetful about meals, less able to recognize hypoglycaemia, and homeostatically and neurologically less tolerant of it.
- Alcohol use must be carefully controlled: it enhances hypoglycaemia and may impair the ability to respond to it; alcohol also dangerously enhances the possibility of lactic acidosis with biguanides; it also causes unwelcome flushing with sulphonylureas, particularly chlorpropamide.
- Some clinicians manage all patients with significant renal impairment (common in diabetics) or hepatic impairment (less common) with insulin.

Selection

Sometimes the first drug tried after dietary failure is **acarbose**. Otherwise, the **sulphonylureas** are often the first group tried, although a **biguanide** is preferable for obese patients and is perfectly satisfactory for others. Patients who fail to achieve blood glucose control or who gain weight on sulphonylureas should try biguanides alone or in combination with a sulphonylurea. Acarbose could be added at any of these stages to improve control.

The role of the **thiazolidinediones** (*troglitazone*) has not yet been established by clinical experience (and they are not available at the time of writing). They are recommended for insulin resistance, but they may come to represent a genuine option for first choice. Theoretically, because they have a different mode of action from the other two groups, various combinations should be synergistic or at least additive, but at present a maximum of two drugs combined is recommended (perhaps different combinations being tried) before moving on to insulin.

The **meglitinides** (*repaglinide*) are also too new for their role to be judged. The hope is that they can replace short-acting sulphonylureas in patients who experience hypoglycaemia between meals. They may also find a place as primary therapy for certain patients, allowing flexible regimens where the oral dose and timing are deliberately varied according to meal size and activity.

In addition to these pharmacodynamic considerations, the choice of an oral antidiabetic drug must take account of:

* Duration of action.
* Mode of clearance.
* Patient age.
* Patient renal and hepatic function.
* Patient preference for number of daily doses.
* Patient tolerance of adverse effects.

The elderly must avoid the longer-acting drugs, while other patients may have particular reasons for preferring more or less frequent dosing. By analogy with insulin regimens, a combination of a single daily dose of a long-acting drug, combined with regular top-up doses of a short-acting one, has been recommended, but is little used. In general there is little to choose between the sulphonylureas, but patients with renal impairment might do better with *gliquidone* (Fig. 9.13).

Some patients cannot be controlled on maximally tolerated doses of combined OADs. This may occur after many years of therapy as the beta-cell function inexorably declines (secondary failure, occurring in up to one-third of patients within 5 years). Alternatively some patients present late, when there has already been considerable degeneration (primary failure). Either way, the situation signifies that there remains insufficient residual beta-cell function, and exogenous insulin supplement becomes mandatory. Sometimes at that stage small doses of insulin are added to OAD therapy. This may delay the onset of full insulin therapy, but this strategy is uncommon and not recommended. When Type 2 patients eventually need to be controlled with insulin they do not of course become Type 1, and they may referred to as **insulin-requiring Type 2 diabetics**.

Insulin

About two-thirds of diabetics are treated with insulin, although not all may be strictly insulin-dependent. Patients on insulin require much finer control of all aspects of management, including diet, activity and dose measurement, than other diabetics. There is less margin for error because patients rely totally on the injected dose.

Aims and constraints

In theory, it should be possible to attain glycaemic control with insulin which closely mimics the natural physiological variations in food intake and metabolic requirement. However, for convenience and despite modern insulin formulations, many patients still match their meals and activity throughout the day to a dose of insulin injected in the morning, perhaps supplemented with an evening dose.

Recall that normal insulin secretion into the portal vein from the pancreas is finely and continuously tuned to variations in blood glucose level (p. 531; *see* Fig 9.4): this is very different from the usual exogenous insulin therapy. An approximation might be attained with frequent, precisely calculated intravenous injections of a rapidly acting soluble insulin, given with all meals. This would resemble the natural pattern, except for the portal delivery to the liver and the supply of a basal level. However, such a regimen is impractical for most patients.

From the more usual subcutaneous injection sites, whether as depot injections or by continuous delivery, absorption in any one patient can vary from time to time and from site to site, particularly with the otherwise more convenient longer-acting preparations. Moreover, whereas exercise inhibits normal insulin secretion, it tends to speed absorption from an injection site by promoting peripheral circulation. It is also likely that subcutaneous injections administered by some patients are effectively intramuscular now that perpendicular injection is recommended, changing absorption characteristics. Furthermore, the clearance of all forms of injected insulin is generally slower than endogenous insulin, the half-life of soluble insulin being about 1 h.

Until the advent of the 'insulin pen' system, the most common compromise was to give a mixture of a fast-acting and a moderately long-acting preparation before breakfast (e.g. soluble plus lente), perhaps with a booster dose of soluble in the evening. With appropriate 'feeding the insulin' throughout the day (p. 548), acceptable control can be achieved. However, this results in relative hyperinsulinaemia, a tendency to hypoglycaemia during the day (especially if a meal or snack is missed) and after midnight, and hyperglycaemia before breakfast (*see* Fig. 9.8).

Insulin types

Developments in insulin technology have produced a range of chemically pure, immunologically neutral preparations of standard strength (100 units/mL in the UK and North America) with a variety of pharmacokinetic parameters.

Pharmacokinetic differences
Formulations of insulin can be divided into four broad groups depending on their duration of action; their times of onset and periods of peak activity also vary considerably (Table 9.18). The fastest action is provided by solutions of insulin.

In solution, insulin molecules normally associate (non-covalently) into hexamers, which are progressively disassociated by dilution in body fluids to the active monomer. This process, which delays onset and prolongs duration, can be accelerated by small rearrangements of molecular structure that affect association characteristics but not pharmacodynamic activity. Increased duration is provided by forming stable suspensions of carefully controlled particle size which gradually dissolve in a uniform manner. A number of pre-mixed formulations provide combinations of properties.

Ultra-short action. By synthesizing an insulin analogue with different amino acids near the end of the B chain (lysine and proline at positions B28 and B29), a molecule is produced which exists in monomeric form with little tendency to associate but which has full activity at insulin receptors. *Insulin lispro* has an onset of about 15 min, reaches a higher peak within half the time of conventional soluble insulin (1 h as opposed to 1.5–2.5 h) and a duration of action little greater than 5 h (as opposed to 6–10 h). Thus, it can be injected 0–15 min before a planned meal; the optimal time will need to be determined for each patient. Other insulin analogues are being developed. The range of applications is still being determined but includes:

- Less imposed delay between injection and food intake (especially breakfast), and/or reduction of postprandial hyperglycaemia if delay not observed.
- Convenient pre-meal bolus doses, as part of basal-bolus regimen (pp. 567–568).
- Easier adjustment for unexpected food intake.
- Reduction of between-meals hypoglycaemia caused in some patients by excessive duration of action on regular short-acting preparations.

Since insulin lispro is still expensive, there may currently be little need to change patients who are satisfactorily stabilized on other preparations. There is no point in using insulin lispro intravenously, and its advantages may be reduced if it is premixed with longer-acting preparations – this possibility is still being evaluated, but at present it should probably not be carried out. Patients who do switch need careful

Table 9.18 Approximate pharmacokinetic parameters of insulin preparations[a]

	Insulin preparation	Duration of activity (h)[b]	Retarding agent
Ultra-short	Lispro		
Short	Neutral/soluble (1)[c]		
	Neutral/soluble (2)		
Intermediate	IZS amorphous (semilente)		Zinc
	Biphasic (1)		Protamine
	Biphasic (2)		
	Biphasic (3)		
	Isophane (NPH)		Protamine
	IZS mixed (lente)		Zinc
Prolonged	IZS crystalline (ultralente)		Zinc
	Protamine zinc suspension		Protamine + zinc

Duration of activity axis (h): 1 2 3 4 5 6 7 8 10 12 14 16 18 20 22 24 36

Legend:
- Duration of biological activity
- Peak activity

[a] Data given are only approximate comparative indications. Activity in patients varies with manufacturer, dose, site and technique of injection, etc. (see Table 9.20).
[b]
[c] Numbers in parentheses indicate different forms available in UK.

IZS, insulin zinc suspension; NPH, neutral protamine Hagedorn; Biphasic, generic name for range of mixtures of short- and medium-acting preparations.

re-education about the relative timing of injection and food intake: the use of insulin lispro might also mean less reliance on foods with a low glycaemic index.

Short action.   Clear solutions of *soluble* or *neutral* insulin act a little less rapidly than insulin lispro and are cleared within 6–10 h. They are useful:

- When intravenous use is required (e.g. for ketoacidosis).
- When titrating a newly diagnosed patient's total daily requirement.
- In a continuous infusion system.
- For intensive, multiple daily dose therapy, including basal-bolus regimens.
- For the temporary insulin therapy of Type 2 patients during pregnancy, surgery or severe illness.

Soluble or neutral insulin are currently used also used where an ultra-short-acting preparation may eventually be preferable, i.e.:

- When a booster dose is needed rapidly.
- For the brittle diabetic who needs frequent injections.

Soluble insulin to cover a particular meal should usually be injected 15–30 min, or occasionally 45 min, beforehand. When newly diagnosed Type 1 patients are being assessed they are usually put on an 'insulin sliding scale' regimen, with 4-hourly soluble insulin doses adjusted according to the current blood glucose level.

Intermediate and prolonged action.   Most patients receive part of their daily insulin dose as a depot injection. This is to provide a continuous basal level of insulin for metabolic activity, independent of postprandial glucose disposal. The choice is dictated partly by life pattern and clinician preference, but ultimately by trial and error. Depot preparations are formulated by complexing insulin with either zinc or protamine, a non-allergenic fish protein. This produces a fine suspension that is assimilated at a rate that is dependent on particle size and injection site perfusion. Being a suspension, it cannot be given intravenously. Available products span a wide spectrum of times of onset, peak activity and duration, allowing considerable flexibility in tailoring regimens (Table 9.18).

The *insulin zinc suspension* range contains an insulin–zinc complex in either crystalline or amorphous form, the latter being more readily absorbed. *Insulin zinc suspension* (*amorphous;* formerly 'semilente') is purely amorphous and combines prompt onset with quite prolonged, but rather variable, action. *Insulin zinc suspension* (*mixed*, 'lente') is 30% crystalline and 70% amorphous, and *insulin zinc suspension* (*crystalline;* 'ultralente') is 100% crystalline, with proportionate increases in duration of activity. *Isophane insulin* containing protamine as the retarding agent also has an intermediate activity.

Protamine zinc insulin and ultralente are the longest-acting preparations available. If an excessive dose of this type is injected, the hypoglycaemic effect is correspondingly prolonged and glucose or glucagon injection may be needed to reverse it. Because the variability in response between different preparations increases with the duration of action, even in the same patient, these very long-acting forms are little used.

A variety of premixed *biphasic* preparations (compatible combinations, usually of neutral and isophane forms) are available to provide further flexibility. Some patients mix specific combinations immediately before injection.

Newer approaches being investigated for prolonging action include different chemical analogues, and acylated insulins which bind to plasma albumin to provide a depot effect. Soluble analogues with a more neutral isoelectric point have been developed that crystallize out at the injection site, providing a predictable, consistently sustained action, and avoiding the variability that a suspension formulation usually entails. (One such product, 'NovoSol Basal', had to be withdrawn owing to local inflammation.)

Purity and antigenicity

There are two significant factors here: chemical, and therefore antigenic, similarity to natural (human) insulin; and contamination with extraneous antigenic material. Originally, all insulin was extracted from ox or pig pancreases supplied by slaughterhouses. (Approval for insulin treatment from these sources has been obtained from most major religions, but strict vegans may present a problem.) Beef insulin differs from the human insulin polypeptide sequence by three amino acids, and porcine by just one. These differences affect antigenicity but not hypoglycaemic potency. As may be expected, porcine is the better tolerated, but neither causes great problems.

Contaminants derived from the extraction process, e.g. pro-insulin, insulin breakdown products and other unrelated proteins, can stimulate the production of insulin antibodies, and allergic reactions used to be quite common. Consequently, chromatographic purification is now used giving *highly purified* or *monocomponent* animal insulins which cause far fewer problems.

Human insulin is made either semi-synthetically, by chemically modifying the single variant amino acid in purified porcine insulin (*emp*, enzyme modified porcine), or biosynthetically (*crb*, chain recombinant-DNA bacterial; *prb*, proinsulin recombinant-DNA bacterial; *pyr*, precursor yeast recombinant). Biosynthesis is becoming the preferred process and human insulin now frequently costs less than animal forms.

Unfortunately, the expectation that human insulin would be vastly superior has not been realized. Anti-insulin antibodies are not significantly less common with human insulin than with the highly purified porcine form, and allergic phenomena still occur – probably due to breakdown products occurring during manufacture, storage, etc. Nevertheless, human insulin is the natural choice in patients with severe allergic problems. Most new patients are started on human insulin.

Human insulin is slightly more hydrophilic than animal forms. Thus, although it has an identical biological action to pork insulin when given intravenously, it is assimilated more rapidly from subcutaneous sites and acts more quickly in otherwise identical formulations. It is also cleared more rapidly, possibly by binding more avidly to those hepatic and renal enzymes that destroy it. These differences are slight and only relevant to patients transferring from one form to the other.

Adverse reactions

The chief adverse effects of insulin are hypoglycaemia, injection site problems, immunological phenomena and resistance. These may be partially inter-related.

Hypoglycaemia

This is the most common complication of insulin therapy and potentially the most harmful; the clinical aspects were discussed on pp. 539–540. Insulin can cause hypoglycaemia either through an excessive (e.g. mis-measured) dose or through an unexpectedly reduced insulin requirement (most commonly, a missed meal).

Human insulin has been associated with an apparent increase in the incidence of hypoglycaemic attacks, including some deaths. This was initially attributed to a reduced hypoglycaemic awareness, i.e. hypoglycaemia is not more common but is permitted to progress more frequently. The autonomic warning symptoms of hypoglycaemia (*see* Table 9.12) seemed to be experienced less intensely or at a later stage when using human insulin, perhaps owing to autonomic (sympathetic) neuropathy.

There is no pharmacodynamic rationale for this phenomenon and it has been suggested that it is only incidentally related to human insulin use. The change to human insulin came at a time when the need for tighter control became apparent and aids to this (e.g. injector pens, home blood glucose monitoring) were developed. Improved control produces lower mean glucose levels and therefore an increased chance of hypoglycaemia. Thus it is not now regarded as a serious problem of human insulin, although it is stressed that great care is necessary in transferring a patient to human insulin. Close monitoring is essential and the daily dose may need to be reduced, particularly when changing from beef insulin or for patients with a higher than average daily insulin requirement.

Injection site lipodystrophy

Some patients develop unsightly lumps (lipohypertrophy) or hollows (lipoatrophy) at frequently used injection sites if they fail to change the site regularly. These are not due to scar tissue but are caused by local disturbances of lipid metabolism. **Lipoatrophy** seems to be an immunological phenomenon; possibly immune complex deposition stimulates lipolysis in subcutaneous adipose tissue. It responds to changing to a purer form of insulin, initially injected around the depression. **Lipohypertrophy** is more common with the newer insulins and may result from enhanced local lipogenesis, a known insulin action. It is reversed when the site is no longer used. Although patients prefer to inject at these easily penetrated, relatively painless sites, such an approach results in delayed and erratic absorption.

Insulin antibodies and insulin resistance

Insulin antibodies (insulin-binding globulins) occur in up to 50% of insulin-treated patients. It might be expected that they would speed the clearance of insulin by forming immune complexes which would be eliminated in the usual way by the monocyte–macrophage system. However, on the contrary, insulin antibodies delay assimilation and prolong the action and so are potentially beneficial. They are otherwise usually harmless, although they may sometimes be responsible for insulin resistance (see below).

Insulin **allergy** ranges from minor local irritation to, very rarely, full-blown anaphylaxis. The less serious reactions commonly remit on prolonged use and are minimized by using the highly purified modern insulin formulations as first choice. The size of the insulin molecule is borderline for antigenicity. Hyposensitization has been used to treat insulin allergy, by injecting extremely dilute insulin solutions at progressively higher concentrations to induce tolerance. Very

occasionally, local steroid injections need to be given with the insulin.

The term **insulin resistance** tends to be used in an ambiguous manner (Table 9.19). In pathogenetic terms, it refers to one of the common underlying problems of Type 2 diabetes, namely reduced receptor sensitivity. As an adverse effect of insulin treatment, it refers to the requirement in some insulin-dependent diabetics for doses of insulin far above the physiological norm.

In this latter sense, insulin resistance occurs only rarely and may be defined as an insulin requirement greater than 1.5 units/kg/day (about 100 units daily in an average patient). There are many possible causes; probably the most common is simply obesity, but poor injection technique may be an unsuspected problem. Insulin resistance is less common now with the use of the monocomponent and human formulations. Treatment involves eliminating any obvious cause and then gradually switching to a highly purified or human insulin. As a final resort, systemic steroids, which are themselves diabetogenic, may be needed.

Administration

Delivery systems

Standard syringe. The multiple use of disposable plastic syringes with fixed needles has become widespread in the UK, despite official

Table 9.19 Some possible causes of insulin resistance

Metabolic	Obesity
	Increased catabolic hormones
	Interacting diabetogenic drugs (e.g. steroids)
Immunological	Anti-insulin antibodies
	Anti-insulin-receptor antibodies
Pharmacokinetic or biopharmaceutic	Poor injection technique
	Increased insulinase activity
	Reduced assimilation from injection site
	• local enzymic degradation
	• scar tissue
	• lipohypertrophy
Genetic	Receptor defect

disapproval. It is has been claimed by some diabetologists and pharmacists that these syringes may be used for up to 1 week without significant contamination of the vial contents (which contain a bacteriostat) and no increase in skin reactions. Patients change the syringe when the needle is blunted or the barrel graduations become unclear. Injection through clothing, long practised by some diabetics, has also been reported to not cause significant problems.

The BDA formerly permitted syringe use up to five times, but now specify compliance with manufacturers' labels, and these always specify single use. Similarly, pharmacists can recommend only the official policy of single use and standard injection method. Patients must also use a safe method of contaminated waste and 'sharps' disposal.

Pen injectors. A significant innovation is the multidose insulin reservoir injector pen. This has up to 300 units (up to 1 week's supply for some patients) loaded in a replaceable cartridge. One form of pen automatically delivers a 2-unit dose for each depression of a trigger, i.e. 2 units per 'click', a situation that is particularly beneficial to visually impaired diabetics; another form permits full doses up to 96 units to be preset visually on a digital scale. The two advantages are ease of correct measurement (and hence less error) and the facilitation of multiple daily dosing, which can provide better control.

Artificial pancreas. The ideal replacement pancreas still resists practicable construction. One experimental approach involves a feedback-controlled, blood-glucose driven 'closed loop' system. An intravenous catheter monitors blood glucose continuously and the results are fed to a microprocessor which calculates the instantaneous insulin requirement. This drives a portable pump, strapped to or implanted in the patient, delivering the appropriate dose. The main problem is designing a suitably sensitive indwelling blood glucose monitor. In another system, an implanted insulin reservoir enclosed in a glucose-sensitive gel membrane permits insulin diffusion in proportion to external glucose concentration. The reservoir is replenished percutaneously.

Other forms. 'Open loop' systems are already available, with pumps (even percutaneously replenished implantable ones) linked to microprocessors that calculate dose according to the independently measured glucose level. If these can deliver insulin into the peritoneal cavity, they have the theoretical advantage of more closely mimicking the natural insulin secretion. Diabetics with advanced nephropathy on continuous ambulatory peritoneal dialysis find it convenient to add insulin to their dialysis fluid. Percutaneous jet injection has also been tried, with some success.

Simple oral administration is impossible because of intragastric enzymic destruction. Systems are being developed which avoid this but do not require the complications of injection. One approach is to incorporate insulin into liposomes that would be taken orally. The lipid coat would act like an enteric coating and the liposomes would be absorbed unchanged from the gut, as are chylomicrons. By analogy with vasopressin (another polypeptide), intranasal administration is being investigated, using a liposomal or polymer vehicle. Another possibility being explored is pulmonary absorption via a metered dose inhaler.

Storage

Insulin should always be kept cool, but is stable at room temperatures for up to 28 days. Newer formulations incorporating polyethylene–polypropylene glycol, specially developed for prolonged reservoir use, are stable for even longer. Thus, insulin may safely be used in pens and continuous subcutaneous infusion, etc. and while travelling. Pharmacy stocks and patients' reserve supplies are refrigerated (**but not frozen**). Before withdrawing a dose, the vial should be warmed to body temperature and gently mixed by inversion or rotation.

Mixing

If a combination of two preparations of different durations is required, specially formulated proprietary mixtures should be used whenever possible, and extemporaneous mixing avoided. The insulin zinc suspension (lente) formulations are intended to be stable after intermixing but others are not, and if so used must be injected within 5 min. One problem is the adsorption of the soluble form onto the retardant from the longer-acting one, which may seriously interfere with the expected rapid action of the former. The order of mixing is important: the soluble form is drawn up first, then the depot form. This prevents contamination of the whole vial of soluble insulin by zinc or protamine.

Injection

Now shorter needles have become available, deep subcutaneous injection perpendicular to the skin is universally recommended (rather than the original 45° into a pinch of skin). Most patients cope well, but instruction and counselling when treatment is started are clearly important, especially with children. The BDA and a number of interested manufacturers produce helpful literature on this and all other aspects of diabetic care.

Equally important is the need to rotate the site of injection regularly so that any one site is only used once in 10–20 injections. Seven general areas are recommended by the BDA (upper arms, thighs, buttocks, abdomen), but within these areas the precise injection site used on one occasion can be avoided on the next; the BDA provides a template to assist such variation. This minimizes skin reactions, especially lipohypertrophy. Patients can also use the slower assimilation sites, e.g. thighs, for the overnight dose. Sites usually covered by clothing are preferred. Factors which may alter absorption from the injection site, possibly upsetting control, are summarized in Table 9.20

Dose regimens

An initial dose titration period on first starting insulin will indicate the total daily dose that the patient requires, but decisions on how this is to be distributed throughout the day require discussion with the patient. A balance must be maintained between the risk of hyperglycaemia (with increased chronic complications) and that of hypoglycaemia (with its threat of coma), while imposing no more restriction on the patient's life than they are prepared to tolerate. This is not easy. Factors to consider are:

* Age.
* Severity of complications.
* Occupation and social habits.
* Ethnic and religious constraints.
* Compliance.
* Physical disabilities.
* Comprehension of disease, prescribed regimen and associated equipment.
* Patient preference.

The choice ranges from multiple daily injections of short-acting insulin closely co-ordinated with eating and activity pattern, to a convenient but very unphysiological single daily dose of a longer-acting preparation (Table 9.21).

Table 9.20   Factors affecting insulin absorption from injection site

Factor	Example	Effect on absorption	
		Slower/reduced	Faster/increased
Pharmaceutical	Incorrect mixing of delayed and rapid forms (especially if injection delayed)	+	–
	Depth of injection	+	+
Local inactivation	Proteolytic enzymes	+	–
	Insulin antibodies	+	–
Local perfusion	Regional differences (abdomen > arm > thigh)	+	+
	Exercise (in limb sites); massage	–	+
	Skin temperature	+	+
	Angiopathy	+	–
	Scar tissue	+	–
	Lipohypertrophy	+	–

Table 9.21   Some examples of insulin regimens

Regimen	Before breakfast	Before lunch	Before evening meal	Bedtime	Examples of patient groups suited to the regimen
1	Long[a] ± short	–	–	–	Insulin-requiring Type 2; Some elderly patients
2	Intermediate + short	–	Intermediate + short	–	Many Type 1
3	Intermediate + short	–	Short	Intermediate	Many Type 1
4	Short	Short	Short	Intermediate	Well-motivated Type 1 Unstable Morning hyperglycaemia and/or nocturnal hypoglycaemia

[a] Duration of action.

Minimum dose regimens

Because of the supposed compliance benefits of few daily injections, this method used to be favoured. However, it imposes inflexibility on activity patterns and mealtimes, or else risks poor control, and so is no longer preferred. The regimen usually consists of morning and evening doses of a combination of short- and medium-acting preparations, the relative doses being determined by trial and error.

There are numerous potential variations. For example, the morning dose could be a mix of about one-third soluble and two-thirds intermediate-acting forms, which covers breakfast and provides a sustained level throughout the day. This may be repeated in the evening – or later in those patients who get serious pre-breakfast hyperglycaemia – or there may simply be a booster dose of soluble before the evening meal. If one of the commercially available combinations can be used it is certainly convenient, especially if a pen is used. More flexibility is provided by individually determined combinations, but then a pen cannot be used.

Alternatively, some patients can be controlled satisfactorily with just a single dose of a long-acting form. These include Type 2 patients with significant residual endogenous insulin production in whom oral antidiabetic drugs have failed, and some elderly patients requiring only symptomatic relief and for whom the threat of long-term complications is less critical.

Multiple injections

These are now favoured for all patients who can manage to self-inject frequent doses of soluble insulin throughout the day, before each food intake. In addition, a morning dose of medium-acting insulin is given for basal needs, and possibly a moderately sustained action formulation overnight for those with morning hyperglycaemia. Within the admitted limitations of regular injections this **basal-bolus** regimen offers the greatest flexibility and most closely mimics the physiological situation.

A multiple injection regimen is especially useful for brittle patients requiring close control, or for temporary transfer of patients to insulin, e.g. Type 2 patients during pregnancy or with serious infections. However, many clinics are starting most new patients on such a regimen, for which injector pens are ideal. Existing patients are also being converted. Many patients can, with experience, finely judge the dose required according to their food intake and exercise.

The improved, more physiological control provided by this type of regimen reduces the development or progression of complications; in some trials they have even remitted. Such regimens can also, if properly used, minimize the risk of hypoglycaemia between meals and of overnight hyperglycaemia.

Continuous subcutaneous insulin infusion

This 'open loop' system is used by some clinics for particularly brittle patients. A portable pump strapped outside the body delivers a continuous basal level of insulin via an indwelling intraperitoneal catheter, with mealtime boosts being manually activated. Although quite successful, these systems are as yet too bulky, expensive and demanding of patients' motivation for general use.

Summary

Diabetes therapy must be individualized following regular close consultation between patients and their clinicians. To a certain extent the optimal result is found by trial and error, but this must be supported by diligent monitoring of blood glucose and reporting of all hypoglycaemic episodes and other disturbances of control.

Monitoring

Diabetics require self-monitoring of their day-to-day biochemical control, and regular assessment by a clinician of the development or progress of long-term complications. The former has recently been much simplified and improved.

Biochemical control

While even moderate control relieves symptoms and prevents serious biochemical abnormalities, very tight control is believed to be essential if complications are to be minimized. In general, diligent monitoring is more important for Type 1 diabetics, but all patients should record all test results.

Glucose

Urine glucose

This has been the traditional way of assessing control. A few elderly diabetics still use the colour reaction based on Benedict's test for reducing substances. It is imprecise, non-specific and cumbersome, even with the ingeniously formulated 'Clinitest' reagent tablets.

Urine glucose estimations can never provide precise information about current blood glucose levels, particularly low, potentially hypoglycaemic ones. Urinary concentrations will vary according to urine volume independently of blood glucose. Furthermore, aglycosuria does not necessarily guarantee normoglycaemia, owing to differences in renal threshold between patients and in the same patient at different times.

Nevertheless, urine testing remains useful as a simple initial screen and for Type 2 patients not prone to hypoglycaemia when tight control is not essential, e.g. the elderly. A trial of testing blood and urine glucose simultaneously may subsequently allow confident prediction of blood glucose from urinary measurements within acceptable limits provided a certain urine level is not exceeded. Some patients may be monitored adequately by regular urinalysis and occasional blood glucose measurements, once the relationship between the two has been established. Others cannot tolerate the regular finger pricking required for blood glucose monitoring.

Urinary glucose measurement also has the advantage that timing is less important than with blood testing because urine concentration reflects control over the previous several hours. Thus, newer glucose oxidase-based urine dipsticks have been developed that are more specific for glucose and far more convenient because they can simply be passed through the urine stream.

Blood glucose

Most patients, especially with Type 1 disease, are now encouraged to measure their blood glucose directly using a drop of blood from a finger prick on a glucose oxidase stick. This provides an immediate measure of glycaemia which is reasonably accurate and reliable, not overly prone to error from poor technique, and easy to read. Most sticks have two scales to cover different ranges. For patients with visual problems, simple colorimeters are available which display the result digitally, and may give audible warnings. Newer devices can store the most recent 100 results, for reporting at clinics. Various spring-operated skin puncture devices may be used to help obtain the blood drop easily and safely, and percutaneous techniques of measurement are being developed.

A few Type 1 patients regularly test four times daily, including fasting and postprandial measures, but this is necessary only in the more erratic, brittle patients, in intensive multiple dose regimens in younger patients, or when previously well-controlled patients start to experience problems. Others will do it randomly a few times weekly and some may perhaps use urine dipsticks daily. The main guideline is to identify a patient's risk times (e.g. between-meal hypos, postprandial hyperglycaemia) and subject those to special scrutiny. Patients who are suitably motivated and educated by the diabetic team will be able to modify their insulin dose on the basis of the results. The occasional fasting blood glucose measurement is usually sufficient in Type 2 patients.

Glycated (glycosylated) haemoglobin

The abnormal, quantitative glycation of systemic protein as a consequence of excess blood glucose (p. 541) applies also to blood proteins, including haemoglobin and albumin, as well as to plasma fructosamine. Because these substances remain in the blood for long periods (120 days for haemoglobin, 7–14 days for the others), their glycation gives a long-term, integrated picture of blood glucose levels over those periods. This can be measured at diabetic clinics and is useful in tracing any problems with control which might not be revealed by patients' tendency to be extra meticulous on the few days before each clinic visit.

The glycated haemoglobin level give the best index of the control needed to minimize complications and is now regarded as the 'gold standard'. Non-diabetics have about 5% of glycated haemoglobin (HbA_{1c}) and the target level for optimal diabetes control is currently below 7%.

Ketones

Regular ketonuria monitoring is unnecessary for Type 2 and most Type 1 patients, but is essential in brittle ketosis-prone diabetics, and in all during periods of stress such as infection or pregnancy. Great accuracy is not required and urine dipsticks are adequate because any ketonuria at all in the presence of glycosuria indicates a dangerous loss of control. Combined glucose/ketone sticks are preferred, especially as heavy ketonuria may interfere with some standard glucose sticks.

Clinical monitoring

In addition to biochemical monitoring, less frequent but regular medical examination is important in the long-term care of diabetics. This will identify as early as possible the development of any of the many possible systemic complications. Table 9.22 lists the factors which need to be monitored at intervals which will vary from patient to patient.

Table 9.22   Regular assessment in diabetic clinic

System	Test or examination
Biochemical	Glycated haemoglobin
	Blood lipids, body weight
Feet	Chiropody; pulses
Eye	Fundoscopy, acuity, cataract
Renal	Proteinuria, creatinine (clearance)
Neurological	Detailed sensory, motor and autonomic neurological examination
Cardiovascular	Blood pressure, ECG, peripheral perfusion (pulses, etc.)
	Symptoms of ischaemia

References and further reading

Alberti KGMM, Defronzo RA, Zimmet P, eds (1997) *International Textbook of Diabetes Mellitus*. 2nd edn. Chichester: John Wiley.

Day JL (1998) *Living with Diabetes. The British Diabetic Association guide for those treated with diet and tablets*. Chichester: John Wiley.

Day JL (1998) *Living with Diabetes. The British Diabetic Association guide for those treated with insulin*. Chichester: John Wiley.

Diabetes Control and Complications Trial Research Group (1993) The effect of intensive treatment of diabetes on the development and progression of long-term complications in insulin dependent diabetes mellitus. *N Engl J Med* **329**: 977–986.

Diabetes in the United Kingdom – 1996 (1995) London: British Diabetic Association.

Nathan DM (1998) Some answers, more controversy, from UKPDS. *Lancet* **352**: 832–833.

Nutrition subcommittee of the British Diabetic Association (1992) Dietary recommendations for people with diabetes: an update for the 1990s. *Diabetic Med* **9**: 198–202.

Watkins PJ (1998) *ABC of Diabetes*. 4th edn. London: BMJ Publishing Group.

10

Pain and its treatment

Pain is a common presenting symptom in primary care and an important cause of morbidity. Patients with mild to moderate pain self-medicate initially, using familiar analgesics or following pharmacist or lay advice. Those with severe pain normally present to GPs or hospitals. The large psychological and cultural components may cause stoics to ignore a pain until the condition is difficult to salvage: doctors have dismissed the pain of their own myocardial infarction as 'indigestion'! Despite its universality and the existence of effective remedies, journal articles frequently discuss the poor management of post-operative, chronic and terminal disease pain.

This chapter discusses the characteristics and pharmacotherapy of various types of pain, to guide best practice. Morphine-like drugs are referred to here as 'opioids', though this term strictly describes only synthetic compounds, 'opiates' being of natural origin. The term 'narcotic' is not synonymous with 'opioid': it describes CNS depressants which relieve pain, producing narcosis (sedation and unconsciousness) at high doses. It is widely used legally for addictive drugs of abuse.

Introduction

Although pain is a universal experience, it is difficult to define. One possible definition is:

> An unpleasant sensory and emotional experience associated with actual or potential tissue damage or described in terms of such damage. It serves biological functions, warning of external danger (e.g. excessive heat or physical trauma) and internal pathology (e.g. inflammation or blockage of a ureter by a kidney stone), enabling avoidance or treatment. It is inherently self-limiting when the provoking source is removed or cured.

This indicates that pain is not simply a physical sensation. Pain perception also depends on the patient's emotional reaction to the stimulus (see below).

Types of pain

Acute pain usually has a definable cause and often performs a protective function, acting as a warning of an external threat or of internal malfunction. Acute pain has a well-defined time of onset, often associated with signs of hyperactivity of the autonomic nervous system, e.g. tachycardia, hypertension and pallor, depending on the severity of the symptoms and how they are interpreted by the patient. The best way of managing acute pain is to diagnose and treat the cause, though temporary relief with analgesics is valuable while healing and recovery proceed.

Pain that has lasted for longer than 6 months is usually considered to be **chronic**. This type of pain often does not signify any immediate danger that requires avoidance and the patient may not interpret such pain as indicating serious disease. Further, adaptation by the autonomic nervous system as the situation develops may lead to the absence of objective physical signs. However, there is often progressive physical deterioration, with sleep disturbance and weight loss. In many cases patients undergo serious affective and behavioural changes, e.g. severe depression.

Essential components in the treatment of chronic pain are the identification of any organic problem, i.e. accurate diagnosis, and recognition of significant affective and environmental factors.

Pain threshold and assessment

The patient's mood, morale and the meaning of the pain for that patient affect their pain perception. Thus if a patient has chest pain and a relative or close friend has recently had a myocardial infarction, the patient may interpret his or her pain as a life-threatening event. Conversely, if another friend with similar pain interprets it as indigestion, this would not be very stressful, the pain threshold would not be lowered, and the pain may be tolerated. Attention must always be paid to factors that modulate the pain threshold (Table 10.1).

Table 10.1 Factors affecting the pain threshold

Threshold lowered	Threshold raised
Insomnia, fatigue	Sleep, rest
Discomfort, pain (presence or fear of recurrence)	Relief of symptoms,
Anxiety, depression, sadness	Sympathy, anxiolytics, antidepressants
Fear, anger, social and mental isolation	Companionship, understanding
Boredom	Diversional activity, occupational therapy

Assessment

Pain is a subjective experience, so only the patient knows its nature and severity: the patient's own assessment and description are vital. Useful clues can be gained from a patient's response to a particular analgesic, e.g. if pain is described as 'severe' but relief is obtained from modest doses of paracetamol (acetaminophen), it is probable that there is a significant emotional component to the pain perception. Careful, sympathetic exploration of this aspect may be more rewarding than the use of increasingly potent analgesics.

The origin of acute pain is usually easy to diagnose, unlike that of chronic pain, which is often of obscure origin, particularly when it is due to non-malignant disease. A careful assessment should be carried out before treatment is started and patients should be re-assessed regularly. The salient features to be elucidated are given in Table 10.2.

Pathophysiology of pain

An understanding of how the sensation of pain is generated is essential to an appreciation of how modification of these pain pathways can ameliorate the pain.

Gate theory

Various theories have tried to integrate the anatomical pain pathways and the psychological and neurological components that contribute to the perception of pain. The generally accepted model is the 'gate control theory', illustrated diagrammatically in Fig. 10.1. This was first proposed by Melzack and Wall in 1965, and has since been modified as knowledge has increased. The theory proposes that neuronal impulses generated by noxious stimuli are modified in the dorsal horn of the spinal cord by a specialized mechanism ('gate'), which can tend either to inhibit or facilitate transmission of the pain impulse from peripheral organs to the brain. The gate is not an 'all-or-none' mechanism, and a balance between opposing factors determines how much of the initial nerve impulse is transmitted through it.

Pain receptors and fibres

Three main groups of skin receptors have been identified:

- Low-threshold mechanoreceptors (which detect light touch).
- Thermoreceptors (which detect heat).
- Nociceptors (which detect injury and noxious (harmful) stimulation). Whereas most skin receptors have a specialized structure, these are simply bare nerve endings in the periphery.

Also, stretch receptors occur in the wall of the gut and the capsules of internal organs.

Three types of nerve fibres are involved in pain transmission. The **A-beta fibres** are large, myelinated, fast-conducting (30–100 m/sec) fibres. They have a low stimulation threshold and respond to light touch. The **A-delta fibres** are

---

Table 10.2   Assessment of pain

The following aspects should be elucidated while taking the history:
- site, distribution, radiation from initial site
- severity (subjective, and score on visual analogue scale)
- nature (dull, sharp, lancinating, etc.)
- mode of onset, duration of episodes, time course of the problem
- aggravating and relieving factors
- response to previous therapy, analgesics used and effective dose
- previous history of similar pain
- meaning of the pain to the patient, e.g. fear of malignancy
- concurrent diseases and treatment

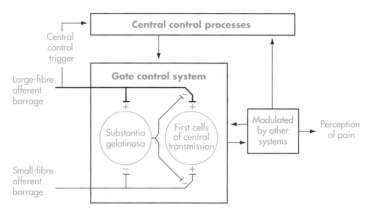

Figure 10.1   Gate control theory of the transmission of pain impulses. +, excitation; –, inhibition.

small, lightly myelinated and slower-conducting (6–30 m/sec). The A-delta fibres respond to pressure, heat, chemicals and cooling, and give rise to the sensation of sharp pain, producing reflex withdrawal or other prompt action. The **C fibres** are small and unmyelinated and therefore slow-conducting (1–2.5 m/sec); they respond to all types of noxious stimuli and transmit more prolonged, dull pain. The last two of these fibres usually require high-intensity stimuli to trigger a response.

According to the gate control theory, A-delta and C-fibres transmit pain signals to the dorsal horns of the spinal cord. Impulses in these fibres can be modulated by A-beta activity which can selectively block impulses from being transmitted to the transmission cells of the **substantia gelatinosa** of the spinal cord. Such blockage prevents upward transmission to the CNS, and no pain sensation is perceived. This explains why rubbing an injured area, or applying a 'counter-irritant', which stimulates the A-beta fibres, can relieve the pain caused by an injury to that area, which stimulates the smaller C-fibres.

The gate control mechanism is believed to operate continuously, even in absence of an apparent trigger, because there is a continuous barrage of impulses from, principally, the C-fibres, whose receptors are continually active and react only slowly to stimuli. The effect is to set a threshold below which there is no effector response. Action subsequent to stimulation depends on the numbers of fibres involved, their firing rate, the proportion of large and small

fibres, and the effect of central control mechanisms. The latter may over-ride the gate control, as occurs under hypnosis. When the complexities of this mechanism have been elucidated, new drugs or techniques of pain control may emerge.

Pathological pain

It has been suggested that peripheral tissue damage, e.g. from trauma, surgery or cancer, causes **central sensitization**, i.e. neuronal changes occur which make the spinal neurones hyper-responsive for a long period to afferent signals that would not normally trigger the gating mechanism. One consequence of this theory is that prophylactic ('pre-emptive') local, regional or opioid analgesia should be given **before** surgery or any predictable moderate to severe pain, to prevent central sensitization occurring. The concept also accords well with our experience of treating severe chronic pain: for effective control it is essential that the pain is not allowed to recur (see below).

New classes of analgesics are emerging, e.g. compounds which block spinal cord receptors for excitatory amino acids such as *N*-methyl-D-aspartate (NMDA). One such drug is *dizocilpine*, which blocks the NMDA ion channel and resembles *ketamine*, but has a much greater potency and is more selective for the receptor. Dizocilpine has been shown to prevent and eliminate central sensitization in animals. Further, recent Swedish research indicates that ketamine is an effective analgesic at concentrations lower than those required to produce anaesthesia, or at which central nervous side effects (hallucinations and other transient psychotic effects) are troublesome. However, UK experience is that few patients can be maintained on *ketamine* for more than a few days. Other general anaesthetics are widely used for the relief of obstetric pain (p. 615).

Neurotransmitters involved in pain

Opioid receptors and endogenous opioids

The important discoveries of stereospecific opioid receptors, of which several sub-types are known, and endogenous opioids further increased our understanding of the biochemical mechanisms involved in pain transmission and perception.

Several families of endogenous opioids have now been identified including the **endorphins**, **enkephalins** and **dynorphins** (p. 581). Each family is derived from a distinct precursor polypeptide and has a characteristic anatomical distribution.

Other transmitters and mediators

Physical or chemical insult can stimulate nociceptors. Inflammation, ischaemia or other pain-inducing stimuli cause the release of noxious chemicals, e.g. bradykinin, histamine and 5-hydroxytryptamine (5HT), in injured tissues. Prostaglandins, although not directly producing pain, appear to sensitize nociceptors to various chemical and pressure stimuli.

Substance P (neurokinin-1), a polypeptide probably released by the small-diameter C-fibres, is believed to be involved in pain transmission in the dorsal horns of the spinal cord. It is probably not the actual transmitter, but initiates a series of events leading to the recruitment of pro-inflammatory agents. The latter release mediators, e.g. prostaglandins, leukotrienes, 5HT, histamine, which stimulate the nerve endings and cause sensitization. Sensitization involves a lowering of the trigger threshold, producing **hyperalgesia**. Excitatory amino acid transmitters, e.g. glutamate, aspartate, may also be involved.

Pain transmission may be blocked if opioid receptors have already been occupied by endorphins at the spinal level. If successful in passing through the gating mechanisms (several are probably involved in the total pathway), the pain impulse is transmitted via the reticular activating system of the pons and midbrain to the thalamus. From there they are directed to the appropriate part of the cerebral cortex where the impulses are perceived as pain. The limbic system, which is anatomically close to these areas, is thought to be responsible for the emotional component of pain (*see* Chapter 7). Transmission of the pain impulse may be modified in the central nervous system by the presence of 5HT and other chemical mediators.

The exact pathophysiology of pain is extremely complex and is still not fully understood. Figure 10.2 shows a simplified concept of the pain pathway and ways in which current treatments are thought to interrupt it.

Principles of analgesic use

The World Health Organization (WHO) recommendation on how to achieve effective analgesia is:

> Dose patients by the mouth, by the clock and by the ladder.

These points, and the general principles which should be employed when using analgesics, are outlined below.

Type and characteristics of pain

Because various types of treatment are available to manage pain (Fig. 10.3), it is important to determine whether the pain is acute or chronic, to diagnose the cause, and to ascertain if any psychogenic component is present before deciding on the appropriate approach to treatment.

Acute pain generally responds well to analgesics, but chronic pain presents a far more complex problem. It often requires a multidisciplinary approach, employing several different modes of therapy. While the main emphasis in

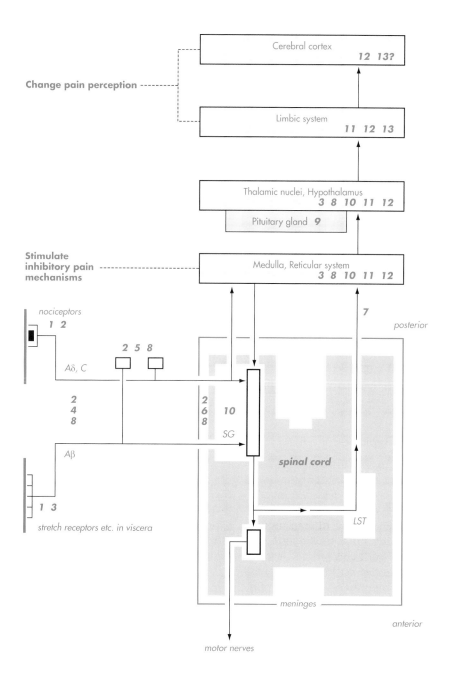

Figure 10.2 Methods of interrupting pain pathways and their possible sites of action. LST, lateral spinothalamic tract; SG, substantia gelatinosa. Aβ, Aδ, C, types of pain fibres; ?, possible effect or site. Bold numbers indicate methods or agents and their sites of action: 1, non-opioid analgesics; 2, local anaesthetics; 3, weak opioids; 4, peripheral somatic nerve block; 5, spinal somatic (extravertebral) nerve block; 6, spinal block; 7, cordotomy (usually in the cervical region); 8, electrical nerve stimulation?, acupuncture?; 9, pituitary gland ablation; 10, opioids (exogenous and endogenous); 11, psychotropic analgesic adjuncts; 12, anaesthetics (inhalation); 13, hypnosis.

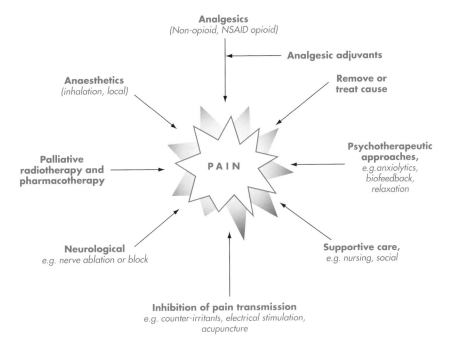

Figure 10.3   Summary of approaches to pain control.

this chapter is on analgesics, alternative methods of pain control will also be discussed briefly, to place them in context.

Choice of analgesic

The type and severity of the pain will usually determine the specific drug or regimen to be used. The appropriate potency of analgesic is found by moving swiftly up the 'analgesic ladder' (Table 10.3) until pain control is achieved. Table 10.3 provides only an outline of the analgesics used, a more comprehensive listing being given in Table 10.4. The use of many of these drugs may be a matter of personal preference or convenience: it is always preferable to learn to use a few drugs well, rather than a wide range indifferently.

Individualization of dosage

Dose requirements are affected by many variables including the severity of the pain, the patient's pain threshold, age, weight and the presence of concurrent disease. Each analgesic should be given an adequate trial by dose titration, i.e. increasing the dose until pain control is adequate or until dose-limiting side effects occur, before switching to another drug.

When using opioids in terminal care patients, the only upper limit is that dose which successfully relieves the patient's pain without causing unacceptable side effects. For example, sedation is only a problem if it becomes coma, but respiratory depression is important, especially if respiratory function is already compromised.

Dosage schedule

Traditionally, pain relief has been given on a 'when required' basis, so that the patient was expected to experience a return of pain before requesting more analgesic. Such an approach may sometimes be useful in acute pain, to see whether the symptoms are regressing, but is inappropriate in treating chronic pain because pain itself is a potent **algesic** (pain promoter): if pain is allowed to recur, a higher dose of analgesic will be required to re-establish pain control.

Table 10.3   The 'analgesic' ladder

Step[a]	Type of analgesic	Preferred analgesic	Possible alternatives
1	Non-opioid ± adjuvants[b]	Paracetamol (acetaminophen)	Aspirin NSAID (diclofenac, flurbiprofen, ibuprofen, indometacin, ketoprofen, naproxen)
If pain persists or increases move to:			
2	Weak opioid Weak opioid ± non-opioid[c] ± adjuvants	Codeine	Dihydrocodeine, dextropropoxyphene (propoxyphene) Ketorolac
If pain persists or increases move to			
3	Strong opioid ± non-opioid ± adjuvants	Morphine	Fentanyl, diamorphine (heroin)[d], hydromorphone, methadone, oxycodone[d], nalbuphine, pethidine (meperidine), phenazocine, tramadol

[a] If drug in one class fails after an adequate dose/time interval trial, move up the ladder: do not use another drug from the same class (*see* Table 10.4).

[b] See p. 591.

[c] Common combinations in the UK are paracetamol (acetaminophen) with codeine (co-codamol), with dextropropoxyphene (propoxyphene) (co-proxamol) or with dihydrocodeine (co-dydramol).

[d] Diamorphine is illegal in the USA. Oxycodone is available in the USA; not generally in the UK.

NSAID, non-steroidal anti-inflammatory drug.

Thus, regular administration of analgesics is essential in chronic pain so that the patient's memory of the pain is reduced and, hopefully, gradually obliterated. This controls the psychological component and associated fear. When the patient has confidence in prescriber and treatment, the pain threshold may be raised, making it possible to reduce the analgesic dose.

The drugs, and their dose level, frequency and routes of administration (see below), must be reviewed frequently to ensure not only that analgesia is adequate but also that doses of concurrent drugs are appropriate and that side effects are minimized and managed suitably.

Routes of administration

In selecting the most appropriate route of drug administration for a patient, factors such as 'nil-by-mouth', gastrointestinal obstruction, limited venous access or reduced muscle mass have to be taken into account.

Oral and sublingual

The **oral route** (per os, PO) is preferred if it is available, though some opioids, e.g. *pethidine (meperidine)*, are poorly absorbed from the gut and bioavailability can vary widely between patients. The peak effect usually occurs 30–60 min after dosing with normal oral formulations. Because peak activity occurs much later with most modified-release preparations, it is inappropriate to initiate pain control with these products. Ideally, the total daily requirement should be determined using a standard-release formulation, i.e. one with maximum bioavailability, preferably in solution form. However, tablets may be used, e.g. with *morphine*, if the solution is disliked. This dose is then translated to an equivalent of a

Table 10.4   Some analgesics in current use

Pain severity[a]	Drug	Class[b]	Routes of administration[c]					
			PO	BC	SC	IM	IV	Re
Severe	Morphine[d]	A	✓	–	✓	✓	sl	✓
	Diamorphine (heroin)[d]	A	✓	–	✓	✓	sl	–
	Hydromorphone	A	✓	–	–	–	–	–
	Levorphanol	A	✓	–	✓	✓	✓	–
	Methadone	A	✓	–	✓	✓	–	–
	Nalbuphine	A	–	–	✓	✓	✓	–
	Phenazocine[d]	A	✓	✓	–	–	–	–
	Dextromoramide[d]	A	✓	–	–	–	–	✓
	Dipipanone	A	✓	–	–	–	–	–
	Fentanyl[e]	A	–	–	–	–	✓	–
	Alfentanil	A	–	–	–	–	✓	–
	Remifentanil	A	–	–	–	–	✓	–
Moderate to severe	Buprenorphine	P	–	✓	–	✓	sl	–
	Pentazocine	PAA	✓	–	✓	✓	✓	✓
	Pethidine (meperidine)	A	✓	–	✓	✓	sl	–
	Meptazinol	P	✓	–	–	✓	sl	–
	Ketorolac	N	✓	–	–	✓	✓	–
	Tramadol	A	✓	–	–	✓	sl	–
Moderate	Nefopam	N	✓	–	–	✓	–	–
	Dihydrocodeine	A	✓	–	✓	✓	–	–
Mild to moderate	Codeine	A	✓	–	–	✓	–	–
	Dextropropoxyphene (propoxyphene)	A	✓	–	–	–	–	–
Mild	Aspirin, NSAIDs (see Chapter 8)	N	✓	–	–	–	–	✓
	Paracetamol (acetaminophen)		✓	–	–	–	–	–

[a] These potency groupings are only approximate. Potency is markedly affected by the dose and route of administration, e.g. IV diamorphine (heroin) has three times the potency of oral morphine.

[b] A, opioid agonist; P, partial opioid agonist; PAA, partial agonist–antagonist; N, non-opioid (see Table 10.5, NSAIDs, non-steroidal anti-inflammatory drugs).

[c] PO, oral; BC, buccal or sublingual; SC, subcutaneous; IM, intramuscular; IV, intravenous (sl = slow injection or infusion); Re, rectal. See also p. 578.

[d] Preferred or alternative analgesic for terminal care: diamorphine (heroin) is illegal in the USA and dipipanone and phenazocine are not licensed there; oxycodone is not licensed in the UK.

[e] Fentanyl is administered with a transdermal patch for chronic pain relief. Alfentanil and remifentanil are rapid-acting and used for induction of anaesthesia. Given IV, all three are short-acting adjuncts to general anaesthetics, used intraoperatively (especially remifentanil).

The duration of action of the drugs is markedly affected by the formulation, route of administration and whether dosing is chronic or single dose. Most opioids have a single-dose duration of action of about 4–6 h, though pethidine (meperidine) is somewhat shorter-acting.

modified-release preparation to reduce the dose frequency.

The **sublingual route** is particularly attractive, because it provides a rapid onset of action and avoids the losses from first-pass metabolism. However, only *buprenorphine* and *phenazocine* are currently available in the UK for sublingual administration.

Parenteral

The **intramuscular route** (IM) is commonly used postoperatively. It has the disadvantages of wide fluctuations in absorption, a 30- to 60-min lag time to peak effect, and a more rapid decline in activity than after oral administration.

In cancer patients, who are often cachectic and thus have reduced muscle mass, intramuscular administration can be painful, and normal doses can give abnormally high peak concentrations. Moreover, because many cancer patients have low platelet counts, IM injection may cause severe bruising. Further, IM injection causes some muscle damage and the release of creatine kinase, so this route must not be used within 48 h of a suspected myocardial infarction (MI) because this enzyme is used as one marker for MI.

A bolus **intravenous** (IV) dose obviously provides the most rapid pain relief. The main determinant of the time taken to achieve a therapeutic effect with a centrally acting drug is its lipid solubility, which determines how quickly the drug leaves the plasma and is distributed into the tissues and the central nervous system.

The **continuous subcutaneous infusion** of opioids is used widely. The IV route does not appear to confer any advantage, and opioid tolerance may occur more rapidly. Virtually constant blood levels are achieved and the IV route enables rapid titration of the analgesic dose in patients with acute, severe pain or an acute exacerbation of chronic pain. The IV infusion of analgesics after major surgery, i.e. providing good postoperative pain control, has been shown to decrease the recovery period and reduce postoperative complications. However, the oral route is equally effective for stable chronic pain unless the patient is unable to absorb oral medications due to vomiting, dysphagia or bowel disease. In such cases subcutaneous infusion is a good alternative to IV administration.

Spinal anaesthesia is used routinely in obstetrics and increasingly for surgery on patients who are unsuitable for a general anaesthetic, postsurgically and for palliative care in terminally ill patients (pp. 615–617).

Rectal

The rectal route (per rectum) is another alternative to oral administration in patients who are vomiting or on a 'nil-by-mouth' regimen, provided that it is not precluded by bowel disease. Several analgesics are available as suppositories (Table 10.4). This route also avoids loss of available drug by first-pass metabolism.

Rectal administration should be avoided in patients with a low platelet count due to cancer chemotherapy or to disease because it is likely to provoke bleeding which is difficult to control.

Transdermal

This route is used currently only with *fentanyl* and *sufentanil*. It is useful if the oral route cannot be used and continuous parenteral infusion is either unavailable or unsuitable. Both fentanyl and sufentanil have a short duration of action if given orally or by parenteral bolus injection, due to their rapid metabolism and tissue redistribution, whereas the transdermal patches provide prolonged dosing.

However, skin reactions may occur with the patches and the *British National Formulary* (BNF) advises application to dry, non-irritated, non-irradiated, non-hairy skin of the torso or upper arm, rotation of application sites every 72 h and avoidance of the same area for several days.

Guidelines for analgesic use

Accurate diagnosis of the cause of the pain is very important.

- Use the oral route whenever possible.
- Only the patient knows if relief is adequate. However, treatment goals should be realistic: complete freedom from pain may be difficult to achieve.
- If an analgesic fails after a trial at adequate dose and frequency, move up the analgesic ladder: a substitute from the same class is unlikely to be more effective.
- If increased activity is required, the dose should be increased but the dosage interval should remain unchanged. Reducing the

- dosage interval below that appropriate for the drug merely makes life more difficult for the patient.
- Pain should not be allowed to recur. Drugs with a short duration of action, e.g. dextromoramide and pethidine (meperidine), are unsuitable for the management of sustained severe pain.
- Opioids are not a panacea: due weight must be given to the use of adjuvants (p. 591), the management of psychosocial aspects and intercurrent disease, and the control of adverse reactions.

- Tolerance to opioids, and dependence on them, is not usually a practical problem when treating severe pain. Many terminal patients remain on a uniform dose throughout most of their illness. Opioid use should not be dictated by a short or poor prognosis, but by the needs of the patient. Physical dependence does not preclude dose reduction if the patient improves or if other treatments relieve the pain.
- Always keep an open mind and review the treatment frequently.

Analgesic drugs and techniques

Opioid analgesics

Mechanism of action

Opioid receptor sites

As discussed earlier, receptor sites exist in the brain, spinal cord and elsewhere where opioids such as morphine bind to produce analgesia (and other pharmacological effects). The body's natural ligands for these receptors are the endorphin, enkephalin and dynorphin peptides. Receptor-binding studies have identified at least three major types of opioid receptors, designated **mu** (μ; two sub-types, μ_1, μ_2), **delta** (δ, two sub-types) and **kappa** (κ; three sub-types), each with distinct roles so that the type of effect, e.g. pain, associated with each receptor is different, as are the effects of the drugs which act at them. These effects are summarized in Table 10.5. About 65% of the amino acid residues of the three receptor types in animals are identical or very similar, as are most of their transmembrane regions and intracellular loops, but most of their extracellular loops differ. A further sigma (σ) receptor has been described, but its role is uncertain because opioid activity there is not antagonized by *naloxone*, a specific opioid antagonist.

Most of the research in this field has been carried out in rats and mice, which sometimes show species differences. A complication is that some of the receptors and their sub-types have been proposed on the basis of drug binding studies, but their pharmacological properties are ill-defined or unknown. Because of these uncertainties and because further receptors and sub-types may exist, it is not currently possible to allocate the actions of drugs with certainty to specific sub-types in man. However, this is an active research field and drugs are likely to emerge which act at specific receptors to achieve analgesia without the unwanted effects.

Morphine and related plant alkaloids have physicochemical configurations which resemble those of the endogenous peptides, and so activate the same receptors. *Methadone*, although chemically unrelated, can adopt a similar configuration. Naturally occurring and synthetic opioid drugs are classified according to the sub-types of receptors to which they bind, and the type of response which they thus evoke (Table 10.5). The available drugs include pure opioid agonists, partial agonists, agonists–antagonists, and pure antagonists. The affinity with which a drug binds to a receptor is important: analgesics with a high receptor affinity, e.g. *buprenorphine*, exert an analgesic action for much longer than their plasma half-life would suggest.

Table 10.5   The selectivity of opioid analgesics and their possible effects at their probable receptors[a]

	Example	Activity at receptor type		
		mu (μ)	kappa (κ)	delta (δ)
Class of drug or agent				
Pure opioid agonist	Morphine	Agonist	Weak agonist	?
	Pethidine (meperidine)	Agonist	Weak agonist	?
Partial opioid agonist	Buprenorphine	Partial agonist	Antagonist	?
Pure opioid antagonist	Naloxone	Antagonist	Antagonist	Antagonist
Endogenous peptide	Beta-endorphin	Agonist	?	Agonist
	Enkephalins	Agonist	?	Agonist
	Dynorphins	Weak agonist	Agonist	Weak agonist
Some effects produced by receptor activation		Supraspinal analgesia Respiratory depression Euphoria Miosis Physical dependence	Spinal analgesia Respiratory depression Sedation Miosis	Analgesia Sedation Hallucinations Reduced gut peristalsis

[a] These results are derived from animal experiments and may not reflect the situation in man.

Opioid agonists and antagonists

Pure agonists (e.g. *morphine*) can, in sufficient concentration, elicit a maximum response from the receptor. However, a **partial agonist**, e.g. *buprenorphine*, can only produce a partial response irrespective of the concentration, and there may even be a decreased response if the optimum concentration is exceeded. The morphine-like opioids are thought to exert their agonist effects primarily at the mu receptor and to a lesser degree at the kappa receptor (Table 10.5). Partial agonists (Table 10.6) bind with the mu receptor and compete with the agonists, both naturally occurring and exogenous. If they are used in combination with a complete agonist, they may act as competitive antagonists and the level of analgesia may be reduced, or as partial agonists, so that they show only limited activity. **Mixed agonists–antagonists**, e.g. *pentazocine*, are antagonists at the mu receptor but are still effective as analgesics through agonist effects at the kappa receptor, the agonist effect being either complete or partial.

At the other end of the spectrum are the **pure antagonists** which are used to reverse respiratory depression postoperatively, to treat opioid poisoning, e.g. *naloxone*, and to prevent relapse in detoxified opioid addicts, e.g. *naltrexone*.

Opioid-sensitive and opioid-insensitive pain

Virtually all acute pain, with the possible exception of labour pain, falls into the opioid-sensitive category, the analgesic effect being related both to the type of agent used (weak or strong opioid) and the dose.

Table 10.6   Classification of partial agonists–antagonists

Morphine-like		Nalorphine-like
Buprenorphine[a] Meptazinol[a] Propiram[a] Profadol[a]	investigational	Butorphanol[b] Nalbuphine[a] Pentazocine[b]

[a] Partial agonist.
[b] Agonist–antagonist.

Opioid-insensitive pains include most headaches and those resulting from muscle spasm and destruction or interruption of afferent (sensory) nerve fibres, i.e. **deafferentation pain**. Pain arising from muscle spasm is best dealt with using muscle relaxants, e.g. *diazepam* and *baclofen*, whereas that caused by deafferentation responds better to anxiolytics, antidepressants and nerve blocks.

Some types of pain may be partially sensitive: that resulting from bone metastases is best treated with a combination of non-steroidal anti-inflammatory drugs (NSAIDs) and opioids. The former may be adequate on their own, e.g. diclofenac suppositories in palliative care or postoperatively when patients are 'nil-by-mouth'. However, opioids may be needed initially or for continuing support. Some other types of cancer pain, e.g. that arising from nerve compression, raised intracranial pressure and extensive tumour infiltration of tissues, may require an opioid plus an **adjuvant**, e.g. a potent anti-inflammatory glucocorticoid with minimal mineralocorticoid activity, e.g. *betamethasone*, *dexamethasone*. Psychogenic pain clearly requires anxiolytics, antidepressants or other psychotropic agents in addition to analgesics. Analgesic adjuvants are discussed on p. 591.

Therapeutic use

Morphine

This has become the standard against which other opioid analgesics are judged and is generally the treatment of choice for chronic severe pain in advanced cancer. No other strong opioid, given orally, is consistently superior.

In addition to its central analgesic action, morphine causes euphoria and a sense of detachment: it also causes drowsiness for up to 7 days after initiating treatment. This profile is clinically useful as it reduces the anxiety and anguish that are commonly associated with severe pain from whatever cause, e.g. myocardial infarction and terminal disease. However, morphine should not be used primarily as a sedative. Occasional patients remain drowsy, in which case coexisting problems should be sought, e.g. renal or hepatic impairment, or concurrent use of other sedatives.

Morphine also aggravates functional gastrointestinal pain, e.g. from colonic spasm and constipation, for which it is unsuitable.

One of the most important advances in the management of chronic pain has been the introduction of modified-release (m/r) oral formulations, which usually give excellent control with once- or twice-daily dosing. These contain morphine bound to an ion exchange resin from which it is released by diffusion of sodium and potassium ions. Because of their slow onset of action, breakthrough pain may occur and is controlled with solution or injections (occasionally normal-release tablets). A long-acting m/r rectal product is likely to be licensed in 2000 and will be useful if vomiting is a problem or patients are unable to swallow.

Papaveretum is a preparation of morphine hydrochloride (85%), papaverine and codeine. It was reformulated in the *British Pharmacopoeia* 1998 to remove noscapine, a centrally acting cough suppressant, which was formerly included because it is a constituent of prepared opium. However, noscapine contributed little, except to side effects and toxicity. It was once used extensively as a routine analgesic, but is now used occasionally for perioperative analgesia. The reformulated product contains a lower weight of the preparation but the same dose of morphine. However, this has created dispensing problems and special care is required. Papaveretum has also been confused with papaverine, which is used to treat male impotence.

The formerly traditional 'Brompton Cocktail' (morphine, cocaine, alcohol and syrup) has no advantages over morphine, and may cause its own unwanted effects. It no longer has a place in treatment.

Another traditional opioid preparation, camphorated opium tincture (paregoric), is occasionally encountered as a constituent of cough mixtures, but has almost completely been replaced by *pholcodine* and *dextromethorphan*. In these days of opioid-addicted mothers it has found a new use in the management of neonatal opioid dependence. Morphine is the antitussive of choice for the treatment of the distressing cough of terminal lung cancer, with methadone as an alternative.

Opium tincture (laudanum), or a similar preparation, was the all-purpose analgesic for thousands of years of galenical pharmacy: the true 'opium of the people', not 'religion', as Karl Marx would have it.

Other pure agonist drugs

Diamorphine (heroin, 3,6-diacetylmorphine)

Opinions differ over the choice between *heroin* and *morphine*. Because of its abuse potential and its disputed benefit, diamorphine (heroin) it is not available (illegal) in the USA and some other countries.

Diamorphine (heroin) itself is not an opioid agonist, but is rapidly metabolized to 6-monoacetylmorphine (6-MAM) and morphine, which are. Because both diamorphine (heroin) and 6-MAM are more lipid-soluble than morphine they penetrate the blood–brain barrier more rapidly and so have a faster onset of action, though the final activity is of the morphine produced on hydrolysis. Diamorphine (heroin) is generally regarded as more potent than morphine on injection, both as a euphoriant and analgesic, and may cause less nausea and hypotension. However, the oral potencies of the two are similar because diamorphine (heroin) given orally is completely hydrolysed to morphine before absorption from the gut.

Diamorphine (heroin) is unstable in solution, so morphine is preferred for oral solutions. However, diamorphine (heroin) is very soluble in water and so is preferred for IM and sub-cutaneous administration as the injection volume is small. This may be important in very emaciated patients. Solutions are prepared from the sterile powder as required and are not stored.

Pethidine (meperidine)

This moderately potent analgesic is most commonly used perioperatively and in obstetric analgesia. Because it is unpredictably absorbed and undergoes significant first-pass metabolism, oral bioavailability is poor and variable, with some trials showing equivalence with paracetamol (acetaminophen). However, some patients obtain satisfactory relief with oral *pethidine (meperidine)*, and saturation of metabolic

pathways may increase bioavailability with chronic use. Given parenterally, pethidine (meperidine) has a swift onset of action as it is highly lipophilic and crosses the blood–brain barrier readily. This property makes it useful for preoperative medication and treating acute pain. The short duration of action, 1–3 h, normally makes pethidine (meperidine) unsuitable for treating chronic pain, as approximately 2-hourly dosing would be required.

The toxic metabolite of pethidine (meperidine), norpethidine, is cleared renally and tends to accumulate with chronic use or in renal impairment. High norpethidine levels have been associated with anxiety, agitation, tremors and seizures.

Pethidine (meperidine) probably causes more nausea, vomiting and hypotension than other opioids, but it may have less effect on smooth muscle and so may be used for renal or biliary colic, though IM or rectal *diclofenac* is more common. Although pethidine (meperidine) produces less euphoria and sedation than morphine, respiratory depression and postural hypotension are common at effective doses. Most of these properties can be corrected by using it with *haloperidol* which potentiates the analgesia and is anti-emetic, sedative and possibly euphoric. However, toxicity limits the maximum dose of pethidine (meperidine) that can be used.

Pethidine (meperidine) interacts with *monoamine oxidase inhibitors* (MAOIs) to cause severe hypertension and hypertensive crisis, and must not be used in patients taking MAOI antidepressants and hypotensives.

Methadone

This agent is well absorbed and well tolerated by mouth and has been used with some success in pain control, particularly in the USA. However, its metabolism and excretion are complex, so the patient's physical, mental and emotional condition need to be monitored closely.

Methadone has a very long elimination half-life on multiple oral dosing, about 25 h, and is very highly bound to plasma and CNS proteins, so that accumulation can occur with chronic use. This leads to drowsiness and confusion and may occasionally be life-threatening. The half-life is extended considerably by renal or hepatic impairment, so methadone must be used with special care in elderly or debilitated patients. Steady-state blood levels are not achieved until at least 4–5 days after the initiation of therapy or a change in dose, so loading doses are sometimes used to overcome this problem. Despite the long half-life, the duration of action is only about 6–8 h, and several daily doses must be given initially, though once- or twice-daily dosing is used when steady-state blood levels have been achieved, because of the risk of accumulation and toxicity.

Although the degree of sedation and respiratory depression reflect the absolute amount of methadone in the body, the total body load does not influence the magnitude of analgesic response, possibly owing to different affinities for the different receptor sub-types.

Methadone is widely used in addiction clinics to help addicts withdraw from opioid abuse, because it may relieve the physical withdrawal symptoms without giving 'highs' for the same length of time. However, methadone may itself lead to a morphine-like dependence and the potential for abuse is similar to that for morphine. Although withdrawal symptoms are less intense than those with morphine, their onset is slower (24–48 h) and more prolonged. Opioid abusers are usually given a very gradually reducing methadone dosage regimen, the level of which is carefully titrated to the patient's needs. However, the value of methadone in opioid withdrawal has been challenged: it is not a cure and is regarded by some workers more as a method of social control, to minimize the criminal aspects of addiction, rather than as therapy.

Levorphanol has similar pharmacokinetics to methadone, being well-absorbed orally and tending to accumulate in long-term use. It is now little used in the UK, having been supplanted by newer drugs, e.g. *tramadol*, but is used in North America.

Dextromoramide

This is equipotent with *morphine* and is less sedating. However, it has a short duration of action (1–2 h) and so is unsuitable for managing chronic pain. Dextromoramide tends to be restricted in use to the cover of painful procedures, e.g. a dressing change. Although it is has been used when patients experience breakthrough pain (pain in between doses of their standard analgesic), this is bad practice: mixing opioids may give unpredictable results, so patients should be maintained on adequate doses of a single drug. If additional analgesia is required, e.g. for a patient taking slow-release morphine, then morphine solution, injection or tablets should be used for the immediate control of breakthrough pain, depending on severity. The dose of slow-release product is then adjusted in the light of the new requirement.

Phenazocine

This very potent analgesic is available as an oral or sublingual formulation. It is the least sedating of all the opioid analgesics and does not increase biliary tract pressure, though it may be more emetogenic than other agents. Sublingual administration has three advantages: it avoids first-pass metabolism, gives a fast onset of action, and is still effective if nausea and vomiting are a problem. Despite these benefits, phenazocine is infrequently used in clinical practice because many clinicians prefer to use more conventional agents.

Hydromorphone

This potent analgesic (about 7.5 times as potent as morphine) is more widely used in the USA and Europe than in the UK. It has a rapid onset of action but a relatively short half-life. Oral dosing is required 4-hourly.

Dipipanone

This agent is usually given orally only, occasionally SC or IM. It should not be given by the IV route because this may produce a dramatic fall in blood pressure.

The only available tablet is formulated with *cyclizine*, an antihistamine, as an anti-emetic. This makes the product unsuitable for chronic use, e.g. in palliative care.

Oxycodone

This is effective orally and is used widely in North America and elsewhere as a modified-release oral product and, combined with aspirin or paracetamol (acetaminophen), for moderately severe pain. In the UK it is available only for rectal use.

Tramadol

This is a newer agent which can be given by almost any route to produce analgesia that is claimed to result from inhibition of noradrenaline (norepinephrine) re-uptake and stimulation of serotonin release at nerve synapses. Tramadol also has actions at opioid receptors. It is comparable to morphine, but appears less respiratory depressant than other opioids. Because tramadol causes less constipation it is often used in the elderly and when toileting difficulties create postoperative problems. There may also be a reduced potential for dependence, but tramadol should not be used if there is a history of addiction or convulsions. It has been used for obstetric and perioperative pain and in myocardial infarction, but is unsuitable for intraoperative analgesia during light anaesthesia.

Side effects are those of the opioids generally, including also occasional hypertension, anaphylaxis, hallucinations and confusion, but tramadol usually causes less constipation.

Fentanyl and its congeners

These agents are used primarily for **intraoperative analgesia**. Opioids are widely used in low doses to supplement general anaesthesia with *nitrous oxide–oxygen* and a neuromuscular blocking agent. The muscle relaxants, e.g. *suxamethonium*, *pancuronium*, *atracurium* (there are many others), relax the diaphragm and abdominal muscles and permit light anaesthesia to be used. In addition, they relax the vocal cords and so facilitate the passage of an endotracheal tube to assist in passing anaesthetic gases or oxygen. Patients who have received a muscle relaxant must always have assisted or controlled respiration during the period of action of the drug.

Alfentanil and *remifentanil* have a rapid onset of action (1–2 min) and are used to reduce the induction dose of an anaesthetic, especially in poor-risk patients. *Remifentanil* can be used intraoperatively as an IV infusion, because it has a very short duration of action and does not accumulate, but for this reason additional analgesia is usually needed postoperatively.

Alfentanil and *fentanyl* are used intraoperatively as IV bolus injections, but these may cause severe respiratory depression, especially with fentanyl. Because respiratory depression may occur for the first time postoperatively, patients who have received either drug need to be observed carefully for some hours after recovery. *Sufentanil* (not licensed in the UK) is used similarly in the USA.

The **side effect** of respiratory depression with alfentanil and fentanyl is used to advantage in intensive care patients on assisted respiration to manage respiration without interference from their endogenous respiratory drive. The opioid effect is reversed with *naloxone* when respiratory depression is no longer required.

Fentanyl and sufentanil are used widely as transdermal patches (Chapter 12) for the control of chronic pain that is unsatisfactorily controlled by conventional opioids. Because it takes about 12 h for the patch to produce adequate analgesia, it should be applied at an appropriate time, e.g. simultaneously with the last m/r morphine dose when transferring from m/r morphine. An intranasal formulation is under trial for breakthrough pain when using patches, as a more suitable alternative to the IV injection.

Partial agonist and agonist–antagonist drugs

These groups of drugs were developed to try to overcome opioid dependence problems. Although not totally devoid of abuse potential, this is less than that of morphine and other similar agonists.

Nalorphine was the prototype of this group but is no longer used owing to an unacceptably high incidence of psychotomimetic side effects. Subsequently, two types of agonist–antagonist have been developed which are classified according to their activity relative to morphine or nalorphine (Table 10.6).

Agents of the nalorphine type characteristically act only as competitive antagonists at the mu receptor but have varying affinities and intrinsic activities at all receptor types. The partial agonist–antagonist of the morphine type have a low intrinsic activity at mu receptors, but a high affinity for them.

Morphine-like opioids

Buprenorphine is a partial agonist which has a 6- to 8-h duration of action and is effective in the relief of moderate to severe pain. Given sublingually, it avoids first-pass metabolism and is often used for acute and postoperative pain, though the sublingual route may be unsuitable for very ill patients who produce little saliva. However, the use of buprenorphine in chronic severe pain is problematic. It has a 'ceiling effect', like pethidine (meperidine), and a low therapeutic index, like pentazocine, so increasing the daily dose above 5 mg is not beneficial. It has been used to manage opioid withdrawal, similarly to methadone.

Side effects. Because of its high receptor affinity, large doses of other opioids may be required to displace buprenorphine from the receptor. This may lead, in those patients who do not obtain adequate pain relief with buprenorphine, to a confused situation of inadequate analgesia, despite a large opioid dose, but enhanced toxicity. If given to a patient receiving other opioids chronically, buprenorphine may precipitate pain and withdrawal symptoms. Thus it is best used either alone or not at all. In common with most other opioids, buprenorphine causes respiratory depression proportionate to its analgesic effect. However, owing to its high receptor affinity this effect is not readily reversed by naloxone, making it more hazardous in overdose, and a respiratory stimulant such as doxapram may be needed. Buprenorphine is highly emetogenic in some patients.

Meptazinol has about one-tenth of the analgesic potency of morphine. Meptazinol is unusual in that it is thought to have two central mechanisms of action: a partial agonist–antagonist effect at opioid receptors, plus effects on central cholinergic receptors. Meptazinol has a rapid but variable onset of action (0.25–3 h orally, 0.5 h rectally), and its duration of action is also variable (2–7 h). Thus dosing is required every 3–6 h, depending on patient response. It undergoes extensive first-pass metabolism, so blood levels after oral dosing are low and this route is better suited to the short-term relief of moderate pain, e.g. perioperatively. For moderate to severe pain, meptazinol is best given by IM or slow IV injection. It is likely to cause nausea and vomiting.

Meptazinol is claimed to cause less respiratory depression than other opioids, possibly because of its cholinergic effects or its preferential action at the mu receptor, and may be a useful analgesic to consider in patients with compromised respiratory function. There is a divergence of opinion on this latter point. Some clinicians advocate the cautious use of morphine, despite its respiratory depressant effects, in patients with compromised lung function, believing that pain itself acts as a respiratory stimulant and reduces the risk of administering a known respiratory depressant. Further, should respiratory depression occur following morphine administration, this can readily be reversed by administering naloxone, whereas complete reversal of the effects of a partial agonist–antagonist such as meptazinol cannot be achieved with naloxone and additional measures, e.g. assisted respiration with oxygen (*see* Chapter 5) and possibly a respiratory stimulant.

The potential for abuse is probably less than that of morphine because its dysphoric effects disappear with increasing dose.

Propiram is not licensed in the UK but is used orally and rectally in the USA and elsewhere.

Nalorphine-like opioids

Pentazocine is a moderately potent analgesic which is used relatively infrequently nowadays in the UK as it shares the hallucinogenic potential of nalorphine and causes a high incidence of confusion and hallucinations. Like buprenorphine and butorphanol, pentazocine may precipitate a withdrawal reaction in patients who are opioid-dependent. It is unsuitable for pain associated with myocardial infarction because, unlike morphine, it can increase the cardiac workload.

The oral efficacy of pentazocine is poor (slightly less potent than codeine) and, due to its low therapeutic index, doses cannot be increased greatly to treat severe pain without also markedly increasing the incidence and severity of **side effects**. However, it is more potent when administered by any parenteral route than both codeine and dihydrocodeine.

Because it is a mixed agonist–antagonist, pentazocine cannot be used to enhance the activity of other opioids.

Butorphanol resembles pentazocine. It is used mostly in North America and continental

Europe for perioperative analgesia, but causes respiratory depression, nausea, weakness, sweating and feelings of unreality. An intranasal spray is available which is useful for treating intractable severe headaches.

Nalbuphine is as effective as morphine but causes less nausea and vomiting and may have less abuse potential, though respiratory depression is similar. It is used primarily for preoperative and perioperative analgesia (p. 614).

Side effects

Actions of morphine other than those described above are usually considered to be side effects.

Nausea and vomiting

Morphine and its derivatives stimulate the chemoreceptor trigger zone (CTZ) and may cause nausea and vomiting, though this tends to be transient, wearing off after a few days of therapy. These effects may be avoided by prophylactic co-administration of an anti-emetic (*see* Chapter 6, p. 332) over this period. Prophylactic anti-emetics are also appropriate in patients who are already vomiting owing to their disease or to the use of a weak opioid or other drug, or who have a history of vomiting with opioids, and may be given initially either rectally or parenterally to bring existing vomiting under control. Anti-emetics are not indicated in patients who are not currently nauseated and so should not be used routinely: good practice is not to prescribe a drug unless there is a positive indication, though it is common to prescribe anti-emetics for use 'as required', in anticipation of need. Consequently, since dipipanone is only available combined with an anti-emetic (cyclizine) it is not recommended for routine terminal care.

Because the incidence of nausea and vomiting is higher in ambulatory patients, it is thought that a vestibular component is also involved. It is often helpful for the patient to lie quietly if this problem occurs.

Constipation

Opioids also cause an increase in gastrointestinal sphincter tone and a decrease in propulsive peristalsis. This causes delayed gastric emptying and, almost inevitably, constipation. The regular co-administration of a stimulant laxative is nearly always used in anticipation of the problem. *Dantron*, as *co-danthrusate* (dantron plus docusate) or *co-danthramer* (dantron plus poloxamer '188'), is probably the most effective agent. *Dantron* is specifically licensed in the UK only for the treatment of constipation in geriatric practice, due to analgesics in terminal care and for patients with cardiac failure or MI, to avoid cardiac stress due to bowel strain. The licence is restricted because studies in rats have indicated a potential carcinogenic risk. Products containing dantron may colour the urine red, and patients should be warned of this apparently alarming effect. Dantron may also cause a rash in the buttock area in incontinent patients.

The equivalent product in the USA is a combination of *casanthranol* (a natural anthracene) and *docusate* (*dioctyl sodium sulphosuccinate*).

Other smooth muscle effects

Morphine also increases the tone in the sphincter of Oddi, which leads to increased pressure in the biliary system and occasional biliary colic. Other actions on smooth muscle include increased urethral tone and contractions and, very rarely, bronchoconstriction after large doses.

Respiratory depression

Morphine and other opioids can significantly depress respiration, and this is usually the cause of death from overdose. Respiratory rate, tidal volume and response to hypercapnia or hypoxaemia are all reduced. However, like many of its other **side effects**, respiratory depression is not usually a limiting factor in patients who are experiencing severe pain: pain is a potent arousal mechanism. Nevertheless, opioids must be used with great care in patients with advanced respiratory disease or otherwise depressed respiratory function. Opioid doses should be reduced if other procedures, e.g. nerve block (Figure 10.2 and p. 597) reduce pain successfully.

The harmful, and beneficial, effects of morphine and other opioid agonists are reversed completely by nalorphine.

Effects on the eye

Stimulation of the oculomotor nerve causes constriction of the pupil, which is often a diagnostic aid in cases of morphine overdose. Thus, opioid analgesics are generally avoided in patients with head injury, because the opioid-induced pupillary changes, nausea and general central nervous system clouding, may mask the signs induced by trauma and confuse the neurological examination.

Cardiovascular effects

The usual doses of opioid analgesics generally do not have major cardiovascular effects in patients with normal cardiac function. However, *morphine* may cause venous pooling and postural hypotension, through its venodilator action. The consequent reduction in cardiac preload (*see* Chapter 3) is an additional benefit (to analgesia and euphoria) immediately following myocardial infarction.

Hypersensitivity

Occasionally, allergic-type reactions occur with opioid agents, and both local reactions at the site of injection and systemic allergic symptoms have been reported. If a patient is hypersensitive to *morphine*, both *codeine* and *diamorphine* (*heroin*) are also contraindicated as they are structurally similar. However, *methadone* and *pethidine* (*meperidine*) are suitable alternatives, being chemically unrelated.

Dependence

Opioid analgesics can produce both physical and psychological dependence, though the latter appears to be a rare event when opioid analgesics are used to relieve pain. If a patient asks for increased dosages of analgesics because their pain has worsened or not been controlled, this should not be perceived as drug-seeking behaviour or evidence of dependence. Physical dependence does occur, and can be avoided by reducing the dose of opioid slowly when it is no longer needed for pain, rather than stopping abruptly.

Naloxone

Adequate doses of this antagonist will reverse completely all the actions of opioid agonists, so it is a complete antidote for both the actions and side effects of morphine-like drugs. However, care should be taken when using *naloxone* to reverse opioid-induced respiratory depression, as patients who have been using opioid agents chronically are extremely sensitive to antagonists and too high a dose of naloxone can precipitate a withdrawal reaction and recurrence of severe pain. Further, it will not fully antagonize the action of partial agonist and agonist–antagonist drugs (p. 586).

The naloxone doses needed to treat respiratory depression in opioid overdose are about 25% of those required to treat opioid poisoning. Because the duration of action of naloxone is shorter than that of morphine and other opioids, repeated injections or IV infusion may be required. The naloxone dose varies widely, being dictated by the patient's condition and response. Oxygen and the respiratory stimulant doxapram may be needed to spare the naloxone dose and so maintain adequate analgesia.

Opioid rotation

Although oral morphine is the potent analgesic of choice, there is a minority of patients in whom their pain is inadequately controlled despite large dose increases. Others develop dose-limiting toxicity that precludes adequate dosing. It is unclear why this situation occurs. Postulated mechanisms are the complex metabolism and pharmacokinetics of morphine, with active metabolites that may accumulate, and down-regulation of receptors or other receptor change.

These patients may benefit from a change in the route or method of administration, e.g. intravenous injection, patient-controlled analgesia (p. 600), nerve blocks (Figure 10.2 and p. 597) or epidural anaesthesia (p. 615).

However, a satisfactory result may be achieved by a change of opioid, i.e. **opioid rotation**. It is preferable to use a pure agonist, e.g. hydromorphone, methadone, sublingual phenazocine (if salivation is adequate) or transdermal fentanyl.

Satisfactory analgesia may be achieved at equipotent doses, sometimes even at smaller doses. The reasons for benefit from rotation are not clear, but include differing metabolism, different receptor sub-type responses and variable sensitivity to side effects.

Opioid rotation is not a universal panacea, and frequent changes are undesirable. It is important to evaluate the reasons for loss of pain control, e.g. new symptoms, intercurrent disease, and to consider alternative approaches to pain control.

Less potent analgesics

These are mainly used for the treatment of acute or chronic pain resulting from trauma, surgery and chronic systemic diseases such as arthritis. They include low potency, centrally acting morphine-like compounds ('weak opioids', e.g. *dihydrocodeine*), and drugs that act on peripheral pain pathways, e.g. *aspirin*, *salicylates*, *NSAIDs* and *paracetamol* (*acetaminophen*) (*see* Chapter 8). Paracetamol (acetaminophen) toxicity is discussed in Chapter 6.

Weak opioids

These drugs have a ceiling to their analgesic effect because of dose-limiting adverse reactions and therefore have a limited efficacy relative to the strong opioids. Therefore combinations of these drugs with *paracetamol* (*acetaminophen*), provided that it is not contraindicated (i.e. liver function is not compromised), or *aspirin* if tolerated, may have an additive, possibly synergistic, analgesic effect. Despite the fact that the BNF states that "... the advantages [of such combinations] have not been substantiated", they are very widely prescribed. Their continuing popularity, with both patients and prescribers, may represent the triumph of experience over theoretical good practice.

Codeine is chemically related to morphine and shares its pharmacological actions, but it is less potent and is thought to have less abuse potential.

Dihydrocodeine is also related to morphine and is mainly used for moderately severe pain. It has a flat dose–response curve, so there is no advantage in increasing the dose above that normally recommended: if analgesia is inadequate, a change to a strong opioid is indicated.

Dextropropoxyphene (*propoxyphene*) resembles methadone structurally, and is less potent than codeine. There has been considerable controversy over its widespread use owing to serious problems if taken in overdose. In the UK, dextropropoxyphene (propoxyphene) is usually taken in combination with paracetamol (acetaminophen) as *co-proxamol*, which is unfortunately used as a common agent for suicide. It has been suggested that as little as 15–20 tablets of this combination can prove fatal, especially if alcohol is implicated. The main cause of death in overdose with *dextropropoxyphene* (*propoxyphene*) is respiratory depression, but in overdose with *co-proxamol* this is compounded with the hepatotoxicity of *paracetamol* (*acetaminophen*) (*see* Chapter 6, p. 373). Acute over-dosage with *co-proxamol* requires prompt administration of naloxone, to antagonize the *dextropropoxyphene* (*propoxyphene*), resuscitation treatment and management of paracetamol (acetaminophen) over-dose. If naloxone is not used, patients may die of cardiovascular collapse before reaching hospital.

Like other opioid analgesics, dextropropoxyphene (propoxyphene) can lead to dependence, the likelihood being about the same as with codeine.

Nefopam is structurally unrelated to the opioids and is sometimes useful when the pain has not responded to other analgesics. Its main advantage is that it does not cause respiratory depression, but its sympathomimetic and antimuscarinic **side effects**, notably restlessness, dry mouth, urinary retention and, less often, blurred vision, tachycardia, insomnia, headache and confusion, may be troublesome. Thus, nefopam must be used with caution in the elderly and if there is evidence of renal or hepatic impairment: it is extensively metabolized in the liver and largely excreted in the urine. Because of its adverse cardiovascular and CNS effects, nefopam is **contraindicated** in MI and if the patient is liable to convulsions.

Non-steroidal anti-inflammatory drugs (NSAIDs)

General properties

NSAIDs appear to act peripherally at the pain receptor level, and so do not produce the physical dependence often associated with opioid analgesia. They are particularly useful in treating patients with chronic disease accompanied by pain and inflammation, e.g. rheumatoid arthritis (*see* Chapter 8) and for the short-term treatment of mild to moderate acute pain, including musculoskeletal injuries. Particular indications include the relief of pain accompanying dysmenorrhoea, and that associated with neoplastic bone metastases. In the latter case, combinations of an opioid with an NSAID are likely to be considerably more effective than an opioid alone.

The **topical use** of NSAIDs is discussed in Chapter 8.

Analgesic adjuvants

Analgesic adjuvants tend to be used primarily in treating the chronic pain of neoplastic disease

(Table 10.7). Their inclusion in a drug regimen may enhance pain relief, or it may be possible to reduce the dose of opioid, and consequently its side effects. Several unrelated categories of drugs are used, e.g. anticonvulsants, antispasmodics, neuroleptics, anxiolytics, tricyclic antidepressants, corticosteroids and antihistamines. The mechanisms by which these agents exert their analgesic effect are not clearly established, but are probably unrelated to the opioid receptor system.

The best results with analgesic adjuvants are often obtained if they are introduced early on in the disease process, e.g. before viral infection or cancer has caused demyelination (destruction or removal of the myelin sheath of nerves). Demyelination may result from infiltration or sustained pressure by a tumour, producing nerve block, slowing of nerve conduction or nerve irritability. These may cause paraesthesias, partial paralysis, painful spasm, etc.

Psychotropic drugs

The modes of action of these agents in the treatment of pain is controversial. It is postulated

Table 10.7 Some types of pain in cancer patients

Pain caused directly by the tumour

Tumour infiltration of viscera, nerves and bone
Nerve compression
Raised intracranial pressure (headaches)

Pain caused by the complication of therapy

e.g. after: • surgery (phantom limb pain, neuralgia, adhesions)
• chemotherapy (peripheral neuropathy caused by vinca alkaloids)
• radiotherapy (fibrosis, myelopathy)
Mucositis
Gastrointestinal distress, constipation
Post-herpetic neuralgia (as a consequence of immunosuppressive treatments)

Incidental pain (unrelated to the tumour)

Pre-existing chronic pain, e.g. arthritis
Bedsores
Headache
Gastrointestinal pain, e.g. due to treatment

that they block the re-uptake of certain neuro-transmitters in the pain pathway, e.g. 5HT and noradrenaline (norepinephrine), thus interfering with pain impulse transmission or modulation. However, their pro-analgesic effect may simply result from their anxiolytic or antidepressant actions, thus raising a pain threshold which had been lowered by the understandable anxiety and depression associated with chronic pain. Some studies have suggested that *tricyclic antidepressants* with an intact tertiary amine group, e.g. *amitriptyline* and *clomipramine*, may be the most effective. Antidepressants are thought to be most effective against the 'burning', deafferentation pain associated with sensory nerve damage, which is unresponsive to opioids.

The benefits of an antidepressant may be further increased by combination with a small dose of a *neuroleptic drug*, such as a *butyrophenone*, e.g. *droperidol*, *haloperidol*, or a *phenothiazine*, most commonly *perphenazine*. *Chlorpromazine* and *promazine* also have an opiate-sparing effect and are anti-emetic, and the use of a neuroleptic with an opioid may produce a state of near indifference to previously severe pain. However, such combinations should only be used by prescribers experienced in their use, because cardiac arrhythmias, postural hypotension, excessive sedation, and enhanced antimuscarinic **side effects** may be a problem. Although neuroleptics are suitable as adjuvants in terminal care, they should be avoided if possible for long-term use in the management of other forms of chronic pain because they may cause tardive dyskinesia (*see* Chapter 11) and dystonias. Further, they may cause myelosuppression and are unsuitable for cancer patients receiving cytotoxic drugs. Because of their extrapyramidal effects, neuroleptics antagonize the action of *levodopa* and exacerbate parkinsonism in the elderly.

Diazepam is particularly useful because it has muscle relaxant properties in addition to its anxiolytic effect, and is frequently used. If anxiety is not a problem and diazepam is too sedating, then *baclofen* is a suitable alternative for muscle spasm.

Stabbing or shooting pains (**neuralgia**) caused by nerve inflammation or damage appear to respond particularly well to anticonvulsant drugs, which are thought to act by suppressing abnormal spontaneous activity in traumatized nerve fibres. *Carbamazepine* is generally the most successful agent, though it is worth trying *phenytoin* or another anticonvulsant if this is ineffective before abandoning this line of treatment. Therapy should be initiated gradually, increasing the dose carefully until relief is obtained or unacceptable side effects are encountered.

Glucocorticosteroids

Glucocorticoids have a wide application in advanced cancer because they reduce the inflammatory swelling around tumours, and hence also the pressure on nerves and in bones, thus alleviating the pain. These actions are additional to any growth-suppressant action on tumour cells, but the effect may only be temporary. Glucocorticoids also suppress the release of mediators such as histamine and kinins and are euphoric, thus raising the pain threshold.

Dexamethasone, and to a lesser extent *betamethasone*, lowers intracranial pressure and is especially useful for relieving the headache and other symptoms of cerebral oedema. Low-dose corticosteroids (e.g. 2 mg dexamethasone) also improve mood and appetite, but co-analgesia requires higher doses – about ten times that dose.

Anabolic steroids (e.g. *nandrolone*, *stanazolol*) have been used to improve food utilization and increase muscle bulk and strength in patients with oesophageal, gastric and small bowel tumours who have problems with swallowing and nutrient absorption. These actions improve patient mood. However, feeding by a nasogastric tube or percutaneous gastrostomy are more usual.

Cannabis and cannabinoids

The use of cannabis as monotherapy or as an adjunct to other analgesics is hotly debated because of its current scheduling in the UK as a Controlled Drug, to which special licensing conditions apply. *Marijuana* is the most widely used, or abused, psychoactive substance. It is regarded by most governments as having no therapeutic uses, though there are numerous anecdotal reports of its benefit, e.g. in relieving spasticity in multiple sclerosis. Clearly, further research is needed. Only one cannabinoid, *nabilone*, is currently in use in the UK, for the management of uncontrolled nausea and vomiting caused by cytotoxic chemotherapy, and this has numerous side effects.

A major barrier to progress is that cannabis smoke contains more than 60 cannabinoids and no standardized product exists. One component, Δ-9-tetrahydrocannabinol (Δ-9-THC),

seems largely to produce the effects of smoking cannabis. However, it would be rash to assume that other cannabis components are not adjuncts or that they do not have potential value as analgesics. The precise effects of Δ-9-THC vary with the immediate environment, dose and route, and the psychological attributes of the user, similarly to alcohol.

Cannabinoid receptors are widely distributed in the brain. Why this is so, and the functions of endogenous ligands, are unknown but are of considerable interest.

Other methods of pain control

Local anaesthetics

Current agents are of two chemical types, depending on whether there is an ester or amide chain linking an aromatic lipophilic group, often a derivative of aniline or benzoic acid, to a secondary or tertiary amine residue. Table 10.8 lists those agents used most frequently.

Morphine has also been reported to be an effective local anaesthetic: low doses (1 mg in 20 mL of saline) injected into the knee joint after arthroscopy were found to be more effective than bupivacaine in preventing postoperative pain.

Mode of action

These agents depend on the ability of the lipophilic aromatic moiety of their molecules to dissolve in and attach to Na^+ channels and penetrate the lipoid nerve membrane. They prevent the large transient Na^+ flux across excitable nerve membranes by interacting directly with the intracellular halves of voltage-gated Na^+ channels. The result is that the excitability threshold rises and nerve conduction slows and eventually fails. Although the drugs also bind to potassium channels and inhibit them at higher concentrations, this is not thought to contribute to their action.

The smaller the nerve fibre, the more sensitive it is to the action of these agents, so there is some selectivity at the concentrations used: they block transmission by small pain fibres but leave inhibitory (large) pain fibres, touch and movement relatively unimpaired.

Local anaesthetics also have important effects on calcium flux across cell membranes, so *lidocaine* (*lignocaine*) is the drug of choice for treating the ventricular arrhythmias that may accompany MI, heart surgery and digitalis intoxication. This effect also contributes to their systemic toxicity.

Use

Except for *procaine*, the penetration of local anaesthetic agents through ophthalmic and mucous membranes is greater than through the skin, permitting effective local anaesthesia in the eye, nostrils, throat, urethra and rectum. This property facilitates the passage of endoscopes, catheters, etc. into body cavities and enables even relatively major operations, e.g. for cataract, to be carried out with minimal trauma as day care procedures.

Except for the use of IV *lidocaine* (*lignocaine*) for treating ventricular tachycardias, local anaesthetics are not normally injected intravascularly.

Table 10.8　Some pharmacokinetic properties of local anaesthetics

Anaesthetic	Onset of action[a]	Duration of action[b]
Ester type		
Tetracaine (amethocaine)	S	+++
Benzocaine	T	+
Chloroprocaine	F	+
Cocaine[c]	F	++
Oxybuprocaine (benoxinate)[d]	F	+
Procaine[e]	F	+
Propoxycaine	F	++
Proxymetacaine (proparacaine)[d]	F	+
Amide type		
Bupivacaine	S	+++
Cinchocaine (dibucaine)[c]	?	+++
Etidocaine	F	+++
Lidocaine (lignocaine)	F	++
Mepivacaine	F	++
Prilocaine	F	++
Ropivacaine	S	+++

[a] S/F, slow/fast onset; T, topical use only.

[b] +/++/+++, short/medium/long duration of effect. Formulation and the use of vasoconstrictors influences these parameters markedly. The action of prilocaine cannot be extended by vasoconstrictors.

[c] Used only in otorhinolaryngology and occasionally in ophthalmology.

[d] Relatively ineffective for topical use.

[e] Seldom used.

However, **intravenous regional anaesthesia** (Bier's block) is used to anaesthetize a limb, intravascular spread being prevented by using a tourniquet. The use of local anaesthetics by IV infusion to produce general anaesthesia is hazardous and requires expert advice, so this route is rarely used. Regional anaesthesia can also be achieved by spinal use (see below).

Skin anaesthesia

This is difficult to achieve through intact skin, owing to poor penetration, though a *lidocaine (lignocaine)–prilocaine cream* may be used under an occlusive dressing (to increase penetration) for 1 h before painful procedures. This is a eutectic mixture which has a low melting point and becomes an oil that is able to penetrate intact skin at normal temperatures. A *tetracaine (amethocaine)* gel can also be used similarly before venepuncture or venous cannulation. These must not be used on wounds, abrasions or inflamed skin because absorption may be rapid and extensive and lead to systemic side effects.

Ophthalmic procedures

Oxybuprocaine (benoxinate) and *tetracaine (amethocaine)* are used extensively. Because tetracaine (amethocaine) produces deeper anaesthesia it can be used for minor surgery. *Proxymetacaine (proparacaine)* and *lidocaine (lignocaine)–fluorescein* eye drops are used for **conventional tonometry** (measuring the intraocular pressure by placing a membrane on the cornea) as one aspect of diagnosing glaucoma. However, non-contact methods, e.g. firing a jet of compressed air at the cornea, are used increasingly. *Oxybuprocaine (benoxinate)* has a similar activity to tetracaine (amethocaine), but is less irritant.

Otolaryngology

Nose, throat and ear procedures are the only ones in which *cocaine* is still used appreciably. It is generally avoided because of its powerful stimulant action and potential for abuse, and its sympathomimetic effects. Because of the latter, cocaine should not normally be used with *adrenaline (epinephrine)* and similar drugs, but some surgeons believe that combination with adrenaline (epinephrine) reduces cocaine absorption and is operatively beneficial. *Cocaine* rapidly produces effective surface analgesia which persists for at least 30 min, depending on the concentration used.

Spinal anaesthesia

Bupivacaine and *ropivacaine* are used to block nerve transmission at any point up to spinal cord level (*see* Fig. 10.2), providing temporary pain relief. This topic is dealt with under 'Chemical nerve blocks' (p. 597).

Prolongation and enhancement of effect

Prolongation and enhancement of local anaesthesia is usually done by **combination with vasoconstrictors**. Most local anaesthetics cause vasodilatation and so are often formulated with *adrenaline (epinephrine)*; this produces local vasoconstriction and so prevents rapid distribution into the surrounding tissues and the circulation.

This effect prolongs the duration of action and potentiates the anaesthetic effect, owing to the increased local concentration of agent. Also, the reduced rate of systemic absorption enables drug metabolism to keep pace, thus reducing any systemic toxicity. Peak plasma concentrations occur after about 10–25 min, so patients should be monitored carefully for 30 min after injection to ensure that no serious side effects arise.

Adrenaline (epinephrine) is **contraindicated** if the anaesthetic is to be used in or near the fingers, toes or other appendages because the vasoconstriction produced may result in **ischaemic necrosis**. *Felypressin*, a synthetic derivative of the antidiuretic hormone vasopressin, may be a suitable alternative to adrenaline (epinephrine) and is used for dental procedures if the latter is con-traindicated in a particular patient. However, vasoconstrictors are themselves toxic and must not be injected into the digits, appendages or terminal arteries because of the risk of ischaemic necrosis. Further, they must not normally be used with *cocaine*, which has intrinsic vasoconstrictor and mydriatic properties. An alternative is to use a viscous vehicle, usually containing *dextran 110*, and this approach has been used to prolong the local action of *lidocaine (lignocaine)* for up to 10 h, though the effect is very variable.

Bupivacaine has a long duration of effect, up to 10 h, and may be useful if adrenaline (epinephrine) or felypressin are contraindicated. However, it has a slow onset of action (30 min), so lidocaine (lignocaine) is usually used initially, followed by bupivacaine if prolonged local anaesthesia is required. The onset of action of bupivacaine depends on the concentration, dose and route used. It is used for peripheral nerve block and infiltration nerve blockade and is the principal drug used for spinal anaesthesia in the UK (p. 597). Bupivacaine is **contraindicated** for use in intravenous regional anaesthesia, because of the risks of its long action, cardiovascular and central nervous toxicity, and because prolonged restriction of the blood supply would be required. Although bupivacaine is widely used for spinal obstetric anaesthesia, the concentration and circumstances of use in this setting require expert advice.

Side effects

As usual, inflammation and trauma increase penetration markedly such that significant systemic absorption may then occur. On occasion, this may lead to toxicity, especially with *tetracaine (amethocaine)*. This drug must never be used on mucous membranes, e.g. before bronchoscopy and cystoscopy: *lidocaine (lignocaine)* is safer. The lidocaine (lignocaine)–prilocaine cream used on the skin is irritant to the eyes and is ototoxic, and so should not be used on or near these organs.

Local anaesthetics are generally very safe, and adverse events are rare when they are used peripherally. However, apart from the use of the *lidocaine (lignocaine)–prilocaine cream* and *tetracaine* (*amethocaine*) *gel* mentioned above, they should generally be avoided for topical application to the skin because sensitization may occur. Systemic complications may also occur, usually when large doses are used to produce nerve blocks in the region of the spinal cord. This is usually from accidental intravascular injection, which is particularly hazardous if injections contain adrenaline (epinephrine).

Hypersensitivity occasionally occurs: compounds of the same chemical type tend to give cross-reactions, but these do not occur between the ester and amide groups (Table 10.8).

Topical agents

Liniments and rubs have a long medical history and were once the only available treatments for localized joint and soft tissue damage. They are mostly essential oil products, e.g. camphor, menthol, methyl salicylate, turpentine, sometimes with capsicum oleoresin or nicotinates.

More recently, several NSAIDs have been presented as gels or creams. These have the advantage that, if only one or two joints are affected they can be applied to those localized areas. This avoids the need to take larger amounts of drug orally and so also avoids some of the associated side effects. Because of this, and possibly because they are involved in the treatment, NSAIDs are liked by patients. Although penetration of the drug into joints and soft tissues has been demonstrated there is little localized effect and the therapeutic benefit is small.

The **modes of action** of most of these, apart from any specific NSAID activity, are alleged to be:

• Increased blood flow to the area, induced by the massage.
• **Counter-irritation**, i.e. stimulation of C neurones inhibits local release of **substance P** and so attenuates the transmission of pain impulses. This mode of action has been demonstrated for *capsaicin cream*, which is used for the alleviation of osteoarthritis and PHN (p. 613).

Physical methods

Traction, to relieve pressure on nerves, and manipulation and mobilization of muscles and limbs are the traditional approaches of osteopathy, chiropractic and physiotherapy (PT), and are of undoubted value in some patients. PT also uses the application of heat (including short-wave diathermy), cold, ultrasound, electrical muscle stimulation and laser therapy. Ultrasound has been advocated for soft tissue injuries, PHN, facial neuritis and phantom limb pain (i.e. that felt in an amputated limb).

Ice packs are widely use in the early treatment of soft tissue injuries, especially sport and similar traumas. The mnemonic, 'RICE', i.e. **R**est, **I**ce, **C**ompression, **E**levation, is used by first-aiders. Care is needed not to cause 'ice burns', by using a cloth between the skin and the cold pack.

Techniques recruiting endogenous inhibitory mechanisms

In addition to increasing the understanding of how conventional analgesics act, the gate theory has stimulated interest in alternative methods of pain relief. The emphasis has shifted from nerve destruction or blocking of pain conduction to the recruitment of the body's own inhibitory systems. This is the principle underlying the use of vibration, percussion, massage, and counter-irritation with rubefacients. The cooling produced by pain-relieving sprays may also stimulate pain trigger points (see below) or, if the cooling is sufficiently intense and prolonged, a degree of local anaesthesia may be produced. However, skin 'burns', or even frost-bite, must be avoided.

These techniques are not always successful, but they may provide acceptable pain relief to some patients with otherwise intractable conditions. Some authorities insist that these simple methods should be used first, and persevered with for several weeks, before either a maximum effect is achieved or the approach is abandoned. Table 10.9 lists the principal alternative methods of pain control.

Table 10.9   Modes of treatment using inhibitory pain mechanisms

Site of action	Treatment mode
Local	Acupuncture, stroking, rubbing, massage, vibration, percussion Counter-irritation, e.g. rubefacient creams (e.g. nicotinates, salicylate esters, capsaicin) Reducing nerve conduction. e.g. pain-relieving sprays, ice packs Transcutaneous electrical nerve stimulation (TENS)
Central	Yoga, hypnosis, meditation, mental training (biofeedback)

Neuromodulation by electrical stimulation

The most commonly used method in this category is **transcutaneous electrical nerve stimulation (TENS)**. This is normally used for the relief of chronic peripheral pain, though it has also been used to relieve acute pain, e.g. of operative incisions. Electrodes are placed on the painful area, or at the periphery of a very sensitive area, though the optimum placing needs to be found by careful trial by the patients themselves. Occasionally, acupuncture sites are used (see below).

Patients wear a battery-driven pulse generator and vary the frequency, pulse width and power, normally to produce a pleasant non-painful tingling sensation. Patients usually know whether the method is going to be successful within 5–15 min. The length and frequency of stimulation varies from three 1-h sessions daily to whole-day use.

The conditions most likely to respond are post-herpetic neuralgia, low back pain, phantom limb pain and postoperative scar pain. The mode of action is believed to be stimulation of the large (inhibitory) A-beta nerve fibres, closing the pain gate in the dorsal horn of the spinal cord and reducing or abolishing upward transmission of the stimulus.

Invasive techniques have also been used occasionally. Electrodes associated with a miniature radio receiver have been implanted around peripheral nerves, near the posterior columns of the spinal cord, or even in the brain, and stimulated by a patient-controlled radio transmitter.

Although complications are rare, electrical neuromodulation is contraindicated for psychoneurotic or emotionally unstable patients, and for opioid addicts.

Acupuncture

Therapeutic acupuncture, i.e. for the relief of chronic pain rather than as an operative anaesthetic, is used both by practitioners who follow the traditional Chinese system, with its over 300 sites for insertion of the needles. Also some Western doctors may follow an empirical system. Needles are inserted to a precise depth and may be left in place for up to 30 min, or rotated, moved up and down, or electrically stimulated.

The mode of action is hotly disputed, but may involve interference with nerve depolarization, stimulation of inhibitory nerve fibres, release of endorphins, enkephalins or 5HT, or hypnotic suggestion. The success of the treatment is certainly influenced profoundly by cultural and psychological factors. One estimate is that about 10% of patients are responders, a further 10% are non-responders, and the remainder experience varying degrees of benefit.

Chemical nerve blocks

Regional nerve blocks

These may be:

- Field blocks, i.e. SC injections at various sites around sensory nerves in the area of the procedure.

- Peripheral blocks involve a similar procedure, but the local anaesthetic is often injected into nerve plexus, e.g. the **brachial plexus**, an intricate network of nerves emerging from the spinal cord at the base of the neck (between the lower cervical and uppermost thoracic vertebrae) which supply the whole arm, or the **pudendal plexus**, which primarily supplies the lower genitalia.
- Central blocks; these can be:
  - **Epidural** (extradural, peridural), outside the spinal cord between the dura mater and the inner wall of the vertebral canal.
  - **Caudal**, in the lumbar or sacral regions of the spinal cord, where it divides to form the cauda equina.
  - **Intrathecal** (subarachnoid), into the cerebrospinal fluid (CSF) between the pia mater and the arachnoid.

With intrathecal anaesthesia the level of the nerve block, and so the area and organs affected, depends on the position of the patient and the specific gravity (SG) of the anaesthetic solution. **Isobaric solutions** have the same SG as the CSF and exert their effect at the level of injection. **Hypobaric** solutions are lighter than CSF and act higher than the injection site, depending on the position of the patient. **Hyperbaric** solutions are heavier than CSF and flow towards the bottom of the spinal cord. They are used primarily for operations in the area of the genitalia and on the legs.

Central and other anaesthetic blocks

Local anaesthetics

These agents (p. 593) may be used to block transmission at any point up to spinal cord level (*see* Fig. 10.2). This provides temporary pain relief or anaesthesia for operations on patients in whom general anaesthesia is unsuitable, e.g. due to cardiac and respiratory problems or when central nervous sedation is undesirable. However, local anaesthetics also block other types of sensation and motor impulses, though usually to a lesser extent. The degree and extent of the anaesthetized area depends on the concentration and volume of solution injected.

Epidural (extradural) and intrathecal *opioids* are sometimes used for the relief of postoperative and chronic pain. Injections are usually given via a catheter located at the correct segment of the spinal cord. The effect is on the sensory, dorsal horn nerves. The release of **substance P** and other neurotransmitters from primary afferent nerves is inhibited by presynaptic opioid receptors and effects on postsynaptic receptors reduce activity in ascending spinal tracts. However, conduction in motor and autonomic nerves is unaffected by opioids, so motor functions and blood pressure are generally not affected by the spinal use of opioids. The analgesia produced is normally insufficient for intraoperative pain so spinal opioids are used as adjuncts to general anaesthetics. Spinal *morphine* may provide 8–16 h of analgesia and can give months of low-dose analgesia in cancer patients without the side effects of oral or parenteral use. *Alfentanil* infusions have also been used.

Such **reversible nerve blocks** are also used in diagnosis and to determine which nerves are involved in a particular pain process and the probable prognosis of a **permanent nerve block**, because the production of the latter by nerve ablation with neurolytic agents can often be inaccurate and may not achieve the desired result.

Cinchocaine (*dibucaine*) is the most potent (and toxic) local anaesthetic available, and has been used intrathecally for this purpose, though *bupivacaine* is more usual in the UK. Once the correct site has been identified, an irreversible block produced by the injection of such agents as alcohol, phenol or chlorocresol, and urethane may provide much longer-lasting relief. Unfortunately, this procedure may be too lengthy for patients who have severe intractable pain.

Alcohol produces total neurolysis, but the extent of blockage produced may be varied by using an appropriate concentration of phenolic agent. These injections may be subarachnoid, extradural, subdural, autonomic or peripheral depending on the site of ablation which provides satisfactory relief.

Permanent nerve blocks

These are most useful in treating patients with well-defined localized pain. As expertise and knowledge increases, a wider range of destructive methods (peripheral, central or autonomic) is becoming available. Because the peripheral nerves are easily accessible, they are often chosen as sites for destruction, though nerve regeneration can occur with consequent return of the pain. Alternatively, the sensory root can be destroyed. This should theoretically result in permanent pain relief, as axonal regeneration should not occur if the nerve fibres are interrupted proximal to the sensory ganglion. Unfortunately, this is not always successful.

The procedures are potentially hazardous, and partial loss of sensation and function, thrombosis, spinal cord infarction, and even death have occurred: a skilled and experienced anaesthetist or neurosurgeon is required to conduct such procedures successfully.

Injection of alcohol can also be used to destroy the pituitary gland in patients who have widespread bilateral cancer pain, especially if the tumour is hormone-dependent. Because the alcohol spreads around the floor and into the cavity of the third ventricle, it is possible that part of the success of this technique is from direct hypothalamic injury. About 70% of patients benefit, more than half of whom obtain complete relief.

Neurosurgical approaches

The most common surgical procedures for pain relief are cordotomy (see below) and insertion of epidural, intrathecal and intraventricular catheters for opioid or local anaesthetic delivery directly to specific areas of the central nervous system. Subarachnoid catheter injection can sometimes be successful in cases where more conventional opioid administration has failed to reach central opioid receptors.

Whereas drug therapy may not completely remove pain, an effective surgical nerve block can do so. The main problem is that it may not be possible to block the appropriate pathway without impairing other sensory pathways.

Cordotomy involves the interruption of the anterolateral quadrant of the spinal cord in the cervical or thoracic region. This may be done percutaneously using a diathermy probe, or sometimes by open surgery, and is most useful in treating unilateral pain below the shoulders. The method is used primarily in patients who have a limited life expectancy (2 years), because the development of alternative nerve pathways often allows pain to return after some time. Thus, cordotomy is used primarily in patients with advanced, irreversible disease and severe intractable pain, of whom over 80% obtain complete relief with such treatment.

Psychotherapy and hypnosis

The role of psychotherapeutic drugs has already been mentioned (p. 591). These behavioural approaches may be effective if there is no organic basis for the pain, i.e. it is psychogenic, if there is a minor cause but the pain is grossly aggravated by psychological factors and if anxiety and depression exacerbate pain significantly.

Meditation and **relaxation training** help patients to divert their attention away from pain and facilitate their tolerance of it. **Hypnosis** sufficient to induce a light trance is a recognized form of treatment and some patients are able to hypnotize themselves. It may relieve pain completely in the (highly suggestible) 20% of responders, and be a useful adjunct to other forms of treatment in many more. Hypnosis is unsuitable for patients with psychiatric illnesses who may be impossible to hypnotize or who behave in a bizarre fashion under hypnosis.

Biofeedback involves linking a patient to equipment which monitors parameters such as heart rate or blood pressure (which are increased by pain) or muscle tension (which may cause pain). The patient is taught techniques for relaxation and sees how this modifies their physiological response and reduces their pain level; thus they learn to control their feelings appropriately.

Patient-controlled analgesia (PCA)

Definition

This is a technique for dosing with *opioids*, and occasionally with *local anaesthetics*, according to the patient's perception of their own needs and pain severity. The method is used for controlling both acute pain, e.g. trauma, postoperative, and chronic pain, e.g. burns patients, cancer.

The equipment usually comprises a microprocessor-driven syringe containing the drug solution, which is administered parenterally via a catheter. This is usually done intravenously, but the SC, IM and epidural routes are also used. When a patient experiences unacceptable pain, they press a button on the control unit and a predetermined dose of drug is administered.

Advantages

The advantages of PCA are as follows:

- Patients are in control of their pain, not vice versa, and feel more secure. This alone improves the quality of analgesia obtained.
- The blood level is maintained more closely within the therapeutic range than can be achieved with injections given on demand. This improves analgesia and minimizes side effects.
- Doses can readily be titrated to cope with wide variations in pain severity and patient needs.
- There is minimal delay between the perception of intolerable pain and obtaining a dose of analgesic. There is also less demand on nursing time and pharmacy provision.

Disadvantages and limitations

The following points are additional to those usually associated with opioid or (local anaesthetic) use:

- Highly trained staff are required to set up the equipment and supervise the patient.
- The method is only suitable for maintenance analgesia. The patient's needs should be established clearly, or readily estimated, and a suitable loading dose given before starting PCA.
- Some patients reject the technique.
- A patient's understanding of how to use the equipment may be limited by:
  - Extreme age.
  - Language or comprehension problems.
  - Sedation or confusion.
- Poorly controlled blood pressure may compromise perfusion of the injection site.
- Changes in renal or hepatic function may cause significant variation in drug availability.

Modes of use

Three arrangements are possible:

- Patient controlled analgesia only.
- Continuous background infusion plus patient-controlled analgesia.
- Continuous background infusion only.

PCA only

PCA is best suited to acute analgesia. If excessive demand is made and the patient becomes sedated, this is a self-regulating situation because the patient then makes less demands for analgesia until the sedation wears off.

Continuous background infusion plus PCA

This is particularly appropriate for chronic pain relief, e.g. severely burned patients, who often need opioids for long periods, can be given 30–50% of their predetermined hourly dose as a background infusion, the PCA being used for breakthrough pain.

Continuous background infusion only

This is not strictly PCA because it is not controlled by the patient. It is more useful in managing chronic pain, especially in patients who may not be able to manage the equipment correctly because they are confused or have little understanding of the equipment and the principles of opioid use. It is less suitable for acute pain because of the inability to manage breakthrough pain, the risk of excessive sedation and other adverse reactions.

Some technical and clinical aspects

Technical and clinical points include the following:

- The bolus dose delivered on demand must be adequate, but must not cause unacceptable side effects.
- The time over which the dose is injected following patient triggering is adjusted according to the route used. Thus, for SC injections the time may need to be lengthened to 5 min to avoid stinging or inadequate clearance from the site. Also the 'lock-out interval', i.e. the time after the end of a dose during which another bolus cannot be obtained, may need to be lengthened. Alternatively, the solution concentration may be increased so that a smaller volume is injected.
- The **lock-out interval** should be long enough to avoid adverse drug reactions. It is usually 5–8 min.
- The **maximum dose** allowed in 1 h, or 4 h, should be controlled, e.g. 30 mg morphine in 4 h.

- **Inadequate analgesia**. If usage is:
  - Two or less doses/hour, counsel the patient about fears of opioid use, etc. and advise more frequent use.
  - More than three bolus doses/hour, increase bolus volume.
  - Also review possibilities, e.g. pain is not opioid-responsive or may be a new complication of the disease and/or surgery.
- **Nausea and vomiting**:
  - Use anti-emetics (*see* Chapter 6, pp. 332–335), e.g. transdermal hyoscine (scopolamine) in patients under 60 years if injections are undesirable (may cause urinary retention and confusion in the elderly).
  - Decrease bolus volume or increase duration of delivery.
  - Change opioid.
- **Urinary retention**: relieve with indwelling or intermittent catheterization.
- **Pruritus**:
  - Change opioid, e.g. to *nalbuphine*.
  - Use a non-sedating antihistamine.
  - Use *naloxone* if intractable, but care is required because the analgesia may be reversed.

Common pain situations

Headache, migraine and facial pain

Epidemiology and aetiology

Headache is probably the most common of all the pain syndromes, and about 80–90% of the population have at least one attack each year. Of these, about 6% experience recurrent episodes which interfere with their normal daily activities, and it is estimated that headaches cause an annual loss of about 70 million working days in the UK.

Peak GP consulting rates occur in the 10- to 40-year age group, the female : male ratio being about 2.5 : 1 overall. Fortunately, most headaches are benign. The principal causes are given in Table 10.10. There are estimated to be over 5 million migraine sufferers in the UK, though at least half have mild to moderate pain and do not consult their doctors.

Analgesic abuse is an important cause of headache, recognition of which requires a high index of suspicion.

Classification

The International Headache Society has issued guidelines classifying headache into 13 categories (Table 10.11). Despite this formidable list, most headaches are benign. Only four types are discussed below, the pain patterns associated with these being illustrated in Fig. 10.4.

Table 10.10   Causes of headache by age

	Children and teenagers	Adults	Elderly
Common	–	Tension headache Migraine	Temporal arteritis[a] Cervical origin
Less common	Tension headache Migraine	Trauma Subdural and subarachnoid haemorrhage Analgesic abuse	Glaucoma Paget's disease
Uncommon	Tumours Subdural and subarachnoid haemorrhage	Glaucoma Paget's disease Cervical origin Tumours	Tension headache Migraine Trauma Subdural and subarachnoid haemorrhage Tumours

[a] See Chapter 8.

Table 10.11   Classification of headache[a]

Tension-type headache[b]
Migraine[b]
Cluster headache[b] and chronic paroxysmal hemicrania
Miscellaneous headaches not associated with structural lesions
Headache associated with:
• head trauma
• vascular disorders
• non-vascular intracranial disorder
• substances or their withdrawal
• non-cephalic infection
• metabolic disorder
Headache or facial pain associated with facial or cranial structures
Cranial neuralgias[b] nerve trunk pain, and deafferentation pain

[a] Based on the classification of the International Headache Society (1988) *Cephalalgia* **8** (Suppl. 7): 1–96.
[b] See text.

Tension-type headaches

Clinical features

These are the most common forms of headache and may arise from sustained muscle contraction in the cervical (neck) region or scalp, stress, or be psychogenic in origin (depression). They may be episodic, i.e. occurring on less than 15 days/month and having no persistent symptoms. However, they are often chronic, present at similar times each day, e.g. on more than 15 days/month for more than 6 months, every morning or evening, or on the same days each week.

The pain is:

• Mild to moderate.
• Typically has a bilateral 'hatband' or more generalized distribution (Fig. 10.4(a)).
• Non-throbbing.
• Not aggravated by movement.

Uncommonly, 'bursting' sensations and **photophobia** and **sonophobia**, light and sound intolerance) may occur. There are few abnormal signs, but the scalp and neck muscles may be tender.

Bilateral pain, infrequency of vomiting and tendency to be chronic rather than episodic distinguish it from migraine (see below), but in North America this syndrome is sometimes called 'minor migraine'.

Management and pharmacotherapy

Treatment of this condition is often unsatisfactory because no specific pathology can be

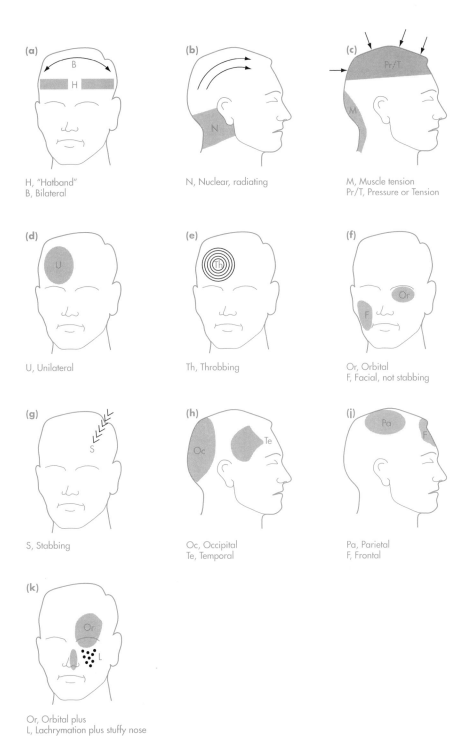

Figure 10.4 Patterns of pain in headache. (a–c) Tension headache; (d–j) migraine; (g) also neuralgia; (k) cluster headache.

identified and it may be difficult or impossible to modify employment, social and personality trigger factors. Management and symptomatic treatment involve:

- Possibly extensive investigations to eliminate serious pathology, e.g. cerebral cancer, stroke, and reassure the patient.
- Avoidance of any identifiable causes, if possible.
- Physical treatments may help, e.g. relaxation therapy, psychotherapy, hypnotherapy, ice packs, cervical manipulation (provided that this has been confirmed as a safe procedure in that patient).
- Analgesics appropriate to severity, e.g. *paracetamol (acetaminophen)*, *aspirin* (in the over-12s, if tolerated) or combinations of these with *dextropropoxyphene (propoxyphene)*, *codeine* or *dihydrocodeine*, but these may be abused.
- Antidepressants or anxiolytics (*see* Chapter 7) if indicated. *Amitriptyline* is widely used.
- *Sumatriptan* (p. 608, 'serotonin agonists') may also be useful.

Treatment is more effective if patients present soon after the initial symptoms occur. Antidepressants are withdrawn gradually after about 6 months' sustained improvement.

Analgesic abuse headache

This may accompany any other form of headache. Because it occurs daily it is frequently associated with tension headaches. The normal pattern is that a patient complaining of headache will manage well initially by self-medicating with simple analgesics as the need arises. There may then be a progression to daily simple analgesic use, seeking advice for 'something stronger', consulting their doctor and regular use of a compound analgesic (*co-proxamol*, *co-codamol* or *co-dydramol* in the UK), even a more potent opioid, without obtaining satisfactory relief. This adds the side effects of the analgesic, i.e. any of the side effects of opioids (see above), to the effects of the headache. Misuse of antimigraine drugs can cause similar problems. Patients with tension-type headache are the most likely headache sufferers to be using opioids.

The correct course is to stop the daily analgesic medication. This may cause rebound exacerbation of headache for 1–2 weeks. Withdrawal symptoms may need to be treated with antiemetics and sedatives. Cognitive therapy (*see* Chapter 7) is usually required, but failure to improve subsequently should prompt a neurological or psychiatric investigation.

Migraine

Definition

There are two main types of migraine:

- *Migraine without aura (common migraine)*. Recurrent moderate to severe, throbbing headache, usually unilateral but sometimes bilateral, accompanied by intolerance of light or noise or nausea and sometimes vomiting. Prostration may last for between 4 h and several days if treatment is unsuccessful.
- *Migraine with aura (classical migraine)*. There may be warning of an impending attack with visual symptoms and sensory and motor limb disturbances, lasting between 4 and 60 min. The headache follows within 60 min, or accompanies these symptoms.

Epidemiology

For epidemiological purposes, migraine patients (**migraineurs**) are defined as having had at least five attacks without aura, or two with aura.

Attacks commence at about 10 years of age and rise to a peak at 14–16 years. There is then a slow rise in women up to age 40 years. Some 10% of the population (female : male ratio = 2.5:1) are 'active migraineurs'; 5% have 18 or more migraine days/year; 1% have one day/week. The average duration of an attack is about 24 h, but may be 2–3 days in 20% of patients.

Aetiology

This has yet to be elucidated in humans. The traditional view that symptoms are simply the result of alterations in cerebral blood flow is probably incorrect. The haemodynamic changes observed during all phases of the attack cannot alone account for the symptoms. Rather, the vascular changes reflect neurological events.

The **anatomy of the cerebral circulation** is complex, probably because:

- The brain is highly active metabolically, consuming about 20% of total blood oxygen at rest.
- There is an absolute requirement for a continuous supply of glucose.
- Even a brief interruption of the blood supply may cause unconsciousness; 1–2 min deprivation impairs brain cell activity and 4–5 min causes permanent damage.

There is a complete circle of interconnecting arteries at the base of the brain (the circle of Willis, derived from the four main ascending arteries, two vertebral, two internal carotid). This minimizes the risk of ischaemia, e.g. due to a small clot, because the circle can be supplied by any of its ascending arteries. The cerebral veins have no valves, have very thin walls, and no muscle layer. Thus they cannot be causal in migraine but can account for the pounding nature of the headache. There are also large venous sinuses which drain pooled venous blood from the brain and skull. Numerous anastomoses connect the arterial circle and this venous system.

There are several pathophysiological theories of migraine symptomatology, reflecting our current uncertainties. Migraineurs probably have a genetically determined, or congenital, reduced CNS excitation threshold, i.e. they fall into an intermediate group between epileptics and 'normals'. Vascular changes can account for the **prodrome** (see below) and the **aura** has been generally accepted as being the result of arteriospasm, reducing cerebral blood supply. However, animal experiments have shown that the aura may be due to **cortical spreading depression** (CSD), a wave of depolarization which travels across the cortex over several minutes, depressing neuronal activity and preceded by a narrow, excitatory front. CSD causes the release of excitatory amino acid neurotransmitters and profound changes in ion flux and cerebral blood flow. Thus the primary changes are neurological. The subsequent headache may result from activation by CSD of the trigeminal ganglion and its vascular branches. CSD and its effects have not yet been demonstrated in humans.

The concept that the subsequent headache is caused by vasodilatation is supported by the fact that potent vasoconstrictors are used for the acute treatment of migraine (p. 608). Theories concerning the headache phase include:

- Opening of arteriovenous anastomoses exposes the cerebral veins to arterial pressures for which they are not designed, causing localized and later widespread venous dilatation and changes in intracranial pressure. This could explain the pounding nature of the headache, because the thin-walled veins would be exposed to the systolic pressure with every heartbeat. They would then expand, putting pressure on the brain, and relax during diastole.
- The arteriovenous anastomoses act as shunts, partially starving the brain of oxygen and glucose.
- Stimulation of cranial nerves, especially the trigeminal, causes neurogenic plasma extravasation in the dura mater and the release of pro-inflammatory mediators from perivascular nerves.
- Dilatation of the carotid arterial circulation causes stretching and thickening of the meninges, producing pain.

Serotonin (5HT), released by vascular nerves or from platelets, is clearly implicated in the pathogenesis of migraine. The recent advances in treatment have been derived from the observation that injection of 5HT can abort migraine attacks, but causes substantial side effects. Additionally, the introduction of a NSAID which is a potent inhibitor of prostaglandin and leukotriene B_4 synthesis has also focused attention on their pathogenetic role. Nitric oxide is also implicated in CNS vasodilatation.

Clinical features

Different patterns occur, ranging from occasional headaches that are almost indistinguishable from tension headache to frequent disabling episodes (Fig. 10.4(d–j)).

Symptoms may mimic those of transient ischaemic attacks (TIAs; these resemble a stroke, but the patient recovers within 24 h) and are clearly associated with cerebral ischaemia. There may be dizziness or partial or complete blindness (**basilar migraine**), partial or complete hemiparesis (one-sided paralysis, **familial hemiplegic migraine**), and paralysis of the eye muscles (**ophthalmoplegic migraine**) or facial muscles. It is important to distinguish these symptoms, which arise gradually, from those of thrombo-embolic TIAs, which are usually of sudden onset, because both treatment and prognosis are very different for the two conditions. These atypical migraines are uncommon but are important because they are associated with ischaemia, so the $5HT_1$ agonists are **contraindicated** for their treatment because they are potent vasoconstrictors. These forms of migraine are now believed to be due to genetically determined abnormalities of the $alpha_1$-subunit (ion-conducting) cerebral calcium channels will not be discussed further here. However, the possibility is raised that migraine is due to an inherited defect of calcium channels.

Migraine is known to be associated with an increased risk of ischaemic stroke, and a recent large European study has found that this risk is increased threefold in young women with migraine. Up to 40% of strokes in this study developed from a migraine attack, and factors such as oral contraceptive use, hypertension and smoking further increased the risk.

Migraine with aura

Triggers for attacks are listed in Table 10.12. There may be three distinct phases to an attack: (i) feelings of well-being, yawning, food rejections or cravings, etc. which may last for up to 24 h (the **prodrome**); (ii) these are followed by an aura; and (ii) finally the headache and associated features.

The aura develops over 5–20 min and may last for 15–60 min or more. The aura is usually visual, including spots (**scotomas**), blurred vision, flashing lights and castellations. 'Pins and needles', facial tingling, speech difficulties and unusual smells may also occur. Nausea may commence.

This is followed by a severe throbbing headache that may start unilaterally and be localized, but may later become more general. Nausea increases and vomiting usually follows. Sufferers are irritable, photophobic and sonophobic and usually retreat to a dark, quiet bedroom. The attack lasts from hours to days and often terminates with sleep, often followed by a longish, variable pain-free period. Because attacks are associated with smooth muscle inhibition there is often a delayed diuresis towards the end of an attack.

Common migraine

This is the most common form of migraine, and affects about 75% of sufferers. The symptoms

Table 10.12   Some trigger factors for migraine

Type of trigger factor	Examples
Foods	Cheese, alcohol (red wine), beans, onions, oranges, chocolate, coffee, tea, Chinese meals
Fasting	
Emotion	Anxiety, tension, stress, depression, fatigue
Hormonal change	Menstrual cycle, puberty, oral contraceptives, pregnancy, menopause
Miscellaneous	Visual (e.g. bright strobe lights, television or computer screen flicker), aural and olfactory stimuli
	Heat or cold
	Sleep disturbance, tiredness
	Allergies?
	Smoking
	Head, neck and eye pain, jaw grinding

resemble those of classical migraine, but tend to comprise only headache, malaise and nausea. Occasionally, aura occurs without other symptoms. There may be considerable difficulty in distinguishing between common migraine and tension headache. The two syndromes may be concurrent or tension headache may exacerbate common migraine at some stage.

Investigation

A typical history and a normal neurological examination is usually conclusive. The presence of atypical features should prompt further examination to exclude meningitis, subarachnoid haemorrhage (SAH), TIAs, sensory epilepsy, stroke and a brain tumour or other serious pathology. A first attack of migraine is very unusual over the age of 60 years: the onset of an exceptionally severe headache unlike any in a patient's previous experience should raise the possibility of significant pathology, even if they are migraineurs. Patients are normal between attacks.

The relevance of all of the factors listed in Table 10.12 should be assessed, possibly with a patient diary.

Because we do not have genuinely specific antimigraine drugs, the response to therapy is not diagnostic.

Management: general aspects

This is as follows:

- Effective treatment of any associated diseases.
- Counselling:
  - For identification and avoidance of possible trigger factors (Table 10.12), especially changing or stopping a combined oral contraceptive in young women.
  - Strong reassurance that the condition is benign (many patients think that they have a brain tumour or are going 'mad').
  - Importance of prompt treatment at the first sign of an impending attack.
  - Rest.

The principles of treatment of are outlined in Table 10.13

Pharmacotherapy of acute attacks

General considerations

Drug absorption from the gut may be compromised with all drugs, especially conventional

---

Table 10.13   A stepped approach to migraine management[a]

Step	Clinical features	Form of management or pharmacotherapy[a]
Step 1 (mild migraine)	Occasional mild symptoms Minimal interference with lifestyle	Simple analgesics, compound analgesics or non-steroidal anti-inflammatory drug Anti-emetic if required
Step 2 (moderate migraine)	Moderate to severe throbbing headaches, one attack a month or less Significant nausea ± vomiting Interferes with lifestyle, e.g. attacks last 2–3 days, quiet rest essential	Compound analgesics Anti-emetic Tolfenamic acid or 5HT$_1$ agonist (second-line drugs if these ineffective)
Step 3 (severe and/or frequent migraine)	More than one severe attack a month Severe nausea ± vomiting Significant interference with lifestyle, e.g. frequent time off work, often unable to carry out tasks of normal living	Treat acute attacks as Step 2 Prophylactic pharmacotherapy[a]

[a] See text.

tablets and capsules, because gastric stasis and generally poor gut peristalsis develops during an attack. Absorption is improved by using effervescent oral formulations and by using an antiemetic and prokinetic drug, e.g. *metoclopramide* or *domperidone*, 30 min before an analgesic. Routes of administration which avoid first-pass metabolism, e.g. buccal dosage forms (sublingual tablets, oral aerosols), nasal sprays and injections, are pharmacokinetically preferable, because many of the drugs used undergo extensive hepatic metabolism. Suppositories are useful if the patient is nauseated and vomiting. Patient dislike of suppositories and repeated injections may be balanced by the rapidity and extent of benefit derived from a product.

It may take experimentation over a few attacks to establish the optimum drugs, dosage and routes of administration. Patients do not always require the same treatment: mild attacks may respond to simple analgesics, while severe ones in the same patient may require specific treatment. The relative responses to different drugs may be different in different attacks, and response to specific treatment seems to be more consistent than that to simple analgesics.

Drugs should not be used during the aura, which is unresponsive to treatment and may not always be followed by headache: they should be reserved for established headache.

Headache recurrence limits the benefits of treatment significantly, not least because patients may regard it as treatment failure. Recurrence occurs in about 35% of responders, for unknown reasons. Generally, **only one repeat dose of a specific antimigraine drug should be used for inadequate relief or a recurrence and non-responders should not repeat the dose.** This is to avoid the potential harm from prolonged vasoconstriction and the risk of analgesic-induced headache. Non-responders will not gain any benefit from a second dose, though the same drug, given by a different route or in a higher dose, may be successful in another attack.

The 'therapeutic gain' (TG) is the response rate to treatment minus the response to placebo or comparator, and is used below. However, trial results are difficult to compare due to different end-points, time of measurement of the response, use of 'escape medication' and comparison in only one attack or over several attacks.

There are two approaches to management: the traditional **stepped-care model** (ladder), i.e. simple analgesic to compound analgesic to ergotamine to a triptan (see below), or to decide on the appropriate treatment for a particular patient depending on their symptoms, the **stratified-care model**. The latter is gaining ground with the introduction of the triptans, which are effective and less toxic than ergotamine.

Simple and compound analgesics

These have been discussed above and in Chapter 8 (p. 478; *see also* **NSAIDs**, p. 489). Effervescent aspirin may be similarly effective to *sumatriptan*.

Non-steroidal anti-inflammatory drugs

Tolfenamic acid is a NSAID that is specifically licensed for the treatment of acute migraine attacks. It has the general properties and side effects of NSAIDs and may also cause dysuria (mostly in men), tremor, euphoria and fatigue, but it seems to be well-tolerated. Tolfenamic acid is reported to be similarly effective to the $5HT_1$ agonists (see below) and is formulated as a tablet which disintegrates rapidly and has good bioavailability.

Serotonin agonists ('triptans')

$5HT_1$ agonists. $5HT_1$ agonists licensed in the UK are *sumatriptan* and the newer *naratriptan* and *zolmitriptan*. Similar drugs, *almotriptan*, *eletriptan*, *frovatriptan* and *rizatriptan* are in late development or already licensed elsewhere. These drugs act highly selectively on specific subsets of $5HT_1$ receptors ($5HT_{1D}$ and, to a lesser extent, $5HT_{1B}$). They have a much lower affinity for other $5HT_1$ receptors and are inactive against $5HT_2$, $5HT_3$, adrenergic, dopaminergic, muscarinic and benzodiazepine receptors.

The role of $5HT_{1D}$ and $5HT_{1B}$ receptors is uncertain. They are believed to be presynaptic 'autoreceptors' which control the release of neurotransmitters at the nerve terminal.

Because of their vasoconstrictor action, $5HT_1$ agonists are likely to aggravate any condition caused by arterial blockage, spasm or inflammation and should not be used in such situations, e.g. ischaemic heart disease, prior MI, atypical angina, uncontrolled hypertension, intermittent claudication, temporal arteritis, Raynaud's disease.

As with all of this group of drugs the dosage regimens are designed to avoid excessively prolonged vasoconstriction, and an adequate interval must be allowed between doses. Non-responders should not take a further dose of any formulation for the same attack because this will increase vasoconstriction and the risk of isch-aemia and thromboembolic stroke, without relieving the migraine. Such patients are more likely to benefit from a change to a different drug class. If a small dose has proved to be inad-equate, a larger dose may help in a **subsequent** attack. Partial responders and those in whom the headache remits and recurs can take a further dose, though the precise details vary with the drug and dosage form.

Although more expensive than previous treat-ments, the cost–benefit ratio is probably no worse than for older drugs. There is less time off work and a better quality of life.

Sumatriptan is active at all stages of the attack. The drug is rapidly but poorly absorbed orally (14% bioavailability) from the tablets, taking 2 h to reach a peak plasma concentration which is 75% of that obtained by SC injection. This is not a suitable route if there is nausea and vomiting, and it clearly gives less prompt relief than the injection. However, some patients who do not wish to inject find it adequately effective (TG 33%, 58% of patients, 100 mg dose). The pre-ferred modes of use are by SC injection, for which an autoinjector device has been produced (peak plasma concentration at 12 min, 97% bioavailability; TG 51%, 71% of patients at 1 h), which avoids first-pass metabolism. An alterna-tive dosage form for those not wishing to inject is the nasal spray. Although this gives rapid absorption, the peak plasma concentration (at 1–1.5 h) is only about 20% of that from the injection, partly due to presystemic metabolism. The terminal elimination half-life is about 2 h.

Side effects include drowsiness, changes in blood pressure (transient increase, reduction), bradycardia or tachycardia and, occasionally, fits. However, these side effects are usually mild and fairly brief. **Caution** is required in renal impairment and, following reports of chest pain and coronary vasoconstriction.

Interactions. Because of the similar mode of action, **sumatriptan must not be used with ergotamine**: nor within 24 h after stopping *ergo-tamine*, which must not be used within 6 h of taking *sumatriptan*.

Use with *MAOIs*, *SSRIs* and *lithium* increases the risk of CNS toxicity, and use of sumatriptan with any of these must be avoided.

Second-generation triptans. These have bet-ter bioavailability, potency at active receptor sites and longer half-lives than *sumatriptan*. Because they are more lipophilic, CNS penetra-tion is also improved and they reduce neuroex-citability, especially in the trigeminal ganglion.

Naratriptan is similarly effective to *sumatriptan*, available as tablets. Used at the lower dose (2.5 mg) it may have fewer side effects than *sumatriptan* and has similar interactions, but the TG is also lower. At the higher dose it resembles *sumatriptan*.

Zolmitriptan is another recent introduction in tablet form, designed to be a potent $5HT_1$ partial agonist and more lipophilic than *sumatriptan*, giving better CNS penetration. It has a slightly higher TG than *sumatriptan* but a higher inci-dence of adverse reactions.

Possible **side effects** include drowsiness and transient hypertension; dry mouth, unpleasant sensory effects and muscle pain and weakness may also occur. Absolute **contraindications** for all of this group include ischaemic heart disease, prior MI, angina and uncontrolled hypertension. Arrhythmias due to accessory cardiac conduc-tion pathways are an **additional contraindica-tion for zolmitriptan**.

Second-line drugs

These include *ergotamine* and *isometheptene mucate*, though low cost has ensured the contin-ued use of *ergotamine*, despite its complex actions and long list of side effects.

Ergotamine tartrate is the oldest antimigraine drug, with ergot preparations having been in use for at least 2000 years. The isolation and phar-macological characterization of the ergot alka-loids in the mid-20th century (pure ergotamine was isolated by Stoll in 1920) was a major event in the development of modern pharmacology. It is an amino-acid alkaloid derived from a lysergic acid nucleus. Preparations contain about 40% of the relatively inactive ergotaminine, due to spontaneous epimerization. Because of its long history, well-conducted controlled trials have not been carried out.

The **actions** of ergotamine include:

- At 5HT receptors ($5HT_1$ and $5HT_2$):
  - Partial agonist in many blood vessels (it is a powerful vasoconstrictor).
  - A mixed agonist/antagonist in the CNS.
  - A non-selective antagonist in many smooth muscles.
- At alpha-adrenergic receptors:
  - Partial agonist/antagonist in blood vessels and smooth muscles (promotes uterine contraction and vasoconstriction).
  - Antagonist in the central and peripheral nervous systems.
- At dopaminergic D_2 receptors:
  - Powerful stimulation of the CTZ, especially with injections.

While the vasoconstrictive effects of ergotamine contribute to its benefit in migraine, these non-selective, wide-ranging actions mean that it also has a formidable array of side effects. These, and the risk of habituation which limits its use to not more than twice per month, have contributed to its second-line rating. It is similarly effective to NSAIDs and somewhat less so than *sumatriptan*.

Ergotamine is available as compound tablets with *cyclizine*, as an anti-emetic, and with caffeine, allegedly to promote absorption. The benefit from caffeine is debatable and it may even cause analgesic headache (see above). Oral bioavailability is poor, about 1–3%, with large interindividual variations in absorption and extensive first-pass metabolism. The use of a buccal aerosol or sublingual tablets may provide improved absorption. Suppositories give about a 20-fold increase in peak plasma concentration, and this is probably the preferred route. Pharmacokinetic data are rather imprecise due to assay difficulties (peak plasma concentrations are only about 10–500 picogram/mL).

Because ergotamine binds irreversibly to receptors it has a longer duration of action than the triptans. This may be beneficial in patients with lengthy attacks or those in whom headache recurs frequently after triptans.

Although injections of ergotamine have been used, they usually contain a mixture of ergot alkaloids. They therefore have numerous side effects and, in addition, are highly emetogenic (20% of patients) and are often poorly tolerated. The **side effects, contraindications**, etc. of ergotamine are given in Table 10.14. **The official dose should never be exceeded and doses must not be repeated at intervals of less than 4**

Table 10.14   Ergotamine: some side effects, cautions and contraindications

Side effects	Gastrointestinal: nausea, vomiting, abdominal pain, diarrhoea
	Cardiovascular: chest pain, angina pectoris, myocardial infarction (rare)
	Respiratory: pleural and peritoneal fibrosis (excessive use)
	Muscle cramps
	Habituation and ergotamine-induced headache may occur
Cautions	Elderly
	Not for prophylaxis
	Peripheral vasospasm: numb or tingling fingers or toes (**stop treatment**; risk of gangrene)
Contraindications	Peripheral vascular disease, Raynaud's syndrome
	Coronary heart disease
	Sepsis
	Severe/uncontrolled hypertension
	Pregnancy, breast feeding

days. Failure to heed these basic procedures have led, fortunately rarely, to a disastrous outcome.

Dihydroergotamine mesylate is a less potent arterial vasoconstrictor than ergotamine and may be helpful if headache recurrence is troublesome. The injection is better tolerated than ergotamine injection, but emesis is still a problem. Dihydroergotamine injection was withdrawn in the UK in 1993, but an intranasal spray – which is effective but slower-acting than the equivalent sumatriptan formulation – has been introduced as an acute treatment. This intranasal formulation provides an ampoule containing four puffs, which is assembled in metered dose nasal spray just before use. Two metered puffs (one in each nostril) are used initially, and a further one or two after not less than 15 min if relief is insufficient. This is the maximum for an attack, the maximum dose being 12 puffs per week. Such treatment may cause a runny or stuffy nose, nausea and vomiting, and flushing. Some patients experience peripheral paraesthesias, chest pain and rarely vascular spasm. The spray is widely used in North America and continental Europe.

Isometheptene, an indirect sympathomimetic agent, is marketed in the UK as an OTC product containing *paracetamol (acetaminophen)*. It may cause circulatory disturbances, dizziness, rashes and, rarely, blood dyscrasias. Its numerous side effects, cautions, contraindications and interactions are considered to outweigh its clinical usefulness.

Prophylactic pharmacotherapy

This may not be necessary if attacks are mild to moderate and are well-controlled and if this situation is well-tolerated by the patient. However, opinion differs as to when prophylaxis should be considered. In the UK, it is often recommended if there is more than one moderate to severe attack a month, whereas in the USA the borderline is drawn at three or more per month. Much depends on what level of pain and disruption to their lives, balanced against side effects, the patient is able to tolerate.

The drugs used comprise:

- **Beta-blockers**: *propranolol, metoprolol,* (possibly *atenolol, nadolol, timolol*).

- **5HT antagonists**: *pizotifen (pizotyline), methysergide.*
- **Tricyclic antidepressants**: e.g. *amitriptyline* (whether the patient shows depressive symptoms or not; unlicensed use; *see* Chapter 7).
- *Sodium valproate* (unlicensed use, *see* Chapter 7).
- *Flunarizine*, a non-selective calcium channel blocker.

The modes of action of these drugs in migraine are unclear, especially because the effects of other beta-blockers, anticonvulsants and calcium channel blockers are similar to those of placebo. Good evidence for the benefit of *pizotifen (pizotyline), methysergide* and *flunarizine* is also lacking.

All of these drugs are, at most, 50% effective in only about half of the patients, but one drug can usually be found to be useful by trial and error. Further, it is difficult to be sure of the true benefit because there is a large placebo effect, up to about 40%. Each of the drugs needs to be tried for at least 2–3 months before it is discarded as ineffective. If the patient responds, treatment should continue, with 6-monthly medication reviews; complete remission is common. It has also been suggested that trials of high-dose *riboflavin* or NSAIDs might be worthwhile. If NSAIDs are used (this is an unlicensed use), the drug selected would have to be relatively free of side effects, e.g. ibuprofen, because long-term use is involved.

Beta-blockers, usually *propranolol*, are usually regarded as the drugs of choice for migraine prophylaxis. Their utility is limited by their side effects (*see* Chapter 3) and, in the past, by their interaction with *ergotamine*, because both drugs cause peripheral vasoconstriction. This interaction is clearly less of a problem if one of the newer 5HT$_1$ agonists is being used to treat attacks.

Pizotifen (pizotyline) is probably the second choice. This also has antihistaminic properties and so causes drowsiness, so the dose should be taken at night and increased gradually. Increased appetite and weight gain often make pizotifen (pizotyline) unacceptable, especially to women. Its weak antimuscarinic properties may cause urinary retention and closed angle glaucoma, so it may not be suitable in middle-aged to elderly patients. Another $5HT_1$ agonist/antihistamine, *cyproheptadine*, is sometimes used in refractory cases.

Clonidine has been used but is regarded as unsuitable in the UK because it may cause or aggravate severe depression. The use of *methysergide* for resistant cases is restricted to hospital consultants in the UK, because of its toxicity.

The highly desirable introduction of more effective prophylactic drugs presumably awaits a better understanding of migraine pathophysiology.

Cluster headache (migrainous neuralgia)

This name derives from the fact that episodes tend to occur in clusters of attacks, lasting several weeks, interspersed by remissions of months to years. Despite its synonym, it is unrelated to migraine, though many of the same drugs are used.

Clinical features

There are abrupt episodes of excruciating, unilateral pain ('suicide headache') which affect the eye, temple or forehead and increase over about 30 min and may last for several hours. The eye waters copiously and there is often flushing of the same side of the face, though this may vary (Fig. 10.4(k)). Attack frequency is between eight per day and one on alternate days, usually once or twice a day for a few weeks or months, often at night and at predictable times. The prodromal signs of classical migraine and the aura do not occur, and the attacks do not usually cause vomiting.

Sufferers are mostly men aged 30–50 years (male : female ratio, 10 : 1), but remission tends to occur by the age of 60 years. There is no persistent major deficit. The cause is unknown, but alcohol may provoke attacks, especially during a cluster.

Pharmacotherapy

Sumatriptan or *ergotamine* are taken in anticipation of an attack, because the timing is usually consistent once a cluster has started. High-dose *oxygen* often provides relief within minutes.

Verapamil or pizotifen (pizotyline) (also *methysergide*, hospital-only) are used for prophylaxis throughout a cluster. *Lithium* (*see* Chapter 7) may help chronic sufferers.

Trigeminal neuralgia

Definition

This is a neuropathy of the fifth cranial (trigeminal) nerve which causes episodes of agonising, lancinating (stabbing) or 'electric shock' pain, usually unilateral, in the face. Each episode lasts for a few seconds.

Clinical features

The trigeminal nerve is mostly sensory and has three branches:

- **Ophthalmic**; carrying fibres from the anterior half of the scalp, forehead, the eye and surrounding structures, the nasal cavity and side of the nose.
- **Maxillary**; contains fibres from the lower eyelid, nose, palate, upper teeth and lip, and parts of the pharynx.
- **Mandibular**; serving the anterior tongue (not taste), lower teeth and jaw, cheek and side of the head in front of the ear.

Trigeminal neuralgia is usually of unknown cause, but it can also occur in multiple sclerosis and due to a fifth nerve tumour. Trigeminal neuralgia may also be a form of post-herpetic neuralgia, when it usually affects the ophthalmic branch. Other neuropathies can affect the trigeminal nerve, but these are usually chronic and distinct from trigeminal neuralgia.

The pain spasms usually affect the mandibular division and may spread upwards to involve the other branches. The characteristics and localized distribution of the pain are diagnostic: no neurological abnormality can be detected.

Spasms may occur several times a day, usually in response to trivial triggers, e.g. cold wind, touching, shaving or washing the face, chewing or tooth brushing. Episodes remit spontaneously for anything from months to years, but always recur. Middle-aged and elderly patients are mostly affected.

Management

Most patients respond to pharmacotherapy with *carbamazepine*, taken at the commencement of an attack. This usually reduces the severity, duration and frequency of attacks and is not beneficial in other forms of headache.

Carbamazepine is a rather toxic, anti-epileptic drug with a long list of side effects and interactions, being a liver enzyme inducer (*see* Chapter 6, p. 379). Consequently, it is usual to start with a low dose in a first attack and build up slowly (fortnightly) until symptoms are controlled. This is especially necessary if dizziness occurs. Like *phenytoin* and some other anticonvulsants, carbamazepine has a narrow therapeutic window, so plasma-level monitoring should be instituted if high doses are used.

Phenytoin may be effective in non-responders. If the side effects of high-dose *carbamazepine* are not tolerated, a combination with *phenytoin* is sometimes used, the doses of each being reduced appropriately. However, these interact and such combinations are rarely justified (*see* Chapter 7).

The dose and build-up in subsequent attacks depend on the patient's reaction and tolerance to the drugs.

Tricyclic antidepressants are more useful in secondary post-herpetic facial neuralgia and in non-specific facial and jaw pain associated with depression.

Surgery or nerve ablation with *alcohol injections* may be required in those not responding to pharmacotherapy.

Post-herpetic neuralgia

Definition

This is a chronic pain syndrome in the dermatome (the skin area served by a single sensory nerve) affected by **herpes zoster**, an acute skin infection (**shingles**) due to reactivation of **varicella-zoster virus** (VZV).

Clinical features

VZV causes **chickenpox**, a common acute skin infection. Most patients (90%) are children aged under 10 years. Infections in older people are generally severe and occasionally fatal, and are usually associated with immunosuppression, e.g. drug treatment (transplant, autoimmune and cancer patients), radiotherapy, some neoplastic diseases (especially lymphomas) and AIDS, or waning immunity in old age.

During recovery from chickenpox the virus tracks up sensory nerve axons to dorsal root ganglia and becomes incorporated in the nuclear DNA as a **provirus**. This location is protected from immunological defence mechanisms, so the provirus persists until it is reactivated by a reduction in host immunity. The virus then tracks back down the nerve axon to cause a skin infection in the area innervated by that sensory nerve. There are usually three distinct phases:

- **Prodromal**, with unilateral nerve pain or paraesthesia lasting 3–5 days (range 1–14 days), the skin being very sensitive to touch, malaise and sometimes mild fever.
- **Active**, vesicles appear over 3–5 days and crust over during several days to 3 weeks, accompanied by nerve and skin pain which seems excessive relative to the skin involvement.
- **Chronic, post-herpetic neuralgia** (PHN) lasting months to years.

Occasionally, the nerve may be affected without any skin eruption.

The affected area is unilateral, sharply demarcated at the mid-line front and back, and may involve a few adjacent dermatomes. The principal sites are the thorax (50% of cases), head and neck (20%) and lumbosacral area (15%). Involvement of the eye or ear requires specialist advice.

Management and pharmacotherapy

Shingles

Mild cases
Only simple or compound analgesics and soothing and drying lotions (*see* Chapter 12) are required.

Moderate to severe cases
These require prompt treatment, especially if the patient is immunocompromised:

- Early *antiviral treatment*, to minimize the risk of PHN and complications, e.g. eye or ear involvement. However, diagnosis may be difficult because the prodromal symptoms may mimic migraine, heart disease or acute abdominal problems. The antivirals used include:
  - *Aciclovir* (*acyclovir*) orally, or by IV infusion in the immunocompromised, plus topical application to the eye or ear if these are affected.
  - Alternatives are *famciclovir* and *valaciclovir*, oral pro-drugs of penciclovir and aciclovir (acyclovir) respectively, with superior bio-availability.
  - *Foscarnet*, occasionally *amantadine*, for resistant strains of VZV (unlicensed uses in the UK).
- Antibacterials for superinfection of the rash (*see* Chapter 13).
- Pain control with:
  - *Analgesics*, including *opioids* if needed.
  - *Local anaesthetics* (p. 593) or *nerve block* (pp. 597–599) if pain is severe.
  - A sedative tricyclic antidepressant at night, as an analgesic adjunct, hypnotic and antidepressant.
- Soothing soaks to the affected skin.

Chronic herpetic neuralgia

Severe pain in the prodromal or early active phases indicates the likelihood of severe PHN, so early aggressive antiviral treatment is indicated. Prolonged PHN requires any of the analgesic treatments listed above (depression is a feature of moderate to severe PHN).

Capsaicin cream, a counter-irritant, is also used **after the rash has healed**. This is very irritant and must not be applied in the early stages until the lesions have healed completely. It should be applied 3–4 times/day, not more or less. If applied less frequently the transient burning sensation may be more severe and prolonged; the skin needs to become habituated. More frequent application also causes skin irritation. Application sites must not be occluded and the hands must be washed immediately after application. The area around the eyes must be avoided.

Non-drug measures, e.g. TENS (p. 597), may help to minimize the dose of analgesic and the risk of opioid dependence. If the patient is otherwise healthy, a short course of oral *corticosteroids* may help. Corticosteroids are **contraindicated** in the acute phase because they may promote widespread viral dissemination.

Prophylaxis

A varicella vaccine is available in the USA, but is not licensed in the UK. Use of the vaccine in non-immune individuals, especially those at risk of varicella infection, may prevent an attack of shingles in later life.

Some special pain situations

Certain categories of patient present particular problems in pain control. This can be from the type of pain itself or may relate to the constraints that their disease state may impose on any choice of therapy.

Opioids and other sedatives in surgery

Premedication

The objectives of pre-anaesthetic medication are:

- To relieve anxiety without excessive drowsiness, so that the patient remains cooperative and the various preparative procedures can proceed smoothly.
- To give an amnesic effect, to avoid unpleasant memories.
- To relieve any preoperative pain.
- To minimize:
  - The dose of the general anaesthetic, usually inhalational.
  - The undesirable effects of anaesthesia, e.g. vomiting, headache, coughing, excessive secretions.
  - Postoperative stress.

Several agents may be required to achieve these ends.

Surgery is often preceded by organic or traumatic pain, and itself obviously causes moderate to severe pain. Even mild preoperative pain interferes with the smooth induction of general anaesthesia and increases the amount of anaesthetic required. Opioids are widely used for premedication, the choice being determined by their duration of action and the incidence of side effects. Premedication with an opioid may reduce the dose of a general anaesthetic required by about 15% and minimizes the occurrence of agitation during recovery.

Morphine or *meperidine* (*pethidine*) are sometimes used if there is moderate to severe preoperative pain, but these have undesirable **side effects**, e.g. prolonged awakening, nausea and vomiting, constipation and urinary retention, bradycardia causing hypotension, respiratory depression (especially in those patients with an asthmatic tendency or frank asthma) and spasm of the bile duct and ureters. Drugs with a rapid onset and short duration of action are now preferred, e.g. *alfentanil, fentanyl, remifentanil* and *tramadol. Remifentanil* can be given by IV infusion, but *alfentanil* and *fentanyl* must be given by repeated bolus injections.

Patients with severe adrenal suppression may have a dramatic fall in blood pressure due to operative stress, so a glucocorticoid is used in anticipation of intraoperative shock and IV during the procedure, as required.

Antimuscarinic drugs, usually *hyoscine* (*scopolamine*) *hydrobromide*, are sometimes used for premedication, often with an opioid. These reduce the excessive bronchial and salivary secretions that occur with some inhalational anaesthetics and are due to intubation. *Hyoscine* (*scopolamine*) produces some sedation and amnesia and reduces vomiting, but may cause undesirable bradycardia and CNS side effects, e.g. excitement, hallucinations, drowsiness, especially in the elderly.

However, modern anaesthetic techniques and the increasing use of day-case surgery largely avoid the need for traditional premedication routines.

Induction agents

Propofol provides rapid recovery without hangover and causes little undesirable muscle activity. Propofol is an oil at room temperature and is injected intravenously, or is given by infusion, as an emulsion which must be drawn up with strict aseptic precautions to avoid bacterial contamination. Propofol is also used as a sedative for short surgical and diagnostic procedures, but there is a significant incidence of bradycardia, allergic reactions and convulsions.

The induction agent *etomidate* also gives rapid recovery (5 min) without hangover, but an opioid may be needed to cover injection pain and *diazepam* will reduce undesirable muscle activity. Nausea and vomiting are common, especially if an opioid has been used.

Obstetric pain

The use of analgesics to control the pain of labour presents several problems and poses risks to both mother and fetus. The ideal agent should meet the following criteria:

- Provide adequate pain relief.
- Interfere minimally with the course and duration of labour.
- Have little effect on fetal vital signs during labour and at birth.

Pethidine (*meperidine*) is the most common obstetric analgesic as it is short acting and generally meets these criteria. However, problems still occur, notably respiratory depression in the neonate, the incidence of which can be reduced by giving the drug early in the course of labour and using the IM route, the IV route being associated with more neonatal depression.

Common alternative forms of analgesia include the epidural administration of local anaesthetics, and the inhalation of sub-anaesthetic doses of 50% nitrous oxide in oxygen.

Palliative treatment of cancer pain

Great advances have been made in this field, and most patients can be maintained virtually free of pain. It is essential to appreciate that pain is not an invariable accompaniment to cancer, and about one-third of cancer patients remain pain-free. A clear understanding of the common pain syndromes associated with neoplasms and their pathophysiological mechanisms, the psychological state of the patient, and the indications and limitations of the available therapeutic approaches, is vital to effective management. Short-acting drugs, e.g. pethidine (meperidine) and dextromoramide, are unsuitable because they require frequent dosing, without additional benefit.

Several different types of pain may be associated with cancer (*see* Table 10.7), and these often exist concurrently, some 80% of patients experiencing two or more types and about 20% four or more types. The pain may be due to the disease itself or to the debility it causes, to co-existing disease or to treatment, and so a combination of therapeutic approaches is often required. Thus, a multidisciplinary approach has been adopted increasingly to form 'pain teams' which take into account the needs of the whole patient. The clinical aspects of cancer and its overall management are discussed in detail in Chapter 11.

Type of pain

Because pain can have many causes, some of which are not directly related to neoplastic activity, especially careful assessment and diagnosis of the pain is essential in cancer patients. Depending on its aetiology, the pain in terminal disease may only be partially responsive to opioid analgesics, so a combination of analgesics with different pharmacological actions is often necessary. Adjunctive agents, radiotherapy or surgical approaches may be appropriate in special circumstances.

Tumour infiltration

Visceral organs
Tumour invasion of the stomach, biliary tract, intestine, uterus or bladder causes intense contraction of the local smooth muscle with increased pressure and local ischaemia. Visceral pain is characteristically increasing, diffuse, unlocalized and constant in intensity. Opioid drugs are the most effective in these circumstances and must be given in adequate doses. A regular laxative is also needed to prevent consti-

pation which would otherwise add to the pain and complicate the picture.

Nerves
Infiltration of local nerves by a tumour, or their compression, may cause a variety of symptoms according to the site of involvement. These include hyperaesthesia (increased sensitivity), dysaesthesia (painful sensation), neuralgia (paroxysmal nerve pain), sensory and motor disturbances and sensory loss. The tumour may cause persistent mechanical stimulation of high-threshold nociceptors, i.e. those not readily stimulated, and partial damage to axons and nerve membranes, resulting in increased sensitivity to sympathetic stimulation and pressure. Standard analgesics are often ineffective in relieving this type of pain, and analgesic adjuvants, nerve blocks or neurosurgical procedures may be more successful.

Bones
Bone pain is common in cancer and may be due either to a primary tumour (e.g. multiple myeloma) or to metastases (e.g. from breast, lung or prostate cancer). Bone tumours stimulate local pain receptors directly and also induce the production of prostaglandins which may cause osteolysis, sensitize free nerve endings and augment pain perception. Inhibitors of prostaglandin release, e.g. NSAIDs, are thus the logical choice to treat bone pain. Although NSAIDs exert their main analgesic action at peripheral sites, there is also a central component. It is worth maximizing the dosage of individual agents and changing drugs if side effects are excessive or the response is poor, because individuals vary considerably, both in their response to different NSAIDs and in the occurrence of side effects. *Bisphosphonates*, e.g. *clodronate* or *pamidronate*, can also help by inhibiting osteolysis.

Opioids are generally not very effective in relieving bone pain and can often be reduced in dose or withdrawn totally after the introduction of an NSAID, though many patients use the combined therapy. If bone pain occurs only at limited sites, a single dose of local radiotherapy is often the treatment of choice, and may have a dramatic analgesic effect.

Morphine in palliative care

Optimal use follows the guidelines given on p. 575 and p. 580. Initially, the oral dose of plain tablets or liquid is given 4-hourly, with rescue medication as required. Doubling the bedtime dose usually enables the patient to sleep throughout the night. With a 4-h duration of action, morphine takes about 24 h to reach steady state, so patients need re-evaluation daily. Once stabilized, the change is made to modified-release tablets (not to be crushed), usually given 12-hourly. If pain increases, the dose should be increased but the dose interval retained, except possibly that for the modified-release preparations which is sometimes reduced to 8-hourly.

If oral dosing is not possible or not tolerated, sublingual, transdermal, rectal (dose equals oral dose) or SC routes (potency relative to oral is 2, as a bolus or continuous infusion) can be used. The choice may depend on the availability of the desired dosage form (*see* Table 10.4) and its suitability, e.g. the sublingual route requires adequate production of saliva and the IM route gives more pain with morphine and should not be used.

A change to diamorphine (heroin) or hydromorphone (in North America or elsewhere that heroin is not licensed) may be needed if high doses are required, because morphine is not very soluble and only smallish volumes can be injected by the SC route. Also, if the SC route is unsuitable due to generalized oedema, coagulation problems, poor peripheral circulation or local adverse drug reactions with the SC route, the IV route may be used (potencies relative to oral morphine: diamorphine (heroin), about 3.5; hydromorphone, about 12).

About 20% of patients fail to respond to these measures. These will need spinal opioids, with local anaesthetics and other adjuncts (see above).

Patients with liver failure

These patients often present a therapeutic dilemma because most of the commonly used analgesics are contraindicated. In particular, the effect of liver failure on the pharmacokinetics and pharmacodynamics of the analgesic has to be considered (*see* Chapter 6, p. 379). Most opioids are significantly metabolized by the liver and will accumulate if dosing intervals are not adjusted. Further, the oral bioavailability of some opioids may be increased owing to reduced first-pass metabolism.

Patients with liver failure are particularly sensitive to the effects of opioids, as to other sedatives, and relatively small doses can precipitate encephalopathy (*see* Chapter 6). Those with cirrhosis are liable to develop oesophageal varices (*see* Chapter 6), and NSAIDs should be used cautiously as the gastrointestinal irritation caused may precipitate catastrophic bleeding. Chronic administration of large doses of hepatotoxic drugs, e.g. *paracetamol* (*acetaminophen*), can further exacerbate the liver failure. Fortunately, the severity of liver failure usually encountered in cancer patients does not require large dosage changes.

In practice, an estimate of the dosage interval required to prevent accumulation occurring is obtained by giving a cautious dose of opioid, the subsequent dose being withheld until the pain reappears. It is particularly important in this situation to use drugs in which the analgesic half-life is similar to the plasma half-life, e.g. *morphine* (plus its active metabolite, morphine-6-glucuronide), because the risk of accumulation is then hopefully avoided, as the loss of analgesic effect should correlate with drug clearance.

Patients with renal failure

Choosing an appropriate analgesic in this group of patients does not usually present a problem. However, some analgesics, e.g. the NSAIDs, can cause nephropathy, so taking a medication history is worthwhile, to determine whether the renal failure may initially have been due to analgesic over-dosage or misuse. NSAIDs may also be contraindicated because they may exacerbate fluid retention and precipitate decompensation in developing heart failure.

Opioid analgesics may present a significant problem in renal failure. *Morphine* and its glucuronide metabolites accumulate, requiring an increased dosing interval or dose reduction.

Fentanyl is said to be safer in renal impairment and can be given intravenously. If injections are not tolerated, then transdermal patches can be used. However, it takes about 24 h after application of the first patch to reach an adequate fentanyl plasma concentration. Further, the long half-life of fentanyl (about 17 h) creates problems if the drug accumulates, and replacement with an alternative must be started at a low dose concurrently with the removal of a patch, and increased gradually thereafter.

Pethidine (*meperidine*) should be avoided as the toxic metabolite norpethidine accumulates in renal failure and can lead to seizures.

References and further reading

Ferrari MD (1998) Migraine. *Lancet* **351**: 1043–1051.

Hawthorn J, Redmond K (1998) *Pain: Causes and Management*. Oxford: Blackwell Science.

McQuay HJ, Moore A (1998) *An Evidence-based Resource for Pain Relief*. Oxford: Oxford University Press.

Melzack R, Wall PD (1989) *The Challenge of Pain*. Harmondsworth: Penguin.

Regnard CFB, Tempest S (1998) *A Guide to Symptom Relief in Advanced Disease*. 4th edn. Hale, Cheshire: Hochland & Hochland.

de Stoutz ND, Bruera E, Suarez-Almazor M (1995) Opioid rotation for toxicity reduction in terminal cancer patients. *J Pain Symptom Manage* **10**: 378–384.

Twycross RG, Lack SA (1990) *Therapeutics in Terminal Cancer*. 2nd edn. London: Churchill Livingstone.

Twycross RG, Wilcock A, Thorp S (1998) *PCF1: Palliative Care Formulary*. Oxford: Radcliffe Medical Press.

Wall PD, Melzack R (1989) *Textbook of Pain*. London: Churchill Livingstone.

Wellchew E (1995) *Patient Controlled Analgesia*. London: BMA Publishing Group.

11

Neoplastic disease

Cancer is a common condition and causes much suffering. It has a high morbidity and a very high mortality, being the second most common cause of death in the developed world. This is mainly because of the tendency to spread to secondary sites and initiate new tumours. Tumours affect health and threaten survival in part simply because of their bulk, but also for more indirect reasons.

Because the causation of cancer is complex and still poorly understood, the prevention of most cancers is currently not possible. Moreover, the natural history of cancer means that it is not usually detected until a late stage when treatment is difficult and, with some exceptions, offers limited success. However, this situation is improving continually and marked benefits may be expected in the medium term.

Classification and epidemiology of cancer

Terminology

Cancer is the general term for a group of disorders caused by the abnormal and unrestricted growth of cells. The term derives from the crab-like histological appearance of an invasive tumour as it seems to extend claws or tentacles into surrounding tissue. Each primary tumour is believed to derive from a single aberrant cell, most probably formed following a mutation.

The term **neoplasm** ('new growth') describes this tendency to excessive, uncontrolled growth. It is synonymous with the less technical 'tumour' (swelling). **Benign** tumours enlarge but do not invade surrounding tissue nor spread beyond their original site (**metastasis**). They are generally much less dangerous than **malignant** tumours, which do invade and do metastasize. However, the term 'benign' can be misleading because a large growth, even if not disseminated, can nevertheless be fatal by interfering locally with a vital organ or function; for example, tumours in the brain or endocrine glands, or those obstructing a major blood vessel.

The nomenclature of cancer is complex and inconsistent (Table 11.1). It attempts to classify three characteristics, all of which have a bearing on prognosis and treatment:

- The tissue of origin (in the histological sense).
- The organ of origin.
- Whether it is benign or malignant.

Table 11.1 Classification of neoplasms, with common examples

Tissue and organ of origin	Examples	
	Benign	Malignant
Haematopoietic	Polycythaemia	–
Lymphoreticular		
Granulocytes	–	Myelocytic leukaemias
Lymphocytes	–	Lymphocytic leukaemias
Lymphoid tissue	–	Lymphomas
Plasma cells	–	Myelomas
Connective tissue		
Bone	Osteoma	Osteosarcoma
Fatty tissue	Lipoma	Liposarcoma
Epithelial tissue		
Glandular	Adenoma	Adenocarcinoma
Squamous	Squamous papilloma	Squamous cell carcinoma
Melanocytes	Moles	Malignant melanoma
Nervous tissue, associated		
Meninges	Meningioma	Meningiosarcoma
Embryonic, germinal	Teratoma	Malignant teratoma
		Choriocarcinoma
		Nephroblastoma

The simple suffix -oma usually denotes a benign tumour, e.g. osteoma (bone tumour), adenoma (gland tumour). Malignant tumours are **carcinomas** (e.g. adenocarcinoma), **sarcomas** (e.g. osteosarcoma) or **leukaemias**. Most malignant human tumours are of epithelial origin (carcinomas), partly because these tissues have the greatest exposure to environmental agents and partly because they usually have a high cell turnover.

Epidemiology

Prognosis in cancer is usually quantified in terms of median survival, i.e. the time after which 50% of patients might be expected to have survived; or as the 5-year survival, which is the proportion of patients expected to be alive after 5 years. Table 11.2 gives some idea of the poor prognosis that still exists for many forms of cancer, despite modern treatment. Taking all forms of cancer together the 5-year survival rate from diagnosis is about 40%. For certain forms, survival is much lower, and while the prospects for breast cancer have improved slowly in recent years (average 5-year survival rate now over 60%), for the second most common tumour, lung cancer, 5-year survival is still below 10%. Ironically, the higher survival rates are often for the less common tumours such as testicular and skin cancer.

Cancer causes 20–25% of all deaths in developed countries, only slightly less than cardiovascular disease. The incidence of the condition started to increase early in the 20th century owing partly to increasing longevity and reduction in deaths from other serious illnesses, which gives tumours more time to develop, and partly to improved diagnosis. Part of the increase is undoubtedly due to environmental features of industrialized life, such as atmospheric pollution, smoking and diet.

There are wide variations in the incidence and prevalence of cancer for different anatomical sites, sexes, ages, and racial, ethnic and geographical groups. These give tantalising but largely unresolved glimpses into the aetiology of different tumours.

Table 11.2 Survival rates for some common tumours (approximate 1981–86)

Site	Approximate 5-year survival rate (%)[a]	
	Male	Female
All sites	35	45
Nasopharynx	30	40
Lung	8	7
Oesophagus	10	10
Stomach	10	10
Large intestine	35	35
Rectum and rectosigmoid	35	35
Liver	4	3
Pancreas	4	4
Skin – malignant melanoma	60	75
Skin – other than melanoma	100	100
Breast	–	60
Cervix	–	60
Uterus[b]	–	70
Ovary	–	30
Bladder	60	55
Prostate	45	–
Testis	85	–
Brain	17	17
Hodgkin's disease (lymphoma)	70	70
Lymphatic leukaemia	30	25

Note: These are the latest figures available.
[a] Proportion of patients alive 5 years after diagnosis.
[b] Carcinoma 'in situ', i.e. locally non-invasive.
Source: Cancer Research Campaign Factsheet 9, 1988.

Site and sex

In developed countries lung cancer is the single most common tumour in men but is falling slowly. The most common tumour in women is breast cancer, but the incidence of lung cancer is increasing. For both sexes, gut tumours, especially of the stomach and colon, are the second largest group, followed by skin cancer (Fig. 11.1).

Age

Cancer incidence generally increases with age. For certain tumours in the very aged the prevalence can be very high, e.g. approaching 100% for prostatic carcinoma in males (although much

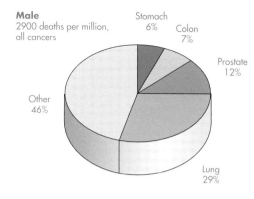

Male 2900 deaths per million, all cancers

Stomach 6%
Colon 7%
Prostate 12%
Lung 29%
Other 46%

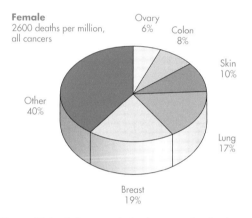

Female 2600 deaths per million, all cancers

Ovary 6%
Colon 8%
Skin 10%
Lung 17%
Breast 19%
Other 40%

Figure 11.1 Relative and absolute mortality for the most common cancers (UK 1994). Source: Cancer Research Campaign Factsheet 1.1 (1994) (excludes non-malignant melanoma).

remains asymptomatic), and rather less for breast cancer in females. However, certain tumours are more common in childhood, such as leukaemia and in the central nervous system (CNS).

The increase with age may be related to the increased chance of an unfavourable carcinogenic event, such as mutation or environmental toxin exposure, the effects of which may be cumulative, and to a reduction in the efficiency of the immune system, which may normally be protective.

Occupation

The first cancers where a definite cause was demonstrated were those associated with exposure to certain industrial chemicals. These included scrotal cancer among chimney sweeps, bladder cancer among azo-dye workers, and bone cancer among watch workers painting luminous dials with radium paints (and licking the brush). Recently, the inhalation of asbestos dust has been linked to an unusual form of lung cancer (mesothelioma). Although such instances represent, as yet, only a small proportion of all tumours, they are important because they are preventable.

Geographic and ethnic variation

Different nationalities have strikingly different incidences for certain tumours (Fig. 11.2). Stomach cancer is far more common in Japan and Chile than in the USA or Israel, while the incidence of colon cancer is particularly low in Asia and Africa. Jewish women, nuns and virgins have a low incidence of cervical cancer. Skin cancer is common in Australia. On the other hand, the prevalence of leukaemia is remarkably constant between nations. Although genetic factors may explain some of these variations, it is often found that immigrants eventually assume the incidence rate of the host population, depending on the extent of cultural assimilation (e.g. Japanese immigrants to the USA have a reduced incidence of stomach cancer). This points strongly to environmental factors such as diet, pollution, etc.

Trends

Changes in incidence and mortality over time reflect a combination of changes in longevity, detection rates, treatment success and exposure to environmental risk factors. Some examples are given in Fig. 11.2. For stomach cancer, because survival is poor, reductions in incidence are significant and produce large reductions in mortality. Although the incidence of testicular cancer has risen, successful treatment has produced significant falls in mortality. For breast cancer, the picture is more gloomy, and although rates are generally lower in the developing world, incidence is increasing in most countries (Fig. 11.3). This probably because of greater longevity and better screening, but treatment is still far from satisfactory. Lung cancer trends are considered below (p. 624).

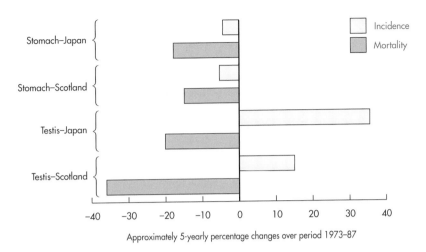

Approximately 5-yearly percentage changes over period 1973–87

Figure 11.2   Trends in incidence and mortality in males for different tumours in Japan and Scotland. Source: Cancer Research Campaign Factsheet 11.3 (1996).

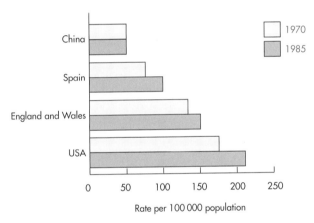

Rate per 100 000 population

Figure 11.3   Trends in incidence of breast cancer in females, 1970–85. Source: Cancer Research Campaign Factsheet 6.1 (1996).

Aetiology

Any theory of the causes of cancer must take into account both genetic and environmental factors. It is unlikely that a single cause accounts for all cancers. Almost certainly, cancers form a heterogeneous group of diseases with multifactorial causes. Individuals may have an inherited predisposition, but this may never be expressed unless an appropriate combination of environmental triggers is met. There are also several steps between initiation and clinical disease, and arrest at any of these will prevent the tumour from developing.

There are two distinct aspects to genetic considerations of cancer. First, the aetiological: to what extent is cancer, or predisposition to cancer, inherited? This is discussed here. Second, to what extent, and by what mechanism, are changes in the genetic code of tumour cells responsible for their neoplastic characteristics? This is discussed on p. 630. Only occasionally, when there are mutations in germ cells, i.e. spermatozoa or ova, do these aspects coincide.

The current consensus is that, although DNA changes are involved in all cancers, hereditary factors contribute only about 20% to the overall causation, while environmental factors contribute 80%. Most known associations between environmental factors and cancer have been discovered empirically: the evidence is epidemiological rather than biochemical. How some of these factors might be encompassed within a unified concept of the pathological mechanism is discussed on pp. 626–631.

The process of causing cancer is called **carcinogenesis**, and material factors (toxins, radiation, etc.) that contribute are called **carcinogens**. The terms 'oncogenesis' and 'oncogenic', although formerly sometimes used in this context, are best avoided because of a potential confusion with the newer concept of the '**oncogene**', which derives from one particular theory concerning the involvement of certain genes in carcinogenesis (p. 629).

Genetic factors

From the viewpoint of natural selection, it is unlikely that genes simply coding for a disease with such a high mortality would survive in the gene pool. Moreover, most cancer patients do not commonly present with a strongly positive family history. However, there is some evidence for genetic links in certain cancers:

- Some chromosomal abnormalities are associated with malignancy (e.g. Down's syndrome with leukaemia).
- Certain rare tumours do run in families (e.g. nephroblastoma).
- There is an association between certain histocompatibility antigens and some malignancies (e.g. HLA-B8 and Hodgkin's lymphoma).
- Certain hereditary tumours are associated with known mutations (e.g. retinoblastoma).

There is a tendency for some common tumours (e.g. breast, ovary, colon) to cluster in family groups. A breast cancer patient's sisters or daughters have a twofold risk of suffering the same disease; this risk is trebled if there are two first-degree relatives with the disease. There is a known association between familial breast and ovarian cancer and mutations of certain genes whose products are crucial to DNA repair mechanisms (the *BRCA* genes). Unfortunately, this has not so far produced a reliable screening method.

With familial tumours it is important to try to differentiate between a shared genetic predisposition and shared environmental factors. In general – and fortunately for the prospects for prevention – most evidence indicates that whatever the importance of genetic predisposition, for common tumours in most people one or more environmental triggers seem to be essential for a cancer to develop.

Environmental factors

Despite the tremendous efforts to identify specific carcinogenic factors, considerable doubt remains about the extent of their contribution. This may reflect a multifactorial causation. A summary of the most likely candidates and their current estimated relative contribution to all cancers is given in Table 11.3. The possible contributions of immunological factors, trauma (e.g. local irritation) and psychology/personality are unknown. Strong circumstantial evidence for the importance of environmental factors comes from the observation that the most common tumours in developed countries (lung, breast, gut and prostate) are rare in many developing countries.

Chemicals

Chemicals seem to be the chief culprits. Most chemical carcinogens are mutagens, i.e. they damage the genes, producing mutations. This provided one of the first clues to the general cause of cancer.

Smoking is by far the largest single contributor, although a wide variety of industrial carcinogens have also been positively identified. The link between smoking and lung cancer is one of the best examples of how the cause of a cancer can be elucidated by epidemiological means. Recent trends in UK lung cancer deaths (Fig. 11.4) can be correlated with evidence of a reduction in the prevalence of smoking among males from a maximum of 65% in 1950 to

Table 11.3 Environmental factors in cancer aetiology: estimates of contribution of various factors to total tumour burden

Factor	Contribution[a]
Chemicals	
• smoking	35
• diet[b]	30
• occupation	3
• alcohol	3
• medicines	1
• hormones	7
Infection (e.g. *Helicobacter*)	10
Radiation	5

[a] Current best estimate of the percentage contribution to the world cancer burden.

[b] High end of the estimated range, and still controversial.

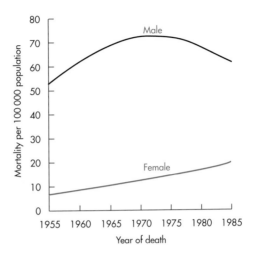

Figure 11.4 Trends in male and female lung cancer deaths (England and Wales). Source: Cancer Research Campaign Factsheet 11.3 (1996).

around 35% in 1991, and, until very recently, the disturbing trend of increasing cigarette smoking among females. And while smoking is currently on the decline in most developed countries, an even more worrying trend is for a dramatic increase in developing ones. This is presumably because legislative and social changes lag behind economic advances (which afford greater access to manufactured cigarettes), aided perhaps by a switch in the focus of a tobacco industry under increasing legislative pressures in the developed countries.

The statistical effort needed to confirm the link between smoking and lung cancer was enormous. Despite the fact that probably 90% of lung cancers (bronchial carcinomas) are smoking related, only one in six heavy smokers is likely to develop the disease. Other common tumours such as breast cancer defy such analysis; recently, links between breast cancer and the intake of fat and alcohol have been claimed. The carcinogenicity of the oestrogens in oral contraceptives is still hotly debated. How much more difficult then to trace the causation of less common cancers with more subtle aetiologies, especially as allowance must always be made for the long lag time between cancer induction and clinical presentation.

Dietary factors are increasingly seen to be important, although the specific carcinogenic constituents remain largely unknown. Excess fats, red meat, food additives, nitrates and numerous other factors have been implicated, as has the insufficiency of fibre or antioxidants; however, strong evidence of any causal link is lacking. Evidence implicating alcohol is growing; for example, it may act synergistically with smoking in oropharyngeal tumours. It has been estimated that dietary factors account for three-quarters of the gut, breast and prostate tumours.

Drugs may cause cancer in a number of ways. The main offenders are the cytotoxics, which may be both mutagenic and immunosuppressant (*see* p. 656). Hormones, especially the sex hormones, e.g. oestrogens, may encourage tumours in hormone-dependent tissues. The relationship between endogenous hormonal activity and such behaviour patterns as breast feeding, age of onset of sexual activity, circumcision, etc. is under intensive investigation.

Other factors

Infection. Although certain viruses cause some animal cancers, this is thought to be uncommon in humans except for a strong association in one or two rare tumours, e.g. Burkitt's lymphoma and Epstein–Barr virus. The discovery of 'viral oncogenes' (p. 629) does not alter this basic view. Recently, evidence has emerged of an association between *Helicobacter pylori* infection and stomach cancer.

Radiation. There are well-demonstrated links between cancer and both ionizing and ultraviolet radiation, which is known to produce genetic damage. Radiation from the nuclear industry, nuclear weapons (early testing and actual use), excessive environmental radon gas in certain geographical areas, and medical equipment (diagnostic and therapeutic) have all produced cancer.

Fair-skinned people in very sunny regions (e.g. Australia, California) have a significantly increased incidence of skin cancer. This is one cause that is understood, quantifiable and avoidable.

Immunological. One possible factor in carcinogenesis is a loss of the body's ability to identify and eliminate cells which have become neoplastic. Normally the immune system is continually checking for the presence of abnormal, non-self cells, a process called 'immunosurveillance'. Neoplastic cells, transformed by genetic mutation, often have altered cell surface structures, and if they are sufficiently different to become antigenic, they are promptly detected and destroyed by the immune system. If the immune system is compromised (owing to e.g. immunodeficiency disorder, immunosuppressant therapy, stress or age) or, alternatively, if the surface changes are minor, then tumour cells are more likely to escape this control.

Trauma. Sometimes chronic irritation seems to initiate tumours, although usually there is an associated infection. This may account for the correlation between oral cancers and ill-fitting dentures and between vaginal cancer and early intercourse or poor genital hygiene. Similarly, chronic inflammation in poorly controlled ulcerative colitis may be responsible for an increased incidence of colon cancer. The explanation may lie in the faster rate of tissue proliferation found in the repair phase of chronic inflammation, which increases the likelihood of a neoplastic mutation.

Psychological. Psychological factors probably do not play a significant part in carcinogenesis, although it has been claimed that people who repress emotions rather than express them are more likely to develop cancer. Nevertheless, major stress often does precede the onset of a tumour, as with many other diseases, possibly because of a related depression of the immune system.

However, psychological factors may significantly affect the course and severity of the disease and thus have a bearing on management. Some of the successes of 'natural' healing methods may be explained in this way. There is also evidence that personality can have an effect on outcome, bearing out the common empirical observation that a positive outlook and 'will to live' may promote longer remissions or even full recovery. One interesting study compared the psychological profiles and outcomes of therapy in a group of women who all had breast cancer at similar stage and received similar treatment. Those who responded to the original diagnosis by aggressively 'fighting' the tumour had the best better survival, while those who were overwhelmed and surrendered did worst. Perhaps surprisingly, those who reacted with 'stoic acceptance' did almost as badly as the overwhelmed group, while 'denial' was almost as favourable as aggression.

Pathobiology

So far, factors involved in the genesis of a neoplasm have been discussed, but not the mechanism. The nature of many carcinogens suggests that the first step is a mutation: a small chemical change in the genetic code. Advances in molecular biology promise eventually to lead to an understanding of how this change transforms a normal cell into a neoplastic one.

In this section, the way that cell growth and proliferation are normally controlled is reviewed and how this might go wrong is examined. The process of single cell division, and the consequences for the whole tissue of normal and abnormal division, are then examined in detail.

Finally, the possibilities for therapeutic intervention in the process are discussed.

Normal cell proliferation

The two important characteristics of normal cellular growth are growth rate and differentiation of function.

Stem cells and differentiation

Each nucleated cell in an organism has within its DNA the potential for performing the function of any cell in the whole organism; (exceptions include, for example, mature red blood cells and platelets, which have lost their nucleus). In mammals, this **totipotency** is suppressed, and effectively lost, early in the embryonic stage. Precursor **pluripotent stem** cells remain; these are less flexible and by **differentiation** are eventually **committed** to one particular function (Fig. 11.5). This process continues through several stages during which the cell becomes progressively less generalized. A final division gives a mature functional **end cell** which performs a specific physiological task but is no longer able to divide.

Capacity for division

During the growing phase of an organism, cell proliferation clearly exceeds cell death, but subsequently cell numbers remain stable throughout life. However, tissues must be able to proliferate in response to either physiological losses (e.g. bone marrow, gut lining) or pathological ones (e.g. injury). Thus, in most tissues there is a reservoir of stem cells which remain dormant until their division is needed to provide either more stem cells or more functional differentiated (end) cells. In the bone marrow there are **multipotent** marrow stem cells which differentiate into more specific stem cell lines, e.g. erythroblasts for erythrocytes, myeloblasts for granulocytes, etc.

The rate of growth of a tissue depends not just on the rate of division of dividing stem cells in that tissue (mitotic activity or turnover rate) but also on the proportion which is dividing. Different tissues have different proportions of stem

cells; the basal layer of the dermis, the gut epithelium, and the bone marrow have the highest. In tissues which are renewed less frequently there is a lower proportion, but the number can increase under the appropriate stimulus. For example, although the liver normally has low cell losses, if part is removed surgically the remainder will regenerate rapidly. On the other hand, nerve and skeletal muscle cells are not replaced (in adults), so presumably no stem cells remain in these tissues.

Ideally, the death of one functional end cell should result in one stem cell dividing to produce another stem cell and a replacement functional one (Fig. 11.5). Furthermore, if the stem cell population is depleted, the remaining stem cells must divide to replace the loss.

Cancer involves uncontrolled division and impaired differentiation, and because stem cells are both incompletely differentiated and still capable of division, neoplasms generally derive from stem cells. These considerations have important consequences for the treatment of cancer: stem cells are the main target of chemotherapy (pp. 645–648).

Control of growth and differentiation

Stem cells need some type of signal to tell them when to divide and to stop, and the daughter cells need to know whether or not to differentiate. This is accommodated by their being in some way responsive to the presence of similar cells immediately surrounding them.

The signals are mediated mainly by cytokines with growth stimulant or growth inhibitory properties. Some cytokines may pass directly from cell to cell, producing negative feedback which inhibits growth in response to increasing population density in the tissue (so-called contact inhibition). Others (paracrines) diffuse through a tissue, establishing a concentration in direct proportion to the number of secreting cells. Another possible factor, unique to neoplastic cells, may be the release of autocrines which act on receptors on the surface of the cell from which they are secreted.

Numerous growth factors specific for particular cell types are known. They are usually peptide regulatory factors, e.g. platelet-derived growth

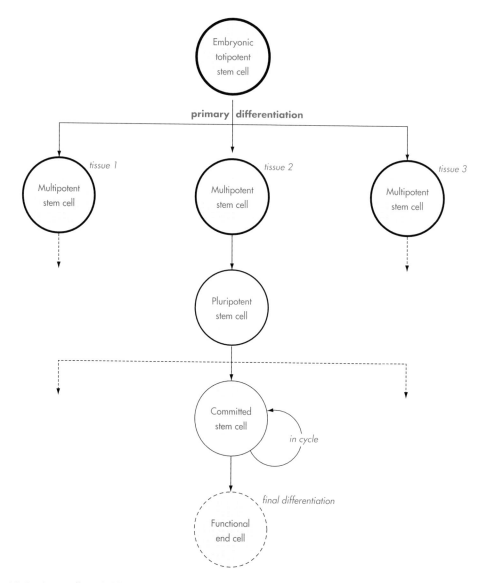

Figure 11.5 Stem cells and differentiation.

factor (PDGF), epidermal growth factor (EGF), erythropoietin, thymopoietin, granulocyte colony stimulating factor (G-CSF, *filgrastim*). Tumours also seem to secrete their own transforming growth factors (TGF), which closely resemble EGF. Generally these are growth stimulants (mitogenic) and are possibly secreted in excess in cancer, although some can act as growth inhibitors and are presumed deficient in cancer. There are also more general, systemic endocrine stimulants such as somatotrophin (growth hormone) and the adrenocorticoids. The sex hormones have a similar, but more specific, role.

The process is well illustrated by the normal reaction to skin injury. The mitotic activity of basal layer stem cells is strongly stimulated and that tissue temporarily becomes **hyperplastic** (see below); it may even overshoot somewhat, causing bulky scars (keloids). Quite soon after the lesion is healed, however, cell turnover returns to normal (*see also* Chapter 2). Another well-known physiological example is the increase in erythropoietin secretion in response to sustained low blood oxygen levels, stimulating red blood cell proliferation in the bone marrow.

Biochemical basis of differentiation

The precise means by which stimulant or inhibitory signals to cell surface receptors control gene expression, and how this affects growth, are still largely unknown. The intracellular mitogenic factors needed to promote cell division could be enzymes whose production is reduced during quiescent, i.e. non-dividing, phases, possibly by repression of the genes controlling their synthesis. Normal cell division is then seen as the expression – by de-repression – of mitogenic genes. Repression and de-repression are well-known processes in the control of cellular metabolism.

Unusual growth patterns

Hyperplasia. This is a form of increased proliferative activity, usually a response to injury. It must be clearly distinguished from neoplasia in that it is:

- Still under control and ceases when the task is accomplished.
- Purposeful: the cells produced are fully developed specific functional cells.
- Restricted to the affected tissue.

Hypertrophy. This involves an increase in cell size, but not cell numbers. An example would be muscle hypertrophy in response to chronic high loading (e.g. myocardial ventricular hypertrophy following untreated systemic hypertension).

Metaplasia. Pluripotent stem cells retain the ability to change their differentiation slightly in response either to normal needs such as the loss of related tissue or to irritant damage. For example, gut epithelial cells can change function and become either glandular or absorptive to compensate for losses after gut surgery. Like hyperplasia, metaplasia is usually protective and controlled. However, exceptionally, it may presage neoplastic change. In *Barrett's oesophagus*, chronic gastric reflux produces metaplastic columnar epithelium which may be pre-neoplastic, and smoking produces some bronchial metaplasia (columnar cells become squamous).

Dysplasia. This term is used to describe an occasional moderate abnormality of differentiation producing a variety of unusual cells (pleomorphism) rather than a uniform cell population. Dysplasia often accompanies hyperplasia, e.g. during inflammation or repair, and as such is transient and insignificant. However, it sometimes represent a preneoplastic condition, especially where there is no evident cause for the hyperplasia. Thus, biopsy samples are examined for evidence of dysplasia when investigating for possible cancers, e.g. cervical smears, gastroscopy specimens.

Abnormal proliferation and differentiation

Insensitivity to local growth control mechanisms, permitting an unnecessary and even self-destructive overgrowth, has long been recognized as a characteristic feature of neoplastic tissue. Usually there is also **de-differentiation**, i.e. reversion to a more primitive cell type which does not perform the normal function of the tissue involved.

Oncogenes

This breakdown in control may involve abnormal secretion of growth factors or an abnormality in growth factor receptors. It is now believed that the genes coding for mitogenic proteins or their receptors become inappropriately expressed. This is based on findings linking the rare human tumour viruses to the far more numerous non-viral tumours. There is now the tantalising possibility of uniting many disparate aspects of carcinogenesis, including the mutagenic nature of many carcinogens, the action of tumour viruses and control of normal cell proliferation. Although viruses seem to be uncommon causes of human cancer, genes resembling tumour virus RNA (i.e. with a similar nucleotide sequence) have been found in all human cells; they are known as cellular oncogenes.

This remarkable discovery implies that viruses cause cancer by mimicking genes which already exist in the host genome. Indeed, the 'viruses' found in some tumours may even be endogenous gene fragments resembling viruses, i.e. the tumour causes the virus, not vice versa. Alternatively, some viruses may have evolved in this way, a survival advantage having been conferred by the acquisition of a gene which promoted clonal expansion, providing a greater potential for further viral replication.

How do oncogenes cause cancer and how are they related to other factors, such as chemical or viral carcinogens? One possible model is as follows. In normal proliferation:

- Human oncogenes are normally present as proto-oncogenes.
- When activated, they code for growth factors, or growth factor receptors, or other mitogenic promoters.
- These factors are essential for a cell's entry into the cell cycle and movement through it as a prelude to cell division (pp. 631–633).
- Expression of oncogenes is strictly controlled and turned off when no further growth is required.

However, neoplastic transformation may result because of one or more of the following reasons:

- A carcinogen causes the inappropriate expression of a human oncogene, often by mutation of a controlling gene (e.g. repressor or de-repressor).
- Viral oncogenes mimic activated human oncogenes.
- An 'anti-oncogene' or tumour suppressor gene malfunctions through mutation, permitting neoplastic transformation.

One promising line of enquiry has been opened by the discovery of a specific gene which controls movement into and through the cell cycle. This *p53* gene is discussed on p. 633.

Role of mutation

Formerly, it was uncertain whether neoplastic change was a chance genetic mutation in a single cell (i.e. a genotypic change, which could explain the action of mutagens) or an abnormality of metabolism or genetic expression which has occurred to a whole group of cells (i.e. a phenotypic change, which could explain its occasional apparent reversibility). The first now seems more likely. Any permanent alteration in the DNA structure of a single cell is passed on to all daughter cells, and a neoplasm is a clone of that first single abnormal cell. However, the majority of random mutations are metabolically so disruptive as to be lethal, preventing proliferation. Moreover, cells have a remarkable capacity for the self-repair of damaged DNA. Thus, only a very small proportion of mutations actually persist to cause cancers.

It may even be that two or more mutations are necessary for complete transformation – the 'two hit' hypothesis. This could explain the long lag times between exposure and disease, and also the occasional familial tumours. Mutations are usually somatic, i.e. not in germ line tissue, but if an initial mutation did occur in a spermatozoon or an ovum, this could be passed on to offspring as a predisposition to the tumour, which would need a further somatic mutation for full expression.

Mutations are usually caused by chemicals or radiation. Other possible causes are random mutations from faulty cell division accumulating in old age, or the introduction of foreign, viral DNA/RNA. The overall process of **neoplastic transformation** probably occurs in several stages. One of the environmental carcinogens identified in Table 11.3 may alone cause the appropriate mutation, or there may be a combination of an initiator and a promoter factor.

Summary

The ultimate cause of cancer is probably that the normal mechanisms which control cell division and differentiation are activated (or suppressed) inappropriately. There is a failure in the processes by which these mechanisms are usually inhibited from functioning during times when they are not needed.

Thus, cancer may eventually prove to be precisely what it has always intuitively seemed to be – a disorder of the controls on cell proliferation.

Nonetheless, the precise mechanisms are difficult to elucidate and it remains to be discovered precisely how differentiation itself is controlled and how this control is lost.

Unfortunately, these concepts cannot yet be applied directly to the prevention or cure of cancer. The present strategies for treating cancer are based on an imperfect knowledge of the growth characteristics of individual neoplastic cells and the neoplasm as a whole. They are directed primarily towards killing every existing neoplastic cell, but with minimum damage to normal host cells. This is insufficiently discriminating and thus crude, unsatisfactory and often unsuccessful. Hopefully, the new understanding of carcinogenesis will lead to a more fundamental approach, such as intervention in the expression or de-repression of oncogenes.

Cytokinetics

In order to control cancer, the condition must either be prevented or differences must be found between neoplastic and normal cells which can be exploited therapeutically. Because of current uncertainty over the aetiology, tumours can rarely be prevented from starting. Nor do tumours have unique biochemical or metabolic processes crucial to their persistence and which can be targeted pharmacologically – as is done successfully when antibiotics are used against microorganisms – because cell division and differentiation in neoplastic cells use essentially the same processes as normal cells.

The only consistent differences between normal and neoplastic cells which we can currently exploit are in the rate of growth and degree of differentiation. Thus, in order to understand how a tumour might be treated, it is necessary to study quantitatively how it grows, i.e. its **cytokinetics**. In the following sections the stages in the life cycle of normally dividing individual cells are first described; this process is then applied to whole cell populations, which leads to a description of natural history of a tumour.

The cell cycle

Phases

Traditional studies of cell division concentrated on the microscopically distinct stages of mitosis, i.e. prophase, metaphase, anaphase and telophase, as described in basic cell biology texts. More relevant for cancer therapy is what happens in the interphase between mitoses. These interphase events, which are common to all dividing cells, can be grouped into several further phases in which there are different types of metabolic activity (Table 11.4). The whole process from one mitosis to the next is known as the 'cell cycle', and cells that are regularly dividing, i.e. active stem cells, are termed 'in cycle'.

On this model, the four traditional stages of mitosis are known collectively as the M phase (Fig. 11.6). Subsequently there is a period of intense protein and RNA synthesis, the G_1 phase (for historic reasons, from 'gap-1'). During this phase the new daughter cells are synthesizing the materials, mostly enzymes, necessary for physical

---

Table 11.4   Phases of the cell cycle

Phase	Approx. duration (h)[a]	Principal synthetic activity[b]
M	1	Spindle protein
G_0	?[c]	None (resting phase)
G_1	480	RNA, protein
S	16	DNA (for replication)
G_2	8	Nucleoprotein

[a] Times for *skin basal layer cells* are given, to show the relative times in different stages. Other tissues may have different patterns.

[b] That is, synthetic activity related to mitosis.

[c] Time in G_0 is extremely variable (see text).

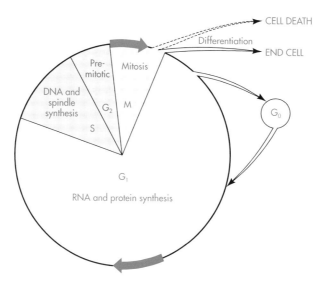

Figure 11.6   Cell cycle.

enlargement. This has the longest but, apart from G_0, the most variable duration.

The time between one M-phase and the next is known as the **intermitotic** or **cell cycle time.** In the example given in Table 11.4 of normal human skin basal layer cells this is about 20 days. For the hyperplastic (but not neoplastic) basal cells in psoriasis it is about one-tenth of this, owing mainly to a shorter G_1 phase. For some bone marrow and gastrointestinal epithelial cells the cell cycle time may be less than 10 h; for liver cells it averages weeks.

G_1 phase
Different cycle times between cell populations or cell types are usually the result of differences in the G_1 phase. However, the G_1 phase in tumour cells is not invariably shorter than that of normal cells' G_1 from the same tissue; often it is longer. It is a popular misconception that neoplasia is simply a more rapid cell division: there is no consistent relationship between cell cycle time and malignancy (*see also* p. 634).

There are a number of possible outcomes to the G_1 phase (Table 11.5). If a cell leaves the cycle, either permanently or temporarily, it is from this phase. Otherwise, it proceeds to the next mitosis.

G_0 phase
Cells in the G_0 resting phase cease all mitotic activity, although of course they continue normal metabolism. It is also likely that DNA repair mechanisms, if needed, are active during this phase. Thus, resting cells enter a reservoir of quiescent stem cells but may be recruited back into the cycle by an appropriate but as yet unknown stimulus.

Tissues which are capable of proliferation or regeneration but only need to do so intermittently (e.g. the liver) probably have a high proportion of stem cells in this phase. The same may be true of certain tumours during periods of remission, such as the leukaemias; they thereby retain the ability to resume the malignant process. Because cells in G_0 are not dividing, they are often insensitive to the usual cytotoxic drugs. Thus resistance to chemotherapy may sometimes occur because there is a high proportion of G_0 cells.

Other phases
During the short S phase the cell is synthesizing new DNA and related proteins in preparation for the next mitosis. There follows a shorter G_2 phase when essential mitotic components such as chromosomal protein are synthesized.

Table 11.5   Possible outcomes to the G_1 phase

A. Cell permanently leaves cycle:
  • a daughter cell may die owing to a defective mitosis
  • the cell may differentiate, maturing into a functional cell after which there will be no further division

B. Cell temporarily leaves cycle:
  • the mitotic cycle is arrested: G_0 phase entered

C. Cycle continues:
  • the cell proceeds to the S phase

Cell death

Cell death is now known to be an organized process rather than merely a wasting away or decline in metabolic functions. Following injury or signals responsible for regulating the cell population, characteristic changes occur which prepare a cell for death and eventual phagocytosis. Termed **apoptosis**, this seems to be a normal and necessary component of the same general control mechanisms that govern the viability of a cell or tissue population which we considered above. Apoptosis includes controlled cleavage of DNA and expression of cell surface receptors which facilitate macrophage activity. As yet this process has not been effectively exploited in chemotherapy, but clearly it is a potential target. If it could be triggered selectively in neoplastic cells this would represent a cytotoxic effect that is highly selective for tumour rather than host (i.e. patient) tissue.

p53 gene

The *p53* gene is emerging as a crucial controller of the cell cycle. Its gene product is a protein which modulates the expression of other genes directly responsible for a variety of aspects of the cycle. In particular, *p53* can halt progress at phase boundaries, e.g. G_1–S. The trigger for such activity seems to be DNA damage: *p53* can allow time for DNA repair mechanisms, thus preventing a potentially harmful mutation to become permanently encoded. It can also trigger apoptosis if a mutation does persist. Thus, *p53* has been dubbed 'the guardian of the genome' and also an anti-oncogene. Even more importantly, at least half of all tumours have been found to have defects in *p53*, implying that if this protection is

lost neoplastic transformation can persist. Furthermore, *p53*-deficient tumours tend to be the more aggressive and more treatment-resistant, perhaps because apoptosis cannot be triggered.

Therapeutic intervention

Cytotoxic drugs and radiation act by interfering in one or more of the active phases of the cell cycle, but are generally ineffective in the G_0 phase. The numerous biochemical events which occur in other phases of the cycle offer a variety of possible pharmacological interventions, e.g. alkylation of nucleic acid or inhibition of protein synthesis, but because the same events occur in all normal dividing cells, these may also be damaged. It important to know in which phase a drug acts so that logical combinations can be chosen; the resultant synergistic effect is well established. It would also be helpful to know when the tumour cells are in particular phases, or the proportions in each phase, but this is impracticable at present. The theoretically attractive strategy of synchronising all cells to the same phase is sometimes attempted, with only limited success.

Cell compartments

The population of cells in any tissue, either normal or neoplastic, divides into a number of different groups or cell compartments (Table 11.6). Some cells will be capable of division, i.e. stem cells, and these may be actively cycling or resting. Most cells will be functional and non-dividing. There will also be some dead cells awaiting scavenging by the reticuloendothelial

Table 11.6   Cell compartments

Cell type	Compartment	Features
Stem cells	Resting	In G_0
	Cycling	Undifferentiated; intense metabolic activity (in G_1, S, G_2 or M phases)
Differentiated ('end cells')	Functional	Main component in normal tissue
	Dead	Variable proportion (usually small, owing to effective scavenging)

system. The relative sizes of these compartments will vary between tissues. Moreover, there are considerable differences in the relative compartment sizes between normal tissue and the neoplastic tissue derived from it, and these are potentially more significant therapeutically than possible differences in intermitotic times (Fig. 11.7 and *see* p. 632).

Measures of tissue growth

Growth rate

What then affects the rate at which a tumour, or any tissue, grows? In normal adult tissue the growth rate is zero, because generally new cell production rate precisely equals cell loss: we have seen that complex feedback mechanisms ensure that this is so. Only in children, or in injured tissues, does growth exceed losses (p. 627). The cell production rate depends directly on the

proportion of cells in the tissue which are dividing (**growth fraction**, representing cycling stem cells) and inversely on the intermitotic time. The cell loss rate (**cell loss fraction**) is dependant on several factors (see below), but is most simply considered as the proportion of dividing cells which survive.

The growth rate of a tissue, especially a solid tumour, is usually expressed as its inverse, the time taken for it to double in size (i.e. number of cells, mass). Thus a greater growth rate means a shorter **doubling time**. The relationship between doubling time and the factors discussed above can be represented empirically as:

$$\text{Doubling time} \propto \frac{\text{Intermitotic time}}{\text{Growth fraction} - \text{Cell loss fraction}}$$

A tumour is by definition a lesion in which cell production rate exceeds cell loss. If the tumour consisted entirely of cycling stem cells and all

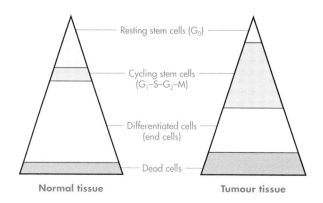

Normal tissue   **Tumour tissue**

Resting stem cells (G_0)
Cycling stem cells (G_1–S–G_2–M)
Differentiated cells (end cells)
Dead cells

Figure 11.7   Relative sizes of cell compartments in normal and neoplastic tissue.

daughter cells survived (and none differentiated), the doubling time would be equal to the intermitotic time and growth would be exponential, i.e. follow first-order kinetics. In this respect, the growth would resemble bacterial growth in optimal conditions, and some young solid tumours do approach this condition. However, generally not all cells in a tumour are cycling stem cells, and a proportion of cells die after division (Fig. 11.7).

In neoplastic tissues the growth fraction is often high. It can be up to 0.9 (90%) in young tumours as more cells leave G_0 and enter the cycle and there is far less differentiation than normal, i.e. daughter cells remain as stem cells. However, the increased number of mitoses in a tumour produces more faulty divisions, resulting in non-viable cells, apoptosis and cell death. Furthermore, a rapidly growing solid tumour often outstrips its ability to grow new blood vessels (**angiogenesis**), so that relatively ischaemic, even necrotic, regions with a high cell loss develop – especially in the centre of the tumour. A further proportion of tumour cells may be destroyed by the immune system. Thus, the cell loss fraction may also sometimes approach 0.9 (90%).

Growth in tumours

It is clear from the above discussion why the intermitotic time of individual cells in neoplasms need not be short. Usually, the main cytokinetic difference between normal and neoplastic tissue is the proportion of dividing cells rather than the rate of division. Moreover, even the doubling time may not be high in a tumour compared with normal tissue, owing perhaps to a high cell loss fraction. Many primary tumours are slow growing. For example, the doubling time in normal leucopoiesis (white cell production) is 2 days, with a growth fraction of about 50%: in acute leukaemia the corresponding figures are 2–10 days and less than 30%. In solid tumours, malignancy derives predominantly from local invasiveness (owing to imperfect differentiation) and metastasis.

As a tumour grows its need for nutrients, and so also for blood vessels to transport them, increases. To facilitate this process the tumour may produce vascular growth factors that promote angiogenesis, or other factors that switch off signals normally inhibiting angiogenesis. This recently characterized aspect of tumour growth offers many possibilities for assessing tumour growth rate, for providing prognostic information, or for therapeutic intervention.

The 'population pressure' produced by these various factors, e.g. increased competition for oxygen and nutrients, may be part of the reason for metastasis: some cells in effect seek a better environment. This tendency is promoted by a greater proliferation of new blood vessels.

Chemosensitivity

Because cytotoxic drugs only act on cycling cells the chemosensitivity of tumours is often closely related to the growth fraction and doubling time (Table 11.7).

Differentiation

Along with its lack of sensitivity to normal feedback inhibition, which is even perhaps partly responsible for this, neoplastic cells often display abnormal differentiation. Such cells may eventually revert to a more primitive form which has little functional capacity beyond replication, i.e. more like a stem cell. There are three ways in which differentiation may be abnormal:

- **Excessive normal function.** This is particularly noticeable with tumours of hormone-secreting cells, e.g. ovarian carcinomas producing high oestrogen levels, or the adrenal adenocarcinoma of Cushing's disease. It may be due to an increased number of secreting cells, but insensitivity to feedback inhibition is also very important. Tumour growth may sometimes be detected and monitored by the abnormal levels of these hormones, or by their effects. Mature tumours however tend to lose this exaggerated normal function and regress (see below).
- **Abnormal differentiation.** The disorganization of genetic expression (abnormal repression or de-repression) may cause the cell to behave like a completely different functional type (a different phenotype), e.g. the secretion of large amounts of antidiuretic hormone by some bronchial carcinomas. Such abnormal

Table 11.7   Cytokinetic parameters[a] of some human tumours

Histological type	Doubling time (days)	Growth fraction (%)	Cell loss fraction (%)	Relative chemosensitivity[b]
Embryonal	25	90	90	++
lymphoma	30	90	90	++
Sarcoma	40	10	70	–
Squamous cell carinoma	60	25	90	+
Adenocarcinoma	80	5	70	+ or –

[a] Approximate values only.

[b] Sensitivity to cytotoxic chemotherapy: ++, very sensitive; +, sensitive; – resistant.

secretions sometimes offer an easy method of detection and objective monitoring.

- **De-differentiation.** The most common pattern is for the neoplastic cell to exhibit no particular function whatsoever: it simply divides. Although often grossly abnormal microscopically, the tumour usually makes its presence felt only by mere pressure of numbers. By this time it is often too late for effective treatment. Some tumours demonstrate their regression by secreting substances that are more usually associated with the embryonic development stage, e.g. alpha-fetoprotein (AFP) and carcinoembryonic antigen (CEA), which may be measured for diagnostic or monitoring purposes.

The natural history of a tumour

Growth curve

Let us assume that a tumour starts as a single cell and continues to divide at a constant rate. Its growth can be traced by plotting its mass or cell number against time (equivalent to the number of doublings; Fig. 11.8). At first, the growth is exponential (the vertical scale in Fig. 11.8 is logarithmic), but the rate falls as the tumour size increases. This decrease is related to a reducing growth fraction and an increased cell loss fraction, and there may also be an increased intermitotic time. In solid tumours these factors, which often make the tumour less sensitive to

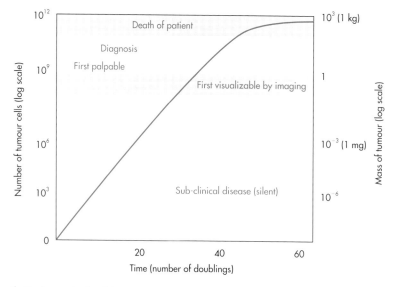

Figure 11.8   Hypothetical growth of solid tumour.

therapy, probably result from relatively poor vascularization.

A vital clinical point is illustrated. The tumour mass will not reach 100 mg until after approximately 30 doublings have produced about 10^8 cells: how long this takes will depend on the doubling time. At this stage, being so small, it will be unnoticed by the patient. There will be no obvious or palpable ('feelable') lump, and it is unlikely to be causing symptoms, except possibly for certain hormone-secreting tumours. Moreover, 100 mg is the smallest size lesion that can be detected on X-ray, so that even mass screening, were it feasible, would miss many significant, slightly smaller tumours. Yet by this stage some tumour types may already have metastasized.

The tumour size would have to increase a further tenfold before becoming palpable, assuming it were superficial, and even then distinct symptoms might not be noticed. Yet there are now 10^9 cells, almost certainly there has been some invasion of local healthy tissue, and some metastases are likely. The task of complete eradication is now daunting, as every last one of these cells must be removed or killed, with acceptable, or at the very least, survivable damage to the healthy host tissues.

Most tumours are diagnosed in the window between 1 g and 100 g, when symptoms become troublesome. This growth pattern explains why many tumours seem to start so suddenly and progress so rapidly. If they are not diagnosed at this stage, or treatment is ineffective, death will usually occur as the tumour burden approaches 1 kg. It can thus be seen why early detection is so important if cancer is to be treated successfully; and, conversely, why successful cancer therapy is generally so difficult to achieve.

Local invasion

As a tumour grows, its bulk (a 'space-occupying lesion') puts pressure on local structures such as nerves, blood vessels, the gut lumen, etc. with predictable symptomatic consequences. Benign tumours tend to be self-contained and have definite margins, so this is their main adverse effect. Malignant tumours, by contrast, partly because of their insensitivity to the presence of other cells and also because of a lower adhesiveness to their basement membrane, are far more invasive. They expand in a very disorganized way, their margin is indistinct and they cause considerable disruption to their environment.

This process is aided by the secretion of proteases (proteolytic enzymes) from tumour cells, which facilitate their passage through basement membranes and the extracellular matrix of connective tissue. Eventually, it is hoped, measurement of the activity of these enzymes might offer an estimate of prognosis (e.g. high levels will predict further growth, metastasis or relapse) and thus a basis for deciding if further therapy is warranted. Inhibition of proteases may have therapeutic potential in limiting tumour spread.

Metastasis

The mechanisms of metastasis are not yet understood. Probably, single cells occasionally detach themselves from the primary tumour mass and are carried away in the blood or lymph, or are shed into a local body cavity, e.g. from abdominal epithelial tumours. Most such cells are destroyed immunologically. Inevitably, however, some will find a new site to colonize and start a new neoplastic clone; well-perfused areas like lung and bone marrow are common.

The rate and pattern of metastasis is partly determined by the site of the primary and its route of local invasion. For example, local lymph nodes – part of whose function it is to trap such debris – are frequent metastatic sites for many types of tumour, e.g. the axillary nodes in breast cancer. The liver is frequently involved in gastrointestinal tumours, which shed cells into the portal circulation.

Even if the pattern cannot be explained by such considerations, it is usually consistent and predictable, e.g. breast cancer commonly causes bone and liver secondary tumours. Knowledge of these patterns is clearly important in treatment and prognosis. The extent of metastasis is part of the basis of 'staging' (p. 642).

Metastases usually grow considerably faster than their parent primary tumour, partly because they are smaller and thus better perfused. Because they are likely to have been exposed to previous chemotherapy they also tend to be more chemoresistant (i.e. survivors have been selected) – this is one reason why disseminated disease is more difficult to treat.

Resistance

The longer a tumour grows, the more likely it is to develop resistance to chemotherapeutic agents, as more cell divisions increase the chances of a mutation favourable to resistance (p. 653).

Summary

Figure 11.9 illustrates in a diagrammatic form some important stages in the growth of a tumour.

Differences between normal and neoplastic tissues

The differences between normal and neoplastic tissues can now be summarized (Table 11.8). Although some of the characteristics, especially the cytokinetics, of a given tumour may be little different from normal, taken together they render a neoplasm unmistakable. They emphasize that the simplistic view of cancer as 'no more than rapid growth' is inadequate.

To illustrate this point, consider why the proliferative skin disorder psoriasis (*see* Chapter 12) is not a neoplastic disorder. Certainly, the cycle

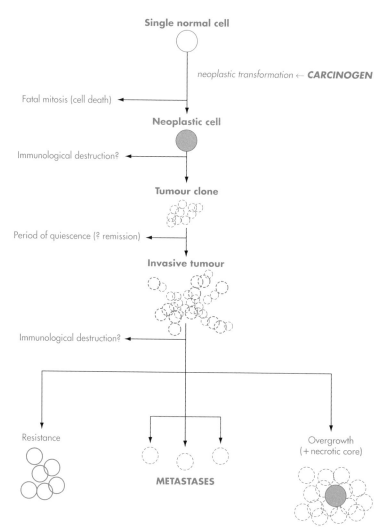

Figure 11.9   Natural history of a solid tumour.

Table 11.8   Some differences between neoplastic and normal tissues

Characteristic	Normal	Neoplastic
Contact inhibition	Present	Absent or reduced
Doubling time	Average for tissue	Low, average or high
Growth fraction	Average for tissue	Average or high
Cell loss fraction	Average for tissue	Average or high
Differentiation	Typical of tissue	De-differentiation (atypical or excess activity)
Invasion of local tissues	Absent	Usual
Spread to distant tissues	Absent	Common

time of the basal cells in a psoriatic lesion is much reduced compared with normal; possibly there is also a greater cell loss fraction. And clearly the hyperplasia is not under full control as it is inappropriate for normal epidermal development. However, the growth is not totally unrestrained. There remains some local inhibition because there is no invasion of the dermis. Moreover, there are no metastases, no primitive basal cell colonies in lymph nodes or bone marrow: in fact, no primitive cells at all. The hyperactive basal cells do more or less what their more sedate cousins, normal basal cells, do: they become prickle cells which move upwards through the epidermis, become keratinized, and are shed. That is to say, they are more or less normally differentiated.

Clinical features

Mechanisms of host damage

Cancer rarely kills because of a functional failure of the primary organ affected. In the case of breast cancer this is obvious, but patients with lung cancer do not usually die of respiratory failure and those with stomach cancer do not die from malabsorption and starvation. Certainly, malfunction of the affected organ can often cause specific symptoms (Table 11.9). However, the clinical consequences of most tumours are generally indirect, being related to their bulk or to the invasion of local or distant tissues. There

is also a diverse group of remote, obscure or secondary effects collectively termed **paraneoplastic phenomena**, some of which may be caused by toxins or other abnormal metabolites released by the tumour, e.g. tumour necrosis factor.

Symptoms and presentation

The range of possible symptoms from cancer is almost unlimited; the condition can mimic almost any other disease on first presentation. The classic story of a 'lump' is not the most common, and even so, lumps may be neither malignant nor even neoplastic. Pain is also an unusual first symptom. Most commonly there is a period of feeling vaguely unwell which is often associated with anorexia and recent significant weight loss.

Table 11.10 lists common symptoms that may be caused by cancer. If these are persistent and unexplained by other circumstances or diseases, then the possibility of cancer must be fully investigated. The presence of known risk factors, such as age, immunodeficiency, environmental exposure, family history, sex or occupation will increase the suspicion. Many symptoms are related to the site of the primary neoplasm, but certain tumours – especially haematopoietic and bone marrow tumours, and also some endocrine tumours – can cause less obvious effects. For example, different marrow neoplasms may cause aplastic anaemia, thrombocytopenia, leucopenia, etc. leading to tiredness, bleeding or infections.

Table 11.9   Mechanisms of host damage by tumours, with examples

Altered organ function

Excessive normal	e.g. ↑ gastrin (in Zollinger–Ellison syndrome)
Diminished	e.g. haemopoietic tumours such as leukaemia
Atypical	e.g. ADH-secreting lung tumours
Abnormal or toxic metabolites	e.g. tumour necrosis factor

Space-occupying lesion

Pressure on local structures	• nerves → pain
	• blood vessels → ischaemia, haemorrhage
	• GI → obstruction
	• brain → neurological symptoms (central and peripheral)
Local invasion	• inflammation
	• ulceration
	• effusion (e.g. pleural, abdominal)
Metastasis: disruption at distant sites	• bone → pain, fractures, hypercalcaemia
	• liver → hepatic failure

Paraneoplastic phenomena

Cachexia: debility, anorexia, wasting	
Depressed immune response	
Anaemia, fever	
Electrolyte imbalance	e.g. hypokalaemia, hypercalcaemia
Metabolic disturbance	e.g. hypoglycaemia
Psychological effects	

GI, gastrointestinal tract.

Table 11.10   Symptoms that may indicate cancer if unexplained and unresponsive to normal treatment

• Lumps
• Dark pigmented skin lesions
• Obvious change in previously stable warts or moles
• Ulceration of skin or mucous membranes
• Anorexia, rapid weight loss, general debility
• Dysphagia, dyspepsia, apparent gastric ulcer
• Persistent unusual constipation, diarrhoea, rectal bleeding
• Persistent bleeding, unusual discharge
• Persistent pain, especially in joints or bones
• Unexplained (pathological) fractures

Specific problems in cancer

Cachexia

The profound debility and wasting that is so typical of advanced cancer probably has a number of causes. Various toxins, metabolites and electrolyte abnormalities, notably hypercalcaemia, doubtless contribute. These may act through anorexia, exacerbated by malabsorption and the patient's depressed mood. Very large tumours may even compete with the host for nutrients. There may also be an abnormality in the regulation of metabolic rate and thermogenesis. A non-specific, hypoplastic, iron-resistant anaemia is also a common feature of many serious chronic diseases. Cachexia may eventually become the predominant feature and often appears to be the main cause of death.

Psychological factors

These are significant as they undoubtedly affect the patient's response to the illness and the rigours of therapy, particularly chemotherapy. Depression is common and requires appropriate treatment. The overall success of treatment may depend on a positive attitude by the patient. Some suffer so severely from the nausea and vomiting of chemotherapy that they decide not to continue with it, and face the consequences, although this is unusual nowadays with the advent of more effective anti-emetic treatments (*see* Chapter 10). On the other hand, in a study already described (p. 626), patients who took a positive, aggressive attitude toward their tumour had a better survival rate.

Pain

This is far less consistent a feature of cancer than is commonly imagined. Most patients with solid tumours experience pain at some time, but many have either little pain or pain only for short periods. Although pain remains the most feared symptom, modern methods of pain control, with their emphasis on active prophylaxis, mean that no patient need suffer unduly (*see* Chapter 10), and about one-third of cancer patients never experience pain. The origin of cancer pain is mainly direct pressure on nerve endings, or the result of the compression against bones causing entrapment neuropathies. Compression within bones from secondary tumours is often one the most intractable forms. There may also be direct stimulation of nerve endings by toxins or abnormal metabolites. Hypercalcaemia is a common feature of many tumours, and this may also cause or exacerbate pain; optimal treatment currently utilizes *bisphosphonates* and rehydration.

Death

The causes of death from cancer are poorly understood. The immediate terminal event may be heart failure, respiratory failure or 'multi-organ failure' but this does not really explain the process. Failure of the organ primarily affected by the tumour is rarely responsible. Often, death seems to be the end result of prolonged cachexia which makes the patient more susceptible to a variety of secondary illnesses, especially overwhelming infection. Immunosuppression is a feature of many cancers.

Investigation and diagnosis

The diagnosis of malignancy is ultimately histological. However, the whole panoply of modern investigative techniques are exploited. The aims of investigation may include:

- Mass screening.
- Locating a suspected lesion.
- Obtaining a biopsy and characterizing it.
- 'Staging' the illness.
- Monitoring the patient's progress.

Screening

Although early detection is highly desirable if the tumour is to be successfully treated, most cancers will have already grown to about 75% of their fatal size before symptoms become apparent. Thus, it might then seem that extensive mass screening should be implemented. However, current techniques are insufficiently sensitive to make a substantial impact.

Programmes currently operating, such as breast screening and the Papanicolaou cervical smear, have not been unequivocally successful. They have been criticised as very inefficient in terms of lives saved in relation to cost; e.g. breast cancer screening in postmenopausal women has not been strikingly successful in reducing mortality. On the other hand, in Scandinavia at least, cervical smears have produced significant falls in uterine cancer incidence and mortality. In Japan, gastroscopy is helping to detect gastric carcinomas earlier, while in the UK, faecal occult blood screening for bowel cancer is being piloted. Intensive screening of high-risk groups such as those with a family history is also being evaluated.

One of the limitations of some programmes is their failure to reach the most at-risk groups. However, there is no doubting that overall these programmes have saved many lives, prevented much suffering and obviated much treatment. Perhaps a fuller understanding of aetiology is required before prevention becomes more generally feasible. Even so, the experience with smoking and lung cancer unfortunately suggests that even positive proof of causation is no guarantee that the public, industry or governments will react appropriately.

Imaging

Some form of imaging is almost always carried out, depending on the suspected location of the lesion. Techniques used include radiology, ultrasound, computed tomography (CT), magnetic resonance imaging (MRI), radioisotope scanning, thermography and fibreoptic endoscopy. Such techniques are also used in mass screening.

Characterization

Biopsy and histological examination are essential to the diagnosis of cancer. Access to biopsy specimens increasingly uses minimally invasive methods such as fibreoptic endoscopy, e.g. for the gastrointestinal, urinary, genital and respiratory tracts, whereas in the past exploratory surgery was required. The histological appearance of the cells will indicate the tumour type, tissue of origin (e.g. epithelial or germ cell), degree of differentiation and extent of dysplasia. From this can be estimated the seriousness of the condition, how advanced it is, its propensity for metastasis, and its likely response to different forms of therapy.

Tumour markers

The presence and extent of the tumour may sometimes be indicated indirectly by the plasma levels of certain specific 'markers' that they produce. Embryonic and fetal substances (e.g. alpha-fetoprotein, chorionic gonadotrophin) can be measured by radioimmunoassay. An elevated level of normal hormones from endocrine tumours, such as levothyroxine (thyroxine) from thyroid or, indirectly, pituitary tumours, or ectopic hormones (e.g. ADH from lung cancer) can readily be quantified.

Staging and monitoring

Staging, an attempt to quantify the severity of a tumour, is essential following diagnosis. Although it varies from tumour to tumour, in general the following qualitative system can be applied to most tumours:

* Stage 1. Tumour confined to original site, with no local invasion ('*in situ*').
* Stage 2. Local invasion.
* Stage 3. Spread to local lymph nodes.
* Stage 4. Metastasis in distant sites.

A more rigorous method, which allows progress or response to therapy to be quantified, is the so-called 'Tumour/Node/Metastasis' or TNM system, where the size of the primary, the number of local lymph node involved and the presence of metastases are determined.

The stage of a tumour has implications for the choice of therapy and for prognosis. For example, the involvement of tissue outside the original mammary lump in breast cancer indicates the extent of surgery required. The 5-year relative survival (i.e. relative to comparable women without cancer) for Stage 1 cervical cancer is 80%, while for Stage 4 it is less than 10%.

Prognosis

Despite sophisticated investigative techniques, empirical and epidemiological means are still important in estimating prognosis. Clinical experience has shown that most primary tumours have a characteristic natural history. Their rate of growth, the degree, rate and pattern of metastatic spread, and their sensitivity to certain types of therapy and even to specific drugs, can often be predicted on this basis.

From these data, and depending on the stage which a patient's tumour has reached, estimates of the prognosis can be made in the form of median survival figures, i.e. 50% of patients at that particular stage usually survive 6 months, 5 years, etc. This is the origin of the much quoted but misguided assertions such as 'the doctors gave him only 6 months to live' (these claims often prefacing enthusiastic accounts of 'miracle cures').

Management: aims and strategy

The three priorities in dealing with cancer are, in order of importance:

- Prevention.
- Early detection.
- Total eradication.

In most cases these are as yet unrealized ideals. Our incomplete knowledge of the causes of cancer, coupled with inadequate methods of screening, usually rule out the first two priorities. Smoking and lung cancer is potentially a major exception. For breast cancer, various preventative techniques including reduced-fat diets (to minimize oestrogen production) and prophylactic *tamoxifen* (an anti-oestrogen) are being investigated. Screening was discussed above (p. 641).

Only occasionally is the third priority achieved. Once diagnosed, the ideal treatment would remove or kill every neoplastic cell, because in theory even a single remaining cell could generate a new neoplastic clone. However, current methods of therapy rarely permit this without unacceptable, even fatal, damage to the patient. On the other hand, when a tumour mass is reduced below a certain size the patient's immune system, by analogy with microbial infections, may mop up the remainder. It must be remembered however that their immune system might well have been compromised by the chemotherapy.

Aims

When therapy is initiated there must be a careful and realistic identification of the therapeutic goals. These may be considered in a hierarchy (Table 11.11). The success of treatment is usually measured in terms of **timed survival**, i.e. the proportion of patients still alive after a given period. A 75% survival rate at 5 years would be considered very good.

Realistic assessment

The most appropriate level in this hierarchy for a given patient will depend on the nature of the tumour, the stage of the disease, and clinical experience. The risks of untreated disease (the prognosis) and the potential benefits of treatment (the likelihood of a response) must be balanced objectively against the predictable risks of treatment (e.g. adverse drug effects). This evaluation must be made in consultation with the patient and his or her family.

The term **cure** is relative: it can never be certain that all metastatic cells have been eliminated. As yet, it can be claimed for only a small number of cancers that a large proportion of patients survive to an extent comparable with disease-free individuals of similar ages. These include some genital tumours (testicular teratoma, chorionic carcinoma), some childhood leukaemias and Hodgkin's lymphoma (p. 646).

For most treatment regimens, in the majority of malignancies induction of remission (a **response**) is the most realistic goal. The aim is to reduce significantly the number of neoplastic cells and hence the bulk of the tumour. In this way patient survival may be improved and symptoms usually reduced. In some tumours, particularly if far advanced at presentation, even this cannot be expected. The aim then is simply palliative, i.e. to deal with any secondary effects that may be causing the patient pain, distress or other serious symptoms. For example, partial surgical excision to reduce pressure on local nerves or blood vessels, or to relieve gastrointestinal obstruction.

Table 11.11   Hierarchy of aims in cancer management

1. Cure	Eradication of tumour and metastases
2. Remission/mitigation	Significant reduction in tumour load
	Increased survival
3. Symptomatic/palliation	Treatment of secondary complications
	Relief of symptoms
4. Terminal care	Improve quality of life
	Optimize symptom control

Terminal care and quality of life

Finally, if treatment fails, strenuous efforts are still made to ensure that the patient's remaining life is as comfortable as possible, with optimal symptom control, optimal nutrition, counselling, attention to psychosocial and spiritual needs, etc. Increasing importance is being attached to the quality of the patient's life with or without therapy. For some patients with advanced disease, even heroic treatment – mutilating surgery, serious adverse effects – may produce only a moderate improvement in survival. In the past there might have been unrelieved therapeutic efforts of increasing toxicity until the patient's death was often secondary to the adverse effects of the therapy, such as overwhelming infection or haemorrhage. Now, clinicians are more realistic and accord the patient a peaceful, dignified and pain-free end: much depends on the attitudes and wishes of the patient and, perhaps, their family.

Modes of therapy

The method of treatment will largely be determined by a realistic assessment of the therapeutic goal. The usual modes used are:

- Surgery (excision of primary tumour).
- Bone marrow transplantation (for some leukaemias).
- Radiotherapy.
- Drugs (cytotoxic chemotherapy, hormone therapy, immunotherapy).

If neoplasms were always benign, simple surgical removal would suffice. Unfortunately, malignant neoplasms invade the tissues surrounding them, making it difficult to determine accurately how much tissue to remove. Furthermore, complete surgical removal of widespread metastatic deposits ('secondaries') is not practicable; besides, many are microscopic and cannot be identified by present techniques. Thus, surgery alone is rarely adequate and some additional form of 'mopping up' of potential secondaries is usually necessary. This is termed **adjuvant** therapy.

The type of adjuvant therapy used depends partly on the likely distribution of presumed secondaries. Local invasion and lymph node spread can be treated by radiotherapy. For disseminated disease, drugs are more suitable because of their potential to reach most tissues in the body. Indeed, for most tumours this is the main role of drug therapy although in certain cases it is the chosen primary therapy.

Two factors generally govern the choice of treatment mode (Table 11.12). The first is empirical clinical experience: some tumours are known to be particularly radioresistant, others are chemoresistant, etc. The second involves practical considerations.

Table 11.12   Principles governing the choice of treatment in cancer

Surgery	Well-defined solid tumour
	Non-vital region (e,g, mastectomy)
	Non-mutilating result (e.g. unsuitable for some head and neck tumours)
	Resection/reconstruction possible (e.g. gut)
Radiotherapy	Diffuse but localized tumour (e.g. lymphoma)
	Vital organ/region (e.g. head and neck, CNS)
	Adjuvant therapy (e.g. post mastectomy)
	Palliation
Chemotherapy	Adjuvant therapy following surgery or radiotherapy
	Neo-adjuvant therapy prior to surgery or radiotherapy
	Widely disseminated/metastasized
	Diffuse tumour (e.g. leukaemia)
	Some primary tumours (e.g. Hodgkin's lymphoma)
	Palliation

Surgery

Surgery is the most appropriate treatment for solid tumours in sites where it would neither threaten a vital function nor be too mutilating, and where reconstruction is possible. However, surgery may inadvertently facilitate metastatic spread, displacing tumour cells and liberating them into the local circulation or lymph. Where lymphatic dissemination is known to occur as part of the natural history of the tumour, local lymph nodes (which may have trapped potential metastasizing cells) are also excised; breast cancer is a prime example. Such **radical surgery** is becoming less common nowadays with the advent of the 'multimodal' approach (see below).

Radiotherapy

Radiotherapy is suitable as primary therapy in some local tumours for which surgery is inappropriate. Also, certain tumours are known to be particularly radiosensitive, e.g. bladder carcinoma and embryonic kidney and nerve cell tumours. Other common applications include adjuvant therapy for diffuse local spread, e.g. after mastectomy or lumpectomy for breast cancer, and 'de-bulking' (size reduction) palliative treatment for inoperable tumours. Thus radiotherapy may be administered in the form of intensive X-radiation from outside the body to administration or implantation of a radioisotope (e.g. radioiodine [^{131}I] for thyroid tumour).

Radiotherapy is often seriously damaging to normal tissue, and strategies have been devised to minimize collateral damage, some of which are analogous to ways of reducing drug toxicity discussed below. These include fractionating the dose and highly specific targeting, which has become much easier with improvements in imaging.

Cytotoxic chemotherapy

As experience with chemotherapeutic agents and knowledge of cytokinetics increase, so more potential roles are found for chemotherapy. Until recently in solid tumours treatment was restricted chiefly to adjuvant therapy, following reduction of the main bulk of the tumour surgi-cally or by radiotherapy. In particular, it is felt that micrometastases, some of which are possibly induced surgically, can be destroyed in this way. One new application even reverses this approach using chemotherapy as the primary debulking procedure, e.g. in breast cancer. This is also known as **neo-adjuvant therapy**.

The other traditional place of chemotherapy was as a desperate last measure in uncontrolled and widely disseminated disease after the failure of surgery and radiotherapy. Small wonder that it gained a poor reputation ('hard cases make bad law'). Nevertheless, palliation may be possible even in such circumstances.

However, intensive chemotherapy at an earlier stage in the disease, perhaps in association with radiotherapy, can be a highly successful treatment of first choice in certain conditions, such as choriocarcinoma, leukaemia and testicular cancer. Many other tumours are now known to be chemosensitive, especially if we also include endocrine therapy, and chemotherapy is becoming far more widely used.

Multimodal therapy

Cancer therapy nowadays usually involves a combination of different modalities. One is used to reduce the bulk of the tumour and another to attempt to eradicate the remainder of the neoplastic cells. In addition, chemotherapy may sometimes sensitize tumour cells to radiotherapy.

Chemotherapy of cancer

It would be satisfying if the theoretical principles discussed in the previous sections, when applied rationally to the selection of drugs, produced a high rate of cure in the majority of tumours. Alas, this is far from true: the overall 5-year survival rate for cancer is presently about 30%. There is still much to be learned about the behaviour and kinetics of neoplastic cells and the design of anti-neoplastic drugs.

Most drug regimens in current use have been devised empirically. Nevertheless, exploitation of what is known will maximize the chances of success, and this section will illustrate the theoretical basis of common practice in chemotherapy, in particular cytotoxic chemotherapy.

Role of chemotherapy

Until the introduction of chemotherapy, surgery and radiotherapy were the sole means of treatment, and the prognosis for cancer had improved little in 150 years. Table 11.13 gives an idea of the changing prognosis for breast cancer, where only in the last 20 years have chemotherapy, and more recently screening programmes, made some impact.

The high failure rates before chemotherapy were usually the result of relapses. Even the most radical surgery or radiotherapy, while it may eliminate the primary tumour, cannot affect metastases. Eventually, in most cases, these caused a relapse and the resultant widespread dissemination was inoperable. Thus the most that could be expected was remission: cure was generally impossible. Adjuvant chemotherapy has brought about significant improvements in some cancer survival rates because of its ability to reach disseminated micrometastases.

Chemotherapy has been gradually refined by:

• The optimization of use, e.g. combination therapy, dose scheduling.
• The development of strategies to minimize toxicity.
• The discovery and controlled clinical trial of more potent and less toxic agents.

Nowadays, the prognosis for a small number of malignancies, especially leukaemia, where the growth fraction is high, is excellent. For some others it has improved significantly, e.g. the cure rate for the rare Wilm's renal tumour was only 20% before chemotherapy but now is 80%. Because leukaemia represents no more than 10% of all tumours, these successes have had only a small impact on overall survival. There are still many malignancies, particularly solid tumours with low growth fractions, that are resistant. The relative chemosensitivity of common tumours is given in Table 11.14. One avenue to exploit potentially is the means of assessing the *in vivo* sensitivity and resistance of tumours in individual patients to specific antineoplastic agents, in a manner analogous to antimicrobial sensitivity testing.

Theoretical basis of chemotherapy

The ideal chemotherapeutic anti-cancer agent would have selective toxicity for neoplastic cells, just as antimicrobial agents are toxic to microbial but not human cells. Unfortunately, save for one minor exception (the utilization of crisantaspase (asparaginase) by some leukaemic cells; see below), human neoplastic cells do not differ in any qualitative biochemical way from normal cells.

Thus, other differences between normal and neoplastic tissue have to be sought and exploited: these are primarily in growth parameters and differentiation (pp. 636–638). The former are currently the most amenable to pharmacological intervention. Cytokinetic differences probably account, in part, for two important observations:

Table 11.13 Approximate survival rates for breast cancer

Year	Overall survival rate(%)		
	5 years	10 years	15 years
1812	50	35	24
1968	60	38	27
1986[a]	80+	65	–

[a] Following the introduction of chemotherapy.

Figures for last period for non-metastasized disease; older figures not based on modern diagnostic techniques, therefore data are not strictly comparable.

Table 11.14   Chemosensitivity of different tumours

Very sensitive (usually responsive)	Leukaemias • chronic lymphoid
	• acute childhood
	• myeloid
	Lymphomas (Hodgkin's, Burkitt's)
	Choriocarcinoma
	Testicular teratoma
	Embryonal tumours
Fairly sensitive (often responsive)	Breast
	Ovarian
	Prostatic
	Head and neck
	CNS
	Lung (rarer 'small cell' form)
Relatively insensitive (occasionally responsive)	Uterus
	Skin (melanoma)
Insensitive (rarely responsive)	Kidney and bladder
	Liver and pancreas
	Colorectal cancer
	Gastric carcinoma
	Lung ('non-small cell')

- Tumours are often more sensitive to agents that interfere with the biochemistry of cell division, a greater proportion of neoplastic cells being affected than those in normal tissue.
- Tumour tissue usually does not recover as rapidly as normal tissue from such interference.

These are the central theoretical principles of cytotoxic therapy; the second is important because it limits toxicity. These differences may be exploited and enhanced clinically, pharmaceutically and pharmacologically by variations in dose scheduling, route of administration, drug combinations, etc.

Selective sensitivity

One reason for the greater sensitivity of neoplastic tissue to cytotoxic action is that it often has a higher growth fraction. There may also be a shorter doubling time and a higher cell loss fraction. The central problem of cytotoxic therapy is that in normal bone marrow there are stem cells in high proportions that are also proliferating very rapidly, and so these may be affected similarly. (This very characteristic is

exploited when using cytotoxic drugs as immunosuppressants.) Less vital tissues similarly at risk are the gut lining and hair follicles.

Thus bone marrow depression (**myelosuppression**) is the main constraint on chemotherapy, and most regimens are designed in an attempt to circumvent or minimize it. Fortunately, there are often significant quantitative differences between the marrow and tumour stem cell populations. Although marrow stem cells have a shorter doubling time than many tumours, 80% are usually in the comparatively resistant G_0 resting phase, so bone marrow has a low growth fraction. It also has a low cell loss fraction. Thus, a single dose of a drug has a disproportionately greater effect on the tumour cell population.

Relative recovery

The slow recovery of tumours is partly because resting tumour cells are recruited more slowly into the cycle. The normal response to the death of a substantial number of cells in a tissue is the recruitment of resting stem cells to replenish the deficit. However, following cytotoxic damage tumour doubling time is not markedly reduced, whereas bone marrow tissue recovers, i.e. repopulates, much more rapidly than the tumour.

Bone marrow recovery

The average lifespan of different blood cells, which is related to the turnover time of their precursors in the marrow, is given in Table 11.15. Thus if there is be a total marrow failure, resistance to infection would be diminished within a few days and coagulation would be compromised within a week but, should the patient survive, anaemia would take months to develop. However, if damage is partial, stem cells are rapidly recruited from the resting (G_0) compartment, the doubling rate is accelerated, and ill-effects are minimized. Three weeks is usually sufficient time for marrow recovery following chemotherapy with most agents in most patients. However, this can vary considerably and treatment is closely monitored by frequent blood counts and levels allowed to return to normal for the individual patient before the treatment is continued.

Pulsed therapy

Because of the need for time for bone marrow recovery, a typical course of chemotherapy is usually given as a series of 21-day cycles of treatment, each of which involves intensive treatment over a few days followed by a rest period.

Figure 11.10 shows various possible outcomes to pulsed therapy depending on the choice of dose, duration of treatment and tumour resistance. One of the many problems of chemotherapy is judging when the tumour has been eradicated. Most commonly, empirical judgements are made on the basis of clinical experience; alternatively, extrapolations can be made from the rate of response while the tumour was

still detectable. This may present the dilemma of having to recommend further treatments with highly toxic drugs, knowing that these will be superfluous, probably unpleasant and possibly harmful for those patients who have already been cured (or responded maximally).

Proportional kill effect

Pioneer work on the tumour cytokinetics in mouse leukaemia, which is a useful model system because the growth fraction approaches 100%, established two further fundamental principles:

- Cell killing by cytotoxic drugs follows first-order kinetics: the proportion of cells killed varies with the dose so that higher doses increase the fractional rather than the total kill.
- A viable tumour can develop from a single neoplastic cell.

Thus, equal doses of drugs kill equal proportions of cells. If a certain dose reduces a tumour population from 10^8 to 10^6 cells, the same dose will, in further reducing the size to 10^4 cells, kill a much smaller absolute number of cells. The same dose is needed repeatedly, no matter how small the tumour has shrunk, until every last tumour cell is killed or the tumour mass is small enough to be eradicated by the immune system.

This is illustrated schematically in Fig. 11.11. However, this assumes no change in growth rate with size, which does not always apply, especially to solid tumours (pp. 631–639). Smaller, younger tumours have a higher growth fraction and a shorter doubling time, and would thus be expected to be more sensitive to chemotherapy. Metastases, however, are often more resistant than the primary from which they arise, which further complicates adjuvant therapy.

Action of cytotoxic drugs

There are two important aspects of the action of the cytotoxic drugs: first, the biochemical mode of action (pharmacological classification); and second, the cell cycle phase or phases when active (cytokinetic classification).

Table 11.15   Average lifespans of blood cells

Neutrophils	24 h
Platelets	7 days
Lymphocytes	Various sub-populations: 10–50+ days
Erythrocytes	120 days

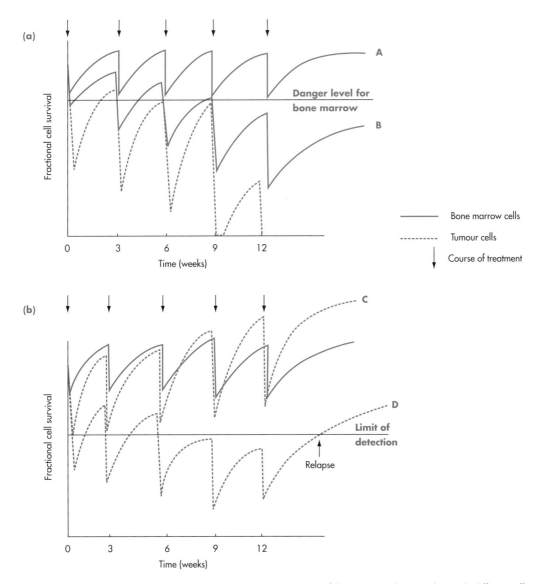

Figure 11.10   Pulsed therapy with marrow recovery phase. (a) Successful tumour eradication, but with different effects on bone marrow. The figure shows the theoretical effect (expressed as fractional survival) of repeated doses of a cytotoxic regimen on tumour and marrow cell populations. Curve A shows successful chemotherapy: the marrow recovers to give acceptable peripheral blood counts after each treatment while the tumour is progressively reduced. Curve B shows what would happen if the treatment required to reduce adequately the tumour cell population was too intense, so that the cumulative marrow effects produced dangerous depression. (b) Different types of unsuccessful chemotherapy. Curve C shows inadequate dosage. Although the bone marrow is spared the tumour regenerates between treatments. Curve D shows what happens if, once the tumour is reduced below the detectable size, treatment is stopped prematurely. Eventually there will be a relapse.

Mode of action

Almost all cytotoxic drugs kill cells by interfering with the production or structure of nucleic acid (or occasionally protein), molecules essential for mitosis and cell growth. It is now believed that cell death following exposure to cytotoxic action (including radiation) is due to the triggering of

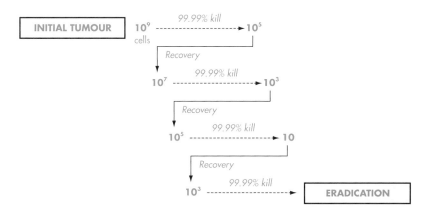

Figure 11.11   Proportional kill effect. The figure shows the theoretical result of successive doses of a particularly effective drug regimen which kills 99.99% of all cycling tumour cells. A reduction in tumour cell number from an initial 10^9 cells occurs after every treatment. However, during the delay between treatments (necessary for marrow recovery) the tumour partially regenerates.

apoptosis, rather than non-specific disruption. Recall that apoptosis is an ordered auto-destructive response to irreparable DNA damage (p. 633).

Cytotoxic drugs are usually classified according to what is believed to be their biochemical mode of action (Table 11.16). The stages in the biochemical sequence of mitosis at which they act are shown schematically in Fig. 11.12. Note that additive or synergistic effects might be expected from logical combinations of agents from different groups.

Phase of action

Because the various reactions with which cytotoxics interfere occur at different phases in the cell cycle, different drugs act at different phases (Table 11.17; Fig. 11.13). Unlike most other cytotoxics, **non-specific agents** act equally on non-dividing cells (non-stem cells and stem cells resting in G_0) and cycling stem cells. Thus, they are highly toxic to normal tissue and are little used nowadays (e.g. *chlormethine (mustine)*). **Cycle-specific agents**, which potentially act on all phases of cycling cells, but not resting cells, are probably the largest group and generally the most useful. However, the phase-specific agents have particular uses if appropriately exploited.

Exploiting cytokinetic differences

The full potential of these differences has yet to be realized, but there have been a number of interesting approaches.

Synchronization. This involves using drugs that arrest the cell cycle at a certain stage (e.g. *dactinomycin* arresting progress from G_1 to S phase); radiotherapy may be used similarly. The drug is then withdrawn and the accumulated cells, which are suddenly 'unblocked', progress to the next phase simultaneously. A drug acting at that next phase is then given, e.g. an *antimetabolite* acting at S phase. If tumour cells have a different intermitotic time from marrow cells, appropriate timing of the second drug should achieve some selectivity. A further intriguing possibility is to synchronize all marrow cells, and then use against the tumour an agent that acts at a different phase, thus providing a measure of protection for bone marrow. Conversely, the new marrow cell colony stimulating factors (p. 660) are being investigated in leukaemia for their potential to increase the proportion of chemosensitive blast cells in the marrow by stimulating them to leave the chemoresistant G_0 phase.

Recruitment. Synchronization would make only a limited impact on tumours with a low growth fraction. Instead, a cycle-specific agent might be used to kill all cycling cells; subsequently, many resting cells return to the cycle to be killed by the next treatment. However, this

Table 11.16   Biochemical mode of action of some cytotoxic drugs

Action	Group	Examples
Alkylating agents (cross-link DNA)	Alkyl sulphonate	*Busulfan*
	Chloroethylamines	*Chlorambucil, melphalan, cyclophosphamide, ifosfamide*
	Nitrosoureas	*Lomustine, carmustine*
	Heavy metal agents	*Cispatin, carboplatin*
Antimetabolites (impair nucleotide base incorporation into DNA/RNA)	Purine analogues	*Mercaptopurine, tioguanine (thioguanine)*
	Pyrimidine analogues	*Fluorouracil, cytarabine*
	Antifolate	*Methotrexate*
Topoisomerase inhibitors		*Topotecan, irinotecan, etoposide*
	Anthracyclines	*Doxorubicin, daunorubicin, epirubicin*
Miscellaneous DNA-RNA inhibitors		*Dactinomycin, hydroxycarbamide (hydroxyurea)*
DNA scission		*Bleomycin*
Mitotic spindle inhibitors (tubulin-binding)	Vinca alkaloids	*Vincristine, vinblastine*
	Podophyllin derivatives	*Etoposide*
	Taxanes	*Paclitaxel, docetaxel*
Precursor depleter	Enzyme inhibitor	*Crisantaspase*[a]
Hormones and anti-hormones	(*See* p. 661 and Table 11.21)	
Uncertain action	Corticosteroids[b]	*Prednisolone*
		Procarbazine[c]

[a] Colaspase, asparaginase.

[b] Possibly act by protein synthesis inhibiton; lympholytic in leukaemias.

[c] Possible alkylating agent.

Agents may act by several mechanisms; it is not always certain which action is rresponsible for clinical effect.

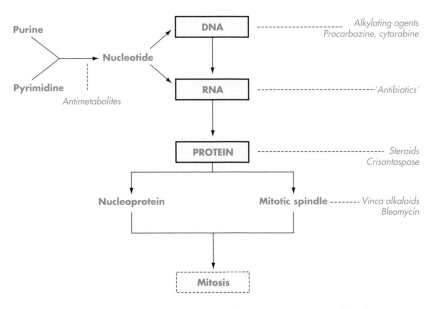

Figure 11.12   Sites of action of some cytotoxic drugs on biochemical pathways of cell cycle.

Table 11.17   Cytokinetic classification of cytotoxic drugs

Phases in which active	Class	Examples
Resting (G₀) plus all cycling cells	Non-specific (Class I)	*Chlormethine (mustine)*
Cycling cells only	Cycle-specific (Class III)	*Alkylating agents*
• all phases		*Anthracyclines*
		Fluorouracil
		Corticosteroids (possibly)
• certain phases only	Phase-specific (Class II)	*Vinca alkaloids*
		Podophyllin derivatives
		Antimetabolites
		Cytarabine
		Hydroxycarbamide (hydroxyurea)
		Procarbazine
		Crisantaspase

Note on common synonyms: phase-specific = 'cell cycle stage-specific' (CCSS); cycle-specific = 'cell cycle stage non-specific' (CCSNS).

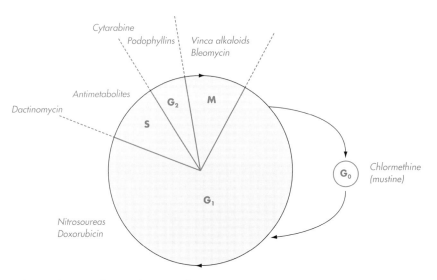

Figure 11.13   Phases of action of some phase-specific cytotoxic agents.

approach is limited by the fact that resting marrow stem cells are also recruited and may eventually be similarly depleted or even eliminated. In another approach, oestrogens can be used to recruit breast cancer stem cells in partial synchrony; these are then attacked with a cytotoxic combination.

Although some success has been reported with techniques such as these, e.g. in leukaemia, the difficulty of ascertaining the detailed cytokinetics of tumour cells in particular patients limits

their application at present. However, experiments in following DNA production through the cell cycle by labelling it with precursor analogues (e.g. *bromodeoxyuridine*) which can be detected by monoclonal antibodies ('flow cytometry') may eventually make this practicable.

Differences in dose–response and toxicity
Unfortunately, the cytokinetic classification of drugs given above is an oversimplification. Some phase-specific drugs are found to act at more

than one phase, and some cycle-specific agents act predominantly at one or two phases only. A distinction of more practical use between the two main classes (II and III) is made on the basis of their dose–response curves; this also helps ensure their correct use. Although both classes need to achieve a minimum threshold plasma level, the consequences of further dose increases vary according to the class.

Phase-specific drugs (Class II).   Both the therapeutic effect, i.e. the tumour cell kill, and the toxicity, i.e. the marrow cell kill, of this class depend mainly the duration of therapy, i.e. they are 'schedule dependent'. This is because the dose–response curve rapidly approaches a plateau as all cells in the affected phase are killed by a single dose (Fig. 11.14). Continued therapy would then kill cells that had initially been at other phases as they come round to the affected phase. As a result, more cells are recruited from the resting compartment. This process can be exploited to maximize cell kill. However, therapy prolonged beyond one or two neutrophil stem cell cycle times (i.e. 24–36 h) may prove disastrous as it will deplete the bone marrow stem cell reserve. This is the main constraint when class II drugs are used either alone or in combination. On the other hand, a single very large dose will not be dangerous because the plateau will already have been reached and no further damage, even to the bone marrow, will be possible.

Cycle-specific drugs (Class III).   Because these drugs act on all phases, their dose–response curve does not plateau: it is exponential for both tumour and bone marrow (Fig. 11.14). Hence, both effectiveness and toxicity are 'dose-dependent', and optimal tumour cell kill is achieved with a single high dose. There is no need to prolong treatment to wait for cells to come round the cycle. However, too high a dose of this class of drug causes excessive myelosuppression. Moreover, if two members of this class are combined the effects will be additive and the toxicity increased, so the doses of each must be reduced.

Non-specific drugs (Class I).   With this class of drugs there is very little difference between the effects on bone marrow and on tumour cells (Fig. 11.14). Thus, they are potentially very toxic and not used unless absolutely necessary.

Resistance

Development of resistance

Although the lack of biochemical specificity is one major problem with chemotherapy, the development of resistance, i.e. an unusually low tumour responsiveness, is equally important. Theoretically, as long as the tumour remains sensitive, suitable adjustment of dosage should preserve marrow function. However, once resistance develops, the chances of a cure diminish rapidly

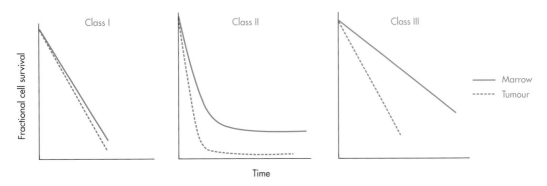

Figure 11.14   Dose-response curves for different cytokinetic classes. Class I drugs (non-specific) show little selectivity for tumour cells and so have a relatively high marrow toxicity. Class II drugs (phase-specific) have non-linear dose-response and dose-toxicity curves, so doses above the minimum effective level are not useful, but prolonged therapy will be. For Class III (cycle-specific) drugs, very high doses may be tolerated, but need not be repeated.

and when the tumour becomes multi-resistant (i.e. to a variety of drugs) then the therapeutic options become very limited (Fig. 11.15).

Unless all tumour cells are killed, resistance will almost invariably develop eventually. Consequently, treatment should be aimed at prompt eradication by early detection and aggressive therapy. Treatment within the 'therapeutic window' before the development of resistance has the best chance of success (Fig. 11.16).

Causes of resistance

In general, resistance is due either to extracellular circumstances that limit drug access to the tumour, or to intracellular pharmacological or biochemical factors that antagonize cytotoxic action (Table 11.18); the latter situation resembles antimicrobial resistance. One of the main aims in devising drug regimens is to prevent or circumvent resistance. Recent studies on the *p53* gene have suggested that treatment resistance may in some cases be associated with defects in this gene, possibly because cytotoxic drug-induced apoptosis is prevented.

Extracellular resistance
Inappropriate dose scheduling or unwanted interactions may result if cytokinetic factors are not taken into account. For example, a methotrexate/crisantaspase (asparaginase) combination is of reduced efficacy because the former arrests cells at the G_1–S boundary, preventing the action of the latter in the S phase. (This is analogous to the antagonism of bactericidal antimicrobials by bacteriostatic ones.) Dose spacing which ignores cell cycle times may also be of reduced effectiveness.

Poor tumour perfusion owing to inadequate vascularization is probably one of the main causes for the resistance of solid tumours to chemotherapy. Poor drug distribution or penetration to micrometastases within **sanctuaries**, e.g. in the brain owing to the blood–brain barrier, also account for some treatment failures. Many of these factors can be minimized by attention to pharmaceutical, pharmacokinetic and cytokinetic aspects of the treatment regimen, e.g. giving a drug intrathecally as 'CNS prophylaxis' in leukaemia if it does not cross the blood–brain barrier.

Intracellular resistance
Neoplastic cells demonstrate a remarkable ability to develop protective mechanisms against cytotoxic drugs. This is one of their few differences from normal proliferating cells: unfortunately, bone marrow cells generally do not become resistant. In some cases cells are intrinsically resistant from the outset. Otherwise, resistance develops as a result either of the increased somatic mutation rate associated with rapid turnover or of adaptive changes in metabolism. Most cytotoxic

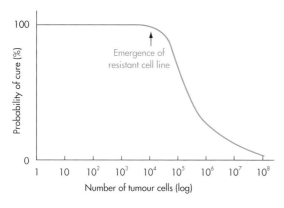

Figure 11.15 Potential survival in relation to tumour cell number. The figure illustrates how the chances of survival fall rapidly once drug-resistant cells have emerged in a typical (hypothetical) tumour.

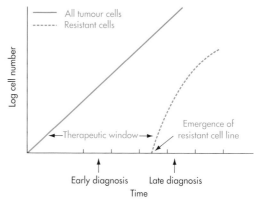

Figure 11.16 'Therapeutic window' before resistance develops. In most primary tumours there will at first be no resistant cells and early diagnosis and treatment during this phase has the greatest chance of effecting a cure. At some stage, resistant cells emerge and if diagnosis is late there will already be a significant population of resistant cells, dramatically reducing the chances of successful therapy.

Table 11.18   Possible causes of resistance to cytotoxic chemotherapy

Extracellular factors	Drug interaction
	Incorrect/inappropriate dosage schedule
	Immune clearance of antigenic drugs
	Poor access to tumour; sanctuaries
	Poor penetration of tumour
	Low tumour growth fraction, large G_0 compartment
Intracellular biochemical factors	
Quantitative	Reduced cellular uptake
	Increased efflux pump activity
	Reduced pro-drug activation
	Increased activity in affected pathway
	Alternative pathway used (block bypassed)
	Increased receptor specificity
	Increased repair of DNA damage
Qualitative (? genetic)	Production of dummy or excess substrate
	Production of drug inhibitors
	Drug inactivation

drugs are also themselves mutagenic. One adaptation is to produce an excess of the drug's target molecule or a 'dummy' target, in effect mopping-up the drug. Chemotherapy exerts a selection pressure that favours the proliferation of resistant cells at the expense of the non-resistant cells, as with antibiotics.

The mechanisms adopted by the tumour cells are often quantitative rather than qualitative metabolic changes, i.e. an inhibited pathway may be avoided or an alternative up-regulated; this may be stimulated by negative or positive feedback. For example, normal DNA autorepair mechanisms may be accelerated to make good any damage. Alternatively, chance novel genetic changes may allow the production of specific inhibitors, antagonists or deactivating enzymes.

The principal therapeutic strategies adopted to prevent or overcome resistance are the use of combination therapy in adequate dosage and a prompt change to different drugs when resistance is suspected.

Multiple drug resistance

An individual cell is highly unlikely to develop multiple resistance by several discrete mutations, yet resistance to a range of structurally unrelated cytotoxic agents is quite common and an extremely serious constraint on chemotherapy. The recent discovery of a non-specific membrane efflux pump for toxins (p-glycoprotein or MDR protein) may provide a clue. This appears to efflux drugs such as etoposide, vincristine and the anthracyclines. The gene coding for this pump has been found in normal cells, and it is presumably expressed when protection is needed from environmental toxins. In multiresistant tumours it may be over-expressed. Certain membrane active drugs, such as the calcium channel blockers, ciclosporin (cyclosporine) and quinidine, appear to inhibit this pump and are being investigated as ways of antagonising multiple drug resistance.

Maintenance therapy and resistance

It is instructive to compare pulsed therapy (p. 648) with earlier approaches that were originally modelled on antimicrobial chemotherapy, this being the only model available for early oncologists to emulate. Tumours were then believed to differ from normal tissue exclusively by a more rapid turnover of all cells; at the same time, the toxicity of the cytotoxic agents was greatly feared. The strategy then was to attempt to achieve a 'minimum inhibitory concentration' with a single drug, i.e. a constant plasma level that caused minimal toxicity. This was maintained until symptoms disappeared or the tumour was no longer detectable.

We now know that such a regimen would merely keep the tumour at bay and the patient asymptomatic. Eventually, as with antimicrobial therapy, resistance developed (Fig. 11.17). A second drug was then used in the same way, and so on, until eventually all possibilities were exhausted and the patient succumbed. Nevertheless, there were a few successes, particularly with leukaemia. Such a strategy is still used for a few such tumours that are difficult to eradicate but rarely become resistant. This strategy is also used with schedule-dependent drugs (e.g. fluorouracil as continuous intravenous infusion in breast cancer), but only in combination with other drugs to limit resistance.

Side effects

The high incidence of severe adverse effects is another important limitation to the success of cytotoxic chemotherapy.

Classification

Side effects can be considered in three main groups (Table 11.19). Almost all agents cause a similar range of cytotoxic and mutagenic effects as a direct result of their intended pharmcodynamic action, i.e. impaired cell division. However, the intensity and rate of onset vary between drugs: some are known to be potent myelosuppressants, others frequently cause hair loss, and so on. The third group comprises the specific idiosyncratic adverse actions of individual drugs. Examples of the clinical consequences of these toxicities are summarized in Table 11.20 and ways of minimizing them on pp. 659–661.

Cytotoxic action

Myelosuppression. Although bone marrow has a smaller growth fraction than most tumours, the intermitotic times of cycling marrow stem cells are usually much shorter. Thus, the marrow is extremely chemosensitive and almost all cytotoxics affect it to some extent. There are two general patterns. Most drugs cause rapid falls in peripheral blood count with a nadir for white cells and platelets at 7 days. A few, however, have a more profound but delayed action, with a nadir at 28 days, e.g. *nitrosoureas, melphalan*. There is also a variation in the intensity of the myelosuppression: e.g. *chlormethine* (*mustine*) almost always produces profound falls, *vincristine* has rela-

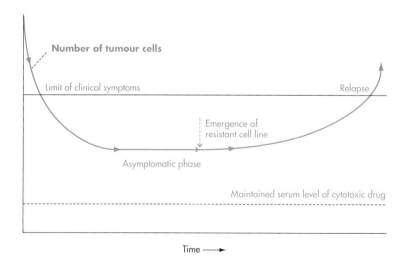

Time ⟶

Figure 11.17 Maintenance therapy and resistance. This illustrates the possible effect of maintaining a single cytotoxic drug continuously at a level sub-lethal to tumour cells. Initially the tumour responds, and symptoms disappear, but resistance eventually develops.

Table 11.19 Side effects of cytotoxics

Cytotoxic action – killing of normal dividing cells

Myelosuppression
Epithelial damage
- gastrointestinal tract
- urinary bladder
- skin and hair
Infertility
Teratogenicity

Mutagenic action – effects of DNA damage

Genetic damage
Carcinogenesis

Miscellaneous

General (many or most cytotoxic drugs)
- emesis
- extravasation
- dangers of handling (preparation, reconstitution)
Specific to particular drugs
Organ systems: e.g. heart, liver, kidney, lungs, bladder, etc.

tively little effect and *bleomycin* (uniquely) almost none.

Leucopenia (reduced white cell count, especially neutrophils) results in immunosuppression and frequent infections, and these are often due to the presence of unusual organisms, e.g. fungi or protozoa. Leucopenia exacerbates the underlying immunodeficiency found in most cancer patients. Thrombocytopenia (reduced platelet count) impairs coagulation, leading to bruising and bleeds, a particular problem as many of these drugs also ulcerate the gastrointestinal tract. Courses are usually too short to produce significant anaemia.

Gastrointestinal tract and bladder. The intermitotic time in gut epithelial cells is not much greater than in bone marrow. Thus, erosion and ulceration are very common, especially in mucous membranes, causing e.g. mouth ulcers or diarrhoea. Certain drugs similarly affect the bladder epithelium, causing haematuria. Although usually less serious than myelosuppression, such symptoms may be more disturbing for the patient.

Table 11.20 Side effects of cytotoxic drugs and their clinical consequences

Organ/system affected	Clinical effect		Examples[a]
Bone marrow	Immunosuppression Bleeding Anaemia		Almost all[b]
Chemoreceptor trigger zone	Nausea and vomiting[c]	• mild	*Fluorouracil, methotrexate*
		• moderate	*Doxorubicin*
		• severe	*Cisplatin, dacarbazine*
GI tract	Mucositis; ulceration; diarrhoea		Many
Metabolic	Hyperuricaemia; gout; nephropathy		Many
Nervous system	Neuropathy – cranial, autonomic, peripheral		*Vincristine*
Heart	Cardiomyopathy		*Doxorubicin*
Liver	Cirrhosis, fibrosis		*Methotrexate*
Kidney	Nephrotoxicity		*Cisplatin*
Bladder	Haemorrhagic cystitis		*Ifosfamide*
Lungs	Pulmonary fibrosis		*Bleomycin*
Hair follicles	Alopecia		*Doxorubicin*

[a] Only limited representative examples given here; *see* References and further reading.

[b] A few agents have mild or almost absent myelosuppression, especially *bleomycin, vincristine*.

[c] Occurs to some extent with most cytotoxic drugs.

GI, gastrointestinal.

The most common gastrointestinal effects, nausea and vomiting, are not the result of direct cytotoxic action (see below).

Skin and hair. The intermitotic time of skin basal layer cells is about 20 days, and so considerably greater than that of marrow; thus serious problems are rare. However, hair loss is quite common and although reversible it is one of the most distressing medium-term complications, especially for women. Regrowth of hair is usually complete once treatment has finished, but the new hair is often subtly different in texture or colour.

Fertility. Spermatogenesis is inhibited and sometimes there may be permanent male infertility, e.g. from the alkylating agents. Female infertility is less common.

Teratogenic action. Cytotoxics are particularly hazardous during the first trimester of pregnancy, i.e. during organogenesis, and the risk seems to be greatest for methotrexate and the alkylating agents. There may be spontaneous abortion, prematurity, gross deformity or delayed growth. The absolute risk is surprisingly low, but strict contraceptive precautions are advisable if chemotherapy is planned.

Mutagenesis

Most cytotoxic agents act by damaging DNA, and the effect of the resultant change in the genome depends on whether somatic or germ cells are affected.

Genetic damage. Heritable defects may be caused if the DNA of spermatozoa or ova is damaged, although most mutations are lethal for the cell. Even exposure *in utero* may affect germ cells, only to be manifested in the subsequent generation. These risks have yet to be fully assessed but are avoided by contraception during treatment.

Carcinogenesis. Cytotoxic drugs are one of the many groups of potentially carcinogenic mutagens. Thus cells may, paradoxically, undergo neoplastic transformation by anti-cancer therapy. Radiotherapy, which likewise damages DNA, has also been associated with an increased incidence of neoplasms; e.g. up to 2%

of ankylosing spondylosis patients treated with X-rays may develop a neoplasm. The long lag time between carcinogenic exposure, mutation and the clinical manifestation of a tumour, and the rather poor prognosis of cancer generally, means that these effects may have been obscured in the past.

Patients on long-term immunosuppressive therapy similarly have a small increased risk of neoplasms, e.g. lymphomas in post-transplant patients treated with *ciclosporin* (*cyclosporine*). This suggests that another possible mechanism for cytotoxic-induced neoplasia is impaired immunosurveillance. Nevertheless, the risk seems to be small. Confirmed cases are few, e.g. second malignancy associated with *etoposide*, and there is currently no alternative to treating the first tumour as effectively as possible. Patients who achieve long-term survival after successful chemotherapy, e.g. following childhood leukaemia, need careful continuous monitoring for subsequent tumour development that is unrelated to the original disease.

Miscellaneous

Nausea and vomiting. The common occurrence of profound nausea, retching and vomiting is what many patients most fear and loathe about chemotherapy. The effects may last for several days after treatment, and are depressing and debilitating, and may even prevent some patients continuing with therapy. The symptoms originate partly from direct stimulation of the chemoreceptor trigger zone (CTZ), which understandably identifies these agents as highly dangerous and rejects them. However, so feared are these effects that 'anticipatory vomiting' before the next treatment is experienced by some patients, so higher brain centres might be involved. There is also probably a local reaction to the damaging effect of cytotoxics on the gastrointestinal epithelium, mediated by 5HT which stimulates the CTZ humorally and via nerve endings in the gut.

Other effects. Each drug or group of drugs has its own characteristic adverse effects on major organ systems. Some important examples are given in Table 11.20. A knowledge of these effects is essential in designing cytotoxic combination therapy, to ensure that no one organ system is overexposed to toxicity.

Secondary hyperuricaemia can occur when the large number of cells killed during treatment release nucleic acid bases that are then degraded to produce an excess of uric acid. This can cause hyperuricaemia, gout and uric acid nephropathy, and is most common in the treatment of lymphomas and leukaemias. Treatment of bone tumours (usually metastatic deposits) may release the large amounts of calcium, causing hypercalcaemia.

Cytotoxic solutions require great care in handling by health workers as they are highly irritant as well as mutagenic. Nowadays they are usually reconstituted centrally in hospital pharmacy departments under strict precautions similar to aseptic technique. For similar reasons, serious local damage to the patient may occur with many cytotoxics if the injection becomes extravasated during administration.

Minimizing side effects

Numerous strategies have been devised to reduce the damage done to normal tissues by cytotoxic drugs (Table 11.21). The aims are either to reduce discomfort, morbidity and mortality or to increase the tolerable dose threshold and thus the dose that can be used. Close monitoring is extremely important, and especially frequent full blood counts. Other investigations will depend on the known particular toxicities of the drugs used, e.g. ECG, neurological or liver function tests, biopsy, etc.

Table 11.21   Strategies for minimizing side effects of chemotherapy

Side effect	Method of minimization	Example
Myelosuppression	Transfusions	Blood platelets
		Granulocytes
		Autologous blood/marrow
		(patient's own)
	Growth factors	*Filgrastim*
	Timing of doses; careful monitoring	
	Isolation in sterile environment	
Nausea and vomiting	Anti-emetics • dopamine antagonists	*Prochlorperazine, metoclopramide,*
	• $5HT_3$ antagonists	*Ondansetron*
	• benzodiazepines	*Lorazepam*
	• corticosteroids	*Dexamethasone*
	• cannabinoids	*Nabilone*
	Hypnosis; suggestion; relaxation therapy	
Mucositis; mouth ulcers	Oral hygiene	Mouthwashes
Subfertility	Sperm banking; in-vitro fertilization	
Hyperuricaemia		*Allopurinol*, hydration
Hypercalcaemia		*Furosemide* (*frusemide*), hydration
Cardiomyopathy	ECG monitoring; cardiac glycosides?	
Hepatotoxicity	Liver function tests (pre and post)	
Anti-folate overdose	(For *methotrexate*)	*Folinic acid* rescue[a]
Nephrotoxicity	Hydration and forced diuresis	
Haemorrhagic cystitis	Hydration and forced diuresis	
	(For *ifosfamide* and *cyclophosphamide*)	*Mesna*[b]
Alopecia	Scalp tourniquet or chilling; wigs	

[a] Bypasses the folic acid synthesis block.

[b] Eliminates bladder-irritant toxic metabolites (see text).

Prevention

Unfortunately, **myelosuppression** can rarely be avoided but is minimized by allowing adequate time for marrow recovery between treatments. Stem cell growth factors, e.g. granulocyte colony stimulating factor (G-CSF, *filgrastim*), given with chemotherapy selectively to enhance marrow proliferation, are starting to be exploited. The possibility of these agents stimulating tumour cells that possess growth factor receptors is being carefully monitored. One technique under investigation is to exploit a naturally occurring, marrow-specific stem cell inhibitor (SCI) to inhibit temporarily marrow cell division during treatment. *Lithium*, which has the usually undesired adverse effect of neutrophilia, has also been tried in this respect.

Forced diuresis is now routinely given with nephrotoxic and bladder-toxic drugs to reduce contact time and urine concentration. This involves modest over-hydration before therapy followed by a diuretic to maintain a high urine output for at least 24 h following therapy. An osmotic diuretic (e.g. *mannitol*) is preferable to loop diuretics, which are frequently nephrotoxic (e.g. *furosemide (frusemide)*). The haemorrhagic cystitis caused by *cyclophosphamide* and *ifosfamide* is due to the metabolite acrolein, which can be rendered harmless by complexation with *mesna* given concurrently.

No universally effective **anti-emetic** regimen has been devised (Table 11.21; *see also* Chapter 6, p. 334). Some patients seem to benefit more than others, and the emetogenic potential of cytotoxic drugs varies. Delayed reactions are especially difficult to prevent and treat. Dopamine antagonists act both centrally and on the CTZ, and high-dose parenteral *metoclopramide* is preferred to the phenothiazines, being less toxic. Metoclopramide is used prophylactically, often combined with a benzodiazepine or a corticosteroid, or both. Benzodiazepines cause both sedation and amnesia, which tends to minimize anticipatory vomiting, and steroids have a euphoriant effect. *Domperidone* is a dopamine antagonist which does not cross the blood–brain barrier; it can be combined with phenothiazines without producing excessive sedation or extrapyramidal symptoms. *Cannabinoids* have not lived up to their early promise.

The discovery that high-dose metoclopramide probably acts partly by antagonising 5HT receptors in the gut and the CTZ has led to a significant advance in the development of specific $5HT_3$ antagonists, that are free from extrapyramidal effects. This group is currently the most effective available and their efficacy is enhanced by combination with corticosteroids.

Remedy or palliation

Transfusions may be the only remedy for patients who react unexpectedly severely to myelosuppression. Autologous blood transfusion is being increasingly performed, using the patient's own blood, which is harvested before the start of treatment. Patients who are severely neutropenic, thrombocytopenic or anaemic may be given cell-specific infusions. The short half-life of neutrophils limits their value in this form, but packed platelets and packed red blood cells are used routinely.

Despite its theoretical advantages, autologous bone marrow replacement in which the patient's marrow is harvested before therapy is still restricted to specialist centres. Ingenious ways have been devised to treat the stored marrow before re-injection, to eradicate contaminating neoplastic cells, especially in leukaemias or lymphomas. For example, monoclonal antibodies to receptors expressed on normal immune cells but not neoplastic ones can be used to facilitate their separation. The technique is gradually gaining acceptance, but has not yet reached routine practice. More recently autologous peripheral stem cell replacement is being exploited, utilizing the finding that significant numbers of marrow stem cells are normally found in blood. This procedure is obviously simpler and engraftment is quicker. Heterologous bone marrow transplants are mainly used in the treatment of leukaemia but may be also used to treat iatrogenic myelosuppression.

Infections in the profoundly immunosuppressed (e.g. after bone marrow transplantation) can be prevented by reverse barrier nursing in sterile conditions. Pharmaceutically, this means that clean precautions have to be observed and original packs used for all drugs.

The use of folinic acid permits the administration of massive doses of methotrexate, subsequently 'rescuing' the patient's marrow (and other tissues) after an appropriate time when a maximal differential neoplastic cell kill has been achieved. In a more general application of the same principle, patients with resistant or widely disseminated disease may be given massive dose chemotherapy, which would normally be fatal owing to myelosuppression, but are subsequently rescued by colony stimulating factors promoting the renewed stem cell activity. This is obviously a high-risk strategy that is only justifiable in certain cases.

For some patients, iatrogenic diarrhoea is antagonized by the opiate analgesics they are taking for pain control.

Other forms of therapy

Endocrine therapy

The growth of certain tissues, especially the sex organs, is hormone-dependent. By manipulating hormone levels the growth of tumours derived from such organs can be reduced, provided that they are still sufficiently differentiated to respond, i.e. they retain hormone receptors.

The effect is to suppress further growth rather than kill cells (analogous to a bacteriostatic antimicrobial drug as opposed to a bactericidal one; *see* Chapter 13.) Thus, although endocrine therapy can never be curative it can provide valuable remissions or can be combined with other treatments to improve their effectiveness. It may also enable cytotoxic therapy to be avoided or delayed in slowly growing tumours. Further, because metastases usually, but not always, have a similar sensitivity to the primary tumour, this treatment can also be used for disseminated, inoperable disease or to delay the development of secondaries following resolution of a primary tumour.

Originally, either the gland secreting the hormone was removed (e.g. the ovaries [oophorectomy]) or else a hormone with a naturally antagonistic action was administered (e.g. androgens to women). More recently, specific synthetic antagonists have been developed (Table 11.22). Most therapy is based on normal endocrine actions but some is partly empirical. This is especially so in breast cancer and is also evident in the widespread use of corticosteroids.

Table 11.22   Hormone manipulation to influence tumour growth

Strategy	Target hormone	Drugs	Tumour
Block synthesis	Steroid	*Aminoglutethimide, anastrozole, letrozole*	Breast
Block secretion	Androgens	Surgery – orchidectomy	Prostate
	Oestrogens	Surgery – oophorectomy	Breast, uterus
	Steroids	Surgery – adrenalectomy	Breast
	Pituitary hormones	Surgery – hypophysectomy	Breast
		High-dose corticosteroid	Various
	Prolactin	*Bromocriptine*	Breast
	Luteinizing hormone	Gonodotrophin releasing hormone analogue – *goserelin, buserelin*	Prostate, breast
	Thyrotrophin	*Levothyroxine* (*thyroxine*)	Thyroid
Block receptor	Anti-androgens	*Cyproterone, flutamide*	Prostate
	Anti-oestrogen	*Tamoxifen*	Breast
Physiological antagonism	Androgens	*Testosterone*	Breast
	Oestrogens	*Diethylstilbestrol*	Prostate, breast[a]
	Progestogens	*Medroxyprogesterone*	Uterus, breast[a]

[a] Primarily postmenopausal women.

These findings suggest that our knowledge of normal hormonal mechanisms is inadequate.

Thyroid cancer

High-dose levothyroxine (thyroxine) has a dual role in patients with disseminated disease for whom thyroidectomy has proved inadequate. It serves as replacement therapy and also inhibits pituitary secretion of thyroid stimulating hormone, which may otherwise promote metastatic growth.

Prostatic cancer

In advanced disease prostatectomy is of limited value. The surgical techniques originally used to reduce androgen output included orchidectomy (castration), adrenalectomy or hypophysectomy (excision of the anterior pituitary) with predictable serious adverse endocrinological and psychological consequences.

Nowadays, 'chemical castration' with progestogens (e.g. *medroxyprogesterone*), anti-androgens (e.g. *cyproterone*, *flutamide*) or, more rarely, oestrogens (e.g. *diethylstilbestrol*) is attempted first. Subsequently, steroid synthesis inhibitors (e.g. *aminoglutethimide*) can be used. Exogenous corticosteroid therapy is then also needed, to prevent reflex ACTH hypersecretion from overcoming the block and to provide the additional advantage of maintenance corticosteroid replacement. Anti-oestrogens (e.g. tamoxifen) have also sometimes been successful. Analogues of gonadotrophin releasing hormone such as *goserelin* and *buserelin* (Table 11.22) have a paradoxical long-term depressant effect on natural luteinizing hormone release, and thus inhibit prostatic growth.

Uterine (endometrial) cancer

Progestogens are used on the assumption that an imbalance between oestrogen and progestogen stimulation, with an excess of the former, may promote endometrial hyperplasia. This has led to some success with metastatic disease.

Breast cancer

Increasing research effort is being directed to finding causes and satisfactory treatments for this, the most common female tumour and the second most common overall cause of cancer death. The reader is referred to the References and further reading section for details.

Nearly every mode of endocrine therapy imaginable has been tried, including both oestrogens and anti-oestrogens (Table 11.22). Treatment is usually given as adjuvant therapy following lumpectomy and/or radiation. The trend is, as with prostatic cancer, first to use chemical rather than surgical techniques (neo-adjuvant). Nevertheless, radical surgery, e.g. oophorectomy, adrenalectomy or hypophysectomy, is still used in the last resort.

Some idea of the complexity of the problem with breast cancer is seen by considering that oestrogens may induce breast cancer in premenopausal women but inhibit it in the postmenopausal: yet the anti-oestrogen and steroid synthesis inhibitors are most successful in the latter group. The explanation lies partly in the fact that after the menopause the adrenals and other tissues still synthesize small amounts of oestrogen so that tamoxifen, aromatase inhibitors or adrenalectomy are still used. Furthermore, in some cases, when a particular hormone therapy stops being successful, withdrawing it will continue the positive response.

Undoubtedly the most useful recent advance has been the discovery of the importance of oestrogen receptors (ER) in tumour tissue. Found in about 60% of cases (ER+), the presence of these receptors favourably predicts both response to endocrine therapy and prognosis, possibly because such tumour cells are not too regressed. Thus, hormone modulation should be considered in all ER+ patients. Other criteria that determine the suitability and likely success of endocrine therapy include age, menstrual status and the stage of the tumour: endocrine therapy is most successful in early, localized tumours but may also be helpful as palliative treatment in advanced cases.

Promising results have been reported recently from a US trial of tamoxifen for breast cancer prophylaxis in high-risk women (e.g. older age, family history, etc.), although the early cessation of this trial because of its apparent success has been felt in the UK to have prejudiced its overall power.

Corticosteroid therapy

Steroids are used in a wide variety of cytotoxic and endocrine regimens. In addition to useful endocrine activity, they have beneficial effects on some complications and some direct anti-tumour action (Table 11.23). Usually, very high doses are needed but often only for a short time, so that adverse effects are limited.

Biological therapies: immunotherapy and gene therapy

Neoplastic transformation almost certainly involves genetic changes. This change in the genotype, as well as being directly responsible for the changes in growth pattern, in turn may cause tumour cells to differ immunologically from normal cells. For example, they may express non-self surface antigens or fail to express self-antigens. Indeed, many potential tumours may normally be aborted by immune mechanisms for this reason (p. 626). This suggests a variety of possible therapeutic approaches (Table 11.24). The immune system could be manipulated, either by actively stimulating it or by using immunoactive substances such as antibodies or immune cells specific for tumour cells (passive immunization). More fundamentally, one could attempt to change the genes involved in the neoplastic process.

Other approaches being tried include inhibiting angiogenesis in tumours, which will inhibit the tumour's growth rather than kill it, and interfering with signal transduction and second messengers (e.g. protein kinases) following gene expression.

Biological therapies offer a very promising line of approach because of the possibility of the holy grail of cancer therapy – selectivity. Few are yet in general use, but all are being vigorously investigated. One recalls admiringly George Bernard Shaw's prophetic exhortation (in a related context): "stimulate the phagocytes".

Immunotherapy

Attempts to stimulate innate active immunity have long been tried (e.g. Bacillus Calmette-Guérin (BCG) vaccine in leukaemia or bladder cancer, *Corynebacterium* in pleural effusions) but are generally unsuccessful. The popularity of the 'immunostimulant' *levamisole* has waxed and waned. A wide variety of natural immunological mediators, usually **cytokines** (lymphokines) are being investigated. The initial over-enthusiasm for *interferon* has generally been disappointed, although it is now used successfully in a small number of tumours, e.g. AIDS-related Kaposi's sarcoma, hairy cell leukaemia. As well as augmenting T and B cell activity, interferons can inhibit cell division and differentiation.

Interleukin-2 (IL-2), a cytokine produced by T-helper cells, generally enhances T cell and natural killer cell activity against tumour cells. IL-2 has been successful particularly in malignant melanoma and renal cell carcinoma. Most adverse effects are mild, e.g. flu-like symptoms, but occasional hypovolaemia caused by widespread

---

Table 11.23   Uses of corticosteroids in cancer therapy

Anti-inflammatory	Symptomatic relief
Euphoriant	Symptomatic relief
Appetite stimulant	
Enhance anti-emetic therapy	
Reduce hypercalcaemia	From bone secondaries
Inhibit secretion of pituitary hormones	GTH, ACTH
Depress DNA/protein synthesis	Antitumour (cytotoxic?) action
Depress haemopoietic cell activity	Antileukaemic action
Inhibit damage from peritumour oedema	e.g. CNS tumours/secondaries; gastrointestinal obstruction

ACTH, adrenocorticotrophic hormone; CNS, central nervous system; GTH, gonadotrophic hormone.

Table 11.24   Potential biological treatments for cancer

Method		Example
Immunotherapy		
Active	Non-specific immunostimulation	BCG
		Levamisole
		Interferon
		Interleukins
	Specific immunostimulation	Killed tumour cells
		Transfected tumour cells
Passive		Monoclonal antibodies
		Polyclonal antibodies
		Sensitized lymphoid cells
Gene therapy		
Immunotherapeutic agent production	Implant HLA gene	
or stimulation	Implant cytokine gene	Interleukin, tumour necrosis factor
Altering neoplastic genotype	Suppress or cancel oncogene	Antisense oligonucleotides
	Replace defective tumour suppressor gene	

BCG, Bacillus Calmette-Guérin.

capillary leakage can lead to acute prerenal failure, especially with IV use.

Yet another approach is to render tumour cells incapable of dividing, yet still capable of eliciting a host immune response. This is analogous to the preparation of antimicrobial vaccines using killed or modified organisms (active immunization). Irradiated leukaemic cells have been tried, but the lack of success possibly stems from the same reason as the growth of the tumour in the first place – an ineffective host immune response to tumour cells. A vaccine which activates a cell surface molecule on breast cancer cells, making them more susceptible to immune attack, is being developed.

A promising approach is to exploit **monoclonal antibodies** (equivalent to passive immunization). None has yet been found which specifically attacks one tumour cell line, but the prospects for their use in detection, monitoring and drug targeting are exciting.

Gene therapy

Cancer is among the first areas of application of this rapidly developing technology, both in facilitating immunotherapy and in changing the neoplastic genome. Cells are being experimentally implanted with a variety of different genes, based on the observation that neoplastic cells may have escaped immunosurveillance because mutation has prevented them from expressing histocompatibility (HLA) antigens. Some tumour cells are implanted (transfected) with appropriate HLA gene sequences and then injected into the patient, to enable a specific immune response to be mounted against the tumour. Alternatively, genes for cytokines such as interleukins and tumour necrosis factor may be implanted. This shortcuts the process whereby HLA normally signals helper T lymphocytes to recruit cytotoxic lymphocytes by secreting such lymphokines.

More direct genetic manipulation involves either inserting normal tumour suppressor genes or disabling the oncogene responsible for the tumour. One technique undergoing development for the latter purpose is to use *antisense oligonucleotides*. Nucleotide sequences are synthesized which mirror and thus bind specifically to oncogene sequences in DNA known to be expressed in certain tumours. In this way they can prevent transcription and thus synthesis of the carcinogenic gene product. This technique could also be exploited to block p-glycoprotein synthesis by preventing expression of *MDR* gene, thus reducing drug resistance. An inversion of this is to transfect normal marrow stem cells *ex vivo* with *MDR* gene and re-implant in the patient, conferring on their bone marrow a degree of resistance to cytotoxic effects and thus reducing adverse effects.

An ingenious technique for drug delivery is being developed using gene therapy: the so-called 'suicide gene' or 'Trojan horse vector'. Certain tumours over-express specific abnormal gene products, e.g. alpha-fetoprotein in liver cancer. The promoters for some of these genes have been isolated and coupled to promoters for genes expressing enzymes that activate a cytotoxic drug. These enzymes are then preferentially activated in tumour cells. For example, if the enzyme cytosine deaminase is released intracellularly it converts the relatively non-toxic flucytosine, given at the same time, to fluorouracil, which then acts as a targeted antimetabolite.

Most of these therapies are still experimental. The main problem is not the identification or preparation of the genetic material itself, nor injection into a genome using retrovirus vectors. The difficulty, as with all gene therapy, is targeting: to be successful, the gene change should be produced in all the neoplastic cells and it is currently not feasible to identify all such cells and to deliver the new gene specifically to them. The potential toxicity of any vector used must also be considered.

Complementary medicine

Forms of alternative medicine which complement or enhance orthodox treatment or replace it when it has little to offer are now widely accepted by cancer care units. Diet, meditation, group therapy and support groups, 'visualization techniques' (where the patient imagines the tumour, for example, as a physical enemy to be combated) and many others, may all have a place. However, care must be taken to ensure that they do not raise falsely optimistic hopes or dissuade the patient from orthodox therapy which could offer a genuine chance of relief or recovery. Cancer patients are especially vulnerable to 'quack' medicine.

There is certainly an increasing acceptance that psychological factors can influence the outcome of cancer. Stress may increase the likelihood of relapse of breast cancer, but doubts remain about whether psychosocial intervention can significantly improve the chances of remission or cure of cancer in general.

Future developments

Some areas of development in cancer treatment include:

* **Chronotherapy.** There may be predictable diurnal variations in the response of tumours to cytotoxic drugs and the body's response to adverse effects. Efforts are being directed to exploiting this to maximize the former and minimize the latter by careful timing of therapy.
* **Photodynamic therapy.** This involves the use of a photosensitive agent that is selectively accumulated by tumour cells and which is converted to a toxic metabolite or free radical by light irradiation.
* **Prostaglandins.** These may be involved in carcinogenesis, possibly through the link with chronic inflammation (p. 626). Chronic aspirin intake has for some time been known to reduce the risk of colon cancer, and cyclo-oxygenase has been found to be over-expressed on breast cancer cells. A potential chemopreventative role for NSAIDs, especially cyclo-oxygenase-2-specific inhibitors, is being investigated.
* **Telomerase.** This is an enzyme found mainly in tumour cells which helps to maintain or repair the ends of chromosome (telomeres) after replication. Agents are being developed which bind to telomeres and inhibit the action of this enzyme, leading to cell death.
* **Tretinoin.** This is a vitamin A derivative with a novel mode of action in haematological malignancy. It appears to induce differentiation in undifferentiated malignant marrow cells, and is currently licensed for the induction of remission in promyelocytic leukaemia. Tretinoin still must be followed by conventional chemotherapy to maintain remission, but its use improves survival, especially in refractory cases.

Rational design of antineoplastic regimens

Many treatment regimens are still derived empirically from clinical experience. Nevertheless, the principles described above do provide a rational basis for designing new regimens, and an explanation for most established ones. The key points are:

• To combine agents with different modes of action.
• To choose agents that are individually effective in the tumour being treated.
• To space drugs to achieve optimum synchronization with the cell cycle.
• To use the maximum tolerable dose of each.
• To use the most effective means of drug delivery to the tumour.

Combinations

The advantages of combination therapy in cancer are similar to those when used in other diseases, especially antimicrobial chemotherapy, but are particularly important with drugs of such a low therapeutic index. Such combinations have additive or synergistic action, reduced toxicity from individual components because lower doses may be used, and a reduced likelihood of resistance.

Each agent in a combination must have demonstrated action alone against the target tumour, and the components should differ as much as possible in their mode of action. Thus they should have different biochemical actions,

come from different cytokinetic classes, act at different phases in the cell cycle, and have different toxicity profiles. The traditional 'MOPP' regimen for Hodgkin's lymphoma (Table 11.25) illustrates some of these principles.

Some combinations may even reduce toxicity, e.g. cytarabine protects against tioguanine (thioguanine) toxicity by preventing its incorporation into DNA, without blocking its therapeutic effect. Other combinations may be antagonistic, e.g. methotrexate and crisantaspase (asparaginase) are both effective individually in leukaemia, but not in combination. Possibly methotrexate, by arresting the cells at the G–S boundary, prevents the activity of crisantaspase (asparaginase) during the S phase.

Dose, scheduling and timing

Although most effective when given early, chemotherapy is still more commonly used as adjuvant therapy after surgery or radiotherapy to 'mop up' micrometastases. However, many oncologists now propose that it be used much earlier or even as sole therapy.

Opinion also varies on the benefits of timing the different components of a combination to take advantage of the different phases at which they act. Some synchronization could be achieved this way. Consider a methotrexate + mitomycin + semustine + vincristine regimen (*see* Fig. 11.13). Methotrexate will arrest the cells G_1–S boundary; then change to mitomycin (S–G_2 boundary), followed by semustine (G_2), then finally vincristine (M).

Table 11.25   MOPP regimen for Hodgkin's lymphoma

Drug	Mode of action	Kinetic class[a]	Main phase of action[b]	Main toxicity
Chlormethine (**M**ustine)	Alkylating agent	I	Several	Marrow
Oncovin[c]	Spindle inhibitor	II	M, S	Neuropathy
Procarbazine	Inhibit DNA synthesis?	II	G_1–S boundary	GI tract
Prednisolone	Steroid (see text)	III	S?	Cushingoid

[a] I, non-specific; II, phase-specific; III, cycle-specific.

[b] *See* Fig. 11.13.

[c] *Oncovin* is a proprietary name for vincristine.

GI, gastrointestinal

Experiments in mice have shown some theoretical justification for this approach, but in man attempts at synchronization have not been very successful. The detailed knowledge of the cell cycle times, needed to determine the intervals between each drug, is often lacking. It is necessary to give each drug long enough for all cells initially at different phases to come to the relevant phase, but this time will vary greatly, both between tumours and between patients.

The general principle of consistently high doses for the optimum time has been well established in a similar way to antimicrobial therapy. In an early experiment with leukaemic mice, a 16-day course of cytarabine given as a 240-mg bolus every 4 days produced no cure, whereas half that dose given as eight 15-mg injections throughout each fourth day produced a 100% cure. In the second regimen the drug plasma level was high enough for long enough so that all cycling cells reached the S phase and were exposed to it. Similarly, intermittent high-dose methotrexate produces better results in human acute leukaemia than continuous low-dose therapy.

Most regimens specify precise intervals. For example, a regimen recommended for lung cancer (Fig. 11.18) uses a 21-day cycle comprising a single bolus of cisplatin on day one, two doses of vincristine a week apart, also starting on day 1, and etoposide on days 3, 5 and 7.

Frequency and pulsing

It has already been shown that an interval of 2–4 weeks between courses of treatment is needed to allow normal marrow cell recovery (p. 648).

Clinical pharmacological factors

Pharmacokinetics

Cancer patients often have grossly disturbed metabolic functions with malnutrition and fluid imbalance (which affects plasma protein level and volume of distribution), and liver and renal impairment (affecting drug clearance). Some drugs, e.g. cyclophosphamide, require hepatic activation. Patients are also likely to be on several other drugs for complications or symptomatic treatment, so there is considerable potential for interactions.

Route of administration and distribution. Cytotoxic drugs are usually given intravenously as a bolus or continuous infusion. This provides predictable plasma levels, whereas oral absorption in cancer patients may be impaired. Moreover, cytotoxics are often poorly tolerated when given orally. Because the usual aim of chemotherapy is the eradication of systemic metastases, methods for selective local administration to a tumour to minimize systemic toxicity are not as useful as might at first be expected. Intra-arterial infusion with the intention of delivering high local drug concentrations into large poorly perfused solid tumours is rarely successful. It causes frequent injection site damage, requires cumbersome arrangements if infusion is to be continuous, and has limited action on metastases. Occasionally, intrathecal administration is used for hydrophilic drugs which do not cross the blood–brain barrier, e.g. methotrexate for potential CNS metastases in leukaemia.

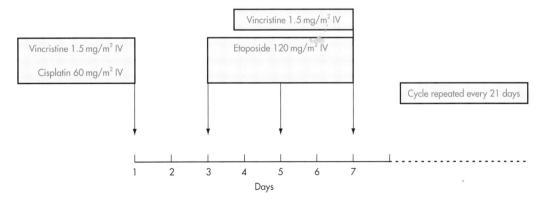

Figure 11.18   A treatment protocol for lung cancer.

Where malignant effusions are troublesome, e.g. in the pleural or abdominal cavities, intracavity instillation may be used palliatively, e.g. with bleomycin.

Clearance. The pharmacokinetics and cytokinetic class of the drugs used need to be considered when deciding dose and duration of therapy. For drugs with such a narrow chemotherapeutic index, which nevertheless need to achieve adequate levels to be effective, more than usual care is needed.

Targeting

Chemotherapy could be optimized if a pharmacological means could be found to limit the action specifically to tumour cells, wherever they were. An early and quite successful example of targeting was the use of *diethylstilbestrol diphosphate* in the endocrine therapy of prostatic cancer. This ester is an inactive pro-drug, allowing high doses which have minimal systemic feminizing effects. It is only activated by dephosphorylation within the tumour cells because they have higher concentrations of alkaline phosphatase than normal cells.

Targeting is potentially one of the most fruitful areas of research. For example, monoclonal antibodies, although they have proved disappointing alone, can be combined with potent toxins (e.g. ricin) or radioisotopes. By specifically locating tumour cells, they potentially allow a very selective toxicity. This promising technique is still under investigation. Another research idea exploits the fact that solid tumours often have large hypoxic areas, which are chemoresistant. By gene manipulation, hypoxia-dependent expression of enzymes that selectively activate cytotoxic pro-drugs in tumour cells only can be arranged.

Principles of chemotherapy: summary

A brief summary of the principles described in this section is given in Table 11.26.

Table 11.26 Principles of cancer chemotherapy

Decision	Principle	Rationale
Treat or not?	Decide realistic goal Assess risk against potential benefit	Prolong life, improve quality of life
When?	Early – when tumour load smallest	Minimize remaining cell number Minimizes resistance Still vascularized Least chance of metastasis
Which drugs?	Drugs with established activity Use effective combinations	Synergy Reduced toxicity and resistance
How much?	Use maximum tolerated doses	Exploit differential sensitivity (tumour/marrow) Reduce resistance
How long?	For short periods	Minimize marrow damage
How often?	Allow time for normal (marrow) cells to recover Repeat treatment as often as necessary or tolerable	Exploit differential recovery Proportional kill effect
What cautions?	Monitor blood counts closely Use appropriate strategies to minimize toxicity Use appropriate supportive therapy	Minimize bone marrow toxicity

References and further reading

Anonymous (1997) Oncology. *Lancet* **349** (Suppl. II):1–30.

Deely TJ, Parish PA (1984) *Cancer and Orthodox Cancer Treatment – a Book for Pharmacists.* Cardiff: Tenovus Cancer Information Centre.

Hancock BW, Bradshaw JD (1990) *Lecture Notes on Clinical Oncology.* 2nd edn. Oxford: Blackwell.

Latchman DS (1997) *Basic Molecular and Cell biology.* 3rd edn. London: BMJ Publishing Group.

Preistman TJ (1989) *Cancer Chemotherapy: An Introduction.* 3rd edn. Berlin: Springer-Verlag.

Price LA, Hill BT, Ghilchik MW, eds (1981) *Safer Cancer Chemotherapy.* London: Bailliere Tindall.

Symington T, Carter RL, eds (1976) *Scientific Foundations of Oncology.* London: Heinemann.

Taussig MJ (1995) *Processes in Pathology and Microbiology.* 3rd edn. Oxford: Blackwell.

Williams C (1989) *Cancer Biology and Management: An Introduction.* Chichester: John Wiley.

12

Skin diseases

The skin is the largest single organ of the body, with an area of about 1.65–1.85 m^2 for an average adult. Because the skin is visible and accessible and gives the first impression from which we judge people, patients are self-conscious about any perceived abnormality. They may expect faster, easier cure of a superficial lesion than an invisible, internal one. The unique skin symptom, itch, can lead to sleep loss and irritability if severe, and can cause emotional problems if associated with a visible, possibly disfiguring lesion.

Dermatological problems comprise about 10% of a general practitioner's case load, and probably more for pharmacists. Diagnosis and treatment leave much to be desired and pharmacists need to learn to diagnose and advise patients confidently. This requires experience. Further, the incidence of atopic dermatitis and skin malignancies has doubled over the past 20 to 30 years: these conditions need to be recognized early.

This chapter deals primarily with eczema and dermatitis, psoriasis, acne, rosacea and urticaria, which comprise most of the dermatological case load. It discusses the general features and management of skin diseases and some special drug classes (corticosteroids, retinoids), and concludes with brief discussions of drug side effects and of transdermal absorption, an important, developing drug delivery system.

There are 16 full colour plates (between pages 684 and 685) to aid diagnosis. Readers are strongly advised to consult one of the specialist books listed in the References and further reading.

Skin anatomy and physiology

Functions

The skin has five principal functions:

- To protect the underlying organs from physical, chemical and mechanical injury.
- To control fluid loss from the body (the skin contains nearly 20% of the total body water).
- To assist in controlling the body temperature by sweating and radiation from the surface.
- To act as an important sensory organ for touch, pain and external temperature.
- To be an organ of emotional expression, as it exhibits feelings by its colour, e.g. flushing, blanching, sweat and odour production.

Anatomy

There skin consists of three principal layers (Fig. 12.1): the epidermis, the dermis and the subcutaneous tissues.

Epidermis

This is the main protective layer of the skin, and therefore of the entire body.

Structure

The epidermis itself is composed of four fundamental layers (Fig. 12.1), most of which (95%) are derived from the **keratinocytes**. These comprise:

- The **basal (germinal) layer**, the deepest part, normally consists of a single sheet of cycling stem cells, most of which divide progressively and mature to form the other three layers of the epidermis. There is a small proportion of resting stem cells which can be recruited into growth to repair damage. The basal cells are joined by intercellular bridges which distribute mechanical stresses more evenly through the skin.
- The **prickle cell layer**, composed of cells also joined by intercellular bridges, is just above the basal layer and contains cells in intermediate stages of development into the **granular layer**. The prickle cell layer also contains Langerhans cells, which are immunologically important dendritic cells that express class 2

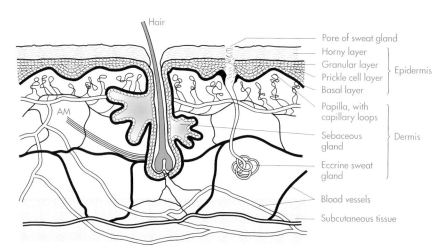

Figure 12.1 The anatomy of the skin. The arrector pili muscle (AM) is shown pulling the hair into the erect position, a reaction to fright or cold: this produces 'gooseflesh' in less hairy areas.

MHC antigens, have receptors for complement (*see* Chapter 2), and are antigen-presenting cells.

- The granular layer comprises a few rows of cells containing granules derived from degenerating nuclei. These cells gradually migrate towards the surface and finally form the outermost **horny layer**.
- This horny layer (**stratum corneum**) consists of keratinized, non-nucleate cells which are shed continuously as small scales from the surface.

There is thus a continual replacement of the hard, keratinized, horny layer from the basal cells. The horny layer varies considerably in thickness, being very thick on those areas which are subject to wear and pressure (palms, soles of the feet) and thinnest in the flexures, e.g. axillae and eyelids. **Keratin** is an insoluble fibrous protein which is the principal constituent of epidermal cells, nails, hair and the organic matrix of tooth enamel.

All of these structures, together with the oily secretions of the glands (see below), serve to protect the underlying tissues from mechanical damage and to control undue water and heat loss.

The **nails** are extensions of the horny layer and consist of solid plates of translucent keratin. Finger nails grow at the rate of approximately 0.1 mm daily, taking 4–5 months for complete replacement. Toe nails grow at about half this rate, so treatment of toe nail conditions needs to be more prolonged than that for finger nails.

Melanocytes form about 5% of the basal layer. They are dendritic cells, forming an irregular network which is very variable in extent. The **melanin** which they synthesize is transferred through their dendrites to other epidermal cells. Exposure to sunlight or ultraviolet (UV) radiation promotes melanin synthesis, the concentration of which in the epidermis influences the basic skin pigmentation of individuals. However, skin colour also depends on the extent of dilatation of the skin capillaries, the amounts of oxidized and reduced haemoglobin in them, and on the presence of yellow carotene pigments in the blood vessel walls and surrounding tissues. Carotenes are present primarily in fatty tissue and are precursors of vitamin A. Dark-skinned people have the same proportion of melanocytes in the basal layer as do the fair-skinned, but they synthesize melanin at a faster rate.

Associated features

These include the hair and the apocrine, eccrine and sebaceous glands.

The **hair** arises in tubular downgrowths from the epidermis, the **hair follicles**. At the base of the hair follicle is a bulb containing the root and the **papilla**. The latter is a projection of the dermis into the bulb and contains blood vessels, nerves and melanocytes. There are three types of hair:

- The **long hairs** of the scalp, beard, moustache, axillae and pubic areas.
- **Vellus** (downy) hair occurring on the rest of the surface; and
- A small amount of short, stiff hairs on the eyebrows and eyelids and in the nostrils and outer ears.

Growth of the long hair is under androgenic control, so hair growth varies with sex, age, during pregnancy, etc. The hair follicles are formed naturally only during embryonic growth and the number is therefore fixed at birth, so hair loss due to follicular degeneration cannot normally be restored. However, it has recently been reported that the expression of two compounds in mouse epithelial cells, beta-catenin and LEF-1, causes adult epithelial cells to revert to an embryonic state and produce new hair follicles. Two problems remain to be solved before this discovery can be translated into treatment for hair loss: whether the results are applicable to humans and elucidating the control mechanisms for this process and so preventing excessive hair growth, and the possible formation of (benign) follicular tumours.

Loss of hair (**alopecia**) or its abnormal increased production (**hirsutism**) may thus be an indicator of endocrine abnormality, systemic disease (Table 12.1) or auto-immunity. All visible hair is dead, and no medical treatment can affect it once it has been formed, though its appearance may be improved (or harmed) cosmetically. Scalp hairs grow continuously for some 2–6 years at the rate of about 10 mm per month before falling out. They are replaced by activation of dormant follicles or by regrowth. All treatments for hair loss are unsatisfactory, though topical *minoxidil* will promote the growth of vellus hair for as long as it is used. High-potency topical or intralesional *corticosteroids* (*see* Table 12.11) and *ciclosporin* (*cyclosporine*) may induce regrowth,

Table 12.1   Some hair disorders

Hair loss

Diffuse
Male-pattern baldness (androgen-dependent)
Telogen effluvium (excessive rate of hair loss due to iron-deficiency anaemia, infections, postpartum, stress)
Hair shaft defects
Endocrine deficiency: hypothyroidism, hypopituitarism, hypoparathyroidism
Systemic lupus erythematosus
Syphilis
Drugs, e.g.:
- cytotoxics: *cyclophosphamide, mercaptopurine, doxorubicin, epirubicin, colchicine*
- anticoagulants: *heparin, coumarins*
- antithyroid: *thiouracils, carbimazole*
- tuberculostatics: *ethionamide*
- vitamins: *vitamin A*
- synthetic retinoids (especially *etretinate*, less common with *isotretinoin*)

Localized
Alopecia areata
Fungal infections
Discoid lupus erythematosus
Lichen planus
Harsh treatments (dyes, permanent waves, bleaches, traction)

Hirsuitism

Endocrine: adrenal, pituitary, ovarian, menopausal
Congenital abnormalities
Idiopathic (hair follicle hypersensitivity to androgens?)
Drugs: *androgens, minoxidil, corticosteroids, ciclosporin (cyclosporine)*

but regression occurs on withdrawal. Oral photochemotherapy (PUVA, p. 700) has been reported to be successful in up to 30% of patients.

There are two types of **sweat glands**:

- The **apocrine glands** are large glands which open into the hair follicles and produce a milky secretion containing carbohydrates, proteins, etc., the production of which is stimulated by emotions such as pain, fright and sexual excitement. These glands develop at puberty.
- **Eccrine glands** occur all over the skin, though their concentration varies enormously with the site, and they play an important role in temperature regulation. Eccrine glands occur as coils of cells in the dermis and open via invisible pores onto the surface where they discharge the sweat, a watery fluid containing 0.5–1% of chlorides, lactic and other acids and nitrogenous compounds, mostly urea.

The **sebaceous glands** are present all over the body, except the palms and soles. They are especially common on the scalp, face, forehead, chin, chest and back, opening into the hair follicles. They do not have ducts, but the cells break down to release the waxy **sebum**. The function of sebum is uncertain, though its waxy nature must influence water movement into and out of the skin. Because sebum production is partly under hormonal control, its odour presumably has a sexual role. Modified sebaceous glands produce wax (**cerumen**) in the ears and form the **meibomian glands** of the eyelids. The latter occasionally become blocked, forming small, benign, irritant cysts (**chalazion**): if troublesome, these cysts are removed surgically.

Chalazion should not be confused with **styes**, which are infections of the hair follicles.

Dermis

The outermost **papillary part** of the dermis lies immediately under the epidermis and rises irregularly into it, producing the **dermal papillae**, that contain blood vessels and nerve elements. The deeper part of the dermis contains a variety of elements:

- Connective tissue (collagen, elastic fibres, etc.), which supports the epidermis, confers elasticity and helps to maintain skin hydration
- Cellular elements: migratory (a few leucocytes; histiocytes, which are phagocytes and also form reticulin fibres) and fixed (fibroblasts and mast cells). These cellular elements are important, since they control the differentiation and function of the overlying epidermal epithelium, resistance to infection and reactions to environmental allergens.
- Blood vessels, which nourish the skin and regulate local tissue temperature.
- Smooth muscle fibres, which erect the hairs and cause 'gooseflesh'.
- Nerves, which are sensory (touch, pain, temperature) and autonomic (controlling the blood vessels and hair follicles).
- Lymphatic vessels.

Subcutaneous tissue

Below the dermis is a layer of loose, **areolar connective tissue**, containing adhesion proteins, nerves and fat, plasma and mast cells, embedded in a semi-solid matrix. This layer has important functions:

- Storage of water and fat, helping to maintain the hydration of surrounding tissues.
- Insulation against heat loss or gain.
- Provision of an access route for nerves and blood vessels to muscles and the dermis.
- Protection of underlying tissue.

Clinical features of skin diseases

Histopathology

The pathological changes that occur in skin due to disease are often not diagnostic, unless invading microorganisms can be recognized. However, there may be characteristic changes in the epidermis in diseases such as **psoriasis** (see below) or **pemphigus**, or in the dermis, e.g. in **scleroderma**. Some structural types of lesions are illustrated in Fig. 12.2, and common pathological changes are listed in Table 12.2.

Many skin conditions are inflammatory or

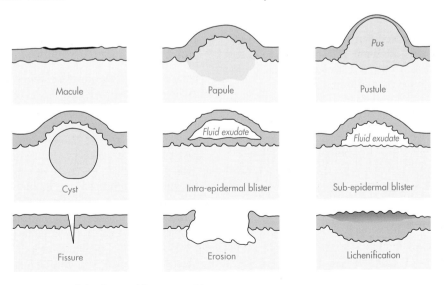

Figure 12.2 Some types of skin lesions (diagrammatic).

Table 12.2   Changes which may occur in the skin due to disease

Descriptive term	Pathology	Examples
Epidermal changes		
Acantholysis	Separation of the epidermal cells from each other, causing splits, vesicles and bullae	Herpes zoster, drug eruptions
Acanthosis	Increased depth of the prickle cell layer	Psoriasis, warts
Hyperkeratosis	Excessive production of the horny layer	Corns, ichthyosis
Inflammation	T cell recruitment, increased blood flow and intercellular fluid	Eczema, psoriasis
Parakeratosis	Incomplete keratinization, with nuclei in the horny layer	Psoriasis
Spongiosis	Intercellular oedema of the prickle layer	Eczema
Dermal changes		
Capillary	Lymphocytic infiltration	Systemic lupus erythematosus
	Sclerosis and obliteration	Scleroderma
Collagen	Sclerosis	Scleroderma
degeneration	Atrophy	Age, corticosteroid treatment
Fibrosis	Hypertrophy	Keloid
Inflammation	T cell recruitment, increased blood flow and intercellular fluid	Eczema, psoriasis

have inflammation (*see* Chapter 2) as a significant component.

Diagnosis

History

The important aspects of the dermatological history (*see also* Chapter 1) are:

- Where did it start? (Fig. 12.3)
- Duration.
- What changes have occurred in the severity?
- The extent when seen, and in the past.
- Features (Tables 12.3 and 12.4): wet or dry, colour, size, itch, distribution (Fig. 12.3).
- Interference with sleep, work, leisure and social contacts.
- Aggravating or relieving factors, e.g. treatments, diet, clothing, light, temperature, seasonal variation, emotional stress, medicines.
- Family history.
- Medication history.
- Occupation and hobbies.
- Cosmetic usage, including hair dyes, perfumes and aftershave lotions, etc.

The last two of these categories, and the patient's own observation, may provide valuable clues as to the cause of contact dermatitis. The emotional response of the patient may also be very important because visible lesions may cause considerable distress even though they are benign, and the associated emotions may aggravate the condition.

Identification of the types of skin changes and of lesions (Figs 12.2 and 12.3, Tables 12.2–12.6) requires a good light and sometimes also magnification.

Psychological features

Patients with skin diseases tend to be more disturbed by their condition, relative to its severity, than are those with other types of illness. This is particularly true if the condition occurs on visible parts of the body. Many common skin diseases, although potentially disfiguring, are completely benign and non-transmissible, e.g. naevi, dermatitis, psoriasis and acne. Patients often experience what has been called the 'leper complex', being at least somewhat rejected by their families, friends and acquaintances, or expecting to be so, and thus becoming miserable and reclusive.

Itching is a common accompaniment to many dermatoses, and may make patients restless during the day and sleepless at night, leading to tiredness, irritability, demoralization and social difficulties.

A clear diagnosis and simple explanation will

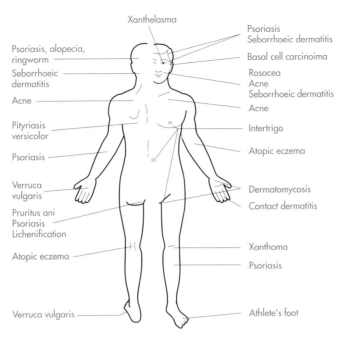

Xanthelasma

Psoriasis, alopecia,
ringworm

Seborrhoeic
dermatitis

Acne

Pityriasis
versicolor

Psoriasis

Verruca
vulgaris

Pruritus ani
Psoriasis
Lichenification

Atopic eczema

Verruca vulgaris

Psoriasis
Seborrhoeic dermatitis

Basal cell carcinoima

Rosacea
Acne
Seborrhoeic dermatitis

Acne

Intertrigo

Atopic eczema

Dermatomycosis

Contact dermatitis

Xanthoma

Psoriasis

Athlete's foot

Figure 12.3   Principal sites of occurrence of some common dermatoses.

Table 12.3   Principal features of some common localized lesions

Clinical features	Disease state
Non-pigmented lesions	
Pearly sheen, often facial, slowly enlarging, usually raised margin with central ulcer, patients usually >50 years of age	Basal cell carcinoma[a] (rodent ulcer)
Usually firm, hyperkeratotic, pin-head to pea-sized, often on hands or soles of feet, epidermal ridges disrupted, pain on lateral pressure	Warts
Firm or hard, deep set, often below knees, patients usually >50 years of age	Histiocytoma
Pigmented lesions	
Collections of blood vessels	
• raised in children, usually paler and flatter in adults; clotting may give bluish pigment	Angiomas, naevi
• solitary, raised red, shiny or eroded, bleeds readily, often presents acutely	Pyogenic granuloma
Uniform, static, even surface, pale to very dark	Mole
Light or dark brown, raised often whitish markings, warty, greasy, patients >50 years of age	Seborrhoeic warts
Usually pigmented (**not always**), enlarging slowly or rapidly, development of satellite lesions, ulceration or bleeding	Malignant melanoma[a]

[a] Malignant, the remainder are benign.

Table 12.4 Some features of scaly rashes

Clinical feature	Possible disease state
NON-INFLAMMATORY	
Mild	Effects of weather, social habits[a]
Present from childhood	Ichthyosis
Adult onset	May indicate systemic disease
Pigmented, ovoid, localized on exposed surfaces, usually elderly	Solar keratoses
Localized, progressive lesions	Possible malignancy
INFLAMMATORY	
Localized	
Non-pigmented, mild to moderate itch	Infestations, tinea, intertrigo, stable plaque psoriasis
Non-pigmented, very itchy	Contact dermatitis
Generalized	
Raised, commonly discrete plaques, slightly itchy, scaling	Psoriasis
Very itchy	Dermatitis/eczema
Discrete lesions, raised border, paler centre	Tinea
Child or young adult, sudden onset with single 'herald patch', mildly itchy, usually on trunk, upper arms and legs	Pityriasis rosea
Itching slight to severe, papules up to 5 mm diameter, shiny violaceous to brown, commonly on wrists, waist, thighs, inside mouth	Lichen planus

[a] Excessive washing, harsh detergents, etc.

often help patients enormously. A readiness to touch non-infectious lesions, demonstrating the conviction of the health care worker or carer that the disease is benign, can be a very effective way of reducing anxiety.

Examination

General aspects

In community pharmacy it may be difficult to gain a sufficiently broad experience, over a long enough time, to be able to recognize even some common skin lesions readily. It is certainly impracticable to learn to do so adequately as a student, though there are several well-illustrated books which can be of great help (see References and further reading). Prior self-treatment, especially with corticosteroids, may alter the appearance of lesions dramatically. There is a temptation to proceed directly to examination of the patient and to form a diagnosis on that basis, because patients often present by showing a readily visible lesion and asking for advice. Although skin symptoms and signs may be pathognomonic, e.g. in acne or stable plaque psoriasis, the history is of prime importance, because the skin has only a limited repertoire of symptoms. Also, the characteristics and severity of lesions may vary widely, even in the same patient with the same disease at different times.

Some general symptom groups and the features which may make it possible to identify the nature of the problem and come to a diagnosis are described below, but the details of the most common diseases are described later in this chapter.

Allergic conditions

These are usually very itchy (itch arises solely in the epidermis). Localized lesions may be due to

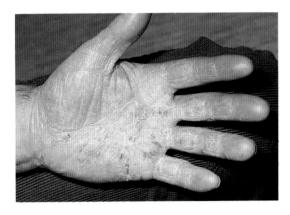

Plate 1 Contact dermatitis. The hands are a common site because they are exposed to a wide range of potential irritants, e.g. detergents and lubricating oils.

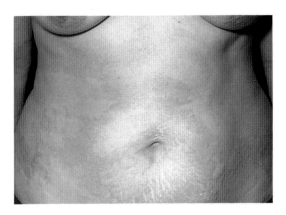

Plate 2 Urticaria. This is a very florid reaction. The raised, itchy weals are surrounded by areas of inflammation. The cause of this reaction was never determined, but common causes are medicines, food additives, animals and plants.

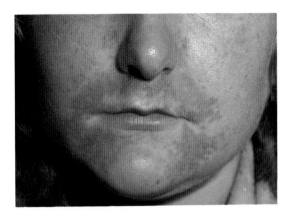

Plate 3 Perioral dermatitis. Note the sparing of the skin immediately around the lips. This reaction was due to a synthetic steroid used to treat an initial reaction caused by cosmetics.

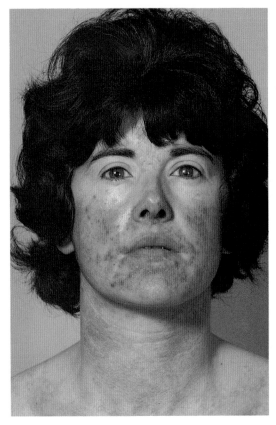

Plate 4 Rosacea. The rash is usually milder and more localized than in this patient. This florid reaction was the result of aggravation by a steroid cream.

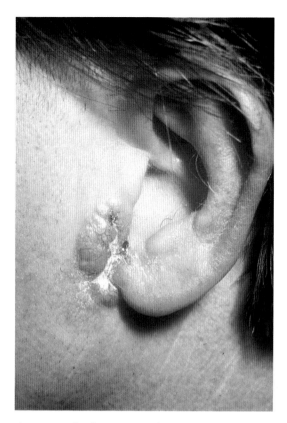

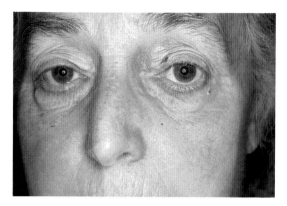

Plate 6 Xanthelasma. Note the large yellowish plaques (cholesterol deposits) on both upper eyelids near the nose and the smaller plaques elsewhere.

Plate 5 Basal cell carcinoma. This is in a typical site, i.e. areas exposed to sunlight. Note the raised, pearly margin, with veins coursing over the surface. Small lesions are uniform but central ulceration may develop with enlargement, as in this example. This patient is rather young, lesions being uncommon under age 40 years.

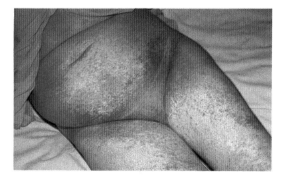

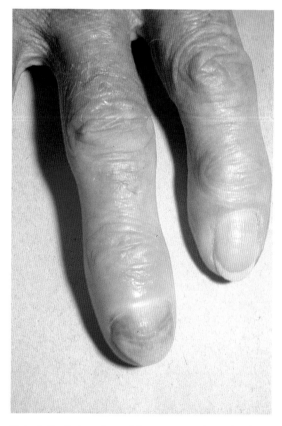

Plate 7 Purpura. This is a florid example of Henoch-Schoenlein purpura, an anaphylactoid reaction often due to medicines or following streptococcal throat infection. In this case, a woman known to be penicillin sensitive took some of her bronchitic husband's amoxicillin capsules.

Plate 8 Psoriatic nails and finger joint arthropathy. Note the pitting, darkening and separation (onycholysis) of one nail. The terminal (DIP) joints are inflamed, swollen and painful whereas they are normally spared in rheumatoid arthritis (see Chapter 8, p. 482).

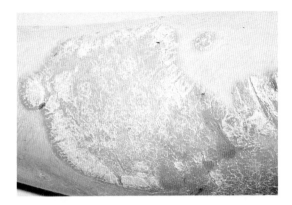

Plate 9 Plaque psoriasis. Note the raised margin and heavy scaling on a pinkish-red ground.

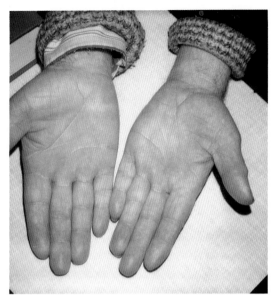

Plate 11 Hyperlinearity of the palms. This is a mild contact dermatitis reaction. Subjects with this sort of skin are particularly liable to react badly to irritants.

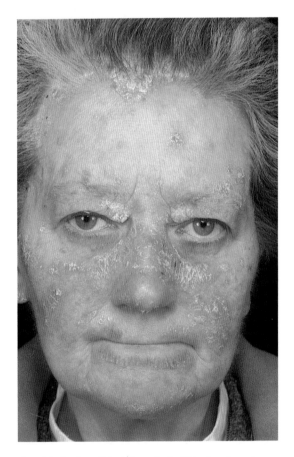

Plate 10 Scalp and facial psoriasis. This chronic rash was particularly noticeable in the hair. Scalp psoriasis does not usually spread far beyond the hair margin and when mild is often mistaken for dandruff.

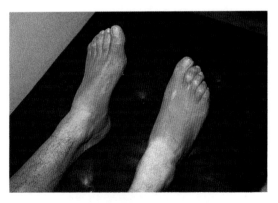

Plate 12 Allergic contact dermatitis. Reactions on the feet may be due to dyes or chrome tanning agents in leather. Plastic footwear may aggravate the problem due to plasticizers or to moisture trapping, giving high humidity and skin maceration. The well-demarcated reaction may subsequently spread widely.

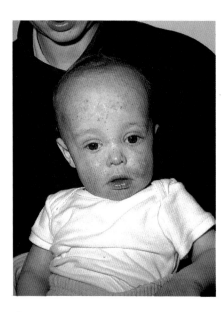

Plate 13 Infantile atopic eczema. The face, especially the forehead, scalp and trunk are usually affected. In older children, the area behind the ears and the flexions of the wrists and knees are often involved symmetrically.

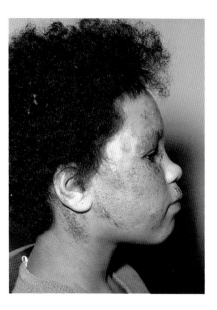

Plate 14 Chronic atopic eczema. This teenager shows the typical dry, scaly, pustular skin and thinning of the outer margin of the eyebrow. Depigmentation may occur in coloured patients.

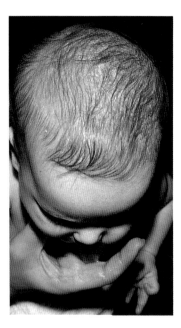

Plate 15 Cradle cap in an infant (3 months of age). This is characterized by coarse, yellowish, greasy, scalp scales. Some children also develop non-irritant erythema and scaling in the body flexures, especially the napkin area, but are otherwise well.

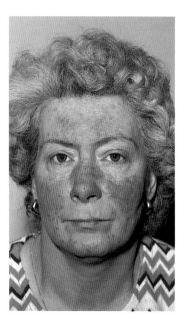

Plate 16 Facial telangiectasis. This irreversible damage was caused by the chronic application of a moderately potent corticosteroid cream. The effect is due to the superficial blood vessels showing through the thinned skin.

contact dermatitis (Plate 1), **atopic eczema** (Plates 13 and 14; *see* p. 701) and **urticaria**.

Rashes

Facial rashes. These are often due to environmental factors, e.g. weather or sunlight, or may be readily recognizable, e.g. acne. If they are due to atopic dermatitis there is often a fairly characteristic appearance: dry, finely scaling skin, facial pallor, swelling or creasing around the eyes and, possibly, a 'creased' pigmentation on the neck. Lesions localized to the eyebrows and perinasal area are usually due to **seborrhoeic eczema** (p. 705), while those around the eyes or mouth may be a **contact dermatitis** from cosmetics, cleansers or medicated creams. Fluorinated corticosteroid creams (*see* Table 12.11), which should never be used on the face, are one regrettable, avoidable cause or aggravator of **perioral dermatitis** (Plate 3).

Areas of inflammation which flush with heat, foods or stress and which tend to become papular are usually due to **rosacea** (Plate 4 and p. 713). Aggravating factors, e.g. corticosteroids, vasodilators, alcohol, hot drinks and hot sunshine, should be avoided. There is possible confusion between acne (p. 707) and rosacea, but there are no comedones (blackheads) with rosacea. If acne is mild it may be left untreated, but topical antibiotics (metronidazole or tetracycline) are usually effective. Oral tetracyclines, or even a retinoid (p. 689) may be necessary in resistant disease: eye involvement requires specialist management.

Other common cause of facial rashes are **seborrhoeic eczema** (p. 705) and, especially in children and teenagers, infections, e.g. **herpes simplex**, **impetigo** (*see* Chapter 13).

Systemic lupus erythematosus (SLE; *see* Chapter 8, pp. 511–514) is a potentially serious disease that may present with a butterfly rash over the cheeks and bridge of the nose, though accompanying symptoms, e.g. arthralgia, fever, are usual. A benign form, **discoid lupus**, causes more limited, well-defined, erythematous plaques on the cheeks.

Scaly rashes. An approach to the identification of scaly rashes is outlined in Table 12.4. Serious problems may arise for the patient if large areas of skin are affected moderately or severely, because temperature and water regulation mechanisms may then be impaired. In severe cases this may lead to hypothermia and dehydration.

Acute generalized rashes. It is to be hoped that patients with lesions of this type (Table 12.5) will consult their doctors promptly. However, patients are frequently reluctant to do this or fail to realize the severity of their condition.

Generalized rashes, especially in childhood, are often caused by **infections**, when there will be associated systemic symptoms (e.g. sore throat, fever, aches, joint pains), possibly with a history of recent case contact. **Guttate psoriasis** (p. 694), with widespread small lesions, may also be triggered by mild infections, especially sore throats.

Localized lesions

The diagnosis of these should always be approached carefully because, although the majority are benign, they are occasionally malignant, especially in older patients. The most common cutaneous malignancy is the **basal cell carcinoma** (BCC, Plate 5), which is much more common in fair-skinned races, especially if there has been prolonged skin exposure in sunny climates. Patients often regard the lesion as a minor, benign 'sore', but must be strongly encouraged to see their doctor as soon as possible, without alarming them unduly, because early treatment carries an excellent prognosis whereas delay can lead to severe damage to underlying tissues.

Table 12.5   Some causes of acute generalized rashes

Cause	Examples
Infections	Measles (rubeola), german measles (rubella), chickenpox (varicella), glandular fever (infectious mononucleosis)
Drugs	Antibiotics (especially penicillins), antirheumatics (e.g. gold), antithyroids, diuretics, morphine-type alkaloids, oral hypoglycaemic agents, psychotropics
Purpura[a]	Drugs, clotting defects, infections
Psoriasis	Following sore throats; relapse of psoriasis after corticosteroid treatment

[a] A rash due to bleeding into the skin (see text).

Moles and **warts** are common and are usually readily recognized, but any change in them should be regarded very seriously. If there is any doubt about the nature of an isolated lesion, prompt medical referral without causing undue alarm is mandatory, though patients are often reluctant to see their doctors. The characteristics of some localized lesions are given in Table 12.3.

Special signs

Koebner's sign is the occurrence of lesions along the track of a skin injury, e.g. a scratch, sunburn or chickenpox lesions, and may be a feature of psoriasis, lichen planus or warts.

Nikolsky's sign is the easy separation of apparently normal epidermis from the dermis by pinching or rubbing. It occurs in **pemphigus vulgaris**, a blistering disease in which there is a loss of cohesion of the outer epidermal cells, though the basal layer remains attached to the dermis.

Investigation

Patch tests for contact dermatitis are done by sticking a strip of a non-allergenic carrier, impregnated at intervals with solutions or gels of different suspected compounds, to a patient's back or arm and observing the occurrence of a reaction after 48 h (Fig. 12.4). Such reactions may persist for 4–7 days. **Prick (scratch) tests** may occasionally be used to identify systemic allergens in atopic subjects, though such procedures carry the risk of severe generalized reactions and should only be carried out where full resuscitation facilities are available.

Other tests include inspection under Wood's light (365 nm UV), to observe hair fluorescence in some types of **tinea**; microscopical examination of skin, hair and nails, or scrapings from the bases of vesicles; blood counts and pathogen culture, serology, etc.; and the biopsy of chronic lesions, especially if there is a possible malignancy.

The **radioallergosorbent test** (RAST, *see* Chapter 5, Fig. 5.16) is used to determine the presence and titre of reaginic antibodies (IgE) when investigating the aetiology of atopic conditions, e.g. dermatitis, urticaria.

Various techniques of **ultrasonography** which provide a two-dimensional picture through the skin are now being used in specialized units.

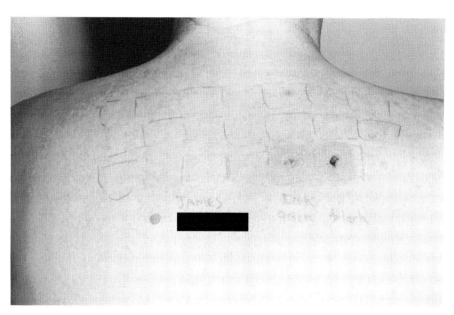

Figure 12.4   Patch testing. This shows the reactions on the back of a young man who was sensitive to black and green printing inks.

The skin and systemic disease

The association of skin lesions with systemic symptoms may indicate the presence of severe underlying disease and must always be taken seriously. Conditions in this group include thyroid and kidney diseases, and renal failure, diabetes mellitus, hyperlipidaemias and malignancies (Table 12.6).

Common associated systemic features include general malaise, muscle weakness, joint pains, fever and weight loss. The dermatological features which may be warning signs of serious disease include the following (some of the possible conditions indicated are given in brackets):

- Acute onset, especially over 50 years of age (cancer, etc.).
- Progressive symptoms (cancer, chronic dieases).
- Blistering and widespread urticaria.
- Erosion of tissue (cancer, ulcers).

- Generalized itching, unrelated to local lesions (liver and renal disease).
- Recurrent boils (diabetes mellitus).
- Xanthomas (yellowish plaques of cholesterol, often around the elbows and knees, indicative of hyperlipidaemias), especially in young adults. When these occur around the eyelids, usually in middle-aged patients, the condition is known as xanthelasma (Plate 6).

A widespread rash following treatment of a sore throat with *ampicillin* is virtually diagnostic for glandular fever. **Purpuras** are rashes due to bleeding into the skin and always require urgent medical referral. They may be distinguished from rashes that are inflammatory in origin because they do not blanch under pressure: a clear plastic spatula or ruler pressed onto the skin compresses dilated blood vessels and so causes blanching of inflammatory rashes but not of purpuric ones. Purpuras may be caused by allergic reactions to drugs, resulting in

Table 12.6 Some dermatological manifestations of systemic disease[a]

Disease	Clinical features
Hyperthyroidism	Hyperhidrosis (sweating); pruritus; production of fine scalp hair, occasional alopecia; pretibial myxoedema (raised red nodules on the legs, often associated with successful treatment for hyperthyroidism)
Hypothyroidism	Coarse, broken scalp hair; hair loss; pruritus; dry skin
Renal disease	Pruritus (due to uraemia); erythema multiforme
Diabetes mellitus	Pruritus; bacterial and fungal skin infections, especially boils; granuloma annulare; necrobiosis lipoidica (firm reddish yellow skin plaques, which may precede the onset of diabetes); leg ulcers, consequent on ischaemia
Cushing's syndrome	Acne vulgaris; hirsutism; striae (stretch marks due to corticosteroid-induced thinning and weakening of dermal and subcutaneous tissue)
Addison's disease	Increased pigmentation
Gastrointestinal disease	Perianal ulceration and pyoderma gangrenosum (Crohn's disease); eczema (malabsorption); dermatitis herpetiformis (gluten enteropathy)
Hyperlipidaemias	Xanthomata; xanthelasma (see text)
Hepatic porphyria	Photosensitivity; hyperpigmentaion; hypertrichosis; blistering
Neoplastic disease	Lymphomas: pruritus, urticaria, herpes zoster, exfoliative dermatitis, ichthyosis (thickening of the skin) Leukaemias: purpura, blistering, ulceration, pruritus, herpes zoster Carcinoid syndrome: flushing Various: skin nodules, adult dermatomyositis

[a] See text and Plates 6 and 7 for further detail.

platelet destruction and clotting failure (Plate 7), to other clotting or vascular defects (p. 716), or to infection (e.g. meningococcal meningitis). Because drugs are a common cause, a medication history may give important clues.

Management of skin diseases

General approach

There are two essential considerations:

- Reassurance of the patient and the reduction of anxiety (see above).
- The avoidance of actual or potential irritants and precipitants.

The range of the latter is very wide and includes soaps, detergents, cosmetics, perfumes, clothing, foods, plastics, rubber, metals (jewellery), lubricating oils, cement, drugs, components of vehicle bases of medicaments, etc. This important aspect requires considerable detailed attention.

An example of the problems involved is provided by the use of rubber gloves: they often do not give adequate protection and are prone to leakage and internal contamination, in turn causing contact dermatitis. If such gloves are used, they should be turned inside out and washed and dried to remove contaminants, preferably after each period of use. Further, plasticizers and other additives in glove materials may themselves cause similar trouble, and extensive trials of different manufacturers' gloves may be needed to find an acceptable brand. It may also be necessary to wear cotton gloves inside the rubber gloves. These problems affect professionals, e.g. dentists, pharmacists working in production units handling *cytotoxics* and making additions to intravenous infusions, as well as housewives and kitchen workers. When handling cytotoxics there is the additional problem of drug penetration through the gloves.

Intensity of treatment

There is a considerable danger of over-treatment and the application of medicaments which are known to have serious potential side effects, e.g. potent local corticosteroid preparations (pp. 687–689). Products may contain unsuspected allergens, e.g. the drug itself, lanolin, preservatives or antioxidants, and may aggravate the original condition or add further problems. If the condition deteriorates while using a product of known effectiveness against it, an adverse reaction should always be suspected, rather than drug resistance. Also, excessively frequent or vigorous application of medicaments, or their removal from damaged skin, may further harm sensitive areas. Minimal treatment with the simplest and mildest effective product should be the rule.

There are five basic target groups of conditions, for each of which a different degree of intervention is appropriate:

- Lesions from which the skin will usually **recover spontaneously** with minimal intervention, e.g. contact dermatitis, many occupational skin diseases, mild acne.
- Conditions which require **protection** of the skin by the application of emollients, barrier creams or 'inert' preparations, e.g. mild nappy rash.
- Conditions which will respond to **active treatment** with anti-inflammatory or other agents, e.g. psoriasis, acne and severe eczema.
- Infections and infestations which require **specific antimicrobial** or **antiparasitic** treatment, e.g. impetigo, scabies.
- Those conditions in which **little can be done** currently to influence their course, e.g. scleroderma.

Medical management is essential in the following situations:

- Lesions affecting more than 10% of the body surface area (BSA, *see* Table 12.7).
- Conditions with associated systemic features.
- Progressive lesions, increasing in severity or size.
- Ulcerating lesions or those which are breaking down centrally.
- Pigmented lesions, other than static ones which are clearly warts or moles.
- Any lesion which has recently changed in character.
- Conditions in which there is a significant inflammatory component.

Table 12.7 Fractions of the body surface area[a] and the approximate amounts of topical product required for application to them

Part of body	Fraction of BSA (%)[a]	Weight[b] for 1 week	Part of body	Number of fingertip units[c]
Scalp (hair)	4	15	Face and neck	2.5
Face	4	15	Arm and forearm	3
Each arm	9	30	Hand	1
Each hand	1	4	Leg and thigh	6
Each leg	18	60	Front of trunk	7
Chest plus abdomen	18	60	Back of trunk	7
Whole of back	18	60	Foot	2
Genitalia	1	4		

[a] BSA, body surface area, approximate figures.

[b] Approximate weight of product (g) required to cover the body part, when applied by a trained operator or patient, assuming two applications per day. The approximate maximum 'safe' weekly doses of topical corticosteroids (p. 687) are as follows: Group III or IV (see Table 12.11), 50 g; Group II, about 30 g, Group I, about 15 g. Use of a high-potency steroid (Group I) for more than 7 days should be undertaken only under the supervision of an experienced dermatologist.

[c] One 'fingertip unit' (FTU) is 'the amount of ointment expressed from a tube with a 5-mm diameter nozzle applied from the distal skin crease to the tip of the index finger.' (Long CC, Finlay AY (1991) Clin Exp Dermatol 16: 444–447). Figures in the table are expressed to the nearest half unit. One FTU covers approximately 312 cm^2 (adult males) and 257 cm^2 (adult females) and is roughly 0.5 g. The hand area (fingers closed) represents 0.76% of the BSA in men and 0.70% in women (Long CC, Finlay AY (1996) Br Med J 313: 690).

Note: The information on the right hand side of the table does not correspond with that on the left hand side.

- Blistering lesions, unless they are known to be due to a minimal insult, e.g. an insect bite, and the patient is otherwise well.
- Conditions which markedly interfere with the patient's lifestyle or occupation.
- Any unidentified lesion which arises acutely in the middle-aged or elderly.

Selection of treatment

Clinical features

Clearly the choice of treatment will depend on:

- The nature, extent and severity of the lesions.
- Whether they are visible and consequently cause the patient considerable anxiety.
- The duration and progression of the condition.
- What is known about the natural history of the condition, i.e. whether it is likely to remit or to have serious sequelae.
- Patient preference, e.g. for a particular formulation or type of emollient.

The patient's perception of their condition is important because steps must be taken to relieve their distress, even though it may be known that the disease is benign and self-limiting: a holistic approach is required.

The general treatment of target symptoms is outlined in Table 12.8.

Type and amount of product

There is sometimes confusion as to when to use ointments and creams, but the simple rule is 'wet on wet, dry on dry'. Thus oil-in-water (o/w) creams are usually used on moist lesions (ointments will not stick anyway), and ointments or w/o creams on dry or scaly lesions to help rehydrate the skin. This may need to be modified according to patient acceptability and the site, e.g. lotions and gels are usually preferred on the scalp.

Table 12.7 gives an indication of the proportion of the BSA represented by various parts of the body, and the approximate amounts of product required for treatment. However, even specially trained dermatology nurses will vary considerably the amounts that they use. A simpler approach is to use the **fingertip unit** of Long and Finlay. Patients using grossly more than the amounts indicated may be using the product excessively.

Table 12.8 The general treatment of dermatological target symptoms

Target symptom	Type of treatment	Examples
Dryness	Hydration	Ointments, occlusive dressings
	Emollients	Aqueous cream, emulsifying ointment
Exudation	Astringents	Aluminium or zinc salts, potassium permanganate
		Wet dressings
	Absorption	Pastes, cellulose/pectin gel, impregnated bandages
	Prevention of adhesion	Paraffin gauze and other non-adherent dressings
Local heat	Cool	Wet dressings, especially alcoholic solutions, calamine lotion (cool by evaporation)
Tenderness	Emollients	Aqueous cream, barrier creams (silicones)
	Lotions, creams	Calamine
Irritation/itch	Antipruritic	Astringent lotions, calamine products, crotamiton, local anaesthetics[a], local antihistamines[a]
Infection	Antimicrobials	Imidazoles, systemic or topical antibiotics[b]; antivirals, e.g. aciclovir (acyclovir); topical antiseptics, e.g. povidone-iodine, potassium permanganate
Sweating	Astringents	Aluminium salts
Localized lesions	Non-spreading	Stiff ointments and pastes
	Highly localized	Very stiff pastes, e.g. Lassar's paste

[a] May cause skin sensitization in some patients.

[b] Topical antibiotics may encourage microbial resistance and cause skin sensitization.

It is important to remember that virtually any product used in treatment may itself be irritant or allergenic to some patients due to components of the base, additives or medicaments. Even *hydrocortisone* has been known to cause rashes. If the condition fails to respond or deteriorates, this may be the result of inappropriate treatment or some component of the medicament.

Targeting symptoms

Dryness

Emollients are invaluable in the management of dry skin conditions, whether they are primary or secondary to other diseases such as eczema, and are the fundamental basis of treatment. Emollients may give substantial relief when used alone and will at least reduce the need for potent medication. A useful routine is given below, but this needs to be tailored flexibly to patient preference to achieve the desired result:

- Avoid soaps and household detergents, which may be irritant or allergenic.
- Use emulsifying ointment (or aqueous cream or a commercial alternative) to wash and bathe, or a bath oil or gel, as the patient prefers.
- Use a 'light' emollient cream (relatively nongreasy and readily absorbed, Table 12.9) after bathing or washing, over the entire affected area. However, in dry skin conditions a greasier product ('heavy cream') may be preferable, because it gives better skin hydration, though it is very uncomfortable if large areas of skin are covered with an oily film. If this cannot be tolerated by the patient, a compromise has to be found. Emollients may also relieve skin tenderness.
- A barrier cream may be used on the hands before work, but may cause its own problems (p. 682).

The skin produces large quantities of a complex mixture of substances, known collectively as **natural moisturizing factor** (NMF), which is

Table 12.9 Characteristics of some emollients

Product	Heaviness[a]	Greasiness[a]
Emulsifying ointment	+++	+++
Hydrous ointment	++	+++
Commercial paraffin-based ointments e.g. DiproBase ointment	++	++
Unguentum Merck	+	++
Hydrous ointment	+	++
Arachis oil-based creams[b], e.g. Oilatum	+	++
Urea-based, e.g. Aquadrate	+	++
Calmurid	+	+
E45	+	+
Paraffin-based creams, e.g. DiproBase, Ultrabase	+	+
Bath additives, e.g. Alpha Keri, Balneum, Oilatum Emollient	+	+

[a] The terms 'heaviness' and 'greasiness' are subjective, and are meant to convey how the products feel when applied to the skin. These impressions will differ considerably between patients. (Modified with permission from Graham-Brown R (1986) Update **33**: 539–544.)

[b] May cause severe allergic reactions in sensitive subjects.

+ → +++, property increases.

believed to be intimately involved in the maintenance, repair and hydration of the epidermis. Some inherited dry skin conditions, e.g. ichthyosis, are presumably the result of an inadequate production of NMF. One component of NMF is *sodium pidolate*, a potent humectant used in some commercial emollients.

Pruritus (itching)

Itch is a symptom that is unique to the skin, and may be caused by a variety of diseases and conditions (Table 12.10). The natural response is to scratch the affected site, but this provides only temporary relief and the itch returns, to be followed by more scratching. If this 'itch–scratch–itch cycle' persists, the skin may become lichenified (thickened and roughened) or even excoriated (scratched sufficiently to cause bleeding), and the skin may become infected or be permanently damaged.

Aqueous cream with 1–2% menthol and *normal saline* are widely used to relieve itching and some bath oils, e.g. Balneum Plus contain antipruritics. Lotions may be cooling, protective, astringent and antipruritic and are often used on inflamed and weeping skin. Although previously widely used, *aluminium acetate lotion* and *calamine lotion* (sometimes with *ichthammol*) are now uncommon. Although there is little objective evidence of effectiveness, *crotamiton lotion* may be preferred

by some patients. *Tar* products may also help to reduce itching. *Calamine lotion* may be too drying and should not be used for scaling dermatoses, for which the oily preparation is preferable.

Provided that there is no infection, occlusive medicated bandages (e.g. *zinc paste* with *coal tar* or *ichthammol*), covered with stockinette or crepe bandage, can be left in place for a week or more. This helps to break the itch–scratch–itch cycle and so allows the skin to heal. Some of these are particularly easy to remove without damaging the skin.

Antihistamines should be given orally as antipruritics and not used topically, because they may cause sensitization. Although many patients use topical antihistamines without any side effects, the patients who need them most are those most likely to be sensitized by them, so they should preferably be avoided.

The sedative antihistamines, e.g. *hydroxyzine, promethazine, alimemazine* (*trimeprazine*), are preferred, with appropriate warnings about drowsiness, driving, etc., and are especially useful at night, when their sedative effect is beneficial in preventing restlessness and scratching during sleep. A particular advantage of *hydroxyzine* is its anxiolytic action.

Because the antipruritic effect tends to accompany sedation, the newer, non-sedating antihistamines may be less useful for this purpose.

Table 12.10   Some causes of pruritus

Pruritic skin lesions

Dermatitis/eczema
Psoriasis
Drug reactions
Allergic reactions, urticaria
Lichen planus
Parasitic infestations, e.g. lice, scabies
Viral and fungal dermatoses e.g. chickenpox
Dermatitis herpetiformis[a]
Psychogenic

Generalized pruritus without skin lesions

Anaemia
Pregnancy
Diabetes mellitus
Thyroid disease
Haematological disease
Anorexia nervosa
Old age
Chronic renal failure
Liver disease
Hodgkin's disease and other neoplasms

Anogenital pruritus

Contact dermatitis, e.g. clothing
Diabetes mellitus
Anal discharge or leakage, faecal soiling
Postmenopausal
Parasitic infestations, e.g. lice, scabies, threadworms
(mostly children)
Psychogenic

[a] *See* Chapter 6, p. 337.

However, these effects are relative and non-sedating antihistamines are often used during the day and sedating ones at night, to avoid the 'hangover' effect that would interfere with schooling, driving, operating machinery, etc. It should be noted that although the newer antihistamines are relatively non-sedating, this does not mean that they are safe under all circumstances, e.g. they may not be licensed for use in children. The doses of *astemizole* and *terfenadine* must not be exceeded, nor the drugs taken together, because serious cardiac arrhythmias may occur. These drugs should be avoided if there is significant hepatic impairment, with hypokalaemia or other electrolyte disturbance. Further, these and *mizolastine* must not be used with anti-arrhythmic agents, e.g. *amiodarone*, *disopyramide*, *procainamide* and *quinidine*, because serious arrhythmias have occurred. Syncope (fainting) in patients taking these antihistamines may indicate an arrhythmia and should be investigated.

Broken and weeping skin
The best initial treatment is still the traditional astringent, mildly antiseptic, *potassium permanganate* soaks (1/8000). Unfortunately, the skin will be stained brown and some patients find this cosmetically unacceptable. Once the skin starts to heal, other medications can be applied. Alternative preparations include *1% ichthammol in calamine lotion* and *normal saline* soaks. If the area is infected, **systemic** *antibiotics* will be required: like the antihistamines, most topical antibiotics are liable to cause skin sensitization and should be avoided whenever possible. Non-adherent dressings should be used if the area needs to be covered, and oily lotions (e.g. oily calamine lotion) are preferred on weeping skin to avoid crusting and the adherence of dressings: this is an exception to the normal 'wet on wet' rule.

There is a large range available of new breathable dressings with good adherence and flexibility. These protect the area, allow oxygen penetration and control moisture loss, so they can be left in place for long periods. They are very useful for incipient pressure sores.

Routes of administration

Topical treatment
Topical treatments are only of value in epidermal (superficial) dermatoses. If lesions are deep-seated, any agent applied to the surface that reaches the dermis will be removed rapidly in the circulation. Thus, dermal disorders require systemic therapy.

Although topical corticosteroids have revolutionized the treatment of many skin diseases the older products still have a place in the first-line treatment of mild to moderate disease. Thus *tar* products are still used in the management of **mild psoriasis** (e.g. 5% *crude coal tar* in a suitable base, or tar paint; p. 698) and may also be helpful in **persistent eczema** and **dermatitis** (p. 701), e.g. 15% coal tar solution in emulsifying ointment applied before bathing. Commercial products are more elegantly formulated than the equivalent official formulary ones and so are usually more acceptable to patients. Although very greasy, a *coal tar + salicylic acid + sulphur + coconut oil ointment* is very useful in treating **scalp psoriasis**.

Magenta paint is still used occasionally for controlling **intertrigo** (eczema of the skin folds, e.g. under the breasts or in the axillae, often macerated and infected with *Candida albicans*) though dry, non-staining antimicrobial agents, e.g. an imidazole, are more acceptable cosmetically. Care must be taken that patients are not sensitive to the products, notably *iodine*, because patients with skin problems tend to be more liable to develop skin sensitization than the general population. In all situations the simplest treatments are best and safest, especially if there is any doubt.

Systemic treatment

This may be required in a variety of situations:

* If there are associated systemic symptoms, e.g. psoriatic arthropathy.
* To control serious conditions, e.g. erythroderma and angioedema (a severe urticarial reaction; p. 715).
* When local treatment might cause skin sensitization, e.g. antibiotics or antihistamines.
* When topical treatment is ineffective or inappropriate, e.g. the use of systemic cytotoxic drugs, corticosteroids, antibiotics and some retinoids, and of evening primrose oil, in psoriasis and eczema.

Corticosteroids in dermatology

Topical corticosteroids are widely used in dermatology. This merits special consideration because their indications, cautions, side effects, etc. differ in important respects from those experienced with systemic corticosteroid use.

Topical use

Selection

This depends primarily on two considerations:

* The **severity** of the condition: clearly, the more severe the damage the greater the potency needed, but this must be tempered by the knowledge that the greater the damage the greater will be the absorption through that site.
* The **site** of application: particularly sensitive sites are the axillae, under the breasts, behind the ears and the genital area, i.e. wherever there are skin folds and delicate skin. It should be clear that greater care needs to be exercised if the face or other exposed areas are to be treated, because any side effects (see below) will then be obvious and very important to the patient.

Potency

These products are classified in the *British National Formulary* (BNF) into four different potency groups (Table 12.11). However, this classification must be regarded as approximate because formulation has a considerable influence on potency. Further, percutaneous absorption depends on the extent of the area of application and the degree of skin inflammation.

The **concentration** of drug used will influence the relative potency. Prescribers frequently order dilutions of commercial products, but it is difficult to see the advantages of this because it should be possible to choose a product of lower potency. Further, extemporaneous dilution has several disadvantages: the product is no longer sterile, it may not be adequately preserved, and injudicious manipulation may impair the uniformity of a carefully formulated and manufactured product. For example, some potent ointments are dispersions of a propylene glycol solution of drug in the base, and excessive manipulation or warming of the product may cause the dispersed droplets to coalesce. A non-uniform product results, even though the correct diluent is used.

Side effects

These will vary with the potency, the amount applied, the area covered, frequency of application and whether the site is inflamed, occluded or particularly sensitive.

Table 12.11 The approximate potencies of some topical corticosteroids[a]

Corticosteroid	Concentration (%, w/w)	Corticosteroid	Concentration (%, w/w)
Group I (Very potent)			
Clobetasol propionate	0.05	Halcinonide	0.1
Diflucortolone valerate[b]	0.3		
Group II (Potent)			
Beclometasone dipropionate[b]	0.025	Fluocinolone acetonide[b]	0.025
Betamethasone dipropionate	0.05	Fluticasone propionate	0.005–0.05
Betamethasone valerate[b]	0.05–0.1	Hydrocortisone butyrate	0.1
Desoximetasone[b]	0.25	Mometasone furoate	0.1
Diflucortolone valerate	0.1	Triamcinolone acetonide	0.1
Fluocinonide	0.05		
Group III (Moderate potency)			
Alclometasone dipropionate	0.05	Fluocinolone acetonide	0.00625
Betamethasone valerate	0.025	Fluocortolone and salts	0.25
Clobetasone butyrate	0.05	Fludroxycortide (flurandrenolone)	0.0125–0.05
Desoximetasone	0.05	Hydrocortisone with urea[c]	1.0
Group IV (Mild potency)			
Fluocinolone acetonide	0.0025	Methylprednisolone	0.25
Hydrocortisone base/acetate	0.1–2.5		

[a] Based on the *British National Formulary* classification.

[b] Potency depends on concentration, lower concentrations may be in Groups III or IV.

[c] Different formulations may vary widely in potency. Some hydrocortisone–urea products fall into Group IV.

Side effects may be local or systemic and are often related to the cytostatic properties of steroids. Thus, repeated application of potent steroids leads to wasting of subcutaneous tissue, due to inhibition of fibroblast maturation and consequent failure of collagen repair in the dermis, similar to what happens in the normal ageing process. This results in thinning of the skin and **telangiectasis**, i.e. a reddening resulting from the disclosure and expansion (they are no longer supported) of the small blood vessels in the dermis (Plate 16). If this effect is severe, the larger vessels will also become prominent and the capillaries will become fragile, so that minor trauma leads to substantial bruising. A similar underlying process may also produce **striae** – permanent disfiguring stretch marks as the dermis and subcutaneous tissues lose elasticity.

Suppression of local non-specific defence mechanisms also occurs due to inhibition of macrophages, neutrophils, etc., resulting in delayed healing and the aggravation of viral and fungal skin infections, notably herpes simplex. Topical corticosteroids are therefore contraindicated if there is any suspicion of viral or fungal infection unless formulated or used with an effective antimicrobial agent. The combination of their cytostatic effects and the suppression of local defence mechanisms means that they are also contraindicated for the management of topical ulcerative conditions, because they may delay healing and promote infection.

Use of the more potent synthetic steroids may result in local erythema, **contact dermatitis** (Plate 12) and **perioral dermatitis** (Plate 3). It is not clear whether the latter condition is due to a true sensitivity to the drug or whether the steroid triggers a latent erythematous tendency.

Corticosteroids will aggravate **rosacea** (p. 713) and, being comedogenic, may exacerbate **acne** (p. 707). Mild skin depigmentation may also occur.

Systemic absorption may be significant, depending on the potency of the steroid and the extent and condition of the affected skin. Inflamed skin permits greater drug penetration than normal skin. The more potent products (Groups I and II) are all capable of producing significant percutaneous **adrenal suppression**, so they must be used with great care, especially in children, whose skin is thinner and whose surface area to body weight ratio is larger than that of adults. Absorbed steroid may also cause some degree of **immunosuppression** due to inhibition of lymphocyte multiplication and maturation.

Patients must therefore be counselled carefully on how to use these products, the major criteria being that they are applied sparingly to the specific lesions and usually not massaged into the skin or occluded. The approximate amounts of products needed for application to various parts of the body are given in Table 12.7. Patients must also be warned that these products are prescribed for treatment of the condition presented, and must not be hoarded to use as panaceas for all skin ailments, or loaned to friends or relatives.

Both patients and some prescribers are wary of steroid use, so that the preparations used may be too weak to control symptoms adequately. A short burst of a potent agent is quite safe: it will often be more effective, and safer in the long run, to control symptoms rapidly with a potent agent and then reduce the potency, rather than to titrate the dose upwards.

Precisely placed **intralesional injections** of poorly soluble forms, e.g. *dexamethasone phosphate, methylprednisolone acetate, triamcinolone hexacetonide*, may be more effective than potent topical products for severe localized lesions, e.g. keloid scars (fibrous, raised and enlarging).

Systemic use

The best estimate of oral corticosteroid usage in the UK is that there are about 250 000 patients, taking an average of 8 mg/day of prednisolone. Most of these are in the 60- to 80-year age group.

In dermatological practice, systemic steroids are indicated only for severe dermatoses. The nor-

mal rules for steroid therapy should be followed, i.e. the minimum dose needed to control the condition should be used, and this should be reduced as rapidly as possible on a sliding scale to the minimum maintenance dose required, preferably nil. However, prednisolone daily doses less than 7.5 mg, or the equivalent of other products, are unlikely to produce significant adrenal suppression and other major side effects in adults. If adrenal suppression does occur during long-term therapy it lasts for up to a year after the cessation of treatment, so corticosteroids must never be withdrawn abruptly in this situation.

Injudicious use of corticosteroids may permanently stunt children's growth. At the other end of life, perimenopausal and postmenopausal women, and some elderly men, are at risk of osteoporosis, the physiological bone loss being increased in proportion to the cumulative dose of corticosteroid. This may lead to peripheral bone fractures following falls, particularly of the neck of femur and wrist, and vertebral crush fractures. Only about 14% of patients receive preventative treatment. In postmenopausal women the treatment of choice is hormone replacement therapy because it also manages symptoms of the climacteric; however, it has its own problems. Otherwise, the best strategy is to ensure an adequate calcium intake (about 1.5 g/day), with vitamin D if sun exposure is limited, plus a **bisphosphonate**, e.g. *alendronate*, cyclical *etidronate*. In the occasional very frail elderly patient **anabolic steroids** (e.g. *nandrolone, stanozolol*) may be appropriate because they have beneficial effects on both bone density and muscle.

Retinoids

Introduction

These compounds are related chemically to vitamin A (*retinol*). The vitamin derived from natural sources is a mixture of isomers of which the most active is *all-trans*-retinol, the form produced synthetically.

Retinol is essential for normal skin formation and keratinization and for proper cell maturation and differentiation generally. However, it has only a moderate activity and an unfavourable

Table 12.12   Some side effects and contraindications of retinoids

Tissue or organ affected	Side effect
Mucous membranes	Dryness and cracking of lips, dryness of mouth, nasal bleeding
Skin	Dryness and hyperfragility, especially palms and soles; dermatitis; erythema; pruritus; shiny, smooth, 'sticky' (sweaty) skin
Hair	Diffuse alopecia (mild)
Nails	Thinning, fragility, paronychia
Eyes	Dryness, irritation, pain, conjunctivitis, abnormal night vision
Hyperlipidaemia[a]	LDLs increased, especially VLDL and triglycerides; HDL cholesterol decreased
Musculoskeletal	Bone abnormalities in children (not suitable for prolonged treatment), arthralgia, myalgia
Liver	Acute hepatitis
CNS (occasionally)	Nausea, headache, malaise, drowsiness

Contraindications

Pregnancy – absolute contraindication, breast feeding
Hepatic or renal impairment
Avoid vitamin A supplementation

[a] (V)LDL/HDL, (very) low-density/high-density lipoproteins.

therapeutic ratio, high doses causing serious side effects on the skin, mucous membranes, liver and CNS. The synthetic retinoids are more potent and have a better therapeutic ratio, though they are still rather toxic compounds with an extensive list of side effects (Table 12.12). Synthetic retinoids should be used only if there are adequate haematological, hepatic and other monitoring facilities available.

The more recently developed compounds ('second-generation', e.g. *acitretin*, *etretinate*) tend to have less serious side effects, especially neurological and hepatic. 'Third-generation' polyaromatic agents (the arotinoids, e.g. *arotinoid ethyl ester*) are some 100–1000 times as potent, but none of these has yet been marketed.

Mode of action

Retinoids bind to inducible nuclear retinoic acid receptors (RARs) which interact with the promoter regions of specific nuclear genes that control the maturation and development of a variety of tissue cells and so regulate their transcription.

Three types of RAR are known, only two of which (RARalpha, RARgamma) are expressed in human skin. RARalpha is present primarily in the basal layer, and its concentration declines progressively as the cells migrate towards the surface. Conversely, RARgamma predominates in the granular layer. Binding of retinoids to these RARs produces specific actions on keratinocyte differentiation.

They also possess antiproliferative and anti-inflammatory actions. They thus have four therapeutic actions:

- Promotion of normal keratinocyte differentiation in the epidermis.
- Blockade of excessive cell proliferation and epidermal growth by down-regulation of ornithine decarboxylase, which is involved in hyperplasia and hyperproliferation.
- Suppression of excessive sebum production.
- Anti-inflammatory, due to inhibition of prostaglandin synthesis and consequent production of pro-inflammatory agents, e.g. HLA-DR and lipoxygenase products and interleukin-6, and modification of both humoral and cellular immune responses.

Apart from their effects on the epidermis, these drugs have powerful effects on general cell maturation. In acute promyelocytic leukaemia (*see* Chapter 11) there is a failure of promyelocytes to differentiate into mature granulocytes. *Tretinoin* and other retinoids cause dose-dependent rapid morphological maturation of these immature cells and have similar effects in other leukaemias.

Pharmacokinetics

The retinoids are lipophilic and so have a relatively low oral bioavailability, so oral dosage forms should be taken with meals to enhance absorption. The currently available compounds cross the placenta and are highly teratogenic. They are excreted in breast milk and so cause skeletal abnormalities in breast-fed infants.

Etretinate is a highly lipophilic aromatic retinoid. It has a large interpatient variability after oral use and has a very long persistence because it is stored in body fat. The effective terminal half-life ($T_{1/2}$) is about 90 days. Although the blood levels of etretinate after stopping are therapeutically inadequate, they may still be teratogenic: it is detectable in plasma up to 2–3 years after stopping chronic dosing. *Acitretin*, a metabolite of etretinate, has a terminal $T_{1/2}$ of only 2 days and does not accumulate in the tissues; however, because it is esterified to etretinate in the liver this benefit is largely nullified.

Isotretinoin is an isomer of *tretinoin*, the acid form of vitamin A, and has a bioavailability of about 25% following oral administration. Peak blood levels are reached in 1–4 h and the elimination $T_{1/2}$ following chronic dosing is of the order of 10–20 h, steady-state blood levels being reached in 3–4 days. Its major active metabolite, 4-oxo-isotretinoin, has a similar terminal $T_{1/2}$ because its formation is rate limited. The shorter $T_{1/2}$ of isotretinoin makes it much safer than *etretinate*.

Tazarotene is a recently introduced esterified pro-drug of the active agent, *tazarotenic acid*, to which it is hydrolysed in the skin. Although used topically, it penetrates skin significantly. In short-term topical use the $T_{1/2}$ is about 18 h. End metabolism of tazarotenic acid yields inactive compounds and appears to be inducible: peak plasma levels after 3 months are about 10% of those seen after 13 days.

In the epidermis, all of these compounds bind to both RARalpha and RARgamma. Vitamin A is transported in the blood by a specific **retinol binding protein** (RBP). Isotretinoin is almost completely protein-bound, but to serum albumin and not to RBP.

The potent aromatic retinoid, *etretin*, is a major metabolite of etretinate and is interesting. Although its terminal $T_{1/2}$ is about 50 h, so that it persists as long as etretinate, isomerization to its inactive *cis*-analogue occurs readily. Thus it is very unstable and very difficult to formulate, and aromatic retinoids have not yet produced useful therapeutic agents.

Adapalene is another recent introduction. This is a synthetic polycyclic, lipophilic retinoid derived from naphthoic acid. Although structurally unrelated to other current retinoids, adapalene is somewhat similar in structure to the arotinoids, although it is very stable. It binds preferentially to epidermal RARgamma and, because skin penetration is very low, it is undetectable in plasma, urine and faeces.

Indications

The retinoids are a potent and interesting group of drugs with great potential. Although there are currently only a few licensed indications, they are known to have beneficial effects in other diseases (Table 12.13) and there are many more for which there is evidence of potential benefit. Further development of this group of drugs will clearly have a profound influence on our understanding of skin diseases and their treatment and of cell maturation processes in general.

Their uses in dermatology derive from the actions outlined previously.

Acne. *Tretinoin* and *isotretinoin* are used topically. *Adapalene* is a topical treatment for mild to moderate acne. *Oral isotretinoin* is used for severe, refractory disease.

Psoriasis. *Tazarotene* is used topically to treat mild to moderate disease limited in area. *Acitretin* is used orally for the treatment of severe, resistant or complicated psoriasis and for some other disorders of keratinization.

Photodamage. Topical *tretinoin* gives a slow improvement (over 3–4 months) of hyperpigmented,

Table 12.13   Some indications for the use of retinoids[a]

Licensed indications[b]

Moderate to severe acne
Psoriasis (all forms)
Congenital disorders of keratinization
Photodamaged skin, including hyperpigmentation
Induction of remission in acute promyelocytic
leukaemia

Indications for which benefit has been demonstrated

Rosacea
Hydradenitis suppurativa (inflammation of abnormal
sweat glands)
Lichen planus
Neoplastic skin diseases: basal cell carcinoma,
squamous cell carcinoma, chemoprophylaxis of skin
cancer in predisposed patients

Potential indications

Chronic discoid lupus erythematosus
Pemphigus (an autoimmune blistering disorder)
Cutaneous manifestations of Reiter's syndrome
Generalized granuloma annulare
Cutaneous sarcoidosis (a chronic, granulomatous
disease)
Basal cell carcinoma

[a] Modified from David M, Hodak E, Lowe NJ (1988) *Med Toxicol* **3**:
273–288 and others.
[b] Licensed in the UK.

wrinkled skin caused by chronic excessive sun exposure.

Other uses.   Because of toxicity, oral *tretinoin* is no longer used for the treatment of psoriasis which, although disfiguring, is rarely life-threatening. However, it is used as a first-line treatment to induce remission in acute promyelocytic leukaemia, after relapse and in resistance to standard chemotherapy. Low-dose *acitretin* has also been reported to reduce skin cancer incidence in renal transplant patients who are on long-term immunosuppressive treatment.

Further details relevant to specific treatment are discussed under the diseases concerned.

Psoriasis

Psoriasis is an hereditary chronic skin disorder, usually characterized by scaly plaques or papules, and often distributed on areas exposed to frequent minor trauma.

Pathology, aetiology and epidemiology

Pathology

Psoriasis is characterized by increased turnover of the basal cells. Their doubling time is reduced from some 20–30 days to about 2–3 days, and there is an increased growth fraction (*see* Chapter 11, p. 634). Further, the three lowest layers of the epidermis are involved in cell germination instead of the normal, single basal layer. Because the resultant cell production considerably exceeds the rate of cell differentiation, the epidermis is thickened (Fig. 12.5) and nucleated cells are present throughout the entire thickness, i.e. the normal granular layer is absent. Even the horny layer contains cells with degenerate nuclei instead of being composed of amorphous keratin.

This increased metabolism causes a full-thickness inflammation of the skin. There is infiltration of neutrophils and activated lymphocytes which release growth-stimulating cytokines. There are dilated, tortuous capillaries high in the dermis and these are present even in the apparently normal skin of patients with psoriasis.

Psoriatic arthropathy (Plate 8) is the consequence of a synovitis which, though very similar to that of rheumatoid arthritis (*see* Chapter 8, p. 480), is believed to be a distinct entity. The condition affects about 7% of patients with psoriasis.

One current theory is that there is an inherited defect of keratinization resulting in abnormal keratinocyte surface antigens. If immunocytes encounter these, e.g. following minor skin trauma, an immunological response is triggered, with consequent stimulation of the basal layer. This is supported by the finding that initiation of psoriasis is accompanied by an influx of CD4+ (helper) T cells into lesions. There may also be an immunological defect because CD8+ T cells are responsible for its maintenance. It has also been suggested that there are genetically abnormal

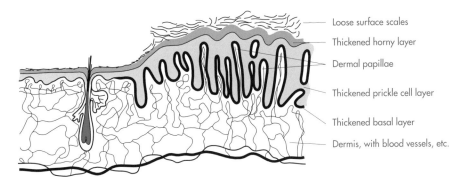

Loose surface scales

Thickened horny layer

Dermal papillae

Thickened prickle cell layer

Thickened basal layer

Dermis, with blood vessels, etc.

Figure 12.5 Comparative anatomy of normal and psoriatic skin. The diagram shows a section through the edge of a psoriatic plaque. The plaque (on the right) shows increased thickness of the basal, prickle cell and horny cell layers, large amounts of surface scale, greatly elongated dermal papillae and increased vascularity/inflammation in the dermis.

fibroblasts which fail to control keratinocyte proliferation.

Aetiology

The precise cause of these changes is not clear. However, there is a polygenic inherited tendency to develop psoriasis. There is an association with certain histocompatibility antigens (HLA-B13, B17, Bw57 and Cw6). HLA-DR7 is associated with both skin and joint disease (p. 694) and HLA-DR4 with the latter only. HLA-B27, which is strongly associated with (seronegative) ankylosing spondylitis (*see* Chapter 8, pp. 503–504), is also linked to psoriatic joint disease and the severe pustular form of psoriasis (p. 694). HLA-B28 is associated with a particularly severe form of psoriatic arthritis.

Environmental factors are implicated in addition to the strong genetic component. Psoriasis occurs more frequently in colder climates in the winter. Known **trigger factors** include:

- Trauma: skin laceration, pressure from belts, brassieres, etc.
- Infections: streptococcal tonsillitis, especially in children; HIV.
- Stress, e.g. marital, bereavement.
- Hormone status: there is an increased incidence in pregnancy and at puberty and the menopause.
- Sunburn or excessive exposure to the sun is harmful in 10% of patients, although sunshine may benefit others, and its lack predisposes to attacks.

- Drugs: alcohol, *antimalarials*, *beta-blockers*, *chlorpropamide*, *lithium*, smoking.

Infants may develop **napkin psoriasis**, which usually responds readily to treatment.

Epidemiology

Psoriasis is very common and affects about 2% of Caucasians, though many more have mild disease for which they do not seek medical treatment. About 30% of patients have a first-degree relative who is also affected. Siblings have an 8% risk, and patient's children have a 16% to 50% risk if one or both parents respectively are sufferers. Identical twins have a concordance rate of about 50%, so environmental factors are important.

The incidence is similar in both sexes. About 75% of cases occur in adults of 15–25 years of age, the condition tending to appear earlier in females than in males. The potential to develop the disease persists throughout life, though the skin may appear normal, so children may develop symptoms before these appear in their parents. The remaining 25% develop symptoms in their mid-fifties.

The disease is less common among Asians, Blacks and Eskimos, and is almost unknown in American Indians. The situation with Eskimos has been taken as circumstantial evidence for an important role of essential fatty acids, present in fish oils, in maintaining epidermal integrity (p. 702).

Clinical features and diagnosis

Onset of psoriasis is usually gradual. In classical **plaque psoriasis** the skin lesions are well defined, raised, reddish ('salmon pink'), slightly itchy plaques of tissue which are covered with large amounts of loose, silvery scales (Plates 9 and 10), surrounded by completely normal-looking skin. If the scales are scratched off there are signs of inflammation: they leave small bleeding points, because the capillaries are near the surface, and this sign is virtually diagnostic for the disease. In dark-skinned people the underlying colour may be much darker, even purplish.

Acute attacks occur most often in early childhood and may be triggered by streptococcal tonsillitis. They often start as evenly scattered small discoid lesions (**guttate psoriasis**) that tend to clear spontaneously within 4 months. A few of these patients develop chronic disease at about 5–7 years of age, when it occurs as large symmetrically disposed plaques (e.g. both knees or elbows), though it may spread to affect 80% of the skin surface (erythrodermic psoriasis, see below). The lesions sometimes heal spontaneously, starting in the centre, and may thus be confused with ringworm.

In **pustular psoriasis** sterile, yellow pustules occur, often at the edges of plaques in severe disease, but sometimes associated with flexural lesions. This form is often very resistant to treatment and is potentially life-threatening if widespread because fluid loss and temperature control are compromised. Chronic brownish pustules on the palms and soles are strongly associated with smoking.

The most **common sites**, in approximate order of frequency, are the elbows, knees, scalp, lower back, chest, face, abdomen and genitalia: all areas exposed to mild trauma from clothing and physical activity. Scalp psoriasis (Plate 10) may easily be mistaken for severe dandruff if mild, or for seborrhoeic dermatitis (p. 705). Diagnostic features are that the plaques on the scalp are raised, as on other areas, and usually isolated, so the margins are palpable and well-defined: the lesions tend to spread somewhat beyond the hair line.

The **course of the disease** is very variable. Psoriasis is normally a chronic, mildly irritant condition. Although some patients have a single episode followed by complete and prolonged remission, it is usually non-progressive, with occasional unpredictable exacerbations. The severity may either increase or decrease with time.

The combination of thimble nail pitting, distal interphalangeal (DIP) arthropathy and nail discoloration (see below) is pathognomonic.

Complications

The nails are affected, usually symmetrically, in about 25% of cases (Plate 8), usually in long-standing psoriasis. They show thimble-like pitting and later thickening, ridging and separation from the nail bed (**onycholysis**). An orange to brown discoloration of the distal lateral margins of the nail bed is characteristic.

Joint pain (**psoriatic arthropathy**) occurs in about 7% of patients. This tends to be asymmetrical, affecting the larger joints and the DIP finger joints (*see* Chapter 8, Fig. 8.5) near affected nails. Psoriatic arthropathy is seronegative (*see* Chapter 8, pp. 503–505) and may precede or follow the skin changes. In contrast, rheumatoid arthritis almost always spares these joints and is characteristically symmetrical and seropositive. Psoriatic arthropathy occasionally leads to severe joint damage and disability.

Erythrodermic psoriasis is a severe, widespread, inflammatory form of the disease. The cause is usually unknown, but it may be triggered by injudicious treatment with potent steroids. If the condition is extensive, serious and possibly life-threatening hypothermia and dehydration may result, because there may be a loss of 90–95% of the normal horny layer. High-output cardiac failure may be precipitated in patients with compensated heart failure, owing to the extensive skin inflammation and consequent increased dermal blood flow.

Management

The two **prime objectives** are to:

- To produce a **complete clearing** of the affected areas: if this is attained, the disease-free intervals between relapses are increased, even in very chronic conditions.

- To **reduce distress**: if lesions are visible, the disfigurement is particularly distressing to juveniles and young adults because it is interpreted by the lay public as a serious and highly infectious disease. However, it is benign except in its severest forms and is certainly not transmissible. Thus, it is important to reduce stress and to reassure patients: a willingness to touch the plaques helps to convince the sufferers of the harmless nature of their condition.

The specific **treatment aims** are:

- To reduce epidermal cell turnover (cytotoxic or cytostatic agents, e.g. *dithranol* (*anthralin*), *corticosteroids*, *methotrexate*, phototherapy; *retinoids*).
- To promote normal maturation of epidermal cells (vitamin D derivatives, *retinoids*).
- To remove scale (keratolytics, e.g. *salicylic acid*, *coal tar*).
- To reduce inflammation and the immunological skin reaction (immunosuppressants, e.g. *corticosteroids*, *ciclosporin* (*cyclosporine*), *methotrexate*).

- To hydrate the skin and reduce itch (emollients).

While this treatment classification is convenient, there is an inevitable overlap between the classes of drugs used. Cytotoxic or cytostatic drugs are also anti-inflammatory, e.g. *methotrexate*, and *corticosteroids* are anti-inflammatory, immunosuppressive and cytostatic.

Factors influencing treatment selection are:

- Age.
- Form of psoriasis (plaque, guttate, localized or generalized, pustular, erythrodermic).
- Site and extent of skin involvement.
- Prior treatment.
- Concurrent disease, e.g. HIV.

Although the course of the disease is highly unpredictable and relapses are common, modern treatments may be very effective and so an optimistic, sympathetic attitude should be maintained. Many patients will need long-term maintenance medication with occasional intensive treatment for exacerbations. A general outline of treatment of psoriasis is given in Table 12.14.

Table 12.14   Management of psoriasis

Aim	Mode	Drugs and techniques used[a]
Reduce cell turnover	Cytotoxics Antiproliferative drugs	Methotrexate, hydroxycarbamide (hydroxyurea) Dithranol (anthralin): high concentration/short time, Ingram regimen Vitamin D analogues: calcipotriol (calcipotriene), tacalcitol Phototherapy[b]: PUVA, tar + UVB (Goeckerman regimen), RePUVA Retinoids: tazarotene, acitretin (Tar)
Reduce inflammation	Immunosuppressants	Corticosteroids[c]: hydrocortisone, clobetasone butyrate Methotrexate Ciclosporin (cyclosporine)
Remove scale	Keratolytics	Salicylic acid Propylene glycol Tar

Hydrate the skin
Reduce itch
	Emollients
	Antipruritics
		Aqueous cream, DiproBase, etc.
		Antihistamines:
		    Daytime: e.g. acrivastine, astemizole, cetirizine
		    Night-time: e.g. azatidine, hydroxyzine, trimeprazine (alimemazine)
		Crotamiton

[a] Also see text. Some drugs fall into more than one class: cytotoxics are also immunosuppressants and both are anti-inflammatory.

[b] PUVA, psoralen + long-wavelength ultraviolet radiation (UVA); RePUVA, retinoid + PUVA; UVB, short-wavelength ultraviolet radiation.

[c] Used only under specific circumstances, not as a general treatment (see text).

Topical pharmacotherapy

Tar preparations, *dithranol* (*anthralin*) and *salicylic acid* have been used safely for many years.

Reducing cell turnover

Dithranol (anthralin)

This is a synthetic agent which has been a mainstay of psoriasis treatment for over 80 years. Although effective, it is now beginning to give way to less irritant and more cosmetically acceptable drugs. Dithranol was preceded by a natural plant product, chrysarobin, introduced in 1877.

Mode of action. This is not known precisely, but dithranol inhibits thymidine incorporation into DNA, mitochondrial DNA replication and repair and ATP supply in epidermal cells, and uncouples oxidative phosphorylation. The combined effects of these leads to inhibition of cell growth.

Pharmaceutical considerations. Major problems with *dithranol* (*anthralin*) are that it is very irritant and chemically unstable, so the extemporaneous preparation of pastes and ointments is unwise. Further, without suitable milling equipment it is difficult to prepare the very fine dispersions that are required for low irritancy, though hospital manufacturing units are usually suitably equipped. Poor dispersions result in highly localized irritation from large particles. Production staff must be made aware of the hazards involved in handling dithranol powder, especially if it gets into the eyes. They must wear suitable protective clothing and wash thoroughly.

Dithranol (*anthralin*) is readily oxidized to brown or purplish pigments, especially under alkaline conditions, which stain skin and fabrics and are difficult to remove. Salicylic acid has been used for stain removal. This chemical instability means that concentrations less than 0.05% are not normally practicable, due to significant loss of potency. The triacetate ester is more stable, because the hydroxyl groups are protected by esterification, the ester being hydrolysed to dithranol (anthralin) in the skin. The ester is used occasionally, being less irritant than dithranol (anthralin), but also less active.

Commercial products provide well-formulated, stable preparations that are cosmetically very acceptable to patients. This has the additional benefit of encouraging patient compliance, thus improving control and hastening the response.

Contraindications to *dithranol* (*anthralin*) treatment are:

* Burning, discomfort, soreness, moistness.
* Spreading of lesions which is anything other than gradual.
* Immediately following topical treatment with steroids.

If reactions occur, a bland preparation (soft paraffin or other emollient) should be used for 14 days before recommencing treatment with a low concentration of dithranol (anthralin) (e.g. 0.05%) and building up slowly once more to the highest tolerated concentration. A moderate-potency corticosteroid, e.g. *betamethasone valerate* 0.025% cream, may be used for dithranol (anthralin) burns. Reactions following corticosteroid use (p. 697) are similarly managed with weaning and emollients.

Phototherapy

Both natural and artificial UV radiation may be beneficial and are often used after tar or psoralen baths (see below). Either UVB (short wavelength, 290–320 nm radiation, responsible for sunburn) is used alone (with emollients) or UVA (long wavelength, 320–365 nm) is used with a drug (photochemotherapy, PUVA; see below). Once the lesions have cleared, mild UV exposure may prolong the period of remission, but over-exposure and burning must be avoided. Patients are usually tested for UV sensitivity by graduated exposure. Although sunlight helps some patients it may trigger attacks in others. Further, hot climates often exacerbate the condition because sweating readily leads to skin maceration. The procedure aggravates erythrodermic and pustular disease.

Retinoids

Tazarotene has recently been introduced for the topical treatment of mild to moderate plaque psoriasis affecting up to 10% of the skin surface (*see* Table 12.7) in adults aged over 18 years. These restrictions derive from insufficient data on the treatment of younger patients and larger areas, though some trials have lasted for a year.

The drug (topical) reduces basal cell hyperplasia via RARalpha receptor binding (p. 690) and promotes normal basal cell maturation and progression to granular cells. Improvement may be seen within a week and a good response occurs in 65% of patients after 12 weeks. The benefit may be maintained for at least 12 weeks after stopping, so pulsed treatment may be appropriate.

As with other retinoids, tazarotene must be used with great care and is suitable primarily for the non-intertriginous areas of the trunk and limbs, provided that the skin is not inflamed or eczematous or covered with hair. Exposure to the sun, UV light or solaria must be strictly limited. Pregnancy and breast feeding are absolute contraindications. The common **side effects** (10–20% of patients) are skin irritation, burning, erythema, contact dermatitis, skin pain and worsening of psoriasis, and are related to concentration and duration of treatment. If severe, these should be managed by cessation of therapy and use of emollients.

Tazarotene is unsuitable for treating pustular and erythrodermic psoriasis.

Promoting cell maturation

Vitamin D analogues

Calcipotriol (*calcipotriene*) reduces excessive epidermal cell proliferation, improves cellular differentiation and strongly inhibits T cell activation by interleukin-1. It is as effective as betamethasone in clearing mild to moderate plaque psoriasis. Despite producing more skin irritation, calcipotriol (calcipotriene) seems to be free from significant side effects and more acceptable to patients than short-contact dithranol (anthralin) (see below). *Calcipotriol* (*calcipotriene*) is currently licensed in the UK for mild to moderate plaque psoriasis affecting not more than 40% of the skin surface. It may be used on the scalp but not on the face or for children under 6 years. *Tacalcitol* is a similar, more recent agent.

All vitamin D analogues may cause hypercalcaemia, so they should not be used if there is any abnormality of calcium metabolism, nor if there is sufficient inflammation or skin damage to permit excessive absorption of the drug. They must be used with caution in pregnancy.

Retinoids

In addition to producing normal keratinocyte maturation, *tazarotene* normalizes final keratinization by interaction with the more superficial RARgamma receptors.

Anti-inflammatory treatment

Corticosteroids are potent anti-inflammatory agents, but have only a limited role in the treatment of psoriasis. Although there is an inflammatory element, and potent steroids may produce a dramatically rapid symptomatic improvement, there may be a substantial rebound effect on withdrawal and subsequent difficulties in treatment. If used as a first-line treatment, corticosteroids may so modify symptoms as to make a definitive diagnosis very difficult. If rebound occurs there may need to be a prolonged weaning period, using progressively less potent preparations and finally an emollient. This may take from 4–8 weeks, depending on the severity of the symptoms, during which time dithranol (anthralin) must not be used.

However, a low- or medium-potency product with low toxicity, e.g. *hydrocortisone* or *clobetasone butyrate* cream, is useful under careful supervision on sensitive sites such as the flexures, ears, face and genital areas. Treatment should be short-term and more potent products avoided, because permanent skin damage may occur rapidly. Scalp lotions may also be useful for short-term treatment if coal tar or coal tar + salicylic acid shampoos are ineffective, or if the scalp preparations referred to above are not cosmetically acceptable.

Methotrexate is also anti-inflammatory and is used systemically (see below). The retinoids also have anti-inflammatory properties and are use topically and systemically.

Skin hydration and antipruritics

Keratolytics

Tar has mild keratolytic, antimitotic and anti-pruritic actions and is thus effective only in mild cases. Although tar is a recognized carcinogen, there are no reports of associated skin tumours over more than 40 years of pharmaceutical use. The crude forms of tar are more effective than refined ones, especially as antipruritics, but the latter and the numerous commercial preparations are more acceptable cosmetically and cause less staining. Tar is used in the form of creams, ointments, pastes, lotions and bath emollients in concentrations of 0.25% to 6%, often prepared from coal tar solutions. Some older *tar* preparations may be unsuitable for use on the scalp or face where they may be irritant or cause folliculitis, and specially formulated commercial shampoos are available.

Tar is sometimes combined with salicylic acid or hydrocortisone, adding an anti-inflammatory effect. It may also be used with UVB radiation (see also PUVA, below), when it presumably acts as a skin sensitizer.

A coal tar + salicylic acid + sulphur + coconut oil **scalp ointment** has been used for many years. Because this is cosmetically unattractive and difficult to prepare, it has largely been replaced by commercial products, e.g. Pragmatar Cream and, more recently, Dovonex Scalp Solution.

Pharmaceutical considerations. Tar is occasionally combined with dithranol (anthralin) However, they are incompatible: the dithranol (anthralin) reacts with tar bases and undergoes a rapid free radical oxidation. Nonetheless, there is one commercial tar ointment which also contains both dithranol (anthralin) and salicylic acid: presumably, the dithranol (anthralin) is protected by the non-aqueous environment and the salicylic acid.

Salicylic acid (2%) is used primarily as a mild keratolytic agent to remove excessive skin scales. It also helps to stabilize dithranol (anthralin) and can be used to remove dithranol (anthralin) staining.

Propylene glycol (50% aqueous solution) is also mildly keratolytic.

Further information on emollients and antipruritics is given above (pp. 683–685).

Topical treatment modes

Scale removal

If the scaling is very thick, e.g. on the elbows and knees, it will hinder the penetration of drugs, so it may be helpful initially to remove excess scale by using 2% salicylic acid ointment on its own for a week or so. Propylene glycol is also used.

Coal tar treatments

Provided that the psoriasis is mild and not too extensive, a correspondingly mild therapeutic approach is appropriate. Ointments or creams containing *coal tar* may be used, in association with tar baths, until the lesions have cleared. Treatment should be started with the weaker preparations, possibly including salicylic acid to help remove excess scale. The scales on the scalp may be especially thick, so this area should be treated with the coal tar + salicylic acid + sulphur + coconut oil scalp ointment, which is left on for 1 h and shampooed out: some patients do not find this cosmetically acceptable. The treatment is unsuitable for young children. The commercial coal tar shampoos are also very useful.

The **Goeckerman regimen** involves the use of topical tar preparations, especially baths, followed by UVB radiation. Coal tar may also be used in conjunction with dithranol (anthralin) (the **Ingram regimen**, see below), though dithranol (anthralin) is the single agent of choice for most patients.

Dithranol (anthralin)

Dithranol (anthralin) is often used as a first choice, with excellent results, especially if the condition is mild to moderate. It is also used if coal tar treatment has not been successful.

The older preparations were rather messy ointments or, for more severe cases, consisted of *dithranol (anthralin) in Lassar's paste*. The purpose of the latter is to provide a stiff vehicle which prevents dithranol (anthralin) spreading from the site of application onto surrounding skin, because it stains and irritates normal skin. This formulation also contains *salicylic acid* which helps to minimize oxidation of the dithranol (anthralin). The *dithranol (anthralin) concentration* used normally varies between 0.1% and 0.5%, depending on the tolerance of the patient's skin (fair skins are the most sensitive) and the response. Although concentrations in the range 0.05% to 4% (even up to 10%) have been used, the higher concentrations require inpatient day care management, at least initially. The paste is applied precisely to the areas of the lesions, usually by a skilled nurse using a spatula, and is covered with talc and stockinette to minimize spreading and staining. Treatment commences with the lowest concentration and the contact time is increased every 3–4 days if there is a response and there are no significant side effects. If a response is not obtained, a higher strength is used. The approach is to find the contact time–strength balance which gives a satisfactory response without burning the skin.

This procedure normally produces some response within 1 week, and many patients will be completely clear, i.e. no palpable lesions, in 2–3 weeks, though chronic cases may take 6 weeks. The purple-brown staining that develops indicates that the lesions are responding to the treatment. This may be ignored because it usually clears spontaneously within a further 2 weeks, to leave 'normal' skin, though the psoriatic potential remains.

Dithranol (anthralin) products are generally unsuitable for application to sensitive areas, i.e. the face, ears, flexures and near the genitalia (but see below). These areas are often treated with steroid creams, with or without coal tar. Clearly, pastes are unsuitable for application to the hair.

Ingram regimen. This common procedure is often used in severe cases as an intensive inpatient routine. It involves:

- Initial patch testing with 0.1% *dithranol (anthralin) in Lassar's paste*, to determine skin tolerance.
- Soaking in a bath containing *coal tar* (coal tar solution or a commercial equivalent).
- Exposure to *UVB* radiation to give a slight erythema, i.e. a mildly damaging dose.
- Application of *dithranol (anthralin) in Lassar's paste* at the desired concentration, leaving for 24 h, removing with oil and bathing as before. A top-up may be necessary after 8–12 h.

Dithranol (anthralin) creams are more acceptable cosmetically than pastes or ointments and are generally less irritant, though they act more slowly. They are more suitable for use by patients at home and can be used on the scalp. A new cream formulation of 1% dithranol (anthralin) in a lipid-stabilized base appears to have low irritancy.

Intensive short contact time regimens. These have been the major advance in dithranol (anthralin) treatment, i.e. '30-minute therapy', rather than the 24 h of the Ingram regimen. These involve the application of higher dithranol (anthralin) concentrations before bathing at night. This has proved to be similarly effective to conventional treatment, though the lesions may take slightly longer to clear, up to 1 month as against 3 weeks. However, there are substantial advantages:

- Less interference with the patient's life style.
- Better patient acceptability and compliance.
- No need for hospital inpatient or day care treatment.
- Less staining of clothes and bed linen.

Higher-potency commercial preparations have been introduced to suit the short contact time approach, with concentrations of up to 2% being used in the community. Concentrations of 8% are sometimes used in hospital.

The lower-strength creams are also suitable for application to delicate areas such as the flexures, provided that no burning or undue local reaction occurs. Shorter contact times may be preferred here. The apparently normal skin at scalp margins and behind the ears must be avoided, because it is very sensitive. Concentrations other than those prepared by the manufacturers are sometimes requested by prescribers, but commercial preparations should not be diluted without careful inquiry because formulations may be critical. It is preferable to use a weaker preparation for a longer contact time or a more concentrated one for a shorter time, depending on patient tolerance, rather than attempt extemporaneous preparation.

Phototherapies

PUVA treatment is used for widespread involvement of the trunk. This involves treating the patient with *methoxsalen (8-methoxypsoralen)*, a phytochemical photosensitizing agent. Patients bathe in a solution of the drug before irradiation in a cabinet with a bank of UVA tubes; alternatively an oral dose is taken 2 h before UVA irradiation. *Trioxysalen (trioxsalen, 4,5′,8-methoxypsoralen)* is a similar drug which is not licensed in the UK but is used in North America.

Dark goggles should be worn during the treatment and for a further 8 h, to minimize the risk of cataract formation.

Combination treatment with a retinoid (*Re-PUVA*) has been used for resistant psoriasis, and is probably the most effective modality. However, the UVA dose must be very carefully controlled.

Many patients will experience long periods of remission with these regimens. The methods are technically simple and can readily be used on an outpatient basis, usually twice weekly for about 5 weeks. They are liked by patients because they avoid the use of messy topical products.

Side effects. Some patients experience nausea and headaches, and burns may occur – even with careful calculation of the UV dose. In the long term, there is premature skin ageing and a slightly increased risk of skin malignancies, so patients under 40 years of age should not be treated unless other approaches are ineffective. Some consultants in the UK still regard PUVA as experimental, though most use it routinely; PUVA is confined to specialist centres.

Narrow band UVB phototherapy appears to be as effective as PUVA and avoids taking psoralens.

Systemic pharmacotherapy

Immunosuppressants and cytotoxics

These potentially very toxic agents are used in psoriasis in lower doses than are used to treat neoplastic disease (*see* Chapter 11) and to prevent rejection of organ transplants (*see* Chapter 4). Because skin diseases are rarely life-threatening there must be careful individualized evaluation of the risk–benefit balance before these drugs are prescribed.

Methotrexate (MTX)

This antifolate agent is very effective but is reserved for the treatment of severe exacerbations or intractable cases because of potentially serious side effects. MTX must be used extremely carefully in the elderly, is unsuitable for children, and is therefore restricted to use by specialists only.

In psoriasis, MTX is usually given orally in low dosage (10–25 mg weekly). Despite this low dose, MTX has caused liver cirrhosis and fatal blood dyscrasias. Deaths have also occurred due to failure to recognize the weekly frequency of dosing. Therefore, the UK Committee on the Safety of Medicines has advised that:

- A full blood count and renal and liver function tests be carried out before starting treatment, and repeated weekly until therapy is stabilized. Patients should then be monitored carefully every 2–3 months.
- Patients should be told to report all symptoms and signs occurring during treatment, especially sore throat.

Blood dyscrasias may occur abruptly and *folinic acid rescue* (*see* Chapter 11, pp. 660–661) may be required. Abnormal liver function tests are a contraindication to starting or continuing treatment, and liver biopsies should be taken if function tests fail to return to normal after stopping MTX treatment.

Renal function tests are also required because MTX is nephrotoxic and accumulates in renal failure.

Analgesics reduce the excretion of MTX and death has occurred with concurrent use of NSAIDs, so such combinations must be avoided in psoriatic arthropathy and patients warned about the risks of self-medication with products containing NSAIDs. Other drugs which may increase toxicity include *penicillins*, *phenytoin*, *pyrimethamine* and *trimethoprim*.

MTX is teratogenic and is absolutely contraindicated in pregnancy and breast feeding. Conception should be avoided for at least 6 months after use in either sex.

Hydroxycarbamide (hydroxyurea, 0.5–1 g daily) has been used in patients who are intolerant of methotrexate or in whom the latter is contraindicated, but it is also myelosuppressive.

Ciclosporin (cyclosporine)

This immunosuppressant has been introduced for the treatment of psoriasis (2.5–5 mg/kg daily), and a very high proportion of patients respond to treatment. It is also very useful for erythrodermic disease. However, the renal toxicity of ciclosporin (cyclosporine) means that it should only be used by hospital consultants. Exposure to UV radiation, e.g. UVB or PUVA (see above), and excessive exposure to sunlight should be avoided.

Retinoids

Acitretin, a metabolite of etretinate (pp. 689–692), is the only member of this group licensed in the UK for the treatment of severe psoriasis. It is especially useful for pustular disease. Because of its toxicity, acitretin is reserved for use in hospitals or under the supervision of hospital consultants for patients unresponsive to other treatments. Acitretin interacts with both alpha and gamma retinoid receptors.

There is considerable interpatient variation in absorption and metabolism, so the dose must be individualized for each patient. Acitretin is often given in 1-year cycles comprising 9 months of treatment followed by a 3-month rest period. Some dermatologists use the drug in low dosage as an adjunct to dithranol (anthralin) or PUVA treatments, if these give inadequate control.

Side effects. Mucocutaneous side effects of acitretin are common, e.g. dryness of the skin, cracked lips and dry eyes. Generalized pruritus, nail problems, nosebleeds and hepatotoxicity may occur, as does slight transient alopecia. Acitretin can cause a rise in plasma lipids and serum triglycerides must be monitored regularly. Concurrent use of vitamin A must be avoided. Because acitretin is highly teratogenic, meticulous contraception must be initiated before treatment and maintained throughout and for at least 2 years after stopping treatment. Hepatic and renal impairment are other contraindications. The drug is rarely used in children because it may cause growth impairment.

Antipruritics

Antihistamines are occasionally used if itching is troublesome, the sedating side effects of the older drugs being useful at night. Anxiolytics may also be useful in some patients to relieve associated stress and anxiety, so *hydroxyzine*, which has sedative, anxiolytic and antihistaminic properties, is often used. However, the most effective approach is adequate counselling and reassurance and effective treatment of the psoriasis.

Other treatments

Corticosteroids are sometimes injected into lesions, to control chronic plaques resistant to other treatments.

Experimental treatments

Improvements in psoriasis have been reported in patients treated with *interferon alpha* and the anti-arrhythmic drug *amiodarone*. The somatostatin analogue, *octreotide*, also has anti-psoriatic activity, possibly because the increased epidermal cell growth is influenced by human growth hormone. However, it is too early to say whether any of these will find a place in routine therapy. Rarely, surgical removal of troublesome plaques has been used and has produced a local cure.

Eczema and dermatitis

Definition and classification

Eczema is an inflammatory, highly itchy, usually chronic epidermal eruption. The terms eczema and **dermatitis** are often used synonymously, but it has been conventional to use the term dermatitis to describe skin reactions due to external agents, and eczema for reactions to endogenous or intrinsic factors in atopic individuals. A classification and some of the characteristics of these types of condition are given in Fig. 12.6. However, it must be emphasized that there is considerable overlap and that atopic patients tend to

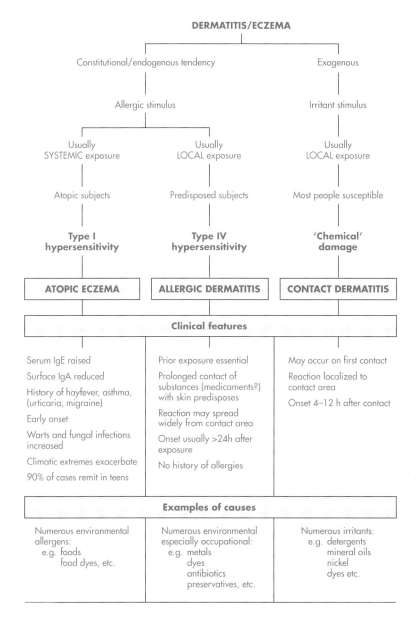

Figure 12.6 Classification of the principal forms of eczema and dermatitis.

develop local reactions, as may patients whose skin is damaged by some other pathological process, e.g. gravitational (varicose) eczema (p. 705).

This group of diseases comprises the largest single group seen in skin clinics and is responsible for about one-quarter of all dermatological referrals.

Aetiology and pathology

Essential fatty acid metabolism

An interesting discovery has been that essential fatty acids (EFAs) are important in the maintenance of epidermal integrity. An example of their nomenclature is arachidonic acid, which is a 20:4n-6 acid, i.e. it consists of a 20-carbon chain with four double bonds, the first of which links carbons 6–7. The composition of the plasma phospholipids is significantly changed in patients with atopic eczema compared with controls, the level of *cis*-linoleic acid being increased, whereas those of its metabolites (including arachidonic acid) are substantially reduced. Since linoleic acid is the major dietary n-6-EFA, this points to a metabolic defect, probably a reduced activity of delta-6-desaturase. This enzyme converts linoleic acid to gamma-linolenic acid, a rate-limiting step. There is also a reduction of alpha-linoleic acid metabolite concentrations in atopic respiratory disease and the same enzyme may be involved.

The **oral** administration of *linoleic acid* and *gamolenic acid* in the form of *evening primrose oil* partially corrects the low n-6 metabolite levels and is reportedly associated with significant, dose-related clinical improvement, but the evidence for this is equivocal. Topical application is not helpful. In a small trial, gamolenic acid has also been shown to be potentially beneficial in the treatment of acne. However, the benefit of gamolenic acid has been challenged and its role in therapy is unclear.

Modification of n-3 metabolite levels would require the administration of fish oils, and circumstantial evidence from the study of Eskimo populations indicates that this may be beneficial in skin diseases, notably psoriasis.

Because abnormal levels of serum fatty acids have also been observed in patients with allergic respiratory disease it seems possible that abnormal fatty acid metabolism is a fundamental feature of atopy, though whether this is a cause or effect remains to be elucidated.

Reactions to external agents

Dermatitis is inflammation of the epidermis. **Contact** (**irritant**) **dermatitis** is usually the result of mechanical or chemical disruption of the horny layer of the skin. Sensitivity varies greatly, and dermatitis is more likely in individuals with an excessively dry skin, in the elderly, and after childbirth. However, almost anyone can develop this form of dermatitis if the insult is sufficiently severe or prolonged. An indication of a tendency to develop such reactions may be given by the presence of thin dry skin showing numerous fine furrows on the palms and palmar surfaces of the fingers (**hyperlinearity**, Plate 11), which is a mild reaction to chronic irritants.

In some patients there is a more severe reaction, with erythema, severe irritation, swelling, vesicle formation and exudation. This may be due to **allergic dermatitis** (Plate 12), in which external agents penetrate the horny layer through minute abrasions or the hair follicles and ducts of the sweat glands. This skin penetration may be the result of low levels of IgA (surface-protective antibody). In some people the allergens bind to antigen-presenting **Langerhans cells** which then sensitize T cells in the regional lymph nodes. Because these sensitized TH cells migrate to all areas of the body via the blood, the entire skin surface becomes sensitive. After a very variable period (days to years), and usually after repeated reinforcement, subsequent contact with the agent elicits a Type IV (delayed) hypersensitivity reaction which may take 24–72 h to develop (*see* Chapter 2).

Almost any substance can sensitize the skin, but the most common agents include:

- Irritants:
  - Soaps.
  - Plants: e.g. *Compositae*, primulas.
  - Solvents (remove protective lipids).
  - Plasticizers in rubber and plastics.
- Allergens and haptens (*see* Chapter 2):
  - Dyes: e.g. hair dyes, clothing, shoes.
  - Fragrances, now included widely in household products.
  - Medicines: e.g. antibiotics, topical antihistamines and anaesthetics, wool alcohols, preservatives and antioxidants, corticosteroids.
  - Metals: e.g. nickel, chromium, cobalt.

Endogenous reactions

In **atopic eczema** there is a skin reaction to presumed systemic antigens. This occurs only in genetically predisposed subjects and is associated with a personal or family history of atopy (allergic rhinitis, hayfever, asthma and, occasionally, urticaria and migraine). It has been estimated that some 10% of the population is susceptible to this form of eczema, though only about half of these actually develop the skin reaction. The fundamental mechanism appears to be a reduced T-suppressor cell activity, and levels of circulating IgE may be increased tenfold. This results in a Type I (immediate) hypersensitivity reaction when the antigen is encountered. Levels of surface-protective antibody (IgA) are low, and this may account for the ability of allergenic substances to penetrate the skin and mucous membranes and produce systemic sensitization.

It is possible that in skin carriers of *Staphylococcus aureus* the bacteria produce superantigens which activate large numbers of T cells and so cause the release of inflammatory cytokines and excessive IgE production.

About 10% of sufferers also have a tendency to develop **chronic lichen simplex**. This causes well-defined areas of dry, roughened, itchy, hyperpigmented skin. The problem starts with attacks of itching provoked by minor stimuli. Scratching causes lichenification and the area becomes very liable to itch, thus provoking a reflex itch–scratch–itch cycle, often leading to excoriation. Infection of the damaged skin is common. The back of the neck, legs, outer forearms, groin, anal and genital areas are most frequently involved.

Food allergies are commonly blamed, though these are far less common than is popularly believed. Such allergies cannot be tested for simply, so the only approach is the use of a rigid, often unacceptable, exclusion diet with gradual replacement of individual foods or food components. This requires dedicated persistence by both dermatologist and patient over a long period. Breast feeding reduces the incidence of the disease, though it is unclear whether this results from the delayed introduction of artificial foods or is a consequence of the protective effect of maternal antibodies.

Clinical features

Contact and allergic dermatitis

The affected area is always itchy and there may be anything from mild inflammation to severe swelling and vesiculation. In **contact dermatitis** (Plate 11) the reaction is confined to the area exposed to the damaging agent. With chronic insult the horny layer disintegrates and the skin becomes thickened, dry and scaly. This leads to loss of the water-retaining property of the skin.

In **allergic dermatitis** the reaction is initially confined to the contact area and is sharply demarcated (Plate 12), though the reaction may spread widely from the original site. Continuing exposure, excoriation or infection may result in the establishment of a chronic state in both conditions.

The conditions are very common, with a prevalence of about 10–20% of occupationally exposed workers, and the condition occurring in twice as many women as men.

Atopic eczema

This often starts in the first few months of life (75% of cases; Plate 13), but may appear for the first time in children or adults. In infants it usually affects the face, scalp and extensor surfaces of the limbs, but in later years it may become more localized and chronic (Plate 14). The course is unpredictable, with occasional or frequent exacerbations and remissions up to 30–40 years of age, sometimes throughout life. In 50% of children there is a slow improvement throughout childhood, with complete remission by puberty. There is usually a personal or family history of hayfever or asthma, i.e. other forms of atopy. In some unfortunate individuals all three conditions may coexist.

Older children and adults often have localized, cracked areas in the flexures (behind the knees, elbows, on the eyelids, neck and wrists). The skin tends to be very dry in most patients, and scratching may lead to chronic lichen simplex.

Although patients with atopic eczema tend not to suffer from allergic dermatitis, exacerbations may be caused by primary irritants, stress, climatic changes and clothing, especially wool. There is an increased susceptibility to skin infections, notably warts and dermatomycoses, and herpes simplex infections may cause serious generalized illness. Acute disease may cause weeping lesions, predisposing to bacterial infection. Long-standing sufferers tend to develop cataracts in early adult life.

Seborrhoeic eczema (seborrhoeic dermatitis)

In infants this occurs as **cradle cap** (Plate 15), with thick encrusted lesions on the scalp and a papular, red eruption of the face. It may also affect the napkin area.

The adult form appears to be unrelated to the infantile one. Onset is gradual with red to yellow scaly lesions and dandruff. It may be otherwise asymptomatic, though there is often a varying degree of itch. The rash occurs mainly on the trunk, but in severe cases the perinasal area, hair line and sternal area may be affected. Facial lesions mostly occur in men. Very rarely, the condition may become more generalized; it has been ascribed to poor diet and hygiene.

Seborrhoeic eczema can be distinguished from atopic eczema in difficult cases because IgE levels and the RAST test are usually normal.

Dandruff is associated with colonization with the yeast *Pityrosporum* (*Pityrosporon*) *ovale*, though whether this is causative or is an opportunistic invader of damaged skin is unclear.

Discoid (nummular) eczema

This is relatively uncommon, with chronic, widespread discoid lesions consisting of confluent vesicles, which ooze and crust. Lesions are more common on the extensor aspects of the arms and legs and on the buttocks.

Pompholyx

This is sometimes called dishydrotic eczema or vesicular palmar eczema. As the latter name implies, the condition has a restricted skin distribution, affecting only the hands (80%) and feet – primarily the palms and soles. The term 'dishydrotic' is misleading because there is no abnormality of the sweat glands. Pompholyx usually occurs in young adults (aged 12–40 years) and may be acute, with no previous history of atopy or skin conditions, chronic or recurrent. Some cases are due to an allergic reaction to active skin disease elsewhere on the body, e.g. **tinea pedis** and **scabies**, with which it may be confused.

Initially there is an itchy or burning vesicular rash. If untreated, the vesicles coalesce to form large, fluid-filled **bullae** (blisters) that may rupture and become infected, causing pain and possibly **cellulitis** and lymphadenopathy. The chronic condition is marked by crusts, dry, cracked skin. Heat or emotion (causing sweating) may precipitate attacks.

'Varicose eczema'

This is also known as **stasis**, **gravitational** or **asteatotic** eczema. It is not a true eczema, because the underlying condition is neither allergic nor irritant, but due to poor peripheral circulation causing pooling of the blood in the lower legs, with resultant oedema. This causes capillary damage, pericapillary deposition of fibrin and poor tissue perfusion. The poorly nourished skin is hyperpigmented and is very friable and readily liable to damage by contact irritants or minor trauma. Varicose eczema is essentially a problem of elderly patients and, because smoking impairs the peripheral circulation, these are mostly men.

The condition responds poorly to treatment, especially because the circulation in the area is so poor. Steroids are largely ineffective, support stockings and occlusive tar bandages or modern absorptive or 'breathable' dressings are usually more useful. Bioengineered skin is now becoming available and apparently gives good healing. There is a tendency to chronic ulceration and infection. If poor circulation is due to atheroma of the femoral or iliac arteries, angioplasty or arterial by-pass grafting may improve the circulation substantially and with it the skin condition.

Complications

Apart from the hazard of secondary infection, the most serious complication of eczema is **exfoliative (erythrodermic) dermatitis**, in which there is a gradual onset of widespread inflammation and scaling. This occurs mainly in middle-aged men. Patients feel generally unwell with hypothermia and rigors due to impairment of temperature regulation consequent on extensive skin damage.

Management

Diagnosis

A **careful history and examination** (pp. 676–678) is essential to identify any possible allergen or irritant. Patch tests may be used to identify or confirm contact allergens in allergic dermatitis. However, in atopic eczema intradermal prick tests and, especially, the **RAST procedure** (*see* Chapter 5, Fig. 5.16) are used.

Because of the limited repertoire of skin reactions there is a possibility of confusion with other skin diseases and, especially, with reactions to serious systemic conditions (p. 681; Table 12.6) such as lymphomas, systemic lupus erythematosus (*see* Chapter 8, pp. 511–514) and skin infestations, e.g. scabies.

Aims

The aims of management are:

- Patient education and reassurance.
- Avoidance of identifiable precipitating or aggravating factors and prevention of recurrence and chronicity.
- Relief of troublesome symptoms, e.g. itch, dry and fissuring skin, moist or weeping lesions, sleep loss.
- Control of the disease.

General principles

The general principles of management are as follows:

- **Patient education and reassurance.** Because there is no specific, curative pharmacotherapy patients may have to learn to manage their symptoms over a long period. A positive, encouraging outlook on the part of the doctor, nurse and pharmacist is important. Patients should also be aware of what it is reasonable to expect from treatment.
- **Avoid precipitants**, especially soaps and detergents, airborne allergens, plants, medicaments and occupational triggers. Minimize vigorous washing in hot water which dries the skin by removing sebum lipids: wash in cool water using an emollient, e.g. aqueous cream (*see* Table 12.9). Complete avoidance is often difficult or impossible, but career choice, e.g. avoiding hairdressing, nursing or contact with lubricating oils, may be important.
- **Control itching** with the liberal use of emollients (*see* Table 12.9), especially for dry skin, and systemic antihistamines, e.g. hydroxyzine. Finding a suitable emollient and using it freely is the cornerstone of eczema management, and will minimize the need for corticosteroids. An emollient alone, used freely, may be adequate in mild disease. Bland topical antipruritics (p. 685) may also help.
- Use drying (astringent) lotions for **moist or weeping lesions** (0.01% potassium permanganate or aluminium acetate lotion). If large areas are affected, potassium permanganate baths can be used (*see* Table 12.8).
- **Control inflammation** with the mildest possible product. Coal tar is used occasionally. However, topical corticosteroids form the essential component of active eczema treatment (p. 687), used in the most appropriate pharmaceutical dosage form (cream, gel, lotion, ointment) for the shortest possible time.
- **Oral corticosteroids.** In **severe disease** with marked systemic symptoms, high doses may be required for a short time to gain control rapidly. The treatment can then be stopped abruptly if it has lasted for less than 3 weeks and relapse is unlikely. Alternatively, the dose can be stepped down rapidly to about 7.5 mg prednisolone (or its equivalent) daily and then more slowly. Careful supervision is needed to avoid relapse. The objective is to move progressively to minimal use of a mild topical corticosteroid or complete discontinuation. If treatment has been more prolonged, follows a longer course within the preceding year or doses greater than 40 mg prednisolone daily have been used, more gradual dosage reduction is necessary. If withdrawal is too abrupt, acute glucocorticoid insufficiency (Addison's disease) may result.
- Pay careful attention to **skin hygiene: control infection promptly** with systemic antibiotics, after taking swabs for sensitivity testing. Multi-resistant *Staphylococcus aureus* (MRSA; *see* Chapter 13) and beta-haemolytic streptococci may be implicated.

It is difficult to be more precise about treatment, because patients vary very widely in their symptoms and in the ways in which they react to medication. Most patients with chronic disease eventually settle down to a particular regimen of emollients and topical corticosteroids which they find suits them best, more vigorous treatment being used to treat exacerbations, as appropriate. A *lithium/zinc ointment* is available for the treatment of seborrhoeic dermatitis and appears to be effective, largely non-irritant and suitable for facial use. However, it must not be used near the eyes or on mucous membranes.

Second- and third-line therapies include:

- Hospital admission for intensive or systemic therapies.
- *Gamolenic acid* (evening primrose oil) may possibly be beneficial at any stage as an adjunct to other therapy, but this is controversial. It is not without side effects, e.g. headache and gastrointestinal discomfort and may even cause pruritus, and must be used cautiously in pregnancy and if there is a history of epilepsy.
- *Phototherapy* or *PUVA* (p. 696).
- **Immunosuppressants**: e.g. *azathioprine* or *ciclosporin* (cyclosporine).

Exfoliative dermatitis is a life-threatening condition. Rest, a high-protein diet to replace the serum proteins lost through the extensively damaged skin, and the use of high-dose systemic steroids comprise the normal treatment mode, plus the specific management of any underlying cause – if one can be identified.

Acne

Definition

Acne is a disorder of the pilosebaceous (hair) follicles and is characterized by excessive sebum production, **comedones** (blackheads), papules and pustules (whiteheads). The lesions occur primarily on the face, but the upper chest, back and arms, etc. may be affected in severe cases – that is, any area where pilosebaceous follicles occur. Only the palms and soles are spared completely.

Epidemiology

Acne affects adolescents of both sexes in industrialized societies, females being affected at a slightly earlier age (10–17 years) than males (14–19 years). The condition is rare in infancy, but the incidence rises sharply with the onset of puberty, and about 80% of the 12- to 18-year age group is affected to some extent. Some 70% of cases remit spontaneously after about 5 years, and most of the remainder improve slowly thereafter. However, acne occasionally persists into late adulthood, affecting five times as many women (5%) as men, though men tend to be more severely affected as a consequence of their higher androgen levels.

Although more common in cold climates and industrialized areas, acne may be aggravated by hot, humid conditions once established.

Pathology and aetiology

The underlying problem seems to be an exaggerated response of the pilosebaceous units to normal levels of circulating androgens, causing increased sebum production.

Because the composition of the sebum is altered, there is hyperkeratosis in the mouth of the follicular duct and outflow of sebum is blocked, causing gross enlargement of the pilosebaceous follicles. Saprophytic bacteria, notably *Propionibacterium acnes*, are trapped in the follicle and produce inflammatory substances from the sebum, so that the follicles become surrounded by inflammatory (polymorphonuclear and lymphoid) cells. Excessive production of free fatty acids in the sebum may initiate blockage of the follicles and maintain the inflammatory response.

Oxidation of tyrosine at the surface of the trapped sebum by tyrosinase and oxygen produces **melanin**, staining the sebum to give the characteristic black comedone – blackheads are not due to dirty skin. Although bacterial activity exacerbates the condition there is no evidence that acne is infective in origin. In some cases rupture of comedones releases their contents into the underlying tissues, causes an intense dermal inflammation (**cystic acne**).

There is a genetic predisposition with a familial association, and the condition is aggravated by stress, hormones (premenstrually) and a hot climate. Certain **drugs** may aggravate acne or cause an acneiform reaction as a side effect (Table 12.15). An environmental or iatrogenic cause is probable whenever acne occurs in an older patient or in an unusual facial distribution.

It has been alleged that acne is due to a poor, fatty diet, but this is without foundation.

Clinical features

Acne is so common and usually has such a characteristic appearance that the diagnosis is seldom in doubt. Onset is gradual, initially with blackheads and whiteheads, progressing to inflamed nodules. The skin and scalp are greasy and dandruff is usually present.

Pustules and deep cysts occur in some patients if the condition is not controlled. Cysts eventually heal to leave permanent, characteristic depressed scars. Cystic acne which is aggravated by a hot climate may be very resistant to treatment and improve only with a move to a more temperate climate.

Because the onset usually coincides with the period of increased sexual awareness, and the lesions are visible and often unsightly, there is always emotional and psychological disturbance, sometimes severe. This may lead to aggressive or reclusive behaviour.

Occasionally there may be a confusion with:

• Rosacea (see below).
• Perioral dermatitis (Plate 3), sometimes caused by the inappropriate use of synthetic topical steroids around the mouth, may also give an inflamed, pustular eruption but comedones and a greasy skin are absent.
• Atopic eczema (p. 704).
• Seborrhoeic eczema (p. 705).

Because the management of these differ from that of acne a firm diagnosis is essential.

Management

Aims

The aims of management are:

• To encourage an optimistic outlook and ensure perseverance and compliance with therapy.

Table 12.15 Some iatrogenic and environmental causes of acne-like eruptions

Iatrogenic

Hormones: *corticosteroids, corticotrophins, androgens, anabolic steroids, gonadotrophins*
Halogenated drugs: e.g. *halothane, hexachlorophane, hyoscine butylbromide, ipratropium bromide, propantheline bromide, bromocriptine* (rarely)
Some antitubercular drugs: e.g. *isoniazid, rifampicin*
Some anticonvulsants: e.g. *phenytoin, phenobarbital, trimethadione*
Psychotropic drugs: e.g. *lithium, maprotiline, chloral hydrate*
Sulphur-containing drugs: e.g. *disulfiram, thioureylenes, thiouracils*
Miscellaneous: *dactinomycin, antibiotics*[a], *cyanocobalamin, ciclosporin* (cyclosporine), *quinine*

Environmental, occupational, etc.

Cosmetics, especially 'heavy' or oily products
Oily sunscreens
Mineral oils
Creosote, pitch, tar
Chlorinated aromatic compounds[b], polychlorbiphenyls, herbicides, preservatives

[a] Due to colonization of lesions with resistant bacteria or *Candida albicans*.
[b] Cause chloracne.

- To prevent disfiguring scarring.
- To unblock the ducts of the sebaceous glands by:
  - Reducing sebum production.
  - Reducing keratinocyte activity in the duct.
  - Loosening the keratin plugs, thus achieving a free flow of sebum.
- To suppress the growth of bacteria which produce inflammatory substances.

General measures

The types of treatment used are outlined in Table 12.16, and a flow chart for the treatment of acne is given in Fig. 12.7.

Patients should be advised sympathetically of an optimistic outcome, because acne can be treated very successfully, though not cured, with safe medication. Complete healing occurs in most cases. However, rapid improvement must not be expected, successful treatment requiring at least 6 months of treatment. The improvement rate is approximately as follows:

- 4–6 weeks, some improvement.
- 2–3 months, 40% improvement.
- 6 months, 75% improvement.

Patients should be taught appropriate self-management. Because most of them tend to have rather sensitive skins, any new treatment should be initiated cautiously at the lowest available concentration. Detergent washes may help by reducing greasiness, but excessively frequent or vigorous treatment is undesirable. Greasy make-up should be avoided.

Good compliance is essential for success, most failures being associated with lack of perseverance or non-adherence to the correct method of use of medication. Initially, once-daily use on a restricted area for 4–5 days will detect the possibility of a severe reaction, before using twice-daily over the whole area. The intensity of treatment can then be increased stepwise.

Patients should avoid squeezing comedones, because this may cause or exacerbate permanent scarring by forcing infected sebum into surrounding tissue, causing intense inflammation. Exposure to sun and wind may be helpful, by promoting skin peeling, but may aggravate reactions to medications.

Topical pharmacotherapy

Skin reaction to treatment
Some degree of inflammation and scaling is inevitable with most treatments (except adapalene), and is desirable because it indicates that they are working. However, inflammation should

Table 12.16   Types of treatment used for acne therapy

Aim	Mode of action	Class of agent	Examples
Reduction of:			
Scarring	Loosening of keratin plugs	Keratolytic	*Benzoyl peroxide* *Salicylic acid/sulphur preparations*
		Retinoid	*Tretinoin*
Keratin production	Antiproliferative	Retinoid	*Isotretinoin*
		Corticosteroid[a]	*Hydrocortisone, methylprednisolone*
Inflammation	Reduce skin flora	Antimicrobial	*Benzoyl peroxide, clindamycin, erythromycin, tetracyclines, potassium hydroxyquinoline sulphate*
Sebum production	Hormonal regulation	Anti-androgens plus oestrogen	*Cyproterone–ethinylestradiol*
	Regulation of cell activity	Retinoids	*Isotretinoin, tazarotene, tretinoin*

[a] Topical corticosteroids should not normally be used for acne, though commercial preparations containing them are available.

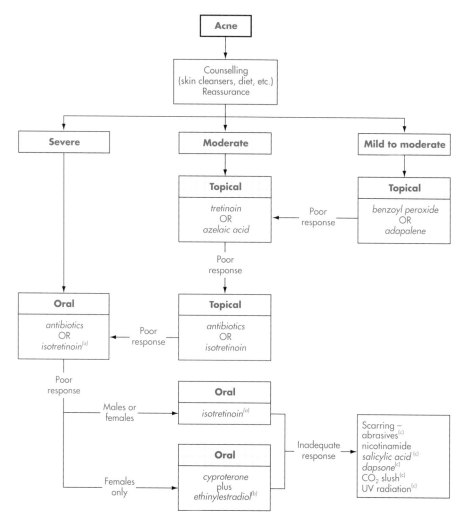

Figure 12.7   Flow chart for the treatment of acne. [a] **Oral** isotretinoin is highly teratogenic. Strict contraceptive precautions are essential. [b] Acts as a contraceptive pill. [c] These agents are of dubious value and are not generally recommended. They are suitable only for specialist use.

not be too severe and it is advisable to have a 1-to 2-day 'drug holiday' after a moderate reaction, before recommencing treatment. An area larger than that currently affected should be treated, but the area around the eyes must be avoided.

Patients using *benzoyl peroxide* or *tretinoin* should avoid bright sunshine and exposure to UV 'sun' lamps, which may produce photosensitive reactions, and there is a possibility of an increased incidence of skin tumours with tretinoin.

Inflamed comedonal lesions

Benzoyl peroxide. This mildly bactericidal keratolytic agent is one of the most effective treatments for mild disease. It is available in a variety of formulations in concentrations of 2.5–10%. Patients with sensitive skins should start with 2.5% once daily, otherwise the 5% products are satisfactory. The aim is to build up to use of the 10% product twice daily, if tolerated. The skin irritation is believed to be associated with the activity of the drug and often subsides as treatment proceeds.

No benefit has been shown for preparations with added sulphur, though products with added antimicrobials, e.g. *erythromycin, hydroxyquinoline, miconazole*, are available (see below).

Patients should be warned that benzoyl peroxide may bleach clothing.

Azelaic acid. This very well-tolerated dicarboxylic acid appears to act by interfering with the mitochondrial function in melanocytes and, presumably, in other basal layer and pilosebaceous cells. It also has antimicrobial properties and is similarly effective to benzoyl peroxide and, additionally, may prevent post-inflammatory hyperpigmentation in dark-skinned patients.

Azelaic acid is not normally used in pregnant or breast-feeding women, and should not be used near the eyes.

Antibiotics. Topical antimicrobial treatment is popular because it avoids the problems associated with long-term systemic use. However, skin sensitization may occur (neomycin is no longer used for this reason) and resistant strains may be encouraged. Because of this it is preferable to use benzoyl peroxide, azelaic acid or adapalene first. Further, antimicrobials are not usually used for longer than 10–12 weeks, though if a response occurs the course may be repeated after a gap of 3–4 weeks, to minimize resistance, which is an increasing problem.

Lotions containing *erythromycin, clindamycin* and *tetracycline* are useful for mild to moderate inflammatory acne. Topical solutions of clindamycin and erythromycin are formulated with alcohol and may not be suitable if benzoyl peroxide is being used concurrently, so some topical solutions are reconstituted as required from powder.

Combinations of erythromycin with benzoyl peroxide or zinc acetate may help to minimize antibiotic resistance.

Retinoids. *Adapalene* is a new topical compound, formulated as a 3- to 10 micron microcrystalline suspension in a gel base. This particle size gives good penetration into the pilosebaceous follicles. Adapalene achieves most of the aims of treatment, having three clinical effects: it is comedolytic, it loosens the keratin plugs and reduces sebum production and the inflammation caused by the irritant effect of sebum on damaged tissue. The specificity of adapalene results in good tolerance. Although adapalene seems to provide a faster response than tretinoin, the overall outcomes of the two drugs appear similar.

An important advantage of retinoids over antibiotics is that retinoids have no effect on *P. acnes* resistance. Further, adapalene does not interact with other treatments and is very stable.

Severe comedonal acne

Because *retinoids* (p. 689) normalize development of follicular keratinocytes they are used when there are numerous comedones. *Tretinoin (all-trans*-retinoic acid) is keratolytic and is available as a cream, gel or lotion in concentrations of 0.01% and 0.025%. The lower of these should be used for patients with sensitive skins, or as a starter dose.

Because it causes photosensitivity reactions, *tretinoin* should not be used with UV lamps, and exposure to sunlight should be minimized. Some patients do better by using this in the morning and benzoyl peroxide at night, but both products should not be applied simultaneously.

Tretinoin is contraindicated in pregnancy (contraceptive precautions should be taken in women of child-bearing age), eczema, on broken or sunburned skin and if there is a history of cutaneous malignancy.

Isotretinoin is an isomer of tretinoin with similar properties. It is available as a 0.05% gel, with or without erythromycin. *Adapalene* is a more recent introduction which resembles the retinoids and is licensed in the UK for treating mild to moderate acne. The contraindications are similar to those for tretinoin. Treatment should be stopped if it causes severe irritation.

Other topical treatments

Nicotinamide gel promotes skin peeling and may be useful. It tends to cause dryness and irritation, and the frequency of application should be reduced if these reactions are not tolerated.

UV radiation is occasionally used to promote skin peeling in resistant acne, but it must be used cautiously if there is any evidence of photosensitivity; in addition, the eyes must be protected. All topical treatments irritate the skin to some extent and make it particularly UV sensitive.

Exfoliation has also been achieved using *glycolic acid* or by swabbing with a solid carbon dioxide–acetone slush.

Corticosteroids are not recommended for use in acne treatment because they aggravate the condition, and the more potent steroids may cause irreversible skin damage (p. 688; Plate 16). Further, *sulphur* and *salicylic acid* preparations, and debridement with mild abrasives, are not considered to be helpful and should no longer be used.

Superficial facial damage has been treated with exfoliating agents and deeper scarring with injections of *collagen*.

Systemic pharmacotherapy

This is required in moderate to severe cases unresponsive to topical treatment. It may be advisable to **continue topical therapy** for up to 1–2 years, **concurrently** with systemic treatment: exceptional cases may need continued topical therapy for some 10–12 years, though this should not be necessary if retinoids or full doses of antibiotics are used.

Antibiotics

If topical antibiotics fail to give significant improvement after 2 months, then systemic antibiotics are used.

For optimal effect, *erythromycin*, *tetracyclines* or *doxycycline* should be used at normal, full antibiotic doses until the lesions have resolved completely. This may take at least 6 months, the dose then being tapered to zero over the ensuing month or two. Although doses lower than those used for normal antibiotic use are common, they are less effective and run the risk of failure due to resistance, although there is less risk of side effects. Antibiotics may occasionally exacerbate acne due to colonization of the lesions with resistant bacteria, usually Gram-negatives or *Candida albicans*. Repeat courses of antibiotics may be needed and do not appear to be commonly associated with problems of bacterial resistance or excessive side effects (*see* Chapter 13).

Tetracyclines should be used with the usual precautions regarding timing of doses in relation to food and other medications. If compliance is a problem, *doxycycline* (once-daily) or *minocycline* (twice-daily) may be preferred; in fact, the latter has been reported to be more effective than tetracycline, possibly because of less resistance problems. However, minocycline may cause a lupus-like syndrome and a bluish/brown skin discoloration: the drug should be stopped immediately if either of these reactions occur. Tetracyclines are unsuitable for children under 12 years of age.

If there is no response after 2 months, or if there is a deterioration or a recurrence during treatment, a change should be made to a second-line antibiotic, e.g. *clindamycin* or *trimethoprim*. Alternatively, if treatment has been initiated in community practice the patient should be referred to a specialist clinic.

Hormone therapy

If an oral contraceptive is being used, a change to one with a higher oestrogen content may be helpful (if tolerated), on order to increase the anti-androgenic activity.

Resistant acne in females may be treated with a *cyproterone–ethinylestradiol combination*, which reduces sebum secretion by 30%. A clear improvement is usually apparent after several months: the product must not be used in males.

Isotretinoin

Patients with pustules or severe cystic acne, or who are unresponsive after 2 months of antibiotic treatment, may need hospital referral. Late-onset acne (at 30–50 years) is also usually resistant to antibiotics. Unresponsive acne usually responds dramatically to *isotretinoin* (p. 691), often with lasting improvement. Isotretinoin causes a marked inhibition of sebum gland activity and complete or nearly complete remission in about 12–16 weeks. Sebum production may remain at low levels for up to a year or so after stopping treatment. Consequently, many acne patients experience long periods of remission with isotretinoin, though men under 25 years of age are more likely to relapse. There is also a secondary anti-inflammatory effect.

There is a long catalogue of side effects associated with isotretinoin (*see* Table 12.12). Because of its toxicity, long-term isotretinoin administration may be unjustified for treating a minor disease state such as acne, although the condition is admittedly potentially disfiguring. Repeat courses are inadvisable. The oral form is available in the UK only through hospital consultants, and through them to named community pharmacies. Sore eyes, cracked lips and dry, peeling skin are common and can be managed with *hypromellose eye drops* and emollients, respectively. Because isotretinoin is teratogenic, fertile women must take strict contraceptive measures, starting 1 month before initiating treatment and continuing for at least 1 month after stopping.

Isotretinoin is contraindicated in pregnancy and in patients with hyperlipidaemia or abnormal liver function.

Other treatments

A small trial of *colchicine* in antibiotic-resistant acne has been reported to produce up to 70% improvement, especially in severe cystic nodular disease. This is the subject of further trial, which will need to demonstrate tolerance of this rather toxic drug, notably the absence of diarrhoea.

Dapsone is used occasionally if other treatments fail.

Rosacea

Definition and epidemiology

Rosacea is a chronic inflammatory condition, characterized by reddish, acneiform lesions of the face and forehead and telangiectases, without comedones. Although less common than acne, rosacea affects about 1% of dermatological outpatients in the UK. In contrast to acne, rosacea is much more common in women, especially during and after the menopause.

Aetiology and clinical features

The pathology of rosacea is unknown, but it may be familial. The condition is provoked by anything causing persistent flushing of the face. The flushing correlates with:

- Perimenopausal incidence, especially if the menopause is prolonged.
- Alcoholism and ingestion of spicy foods.
- Exposure to bright sunshine and high winds (there is a high incidence in outdoor workers).

Unlike acne, rosacea occurs only on the face and in an older age group. Although there are no comedones, there is more generalized inflammation and the skin is dry. New facial capillaries develop and these dilate to form **telangiectasia**. Hypertrophy of the sebaceous glands may cause **rhinophyma**, with a bulbous, reddened nose, primarily in male alcoholics. **Ocular involvement** is a serious complication.

Pharmacotherapy

Mild rosacea may not require treatment unless it is causing psychological distress. Mild to moderate disease is treated empirically with topical *metronidazole* gel or cream, or any of the topical antibiotics used for acne. However, those with an alcoholic base may aggravate flushing. Emollients may be useful.

Moderate to severe rosacea and resistant disease requires the use of high-dose *antibiotics*; e.g. 1–2 g/day of *erythromycin* or *tetracycline*, 100–200 mg/day *minocycline*. Topical agents should be continued. The benefit of antibiotics is probably due their mild toxicity to epidermal cells.

Antibiotics may be ineffective against erythema and flushing: a *beta-blocker* can help with the former and, paradoxically, 4% topical *nicotinamide* with the latter, but this may be very irritant. Low-dose *clonidine* (25 micrograms, twice-daily) may also help to control flushing, but has potentially serious side effects including depression. This is clearly undesirable in a patient who is already depressed because of their condition.

Ocular involvement requires specialist ophthalmological management. **Rhinophyma** is dealt with by plastic surgery, nowadays usually by high-frequency diathermy or laser therapy, which may give long-term benefit.

Urticaria

Definition

The condition involves transient, pruritic, chronic or recurrent inflammatory weals, plaques and papules. It is also known as **nettlerash** and, mostly in North America, as hives.

The weals are raised, oedematous lesions, that are very variable in size and extent. Hereditary **angioedema** (angioneurotic oedema) involves larger areas of the subcutaneous tissues and dermis, producing gross swelling.

There is an arbitrary distinction between **acute and chronic urticaria**. The acute form persists for <30 days before remission occurs, with recurrences after variable periods, whereas chronic urticaria involves episodes lasting for >30 days.

Pathology and aetiology

The condition can have various causes (Table 12.17):

- Immunological, mediated by IgE, complement components or immune complexes (*see* Chapter 2).

- Physical, caused by several external agents, including drugs.

Whatever the mechanism, the final result is gross dilatation of the skin capillaries, allowing the escape of fluid, and sometimes leucocytes and less frequently erythrocytes, from the circulation into the dermis, i.e. localized oedema. The escape of erythrocytes causes a purpuric rash (p. 681) which may leave residual pigmentation.

Acute urticaria is usually due to a Type I (allergic) reaction in atopic subjects, which releases histamine from mast cells. This can be due to numerous stimuli (Table 12.17).

The underlying mechanisms in **chronic urticaria**, i.e. urticaria persisting for more than 6 weeks, are unknown in 80–90% of cases, but may be:

- Immune complex disease (*see* Chapter 2) coupled with a defective complement cascade, e.g. lack of inhibition of C3a by carboxypeptidase B permits an ongoing reaction.
- Abnormalities of the arachidonic acid–eicosanoid pathway (*see* Chapter 8), evidenced by sensitivity to *salicylates* and *indometacin*.
- Chronic infection, e.g. *Helicobacter pylori* (*see* Chapter 6).

Table 12.17   Aetiology of urticaria

Immunological reactions

Hypersensitivity:
Mediated by IgE
Foods: meat, shellfish, eggs, nuts (especially peanuts), wheat gluten, strawberries, additives (benzoates, tartrazine)
Environmental allergens: house dust (mites), feathers
Drugs releasing histamine: especially *aspirin* and *salicylates, indometacin, codeine, morphine, penicillins*, radiocontrast agents
Parasitic infestations (intestinal worms, fleas, lice)
Chronic diseases: infections (sinus, urinary), thyrotoxicosis, systemic lupus erythematosus, lymphomas

Mediated by complement (especially hereditary angioedema)
Antibodies (sera, immunoglobulins), blood products

Physical

Cold, heat, sunlight, pressure (clothing), rubbing, vibration, vigorous exercise

Psychogenic, idiopathic

- Autoimmune disease:
  - IgG auto-antibody reacting with IgE cross-linked to receptor sites.
  - There is a linkage between autoimmune mast cell disease and autoimmune thyroid disease in about 15% of patients, so thyroid function tests may be indicated.
  - Some patients with systemic lupus erythematosus and Sjögren's syndrome (*see* Chapter 8, pp. 511–515) have an urticarial vasculitis.

Hereditary angioedema is a severe, episodic, autosomal dominantly inherited disorder that affects the face, larynx, extremities and gut. It is associated with an abnormal or deficient C1 esterase inhibitor, allowing excessive bradykinin formation. The condition is sometimes associated with perivascular leucocytosis and eosinophilia in the area of lesions. Chronic urticaria may coexist with angioedema.

Clinical features and diagnosis

Acute urticaria is described by the symptoms. There are transient (hours) pruritic weals, which may vary in size from 1–2 mm to 10–80 mm or be widespread; these may be oval, annular or may follow bizarre shapes and patterns. The weals are usually pink, though larger lesions have a light central area with an erythematous margin. The weals occur commonly on pressure areas, hands, feet and trunk, especially exposed areas.

Hereditary angioedema affecting the lips, tongue and neck is one of the few dermatological emergencies because it may compromise respiration. The weals characteristic of other forms of urticaria do not occur, but tissue swelling may be moderate to gross; in some cases the patient becomes completely unrecognizable. Abdominal involvement causes severe pain.

About 25% of sufferers have **chronic urticaria**. This occurs in the age range 10–50 years, most commonly in the 20- to 40-year group, and about twice as many women as men are affected. The symptoms are similar to those of the acute form, though some patients have symptoms lasting 20 years or more. Patients tend to be intolerant of salicylates and benzoates. Some aetiologies can be determined by simple challenge tests:

- Cold: application of an ice cube for 10 min gives a weal within 5 min of removal.
- Solar: exposure to an UV or powerful sun lamp for 30–120 sec gives weals within 30 min.
- Cholinergic: a hot shower produces weals on the neck, limbs and trunk.
- Pressure: firm pressure perpendicular to the skin gives a persistent weal after 1–4 h.

Apart from pressure-related forms, these tend to be associated with angioedema, so prompt treatment needs to be available.

Management

The management of urticaria involves:

- Avoidance of known precipitants.
- *Antihistamines* (both H_1 and sometimes H_2 blockers), e.g. *astemizole, cetirizine, fexofenadine* or *mizolastine* during the day, *hydroxyzine* or another sedating antihistamine at night (*see* pp. 685–686 for side effects): *ranitidine* may also help. *Doxepin* has both antihistaminic and antidepressant properties and is useful for patients depressed by their condition.
- *Corticosteroids:*
  - A moderate potency topical steroid for most patients.
  - Oral *prednisolone*: for severe reactions, especially angioedema. The very severe throat swelling of those suffering from **hereditary angioedema** needs IV *hydrocortisone* and SC *adrenaline* (*epinephrine*).
- Severe resistant urticaria may respond to *ciclosporin* (*cyclosporine*) or to *human immunoglobulin.*
- *Danazol* may be helpful for the long-term treatment of hereditary angioedema (unlicensed indication in the UK).
- Whole fresh plasma, C1 esterase inhibitors and plasmapheresis: these methods are successful with the immune complex form of urticaria because they remove circulating antigen–antibody complexes.

Drug-induced skin disease

Skin eruptions are one of the most common manifestations of systemic or topical drug therapy (Table 12.18). Probably every pharmaceutical product has the potential to cause dermatoses – even topical steroids – though this is very unlikely with hydrocortisone. The reactions may be immunological in character and cover the whole range of skin manifestations.

The systemic use of drugs may cause lesions that may be:

* Bullous or vesicular, e.g. *sulphonamides*.
* Erythematous, e.g. *antisera*.
* Lichenoid, e.g. *antimalarials, gold, phenothiazines*.
* Photosensitive, e.g. *chlorpromazine, sulphonamides*.
* Pruritic, e.g. *tetracyclines*.
* Purpuric, e.g. *barbiturates, chloramphenicol, aspirin*.
* Urticarial (see above).

One rather unusual type of response is the **fixed drug eruption**, which is characterized by a skin reaction in the same localized sites on each occasion that the drug is taken. If the reaction occurs repeatedly, there may be persistent pigmentation of the site – even in the absence of the drug and of an overt skin reaction. Common causes are barbiturates and phenolphthalein.

Serious systemic reactions may occur, such as **Stevens–Johnson syndrome**, with a severe rash, high fever, joint pains and painful involvement of the mucous membranes. This needs expert diagnosis and management, using rest, antibiotics and high-dose corticosteroids.

Topical manifestations include any of those described above under 'eczema and dermatitis' (p. 703).

The skin as a route for systemic drug delivery

Transdermal (percutaneous) administration is a technique for delivering drugs systemically at a controlled rate over a relatively prolonged period: it is not used for the topical treatment of

---

Table 12.18   Some side effects of drugs on the skin[a]

Side effect	Examples of drugs which may cause the adverse reaction
Exanthematous eruptions (erythemas or widespread macular rashes)	*Amitriptyline, barbiturates, diuretics, gold salts, suphonylureas, penicillins (especially ampicillin), penicillamine, suphonamides*
Urticaria	*Antisera, aspirin, cephalosporins, penicillins,* X-ray contrast media
Fixed drug eruptions	*Barbiturates, chlordiazepoxide, metronidazole, phenolphthalein, sulphonamides*
Acneiform reactions	*Androgens, anti-epileptics, antitubercular drugs, bromides, corticosteroids, iodides*
Photoallergic and phototoxic reactions	*Antibiotics, chlorpromazine, sulphonamides, sulphonylureas, thiazides*
Eczematous reactions	*Anaesthetics* (local), *antibiotics, antihistamines* (topical), *methyldopa*
Exfoliative dermatitis	*Carbamazepine, gold salts* and heavy metals, *isoniazid, phenindione, streptomycin*
Purpuras	*Indometacin, quinine, sulphonamides, thiazides*

[a] Systemic use, except where indicated. Excludes reactions to vehicles, antioxidants, preservatives, etc.

skin diseases. Details of this subject concern the formulation pharmacist and are not pertinent here (*see* References and further reading).

The principal barrier to drug penetration of the skin is the horny layer. 'Shunt routes' through the hair follicles and sweat glands are significant in the early stages after application, but only for some electrolytes and highly polar corticosteroids and antibiotics, which penetrate keratin poorly. These shunt routes are important because they probably represent the principal routes of penetration and systemic absorption of the topical corticosteroids, though they contribute only marginally to the steady-state flux across the epidermis for many agents. Once past the horny layer, the drug molecules rapidly penetrate the living tissues of the epidermis and dermis and are swept away into the circulation.

The skin also acts as a drug reservoir, due to:

- Binding by proteins in the horny layer, giving a persistence of up to 2–3 weeks after application has ceased.
- Concentration of lipophilic agents in the fatty tissues in the dermis, from which they leach gradually into the circulation. However, this mechanism contributes little to any effect that the product may have on most skin problems, which are generally epidermal in origin.

Factors relevant to penetration include:

- Concentration of the drug.
- Formulation of the product.
- Mode of use (occlusion and greasy vehicles enhance skin penetration).

- Contact time.
- Site of application (the skin behind the ears is very thin and may be the preferred site).
- Patient age: young children and the elderly have readily penetrable skin.
- Features of the disease state, e.g. inflammation enhances drug penetration.

Factors affecting possible side effects are the skin type (fair-skinned people are more likely to suffer an adverse reaction) and the potential of the formulated product to cause skin problems, e.g. rashes due to the drug, preservatives, adhesives, plastics, etc.

Finally, patients have to find the patches cosmetically acceptable.

References and further reading

Breathnach SM, Hintner H (1992) *Adverse Drug Reactions and the Skin.* Oxford: Blackwell Science.

Chien YW (1992) Transdermal drug delivery and delivery systems. In: Chien YW (ed.) *Novel Drug Delivery Systems.* New York: Marcel Dekker.

Fitzpatrick TB, Johnson RA, Wolff K, *et al.* (1997) *Color Atlas and Synopsis of Clinical Dermatology.* 3rd edn. New York: McGraw-Hill.

Hallworth RB (1998) Prevention and treatment of postmenopausal osteoporosis. *Pharm World Sci* **20**: 198–205.

Mackie RM (1996) *Clinical Dermatology: An Illustrated Text.* 4th edn. Oxford: Oxford University Press.

Solomons B (1996) *Lecture Notes on Dermatology.* 7th edn. Oxford: Blackwell Science.

13

Infections and antimicrobial therapy

At some point in their life, everybody is likely to suffer an infection that will require treatment with antimicrobial agents. However, such an infection is unlikely to prove fatal unless there is some underlying chronic condition or complication. Yet, only 50 years ago death from acute infection was common and antimicrobial chemotherapy was still in its infancy.

Antimicrobial chemotherapy began with the introduction of the sulphonamides in the 1930s, and this was followed closely by penicillin in the 1940s. The original *benzylpenicillin* (penicillin G) had the largest impact on the early therapeutics of infection, but now has only limited applications. This illustrates the important principle that the therapeutics of infectious disease must be developed continually in order to remain effective. Compare this situation with that of diabetes, for example, in which the major therapeutic advance was made in the 1920s with the introduction of insulin. Essentially the same treatment has been in use up to the present day. The disease itself has neither changed nor 'adapted' to the treatment. By contrast, the staphylococcal organism against which *benzylpenicillin* was originally so dramatically effective is now almost universally resistant to antibiotics.

Introduction

The constantly changing pattern of organism sensitivity has been the principal factor contributing to the proliferation of antimicrobial agents. Most of this chapter is devoted to the treatment of bacterial infections but similar principles apply to the treatment of fungal and viral infections. We use the term **antimicrobials** when describing chemotherapeutic agents generally, and **antibacterial**, **antifungal** and **antiviral** for those used specifically to treat bacterial, fungal or viral infections. The older term, antibiotic was applied only to those agents derived from living organisms, usually fungal or bacterial. The chemotherapy of neoplastic disease is discussed in Chapter 11.

Although there is a very wide range of antibacterials available, patients may commonly be prescribed agents from among the penicillin, cephalosporin, macrolide, tetracycline or quinolone groups. Yet a lower urinary tract bacterial infection is most likely to be due to *Escherichia coli* – an organism against which only some of these agents are effective. How can the prescriber choose the most appropriate antimicrobial treatment for a particular infection? The first part of this chapter describes the various groups of antimicrobial agents, and then discusses the principles of selection by considering the various steps in the decision-making process that should be taken when diagnosing and treating an infection. The final part of the chapter will consider the application of these principles in the treatment of some important infections.

Before considering individual agents, we should review a simple classification system for microorganisms and examine the concept of minimum inhibitory concentration.

Classification of microorganisms

Bacteria may variously be classified as described in Table 13.1: **Gram-positive** or **Gram-negative** (depending on whether the bacterial cell wall retains the Gram stain used for microscopical investigation); **aerobic**, **anaerobic** or **facultative** (depending on metabolic processes); and the bacterial shape. *Escherichia coli* is therefore described as an aerobic, Gram-negative rod. Refinements of classification include whether a stain

Table 13.1   Some ways of classifying bacteria

Classification method	Criterion	Classes	Examples
Gram stain	Retention of stain by cell wall	Gram-positive	*Staphylococcus aureus*
		Gram-negative	*Pseudomonas aeruginosa*
Metabolism	Oxygen requirements	Anaerobe	*Bacteroides* spp.
		Aerobe	*Streptococcus pneumoniae*
		Facultative anaerobe	*Staphylococcus* spp.
Morphology	Microscopic appearance	Rod	*Escherichia coli*
		Coccus	*Neisseria meningitidis*
		Spirochaete	*Treponema pallidum*
Source	Resident in GI tract	Enterobacteria	*Escherichia coli*
Structure	Cell wall	Most bacteria	
	No cell wall	Mycoplasmas	*Mycoplasma pneumoniae*

GI, gastrointestinal.

cannot be removed by acid (acid-fast) or if they are found in the human gastrointestinal tract (e.g. *Enterobacter*). This will enable the prediction of likely sensitivities to antibacterials.

In general, it is more difficult for antibacterials to penetrate the cell wall of Gram-negative organisms than Gram-positive ones.

Antibacterials that are predominantly effective against a restricted range of either Gram-positive or (less commonly) Gram-negative organisms are said to posses a **narrow spectrum** of activity, whereas those that are effective against a range of both types of organism are termed **broad spectrum**. Anaerobes may be either Gram-positive (e.g. the clostridia) or Gram-negative (e.g. *Bacteroides* spp.) and usually require special groups of agents. Only very narrow-spectrum agents are effective against other classes of microorganisms such as viruses, fungi or protozoa. This is particularly true of antiviral agents, e.g. *aciclovir* (*acyclovir*) is only effective against herpes virus.

Minimum inhibitory concentration

For an antimicrobial to be effective in treating a particular infection it must be able to inhibit the growth of the causative organism. The **mini-mum inhibitory concentration (MIC)** is the minimum concentration of an antimicrobial that is capable of inhibiting the growth of an organism. The MIC for a resistant organism is higher than the concentrations which can reasonably be achieved *in vivo*. Thus, an antimicrobial agent will possess a spectrum of activity, those organisms inhibited at low MIC being termed **sensitive** and those inhibited only at a high MIC being **resistant**. Table 13.2 gives the MICs of some penicillins against selected organisms and shows that, provided that high enough concentrations are achieved, even organisms normally considered resistant will be inhibited, although this would require prohibitively high doses.

In some diseases, e.g. bacterial endocarditis, it is essential that the organisms be killed, not merely inhibited, in order to prevent relapse. In such cases, the **minimum bactericidal concentration (MBC)** is more relevant.

Classification and properties of antimicrobials

Antimicrobials may be classified by their chemical structure, mode of action or spectrum of activity.

Table 13.2   Minimum inhibitory concentrations (MIC) of some penicillins

	MIC (mg/L)			
	Benzylpenicillin	Ampicillin	Flucloxacillin	Piperacillin
Gram-positive species				
Staphylococcus aureus (not penicillinase-producing)	0.03	0.1	0.1	0.5
Streptococcus pneumoniae	0.01–0.03	0.03	0.25	0.03
Streptococcus faecalis	2	0.5	16–32	2
Gram-negative species				
Bacteroides fragilis	32	32	R	8
Neisseria gonorrhoea	0.01–0.03	0.1	0.1	<0.01
Escherichia coli	64	4	R	2
Klebsiella pneumoniae	R	R	R	16
Haemophilus influenzae	1	0.5	8–16	0.03
Pseudomonas aeruginosa	R	R	R	2

R = MIC > 128 mg/L.

Chemical structure

For the pharmacist, the most convenient method of classifying an antimicrobial is by its chemical structure (Fig. 13.1). The antibacterials are usually classified according to the chemical nucleus of the original (parent) drug. Different side chains attached to this basic nucleus form the various members of the group, which often possess properties different to those of the parent compound. Such derivatives may have an extended spectrum of activity, the ability to overcome resistant organisms, improved bioavailability, or fewer adverse effects.

Mode of action

The mode of action of antimicrobials is of little practical therapeutic relevance, though it may

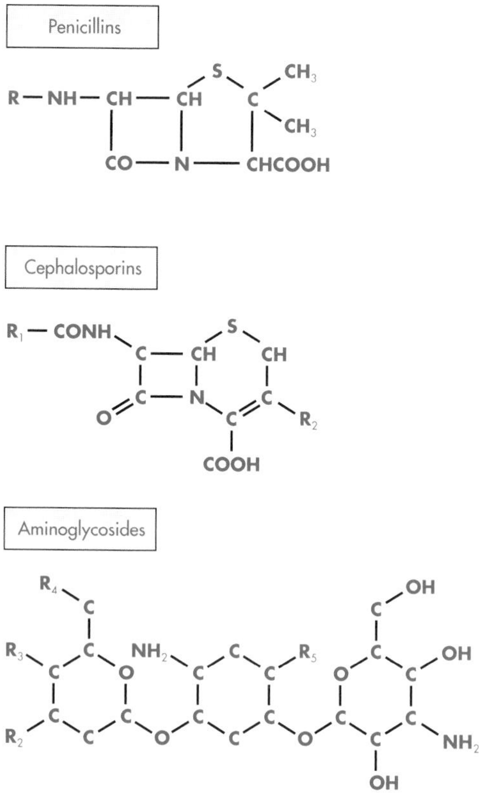

Figure 13.1   Structures of some important antimicrobials, showing the parent nucleus. R_1–R_5 represent various side chains.

determine the spectrum of activity. However, it may be useful to distinguish between **bacteriostatic** agents, which inhibit replication of microorganisms and allow the body's defence system to clear up the infection, and **bactericidal** ones, which kill organisms outright under suitable conditions. Tetracyclines, sulphonamides and low doses of erythromycin are examples of bacteriostatic agents. The penicillins and most other antibacterials are bactericidal. A bacteriostatic agent might be expected to have a slower therapeutic effect, but otherwise the terms imply an unrealistic distinction because the difference may be simply the effect of concentration, a low concentration being inhibitory and a high concentration lethal. Furthermore, host defence mechanisms play an important part in eliminating an infection, even in the presence of a bactericidal agent.

Table 13.3 shows that antimicrobials have a variety of modes of action, although this usually has little bearing on the choice of antimicrobial agent, because monotherapy with the single most effective narrow-spectrum agent is the usual aim. The ability to use antimicrobials effectively to cure human disease relies on structural or metabolic differences between the microbial and host (mammalian) cells. Thus, because penicillins specifically inhibit a step in the formation of bacterial cell walls, which are not present in mammalian cells, they are virtually non-toxic to animals. However, the aminoglycosides (e.g. gentamicin) interfere with bacterial ribosomal activity; thus, because there are ribosomes in animals as well as bacteria these antibiotics – when present in sufficient concentration – are particularly toxic to man.

Spectrum

The problem faced by the prescriber is to decide which agent from a selection of many antibacterials will be the most effective against the organism responsible. In the absence of sensitivity testing and identification (i.e. treating **blind**) this decision must be based on a knowledge of spectrums of activity of available antimicrobials and a knowledge of the most likely infective agent in the particular patient.

Table 13.3 The modes of action of some antimicrobial agents

Mechanism	Examples
Inhibition of cell wall synthesis	Penicillins
	Cephalosporins
	Macrolides
	Vancomycin
Interference with bacterial protein synthesis	Aminoglycosides
	Tetracyclines
	Chloramphenicol
Interference with bacterial DNA replication	Quinolones
Inhibition of bacterial folate synthesis	Sulphonamides, trimethoprim
Alteration of cell membrane permeability	Antifungals
Incorporation into nucleic acid side chain	Aciclovir (acyclovir)
Reverse transcription inhibitor	Zidovudine

Penicillins

Chemical structure

The penicillins possess a **beta-lactam** group as part of the parent nucleus (6-amino-penicillanic acid; Fig. 13.1). The cephalosporins, monobactams and carbapenems are also beta-lactam antibacterials. The substitution of different side chains on the parent nucleus has produced compounds with an extended spectrum of activity, the ability to overcome resistance, and improved bioavailability.

Spectrum of activity

The original *benzylpenicillin* was active only against Gram-positive organisms and Gram-negative cocci. However, this drug remains the most effective agent for the treatment of streptococcal infection, and resistance is rarely a problem except for *Streptococcus faecalis*. Benzylpenicillin also remains the first-line treatment for both meningococcal and gonococcal infections, although resistance is beginning to limit its use as a sole agent for the latter. Other Gram-negative organisms are resistant.

Beta-lactamase-resistant penicillins

Staphylococcus aureus, one of the most important wound pathogens, was initially satisfactorily treated with benzylpenicillin. However, 90% of isolates now produce the enzyme beta-lactamase (penicillinase) which splits the beta-lactamase nucleus, and so they are resistant. Indeed, most beta-lactam antibacterials could potentially be inactivated by beta-lactamase. Penicillins have been developed which are resistant to beta-lactamase; these include *methicillin* and *flucloxacillin*. The latter is now the most widely prescribed owing to its superior oral bioavailability. However, as a result of gaining beta-lactamase stability, the spectrum of this group is narrowed. Even though *flucloxacillin* retains activity against streptococci, its MIC is greater than that of *benzylpenicillin*. *Flucloxacillin* is therefore restricted to the treatment of *Staph. aureus* infection. If any other organism is suspected in a particular infection, another antibacterial must be added. Alternatively, a beta-lactamase inhibitor (e.g. *clavulanic acid, tazobactam*), may be used in combination with a broad-spectrum penicillin, e.g. *amoxicillin, ticarcillin* and *piperacillin*.

Broad-spectrum penicillins

Ampicillin was the first broad-spectrum penicillin developed and extended the Gram-negative range of penicillins to include *Haemophilus* and *E. coli* species. Unfortunately, many strains of these organisms are now resistant to ampicillin, its activity against many other Gram-negative organisms is unimpressive and it is completely ineffective against *Pseudomonas*. The newer *amoxicillin* has better bioavailability (see below) but a similar activity spectrum.

Carbenicillin was the first antipseudomonal penicillin, but this has now been superseded by the ureidopenicillins, e.g. *azlocillin, ticarcillin* and *piperacillin*. There is little to choose between these: *azlocillin* possibly has the greater antipseudomonal activity. Although the ureidopenicillins are active against Gram-positive organisms, the older type of penicillins are usually used against these infections because they are often effective at lower concentrations, cheaper, and may be administered orally.

A common observation is that as the spectrum of activity of an antimicrobial is extended into the Gram-negative range, so its usefulness against Gram-positive organisms diminishes. As well as the blind treatment of septicaemia, the ureidopenicillins are also used prophylactically in certain surgical procedures or in immunocompromised patients. However, they are susceptible to beta-lactamases and may need to be administered together with other agents (e.g. *clavulanic acid*) if the sensitivity of the pathogen is unknown.

The data in Table 13.4 may be taken to imply that most infections could be adequately treated with a ureidopenicillin, and that there could be little reason to prescribe any other type of penicillin. We shall see later that other general factors (e.g. drug concentration at the site of infection, cost, ease of administration and resistance) may affect antimicrobial choice in addition to spectrum of activity.

Bioavailability and formulation

A particular problem of benzylpenicillin is that it can only be administered parenterally because it is inactivated by gastric acid. The substitution of a phenoxymethyl group (giving *phenoxymethylpenicillin* or *penicillin* V) confers improved acid stability and absorption. Oral bioavailability is improved still further by synthesizing a pro-drug ester (e.g. *pivampicillin*), which is acid-stable, well absorbed orally and hydrolysed to the active compound in the bloodstream. It is sometimes advantageous to administer a single high dose of penicillin intramuscularly using *procaine penicillin*, which is only slowly absorbed.

Table 13.4 The spectrum of action of some penicillins

	Benzylpenicillin	Ampicillin	Flucloxacillin	Piperacillin
Gram-positive species				
Staphylococcus aureus	+++	+++	+++	+++
Staphylococcus aureus (penicillinase-producing)	R	R	+++	R
Streptococcus pneumoniae	+++	+++	++	++
Streptococcus faecalis	++	+++	+	++
Gram-negative species				
Bacteroides fragilis	+	+	R	++
Neisseria gonorrhoea	+++	++	+	++
Escherichia coli	R	++	R	++
Klebsiella pneumoniae	R	R	R	++
Haemophilus influenzae	R	+++	R	++
Pseudomonas aeruginosa	R	R	R	++

+++, Sensitive, first-line therapy.

++, Sensitive, but not often first-line therapy.

+, Rarely or never used; many resistant strains, poor activity (high MIC but less than 128 mg/L) or otherwise inappropriate (see text).

R, Resistant.

Side effects

The penicillins have a very wide therapeutic range, i.e. blood levels much higher than those required for treatment need to be attained before dose-related side effects occur.

A disadvantage they share with many broader-spectrum oral antibacterials is the tendency to cause **diarrhoea** owing to an alteration in gut flora. This is particularly true of the less well-absorbed types, such as *ampicillin*. *Pivampicillin* and the well-absorbed *amoxicillin* tend to cause far less diarrhoea.

The main problem associated with penicillins is **hypersensitivity** reactions. These result from their action as haptens (*see* Chapter 2), and hypersensitivity developed to one member of the group may preclude the use of all other related compounds. The further from the basic penicillin structure a molecule is, the less the chances of a cross-reaction. An individual who has a hypersensitivity reaction to a penicillin has a 10% chance of reacting similarly to a cephalosporin (*see* Fig. 13.1). The chances of developing a cross-reaction to a monobactam (*see* p. 728) would be slight.

The hypersensitivity reactions vary; the most serious form is **acute anaphylaxis**, but a pruritic rash of delayed onset is much more common. Other reactions include urticarial rash (Chapter 12), fever and organ damage. Although a patient presenting with a mild hypersensitivity reaction need not necessarily develop a life-threatening reaction on subsequent treatment, it is good practice not to prescribe penicillins if there is any previous history of allergy to them. A careful history of such allergy should be taken, as patients may confuse true allergy with non-allergic side effects such as diarrhoea. If hypersensitivity is a problem it is usually safer to choose a different class of antibacterial completely, such as a macrolide. Indeed, from a therapeutic standpoint the main advantage to the structural classification of antimicrobials is to be able to predict and avoid the hypersensitivities or adverse drug reactions associated with a particular group.

There has been recent concern over the occurrence of cholestatic jaundice associated with the use of flucloxacillin, and possibly to a greater extent with clavulanic acid combinations. This reaction is rare, reversible and more likely in older patients.

Cephalosporins

Chemical structure and mode of action

These are the antibiotic group most closely related structurally to the penicillins, as they also possess a beta-lactam ring. As with the penicillins, substitutions on the parent nucleus (7-amino-cephalosporinic acid) produce agents with differing pharmacokinetic profiles, spectrums of activity and adverse effects. Cephalosporins are classified in terms of generations, three to date, with each new generation producing members with improved Gram-negative activity. The cephamycins are closely related to the cephalosporins, *cefoxitin* being the only member in clinical use in the UK. All have the same mode of action as the penicillins.

Spectrum of activity

The first-generation cephalosporins (*cefradine, cefalexin, cefaloridine* and *cefalotin*) have a similar spectrum of activity (Table 13.5) to ampicillin. Although they are more stable to staphylococcal beta-lactamase, they are not completely resistant to it, so *flucloxacillin* would be a more rational choice for treating staphylococcal infection. Gram-negative organisms also inactivate many of the early cephalosporins by the production of beta-lactamases. Thus, the first-generation cephalosporins are now used mainly as second-line agents.

The second-generation cephalosporins are far more stable to Gram-negative beta-lactamase and therefore have a wider spectrum of activity. *Cefuroxime* and *cefadroxil* are the most important members of this group and are often used in the treatment of exacerbations of chronic bronchitis due to *H. influenzae*. However, activity against Gram-positive organisms is reduced so these are not the antibacterials of choice for such infections. *Cefoxitin* is often classified together with

Table 13.5 Spectrum of action of cephalosporins

	1st Generation	2nd Generation	3rd Generation
Gram-positive species			
Staphylococcus aureus (penicillinase-producing or not)	++	++	+
Streptococcus pneumoniae	++	++	+
Streptococcus faecalis	R	R	R
Gram-negative species			
Bacteroides fragilis	R	+	+
Neisseria gonorrhoea	+	+++	++
Escherichia coli	++	++	++
Klebsiella pneumoniae	+	++	+++
Haemophilus influenzae	+	+++	+++
Pseudomonas aeruginosa	R	R	+++

+++, Sensitive, first-line therapy.

++, Sensitive, but not often first-line therapy.

+, Rarely or never used; many resistant strains, poor activity (high MIC but less than 128 mg/L) or otherwise inappropriate (see text).

R, Resistant.

the second-generation cephalosporins as the spectrums are similar; however, it is also effective against anaerobes.

The parenteral third-generation cephalosporins (e.g. *ceftazidime* and *ceftriaxone*) extend the Gram-negative spectrum still further to cover pseudomonads. *Cefpirome* has the greatest beta-lactamase stability of the third-generation cephalosporins and greater activity against pseudomonads. As with the penicillins, this extended activity in the Gram-negative range makes them correspondingly less effective against Gram-positive organisms (especially *Staph. aureus*) than the second-generation agents. However, *ceftriaxone* has useful activity against both Gram-positive and Gram-negative organisms, but poor activity against *Pseudomonas aeruginosa*. Its main application is in the management of bacterial meningitis (*see* pp. 742–745), and its long half-life also allows for just twice-daily dosing.

As a further complication to this somewhat awkward classification system, there are now third-generation oral cephalosporins available with an improved Gram-negative activity compared with those of the second generation (e.g. *cefixime* and *ceftibuten*). However, they are ineffective against pseudomonads.

Therapeutic role

This is much debated as the spectrum of action of cephalosporins can be covered by various penicillins and other cheaper antibacterials. The use of intravenous cephalosporins as first-line agents is often determined by the local antibiotic policy, where recommendations for antibiotic prescribing in a particular area is determined by local patterns of resistance as monitored by a hospital microbiology department. For instance, a hospital might employ *ceftazidime* as first-line therapy for life-threatening *Pseudomonas* infection, often in combination with an aminoglycoside, in preference to an aminoglycoside–ureidopenicillin combination, despite the possible cost implications. Other possible applications for first line use may include surgical prophylaxis, exacerbations of chronic bronchitis if *H. influenzae* is suspected, or pyrexia of unknown origin (PUO), but most of these uses can be covered by other cheaper antibacterials.

Cefadroxil and the oral pro-drug of *cefuroxime axetil* (*cefuroxime*) both have poor oral bioavailability, but are useful in the treatment of *H. influenzae* chest infections that are resistant to ampicillin. However, it is doubtful whether they should be used as first-line agents in the community on grounds of cost and the danger of development of cephalosporin-resistance.

Side effects

Although the very early cephalosporins (*cefalotin* and *cefaloridine*) caused significant renal damage, this does not occur with other members of the group. Hypersensitivity reactions (analogous to those with the penicillins) are the only major problems encountered.

Aminoglycosides

Chemical structure and mode of action

Streptomycin, first isolated from the fungus *Streptomyces griseus* in 1944, revolutionized the treatment of tuberculosis. The class name describes the structure of this group: glycosidically linked aminosugars.

The most widely used are *tobramycin* and *gentamicin*, which are both members of the kanamycin group. Despite the availability of numerous derivatives, the properties of the kanamycin group vary little. The other aminoglycosides have few clinical applications.

The aminoglycosides act by interfering with bacterial protein synthesis via actions on bacterial messenger and transfer RNA (mRNA, tRNA). Miscoding causes incorrect amino acid insertion into peptide chains, suppressing cell growth and eventually causing cell death.

Spectrum of activity

Gentamicin is the most widely prescribed aminoglycoside. The other clinically useful members of the *kanamycin* group (*tobramycin, amikacin* and *netilmicin*) have very similar activity against a wide variety of Gram-negative bacteria (Table 13.6), particularly pseudomonads, and there is little to choose between them. *Amikacin* is claimed to have greater stability to inactivating enzymes produced by *Pseudomonas*, but this rarely affects clinical choice. All aminoglycosides are active against *Proteus*, but anaerobic bacteria are resistant.

Gentamicin is useful for treating staphylococcal infections but has only moderate activity against streptococci. It is synergistic with penicillin against this species, possibly by increasing cell permeability to penicillin.

Other aminoglycosides have more specific uses. *Spectinomycin* is highly effective against gonococci but is inactive against other organisms, so it is only used for the treatment of penicillin-resistant gonorrhoea. Because of problems with toxicity and resistance and because it can only be administered intramuscularly, *streptomycin* is used primarily as a second-line drug for the treatment of tuberculosis. It is also used for the treatment of plague and, occasionally, for resistant coliform infections.

Pharmacokinetics

The aminoglycosides are highly polar, not significantly absorbed orally, and are largely excreted unchanged via the kidney. Thus they are usually administered parenterally unless intended for local or topical (e.g. ophthalmic) use. *Neomycin* if given orally retains its antibacterial activity in the gut lumen and has been used for 'sterilization' of the gut before gastrointestinal surgery.

They are generally well distributed in the tissues after parenteral administration, but penetrate the cerebrospinal fluid poorly.

Toxicity

The aminoglycosides are among the most toxic antimicrobials, the main problems being renal and eighth cranial nerve toxicity (ototoxicity). Nephrotoxicity is rare, except in patients with previous renal impairment, but more commonly ototoxicity may lead to hearing impairment. These effects are related to plasma levels, although it has been suggested that some ototoxicity may occur even with careful control of gentamicin dosage, if this is given for longer courses. Other rare side effects include hypersensitivity reactions and neuromuscular block.

As toxicity appears associated with sustained

Table 13.6   Spectrum of action of some other antibacterial agents

	Aminoglycosides	Erythromycin	Ciprofloxacin	Trimethoprim
Gram-positive species				
Staphylococcus aureus (penicillinase-producing or not)	+++	+++	++	++
Streptococcus pneumoniae	+	+++	+	++
Streptococcus faecalis	+	R	++	++
Gram-negative species				
Bacteroides fragilis	R	+	+	+
Neisseria gonorrhoea	+	+	++	R
Escherichia coli	++	+	+++	+++
Klebsiella pneumoniae	++	R	+++	++
Haemophilus influenzae	+	++	+++	++
Pseudomonas aeruginosa	+++	R	+++	R

+++, Sensitive, first-line therapy.

++, Sensitive, but not often first-line therapy.

+, Rarely or never used; many resistant strains, poor activity (high MIC but less than 128 mg/L) or otherwise inappropriate (see text)

R, Resistant.

trough levels rather than the peak attained immediately post-dose, only once-daily dosing of an aminoglycoside may be appropriate in many situations. Thus, a single daily dose of 4.5 mg/kg of gentamicin would produce blood levels of 12–14 mg/L, well above the 10 mg/L required to treat *Pseudomonas* infection. By administering gentamicin just once a day, accumulation should be avoided, allowing trough levels to fall below the 2 mg/L known to be associated with both ototoxicity and nephrotoxicity. The value of this regimen is supported by the observation that aminoglycosides have a persistent effect against *Pseudomonas*, i.e. growth inhibition is present for some hours after plasma levels fall below the MIC. Regular blood level monitoring would still be prudent.

Other antimicrobial agents

The penicillins, cephalosporins and aminoglycosides are the most widely used groups of antibacterials, and one or other of them are first-line agents for the treatment of many infections. The groups discussed next are older agents whose use is diminishing (e.g. sulphonamides), recent introductions whose full potential has yet to be realized (e.g. new beta-lactams), or groups represented by only a few related agents in clinical use (e.g. macrolides).

Other beta-lactams

Two new classes, the carbapenems and monobactams, have widened the choice. *Imipenem* is a very broad-spectrum carbapenem which is active against most Gram-negative organisms, including *Pseudomonas*, and it also has useful activity against a range of Gram-positive bacteria. Two major disadvantages initially associated with *imipenem* were that nephrotoxic metabolites were formed by the action of renal dihydropeptidases, and that this renal metabolism tended to shorten the half-life of the antibiotic considerably. These problems have been overcome by co-administration with cilastatin, an alpha-dihydropeptidase inhibitor. However, this combination has been largely superseded by *meropenem*, which does not require the co-administration of cilastatin because it is not metabolized in the same way.

Aztreonam is the only monobactam in current use in the UK. It is only active against aerobic Gram-negative organisms, notably *Ps. aeruginosa*, and must be given parenterally.

Macrolides

The most important member of this group is *erythromycin*. Other macrolides, such as *clindamycin* and *lincomycin*, are now less used in the UK owing to their associated incidence of antibiotic-associated colitis (*see* p. 750). *Clarithromycin* and *azithromycin* are recent additions with superior bioavailability to erythromycin.

Erythromycin is bacteriostatic at the serum levels achieved with usual oral doses, but the higher levels achieved with intravenous use are bactericidal. The antibiotic interferes with bacterial protein synthesis by inhibiting the transfer of amino acids from tRNA to the peptide chain. It is particularly effective against Gram-positive organisms (Table 13.6) and is a very useful alternative for patients who are hypersensitive to penicillin. Erythromycin has limited application in the treatment of Gram-negative infection because cell wall penetration is poor, although some *Haemophilus* strains are sensitive. Activity is particularly good against bacteria which do not have a cell wall, such as mycoplasmas, and erythromycin is the agent of choice for treating *Legionella*. The most common adverse reaction to erythromycin is gastric upset, but this is reported to be far less of a problem with *clarithromycin* and *azithromyicin*.

A further important advantage of both *clarithromycin* and *azithromycin* is enhanced activity against *Haemophilus* spp. A major distinction between these two agents is that while *azithromycin* may have superior tissue penetration it achieves poorer sustained blood levels compared with *clarithromycin*. Thus, *azithromycin* has a theoretical disadvantage if septicaemia is likely to be a problem, so *clarithromycin* is more widely used. The main indication for *azithromycin* is as a convenient single-dose therapy for treating *Chlamydia trachomatis*.

Chloramphenicol

This synthetic antibacterial is mainly bacteriostatic with a very wide spectrum of activity. The mode of action is by inhibition of bacterial protein synthesis, although the exact mechanism is not understood. Major drawbacks to its use include toxicity and the development of resistance. Being among the cheapest of broad-spectrum agents, chloramphenicol is used extensively and often inappropriately in the Third World for treating many types of infection. Thus, this very useful agent has become virtually ineffective in the treatment of various endemic infections (e.g. typhoid fever) in certain countries.

The incidence of aplastic anaemia associated with *chloramphenicol* has led to the general recommendation that it should only be used systemically for severe infections. Owing to the development of many safer broad-spectrum antibacterials, the principal systemic indication for chloramphenicol is the treatment of meningitis, although even here it is being replaced by third-generation cephalosporins. Chloramphenicol still has valuable topical use in the treatment of eye infections, e.g. conjunctivitis, though recent occasional reports of aplastic anaemia associated even with the eye preparations has led some physicians to advise against its use for bacterial conjunctivitis. However, there is little direct evidence of a causal relationship and the incidence of such reactions seems no greater than that observed for aplastic anaemias in the general population.

Tetracyclines

Like chloramphenicol, and introduced at the same time, the tetracyclines are broad-spectrum bacteriostatic agents which inhibit bacterial protein synthesis. Their Gram-negative activity is unimpressive because many organisms including *Pseudomonas* and *Proteus* were originally resistant, and resistance has emerged with *Haemophilus*. Even in Gram-positives, acquired resistance has led to a reduction in the use of tetracyclines.

Their low toxicity still makes this group a

popular choice for the treatment of chest infections in the community. Interestingly, it has been claimed by some that the fall in popularity of the tetracyclines has resulted in a decline in certain resistant strains of bacteria. The tendency to cause an irreversible staining of teeth in children from deposition in the developing bone contraindicates their use in pregnancy and in children under 12 years of age.

The group contains a number of closely related compounds, all of which have a very similar spectrum of activity but different pharmacokinetic profiles. *Oxytetracycline* has largely replaced tetracycline for oral use owing to its superior bioavailability. The long half-life of *doxycycline* allows once-daily dosage. *Minocycline* is another long-acting agent, with twice-daily dosage, that has been used principally for mixed gonorrhoea/chlamydial infection and for prophylaxis against meningococcal meningitis. In addition, *doxycycline* and *minocycline* are the only tetracyclines that can be safely administered in renal impairment. Tetracyclines are still widely used for the treatment of acne when they are given orally for courses lasting many months. Occasionally, they are applied topically for infections of the skin or eyes, and for acne.

Sulphonamides and trimethoprim

Sulphonamides were the earliest synthetic antibacterials to be used, but have been largely replaced by more effective agents. They are bacteriostatic, acting by inhibition of bacterial folate synthesis. Determining true MICs for sulphonamides is difficult as their action is markedly affected by the culture media used. Because many previously susceptible strains are now resistant it is difficult to be sure of their true spectrum of activity.

Sulphonamides have been used in the treatment of a variety of infections, and both Gram-negative and Gram-positive organisms may be sensitive, so the theoretical spectrum is quite wide (Table 13.6). Their slow onset of action, high incidence of side effects (e.g. renal/hepatic damage, hypersensitivity and blood dyscrasias) and pattern of resistance have greatly limited their use. Until recently, the only widely used

member of the group was *sulfamethoxazole*, usually in combination with another folate synthetase inhibitor *trimethoprim* (as *co-trimoxazole*). Although synergism was claimed for these two agents which act at different points in the folate synthetic pathway, *trimethoprim* alone is equally effective in most situations. Recent fears over the incidence of bone marrow suppression have further limited indications for *co-trimoxazole*. The most important remaining indication is the control of *Pneumocystis carinii* pneumonia in AIDs sufferers.

Nitroimidazoles

The principal agent in this group is *metronidazole*, originally employed successfully in the treatment of trichomoniasis, and now a widely used antiprotozoal agent, e.g. for amoebiasis and giardiasis. It is also effective and frequently used in the treatment and prophylaxis of anaerobic infections, caused by either *Bacteroides fragilis* or clostridia. Resistance is uncommon. The use of metronidazole is limited by gastrointestinal disturbance, the occurrence of an 'antabuse-like' reaction in patients drinking alcohol, central nervous effects (e.g. dizziness, headache, epileptiform seizures) and peripheral neuropathy. The newer compound *tinidazole* offers few clinical advantages over *metronidazole*.

Quinolones

The prototype of the class, *nalidixic acid,* has the disadvantage of low activity, poor tissue concentration and the rapid development of acquired resistance, and so is now rarely used.

The more recently introduced fluoroquinolones have wider therapeutic applications. *Ciprofloxacin*, the first to enter clinical use, is active against Gram-negative and, to a lesser extent, Gram-positive organisms (Table 13.6). Important exceptions include *Bacteroides*, some pseudomonads, *Clostridium difficile*, *Strep. faecalis*, and *Strep. pneumoniae*. The main indication for *ciprofloxacin* is therefore in the treatment of aerobic Gram-negative infections. Its principal advantage over other agents is that it is the only orally active antipseudomonal. *Ofloxacin* has the same spectrum of activity as ciprofloxacin but may be administered once a day as opposed to the twice-daily dosage of ciprofloxacin. Quinolones act by interfering with bacterial DNA gyrase, responsible for the supercoiling of DNA. The resultant aberrant DNA cannot fit the bacterial cytoplasmic space, resulting in a rapid cell death. This mode of action has the advantage of preventing plasmid formation and therefore plasmid-mediated resistance, although resistance can still develop by chromosomal mutation.

Levofloxacin and *grepafloxacin* are recent additions to this group, with the important advantage of greater activity against Gram-positive pathogens.

Rifamycins

The chief member of this group, *rifampicin*, will be considered in greater detail in the treatment of tuberculosis (p. 750). It is also active against staphylococci, various mycoplasmas, meningococci and *Legionella pneumophila*, although its wider application has been limited by fears of development of resistance by *Mycobacterium tuberculosis*. However, it is used for prophylaxis in close contacts of meningococcal meningitis and in combination with other drugs (e.g. *fusidic acid*) for the treatment of infections due to resistant *Staph. aureus* (MRSA).

Vancomycin

This glycoprotein, which inhibits cell wall synthesis, is only active against staphylococci (including beta-lactamase-producing strains), streptococci and clostridia. It is particularly useful systemically as a treatment for multi-resistant *Staph. aureus* infection (MRSA), and orally for antibiotic-associated colitis due to *Clostridium difficile* bowel infection (when its poor oral absorption is advantageous). Although relatively expensive and somewhat nephrotoxic there is often little alternative when treating MRSA, but resistance to vancomycin has been reported recently. *Teicoplanin* is similar and is also indicated for the treatment of MRSA.

Sodium fusidate

This is the only member of a group of antibacterials of steroidal structure in clinical use. Its only indication is the treatment of staphylococcal infection in conjunction with either *penicillin* or *erythromycin* because resistance is likely to occur if used alone. Such combinations are often employed in the treatment of infective osteomyelitis, which is usually due to staphylococcal infection. Sodium fusidate is used topically for staphylococcal skin infections, and the ocular preparation has gained in popularity for the treatment of conjunctivitis owing to the fears about chloramphenicol, described above.

Peptide antibiotics

Included in this group are *bacitracin, polymyxin* and the related compound *colistin*. These act by interfering with cell membrane function. Being highly polar, they are not absorbed orally and when given parenterally can lead to serious neurotoxicity and nephrotoxicity. Thus they are only used topically.

Colistin is active against many Gram-negative organisms, including *Ps. aeruginosa*, and is sometimes used orally for gut sterilization in immunosuppressed patients. Bacitracin is active against Gram-positive species but has few clinical applications. They have been used topically often in combination to treat infected wounds and in eye and ear drops, but the use of any topical antibacterial for wounds is to be discouraged owing to problems with acquired resistance and skin sensitization.

Antifungal agents

Included here are agents active against true filamentous fungi (e.g. *Aspergillus*) and those used for treating yeast infections (e.g. *Candida albicans*). Fungal infections require quite separate agents from those effective against bacteria.

Candidal infections (e.g. oropharyngeal and vaginal **thrush**) are among the most common and troublesome, and two principal groups of agents are used in their treatment: the *polyene* *antibiotics* and the *imidazoles*. Another common fungal infection in humans is **tinea**, caused by filamentous fungi known collectively as the dermatophytes. Tinea may affect various areas of the body surface, the skin infection known as ringworm being an example. Fungal infections of the skin and nails are usually difficult to eradicate, and therapy is often prolonged. More serious systemic infections such as pulmonary aspergillosis or *Cryptococcus* are usually opportunistic infections in immunocompromised patients, and require parenteral therapy.

Imidazoles

Clotrimazole, miconazole and *niridazole* are all used topically in the treatment of vaginal thrush. *Miconazole* gel is a useful alternative to *nystatin* for the treatment of oropharyngeal thrush. The newer imidazoles are well absorbed. The first of the orally active agents was *ketoconazole*, but this is associated with severe hepatotoxicity if administered at high doses or in long courses. Newer, less toxic agents, e.g. *fluconazole*, are now available and are useful for the treatment of candidiasis. Parenteral miconazole is less toxic than amphotericin, although it is usually not as effective.

Polyene antibiotics

Examples of these are *amphotericin* and *nystatin*, which act on the fungal cell membrane to cause cytoplasmic leakage. They are not absorbed orally and may be administered as lozenges or mouthwashes for treating oropharyngeal thrush. For vaginal thrush, nystatin is administered as a pessary but has largely been replaced by the imidazoles. Amphotericin is administered parenterally for serious systemic fungal or yeast infections, but may cause severe renal damage even at low doses – a problem now largely overcome by the introduction of liposomal formulations.

Other antifungals

Fungal infections of the scalp and nails respond well to oral *griseofulvin*, which accumulates in those tissues, although this may need to be administered continuously for up to 6 months.

Shorter courses of treatment and better cure rates are achieved by using more modern agents such as *terbinafine*. Tinea pedis (athlete's foot) may respond to topical antifungals such as *tolnaftate* or an *undecanoate*, but is now often treated with topical imidazoles. In the treatment of systemic candidiasis, amphotericin may be used in combination with *flucytosine*, an anti-metabolite of cytosine that has no action on the filamentous fungi.

Antivirals

The search for useful antiviral drugs has intensified since the emergence of AIDS. As the life cycle of the virus is intimately intertwined with that of the host cells, it is difficult to find agents that inhibit virus replication without affecting mammalian cells. However, there are certain events in the synthesis of viral DNA and RNA which differ from those of the host, and these have been exploited with the nucleoside group of antivirals. These act either by interfering with DNA/RNA polymerase or by incorporation into nucleic acid to form 'nonsense' nucleotide sequences. One of the first nucleoside antivirals, idoxuridine, is active against herpes simplex (cold sores, genital herpes) and herpes zoster (shingles), but it is too toxic for systemic use. *Aciclovir (acyclovir)* and its congeners have largely replaced idoxuridine and can be administered both topically and systemically.

Zidovudine (AZT) will prolong life expectancy in AIDS patients, but is not a cure for the disease. Human cytomegalovirus infection is a secondary complication in AIDS and has been successfully treated with *ganciclovir*, a nucleoside analogue. The treatment of AIDS and AIDS-related infections is a fast-expanding specialist field which will not be discussed further here.

Interferons are the body's own natural antiviral agents (*see* Chapter 2), and recombinant genetic engineering techniques have now produced these in commercially useful quantities. The interferons are proving useful in the management of viral hepatitis A and B. *Amantadine* is indicated for the treatment and prophylaxis of influenza A infections in especially at-risk patients, but this strain is not always implicated in epidemics.

Therapeutic decisions in antimicrobial therapy

Simply possessing a knowledge of the organism involved and spectrum of activity of various antimicrobials is usually insufficient to treat suspected infections effectively. The full therapeutic decision making process is summarized in the flow diagram (Fig. 13.2) and will be discussed below.

General clinical features of infection

The first decision to be made is whether the symptoms are indeed caused by microbial infection.

Local infection

Any tissue injury causes inflammation (*see* Chapter 2). Injury due to microorganisms is no exception and any localized infection, whether on mucous membranes (e.g. sore throat) or the skin surface (e.g. impetigo), will result in the cardinal signs of inflammation: i.e. redness, heat, swelling and pain. However, localized inflammation can have origins other than infection: contact dermatitis, for instance, may often be restricted to a particular area of skin. Non-infective inflammation can be complicated further by the

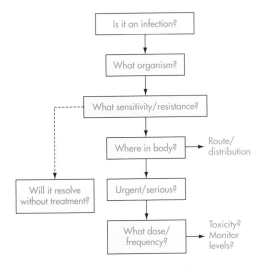

Figure 13.2   Flow chart for decision-making in antimicrobial therapy.

presence of a secondary (opportunistic) infection invading the damaged issue and increasing the degree of inflammation. The formation of **pus** usually indicates the presence of a localized bacterial infection, and is most commonly associated with staphylococcal infections. However, provided that the infection does not penetrate the deeper layers of the skin or traverses a mucous membrane, the patient is unlikely to suffer much harm, e.g. a sore throat will often resolve spontaneously if the individual is otherwise healthy.

Systemic infection

The physician needs to be particularly vigilant for the signs of progressive or systemic infection. An initially localized infection may sometimes progress to become more generalized and even life-threatening. In the case of skin infections, problems arise when organisms penetrate the dermis or deeper subcutaneous layers to produce a widespread inflammation, resulting in **cellulitis**. If the organism responsible, usually a streptococcus, reaches the lymphatic system (causing **lymphangitis**), the subsequent spread can be very rapid. In the absence of effective antibiotic therapy, amputation of the infected limb may be necessary to prevent severe septicaemia. Similarly, in the case of a streptococcal sore throat, long-term complications such as rheumatic fever, endocarditis and glomerulonephritis, may ensue if the organism reaches the general circulation.

The early signs of a systemic infection tend to be non-specific: lethargy, tiredness, muscular aches and chills are common. The cardinal sign of systemic infection is **fever** (raised body temperature). However, this does not always indicated the presence of living organisms in the bloodstream because **pyrogens** derived from Gram-negative bacteria and white blood cells also cause pyrexia. The biological advantage to the host of an increase in body temperature is obscure. Possibly a slight rise in temperature may be less favourable to the growth of the invading organism, or it may stimulate host defence mechanisms.

Many systemic inflammatory diseases, e.g. rheumatoid arthritis, may cause fever during acute exacerbations, and the growth of some tumours may present with fever as a non-specific symptom. Body temperature can be raised following severe trauma. Drugs may also be implicated, e.g. *rifampicin* can give rise to influenza-like symptoms. All these possibilities must be considered before infection is diagnosed and antimicrobials are prescribed.

Some signs of systemic infection can be determined from blood samples. The erythrocyte sedimentation rate (ESR) will be raised, but this will also occur for any systemic inflammatory process. The white blood cell (WBC) count has a greater diagnostic value, and may be extremely high in severe bacterial infection. In addition, the appearance of WBCs in normally sterile body fluids, e.g. urine or cerebrospinal fluid, may indicate the presence of an invading organism. Severe septicaemia can lead to septic shock (*see* Chapter 2, p. 48), with hypothermia and life-threatening hypotension. Finally, if a particular organ is affected owing to systemic or local infection it may become painful and inflamed and eventually may malfunction.

Almost any organ can become infected, from parts of the gastrointestinal tract, e.g. the appendix, to vital organs such as the heart, kidney, brain or liver. In extreme cases these organs may fail completely in the absence of effective treatment, leading to death.

Laboratory culture and sensitivity testing

In hospital, the identity of any suspected infecting organism and its sensitivity to a representative range of antibacterials, are usually determined routinely. Thus swabs will be taken from infected wounds and urine is sampled or the cerebrospinal fluid tapped by lumbar puncture if urinary tract infection or meningitis are suspected. Samples are then inspected microscopically and cultured in appropriate media and the organism is provisionally identified. Filter papers impregnated with different antibacterials are placed on an agar plate inoculated with the organism, and its sensitivity is determined by observing growth inhibition. Wherever possible, culturing and sensitivity testing are performed **before** antibacterial treatment is initiated because the presence of antibacterials in the

sample, or the effect of treatment on the organism, may inhibit the test culture sufficiently to give negative or inconclusive results. Sometimes, the laboratory will carry out detailed identification and typing, to assist treatment and to support epidemiological monitoring, e.g. to trace the origin of a food poisoning outbreak.

Limitations of culturing and sensitivity testing

Not all sites of infection are amenable to culturing and sensitivity testing. Areas that are heavily colonized with commensals, such as the skin or gastrointestinal tract, often yield unhelpful results as a large variety of organisms will invariably be cultured, including organisms which are potentially pathogenic but are unrelated to the current infection. *E. coli* is a ubiquitous enteric commensal, only certain toxigenic or enteropathogenic strains of which are responsible for gastrointestinal upsets.

Similarly, identification of *Staphylococcus epidermidis* in a wound swab does not necessarily mean that antibacterial therapy should be given. It is only when the patient's immunity is compromised or a particularly heavy infection leads to cellulitis or septicaemia that treatment is required. In some cases of gastrointestinal or urogenital infections, the use of antibacterials – especially those with a broad spectrum of activity – can permit over-growth and infection by resistant but normally non-pathogenic organisms.

Treating in the absence of sensitivity tests

Culturing and sensitivity testing can take days, or sometimes even weeks (e.g. tuberculosis, p. 750), and in some cases treatment may have to be started blind on a 'best guess' about the likely organism. This is usually arrived at by considering the epidemiology of the disease, the site of infection, and local experience. Table 13.7 lists some organisms most commonly associated with different infections. However, organisms other than those described may be responsible: e.g. *E. coli* causes 95% of urinary tract infections, but other Gram-negative organisms, such as *Klebsiella aerogenes* and *Ps. aeruginosa* or *Proteus* spp. may be responsible (*see* p. 753). After deciding on the most likely organism, knowledge of the

Table 13.7   Some common infections and likely responsible organisms

Infection	Likely organism[a]	Suitable antimicrobial[b]
Ear, nose and oropharynx		
Sore throat	2/3 cases are viral	None
Tonsillitis	*Streptococcus pyogenes*	*Penicillin V*
Otitis media (in infants)	*Haemophilus influenzae*	*Amoxicillin* or a *cephalosporin*
Respiratory tract		
Chronic bronchitis (exacerbations)	*Haemophilus influenzae*	*Amoxicillin* or *trimethoprim*
Pneumonia (uncomplicated)	*Streptococcus pneumoniae*	*Amoxicillin* or *erythromycin*
Urogenital		
Cystitis	*Escherichia coli*	*Trimethoprim* or *nitrofurantoin*
Vaginitis	*Candida*	*Clotrimazole* (topical)
	Trichomonas	*Metronidazole*
Skin		
Cellulitis	*Streptococcus pyogenes* and/or *Staphylococcus aureus*	*Penicillin V* + *flucloxacillin* or *co-amoxiclav*

[a] Other organisms may be responsible.

[b] Antibacterials other than those indicated may be suitable.

spectra of activity will then determine the choice of antimicrobial, though strain resistance may confound even the most astute choice.

Antimicrobial resistance

The high incidence of bacterial resistance makes culture and sensitivity testing of great importance, especially in hospital. The problem in the community is less, although here cultures are taken far less frequently so the true scale of the problem is unknown. Knowledge of patterns of resistance is therefore important especially when treating 'blind'.

Mechanisms of resistance

An organism may protect itself from antimicrobial attack in a number of ways (Table 13.8), enzyme degradation being the most important. Extracellular beta-lactamases tend to be produced by Gram-positive organisms, whereas intracellular lactamase may be found in the periplasmic space of Gram-negative organisms. Prevention of access to the target due to decreased penetration is more likely to be found in Gram-negative organisms, and binding of antibiotics in the periplasmic space is a particular problem for beta-lactam antibiotics. A further mechanism is efflux resistance, where an antibiotic is actively extruded from the bacteria.

Resistance develops primarily by selection from a small population of genetically resistant strains under the selective pressure imposed by the antibacterial, so the 'fittest' organisms survive. Mutation during treatment, with a genetic change conferring resistance, is rare.

Plasmid transfer, whereby resistant genes are transferred from one bacterium to another, plays a key role in spreading resistance rapidly through a microbial population. Less commonly, DNA can be transferred by two further mechanisms: transduction by viral bacteriophages, and transformation by uptake of free DNA material.

Patterns and causes of resistance

The development of resistance by previously sensitive organisms has been a problem ever since the introduction of the sulphonamides in the 1920s. A number of factors are involved in

Table 13.8 Mechanisms of resistance

Process	Example
Enzymic degradation	Beta-lactamase
	Aminoglycoside inactivators
	Various specific enzymes
Modification of target enzymes	Non-binding of trimethoprim to dihydrofolate reductase
Prevention of access to target	Resistance of some strains of *Staphylococcus aureus* to tetracycline

this phenomenon, with resistance by organisms responsible for **nosocomial** (hospital-acquired) infections playing a central role.

The emergence of resistance in the community and the hospital are closely inter-related. Recent problems with resistance in the community by organisms such as streptococci and staphylococci may have contributed to the level of resistance of these bacteria in nosocomial infections after entering the hospital pool. Also, the use of antibiotics in animal feeds may have contributed to the prevalence of community-acquired resistance. Of particular concern is the emergence of penicillin-resistant pneumococci in community-acquired pneumonia. In this case it has been suggested that the problem can largely be overcome by administering higher than standard doses. However, hospitals and nursing homes are responsible for much of the resistance seen today. A major factor in this is the use of prophylactic antibacterials in surgical and other procedures, which may bring patients into contact with pathogenic organisms such as *Pseudomonas*, e.g. during catheterization.

Immunocompromised patients, for example those having cytotoxic treatment or high doses of steroids, the frail and elderly, cancer patients and AIDS sufferers, will often require prolonged and intensive treatment for any nosocomial infection. Additionally, sub-therapeutic antibacterial concentrations occur in the general hospital environment from the indiscriminate use of topical antibiotics and from lack of care in handling parenteral forms. Therefore, resistant organisms cause particular problems in intensive therapy units where antibiotic use is high, where there are many staff with direct patient contact, and where patients have impaired resistance.

The resultant high level of antibacterial environmental contamination in hospitals greatly increases the chance of the emergence of resistant strains.

Patterns of resistance vary on the national and the international scale. For instance, the incidence of beta-lactamase-producing *H. influenzae* is far lower in the UK (6.2%) than in the USA (>30%). Local changes in the resistance of *E. coli* to trimethoprim and ampicillin have been observed within the UK. Resistance can also develop within an individual either quite rapidly or some time after commencing treatment. Those receiving higher doses of antimicrobials for prolonged courses are the most likely to suffer. Individual resistance is a particular problem in intensive care and burns units where staphylococcal, coliform, pseudomonad and *Haemophilus* infections are often implicated. As well as resistant organisms occurring in an individual they can be transferred from patient to patient unwittingly by health workers.

Resistance usually starts to be reported quite soon after the introduction of a new antibacterial into clinical use. For example, resistance to ciprofloxacin was observed only a year after its introduction despite the fact that it is said to inhibit plasmid replication. Certain organisms tend to cause more problems than others. *Ps. aeruginosa* has a particularly high tendency to develop resistance, and there have been reports of cross-resistance of this organism to both ciprofloxacin and ureidopenicillins. Another Gram-negative organism causing great concern is *Klebsiella*. After a period during which staphylococcal resistance appeared to stabilize, *Staph. aureus* has re-emerged recently in the form of **multiple (or methicillin) resistant strains**

(MRSA). Once these occur in a hospital ward the most stringent infection control measures are required.

Overcoming resistance

Several means are used to counteract the problem of resistance. One method is to find new antimicrobials to which resistant organisms are sensitive, or to use compounds capable of neutralizing any enzymes produced by the bacteria, e.g. clavulanic acid for penicillinase. However, it is less costly to prevent resistance occurring in the first place, by controlling the way in which these agents are used, particularly in the hospital, through the introduction of **antibiotic policies**. This involves measures such as periodically changing the antimicrobials in common use for certain organisms, preventing inappropriate prescribing, and ensuring the prescribing of full courses at adequate doses. Full courses are particularly important to the individual as they will prevent the re-emergence of an infection with potentially resistant organisms, which might follow incomplete kill.

A further method is to use **combinations of antimicrobials**. This is an essential element in the treatment of tuberculosis and endocarditis, but there are few other applications.

Combination therapy

Apart from attempting to avoid resistance there are a few other instances when combinations of antimicrobials might be indicated. These may be used:

- To achieve synergy, e.g. the concurrent use of an aminoglycoside and a ureidopenicillin in the treatment of pseudomonal infection.
- In life-threatening infections, e.g. meningitis or septicaemia, when a combination may be used until sensitivity testing has been performed.
- When the immune system is compromised, as in the chemotherapy of leukaemia, where very broad prophylactic cover is required using a combination of both antibacterial and antifungal agents.

The problems of tuberculosis are dealt with below.

Penetration to the site of infection

Even if the responsible organism is sensitive to an antimicrobial agent, the drug must reach the site of infection in order to be effective. Factors which affect the achievement of adequate local antibacterial concentrations include:

- Perfusion problems.
- Internal barriers.
- Route of elimination.

Perfusion problems

Any systemically administered drug must be transported in the blood to the desired site of action before it can have an effect. Thus, well-perfused tissues will be the most accessible to systemic antimicrobials. The alveoli of the lung are particularly well perfused in that they receive the whole of the cardiac output. Thus if they become infected (pneumonia, p. 745), appropriate antibacterial therapy is almost invariably successful provided that the patient is otherwise healthy. Conversely, an infection within the poorly perfused pleural cavity (e.g. in **empyema**) may require longer courses of treatment and higher doses.

The treatment of **wound infections** can be made particularly difficult when the peripheral circulation is impaired. This is important in diabetics (*see* Chapter 9), in whom atherosclerosis and capillary damage to the microcirculation of the skin slows wound healing and impairs the penetration of antimicrobials. The elderly also tend to have a poor peripheral circulation; this predisposes them to pressure sores and venous ulcers and makes such lesions very difficult to treat should they become infected.

Infection of **connective tissue** is similarly problematical, e.g. staphylococcal bone infections (**osteomyelitis**) can be very difficult to treat if the organism becomes sequestered following orthopaedic surgery or a compound fracture. A combination of antibacterials is then needed e.g. *sodium fusidate* plus *flucloxacillin* and/or *gentamicin*.

Internal barriers

In several circumstances infections may occur in body sites that are not easily accessible to antimicrobials. In others, the infection itself will create a barrier to penetration.

If large amounts of infected **sputum** are produced in pulmonary infections, as in bronchiectasis and cystic fibrosis, the mucus prevents ready access by antimicrobials, necessitating frequent high-dose treatments. Although, it has been claimed that *amoxicillin* is better than *ampicillin* in treating chest infections owing to a superior penetration into sputum, the difference is probably of minor clinical significance provided that adequate blood levels of *ampicillin* are attained. Similarly, when the infection results in the formation of large quantities of pus, as in a staphylococcal boil or abscess, the bacterial coagulase causes a fibrin clot to be formed around the lesion which inhibits penetration of the antibacterial: surgical drainage must precede antimicrobial therapy. A cyst (which is not surrounded by a fibrin clot) is far more amenable to antibacterial therapy.

Penetration of the **CNS** by antimicrobials is also extremely variable due to the 'blood–brain barrier' which usually prevents the penetration of hydrophilic molecules. Fortunately, both *benzylpenicillin* and cephalosporins, when given intravenously, are able to attain therapeutic concentrations in the cerebrospinal fluid and cure bacterial meningitis (p. 742). This is because meningeal inflammation opens the tight cell junction of the blood vessels that form the barrier and so permits antibiotic penetration.

Route of elimination

This is of particular importance when dealing with **urinary tract infections** (UTIs, p. 752). *Nitrofurantoin* is excreted unchanged in the urine in concentrations which exceed the MIC for likely urinary pathogens, even though the plasma concentration is inadequate to treat a systemic infection. Indeed, adequate antimicrobial plasma levels would cause unacceptable side effects. In contrast, penicillins are excreted unchanged in the urine and adequate plasma levels are also achieved for systemic infection.

With biliary tract infections it is essential that a sufficient amount of the unchanged antimicrobial is eliminated by biliary excretion to obtain therapeutic levels. This occurs with penicillins and cephalosporins, which consequently may be effective in the treatment of infective cholecystitis.

Indications for antimicrobial therapy

Before antimicrobials are prescribed it is important to consider whether this is the most appropriate therapy: there may be very positive indications, or they may be valueless. Thus, most **viral** infections – especially the respiratory ones – do not respond to currently available antiviral therapies. The major exceptions to this are the herpes infections which can be treated in the early stages with aciclovir (acyclovir).

Even if the organism is responsive, treatment may still not be worthwhile if the infection is **self-limiting**, e.g. mild streptococcal throat infection or mild staphylococcal skin infection. In an otherwise healthy individual such infections will be overcome by host defences in 2–3 days. Salmonellosis (p. 748) of the gastrointestinal tract does not respond well to treatment, and some antimicrobials may actually prolong the carrier state (the time during which the organism will be found in the stools).

Recall that indiscriminate use of antimicrobials, even if they do not cause serious toxicity, increases the risk of resistance developing.

Severe and systemic infection

Many systemic infections require **prompt treatment** owing to the danger of spread to vital organs or the development of septicaemia and, in extreme cases, septicaemic shock. Clinical judgement of severity is important and the physician must consider:

- The degree of pyrexia and other symptoms associated with fever, e.g. fits in young children, rigor and malaise.
- The time course of the infection.
- The patient's immune status.

Impaired resistance to infection is encountered in a number of diseases. Major inherited disorders of the immune system, e.g. hypogammaglobulinaemia, may predispose to infection but are rare. A more common problem occurs in the management of leukaemia, where the WBCs, although produced in large numbers, are ineffectual in combating infections. The use of cytotoxic agents further compromises the immune system. The leukaemic patient is thus prone to infection by a variety of organisms, some of which are opportunistic. Even commensals normally resident in the gut may cause opportunistic superinfections under these conditions, and any infection occurring in such a patient must be treated vigorously.

Immunosuppressive therapy is given to prevent rejection following an organ transplant, so antimicrobial therapy and barrier nursing are employed prophylactically until the danger of early rejection of the organ has passed. Immunodeficiency associated with disease is now a world-wide problem owing to HIV infections (AIDS), in which suppression of cell-mediated immunity exposes the patient to a variety of unusual infections. One of the most common and serious of these is *Pneumocystis* pneumonia, which is treated with high-dose *co-trimoxazole* or *pentamidine*. Additionally, nebulized *pentamidine* is administered prophylactically.

Elderly debilitated patients are also at risk, and prompt treatment may be indicated for even a mild infection in such cases. This occasionally raises ethical problems, because the prognosis may be extremely poor owing to other medical conditions, and treating such an infection may prolong a life of greatly reduced quality.

Prophylaxis

Antimicrobial prophylaxis is contentious. Inappropriate prophylaxis can not only lead to increased resistance but also add significantly to the hospital drug budget. However, prophylaxis against infection may sometimes be appropriate.

In some **surgical procedures** prophylaxis is essential, particularly 'dirty' surgery involving the gastrointestinal tract, when the antimicrobials used must protect against opportunistic infection by gastrointestinal commensals. A combination of cephalosporins to cover coliforms and *metronidazole* for anaerobic bacteria is usual. The aim is to prevent such organisms from causing a systemic infection if they should reach the patient's bloodstream and to prevent sepsis along a suture line. The practice of oral presurgical gut 'sterilization' using neomycin or a nonabsorbed sulphonamide is now rarely employed; antimicrobials are preferably given intravenously just before surgery and perhaps for a day or so after. A further example is in dental surgery, where those with a history of heart valve disease may require prophylaxis before any procedures are carried out.

Prophylaxis may sometimes be required over longer periods. Those with sickle cell anaemia can suffer an extremely painful, and sometimes fatal, sickling crisis as a result of infection. As streptococci are often implicated, continuous low-dose penicillin prophylaxis is often prescribed.

Cystic fibrosis patients may also require continuous, lifelong prophylaxis in order to prevent the chest infections that are a major feature of this disease. As *Pseudomonas* is usually implicated, courses of inhaled aminoglycosides are often prescribed.

Finally, prophylaxis is often indicated when there has been contact with certain virulent infections, e.g. meningococcal meningitis (p. 744). Close contacts require only fairly short courses of rifampicin in such cases.

Side effects

Hypersensitivity is a major contraindication to using a particular antimicrobial. This is well recognized with the penicillins, but can occur with any agent. Close questioning is necessary to ascertain the status of claimed hypersensitivity reactions because patients sometimes confuse these reactions with other adverse effects such as a mild gastric disturbance, reporting that they are 'allergic' to a particular antimicrobial. Taken at face value this precludes the administration of an otherwise useful drug because unless no suitable alternative is available, prescribers will always avoid the possibility of a major allergic reaction – however unlikely it seems to be from the history. If essential or when an antimicrobial is given intravenously for the first time, it is common practice to prepare for the possibility of an anaphylactic reaction by having injections of *adrenaline (epinephrine)*, *hydrocortisone* and an antihistamine readily available. Penicillin desensitization, whereby the patient is exposed to gradually increasing concentrations of penicillin, is rarely employed as it is a perilous procedure and it is usually possible to choose an alternative antibacterial.

Some adverse effects, such as the renal toxicity and ototoxicity associated with aminoglycoside therapy, are **dose related** (see below). Other adverse effects may be more difficult to predict and may not resolve on discontinuation of treatment, e.g. the bone marrow toxicity associated with *chloramphenicol*. Table 13.9 summarizes some of the most common adverse reactions to antimicrobials. Apart from these there are various rare idiosyncratic and unpredictable reactions, such as the lupus syndrome with isoniazid and blood dyscrasias with cephalosporins. Gastrointestinal adverse effects are discussed on p. 750.

Interactions

Consideration should also be given to potential interactions between antimicrobials and other drugs, although these are relatively few. The use of *gentamicin* and a loop diuretic has been reported to increase the incidence of ototoxicity. Similarly, the combination of a cephalosporin and a loop diuretic may increase nephrotoxicity although this is a major problem only with the early first-generation cephalosporins, e.g. cefaloridine.

There is a theoretical interaction between bactericidal and bacteriostatic agents because bactericidal agents can only act on dividing cells and their effectiveness may be reduced by agents that inhibit cell division. However, such combinations are rarely necessary. Where they are used together, e.g. in the treatment of a suspected atypical chest infection when ampicillin and oral erythromycin may be given in combination, the interaction does not seem to present any particular problems.

The potential of certain antimicrobials to alter the activity of liver enzymes is well recognized. *Rifampicin* is an hepatic enzyme inducer which causes problems if it is administered with drugs that are eliminated predominantly by hepatic metabolism. Cases have been reported of failure of the contraceptive pill after women had taken short courses of *rifampicin* for prophylaxis against meningococcal infection.

Erythromycin will inhibit the metabolism of certain other drugs, notably *theophylline* and *warfarin*. This effect tends to make it difficult to maintain control of serum levels of affected drugs during courses of *erythromycin* treatment, because plasma levels will rise during therapy

---

Table 13.9   Some adverse effects of antimicrobials

System	Severe	Mild
Gut	Clindamycin	Most broad-spectrum agents
Renal	Aminoglycosides	
	Amphotericin	
	Some sulphonamides and cephalosporins	
Liver	Rifampicin	
	Ketoconazole	
	Co-amoxiclav	
Ear	Aminoglycosides	
Bone marrow	Chloramphenicol	
Hypersensitivity	Penicillins[a]	Penicillins
	Sulphonamides	Sulphonamides

[a] Especially ampicillin (rashes).

and then fall again when the course has finished. A similar interaction has been observed between *ciprofloxacin* and *theophylline*

Dose and frequency

These parameters are often determined on the usual age and weight basis, and with due regard to renal and liver function. Precise dose calibration is not particularly important with the penicillins, which have a wide therapeutic window, but close monitoring is essential for agents possessing a narrow therapeutic window, e.g. *gentamicin*. Antimicrobials such as the aminoglycosides and quinolones, where high plasma levels are limited by safety, exhibit a concentration-independent lethal profile, so it is only necessary to exceed the MIC for a short space of time to kill the organism. Conversely, beta-lactams exhibit a concentration-dependent killing profile, where levels need to be sustained above the MIC for most of the interval between doses.

The aminoglycosides are eliminated via the kidneys, and gentamicin clearance correlates well with glomerular filtration rate (estimated from plasma creatinine). However, with longer courses it is necessary to monitor plasma levels directly because the volume of distribution can vary markedly between individuals. Also, the toxic effects (especially ototoxicity) are more likely if trough levels remain above 2 microgram/mL. Therefore the size and frequency of gentamicin doses are calculated to allow trough levels to fall below 2 microgram/mL, but to achieve peak levels of 6 microgram/mL after administering a dose, in order to exceed the MIC for *Pseudomonas*.

Antimicrobials eliminated by hepatic metabolism can accumulate in liver failure, but the degree of accumulation is difficult to predict or calculate. The best advice is to avoid giving antimicrobials such as erythromycin and rifampicin if liver dysfunction is suspected.

The frequency of administration is important, not least because of the level of non-compliance associated with this group of drugs. Patients tend to stop in the middle of a course if the regimen proves too irksome or they feel better – as they often do after 24–48 h of antimicrobial therapy. Therefore, the fewer the doses that must be taken each, day the greater the compliance.

The half-lives of the penicillins and many cephalosporins are only a few hours. Ideally, doses should be timed to the half-life of the drug, but this would be impractical in most cases of penicillin therapy. Therefore, with these less toxic antimicrobials doses are chosen that achieve plasma levels several times greater than the MIC. In this way the frequency of administration can then be reduced, as the plasma level will still exceed the MIC before each subsequent dose. Antimicrobials that can be given just once a day, such as ofloxacin and cefixime, may offer advantages for patient compliance.

Duration of therapy

A balance must be achieved between eliminating pathogens completely in order to limit the growth of resistant organisms, and giving too long a course, with which the patient is unlikely to comply and with the risk of increased adverse effects.

The usual recommended course for most antibiotics is 7–10 days, but there is much debate and there are a number of exceptions to this empirical generalization. Urinary tract infections for example, are usually adequately treated with 3-day courses. It is common practice to treat upper respiratory tract infections, in the absence of any chronic lung disease, with a 5-day course. *Chlamydia* infection can be treated with a single dose of *azithromycin*. Other treatments may require weeks (e.g. endocarditis) or months (e.g. tuberculosis) of antimicrobial treatment.

Failure of therapy

Even after the most diligent choice of antimicrobial, therapy may still fail. Table 13.10 summarizes the possible reasons for such failure and reflects the main points made in this section regarding appropriate therapeutic choice.

Table 13.10   Possible reasons for the failure of therapy[a]

1. Diagnosis	• no infection; viral
	• non-responsive condition
2. Drug	• non-sensitive organism
3. Dose	• age, site
4. Distribution	• in CSF, pus, urine, bile
	• nausea, food, compliance
5. Duration	• early resolution → non-compliance
	• impatience
6. Disease	• underlying serious disease, e.g. tumour, chronic bronchitis
7. Drugs (other)	• immunosuppressives, e.g. steroids, cytotoxics
8. Drug resistance	• selection from original population
	• supra-infection
	• mixed infection from start

[a] Failure may arise because of wrong decision in factors 1–6, or failure to appreciate factors 7 or 8.
CSF, cerebrospinal fluid.

Some important infections

Meningitis

Pathology and aetiology

The brain and spinal cord are surrounded by three membranous layers known collectively as the **meninges**. The outermost layer, the **dura mater**, is in intimate contact with the skull and vertebral column. The innermost **pia mater**, is in contact with the brain and spinal cord. Sandwiched between these is the arachnoid. Between the **arachnoid** and **pia mater** is the subarachnoid space which contains the **cerebrospinal fluid** (CSF). This has little intrinsic immunological activity, containing only small numbers of WBCs; thus, if even a few organisms reach the CSF via the bloodstream, they proliferate very rapidly.

A primary bacterial infection caused by *Neisseria meningitidis* in the nasopharynx, which may be transported via the bloodstream to the subarachnoid space, produces meningeal inflammation. As with any acute inflammation, WBCs and protein then pass from the bloodstream into the CSF, and if the CSF is examined (following lumbar puncture) it appears turbid instead of clear. Most of the damage to the CNS is not actually due to the microorganism, but to the host response via the inflammatory process, whereby vascular leakage results in a raised intracranial pressure.

Secondary bacterial meningitis can occur following a skull fracture which damages the meninges, or by an ascending infection from the middle ear.

Viral meningitis is the most common type, but it is usually mild. Unlike bacterial meningitis, there may be no changes in the appearance of the CSF and for this reason it is sometimes erroneously termed aseptic meningitis. Other rarer forms of meningitis are caused by fungi (especially in immunocompromised patients), mycobacterium and protozoa.

Clinical features

Characteristically, with primary bacterial meningitis an ear or upper respiratory tract infection is followed abruptly by only mild generalized malaise and possibly drowsiness, so diagnosis in the early stages is difficult. Later, a high fever together with symptoms indicating CNS involvement (headache, photophobia, neck stiffness and other neurological signs) will confirm the diagnosis, although the classical diagnostic neurological features are seen in only 50% of cases. Meningococcal infection is often accompanied by the appearance of a haemorrhagic (purpuric) skin rash within the first 18 h.

The progress of the disease can be very rapid,

particularly in fulminating (explosive) meningo-coccal infection. In this case there are severe systemic complications (shock, disseminated intravascular coagulation and renal failure) and death may occur within 24–36 h. These compli-cations of meningococcal sepsis are believed to result from endotoxin production. Patients may occasionally deteriorate rapidly on initial treat-ment with antibiotics owing to a release of these endotoxins from killed bacteria. If prompt appropriate treatment is given, healthy adults will suffer no permanent CNS damage. In chil-dren however, neurological sequelae such as blindness and mental retardation may occur in up to 30% cases, despite antibacterial therapy.

Epidemiology

Localized outbreaks of meningococcal infection in the UK often gain media attention, particu-larly as the younger population tend to be the most affected. In fact, most mortality is due to a meningococcal septicaemia rather than a meningitis. About 5% of the population are nasopharyngeal carriers of meningococci. Quite why these local outbreaks occur, or how meningococci find their way into the CSF, is not known.

Although nasal carriage of *N. meningitidis* is common, the annual incidence of meningitis in the UK is only about 10 per 100 000. Occasional local epidemics are caused by the group B serotype. More widespread epidemics take place in the Third World due to the group A and C serotypes.

Table 13.11 summarizes the probable pathogens which can usually be deduced from the age of the patient. Of the organisms listed, *N. meningitidis* is the most likely in an adult. For the elderly, streptococcal infection is the more common as it may accompany a pneu-mococcal chest infection (i.e. pneumonia) to which this age group is particularly prone. There has been much concern regarding the incidence of penicillin resistance to pneumo-cocci, but as yet this is currently no great problem in the UK

Haemophilus influenzae meningitis was formally one of the main causes of childhood meningitis, but since the introduction of an effective vaccine (Hib), the condition is comparatively rare in the UK. *Listeria* meningitis is occasionally found in both neonates and the elderly. A completely dif-ferent group of Gram-negative bacteria is usually implicated in neonatal meningitis.

A secondary infection, e.g. following a fracture of the skull, may allow organisms that are resi-dent on the skin surface to come into contact with the meninges. Staphylococcal and strepto-coccal organisms are likely pathogens in such cases, but occasionally *Pseudomonas* may cause problems.

Table 13.11 Aetiology and treatment of meningitis in the UK

Age group	Likely organisms	Initial therapy
Adult and children	*Neisseria meningitidis* *Streptococcus pneumoniae*	Cefotaxime
Elderly	*Neisseria meningitidis* *Streptococcus pneumoniae* *Listeria monocytogenes* Aerobic Gram-negative bacilli	Cefotaxime plus ampicillin
Neonate	Group B Streptococci *Escherichia coli* Other Gram-negative bacilli *Listeria monocytogenes*	Cefotaxime plus ampicillin or ampicillin plus aminoglycoside

Pharmacotherapy and its problems

Wherever possible, a lumbar puncture is performed before initiating therapy and the CSF is examined by direct Gram staining, culturing, sensitivity testing and immunoelectrophoresis (for antigens). Prior treatment usually results in negative CSF findings. If there is a delay of more than about 1 h before a lumbar puncture can be performed, then intravenous blind antibacterial therapy is usually administered immediately because meningitis can develop very rapidly. If meningitis is suspected GPs are now recommended to administer an initial dose of *benzylpenicillin*, after obtaining a blood sample. Diagnosis is still possible through serological findings and bacterial antigen tests of the CSF.

Due to the low intrinsic immunological activity of the CSF, some time will elapse after the invasion of the organism before an effective immunological response can be mounted, and this can lead to an overwhelming infection. Therefore, it is important to achieve high CSF concentrations of antibiotics promptly. As discussed, a limiting factor in the choice of antibacterials is their ability to cross the blood–brain barrier sufficiently to achieve sufficiently high CSF levels. Some antibacterials (e.g. *chloramphenicol*, antitubercular drugs and *amphotericin*) readily cross into the CSF, whereas others (e.g. cephalosporins, penicillins) will provide high CSF levels only if the meninges are inflamed. The more polar antibacterials (e.g. aminoglycosides, fusidate) always achieve only poor CSF concentrations, and if needed must be administered intrathecally. This procedure requires careful aseptic technique and is technically difficult to perform on neonates.

Acute infection

The initial treatment will depend to some extent upon the age of the patient and the results of direct CSF examination (Table 13.11). The third-generation *cephalosporins*, e.g. cefotaxime and ceftriaxone, are broad-spectrum agents widely used in the initial management of meningitis. Their spectrum of activity offers a more certain alternative to the previously used *chloramphenicol–benzylpenicillin* combination. The cephalosporins are active against *N. meningitis*, streptococci and the Gram-negative organisms that may be responsible. If *Listeria monocytogenes* is suspected, e.g. in the young and elderly, it would be wise to add ampicillin to the regimen. If penicillin-resistant strains of pneumococci are suspected, then the addition of vancomycin has been suggested.

The place of corticosteroids in limiting the inflammatory response caused by endotoxin release associated with antibiotic-induced bacterial lysis and in lowering CSF hydrostatic pressure is debatable. The only convincing clinical data support the use of corticosteroids in meningitis of *H. influenzae* type B.

Treatment of neonatal meningitis is more problematic than that of other age groups owing to the variety of possible pathogens, and initial therapy is often a matter of local policy. The combination of *ampicillin* and a third-generation cephalosporin is effective against a wider range of Gram-negative organisms, while providing adequate cover against streptococci. *Gentamicin* is sometimes added but would need to be given intrathecally: this needs expert advice and careful monitoring for neurotoxicity.

Once the results of a lumbar puncture have been obtained, therapy can be continued for the specific organism, e.g. *benzylpenicillin* for *N. meningitidis*.

Following a head injury, the danger of a secondary meningitis may require treatment using different antimicrobials. Thus, a high-dose regimen of flucloxacillin and ampicillin would be required to cover staphylococci and streptococci. Occasionally, an anaerobic organism may be implicated and *metronidazole*, which crosses readily into the CSF, is used.

Prophylaxis

Meningococci are highly transmissible, so prophylaxis is advised for close family contacts or for those living in closed communities such as boarding schools and prisons. *Rifampicin* has replaced sulphonamides as the drug of choice owing to an increased incidence of sulphonamide resistance. *Minocycline* is also used, but is somewhat less effective.

Vaccines have been developed to the A and C strains of meningococci and are recommended as routine prophylaxis for travellers to endemic areas. No vaccine is currently available against the B strain.

Summary

The treatment of meningitis illustrates the following general points:

- This type of infection is a medical emergency. Prompt blind treatment with an appropriate antimicrobial is essential.
- Samples for culturing and sensitivity testing should be obtained **before** initiating therapy but treatment must not await results. Immediate microscopical examination of Gram-stained CSF may provide valuable clues to appropriate therapy.
- Factors besides the site of infection may indicate the most likely organism involved. In meningitis, age is the most important determinant.

Pneumonia

Definitions and epidemiology

Despite the availability of effective treatments and the continuing sensitivity of the organisms to antimicrobials, the absolute mortality from pneumonia in the UK is greater than for any other type of infection. This is largely a reflection of the type of patient most susceptible: the elderly and the very young. In the UK, pneumonia accounts for 50 000 hospital admissions per year, the majority of these patients being elderly. The mortality rate is between 16% and 40%. Pneumonia is also liable to prove a greater problem in the chronically ill, frail or those with otherwise impaired immunity, e.g. lymphomas, AIDS and those taking immunosuppressants, in whom it is a common secondary complication.

The term pneumonia refers to inflammation of the lung alveoli. This is usually due to infection, but it may be caused by any physical, chemical or allergic irritant, e.g. **lipoid pneumonia** caused by accidental aspiration of liquid paraffin from laxatives or nose drops. In most cases the cause is aspiration of microorganisms from the upper respiratory tract into the lower respiratory tract and alveoli.

The term 'chest infection' is often used to indicate an infection of the lower respiratory tract, i.e. bronchioles and/or alveoli. It is important to distinguish signs of pneumonia, as in many cases it is unnecessary to treat uncomplicated lower respiratory tract infections not involving the alveoli with an antibiotic. In general, physicians will examine for signs of lung consolidation, e.g. crepitations and sudden shortness of breath to reach a diagnosis of pneumonia.

Traditionally, pneumonia has been classified by its old anatomical terms, bronchopneumonia and **lobar pneumonia**, but these terms are of little clinical relevance. The usual classification is aetiological (Table 13.12). This is another example of a disease which, like meningitis, may be life-threatening, and which is treated on a best-guess basis before results from sensitivity testing are known.

Diagnosis

Diagnosis is based primarily on clinical symptoms and signs. In severe infections with an at-risk patient, or in hospital-acquired infection, appropriate investigations must be carried out immediately, e.g. chest X-ray and sputum for culture and sensitivity testing. The classical signs and symptoms, i.e. cough, haemoptysis, pleuritic chest pain (pain on coughing), acute dyspnoea and fever, may not all be present. *Legionella pneumophila* infection is often associated with a non-productive cough. In 60% of *Mycoplasma* infections there are minimal respiratory signs. Furthermore, the elderly may show no signs of fever and present with confusion. Treatment must be commenced immediately, and if there is any indication of serious systemic disease such as sepsis, confusion, raised respiratory rate or a fall in blood pressure suggestive of septic shock, then treatment must be aggressive.

Aetiology

In community-acquired infection the most likely organism is *Streptococcus pneumoniae* (pneumococcal pneumonia). If bacteraemia develops as a complication, there is a 25% mortality rate. Influenza A is an occasional cause of viral pneumonia and although this will not respond to

Table 13.12　Classification and aetiology of pneumonia

Class	Aetiological agents	Percentage of cases
Community-acquired	*Streptococcus pneumoniae*	60–75
	Mycoplasma pneumoniae	5–18
	Legionella pneumophila	2–5
	Viral	2–8
	Haemophilus influenzae	4–5
	Staphylococcus aureus	1–5
Hospital-acquired	Gram-negative organisms, e.g.	50–60
	Klebsiella	
	Pseudomonas	
	Proteus spp.	
	Gram-positive organisms	10–20
Opportunistic[a]	*Pneumocystis carinii*	
	Aspergillus	
	Candida	

[a] In compromised or immunosuppressed patients, e.g. AIDs.

antibacterial therapy, opportunistic superinfections may require antibacterial treatment.

Atypical community-acquired infections, e.g. *Mycoplasma pneumoniae* and *Legionella pneumophila* must also be considered: the former is probably the second most common cause of pneumonia, with epidemics occurring in 4-yearly cycles. *Legionella* is now recognized as originating from water-cooled air-conditioning systems. The term atypical derives from the unusual signs on chest X-ray, combined with a normal WBC count and the symptom of a dry cough. These are all examples of **primary infections** where the initial infecting organism alone is responsible for the illness.

Common examples of **secondary pneumonias** are those that occur as complications of chronic bronchitis. *Haemophilus influenzae* may be aspirated from the upper respiratory tract of chronic bronchitics, although pneumococci may also be implicated. Aspiration pneumonia following the inhalation of stomach contents or vomit can be caused by staphylococci, streptococci and, rarely, anaerobic organisms. Staphylococcal pneumonia is often associated with an underlying influenzal infection and carries a very high mortality.

A different range of organisms is likely to be responsible for hospital-acquired respiratory tract infections. These are usually due to Gram-negative organisms that have been aspirated from the upper respiratory tract. Immobility and reduced consciousness may contribute to the risk of such aspiration.

Yet another group of organisms are encountered in immunocompromised patients. Cytotoxic chemotherapy renders patients susceptible to pneumonias caused by *Klebsiella pneumoniae* or, particularly seriously, fungi such *Aspergillus*. AIDS patients may contract pneumonias which previously were rarely seen. *Pneumocystis carinii* is one such organism which carries a high mortality and was previously seen only in some patients with abdominal cancer. Other types of pneumonias contracted by AIDS patients include those caused by *Mycoplasma pneumoniae* and cytomegalovirus.

Pharmacotherapy

Many countries, including the UK, now have official guidelines for the treatment of community acquired pneumonia. High-dose *amoxicillin* is felt to be sufficient to deal with the pneumococci responsible for most mild to moderate cases. In other countries, where penicillin resistance is a greater problem, other antibiotics such as a macrolide or *tetracycline* might be given as first-line therapy. A macrolide is also suitable for those with penicillin allergy. For a more severely ill patient not requiring hospital admission, intramuscular *benzylpenicillin* could be administered initially before continuing with *amoxicillin*.

The regime is occasionally varied in those who have co-morbidity, e.g. chronic lung disease, diabetes or renal/hepatic failure, to cover the possibility of encountering resistant organisms. In such cases *co-amoxiclav* or *clarithromycin* are used by some physicians, due to a potential problem with beta-lactamase-producing *H. influenzae*. Penicillin-resistant pneumococci are rare in the UK and less than 20% of *H. influenzae* are resistant. Therefore empirical treatment of mild to moderate pneumonia with antibiotics other than amoxicillin remains controversial.

For seriously ill patients who cannot be managed at home, intravenous antibiotic therapy should be instituted as soon as possible. The suggested regimen is to use a second-generation cephalosporin (e.g. *cefuroxime*) which would provide good cover against *H. influenzae*, combined with *erythromycin* in atypical infection. *Flucloxacillin* may be added if staphylococcal infection is suspected. If a pneumococcal infection is confirmed, *benzylpenicillin* should be used. Provided that the patient responds, oral therapy may be substituted after a few days. Treatment will usually continue for 7 days, or up to 3 weeks in cases of staphylococcal pneumonia or *L. pneumophila*.

If the infection was acquired in a hospital, treatment using agents effective against Gram-negative organisms is indicated; the choice will often depend on the prevailing antibiotic policy. A third-generation cephalosporin or a ureidopenicillin (with or without the addition of an aminoglycoside) can be used.

Other antibacterials are occasionally indicated for certain atypical infections. Mycoplasmas respond to *tetracycline* and *Pneumocystis carinii* to *co-trimoxazole*.

Summary

Treatment of pneumonia can thus be summarized as follows:

- A 'best-guess' of likely organisms dictates the initial antimicrobial therapy.

- The environment in which the infection was contracted (hospital or community) and the immune status of the patient determine the most likely organism.

Infections of the gastrointestinal tract

The human bowel, being in contact with the external environment, contains a range of commensals that might be pathogenic were they present in any other part of the body. Anaerobes such as *Bacteroides fragilis* predominate, and there are also coliforms (e.g. *Klebsiella*), *Strep. faecalis* and *Proteus*. Problems arise when the balance between these organisms, or between them and their host, is upset or an unusual organism is introduced.

The term **gastroenteritis** is often applied nonspecifically to a bowel infection resulting in diarrhoea, the aetiology and causative organisms tending to be different for adults and infants. Other groups of organisms are responsible for specific infection of the gastrointestinal tract, e.g. cholera and typhoid. This section deals only with acute infective diarrhoeas; chronic diarrhoeas and those of other origins are dealt with in Chapter 6.

Acute diarrhoea in children (infantile gastroenteritis)

This is rarely fatal in otherwise healthy children, but with malnourishment and poor housing there is a high risk of mortality. Viruses (especially rotavirus) are usually responsible. An important feature of infantile gastroenteritis is the depression of gastrointestinal luminal disaccharidase levels, resulting in an osmotic diarrhoea (*see* Chapter 6). Oral rehydration therapy is the mainstay of treatment, as the young are particularly vulnerable to becoming dehydrated. Antimicrobial therapy is likely to be useless and may prolong symptoms by causing further disturbance to the gastrointestinal flora.

Bacterial gastroenteritis in infants is often caused by auto-infection with enteropathogenic strains of *E. coli*. These either produce an exotoxin that increases gastrointestinal fluid secretion resulting in the production of a watery diarrhoea, or cause damage to the mucosa that results in a bloody diarrhoea. *E. coli* infections are usually self-limiting and require simple rehydration therapy. However, certain rare enterotoxigenic strains, e.g. 0157, can cause a more severe or even fatal outcome. This has occurred in recent incidences of food poisoning where this strain resulted in a high incidence of complications, including renal failure

Both the viruses and bacteria are transmitted via the faecal/oral route. *Campylobacter fetus* (ssp. *jejuni*) may be ingested from dog faeces, often through children playing in contaminated soil. This will result in severe abdominal pain, and if septicaemia develops then antibacterial treatment may be required. As with many gut infections, the antibacterial response is variable, but *erythromycin* is usually the first choice.

Other gut infections, e.g. shigellosis or giardiasis, which are rare in the West, require treatment with specific antimicrobials as in adults (see below).

Adult diarrhoea

Acute infective gastroenteritis is usually attributed to 'food poisoning' or 'travellers' diarrhoea' in the lay mind. Table 13.13 shows that a variety of organisms may be responsible, but antimicrobial therapy is rarely indicated. In other cases, e.g. dysentery, typhoid or giardiasis, the specific sensitive organism responds to antimicrobial therapy.

Salmonella infections

Infection by *Salmonella* spp. (but not *S. typhi*) is overall the most common cause of food poisoning, although *Campylobacter* infections are of equal or greater importance in developed countries. *Salmonella* is found in the bowels of many animal species and may be passed to humans from undercooked contaminated foodstuffs. Symptoms usually last for a few days, rarely a week, and range from a watery stool to a severe diarrhoea with abdominal pains, vomiting and fever. Even for the most severe form, healthy adults require only oral rehydration. Indeed, antibacterials may prolong the duration of intestinal carriage. However, if there is severe sepsis or the patient has some other underlying problem, for example is immunocompromised, then antibacterials would be indicated. *Ciprofloxacin* may be used to treat the general systemic infections in these patients, and rehydration therapy will still be required.

Traveller's diarrhoea

This may be caused by a variety of organisms, depending on local conditions, although enteropathogenic *E. coli* is usually responsible. If

Table 13.13 Diarrhoea in adults

Common name	Likely organisms
Food poisoning, traveller's diarrhoea	*Salmonella* spp.
	Clostridium welchii
	Yersinia enterocolitica
	Escherichia coli
	Campylobacter jejuni
	Staphylcoccus aureus
	Brucella spp.
	Bacillus cereus
Dysentery	*Shigella* spp.
	Entamoeba histolytica (amoebic dysentery)
Giardiasis	*Giardia lamblia*
Cholera	*Vibrio cholerae*
Typhoid	*Salmonella typhi*/*S. paratyphi*
Antibiotic-induced	Non-specific
	Clostridium difficile

the symptoms are severe (nausea, vomiting and blood in stools) prolonged, or signs of septicaemia are present, *ciprofloxacin* may lessen the severity and reduce duration of symptoms from about 5 days to 24 h. The prophylactic use of sulphonamides is undesirable as the chance of infection is only reduced by 50% and adverse effects are common.

Typhoid fever

In contrast to foodborne salmonellosis infection, *Salmonella typhi* infections require antimicrobial treatment. Infection is usually spread by sewage-contaminated water.

Typhoid fever is not always associated with diarrhoea. Patients may have constipation in the early stages, and the systemic complications rather than local gut symptoms are more important. This is because the organism can penetrate the gastrointestinal mucosa and proliferate within the local reticuloendothelial cells before spreading throughout the body. The gut wall is therefore weakened and after about 3 weeks may be sufficiently damaged to cause initial symptoms, e.g. dehydration, fever and confusion. The most serious complications are gastrointestinal haemorrhage and perforation.

Broad-spectrum antibacterials (*ampicillin*, *sulphonamides* and *chloramphenicol*) are active against some strains of *S. typhi*, but ciprofloxacin is the treatment of choice. Although resistance is a problem, treatment is effective provided that there is early diagnosis and sensitivity testing.

Cholera

The insidious onset of typhoid contrasts markedly with infection by *Vibrio cholerae*. This organism does not invade the gut wall and the tissues, but produces a toxin which rapidly acts on the bowel to induce an intense watery diarrhoea, resulting in dehydration. Over the years cholera has tended to become less virulent than the 'classic cholera' encountered earlier in the century, when diarrhoea and death from dehydration could follow quite rapidly. In otherwise healthy people the course is often mild; cholera is very rare in Western travellers to regions where it is endemic, and may even pass as a bout of simple travellers' diarrhoea. However, present-day cholera, which tends to cause epidemics when sanitary conditions are very poor, does cause many fatalities amongst the young, elderly or malnourished. Oral rehydration can therefore be life saving; intravenous fluids are needed only in very ill patients. The disease is otherwise self-limiting.

Antimicrobial therapy plays only a small part in the management of cholera. Antibacterials such as the tetracyclines will reduce fluid loss to some extent, but availability is limited in countries where cholera is endemic and resistance is a problem.

Dysentery

Bacillary dysentery (shigellosis) is an example of a gastrointestinal infection requiring antimicrobial therapy in severe cases. *Shigella* spp. are only found in the bowel of man and the higher primates. The disease is associated with overcrowding and poor sanitation. Invasion of the colon wall causes a diarrhoea containing inflammatory exudate, WBCs, blood and mucus. Systemic symptoms (fever, malaise) will also be present and arthritis and renal damage may occur.

Treatment with antidiarrhoeals (*loperamide*, *diphenoxylate*, opioids) should be avoided as this will tend to retain inflammatory exudate in the bowel and prolong symptoms. *Ampicillin, tetracyclines* and *chloramphenicol* are often effective, although multiply resistant strains are sometimes encountered.

Ciprofloxacin is again the treatment of choice, but there have been reports of resistance even to this antimicrobial, so sensitivity testing is an essential guide to therapy in severe disease.

Amoebic dysentery, caused by the protozoon *Entamoeba histolytica*, has similar symptoms to shigellosis but systemic effects are uncommon. The condition tends to be longer-lasting than shigellosis, and the treatment of choice is *metronidazole* in high doses. *Diloxanide furoate* may needed to eradicate resistant cysts.

Giardiasis is caused by *Giardia lamblia* (another protozoon), and results in diarrhoea of long duration – sometimes months if not treated. In this case there is no blood present in the stools, but owing to malabsorption a frothy foul-smelling diarrhoea with much flatulence (steatorrhoea) may result. *Metronidazole* is the treatment of choice and can be given as a short 3-day course.

Antibacterial-induced diarrhoea

The use of oral broad-spectrum antibacterials, particularly if poorly absorbed, can lead to over-growth in the gut lumen of organisms resistant to that agent. This may cause a mild diarrhoea that resolves on discontinuation of treatment. In some cases the disturbance is drug-specific; *erythromycin* causes an increase in drug transit time and *tetracyclines* can inactivate lipases.

Antibiotic-associated colitis (AAC) is more serious and is the result of overgrowth of *Clostridium difficile*. This organism releases an exotoxin which causes a local inflammation and formation of a membrane of necrotic tissue over the bowel wall, which in about 20% of cases leads to a form of chronic diarrhoea called **pseudomembranous colitis**. This is an intense, potentially fatal diarrhoea that requires oral treatment with *vancomycin* or *metronidazole*.

Summary

In summary:

- Most cases of diarrhoea will not require antimicrobial treatment. Exceptions to this are:
  - When systemic effects are present.
  - When the patient is either very young or elderly.
  - When there is some other debilitating condition.
- Oral or intravenous rehydration are the most important factors in the management of persistent diarrhoea.
- Infection caused by certain specific organisms may benefit from antimicrobial therapy, particularly when there are systemic complications. While the 4-quinolones are the treatment of choice for bacterial infections, *metronidazole* can be used to treat giardiasis or amoebic dysentery.

Tuberculosis

During the 19th and early 20th centuries, tuberculosis (TB) was a major cause of death and morbidity in the UK. However, today it is far less common, affecting 5–10 per 100 000 of the native population, though it has a higher prevalence among some immigrant groups. Although the fall over the century in the incidence of TB can be linked to general improvements in living standards, immunization and chemotherapy has played an important part since the 1950s, so that death from TB infection is now rare in the West.

In recent years however, tuberculosis has once again become a serious world-wide health issue. It is now estimated that TB is responsible for 3 million deaths per year, and this is expected to rise to over 4 million by 2004. TB is the major cause of death from infectious illness among those over 5 years of age. The World Health Organization has declared the disease a global emergency. Much of the problem is related to the emergence of HIV, which renders the affected individual much more susceptible. Approximately 10% of cases, rising to 20% in certain African countries, are related to HIV infection.

Aetiology

Pulmonary tuberculosis is caused by *Mycobacterium tuberculosis* transmitted via airborne droplets coughed or sneezed by infected individuals. Rarely, **bovine tuberculosis**, transmitted via cow's milk, causes tuberculosis of the gastrointestinal tract. The organism is unusual in that it possesses an outer waxy coat which makes it particularly resistant to the host's defence mechanisms. The bacterium becomes a focus for chronic inflammation, and granuloma (**tubercle**) formation (*see* Chapter 2) is a particular feature of this infection.

Pathogenesis

The pathogenesis of TB is summarized in Fig. 13.3. Following **primary infection**, usually in the lungs, neutrophils are attracted to the site of

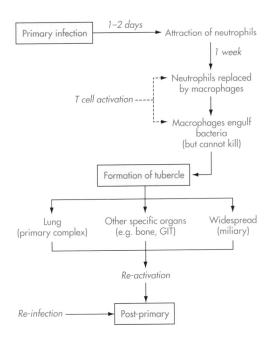

Figure 13.3 Pathogenesis of tuberculosis. GIT, gastrointestinal tract.

infection and replaced by macrophages after about a week. The latter engulf and attempt to digest the organisms, which however usually remain unharmed and viable owing to their waxy coat. T cells are also activated and their lymphokines attract and maintain the population of macrophages around the focus of infection. Two groups of T helper cells are known to be involved in this immune response; the T_{H_1} and T_{H_2} cells are distinguished by the different cytokines that they release. It is believed that T_{H_1} activity is responsible for macrophage activation, but that T_{H_2} or a mixed T_{H_1}/T_{H_2} activity renders cells highly susceptible to killing by tumour necrosis factor. It is the activity of the immune system and its cytokines that is responsible for much of the lung damage associated with TB. This process eventually leads to the formation of tubercles, which may heal completely leaving a small scar, or alternatively spread via the lymphatics into the lymph nodes, where they form a more widespread primary complex. Occasionally, and usually in immunosuppressed patients or the elderly, mycobacteria spread via the bloodstream to form small tubercules in various tissues (e.g. the lung, spleen, liver and kidneys), a condition known as **miliary tuberculosis.** Bacteria may also reach the central nervous system (**tuberculous meningitis**) or become sequestered in bones (usually the spine) where they become centres for granulomatous lesions and cause deformity.

The major complications usually occur on reactivation of the disease (**post-primary tuberculosis**). Infected individuals become sensitized to bacterial proteins, displaying a local hypersensitivity (Type IV) reaction which causes further tissue damage. This post-primary infection of the lung produces the typical symptoms of pulmonary TB, the primary infection being mild or asymptomatic. Re-infection is another uncommon cause for the gradual spread of a primary infection.

Clinical features

The classic respiratory symptoms of a post-primary infection include cough, haemoptysis and purulent sputum. There may also be chest wall pain, dyspnoea and wheeze. Other non-specific signs are fever, weight loss and night sweats. Without adequate therapy, lung damage will lead to progressive disability and a slow, lingering death.

Immunization

In the UK, Bacillus Calmette-Guérin (BCG), a live attenuated vaccine against tuberculosis, is offered to all non-immune children aged 10–13 years, so reducing the risk of contracting TB by up to 75%. In other countries efficacy may be much lower. In addition, immunity may be lost in later life, but the efficacy of BCG in older adults has been less well studied.

Pharmacotherapy

The purpose of chemotherapy is to eradicate the organism completely, but there are major problems associated with this. It can take 6–8 weeks to culture the slow-growing *Mycobacterium*, and a further similar period for sensitivity testing. However, newer DNA probe techniques are being developed which reduce this to less than a week. This means that therapy must be started blind.

M. tuberculosis is resistant to the usual antibacterials owing to poor cellular penetration of the agent. Moreover, resistance is inevitable if a single agent is used (p. 735). During active disease, the growing bacteria must be dealt with quickly, but there will also be dormant or semi-dormant bacteria that require protracted therapy.

These problems are dealt with by using antitubercular drugs. These are often rather toxic, and must be used long term; both of these factors will tend to reduce compliance. In addition, compliance is often poor as patients tend to feel much better soon after initiating chemotherapy. Poor compliance results in an incomplete kill of the organisms and, almost inevitably, future reactivation of drug-resistant disease.

There has been much interest in finding ways of improving compliance. Uniquely this has become very much a public health issue, where it has been shown that good compliance to a regimen actually reduces the rate of TB notification. A useful strategy would be to monitor urine levels of the various agents. A direct observation therapy scheme (DOTS) has also been tried successfully, inviting patients to attend clinics three times each week, the dosages being adjusted accordingly to allow for the increased interval between them.

Figure 13.4 shows the current recommendations made by the British Thoracic Society for the treatment of pulmonary TB. In order to minimize resistance, a combination of *isoniazid, rifampicin* and *pyrazinamide* is given for the first 2 months. *Isoniazid* and *rifampicin* are then usually given for another 4 months, if laboratory results indicate that these two agents are effective. It is important to continue with all three agents until such results are available. *Rifampicin* and *isoniazid* are somewhat more rapidly acting than *ethambutol* or *pyrazinamide*. All drugs are administered as a single daily dose, 30 min before breakfast, in order to improve compliance.

Rifampicin, isoniazid and *pyrazinamide* can all cause liver damage, so liver function must be monitored throughout treatment. *Ethambutol* at high doses has been associated with retinal damage and should be discontinued if visual disturbances are apparent. Isoniazid-induced peripheral neuropathy can be avoided by giving pyridoxine. *Rifampicin* can turn urine or tears an orange-red colour, the latter effect potentially causing staining of contact lenses.

Isoniazid may also be used for the **prophylaxis** of close contacts. If such contacts are to be immunized using BCG, an isoniazid-resistant strain of the vaccine must be used.

Multiple resistance

There has been recent concern over the emergence of multiple drug resistance strains of TB. In the UK, resistance to *isoniazid* alone occurs in 3% of isolates, and dual resistance to *isoniazid* and *rifampicin* in 0.6%. Resistance may be primary, where a person has been infected by resistant strains, or secondary where a resistant strain has emerged owing to incomplete treatment. If *isoniazid* resistance is suspected (e.g. if immuno-compromised or previously treated), then *ethambutol* should be added to the initial standard regimen. Once *isoniazid* resistance has been confirmed, treatment should continue with *rifampicin* and *ethambutol* for a year.

Rare in the UK, but increasingly common in some other counties, are strains of TB that are resistant to the usual first-line drugs. In such cases, second-line drugs such as *cycloserine*, which is neurotoxic, are required. Encouraging results with 4-quinolones have been obtained when used to treat such multiply resistant strains.

Summary

The treatment of TB illustrates the following:

- A need for multiple agents to overcome drug resistance of the organisms.
- The importance to patients of completing courses of treatment.
- The problems of poor compliance associated with prolonged courses of treatment with agents that have serious side effects.

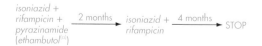

Figure 13.4 Standard treatment of tuberculosis. [a]Add if isoniazid resistance is likely.

Urinary tract infections

Signs, symptoms and aetiology

Infection of the lower urinary tract (Fig. 13.5) occurs either in the bladder (**cystitis**) or the urethra (**urethritis**), and is estimated to occur in up to 50% of women at some time in their life. The symptoms of dysuria and frequency, though not life-threatening, may be extremely uncomfortable. In addition, the urine may appear turbid due to the presence of pus, and may have a fishy smell due to the existence of bacterial metabolites.

Diagnosis and treatment may be confused by symptoms being present even if the urine is sterile, a condition known as **abacterial cystitis**, which can occur in up to 50% of cases. Conversely, because bacteria are often isolated from the urine in the absence of any overt symptoms (**covert bacteriuria**), the diagnostic criterion for **significant bacteriuria** is normally taken to be more than 10 organisms per mL. More vigorous treatment may be indicated for certain groups of patients, particularly in the presence of recurrent or ascending infections: this includes pregnant women, children and all men. The elderly may also be prone to complications, which may present as confusion in the absence of the usual signs of infection.

The full spectrum of renal tract infection, including pyelonephritis, is discussed in detail in Chapter 4. Here, we will discuss only the treatment of cystitis.

Organisms responsible

The majority (90%) of acute uncomplicated urinary tract infections (UTIs) are due to auto-infection with *E. coli*. Other Gram-negatives (*Proteus, Klebsiella, Pseudomonas*) may be implicated, particularly if the infections are of a chronic nature. Infections due to staphylococci are the second most common in the community but are less usual in hospital. Organisms other than *E. coli* are also more likely in hospital-acquired infections, especially in catheterized patients. In cases that fail to respond to treatment, organisms such as *Chlamydia* or *Candida* should be considered.

Investigation

A urine specimen that is uncontaminated by commensals from the genitalia is necessary for

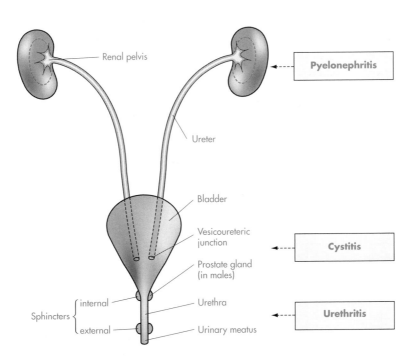

Figure 13.5   Sites of urinary tract infections.

culturing and sensitivity tests. This is obtained through a midstream urine (MSU), usually collected at home by the patient: the genital area is washed with mild soap, dried and the first and final parts of urine are rejected. The sample is collected first thing in the morning when the bacterial count is likely to be highest due to undisturbed overnight growth. However, an uncontaminated sample is difficult to collect in some circumstances, e.g. young children and elderly, and a more reliable method is via a catheter, although this may itself introduce infection into the bladder. Rarely, suprapubic bladder aspiration with a syringe may be required when it is difficult to collect a sample, e.g. from a young infant.

Apart from culturing, which may take some time, other changes in the urine can indicate the presence of microorganisms. Reagent strips can be used to detect the presence of nitrite produced as a result of bacterial metabolism. The pH of the urine may be low in the presence of *E. coli* or high if due to *Proteus* spp. or other urease-positive (ammonia-producing) species.

Further investigations for potential complications are indicated in all cases of male or childhood UTI, in women with recurrent or persistent symptoms, or when sterile urine has not been achieved after standard therapy (*see* Chapter 4, p. 205).

Management

Aims

The immediate aim of treatment, from the patient's view, is the rapid relief of uncomfortable symptoms. This is best achieved by the eradication of the responsible organism using a short course of an appropriate antibacterial. The prevention of recurrent and chronic infections and of subsequent renal damage is a further aim that may require longer courses of treatment.

Choice of antibacterial

As *E. coli* is the most likely organism, the initial antibacterial choice is relatively simple. The final decision will depend on known patterns of resistance. *Trimethoprim* may be appropriate for blind treatment and achieves high urine concentrations. Resistant strains of bacteria are becoming increasingly common in hospitals and, to a lesser extent, in the community, and *first-generation cephalosporins* are a useful alternative. *Nitrofurantoin* is also suitable, although its use is limited by toxicity and *Proteus* spp. are resistant. The *4-quinolones* are active against a wide range of organisms including pseudomonads, but should be reserved for infection of proven sensitivity which are resistant to other agents or treatment failures. The quinolone *norfloxacin* is restricted to treating UTIs because it achieves sub-therapeutic blood levels, but a high concentration in the urine.

The last dose of the day should be taken just before going to bed in order to achieve high urine concentrations when bacterial count is likely to be maximal. Symptoms should begin to clear within 48 h, and a 3-day course is usually sufficient for uncomplicated cystitis.

Chronic or recurrent infections

Frequent UTIs may require prophylactic use of antibacterials. In children, low-dose *trimethoprim* can be used, given last thing at night for many months. In adults, prophylaxis with low-dose *nitrofurantoin* is an alternative and rarely causes problems.

Other modes of treatment

Alkalinization of the urine with potassium or sodium citrate or sodium bicarbonate may provide some symptomatic relief if the urine is very acid, and will inhibit growth of *E. coli*. Raising the urine pH will also inhibit the precipitation of any sulphonamide used in treatment. However, the use of potassium or sodium citrate may be hazardous in elderly patients and others with impaired renal function owing to cardiovascular effects of accumulated sodium or potassium. Moreover, *Proteus* spp. thrive in a high pH, but not under acid conditions, so acidification of the urine with ammonium chloride may be appropriate in such infections. Thus, simple pH testing with indicator paper should guide this type of treatment.

Advice should always be given to increase fluid intake and to ensure regular voiding in order to obtain maximum washout of organisms from the bladder. Pushing fluids (200 mL three times an hour for several hours) may abort an infection without the need for antimicrobial treatments, provided that it is started promptly when symptoms occur. It is also important to void completely in order to leave the minimum of infected urine in the bladder.

Summary

Treatment of UTIs illustrate the following general principles:

- *E. coli* is responsible for the majority of acute UTIs, so initial therapy can be chosen with a high degree of confidence.
- Local patterns of resistance will indicate which of a number of possible agents should be used.
- The antimicrobial must be present in high concentrations at the site of infection. Therefore, only those agents that are rapidly excreted unchanged in the urine are suitable for the treatment of UTIs.

References and further reading

Anonymous (1995) Drug-resistant tuberculosis. *Drug Ther Bull* **33** (4): 28–29.

Anonymous (1997) The management of urinary tract infections in women. *Drug Ther Bull* **35** (9): 65–69.

Finch RG, Woodhead MA (1998) Practical considerations and guidelines for the management of community-acquired pneumonia. *Drugs* **55**: 31–45.

Infections (1996) *Medicine International Series* **24** (7): Parts 1–3.

O'Grady F, Lambert HP (1997) *Antibiotic and Chemotherapy*. 7th edn. Edinburgh: Churchill Livingstone.

Shanson DC (1999) *Microbiology in Clinical Practice*. 3rd edn. Oxford: Butterworth-Heinemann.

The British Thoracic Society, London (1993) Guidelines for the management of community-acquired pneumonia in adults admitted to hospital. *Br J Hosp Med* **49**: 346–350.

Tunkel AR, Scheld WM (1995) Acute bacterial meningitis. *Lancet* **346**: 1675–1679.

Index

Drug names and their salts are in **bold** type. Page numbers in *italics* refer to tables or figures.